Alveolar Gas Exchange and Pulmonary Circulation

Main Symbols

C	concentration in a liquid
Cap	capacity
D	diffusing capacity
f	respiratory frequency
F	fraction
G	conductance
P	pressure, total or partial
Q	volume of liquid
$\dot{Q}$	flow of blood, perfusion
R	gas-exchange ratio
S	saturation
V	gas volume
$\dot{V}$	ventilation
β	slope of a dissociation curve
θ	reaction rate

Modifiers

a	arterial
A	alveolar
B	barometric
c	capillary
DS	dead space
e	effective
E	expired
I	inspired
la	left atrial
m	membrane
p	plasma
pa	pulmonary arterial
pc	pulmonary capillary
pc′	pulmonary end capillary
pv	pulmonary venous
pw	pulmonary wedge
s	shunt
t	time *t*
T	total
ti	tissue
v	venous
$\bar{v}$	mixed venous
va	venous admixture
0	(zero) initial value

Special Symbols

ATPD	ambient temperature and pressure, dry
ATPS	ambient temperature and pressure, saturated
BTPS	body temperature, ambient pressure, saturated with water vapor
STPD	standard temperature and pressure, dry

Examples of Combinations

$C\bar{v}_{O_2}$	concentration of O_2 in mixed venous blood
O_2Cap	O_2 capacity
Pa_{O_2}	partial pressure of O_2 in arterial blood
$PA_{O_2} - Pa_{O_2}$	alveolar-arterial difference in partial pressure of O_2
P_{O_2}	partial pressure of O_2
$\dot{Q}T$	cardiac output
Sa_{O_2}	saturation of hemoglobin with O_2 in arterial blood
$\dot{V}A/\dot{Q}$	ventilation-perfusion ratio
$\dot{V}E$	expired minute ventilation
$\dot{V}max_{O_2}$	maximum O_2 consumption (also $\dot{V}_{O_2 max}$)

Control of Breathing

$Pm_{0.1}$	mouth occlusion pressure 0.1 s after onset of inspiration
TE	expiratory time
TI	inspiratory time
TT	total respiratory cycle duration

See Symbols and Abbreviations, p. ix.

HANDBOOK OF PHYSIOLOGY

SECTION 3: The Respiratory System, VOLUME IV

Laurie S. Chambers, Elizabeth M. Cowley,
Susie P. Mann, *Editorial Staff*

Brenda B. Rauner, *Production Manager*

Constantine J. Gillespie, *Indexer*

HANDBOOK OF PHYSIOLOGY

A critical, comprehensive presentation
of physiological knowledge and concepts

SECTION 3: **The Respiratory System**

Formerly SECTION 3: Respiration

VOLUME IV.
Gas Exchange

Section Editor: ALFRED P. FISHMAN

Volume Editors: LEON E. FARHI
S. MARSH TENNEY

Executive Editor: STEPHEN R. GEIGER

American Physiological Society, BETHESDA, MARYLAND, 1987

Library of Congress Catalog Card Number 84-24381

International Standard Book Number 0-683-03039-6

Printed in the United States of America by Waverly Press, Inc., Baltimore, Maryland 21202

Distributed by The Williams & Wilkins Company, Baltimore, Maryland 21202

Preface to the Section on Respiration

The intent of this *Handbook* section is to provide a scholarly, comprehensive, and critical view of contemporary respiratory physiology within the framework of respiratory biology. This has been no simple task; in the 20 years since the first edition, respiratory physiology has extended far beyond its original bounds while becoming more deeply rooted within traditional confines. In large measure this flourishing of respiratory physiology is attributable to the biochemists, anatomists, pharmacologists, pathologists, and bioengineers who have entered the field and enriched it with their approaches, knowledge, concepts, and techniques. During this period the growth of ideas, advances in technology, and accumulation of facts has been steady, with occasional punctuation by scientific upheavals that have reoriented thinking and opened new directions for exploration. To accommodate the expanded body of knowledge and its conceptual framework requires four volumes instead of the three volumes originally planned.

The increase in content, the new direction, and the broader horizons are reflected in the title of this section. The 1964–1965 edition was simply designated *Respiration*; this edition is entitled *The Respiratory System*. This change is a reminder of the complexity, organization, and integration that make respiration possible. Other parts of the body have the same characteristics, but probably in no other component are these characteristics so striking because of the phasic nature of the breathing process, the automatic adjustments of breathing to changing metabolic states, and the many provisions for interruptions in the phasic process by episodic events, such as eating, talking, coughing, straining, and vomiting.

One fruitful way to regard the living organism is to view it as a system of interrelated functional hierarchies. From this vantage a hierarchy or its components can be probed in great detail, always within the larger framework of the whole animal. In this section, one large hierarchy—the respiratory system—and its component parts are put under the microscope, leaving other large and related units, such as the circulatory system, to be considered elsewhere.

The hierarchical approach has broad implications. First, the predominant concern is with function rather than anatomy; boundaries, orderliness, and self-containment are more a matter of feedback mechanisms than of structural restraints. Second, within the framework of the whole body a hierarchy may be involved in more than one function; a single hierarchy (such as the arachidonic acid cascade) generates some substances that act locally and others that behave as circulating hormones and exert their biological effects in remote corners of the body. Third, large systems (such as the respiratory and circulatory systems) are closely interlinked and interdependent; as a rule the larger systems modulate the activities of smaller hierarchies within them. Fourth, at the level of the cell and organelle, hierarchies are exceedingly minute, yet they retain complexity and integration as cardinal features; in this realm, structure gives way to molecular interactions as the basis for function. Finally, the living body could not operate effectively as a conglomeration of hierarchies without sophisticated methods for information transfer to ensure integrated performance.

Currently much physiological experimentation is concerned with information transfer and control mechanisms. Not very long ago this aspect of physiology dealt almost exclusively with nerves and neurohumoral transmitters. Visionaries such as Bernard, Cannon, Barcroft, Henderson, and Sherrington constructed grand schemes to explain the complicated biological interplays that automatically adjust the body at rest, during exercise, on exposure to unsettling environments, and during the fight-or-flight reaction. Their legacy is a body of monumental concepts epitomized by rubrics such as "Homeostasis," "The Architecture of Physiologic Function," and "The Wisdom of the Body."

Although the integrated responses of the whole body continue to be intensely researched, within the hierarchies of the body there is apparently much more to information transfer than nerves, neurohumoral substances, and feedback mechanisms. Individual cells could not do their job without self-replenishing receptors at their surfaces for signal transduction, which triggers biochemical events that activate and regulate the activities of the cells. Endothelial cells that line blood vessels communicate by elaborate biological machinery with smooth muscle cells in the vascular walls. Electrical stimuli conveyed by nerves link events at the cellular level with humors in the central nervous system. An elaborate system for maintaining acid-base balance ensures a background of stability in hydrogen ion concentration so that background noise does not interfere with message centers or media in a hierarchical system that relies so heavily on uninterrupted information transfer for its survival, operation, and propagation.

The respiratory system is currently being explored as a component of the entire organism and in terms of its constituent parts: the perspective of overall integration is exemplified by the exploration of the control of breathing; that of molecular biology is exemplified by the study of macromolecular transport across special domains on the plasma membrane of the pulmonary capillary endothelial cell. The broad sweep of research on the respiratory system and its components and the ways in which the system relates to other systems during rest, activity, stress, and adaptation are the mainstays of this *Handbook* section.

For convenience the section has been subdivided into four volumes: *Circulation and Nonrespiratory Functions, Control of Breathing, Mechanics of Breathing*, and *Gas Exchange*. The hierarchies vary from chapter to chapter in size, complexity, regulatory mechanisms, and machinery for information transfer. The volumes devoted to the circulation and nonrespiratory functions of the lungs and gas exchange give high priority to organization and operation at the cellular level. Those concerned with the control and mechanics of breathing are more inclined toward integrating mechanisms at the level of the whole body. Full understanding of the respiratory system requires reconciliation of its materials and design with its effectiveness in performance under ordinary and under trying conditions. No matter how meticulously and successfully each component of the system is probed, in the last analysis the responsibility of physiology is to restore the isolated component to its proper place in the operations of the respiratory system and to reconcile the respiratory system with the other inner workings of the entire organism.

My debt to the volume editors and authors is self-evident: without them there would be neither content, organization, nor style (in fact, no books). Less evident is my obligation to those in my organization, particularly Jayne Pickard, who managed—by prompting and cajoling authors and editors and by unremitting devotion to the cause—to ensure proper review in my office while maintaining an uninterrupted flow of manuscripts to the Society's publications office.

This was a large effort. One can only hope that the product lives up to the expectations and needs of the readers.

ALFRED P. FISHMAN
Section Editor

Preface

The fourth and last volume of the *Handbook of Physiology* section on the respiratory system deals with the ultimate goal of the system, gas exchange. To fulfill this role the lung cyclically expands and contracts and the alveoli are perfused; the regulatory function is geared to optimize the exchange of oxygen and carbon dioxide. Like other areas of respiratory physiology, the study of gas exchange has made giant strides since the first edition of the *Handbook* was published. Much of what was written then remains important and serves as a basis for the more recent developments. Consequently, like all good reviews, this volume includes "something old and something new, something borrowed and something true."

Although logic and didactic practice dictate the chapter order, from the description of basic physical principles to their application under both normal and unusual conditions, some changes in representation have been introduced. For example, the fundamental gas laws, instead of following the usual cut-and-dried presentation, are developed in their historical context.

By its nature a book written by many specialists dealing with overlapping topics must contain some duplication. Although the goal was to minimize repetition, we deemed it more important to maintain the integrity and continuity of each chapter and did not request the authors to cripple their contributions by deleting all that was to be found elsewhere. Finally, progress in science often results from divergence of opinion and controversy. The authors are complimented for giving both sides of the argument whenever possible and excused for occasionally allowing their biases to show.

With a mixture of pride and relief we present this book, hoping that it will serve its public as well as the first edition has for so many years.

LEON E. FARHI
S. MARSH TENNEY

Symbols and Abbreviations

In the summer of 1977 at the International Union of Physiological Sciences Congress in Paris, the Commission on Respiratory Physiology established a committee to improve the glossary of terms and symbols used in respiratory physiology. Shortly thereafter the American Physiological Society decided to publish the new *Handbook* series on respiratory physiology. To incorporate the IUPS symbols into these books, a committee consisting of one of the editors of each *Handbook* was established, namely Leon E. Farhi, Alfred P. Fishman, Peter T. Macklem (chairman), and John G. Widdicombe, along with Curt von Euler and Peter Scheid. The symbols and abbreviations chosen by this committee were approved by the Commission on Respiratory Physiology at the Budapest Congress in 1980 and subsequently approved for publication in the *Handbook of Physiology* by the Publications Committee of the American Physiological Society.

SYMBOLS IN RESPIRATORY PHYSIOLOGY

Main Symbols

The main symbol indicates the nature of the variable and usually appears in the form of a single large capital letter. More rarely it is denoted by a Greek letter, a lowercase letter, or a combination of capital and lowercase letters. Exceptions are the subdivisions of lung volume and symbols for measurements of forced respiratory maneuvers for which accepted usage has been followed.

The main symbol can be modified by a character that appears over the symbol itself (bar for a mean or average value, single dot for the first time derivative, two dots for the second time derivative).

Modifiers

Main symbols are further clarified by the addition of one or more modifiers, usually small capitals for the gas phase, standard chemical symbols for the chemical species, and lowercase letters in most other instances. Modifiers denote locations, anatomic structures, media in which the measurements are made, respiration phases, types of resistance to motion, chemical species, and so forth. The first modifier appears directly after the main symbol. Subsequent modifiers are either separated from the other modifiers by commas or more rarely appear as subscripts. Chemical species always appear as subscripts and follow all other modifiers used (the only exception is the symbol for capacity of a gas). Modifiers denoting time (t or 1.0 s) or numerical designations (0, 1, 2, 3, . . .) appear as subscripts.

The symbols have been divided into three main groups: *1*) respiratory mechanics, *2*) alveolar gas exchange and pulmonary circulation, and *3*) control of breathing. Rather than introduce entirely new symbols to replace those that have gained widespread acceptance, the committee that prepared this guide feels that greater clarity is achieved by some symbols having different meanings and some words more than one symbol. Thus $\dot{V}$ in respiratory mechanics usually means flow, whereas in gas exchange it usually means ventilation. The symbol C can have one of three meanings: compliance in mechanics of breathing, capacity in the subdivisions of lung volume, and concentration in a liquid in gas exchange. In gas exchange, capacity is represented by the symbol Cap. The symbol R signifies respiratory exchange ratio or resistance. The meaning of the symbols should be clearly understood from the context. (*See* endpapers.)

PETER T. MACKLEM

Contents

An overview of gas exchange

ARTHUR B. OTIS | *Department of Physiology, University of Florida College of Medicine, Gainesville, Florida*

CHAPTER CONTENTS

A GLOBAL OVERVIEW of respiratory gas exchange might start with the photosynthetic production of O_2, follow the pathways of O_2 flow from the atmosphere to the mitochondria of myriads of living organisms, examine the mechanisms and energetics of this movement, and finally trace the flows and fate of the CO_2 and H_2O released by metabolic processes into which O_2 temporarily vanishes only to reappear at the beginning of the cycle. The picture presented here is a more modest scheme for considering some aspects of the flow of O_2 from the atmosphere to the tissues of human beings. A similar scheme could be constructed for the simultaneous flow of CO_2 in the opposite direction.

The framework of this presentation is not original. It is largely based on concepts already stated by others, e.g., Fenn (5), Dejours (3), Piiper et al. (11), Haab (6), Taylor and Weibel (13), and Weibel et al. (16, 17). [See also Holmgren (7).]

GAS-EXCHANGE SYSTEM: A SERIES OF CONDUCTANCES

As a highly simplified conceptual approach to the problem of O_2 transport, the gas-exchange system in the human can be visualized as five major compartments: *1*) inspired gas, *2*) alveolar gas, *3*) pulmonary capillary blood, *4*) tissue capillary blood, and *5*) tissue.

These compartments are connected in series to form a continuous pathway along which there is a net flow ($\dot{M}$) of O_2 from compartment 1 to compartment 5, where it enters into chemical reactions and disappears as a separate entity (Fig. 1).

For this simplistic analysis, assume that the partial pressure of O_2 (P_{O_2}) within each compartment is uniform throughout that compartment. This is generally true for compartment 1 and approximately so for compartment 2, at least for normal lungs. In the capillaries of the lung and of the tissues, partial pressure varies along the length of each capillary. Nevertheless a mean partial pressure can be conceptualized, which, if it existed throughout the capillary, would allow the same rate of O_2 flow as actually occurs. Likewise a mean value that characterizes the P_{O_2} in the tissues of the body can be imagined.

The connecting elements between compartments can be regarded as conductances or resistances. Flow along these pathways is associated with a loss of partial pressure, just as the flow of electric current through a resistance is associated with a drop in potential (Ohm's law), or a flowing stream with a loss of hydrostatic pressure head (Poiseuille's law).

In the study of gas exchange we are concerned with transfer of an amount M of a given gas species between two designated locations. The rate of transfer ($\dot{M}$) is given by the product of the conductance (G) of the pathway and the difference in partial pressure between the two locations

$$\dot{M} = G\Delta P \tag{1}$$

Conductance is a property of the system or of an element of the system. The concept of conductance does not necessarily imply any particular mechanism. It merely states a relationship; hence its application is general.

The reciprocal of conductance, 1/G, is a resistance (R)

$$\dot{M} = \Delta P/R \tag{2}$$

Thus conductance and resistance are manifestations of the same basic properties of a system. Conductance connotes ease of transfer; resistance implies opposition. One can think of conductance as amount transferred per unit time (t) when ΔP is unity, and resistance as the time required to transfer unit amount when ΔP is unity or as the ΔPt product required to move unit amount. A unit change in resistance does not produce the same change in rate of transfer as does a unit change in conductance, because conduct-

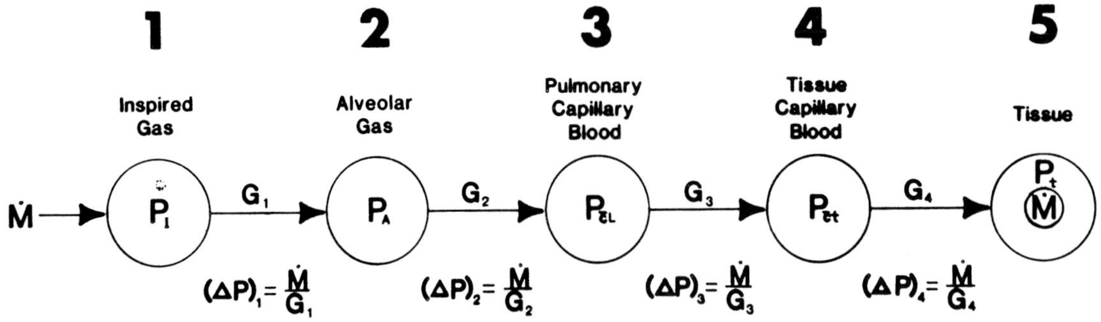

FIG. 1. Gas-exchange system for O_2 considered as 5 compartments and 4 conductances. Each conductance is characterized by a partial pressure, P. Oxygen flows along the system at rate $\dot{M}$. Each conductance is defined as $G = \dot{M}/\Delta P$.

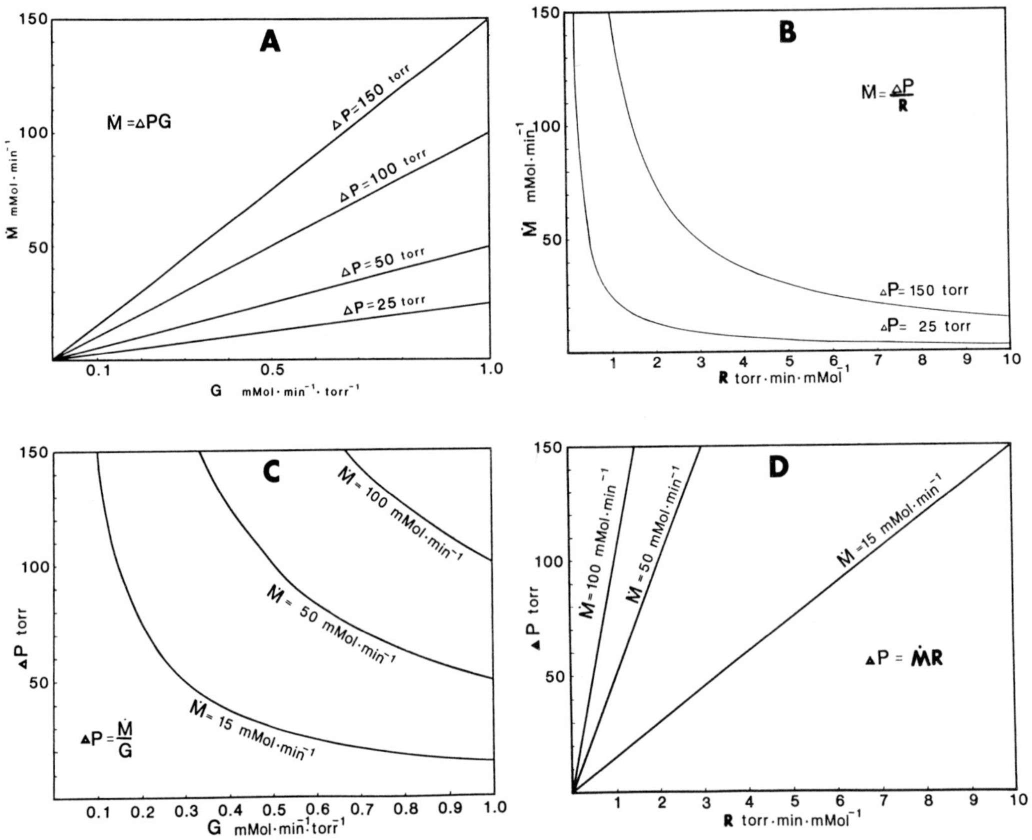

FIG. 2. Relationships between O_2 flow, M; conductance, G; resistance, R; and pressure drop, ΔP. *A*: O_2 flux as a function of conductance at different pressure drops. *B*: O_2 flux as a function of resistance at different pressure drops. *C*: pressure loss as a function of conductance at different O_2 fluxes. *D*: pressure loss as a function of resistance at different O_2 fluxes.

ance and resistance are logarithmically rather than arithmetically related

$$\log R = -\log G \tag{3}$$

A doubling of resistance is the same as a halving of conductance; a 10-fold increase in resistance is a reduction of conductance to 1/10 its initial value. For any constant ΔP, the rate of transfer is a linear function of conductance but is hyperbolically related to resistance. For any constant value of $\dot{M}$, however, the relationship between ΔP and conductance is hyperbolic, whereas ΔP and resistance are linearly related (Fig. 2). Because a straight-line function is generally easier to comprehend, it is useful to think in terms of conductances for some problems and in terms of resistances for others.

Although the notion of the respiratory gas-exchange system as a series of conductances or resistances is an abstraction that may seem to ignore reality, it does serve as a basis for an overview of the physiology of the system and as a coherent framework on which to assemble factual information. As Wallace Fenn (5) so nicely stated:

> With this concept for steady state conditions, one can write a series of equations in each of which the rate of oxygen consumption or the current of oxygen is equated to the product of two factors, a gradient of partial pressure, and a conductivity or diffusion capacity or reciprocal resistance.... It is impressive to consider what an intricate problem it is for the mathematical wisdom of the body to see that all these equations are balanced at once. Moreover, this concept emphasizes the fact, not often stated explicitly, that the total partial pressure of oxygen in the ambient air must be divided between the series of resistances existing between the mitochondria and the air and that no part of this can really be used twice. The mean pressure in the pulmonary capillaries can never be the same as the mean pressure in the tissue capillaries unless the circulation rate is increased to infinity.

The utility of this approach can be demonstrated by applying it to the O_2 flux in a hypothetical human (see Fig. 1). Let the P_{O_2} in compartment PI (PI, partial pressure of inspired gas) be 150 Torr. The values in the remaining compartments will be determined by $\dot{M}$ and the conductances G_1, G_2, G_3, and G_4. Suppose that initially $\dot{M} = 0$ and that each conductance has some value >0. The steady-state P_{O_2} at all points in the system will be equal: i.e., $P_I = P_A = \bar{P}_{c,L} = \bar{P}_{c,ti} = \bar{P}_{ti}$, where PA is alveolar P_{O_2}; $\bar{P}_{c,L}$ is mean pulmonary capillary P_{O_2}; $\bar{P}_{c,ti}$ is mean tissue capillary P_{O_2}, and $\bar{P}_{ti}$ is mean tissue P_{O_2}. Suppose that $\dot{M}$ is now changed to some finite value. Oxygen will begin to flow and a new steady state will develop in accordance with the relationship

$$\begin{aligned}\dot{M} &= G_1\Delta P_1 = G_2\Delta P_2 = G_3\Delta P_3 = G_4\Delta P_4\\ &= \Delta P_1/R_1 = \Delta P_2/R_2 = \Delta P_3/R_3 = \Delta P_4/R_4\\ &= (\Delta P_1 + \Delta P_2 + \Delta P_3 + \Delta P_4)/\\ &\qquad (R_1 + R_2 + R_3 + R_4)\\ &= (P_I - \bar{P}_{ti})/R\\ &= G(P_I - \bar{P}_{ti})\end{aligned} \tag{4}$$

where R and G are respectively the total resistance and conductance of the system. The total pressure drop across the system is the product $\dot{M}R$. The pressure drop across any element of the system is the same fraction of the total pressure drop as the resistance of that element is of the total resistance of the system. If the magnitudes of the conductances (or resistances) are fixed, the pressure drop across any element changes in direct proportion to any change in $\dot{M}$, the metabolic rate of O_2 consumption. Hydraulic and electrical analogues are shown in Figures 3 and 4.

Data for the hypothetical resting human that will enable us to calculate conductances and to make a few physiological inferences are now tabulated. Then the physiological determinants of the several conductances are considered and possible physiological changes that may occur in response to stress are examined.

The first column of Table 1 lists values for P_{O_2} in each of the five compartments. The value for PI can be measured with great accuracy, but as we go down the list the margin of error in the estimates becomes progressively greater; the reader is cautioned not to regard these values as exact. Indeed, the estimate of

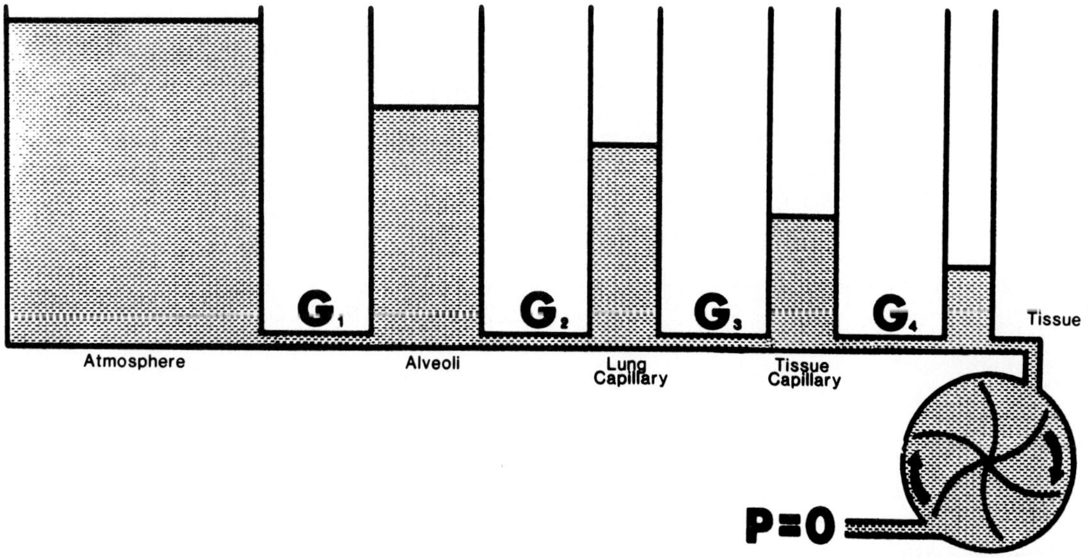

FIG. 3. Hydraulic analogue of O_2-transport system. Height of water in each rectangular compartment represents the partial pressure of O_2 (P_{O_2}) in that compartment. Last, circular compartment represents participation of O_2 in metabolic energy generation, a process in which P_{O_2} is reduced to zero. In any given situation atmospheric P_{O_2} is considered constant; the height in the 4 succeeding compartments is determined by O_2 flow and 4 conductances. Volume of compartment is immaterial in steady state but is of great importance in transient events.

TABLE 1. *Oxygen Cascade in Resting Human at Sea Level*

	P_{O_2}, Torr	ΔP_{O_2}, Torr	G, mmol·min^{-1}·Torr^{-1}	R = 1/G	Energy Loss, J/mmol	Rate of Energy Loss	
						W	W/Torr
P_I	150						
		50	0.30	3.33	1.04	0.26	0.005
P_A	100						
		15	1.00	1.00	0.42	0.10	0.007
$\bar{P}c,L$	85						
		30	0.50	2.00	1.12	0.28	0.009
$\bar{P}c,ti$	55						
		15	1.00	1.00	0.82	0.20	0.014
$\bar{P}ti$	40						
Total		110	0.14	7.33	3.40	0.85	0.008

Resting O_2 consumption, 15 mmol/min. ΔP_{O_2}, changes in partial pressure of O_2 between adjacent compartments; G, conductance; R, resistance (reciprocal conductance); P_I, P_{O_2} of inspired gas; P_A, alveolar P_{O_2}; $\bar{P}c,L$, mean P_{O_2} of pulmonary capillary blood; $\bar{P}c,ti$, mean P_{O_2} in tissue capillary blood; $\bar{P}ti$, mean P_{O_2} in tissue.

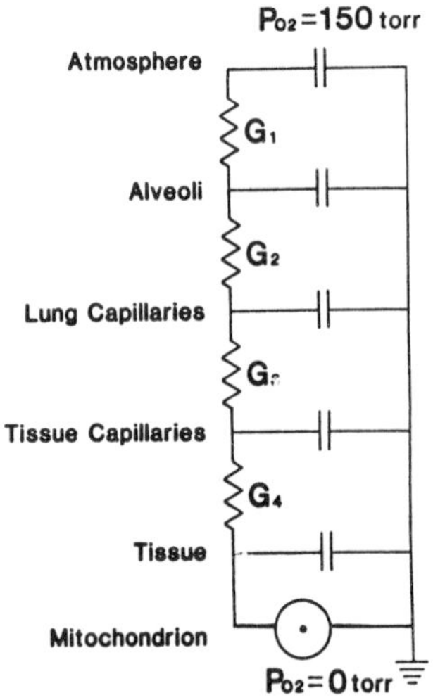

FIG. 4. Electrical analogue of O_2-transport system. Each compartment is represented as a capacitor and each conductance (G) as a resistor. At any given metabolic rate the mitochondria constitute a constant current device in which the potential is reduced to zero ground level.

$\bar{P}ti$ is little more than a guess. However, the listed values are reasonable for purposes of illustration.

What is the highest possible O_2 flow with the conductances listed in Table 1? Suppose that $\dot{M}$ is increased until the mean P_{O_2} in the tissue ($\bar{P}ti$) reaches a lower limiting value of zero. The conductance of the total system is 0.14 mmol·min^{-1}·Torr^{-1}. Thus the maximal rate of O_2 flow ($\dot{M}_{O_2}$) is 0.14 × 150 = 21 mmol/min. This is an overestimate, because $\bar{P}ti$ cannot be zero. Some regions of the tissue must have positive P_{O_2} values, and negative values are impossible; hence $\bar{P}ti$ must be positive. Suppose the minimal possible steady-state value of $\bar{P}ti$ is 10 Torr; then the maximal $\dot{M}_{O_2}$ with the conductances given is 0.14 × 140 = 19.1 mmol/min. This is an increase of only 27% over that initially assumed. Any greater increase in $\dot{M}_{O_2}$ requires an increase in one or more of the conductances. The smallest conductance is that between P_I and P_A; suppose it is increased to infinity, i.e., R_1 is reduced to zero. This makes P_A = 150 Torr and reduces the total resistance of the system to 4 (increases the conductance to 0.25); with a $\bar{P}ti$ = 10, the maximal $\dot{M}_{O_2}$ is 0.25 × 140 = 35 mmol/min. This is little more than a doubling of the original resting value of 15 mmol/min. Thus to allow increases in $\dot{M}_{O_2}$ greater than about twofold, an increase in more than one of the conductances is necessary.

The last three columns in Table 1 emphasize the fact that the loss of partial pressure as O_2 flows down the cascade implies a loss of physical energy. These energy losses have been calculated from the equations

$$\text{energy loss per mmol} = 0.001RT \ln(P_1/P_2) \quad (5)$$

and

$$\text{rate of energy loss} = \text{energy loss per mmol} \times 0.25 \text{ mmol/s} \quad (6)$$

where R is the universal gas constant and T is absolute temperature.

The last column of Table 1 shows the rate of energy loss per torr as O_2 flows from one compartment to another. It may also be thought of as the rate that work would have to be done per torr to restore the P_{O_2} in a given compartment to that in the compartment where the gas previously resided. As partial pressure decreases, the cost of restoring it by a given increment to a higher value increases. In other words, for a given pressure loss the energy loss is greater the lower the initial pressure. This is implicit in Equation 5 and is illustrated in Figure 5. Note that this refers only to physical energy available for O_2 transport and not to the energy released when O_2 enters into chemical reactions within the cell. In the latter case the P_{O_2} becomes zero and no purely physical process can restore it to a finite value.

For comparison with Table 1, Tables 2–4 have been constructed for more stressful conditions. Except for P_I the partial pressures listed in the first column of these tables are for the most part even more conjectural than those in Table 1. They serve, however, to illustrate some general points. Note that the system conductance in each case is at least double that for the condition of Table 1. Clearly the system conductance of 0.14 $mmol \cdot min^{-1} \cdot Torr^{-1}$ shown in Table 1 would not suffice for any of these more stressful conditions. Exercise of the magnitude indicated would, with no increase in conductance, require an O_2 pressure gradient of $(100\ mmol \cdot min^{-1})/(0.14\ mmol \cdot min^{-1} \cdot Torr^{-1}) = 714$ Torr, which is not possible with air as the inspired gas. Furthermore, breathing pure O_2 would not be much help. The altitude conditions would, with a conductance of 0.14 $mmol \cdot min^{-1} \cdot Torr^{-1}$, require a gradient of 110 Torr, which is clearly not available, although in this case the breathing of pure O_2 would be of great value. The minimal conductances consistent with the conditions specified and with the stipulation that mean tissue P_{O_2} be no lower than 10 Torr are tabulated in Table 5.

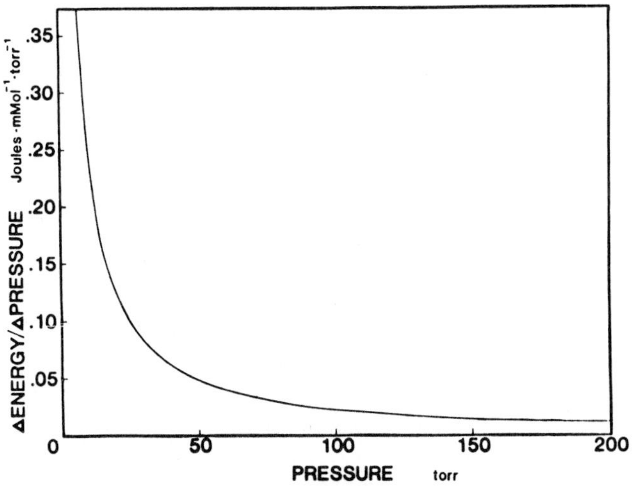

FIG. 5. Relationship showing physical energy loss per unit pressure drop as a function of pressure. Loss is greater at low than at high pressures. Thus raising the partial pressure of a mole of gas by a given increment is more costly when the initial pressure is low than when it is high.

PHYSIOLOGICAL COMPONENTS OF CONDUCTANCE

Inspired Gas to Alveolar Gas

The basic physiological variable comprising G_1 is the alveolar ventilation ($\dot{V}_A$). Assuming for simplicity a respiratory exchange ratio of unity

$$\dot{V}_{O_2} = (F_{I_{O_2}} - F_{A_{O_2}})\dot{V}_A \tag{7}$$

where $F_{I_{O_2}}$ and $F_{A_{O_2}}$ are respectively the fractions of O_2 in inspired and alveolar gas; $\dot{V}_{O_2}$ is the O_2 flow and $\dot{V}_A$ the alveolar ventilation, both at BTPS (body temperature, ambient pressure, saturated with water vapor) conditions. External sources of inspired gas may vary considerably in temperature and humidity, but by the time the inspirate has reached the tracheal bifurcation, it is usually considered to have warmed to body temperature and become saturated with water vapor.

TABLE 2. *Oxygen Cascade in Exercising Human at Sea Level*

	P_{O_2}, Torr	ΔP_{O_2}, Torr	G, $mmol \cdot min^{-1} \cdot Torr^{-1}$	R = 1/G	Energy Loss, J/mmol	Rate of Energy Loss: W	Rate of Energy Loss: W/Torr
PI	150						
		50	2.0	0.50	1.04	1.74	0.034
PA	100						
		35	2.9	0.35	1.11	1.85	0.052
P̄c,L	65						
		30	3.3	0.30	1.59	2.65	0.088
P̄c,ti	35						
		10	10.0	0.10	0.87	1.44	0.144
P̄ti	25						
Total		125	0.8	1.25	4.61	7.68	0.061

O_2 consumption, 100 mmol/min. See Table 1 for symbols. [Data in part from Astrand and Rodahl (1).]

TABLE 3. *Oxygen Cascade in Resting Human at 5,365 m*

	P_{O_2}, Torr	ΔP_{O_2}, Torr	G, $mmol \cdot min^{-1} \cdot Torr^{-1}$	R = 1/G	Energy Loss, J/mmol	Rate of Energy Loss: W	Rate of Energy Loss: W/Torr
PI	71						
		29	0.52	1.93	1.35	0.34	0.012
PA	42						
		6	2.50	0.40	0.40	0.10	0.017
P̄c,L	36						
		4	3.75	0.27	0.30	0.08	0.019
P̄c,ti	32						
		7	2.14	0.47	0.64	0.16	0.023
P̄ti	25						
Total		46	0.33	3.07	2.69	0.68	0.015

O_2 consumption, 15 mmol/min. PB (barometric pressure) = 386 Torr. See Table 1 for symbols. [Data in part from Dill et al. (4).]

TABLE 4. *Oxygen Cascade in Resting Human on Peak of Mount Everest*

	P_{O_2}, Torr	ΔP_{O_2}, Torr	G, mmol·min^{-1}·Torr^{-1}	R = 1/G	Energy Loss, J/mmol	Rate of Energy Loss	
						W	W/Torr
PI	43						
		8	1.88	0.53	0.53	0.13	0.016
PA	35						
		5	3.00	0.33	0.40	0.10	0.019
$\bar{P}$c,L	30						
		3	5.00	0.20	0.27	0.07	0.026
$\bar{P}$c,ti	27						
		7	2.14	0.47	0.77	0.19	0.028
$\bar{P}$ti	20						
Total		23	0.65	1.53	1.97	0.49	0.021

O_2 consumption, 15 mmol/min. PB = 253 Torr. See Table 1 for symbols. [Data in part from West et al. (18).]

TABLE 5. *Minimal Conductance or Maximal Resistance Consistent With Specified Values*

Condition	$\dot{M}_{O_2}$, mmol/min	PI_{O_2}, Torr	$\Delta Pmax_{O_2}$, Torr	Gmin, mmol·min^{-1}·Torr^{-1}	Rmax, min·Torr·mmol^{-1}
Rest, sea level	15	150	140	0.11	9.33
Exercise, sea level	100	150	140	0.71	1.40
Altitude, 5,365 m*	15	71	61	0.25	4.06
Mount Everest†	15	43	33	0.45	2.20

$\dot{M}_{O_2}$, rate of O_2 consumption; PI_{O_2}, inspired P_{O_2}; $\Delta Pmax_{O_2}$, maximum P_{O_2} difference; Gmin, minimum conductance; Rmax, maximum resistance. * PB = 386 Torr. † PB = 253 Torr.

By use of the universal gas law, $n/V = P/RT$ (where n is the number of moles and V is volume), $\dot{V}_{O_2}$ can be converted to molar units

$$\begin{aligned}\dot{M}_{O_2} &= (1/RT)(P_B - 47)(FI_{O_2} - FA_{O_2})\dot{V}_A \\ &= (PI_{O_2} - PA_{O_2})(1/RT)\dot{V}_A\end{aligned} \quad (8)$$

where PB is barometric pressure. The conductance is

$$G_1 = \dot{M}/(P_I - P_A) = (1/RT)\dot{V}_A \quad (9)$$

The expression $1/RT$ is the molar concentration of a gas per unit partial pressure and is sometimes designated β_g (11). At body temperature β_g has a value of 0.052 mM/Torr, and

$$G = 0.052\dot{V}_A \quad (10)$$

or

$$G = 0.052f(V_T - V_{DS}) \quad (11)$$

where f is frequency of breathing, VT is tidal volume, and VDS is dead space volume; these three physiological variables determine $\dot{V}$A and hence G_1. Reference to Figure 2*C* makes it apparent that the amount of $\dot{V}$A (and hence work of breathing) required per torr increase in PA becomes greater the closer PA approaches PI.

Alveolar Gas to Pulmonary Capillary Blood

By definition $G_2 = \dot{M}/(P_A - \bar{P}c,L)$, which is also the definition of what is usually called the diffusing capacity or transfer capacity of the lungs (DL) (8). The reciprocal conductance (resistance) between alveolar gas and blood can be subdivided into two components: a true diffusion barrier, 1/Dm, where Dm is the diffusing capacity of the membrane, and a virtual barrier that depends on the reaction rate (θ) of O_2 with hemoglobin and on the volume of blood in the pulmonary capillaries (Vc). Thus

$$1/G_2 = 1/Dm + 1/\theta Vc \quad (12)$$

or

$$G_2 = (Dm\theta Vc)/(Dm + \theta Vc) \quad (13)$$

This conductance could be further analyzed into such factors as length of diffusion pathways, surface area available, solubility of gas in tissue, and tissue viscosity (16). For a discussion of the roles of chemical reaction and diffusion in pulmonary gas exchange see the review by Wagner (15).

Pulmonary Capillary Blood to Tissue Capillary Blood

This conductance (G_3) is defined as $\dot{M}/(\bar{P}c,L - \bar{P}c,ti)$. By the Fick relationship

$$\dot{M} = (Ca - C\bar{v})\dot{Q} = (Pa - P\bar{v})\beta_b\dot{Q} \quad (14)$$

where Ca and $C\bar{v}$ are the concentrations, and Pa and $P\bar{v}$ the partial pressures of O_2 in arterial and mixed venous blood, respectively, and β_b is the slope of the O_2 dissociation curve between Pa and $P\bar{v}$. Thus

$$G_3 = (Pa - P\bar{v})\beta_b\dot{Q}/(\bar{P}c,L - \bar{P}c,ti) \quad (15)$$

The independent physiological variables determining G_3 are blood flow ($\dot{Q}$) and β_b. Cardiac output is capable of a severalfold increase over the resting value. The value of β_b depends on the location of the arterial and venous points on the dissociation curve and on the O_2-carrying capacity of the blood and thus may vary over a wide range of values. It is clear that the ratio

TABLE 6. *Oxygen Conductances*

Pathway	Physiological Variables	Quantitative Relationships
Inspired gas to alveolar gas	Tidal volume Breathing frequency Dead space	$G_1 = \frac{\dot{M}}{P_I - P_A} = \beta_g\dot{V}_A = \beta_g f(V_T - V_{DS})$
Alveolar gas to pulmonary capillary blood	Alveolar-capillary membrane Capillary blood volume Hb-O_2 kinetics Ventilation/perfusion distribution	$G_2 = \frac{\dot{M}}{P_A - \bar{P}_{c,L}} = D_L = \frac{D_m\theta V_c}{D_m + \theta V_c}$
Pulmonary capillary blood to tissue capillary blood	Rate of blood flow Slope of O_2 dissociation curve	$G_3 = \frac{\dot{M}}{\bar{P}_{c,L} - \bar{P}_{c,ti}} = \frac{(P_a - P_{\bar{v}})\beta_b\dot{Q}}{\bar{P}_{c,L} - \bar{P}_{c,ti}}$
Tissue capillary blood to tissue	Capillary geometry Hb-O_2 kinetics	$G_4 = \frac{\dot{M}}{\bar{P}_{c,ti} - \bar{P}_{ti}} = D_{ti}$

See Equations 1–16 for symbols.

$(P_a - P_{\bar{v}})/(\bar{P}_{c,L} - \bar{P}_{c,ti})$ must be a number greater than unity because $\bar{P}_{c,L}$ must be $<P_a$ and $\bar{P}_{c,ti}$ must be $>P_{\bar{v}}$. For any constant value of $\dot{M}$ the arteriovenous difference $(P_a - P_{\bar{v}})$ varies inversely with $\beta_b\dot{Q}$; thus, as $\beta_b\dot{Q}$ increases, both $P_a - P_{\bar{v}}$ and $\bar{P}_{c,L} - \bar{P}_{c,ti}$ decrease and both approach zero as $\beta_b\dot{Q}$ approaches infinity.

Tissue Capillary Blood to Tissue

This conductance (G_4) is defined as the O_2 flow divided by the difference between the mean partial pressure of O_2 in the tissue capillaries and that in the tissues. This may be regarded as a diffusing capacity for the tissues (Dti) analogous to that for the lung

$$G_4 = \dot{M}/(\bar{P}_{c,ti} - \bar{P}_{ti}) = D_{ti} \quad (16)$$

The principal physiological variables determining G_4 are the kinetics of oxyhemoglobin dissociation and the geometry of the capillaries perfusing the metabolizing tissues. The former is subject to modulation by such factors as the Bohr effect, concentration of 2,3-diphosphoglycerate (DPG), and temperature. The latter can be varied widely by neural and humoral mechanisms under either local or central control.

The relationships describing the four conductances, their physiological components, and modulating influences are summarized in Table 6. The primary mechanism in G_1 and G_3 is convection (bulk flow); in G_2 and G_4 it is diffusion (Fig. 6).

The use of the virtual mean partial pressures of O_2 ($\bar{P}_{c,L}$ and $\bar{P}_{c,ti}$) simplifies analysis of the flow of O_2 between lung and tissue, but it conceals the interaction of perfusion and diffusion involved in the transport mechanism. Some aspects of this are illustrated by the electrical analogue shown in Figure 7, which is in principle similar to the model proposed by Piiper and Scheid (12; see also ref. 10). This model assumes a linear relationship between partial pressure and gas content of blood, and hence applies only approximately for the carriage of O_2.

A central feature of the model shown is the representation of the circulating of blood as an assembly of capacitors mounted on an endless belt, which continuously rotates in the direction indicated. As each capacitative element enters the pulmonary capillary, one terminal makes contact with a conductor connected to a large capacitor (representing the alveoli) that is kept charged (by $\dot{V}_A$) at a constant potential P_A. During their passage through the pulmonary capillary, the capacitative elements become charged at a rate dependent on the resistance, $R_L = 1/D_L$, and on the capacitance, $\beta_b V_c$, of the blood in the capillary at any moment. The time constant (τ) for charging the capacitors is $R_L\beta_b V_c = \beta_b V_c/D_L$. The time spent in the capillary is $V_c/\dot{Q}$. A time $= 6\tau$ is required for charging to be essentially complete (99.75% of equilibrium). If the time spent in the capillary is small relative to the time constant, i.e., if $D_L/\beta_b\dot{Q} < 6$, the charge on the capacitors will not be complete when they leave the pulmonary capillaries. In other words,

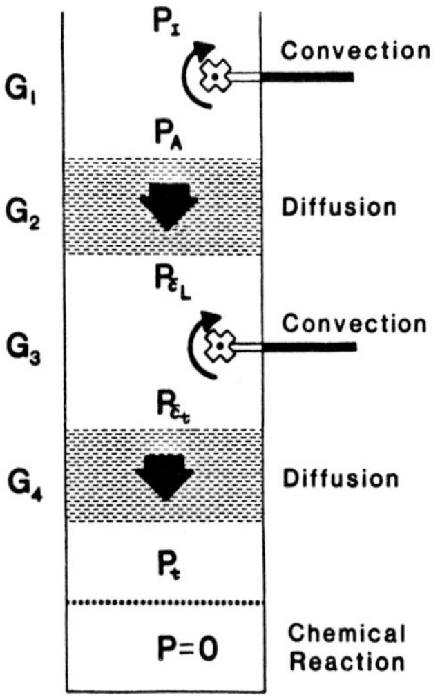

FIG. 6. Oxygen cascade as 2 diffusive and 2 convective conductances. Difference, ΔP, between 2 successive regions is determined by the metabolic O_2 consumption and the conductance between the 2 regions. Convective conductance may be regarded as the mixing of the 2 extreme regions of a conductive element by stirring (alveolar ventilation or blood flow). The faster the stirring the smaller the $P_I - P_A$ or $\bar{P}_{c,L} - \bar{P}_{c,ti}$. P_I, partial pressure of O_2 (P_{O_2}) in inspired gas; P_A, P_{O_2} in alveolar gas; $\bar{P}_{c,L}$, mean P_{O_2} in pulmonary capillary blood; $\bar{P}_{c,t}$ ($\bar{P}_{c,ti}$), mean P_{O_2} in tissue capillary blood; Pt (Pti), P_{O_2} in tissue.

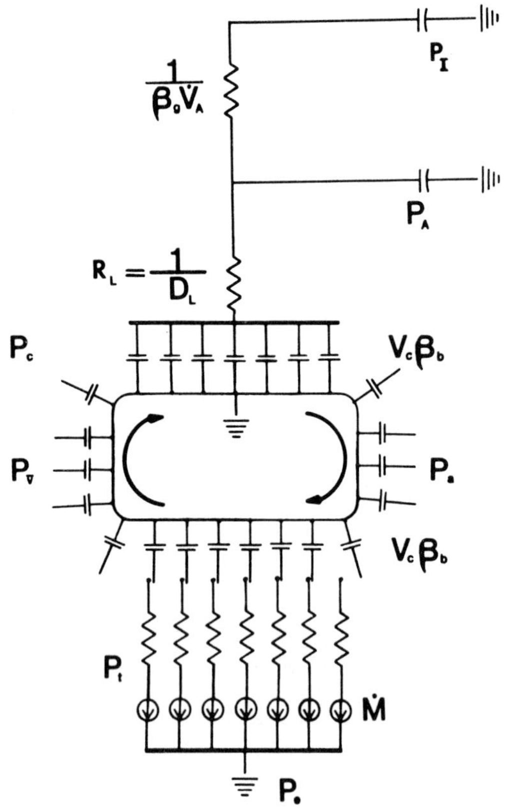

FIG. 7. Electrical model of O_2 transport system to demonstrate factors determining the rate of O_2 transfer into pulmonary blood and out of tissue capillary blood. Blood is represented as an assembly of capacitors mounted on an endless belt rotating at a rate $\dot{Q}$. Rate of charging of capacitors in the lung is determined by DL (diffusing capacity of the lung) and PA − $\bar{P}$c,L (PA, alveolar P_{O_2}; $\bar{P}$c,L, mean P_{O_2} in pulmonary capillary blood). Rate of discharge in the tissue is determined by $\dot{M}$ (use rate). β_g, Molar concentration of a gas per unit partial pressure; $\dot{V}$A, alveolar ventilation; PI, inspired P_{O_2}; RL, pulmonary resistance; Pc, capillary P_{O_2}; Vc, capillary volume; β_b, slope of the O_2 dissociation curve; P$\bar{v}$, mixed venous P_{O_2}; Pa, arterial P_{O_2}; Pt (Pti), tissue P_{O_2}; P_0, $P_{O_2} = 0$.

there will be an alveolar-arterial gradient. This can occur either because of a diffusion impairment, a high flow, or a high capacitance. In this case the rate of transfer from lung to blood is said to be diffusion limited. On the other hand, if $D_L/\beta_b\dot{Q}$ is ≫6, the blood will be essentially in equilibrium with alveolar gas before the end of the capillary is reached and the rate of transfer will be limited by the rate of blood flow; i.e., the system is perfusion limited (12).

Further understanding can be gained by deriving a mathematical description of the model.

At any distance x along the pulmonary capillary

$$\Delta P = P_A - P_{c,L} \quad (17)$$

where PA is the partial pressure in the alveoli and Pc,L is the partial pressure in the blood at distance x along the capillary.

The rate of change of ΔP with time is proportional to ΔP

$$d\Delta P/dt = K\Delta P \quad (18)$$

where K is the rate constant. Integrating with respect to time gives

$$\Delta P = Ae^{-kt} \quad (19)$$

where A is a constant of integration that is readily evaluated because when $t = 0$

$$A = \Delta P = P_A - P_{\bar{v}} \quad (20)$$

Furthermore

$$K = \frac{D_L}{\beta_b V_c} \quad (21)$$

and

$$V_c = \dot{Q}t' \quad (22)$$

where $\dot{Q}$ is the blood flow through the capillary and t' is the total time an element of blood spends in the capillary. Thus

$$\Delta P = P_A - P_c = (P_A - P_{\bar{v}})e^{\frac{-D_L}{\beta_b\dot{Q}}\cdot\frac{t}{t'}} \quad (23)$$

or

$$\frac{P_A - P_c}{P_A - P_{\bar{v}}} = e^{\frac{-D_L}{\beta_b\dot{Q}}\cdot\frac{t}{t'}} \quad (24)$$

The ratio (PA − Pc)/(PA − P$\bar{v}$) is the difference in partial pressure between alveolar gas and capillary blood expressed as a fraction of the initial difference at time 0 when the blood first enters the capillary.

The change of this value with time is shown for various values of $D_L/\beta_b\dot{Q}$ in Figure 8. Similar in-

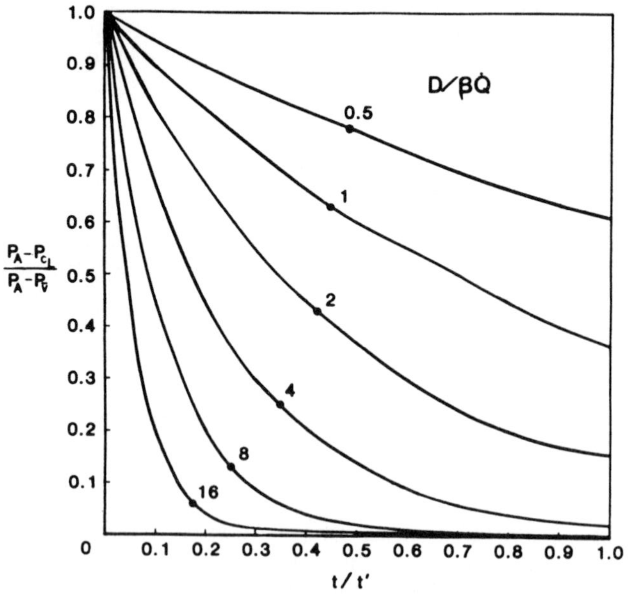

FIG. 8. Change in alveolar–pulmonary capillary P_{O_2} with time (t) (or distance) along a pulmonary capillary at different values of $D/\beta_b\dot{Q}$. D(DL), diffusing capacity of the lung; β_b, slope of the O_2 dissociation curve; $\dot{Q}$, blood flow; PA, alveolar P_{O_2}; Pc,L, P_{O_2} in pulmonary capillary blood; P$\bar{v}$, mixed venous P_{O_2}; t', total time. ●, Mean ΔP_{O_2} for indicated $D/\beta_b\dot{Q}$.

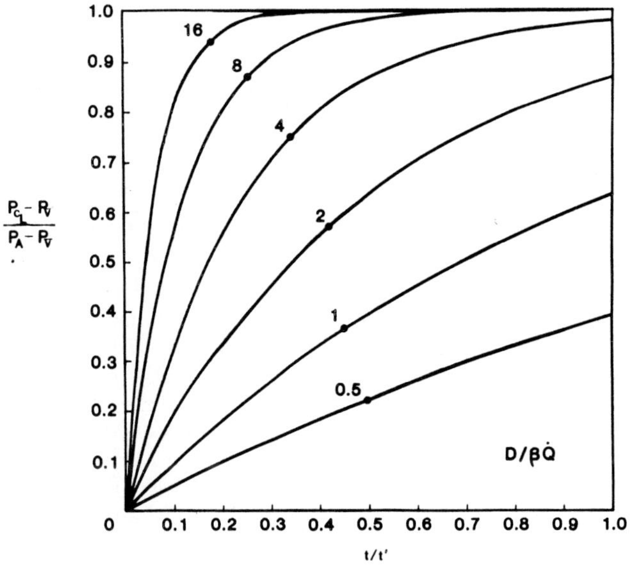

FIG. 9. Increase in pulmonary capillary P_{O_2} with time (or distance) along a pulmonary capillary at different values of $D/\beta_b\dot{Q}$.

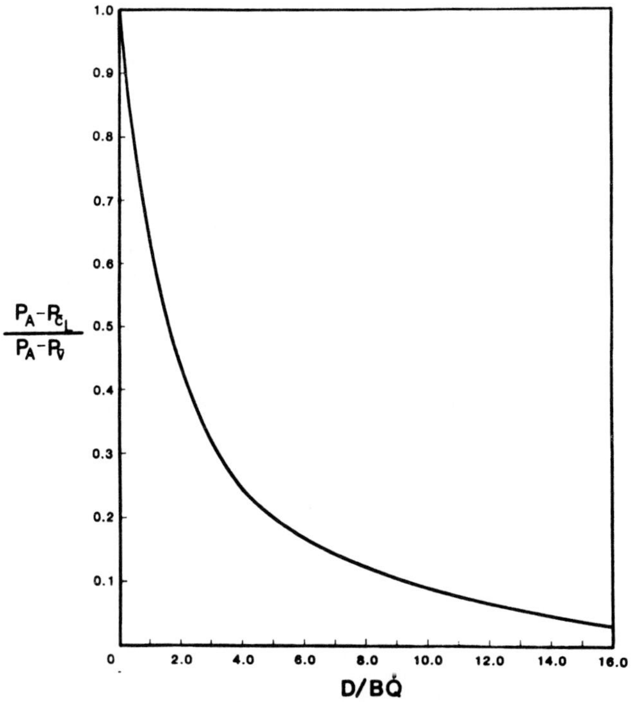

FIG. 10. Mean alveolar–pulmonary capillary P_{O_2} difference as a function of $D/\beta_b\dot{Q}$.

formation is shown in Figure 9 where $(P_{c,L} - P_{\bar{v}})/(P_A - P_{\bar{v}})$, i.e., the increase in $P_{c,L}$ expressed as a fraction of $P_A - P_{\bar{v}}$, is shown as a function of time. Also on these graphs are points showing the $\bar{P}_c$ values for each value of $D_L/\beta_b\dot{Q}$. These values may be derived as follows

$$\dot{M} = D_L(P_A - \bar{P}_{c,L}) = \beta_b\dot{Q}(P_a - P_{\bar{v}}) \quad (25)$$

$$(P_A - \bar{P}_{c,L}) = (P_a - P_{\bar{v}})/(D_L/\beta_b\dot{Q}) \quad (26)$$

Normalizing gives

$$\frac{P_A - \bar{P}_{c,L}}{P_A - P_{\bar{v}}} = \frac{1}{D_L/\beta_b\dot{Q}}\left(\frac{P_a - P_{\bar{v}}}{P_A - P_{\bar{v}}}\right) \quad (27)$$

or

$$\frac{\bar{P}_{c,L} - P_{\bar{v}}}{P_A - P_{\bar{v}}} = 1 - \frac{P_A - \bar{P}_{c,L}}{P_A - P_{\bar{v}}} \quad (28)$$

Graphs showing $(P_A - \bar{P}_{c,L})/(P_A - P_{\bar{v}})$ and $(\bar{P}_{c,L} - P_{\bar{v}})/(P_A - P_{\bar{v}})$ as a function of $D_L/\beta_b\dot{Q}$ are plotted in Figures 10 and 11.

It is apparent from Figures 8–11 that as $D_L/\beta_b\dot{Q}$ increases, equilibration of Pc with P_A is approached earlier during the passage of blood through a pulmonary capillary. It is also evident that as $D_L/\beta_b\dot{Q}$ decreases, the locus of $\bar{P}_c$ moves farther from the entrance of the capillary and approaches a limit halfway along the capillary.

In the tissue capillaries of our model, the mean partial pressure is midway between the arterial and mixed venous values. This is because the rate of flow of O_2 out of a capillary is considered to be constant along its length, since it is governed by the rate of O_2 uptake by the mitochondria. Thus in the model

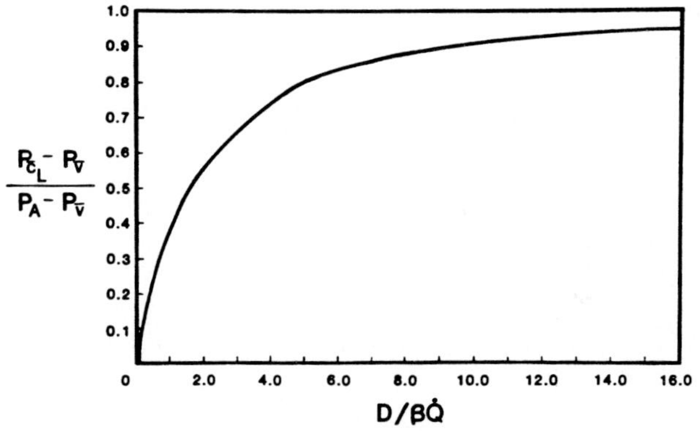

FIG. 11. Difference between mean pulmonary capillary P_{O_2} and mixed venous P_{O_2} as a function of $D/\beta_b\dot{Q}$.

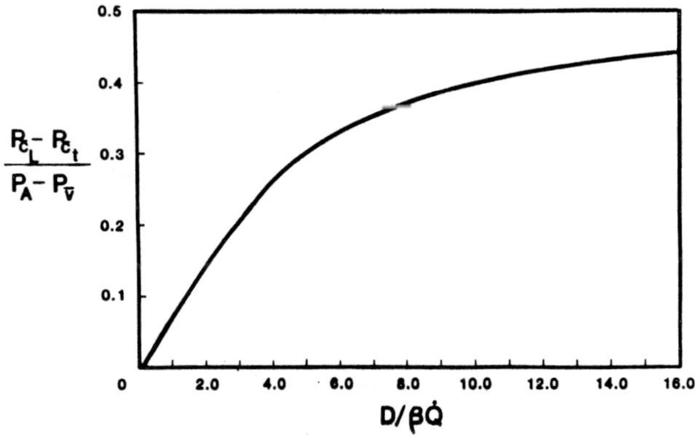

FIG. 12. Difference between mean pulmonary capillary P_{O_2} and mean tissue capillary P_{O_2} as a function of $D/\beta_b\dot{Q}$. Upper limit for this difference is half the alveolar–mixed venous difference.

$$\bar{P}c,ti = (Pa + P\bar{v})/2 \qquad (29)$$

Because Pa cannot exceed PA, the upper limit for $\bar{P}$c,ti is halfway between PA and P$\bar{v}$. The upper limit for $\bar{P}$c,L is PA. Thus the upper limit for ($\bar{P}$c,L − $\bar{P}$c,ti)/(PA − P$\bar{v}$) is 0.5.

In Figure 12, the difference ($\bar{P}$c,L − $\bar{P}$c,ti) between mean pulmonary capillary and mean tissue capillary P_{O_2} is shown as a function of $D_L/\beta_b\dot{Q}$, and in Figure 13 relative values of Pa, $\bar{P}$c,L, and $\bar{P}$c,ti are shown with reference to PA and P$\bar{v}$. Changes occurring with time in lung capillaries and in tissue capillaries during a circulatory cycle are shown in Figure 14 for two values of $D_L/\beta_b\dot{Q}$. Finally the changes of P_{O_2} along a tissue capillary are shown in Figure 15 with the parallel changes presumed to occur in the tissue (9). Note that these representations, like earlier ones, depend on the assumption of a linear O_2 dissociation curve. For a discussion of factors influencing $\bar{P}$c,ti and $\bar{P}$ti, see Tenney (14).

In conclusion, this highly simplified model of gas exchange ignores obvious facts and omits important details. The representation of gas exchange as a series of conductances seems basically valid, but keep in mind that, in both lungs and tissues, millions of parallel units have, in effect, been lumped into single entities. Thus the problem of inequalities of ventilation/perfusion ratios in the lungs has been ignored (2). Likewise I have ignored the fact that tissue is not a single homogeneously perfused structure but that it consists of a multitude of separate parallel units, each with its own demand for O_2.

Furthermore the model ignores such realities as the nonlinear relationships between P_{O_2} and O_2 content of blood and the effect of such factors as CO_2, pH, DPG, and temperature on this relationship.

This chapter deals only with steady states and not the transient effects that occur whenever the system

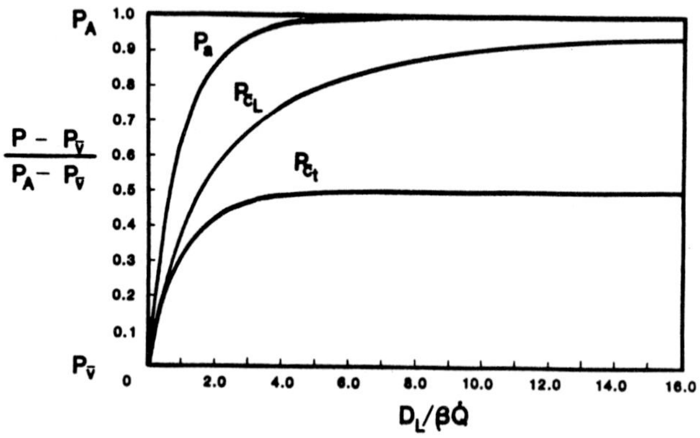

FIG. 13. Arterial, mean pulmonary capillary, and mean tissue capillary P_{O_2} as a function of $D/\beta_b\dot{Q}$.

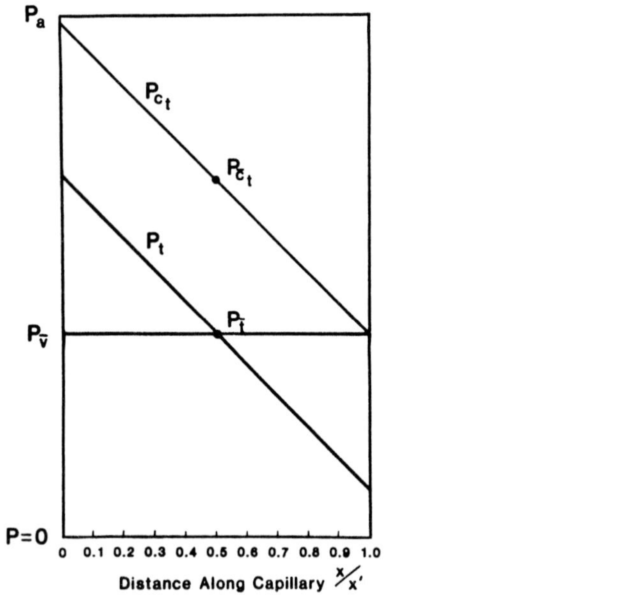

FIG. 15. Changes of P_{O_2} in a tissue capillary and in tissue as a function of distance (x) along the capillary.

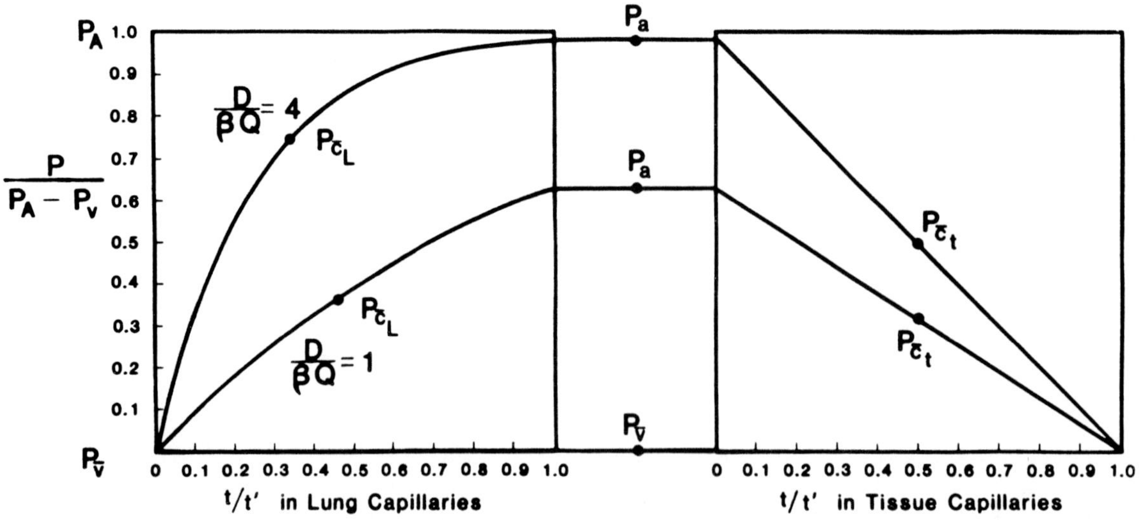

FIG. 14. Changes in P_{O_2} along lung capillaries and along tissue capillaries at 2 different values of $D/\beta_b\dot{Q}$. ●, Mean P_{O_2} values in each region.

is perturbed. The remarkable physiological control system, composed of elements both neural and chemical, that regulates the conductances so as optimally to apportion O_2 flow to the various parts of the body in accord with the needs of the separate tissues and of the body as a whole, is also not examined. This overview has been painted with a broad brush; the result is a blurred approximation of reality. It is hoped that the inexactitude of detail is offset by a clearer emergence of general concepts that can serve as a basis for dealing with problems of gas exchange. Many of the missing details appear in subsequent chapters of this *Handbook*. Some future author supplied with more complete and accurate information will, with computer assistance, be able to compose a more satisfactory picture.

REFERENCES

1. Astrand, P., and K. Rodahl. *Textbook of Work Physiology.* New York: McGraw-Hill, 1970.
2. Chinet, A., J. L. Micheli, and P. Haab. Inhomogeneity effects on O_2 and CO pulmonary diffusing capacity estimates by steady-state methods. Theory. *Respir. Physiol.* 13: 1–22, 1971.
3. Dejours, P. (editor). *Principles of Comparative Respiratory Physiology.* Amsterdam: North-Holland, 1975, 253 p.
4. Dill, D. B., J. H. Talbott, and W. V. Consolazio. Blood as a physicochemical system. Man at high altitudes. *J. Biol. Chem.* 118: 649–666, 1937.
5. Fenn, W. O. Introduction. In: *Oxygen in the Animal Organism*, edited by F. Dickens and E. Neil. New York: Pergamon, 1964, p. xi–xvii.
6. Haab, P. Systématisation des échanges gazeux pulmonaires. *J. Physiol. Paris* 78: 108–118, 1982.
7. Holmgren, A. Introduction to panel discussion: the 'oxygen conduction line' of the human body. *Proc. Int. Symp. Cardiovasc. Respir. Effects Hypoxia, Kingston, Ontario, 1965.* New York: Hafner, 1966, p. 391–400.
8. Meyer, M., P. Scheid, G. Riepl, H.-J. Wagner, and J. Piiper. Pulmonary diffusing capacities for O_2 and CO measured by a rebreathing technique. *J. Appl. Physiol.* 51: 1643–1650, 1981.
9. Otis, A. B. Some simple models for the diffusion of oxygen from blood to tissue. In: *Physical Bases of Circulatory Transport*, edited by E. B. Reeve and A. C. Guyton. London: Saunders, 1967.
10. Piiper, J. Theoretische Untersuchung der alveolär-capillären O_2-Diffusion bei verschiedenen Annahmen über die Lage des Diffusions-widerstandes. *Pfluegers Arch.* 275: 173–192, 1962.
11. Piiper, J., P. Dejours, P. Haab, and H. Rahn. Concepts and basic quantities in gas exchange physiology. *Respir. Physiol.* 13: 292–304, 1971.
12. Piiper, J., and P. Scheid. Blood-gas equilibration in lungs. In: *Pulmonary Gas Exchange. Ventilation, Blood Flow, and Diffusion*, edited by J. B. West. New York: Academic, 1980, vol. 1, p. 131–171.
13. Taylor, C. R., and E. R. Weibel. Design of the mammalian respiratory system. I. Problem and strategy. *Respir. Physiol.* 44: 1–10, 1981.
14. Tenney, S. M. A theoretical analysis of the relationship between venous blood and mean tissue oxygen pressures. *Respir. Physiol.* 20: 283–296, 1974.
15. Wagner, P. D. Diffusion and chemical reaction in pulmonary gas exchange. *Physiol. Rev.* 57: 257–312, 1977.
16. Weibel, E. R. *The Pathway for Oxygen. Structure and Function in the Mammalian Respiratory System.* Cambridge, MA: Harvard Univ. Press, 1984.
17. Weibel, E. R., C. R. Taylor, P. Gehr, H. Hoppeler, O. Mathieu, and G. M. O. Maloiy. Design of the mammalian respiratory system. IX. Functional and structural limits for oxygen flow. *Respir. Physiol.* 44: 151–164, 1981.
18. West, J. B., P. H. Hackett, K. H. Maret, J. S. Milledge, R. M. Peters, Jr., C. J. Pizzo, and R. M. Winslow. Pulmonary gas exchange on the summit of Mount Everest. *J. Appl. Physiol.* 55: 678–687, 1983.

CHAPTER 2

Laws of physics pertaining to gas exchange

RALPH H. KELLOGG

Department of Physiology and Department of the History of Health Sciences, University of California, San Francisco, California

CHAPTER CONTENTS

THE CHAPTER BY RADFORD (114) in the 1964 edition of the *Handbook* section on respiration provided a comprehensive summary of the physics of gases. This chapter describes the historical development of the gas laws and explains their practical application to pulmonary gas exchange. It begins with a familiar equation that illustrates applications of the gas laws to pulmonary gas exchange and then summarizes the history of each physical concept or law involved and the practical aspects of its use. The historical development should explain why some rather illogical expressions have become customary. The chapter ends with a recommendation for replacing these anachronisms with modern units.

For historical identification of each person when first mentioned, the full name is spelled out. Where a person is not ordinarily known by his first name, all given names except that usually used are enclosed in brackets. Dates of birth and death (where known) are also given, except that the birth dates of living persons are omitted to avoid calling unnecessary attention to their ages. The references cite the original publication whenever I have seen it directly or in photocopy. A reprint or translation is also cited if considered helpful.

Because in this chapter I need to distinguish between millimeters of mercury as a unit of pressure and millimeters of mercury as the actual length of a column of mercury, I have deviated from the usual *Handbook* style. Instead, I use the abbreviated term *mmHg* when I refer to the unit of pressure, which is the most common use of this abbreviation, and I spell out the words *millimeters of mercury* when I use them in their nontechnical sense as the actual length of a column of mercury, where millimeter is the unit, not millimeters of mercury.

FAMILIAR EQUATION ILLUSTRATING APPLICATION OF GAS LAWS

One of the most fundamental and widely used relationships in pulmonary gas exchange (115) is commonly summarized by the equation stating that, in the steady state and when inspired CO_2 is negligible, the alveolar partial pressure of CO_2 ($P_{A_{CO_2}}$) is proportional to the ratio of the rates of CO_2 elimination ($\dot{V}_{CO_2}$) and alveolar ventilation ($\dot{V}_A$)

$$P_{A_{CO_2}} = 863(\dot{V}_{CO_2}/\dot{V}_A) \tag{1}$$

This equation illustrates the importance of several fundamental gas laws.

$P_{A_{CO_2}}$. Whenever alveolar gas samples are analyzed in terms of the percentage of CO_2 in dry gas, Dalton's law of partial pressures must be used to calculate the partial pressure of CO_2 from the percentage composition, the vapor pressure of water at body temperature, and the barometric pressure. The partial pressure of CO_2, rather than the percent CO_2, is the significant variable physiologically because of Henry's law of solubility: the concentration of a gas physically dissolved in a liquid is determined by its partial pressure in the gas phase with which it has equilibrated.

863. This peculiar number is the body temperature (310°K) multiplied by the ratio of the standard pressure and standard temperature (760 mmHg/273°K) adopted to express moles of CO_2 in terms of volumes at standard temperature and pressure, dry (STPD). Because the units of temperature cancel, 863 has the

units of mmHg, matching the units of PA_{CO_2}. The fact that most physiologists still tend to express pressure in terms of mmHg, the linear height of a mercury column (suitably corrected for density and gravity), or its more recent equivalent, torr, reflects the introduction of mercury columns for measuring pressure before it was generally recognized that pressure should have the dimensions of force per unit area. The International System of Units (SI) recommends the more logical expression of force per unit area in newtons per square meter, which are called pascals and symbolized Pa in SI units. Some authors are already using pascals. I use mmHg in this chapter for its historical significance, but values can readily be converted to pascals by remembering that 7.5 mmHg = 1 kPa, or more precisely, 7.5006 mmHg = 1 kPa.

$\dot{V}_{CO_2}/\dot{V}A$. Both of these values are commonly based on gas volumes measured at ambient temperature and pressure, saturated with water vapor (ATPS), as in a spirometer. The rate of CO_2 output ($\dot{V}_{CO_2}$) must be converted to the corresponding volume at STPD by using the laws of Boyle and Charles for ideal gases, whereas the rate of alveolar ventilation ($\dot{V}A$) must be converted to the volume the expired gas had at body temperature and pressure saturated with water vapor in the lungs (BTPS). Why should these two volumes be expressed at different conditions in the same equation? This anomaly has arisen because of the way in which knowledge of barometric pressure and the gas laws developed.

BAROMETRIC PRESSURE AND ALTITUDE

This account of the development of our modern understanding of gas pressures begins with Evangelista Torricelli (1608–1647), who had been a pupil of Galileo Galilei (1564–1642). In the middle of the seventeenth century, Torricelli and his associates in Florence made the first mercurial barometer (96), a long glass tube completely filled with mercury and inverted into a dish of mercury. It was immediately apparent that in sufficiently long tubes the mercury fell when the tube was inverted, leaving a space above the mercury. Tubes set side by side showed the same height of mercury column, even when the diameter or the volume of space left above the mercury differed from tube to tube. Some observers considered that this was evidence that the column of mercury (i.e., the mercury that is in the tube and above the level of mercury in the dish) was supported by the weight of the atmosphere pressing down on the surface of the mercury in the dish, but others disputed this idea. Torricelli's observations with the mercurial barometer were disseminated in the form of his letter of June 11, 1644 to his young friend Michelangelo Ricci (1619–1682) of Rome, who had also been a pupil of Galileo and later became a cardinal. Ricci sent copies around Europe to other scholars with whom he maintained correspondence (96).

Blaise Pascal (1623–1662) in France heard about Torricelli's interesting experiments and realized that if the height of the mercury column were determined by the weight of the atmosphere, it should be less at higher altitude. In 1648, Pascal had his brother-in-law, Florin Périer (1605–1672) of Clermont-Ferrand, carry a barometer up the Puy de Dôme, a 1,465 m mountain near Clermont-Ferrand in south central France, to establish this point. Pascal confirmed the relationship by observing the height of the mercury column at the surface of the Seine in Paris and at the top of a nearby tower (103, 104).

Realization that barometric pressure varies with altitude led to progressively more refined attempts to determine altitude from observed barometric pressure; however, this long history is not discussed here because the results are inevitably inaccurate. Pressure varies from several factors, including the weather. Nevertheless the general form of the theoretical relationship in terms of the temperature and density of the atmosphere, the acceleration of gravity, etc., can be expressed by a complicated logarithmic expression, and a "standard atmosphere" based on assumed values for the important variables can be calculated. Currently the international standard is the ICAO Standard Atmosphere, most recently revised in 1964 by the ICAO, the International Civil Aviation Organization (64, 143). The pressure predicted by the ICAO Standard Atmosphere for any particular altitude from 0 to 11 km above sea level (the troposphere where temperature varies with altitude) can be calculated to within 0.1 mmHg by the following formula, which I have simplified from the equations in the ICAO *Manual* (64)

$$PB = 760[288.15/(288.15 - 6.5H)]^{-5.256} \qquad (2)$$

where PB is the predicted barometric pressure in mmHg and H is the altitude in kilometers. For the isothermal layer from 11 to 20 km, the corresponding formula is

$$PB = 169.8 \exp[-0.1577(H - 11)] \qquad (3)$$

Contrary to popular belief, the ICAO Standard Atmosphere does not reliably indicate even the mean barometric pressure to be expected at any particular point of known altitude on the earth's surface. Mountains tend to introduce peculiarities in their immediate vicinity, and the variations of temperature and air density with altitude in equatorial regions are quite different from those in the temperate zone, for example. The first measurement of the barometric pressure on the summit of Mt. Everest, 8,848 m above sea level, made by Christopher James Pizzo, M.D., on October 24, 1981, showed that the pressure was about 15 mmHg higher than that predicted from the ICAO

Standard Atmosphere (145), a difference that is probably crucial for the ability of acclimatized man to climb to the summit without O_2 equipment. Because the important variable affecting physiological processes such as blood oxygenation is pressure rather than altitude, the actual barometric pressure should always be specified in proper pressure units when reporting respiratory experiments, even if the actual altitude or the equivalent altitude determined from the ICAO Standard Atmosphere is mentioned.

PRACTICAL USE OF MERCURIAL BAROMETERS

The theory of mercurial barometers has greatly advanced since Torricelli's time (96). It is now recognized that the atmospheric pressure or absolute force per unit area equals the product of three factors: the height of the mercury column, the density of the mercury, and the acceleration of gravity. The length of the measuring scale and the density of the mercury vary with the temperature of the barometer, whereas gravity varies with latitude. Therefore these three factors must be standardized to specify a pressure in mmHg or torr. The necessary corrections are discussed next.

If the height of the mercury column is to be read accurately, the barometer and its scale must be exactly vertical and the mercurial surface in the reservoir must be adjusted to the zero of the scale. In the common precision instruments of the Fortin or similar designs adopted as standards by the U.S. Department of Commerce Weather Bureau (91), this is accomplished by adjusting the bottom of the mercury reservoir until the surface of the mercury in it just barely contacts the tip of the ivory point without being dimpled by it. The level of the other surface, exposed to the Torricellian vacuum, is then read by sighting across the highest point of the meniscus (i.e., the point farthest from the walls that depress the mercurial surface by capillarity). A vernier device is commonly provided to read the scale to 0.1 mm or 0.1 in without parallax.

Because barometer scales change length with temperature, a scale reading represents the true length from its zero only at the temperature for which it was calibrated. At all other temperatures, the scale reading must be corrected for the thermal expansion of the scale. By a curious convention, barometer scales reading in English units are calibrated to be correct at 62°F, whereas all metric scales are calibrated to be correct at 0°C (32°F). Thus a thermal-correction formula or table designed for English units must be used to correct the reading of a barometer scale marked in inches to the true distance. Similarly, a thermal-correction formula or table designed for metric units must be used to correct the reading of a barometer scale marked in metric units to the true distance. In either case, the scale reading must be converted to true distance by the appropriate thermal correction before the distance can be correctly converted to the equivalent value in the other system of units.

Because the density of mercury varies inversely with temperature, the true height of the mercury column must be corrected for this change in density from its value at 0°C, the standard for both English and metric units. The usual thermal-correction tables for barometers correct for the thermal change in length of the scale as well as in density of the mercury; thus the table selected must conform to the scale's material and units.

Gravity does not result simply from Newton's law of gravitation. The rotation of the earth produces an opposing centrifugal force, which is greatest at the equator and decreases to zero at the poles. After the barometer reading has been corrected for the deviation of temperature from its standard value, the result must be further corrected for the deviation of gravity from its standard value, which is the combination of gravitation and centrifugal force at a latitude of 45° from the equator. The centrifugal force is also greater on a mountain than at sea level, because of the greater radius of rotation, but this further correction is negligible.

Physiologists, unlike meteorologists, should not reduce barometric pressure readings to sea level. Wind and weather are influenced by horizontal differences in the gradient of pressures above the earth's surface. Thus meteorologists compare barometric pressure readings predicted for a single altitude (sea level) by assuming the weight of an air column that might exist between the barometer and sea level if the intervening space were occupied by air rather than solid ground. Physiological effects, however, depend on the actual barometric pressure at the subject, which may be quite different from the value cited in a weather report.

A small altitude correction may be needed if the nearest barometer is at a different altitude from the physiological experiment being conducted, for example on a different floor of a multistory building. The ICAO Standard Atmosphere indicates the difference in ambient pressure to be expected between the altitude of the barometer and that of the experiment, if the only cause of that pressure difference is the weight of the intervening column of air. That difference cannot be used for correction, however, if some other agent, such as a ventilating fan, could be contributing to the difference in pressures at the two points. Because the adjustment per meter becomes progressively less as one goes above sea level, the correction must be worked out separately for each altitude.

Brass scales expand 0.0000184 per °C from 0°C. Mercury expands $(181{,}792 + 0.175t + 0.035116t^2) \times 10^{-9}$ per °C, where t is the temperature in °C (143). The conventional equation (137) predicts that gravity in centimeters per seconds squared at any latitude is equal to $978.03184558(1 + 0.0053024\sin^2\phi - 0.0000059\sin^2 2\phi)$, where ϕ is the north or south latitude. Conversion tables for thermal correction with brass or glass scales in English or metric units and separate tables for the value of gravity as a function of latitude are readily available (143). Those using programmable calculators or a computer may prefer to use the following formula, which I have simplified from the above relationships to correct the reading of a mercurial barometer with a brass millimeter scale for latitude and for temperatures between 0°C and 40°C with an accuracy within 0.1 mmHg

$$P_B = S/[(1 + 0.0001634t)k] \quad (4)$$

where P_B is the corrected barometric pressure in mmHg or torr, S is the brass scale reading in millimeters, t is the barometer temperature in °C, and k is a constant that depends only on the latitude and therefore needs to be calculated only once for any given barometer location

$$k = 0.99736 + 0.00529\sin^2\phi \quad (5)$$

The local barometric pressure corrected by Equations 4 and 5 to standard mmHg or torr can be converted to precise absolute units of force per unit area by using the standard density of mercury at 0°C (13.595 g/cm^3) and the standard value of gravity at 45° latitude (980.6 cm/s^2) or by recalling that 7.50 mmHg = 1 kPa = 1,000 N/m^2.

Detailed instructions for mercurial barometers are available (91), but a few words about preserving the Torricellian vacuum may be useful. When the Chamonix physician Michel Gabriel Paccard (1757–1827) made the first ascent to the summit of Mt. Blanc in 1786, he carried a mercurial barometer to measure the atmospheric pressure at various points along the way. His data show that when he fell while crossing a crevasse he must have introduced a small bubble of air into his Torricellian vacuum; from that point on his pressure readings were systematically too low (51). To avoid that and other mishaps (e.g., letting the inertia of the mercury break out the top of the barometer tube), a special procedure in five successive steps is necessary whenever a mercurial barometer is to be moved (91). *1)* The bottom of the reservoir is raised until only a small bubble of air (to allow for slight thermal expansion of the mercury) is left in the reservoir. *2)* The reservoir is then closed from the atmosphere if possible. *3)* The bottom of the reservoir is raised further until the mercury is almost at the top of the tube. *4)* The barometer is slowly tilted from the vertical so that the mercury slowly rises to the top of the tube, making a tiny click when it obliterates the Torricellian vacuum, without breaking the glass. *5)* The barometer is turned completely upside down and transported with the reservoir uppermost. The process is reversed to make the barometer usable in its new location.

If air is admitted or if a barometer becomes dirty and needs cleaning, repairs should be attempted only by a well-equipped expert. Mercury does not wet glass and thus tends to trap air molecules that eventually rise to ruin the Torricellian vacuum. The complicated procedures needed to avoid this (91) commonly include boiling the mercury in the inverted barometer tube to carry off trapped air molecules in the escaping mercury vapor, which is highly toxic.

BOYLE'S LAW (MARIOTTE'S LAW)

Shortly after Torricelli's original experiments with a mercurial barometer, Otto von Guericke (1602–1686) invented a pump that would draw air out of a vessel. Gaspar Schott (1608–1666) included a description of von Guericke's air-pump experiments at Magdeburg in his 1657 treatise (128), which came to the attention of Robert Boyle (1627–1691).

Boyle was a younger son of the first Earl of Cork, wealthy enough that he could live in Oxford on the High Street near University College and pursue his own scientific interests (85). During this time he employed a young assistant, Robert Hooke (1635–1702/3)[1], who was clever at mechanical things and later made many important contributions in his own name (53, 146). Boyle had Hooke build an improved air pump. To establish whether it was atmospheric pressure that supported the mercury column of a barometer, they put one into a suitable vessel and then proceeded to pump some of the air out of the vessel. The mercury column descended as they did this, proving that it was indeed the pressure of the air that supported the mercury column. In 1660 Boyle published the first edition of his famous book, *New Experiments Physico-Mechanicall, Touching the Spring of the Air . . .* (10), which describes these and other experiments agreeing with those who believed that the space above the mercury was a vacuum.

[1] The slash indicates dates by both Julian and Gregorian calendars. Hooke died in London on March 3, 1702 by the Julian calendar that was still in use in England (53, 146). By this calendar March 25th was the start of the New Year. Thus he died 22 days before 1703 would start in England, although it had been 1703 for several weeks by the Gregorian calendar already in use throughout Roman Catholic countries and some Protestant countries. England shifted to the Gregorian calendar half a century after Hooke's death, by making September 2, 1752 "Old Style" be followed by September 14, 1752 "New Style," eliminating the 11-day phase lag that had accumulated in the Julian calendar because of the inaccuracy of the Julian leap-year correction. The year 1753 was started on the next January 1 to bring the numbering of years into phase. Thus the year 1752 in England lasted less than nine months. Several countries adhering to the Eastern Orthodox faith did not adopt the Gregorian calendar until about 1912–1923. This illustrates that it was not merely weights and measures but even time that was confusingly measured in different places until people sacrificed their own convenience to learn a new, universal system of measurement for the benefit of future generations. Despite progress, we are still fighting the battle for better international units.

Franciscus Linus (Francis Line, 1595–1675) attacked Boyle's work and particularly this aspect of it, expressing his own view that there was something invisible above the mercury that was holding it up (81). When Boyle published the second edition of his book in 1662, he included as an appendix a defense of his ideas against Line's attack (11). He knew of the unpublished experiments of Henry Power (1623–1668) and Richard Towneley (1629–1706/7), who had put some air above the mercury in a barometer and carried it up and down a hill, concluding that the volume of the air changed reciprocally with pressure (144). Boyle improved on this by quantitative measurements of air trapped over mercury in a U tube. When he poured additional mercury into the open end of the U tube, the volume of the trapped air decreased in exact proportion to the increase in its absolute pressure, determined as the sum of the current barometric pressure of the atmosphere and the difference in the heights of the mercury in the arms of the U tube. Conversely, when the pressure on the trapped air was reduced below atmospheric, its volume increased in direct proportion to the decrease in its absolute pressure. Thus Boyle established the relation that we today call Boyle's law: at constant temperature the volume of a given mass of gas varies reciprocally with its absolute pressure [i.e., the product of volume and absolute pressure is a constant (11)].

In France this law is commonly known as Mariotte's law, because Edme Mariotte (?–1684) came to the same conclusion and presented it to the Paris Academy of Sciences in 1679, when Boyle's work had largely escaped notice on the Continent (see p. 150–155 in ref. 90). Although Mariotte makes no reference to Boyle, he probably was influenced by Boyle's work (92). Certainly, however, it was Mariotte who disseminated the law throughout Europe, for during the next several decades most writers on the Continent referred to Mariotte as if he were the discoverer of the law.

CHARLES'S LAW

Although the quantitative effect of pressure at constant temperature became known in the middle of the seventeenth century, it was not until the early nineteenth century that the effect of temperature on gas volume was understood in a similarly quantitative way. The first attempt was reported in 1699 by Guillaume Amontons (1663–1705), a physicist and inventor in Paris, who wanted to harness the heat of fire to move machinery (2). His idea involved heating air so that its expansion would push water from the bottom to the top of a water wheel. To calculate the power that could be produced, he measured the increase in pressure of air trapped in vessels of different sizes when the vessels were suddenly immersed in boiling water. He concluded that the temperature of water could not be raised above that at which it boiled, that unequal masses of air would increase their pressure equally by about 10 Paris inches (pouces) of mercury (271 mmHg in today's units) (150) when heated to the temperature of boiling water at constant volume, and that if allowed to expand at constant atmospheric pressure, in accordance with Mariotte's law the volume of any given mass of gas would increase in volume by about one-third. In a subsequent paper, he recognized that the decrease in pressure of gases with decreasing temperature could be extrapolated to the temperature at which a gas might exert no pressure at all, the origin of the concept of absolute zero (0°K) (3). Unfortunately, several investigators over the succeeding decades were unable to confirm Amontons's observations on the thermal expansion of gases. Instead they disagreed among themselves as to the coefficient of expansion for air and they failed to find equal thermal expansion for different gases (43, 117).

The reason for these discrepancies remained unclear for a long time. Philippe de la Hire (1640–1718) had pointed out in 1708 that a gas had to be dry if consistent results were to be obtained (73). Unfortunately, investigators were not careful enough. Even John Dalton (1766–1844) was not able to convince others of his finding, which was presented to the Manchester Literary and Philosophical Society in October 1801, that all gases expand equally for any given rise in temperature (26). It is now understood that when a gas is in contact with liquid water, heating the system not only expands the gas already present but adds an additional mass of gas by evaporation from the liquid water, because the vapor pressure of water increases with temperature. Similarly, when a moist gas is cooled below its dew point, some water condenses, reducing the mass present in the gas phase. Thus the results are confusing unless the evaporation and condensation of water can be avoided or taken into account.

The confusion was cleared up by Joseph Louis Gay-Lussac (1778–1850). After graduating from the École Polytechnique in Paris in November 1800, when not quite 22 years old, Gay-Lussac entered the distinguished civil engineering school, the École Nationale des Ponts et Chaussées (23, 24). By the following winter he had made such an impression that the prominent chemist Claude Louis Berthollet (1748–1822) made him his laboratory assistant at his country house in Arceuil. With the encouragement of Berthollet and Pierre Simon de Laplace (1749–1827), Gay-Lussac undertook a restudy of the thermal expansion of gases as his first research project. Realizing the problem with water, he took great pains to dry his gases, manipulating them over dry mercury. With these precautions, all the dry gases he tested followed the same quantitative law, expanding and contracting equally for equal increases and decreases in temperature. Changing the temperature from that of melting ice to that of boiling water, he found that all gases expanded by 37.5%, a coefficient of thermal expansion from 0°C of 0.00375 or 1/266.7 per degree Celsius. (This corresponds to a predicted absolute zero of −266.7°C.) Furthermore, he showed that a wet gas follows this law if it is kept above its dew point and out of contact with any liquid water. In other words, as long as evaporated water stays in the gas phase, it acts like any other gas. He published these important results in 1802, when he was not quite 24 years old (43, 117).

After completing his own experiments, Gay-Lussac discovered by chance that Jacques-Alexandre-César Charles (1746–1823) had attempted similar experiments about 15 years earlier (approximately 1787) but had never published them. Charles was the physicist who first used H_2 to improve on the Montgolfier brothers' invention of the hot-air balloon (47). When Gay-Lussac wrote up his own work, he reported that Charles had previously found that water-insoluble gases expanded equally with an equal rise in temperature but that each water-soluble gas seemed to Charles to have its own thermal coefficient of expansion, unlike Gay-Lussac's findings. Moreover Gay-Lussac pointed out a flaw in the design of Charles's apparatus that made his quantitative values for the thermal coefficient of expansion incorrect. Despite these flaws in Charles's unpublished work, Gay-Lussac's honesty in mentioning it led to the ironic result that most people refer to the law of thermal expansion of gases as Charles's law rather than Gay-Lussac's law, although the latter name is also used. This custom avoids ambiguity, because Gay-Lussac's name is also applied to his law of combining volumes, i.e., gases combine chemically in volumetric proportions (STPD) that are small whole numbers (44, 45).

The development of our modern formulation of the ideal gas law that combines both Boyle's (Mariotte's) law and Charles's (Gay-Lussac's) law can be concisely summarized by referring to the formulations used in the classic papers on thermodynamics. [Nicolas Léonard] Sadi Carnot (1796–1832), in writing his seminal monograph (17, 18) describing the Carnot cycle in 1824, had to deal with the effect of changing combinations of pressure and temperature on the volume of a fixed mass of gas in the sealed cylinder of an ideal engine. He combined the laws by saying that $v = c(267 + t)/p$, in which v is volume, t is temperature in °C, p is pressure, and c is a constant that depends on the weight of the gas and the units used. At that time, 267 was believed to be the number needed to convert degrees Celsius to absolute temperature. Ten years later, [Benoit-Pierre] Émile Clapeyron (1799–1864), in bringing Carnot's ideas to the attention of other physicists (18, 20), defined all the possible combinations of pressure and volume that might be derived from an initial combination by the equation $pv = p_0v_0(267 + t)/(267 + t_0)$. He then proposed, for simplification, to let the initial values $p_0v_0/(267 + t_0) = \mathrm{R}$, making $pv = \mathrm{R}(267 + t)$. When Rudolf Clausius (1822–1888) in 1850 developed Clapeyron's ideas further (18, 21), he followed Clapeyron's formulation but added the comment that R (which Clausius italicized although Clapeyron had not), varied from gas to gas in such a way as to be inversely proportional to the specific gravity. Because for any given pressure, volume, and temperature the specific gravity of a gas is directly proportional to its molecular weight times the moles per unit volume, it was a short step to the formulation used by Johannes Diderick van der Waals (1837–1923) at the end of the 1800s to replace R by $\mathrm{n}R$, where n is the number of moles, making R a universal gas constant, the same for all ideal gases (140, 141, 143).

DALTON'S LAW AND THE VAPOR PRESSURE OF WATER

The laws of Boyle and Gay-Lussac relate pressure, temperature, and volume changes correctly only if the mass of the gas remains constant. When the gas can equilibrate with liquid water, Dalton's law of partial pressure and the effect of temperature on the vapor pressure of water must also be used. Dalton's law, however, because it deals with specific molecular species in a mixture of gases, could hardly be envisaged until it was recognized that gases could exist as physical mixtures of materials of different chemical composition. This became conceivable in the latter half of the 1700s with the recognition that O_2, CO_2, and N_2 are different gases (102), but it was not immediately obvious that these gases mixed physically rather than somehow combining chemically with air.

Although Dalton was excluded as a Quaker from attending Oxford and Cambridge, which required conformity to the Church of England, he managed to obtain a good education that was especially strong in mathematics and natural philosophy (134). In 1793, when he had become Professor of Mathematics and Natural Philosophy at the New College founded by the dissenters in Manchester, he published his first book, *Meteorological Observations and Essays* (25). In "Essay Sixth: On Evaporation, Rain, Hail, Snow, and Dew" he asserted that water was ordinarily present in the atmosphere, dispersed among the particles of other gases. With this in mind, he measured the vapor pressure of water as a function of temperature and the temperature of boiling water as a function of the absolute pressure. He concluded that air takes up water physically, not chemically, and that it takes up more water at higher temperatures. His evidence was that the amount of water that evaporated into a gas at a given temperature depended only on the volume into which it was evaporating, regardless of the pressure and hence of the mass of gas already present. This was inconsistent with what was already known about chemical combinations of gases. His book does not seem to have attracted a great deal of attention, and Dalton continued thinking about such problems while continuing to investigate related meteorological matters.

In October 1801, however, Dalton read a series of essays to the Literary and Philosophical Society of Manchester, publication of which in the Society's memoirs in 1802 (26) attracted widespread attention. Here he clearly spelled out his conviction that when two gases are mixed there is no mutual repulsion among the particles; the particles of one gas exert the same pressure as they would if the other were not present, and the total pressure is the sum of the partial pressures. He based his ideas of physical mixing on the fact that when different gases, such as O_2 and N_2, are mixed at constant pressure, the volume of the mixture equals the sum of the two initial volumes and there is no sign that they combine into a denser material of different chemical properties, such as happens when O_2 and NO combine to form NO_2. Although different gases have different densities, there is no sign that they remain separate, the lighter one layering above the denser one. Furthermore, he noted that when a liquid evaporated into a fixed volume of a gas, the pressure increased by an amount that was determined solely by the temperature and hence the vapor pressure of the liquid, regardless of the volume and pressure of the gas already present. Moreover, when atmospheric air saturated with water vapor was compressed, it did not follow Boyle's law exactly, because of the condensation of water vapor to keep its partial pressure constant at the value determined by the temperature. Dalton confirmed that dry gases, of course, did follow Boyle's law. Dalton also studied the evaporation of ether and spirit of wine to confirm the generality of these conclusions. It follows from all this that the total pressure of a gas mixture could be divided among the partial pressures of the components in the mixture in proportion to what we would now call the mole fraction of each gas.

These ideas meshed well with those of Gay-Lussac (referred to in CHARLES'S LAW, p. 17) that were published at about the same time (43). When a gas is heated while in equilibrium with liquid water and at a fixed total gas volume, the total pressure is the sum of the pressure of the variable mass of water in the gas, determined solely by the vapor pressure of the water at that temperature, and the pressure of the fixed mass of nonwater molecules, which rises in accordance with Charles's law.

HENRY'S LAW

While defending his controversial ideas about gases, Dalton looked at some aspects of their solubility in liquids. It was probably this study that stimulated his close friend William Henry (1774–1836) to start working on the same problem; Dalton's ideas certainly influenced Henry's interpretations of his observations. William Henry (60) was the son of Thomas Henry (1734–1816), a physician of Manchester who had helped found the Manchester Literary and Philosophical Society and, in 1794, had sponsored Dalton for membership (134). William Henry studied medicine in Edinburgh, where his chemistry teacher in 1795–1796 was Joseph Black (1728–1799), the discoverer of "fixed air" (i.e., CO_2) (102). Although Black published very little himself after his famous dissertation on CO_2, he was a stimulating teacher who continued to contribute through the discoveries of his students (William Henry is a good example). William Henry joined his father in medical practice in Manchester; thus he is one of several physicians who have made important contributions to the physical sciences. He was aware that Joseph Priestley (1733–1804) had reported to the Royal Society in 1772 that heat or a vacuum would extract CO_2 from Pyrmont mineral water and that he had suggested using pressure to impregnate water with CO_2 (112). William Henry wished to determine the quantitative relations. At first he resisted Dalton's idea of the independent partial pressures of gases in mixtures, but later he realized that it would help explain his observations.

On December 23, 1802, just 14 months after Dalton had presented his great paper in Manchester, William Henry reported to the Royal Society of London that the quantity of CO_2 absorbed by water at 55°F (12.8°C) increased in direct proportion to its absolute pressure, which he raised to about 3 atm with a mercury column (59). He noticed, however, that when the CO_2 was diluted by some residual air in his apparatus, less CO_2 dissolved. Investigating this, he found that CO_2 dissolved in proportion to its partial pressure in the mixture. He also showed that the solubility of CO_2 decreased by about $1/14$ for each 10°F (5.6°C) increase in temperature. He found that other gases also dissolved in proportion to their partial pressure, although with different solubility coefficients for each gas; however, he was unable to make satisfactory measurements of the effects of temperature on their solubilities (59). Henry's law, therefore, is simply that, at constant temperature, any gas physically dissolves in a liquid in proportion to its partial pressure, although the solubility coefficient decreases with increasing temperature and differs from one gas to another. Of course this law applies only to physical solution and ignores any amount of gas that may chemically combine, as CO_2 combines with an alkaline solution or as O_2 combines with hemoglobin.

GRAHAM'S LAW

Thomas Graham (1805–1869) was educated at the Universities of Glasgow and Edinburgh and became a professor of chemistry in Glasgow and subsequently in London. He first published on the subject of gaseous diffusion in 1829 (68). His attention had been attracted by a chance observation of Johann Wolfgang Doebereiner (1780–1849) that H_2 would leak out of a glass jar with a small crack, whereas other gases failed to do so (30). This led Graham to study gas diffusion through porous materials such as unglazed Wedgwood stoneware, plaster of paris, and compressed graphite similar to that used for pencils but prepared in the form of a porous disk (48). He found that bulk flow of gas through the disk was directly proportional to the difference in total gas pressures on the two sides and inversely related to the porosity [as one would predict from the law of another physicist-physician, Jean-Léonard-Marie Poiseuille (1797–1869), for the flow of fluids through small capillaries (111)], without distinction between the components of the mixture of gases. When Graham placed two different gases at equal barometric pressure on the two sides of the disk, however, each gas diffused through at its own rate, which was inversely proportional to the square root of its density. Hydrogen, having the lowest density, diffused fastest. In 1833 Graham was able to publish definitive evidence of what we now call Graham's law (48): the rate of diffusion of a gas is inversely proportional to the square root of its density. Today this makes sense, because we believe that at any temperature the mean kinetic energy ($mv^2/2$) is the same for molecules of all molecular weights or masses (m). The mean velocity (v) determining the diffusion of molecules must therefore be inversely proportional to the square root of their mass, which directly determines the gas density. Graham later showed that his law also applies to the free diffusion of gases without any porous barrier (50), and he applied similar analysis to his measurements of the diffusion of solutes in a liquid (49), which helped Adolf Fick develop his law of diffusion.

FICK'S LAW

Adolf Fick (1829–1901) was still another physician by training who made important contributions to physical science, although in his case he worked as a physiologist rather than as a clinician. Fick demonstrated that the diffusion of molecules follows the same law as the conduction of heat described mathematically by [Jean Baptiste] Joseph Fourier (1768–1830) three decades earlier (40, 41). Fick's law of diffusion states that the transfer of solute by diffusion is directly proportional to the cross-sectional area available for diffusion and to the difference in concentration per unit distance perpendicular to that cross section (38). The concentration of a dissolved gas, from Henry's law, is the product of its solubility and its partial pressure. For a very soluble gas such as CO_2, a given partial pressure difference provides a greater concentration difference to drive its diffusion than for a less-soluble gas such as O_2. In 1875 Franz Serafin Exner (1849–1926), while working with diffusion of gases through soap bubble films, combined this principle with Graham's law to demonstrate that the relative diffusional transfer of two gases, x and y, through a liquid barrier is directly proportional to the ratio of their solubilities and inversely proportional to the ratio of the square roots of their molecular weights (36)

$$\frac{\dot{V}_x}{\dot{V}_y} = \frac{(P'_x - P_x)(\alpha_x)(\sqrt{MW_y})}{(P'_y - P_y)(\alpha_y)(\sqrt{MW_x})} \tag{6}$$

where $\dot{V}$ is the volume of x or y diffusing through the barrier per unit time, P' and P are the partial pressures of x or y on the two sides of the barrier, α is the solubility of x or y in molar concentration per unit partial pressure, and MW is the molecular weight of x or y. This relation formed the basis for the classic estimation of the pulmonary diffusing capacity for O_2 from measurements made with carbon monoxide (71).

DEVIATIONS FROM IDEAL GAS LAWS

Once the general principles representing the behavior of ideal gases were known, there remained the need for obtaining precise values for the coefficient of thermal expansion of gases, the vapor pressure of water as a function of temperature, etc. When these values were measured more precisely, their deviations from ideal behavior became more apparent.

Although Amontons (3) suggested the concept of an absolute zero temperature where gases would no longer exert any pressure, other investigators preferred to avoid any such hypothetical assumption by expressing thermal effects in terms of the fractional increase in pressure or volume (which were assumed to be interchangeable in accordance with Boyle's law) when a gas was heated from the freezing point to the boiling point of water. The latter, of course, is the temperature at which the vapor pressure of water equals the barometric pressure, which varies with weather as well as with altitude, making the boiling point not as reproducible as was at first supposed. Gay-Lussac obtained a value of 0.375 for the fractional expansion of dry air for this 100°C interval, or 0.00375 per degree Celsius from 0°C (43, 117). (Because the reciprocal of this fractional increase per degree Celsius is the number that must be added to degrees Celsius to obtain the absolute temperature in degrees Kelvin, I provide the fractional equivalent of the decimal, in this case 1/266.7, for comparison with the modern value of 1/273.16.) Gay-Lussac's value for thermal expansion agreed adequately with that obtained by Dalton. In 1816–1817, Pierre Louis Dulong (1785–1838) and Alexis Thérèse Petit (1791–1820) also confirmed Gay-Lussac's value (34, 35). Hence that value was generally accepted until 1837, when Fredrik Rudberg (1800–

1839) of Uppsala challenged it on the basis of his own measurements (125, 126), which indicated that the correct value should be 0.3646 (= 1/274.3 per °C from 0°C). Gay-Lussac and his contemporaries had measured the increase in volume at constant pressure, but Rudberg measured the increase in pressure at almost constant volume (there was some thermal expansion of his glass container), which should be identical by Boyle's law. [Heinrich] Gustav Magnus (1802–1870) in Berlin and [Henri] Victor Regnault (1810–1878) in Paris each noticed Rudberg's report and independently each began to reinvestigate the matter. Their results (87–89, 119, 120) appeared so nearly simultaneously in 1841–1842 that they jockeyed for priority (89).

In his studies of the thermal expansion of gases, Magnus (87, 88) found problems with mercurial calibration of volumetric apparatus and copied Rudberg in measuring pressure increase at constant volume, obtaining a thermal coefficient for air of 0.366508 per 100°C (= 1/272.9 per °C from 0°C) and for H_2 of 0.365659 per 100°C (= 1/273.5 per °C from 0°C). These values were in reasonably good agreement (and much closer to today's values than Gay-Lussac's value of 1/266.7 per °C from 0°C had been) but Magnus's value for CO_2 (0.369087 per 100°C or 1/270.9 per °C from 0°C) was significantly different. He attributed this to failure of CO_2 to obey Mariotte's law.

Regnault at first obtained values of 0.3665 per 100°C (= 1/272.9 per °C from 0°C) for air and 0.36896 per 100°C (= 1/271.0 per °C from 0°C) for CO_2 (119, 120), agreeing well with Magnus. Thus there seemed to be a systematic difference between CO_2 and air. These first results led Regnault to undertake a major reinvestigation of the thermal properties of gases, the work for which he is best known. This would have been prohibitively expensive with only the resources available to him as professor of chemistry at the École Polytechnique, where he succeeded Gay-Lussac in 1840, and as professor of physics at the Collège de France, where the work was done (42). However, beginning in 1842 he received massive financial support from the French government because of the importance of these matters for the precise design and performance of steam engines. For nearly 30 years he devoted himself primarily to these experiments in painstaking detail, measuring the small differences in the thermal coefficients of different gases, their precise deviations from Boyle's law, their vapor pressures under a wide range of conditions, and related matters. His most important findings for our purposes (121) filled volume 21 of the *Mémoires de l'Académie Royale des Sciences* in 1847, and additional material filled volume 26 in 1862 and volume 37 in 1868, for a total of 2,641 pages. (What editor today could afford to provide so much space in his journal!) These monumental studies provided the most precise and extensive tables of experimental values available for many years, but Regnault left theoretical or otherwise creative interpretation almost entirely to others.

TEMPERATURE SCALES

The freezing and boiling points of water are by themselves insufficient to define a temperature scale (97). Magnus, for instance, had taken as his standard the boiling point of water at 760 mmHg, whereas Rudberg had adopted the boiling point of water at 28 Paris inches (pouces) of mercury, which converts to 757.96 mmHg. Before adoption of the metric system, the Paris inch was 27.07 mm, the British Imperial inch was 25.4 mm, the Swedish inch (tum) was about 30 mm, and the German inch (Zoll) varied from place to place, ranging from 24 mm in Bavaria to 30 mm in Baden (149), although sometimes a scientist in one region would express his measurements in the units of a more important center. Comparison of observations between one laboratory and another was certainly difficult before the metric system provided international standards.

The first reproducible liquid-in-glass thermometers calibrated by the freezing point and boiling point of water with the interval subdivided into equal units of thermal expansion appear to have been those made with alcohol by the Danish astronomer Ole Christensen Rømer (1664–1710) in 1702 (97). Daniel Gabriel Fahrenheit (1686–1736) of Danzig visited Rømer in 1708 and then began to develop the scale that is still widely used in English-speaking countries and that divides this interval into 180°F. The scale named for René-Antoine Ferchault de Réaumur (1683–1757) that became popular in France divided the interval into 80°R, whereas Anders Celsius (1701–1744) in Sweden chose 100 divisions, although he first put his 100° at the freezing point and his 0° at the boiling point of water. Actually he used the boiling point of water when the barometer read 25.25 Swedish inches (751.16 mmHg), corresponding to 99.67°C today. The botanist Carl von Linné (Linnaeus; 1707–1778) was probably instrumental in interchanging the top and bottom of that scale to correspond to the Celsius scale that is now in use (97). In English-speaking countries this scale was commonly called the centigrade scale until, by international agreement in 1948, it was renamed the Celsius scale to avoid confusion in France, where centigrade already referred to the division of a right angle into 100 parts (58).

How should this interval be subdivided into equal intervals of temperature when mercury, alcohol, and gases all expand alinearly when compared with each other? When this problem became abundantly clear from Regnault's work, William Thomson (1824–1907; later known as Lord Kelvin) was in the process of developing the principles of thermodynamics (13, 133), after being stimulated by Carnot's ideas about idealized heat engines (17, 18). In 1848 he proposed an absolute thermodynamic temperature scale based on equal amounts of energy per degree that would be independent of the expansion of any particular substance (135), developing it further with the help of James Prescott Joule (1818–1889) and using Regnault's experimental data (66). This is why absolute temperature is expressed in degrees Kelvin today.

VAN DER WAALS'S EQUATION

These developments of thermodynamic theory and precise experimental data led Johannes Diderik van der Waals (1837–1923) of the Netherlands to try to refine the theory involved (113). Dalton's idea of individual gas particles each acting as if no other particles were present could not be quite correct. In van der Waals's doctoral dissertation, which was later translated into German and then English with some revisions (140, 141), he was able to link the pressure, absolute temperature, and volume of any gas more precisely by a relation that can be expressed as $(P + n^2a/V^2)(V - nb) = nRT$, where a relates to the attractive force between molecules and b relates to their volume, which is not negligible. Both of these "constants" are now known to vary somewhat with temperature. The number of moles of gas present is represented by n, and R is the universal gas constant that links the various units used for the other variables. Following Dejours (29), I italicize R to distinguish it from R, the standard symbol for the respiratory exchange ratio; R has the value 62.3656 liters mmHg per mole degree and T is in degrees Kelvin. In pulmonary gas exchange, a and b are usually assumed to be zero and PV/T is assumed to equal nR. This indicates that one mole of any dry gas at 0°C and 760 mmHg should occupy 22.4 liters. In fact, although this is true for most gases we breathe, the volume of a mole of CO_2 or of N_2O is 22.26 liters, whereas the volume of a mole of krypton is 22.6 liters (114, 143). Van der Waals's refinements to the ideal gas equation are important primarily when gases are under high pressures or at high density. Further refinements of theory and experimental data (114) can usually be neglected in dealing with pulmonary gas exchange.

PRACTICAL CONVERSION FORMULAS BASED ON IDEAL GAS LAWS

To summarize, the problem of changing the temperature of gases in contact with liquid water is that the total number of molecules of gas present does not stay constant. However, if n in the equation $PV = nRT$ is made to represent the moles of nonwater molecules, which is constant, by using only the pressure exerted by the nonwater molecules [total pressure minus the vapor pressure of water (P_{H_2O}) in the gas], temperature and pressure conversions can be made by using the equation $(P - P_{H_2O})V/T = nR = (P' - P'_{H_2O})V'/T'$. Applying this to the usual conversions between BTPS, ATPS, and STPD conditions, one obtains

$$\frac{(P_B - Pbt_{H_2O})(V_{BTPS})}{(273 + bt)} = \frac{(P_B - Pt_{H_2O})(V_t)}{(273 + t)} = \frac{(760)(V_{STPD})}{(273)} \tag{7}$$

In these equations, bt is the body temperature, t is the ATPS temperature in degrees Celsius, and 273 (more precisely 273.16) is the amount that must be added to them to express the absolute temperature in degrees Kelvin. Converted to the most commonly used forms, when bt = 37°C

$$V_{STPD} = V_{ATPS}\,\frac{(P_B - Pt_{H_2O})\ (273)}{(760)\ (273 + t)} \tag{8}$$

$$V_{BTPS} = V_{ATPS}\,\frac{(P_B - Pt_{H_2O})\ (273 + 37)}{(P_B - 47)\ (273 + t)} \tag{9}$$

PRACTICAL USE OF VAPOR PRESSURE

Physiologists commonly look in a table (143) for the vapor pressure of water to use in Equations 7–9. Computers and hand-held programmable calculators make it easy to compute values from an equation such as that of Duclaux (33) or of Keyes (70), instead. For the purposes of this chapter, I have simplified Duclaux's equation to the form

$$P_{H_2O} = 760e^z \tag{10}$$

where P_{H_2O} is the vapor pressure of water accurate within 0.1 mmHg for temperatures between 0°C and 50°C, e is the base of natural logarithms, and

$$z = (13.96 - 0.0076t + 0.000012t^2)\,\frac{(t - 100)}{(t + 273)} \tag{11}$$

The effect of solutes on vapor pressure is summarized by Raoult's law. In 1887 François Marie Raoult (1830–1901) found that at any temperature the vapor pressure of a solvent is depressed in proportion to the mole fraction of nonvolatile solute present (65, 118). Because the mole fraction of solute in plasma, with which other body fluids equilibrate osmotically, is ordinarily about 0.5%, at 37°C its vapor pressure should be about 46.83 mmHg compared with 47.07 mmHg for pure water (143), a negligible difference. The fluid lining the alveoli presumably equilibrates osmotically and hence should be similar. The large surfactant molecules on the alveolar surface are so insoluble in water that they would be expected to act only as a resistance to potential water flow that would not change alveolar vapor pressure under normal circumstances (J. Goerke, personal communication).

The effect of a change in body temperature on the vapor pressure of water is somewhat larger. For example, at a febrile temperature of 40°C, the vapor pressure of water is 55.32 mmHg. Assuming 37°C in converting to BTPS at sea level for such a patient would make a calculated lung volume too low by about 2.1%.

In 1872 William Thomson (by this time Sir William Thomson) pointed out as a result of very ingenious armchair reasoning that the vapor pressure must be lower above a concave surface than it is above a plane surface (136). A simple calculation based on his equations, however, indicates that this effect would be negligible even at the microscopic radii of curvature to be expected in alveoli.

When a gas is analyzed by measuring the decrease in its volume due to absorption of a component by an aqueous reagent, such as CO_2 by 10% KOH and O_2 by pyrogallol, water is condensed from the gas phase in proportion to the CO_2 or O_2 absorbed, because temperature and vapor pressure stay constant while the gas volume decreases. This is the principle of the classic analytical method devised by John Scott Haldane (1860–1936) of Oxford (54) and modified by Per Fredrik Scholander (1905–1980) (127). Thus, although these methods analyze wet gas, the fractional decrease in volume exactly equals the fraction of CO_2 or O_2 in dry gas represented by the standard symbols F_{CO_2} or F_{O_2} (32, 101). The early use of wet absorption is probably one reason for gas analyses to be customarily expressed this way, but it is also particularly convenient when dealing with a gas that may change in water content, as is usually the case in respiratory systems. Earth's atmosphere, for example, has a variable amount of moisture in it, but O_2 is always 20.95% of dry air. For any inspired gas, its partial pressure is conventionally expressed in terms of the gas flowing into the alveoli after being saturated at body temperature in the airway. The inspiratory partial pressure of O_2 ($P_{I_{O_2}}$) is therefore calculated from Dalton's law by subtracting the vapor pressure of water at body temperature from the barometric pressure before multiplying by 0.2095. Alveolar partial pressures are calculated from alveolar gas composition in the same way (32). The relative humidity of inspired and expired gases becomes important only in evaluating respiratory water exchange (142).

When analyzing a gas by physical methods such as infrared absorption or paramagnetic properties, one commonly has a compressed (and therefore dry) gas to standardize an instrument that will be used to measure a moist respiratory gas. In this case calibration must take into account not only that water vapor dilutes the CO_2 or O_2 but also that water vapor itself may affect the reading obtained from the instrument. A well-known example is the pressure-broadening effect of many gases including water vapor on infrared spectra (132).

HISTORICAL USE OF STPD CORRECTIONS IN RESPIRATION

Elucidation of the gas laws by physicists did not guarantee that they would be properly applied by physiologists. It is instructive to review the history of the introduction of the gas laws into respiratory physiology to make STPD and BTPS corrections.

In respiratory physiology, STPD corrections are most commonly used in measuring O_2 consumption and CO_2 production and in specifying O_2 and CO_2 concentrations in blood. Representative examples from significant papers illustrate how these corrections came into general use. In 1777 Antoine-Laurent Lavoisier (1743–1794) read his first paper recognizing the role of O_2 in respiration (75); in the next few years he undertook with Laplace to measure O_2 consumption quantitatively in animals and compare it with the heat production measured in their new ice calorimeter (76). Lavoisier and Laplace recognized the necessity of correcting their gas volumes to a specified pressure and temperature and chose 28 pouces of mercury (758 mmHg) and 10°R (12.5°C), using the relation that gases at about that temperature expanded 1/215 for each degree Réaumur (1/256 per degree Celsius from 0°C). They clearly recognized the need for correction, although, before Gay-Lussac's 1802 paper (43), they could not do it correctly. Lavoisier followed this same procedure in making the first measurements of human O_2 consumption (77, 131), using as subject his collaborator at that time, Armand Séguin (1767–1835). In 1808, after Gay-Lussac's publication, William Allen (1770–1843) and William Hasledine Pepys (1775–1856) also reported O_2 consumption and CO_2 production (1). They converted their volumetric measurements to a standard 30 in of mercury (762 mmHg) at 60°F (15.6°C) without any consideration of water vapor. They then used a value for density to convert to grams of dry gas. Thus they were aware of the need to specify the mass of gas even if their volumetric correction was not quite right.

The other common use of STPD correction is to specify O_2 and CO_2 concentrations in blood. In 1837 Gustav Magnus was the first to report such measurements, but this was before he began studying the thermal expansion of gases and I see no sign that he made any temperature or pressure correction to the volumes he reported (86). In the following year John Davy (1790–1868), a physician and the younger brother of Humphry Davy (1778–1829), likewise made no corrections when reporting his attempt to measure blood gases (28). By 1842, however, Magnus had published his careful measurements of the coefficient of thermal expansion of gases (87–89). The following year, 1843, Carl Emanuel Brunner (1796–1867) and Gabriel Gustav Valentin (1810–1883) showed that they understood how to correct for water vapor and used Magnus's new value for the coefficient of thermal expansion, but they avoided analytical problems by gravimetric determination of O_2 and CO_2 absorbed in a dry system (12). In 1844 Carl Vierordt (1818–1884) quoted the coefficients of thermal expansion of both Regnault and Magnus and converted his gases to a pressure of 336 Paris lines (758 mmHg) and 37°C (138). He dried his gases with calcium chloride first, making a water vapor pressure correction unnecessary. In their extensive 1849 study of metabolism (122), Regnault and Jules Reiset (1818–1896) converted their gas volumes to 0°C and 760 mmHg and then expressed all results in grams of O_2 and CO_2, as might be expected from a careful physicist. Georg von Liebig (1827–1903), the son of the famous chemist Justus von Liebig (1803–1873), while working in the laboratory of Gustav Magnus, also handled his conversions correctly in his 1850 paper on respiration of muscle (78). In fact he spelled out carefully how he subtracted the vapor pressure of water from the barometric pressure and then converted to a standard 760 mmHg and 0°C.

After 1857 practically everyone corrected gas and blood gas measurements to STPD or to grams, following the precise instructions of Robert Wilhelm Eberhard Bunsen (1811–1899), who published his influential book on gasometric methods in that year with simultaneous editions in German and English and with a French edition the following year (14–16). However, there still was confusion about standard conditions. The standard temperature was 0°, which fortunately was the same on both Celsius and Réaumur scales. Bunsen, however, recommended a standard pressure of 1,000 mmHg, instead of the 760 mmHg that had been coming into common use. This caused amusing inconsistencies for several decades. For example, in his famous 1857 paper on blood gas analysis, which first showed that O_2 was held in blood by something besides simple solution (95), [Julius] Lothar Meyer (1830–1895) published tables in which some data were reduced to 760 mmHg and other data in the same table were reduced to 1,000 mmHg. He had studied in Zürich with Carl Ludwig (1816–1895) and also in Würzburg before moving to Heidelberg to study with Bunsen, so perhaps he became confused by differing customs. In 1877, 20 years after the appearance of Bunsen's book, Eduard Friedrich Wilhelm Pflüger (1829–1910) used 1,000 mmHg in his paper on the influence of pulmonary mechanics on metabolism (109), while his own laboratory assistants used 760 mmHg in their adjoining paper on the same subject (39), in the journal of which Pflüger was editor. The use of 1,000 mmHg persisted in some laboratories at least until 1898 (98).

When clinicians became more interested in measuring the basal metabolic rate of patients, tables for reducing gas volumes to STPD became popular. Such a table gives correct results only if it was calculated from assumptions that are correct for the particular application. Thorne Martin Carpenter (1878–1971), long-time associate of Francis Gano Benedict (1870–1957) at the Nutrition Laboratory of the Carnegie Institution of Washington in Boston, published a volume of such tables in 1921 that was reprinted in 1924, 1939, and 1948 with minor additions (19). Although all these editions included a table for correcting saturated gas (ATPS) to STPD, Carpenter continued to specify instead the dry-gas table ignoring water vapor (ATPD to STPD) for correcting Benedict-Roth metabolism measurements, even though the 1922 paper by Paul Roth (1871–1946), which improved on Benedict's apparatus, included evidence that the expired gas passing through the best CO_2-absorbing chemical had a high humidity (124). Examination of a table for reducing Benedict-Roth metabolism measurements to STPD that was printed on the back of the recording paper for the Benedict-Roth apparatus made by Warren E. Collins, Inc., suggests that it may have been calculated from the assumption that spirometer gas had 80% relative humidity. John Punnett Peters (1887–1955) of Yale and Donald Dexter Van Slyke (1883–1971) published a table in their widely used 1932 book on methods that combined the temperature correction for a mercurial barometer with that for converting ATPS to STPD (108). Unfortunately such a table can be correct for only one type of scale, a particular latitude, and situations where barometer and spirometer are at the same temperature. It is useless with an aneroid barometer. All such special-purpose tables unfortunately invite the unwary to apply them improperly, simply because the individual factors in the corrections are not considered explicitly. Despite such minor problems, the record on STPD conversions is remarkably clean, compared with the handling of BTPS corrections.

HISTORICAL USE OF BTPS CORRECTIONS IN RESPIRATION

Corrections to BTPS are usually necessary when measuring lung volumes, especially the vital capacity, histories of which have already been published (4, 99). Although Giovanni Alfonso Borelli (1608–1679) is thought to have been the first to measure the volume of a breath, I can find no indication that he made any correction for temperature or pressure (9). A British physician, James Jurin (1684–1750), was probably the first to correct his lung volume measurements for cooling, pressure, and vapor, but I do not see any experimental basis for the values he used (67).

The Reverend Stephen Hales (1677–1761) is well known as the first (in 1733) to measure the arterial pressure (57). Less well known is the fact that his 1727 book *Vegetable Staticks* ... (56) included attempts to measure lung volume, tidal volume, and gas exchange. He clearly understood the effect of pressure on volume (Boyle's law) and that gases shrink when they cool (56), but in practice he merely cited his measurements at ambient conditions without numerical corrections.

In 1788 Edmund Goodwyn (1756–1829) was much more meticulous (46), as might be expected of another student of Joseph Black. When he attempted to measure the average inspiratory tidal volume of three normal subjects for his dissertation, he realized that the volume of air removed from his ingenious pneumatic vessel (drawing in water that could be weighed) would expand as it went into the warmer lungs. Not knowing how to predict such expansion quantitatively, he enclosed a similar volume of air in a graduated cylinder inverted over water and then heated this entire system from his room temperature of 69°F (20.5°C) to an estimated body temperature of 98°F (36.7°C). He found that this air expanded by ⅙ or 16.7%. He used this to correct his tidal volume measurement of 12 in^3 (197 ml) to 14 in^3 (229 ml). This value seems small for mean tidal volume of normal subjects, and his thermal correction is unduly large; nevertheless I think that his rational empirical approach deserved a prize. The Humane Society did in fact award him a medal for the book, although probably for other reasons.

Another important paper on lung volumes is the 1790 doctoral dissertation of Robert Menzies, still another student of Joseph Black at Edinburgh (93, 94). Menzies immersed his subject up to the neck in a barrel of water and then measured the actual increase in lung volume by water displacement, a method that requires no correction. However, from these actual changes in lung volume he calculated the smaller volume of room air that must have been inspired to fill this expanded lung volume, assuming that air would be warmed by 40°F (22.2°C) and that the thermal coefficient of expansion was 1/472.5 per degree Fahrenheit (1/262.5 per °C), without any correction for water vapor.

The next landmark in the field of lung volumes was the 1800 measurement of residual volume in man by Humphry Davy (1778–1829) using H_2 dilution (27). Davy realized that his allowance for the decrease of gas volume on cooling was only an imperfect approximation, because the thermal coefficient of expansion was still uncertain, especially for mixed gases into which water was evaporating.

Edward Kentish (?–1832) was probably the first person to advocate the routine measurement for diagnostic purposes of what is now called the vital capacity (4). About 1814 Kentish (69) described the use of his "pulmometer" for this purpose, in an appendix to his proposal to establish a "Madeira-House" in Bristol that would reproduce by central heating the climate of Madeira, which was supposed to benefit cases of pulmonary tuberculosis. In addition to its use to evaluate patients, he proposed that the "lung power" (now called vital capacity) measured by his pulmometer would be a better criterion for selecting infantrymen than their height, which was then used for that purpose. He supported this view by case reports showing diminished vital capacity in disease. His pulmometer actually consisted of a glass jar filled with two quarts of water and six quarts of air, inverted in a water trough, and fitted with a breathing tube at the top. Because the jar appears to have been stationary, inspiration would have required subatmospheric pressure to raise the column of water in the jar, but he does not seem to have considered the effects of pressure or temperature on his measurement, even though his paper appeared a dozen years after that of Gay-Lussac (43).

Fourteen years later, Ernst Friedrich Gustav Herbst (1803–1893) of Göttingen published an extensive review of lung capacity measurements (61) that mentioned the corrections used by Jurin. Like Kentish, however, Herbst made no corrections himself. Several German respiratory papers in the early 1840s all show that their authors knew how to make temperature and pressure corrections properly (12, 129, 138). Unfortunately, however, this was not the case with the very influential paper written by Hutchinson.

John Hutchinson (1811–1861) was an English surgeon who wrote a 116-page paper in 1846 popularizing the counterbalanced water-sealed spirometer for measuring vital capacity and reporting his very large series of normal values as a function of height and weight to serve as diagnostic standards (62). Perhaps he was merely looking for a simple clinical index rather than an absolute measurement, or perhaps he did not understand the effect of the changing vapor pressure of water. Whatever his reason, he simply corrected his spirometer measurements (ATPS) to his average room temperature of 60°F (15.6°C) by a calculation that would be correct only if the gas were dry. He assumed that in this range the thermal coefficient of expansion would be 1/500 per °F (= 1/262.2 per °C from 0°C). This is closer to Gay-Lussac's 1802 value for dry gas (= 1/266.7 per °C from 0°C) than to the improved values for dry gas published by Rudberg (125, 126), Magnus (87–89), and Regnault (119, 120) just a few years earlier, of which he may have been unaware. The large effect of temperature on vapor pressure would have increased thermal expansion by about one-third in this range, but his major blunder was that he failed to correct to body temperature. Thus all his data differ from the vital capacity, the true volume change in the lungs that he was interested in, by an amount that depended on the temperature and barometric pressure in his laboratory and would be different elsewhere. This made his much-admired set of standards invalid in other laboratories, a fact that unfortunately was not recognized at the time.

Hutchinson's paper was soon translated into German (63), and its English and German versions attracted a great deal of attention from clinicians in Europe and America. In the next decade many publications of vital capacity measurements specified that Hutchinson's methods had been followed (31, 37, 72, 107). Then in 1854 M. Anton Wintrich (1812–1882) of Erlangen in Bavaria published a 384-page monograph on this subject, including his own data on some 3,500 subjects and 500 patients (147). Presumably to improve on Hutchinson, Wintrich not only reduced his values to his own average temperature of 18°C but also to his own mean barometric pressure of "27 Zoll und 3 Linien." If Wintrich was using the Prussian value for the Zoll (26 mm) rather than the traditional Bavarian value of 24 mm (149), this converts to 728 mmHg, about the right value for the altitude of Erlangen. It seems odd that he expressed his barometric pressure in Zoll when he expressed his gas volumes in cubic centimeters. Wintrich used a better value for dry-gas temperature conversion than Hutchinson, but his pressure conversion made things worse. The ambient barometric pressure (over the small range of weather fluctuations at any one altitude) makes only a small difference in the correct conversion from ATPS to BTPS, because the same value (before subtraction of vapor pressure) occurs in both numerator and denominator of Equation 9. Converting to any standard barometric pressure, however, makes weather fluctuations and differences in altitude influence the results. Values would tend to correlate with the moles of gas expired from the lungs rather than with the volume changes that would be significant for alveolar ventilation and for diagnostic evaluations. Fortunately he chose as his standard the average barometric pressure where he worked rather than a sea-level barometric pressure such as 760 mmHg, which would have made all his vital capacities much too low relative to the values reported for near sea level.

In France, Nestor Gréhant (1838–1910), a pupil of Claude Bernard (1813–1878), in his 1864 measurements of functional residual capacity by H_2 dilution, converted to BTPS correctly except that he used 35.5°C, the temperature of gas expired from the mouth, instead of body temperature (52). Because the gas in the alveoli is undoubtedly at core body temperature, its subsequent loss of heat to the walls of the respiratory tract, which are cooled during inspiration (142), is quite irrelevant. Nevertheless, Gréhant was much closer than Rudolph Ritter von Vivenot (1834–1870), whose father was the prominent physician Rudolph Ritter von Vivenot (1807–1884). The son was a physiological climatologist in Vienna who was interested in high and low pressures. He corrected his lung capacity measurements of 1865 by the thermal coefficient of expansion for dry gas (139). Georg von Liebig performed his STPD conversions correctly in 1850 when working in Magnus's laboratory (78). In his hyperbaric chamber study of 1869, Liebig followed Gréhant in correcting his expired gas volumes to 35.5°C or later to 35.0°C saturated with water vapor (79, 80); clearly he thought that the temperature of expired gas was the crucial criterion. Liebig recognized that failure to correct for both temperature and vapor pressure would give a false value for the actual volume of breathing. In fact he calculated an example to show how different the effect of water vapor on the BTPS correction is at different ambient barometric pressures. In his 1882 review, Isidor Rosenthal (1836–1915) merely noted that the temperature and the water vapor must be taken into account in calculating the volume of expired gas (123).

Despite these clear and essentially correct expositions of BTPS corrections, when Wilhelm August Ernst Friedrich Schumburg (1860–?) and Nathan Zuntz (1847–1920) published their observations on man at high altitude in 1896, they reported expired volumes either corrected to STPD (for calculation of O_2 consumption and CO_2 production) or uncorrected at ATPS (130). Specifically they measured vital capacity with a gas meter and reported it uncorrected. On this basis they concluded that the vital capacity was reduced at high altitude. Adolf Loewy (1862–1937) in his hypobaric chamber studies in 1895 made the same mistake (82). Angelo Mosso (1846–1910) of Turin and the Monte Rosa laboratory vacillated somewhat but became convinced that breathing was depressed by the low alveolar partial pressure of CO_2 at high altitude because the expiratory minute volume converted to STPD was lower on Monte Rosa than in Turin, although his raw data show that the actual expiratory minute volume (i.e., corrected to BTPS) was higher on Monte Rosa than in Turin (98).

Christian Bohr (1855–1911) of Copenhagen is famous not only as the father of Nobel Prize physicist Niels Henrik David Bohr (1885–1962) and grandfather of another Nobel Prize physicist, Aage Niels Bohr (b. 1922), but also as the founder of a whole school of Danish respiratory physiologists. As a student under Carl Ludwig (1816–1895) in Leipzig, Christian Bohr developed his life-long interest in blood O_2 transport. Among his first papers in this field was a study of the deviations from Boyle's law shown by O_2 (5, 7) and measurements of the solubility of O_2 in water (6). With this background in the physical properties of gases, it is hardly surprising that he made proper BTPS corrections when he came to measure lung volumes (8). Those influenced by him [e.g., John Scott Haldane (1860–1936) of Oxford] did likewise (55). Even in the most prestigious American laboratories, however, many continued to follow the incorrect example of Schumburg and Zuntz (130), correcting O_2 to STPD while leaving lung volumes uncorrected (83, 84, 105, 106). Indeed, even the abbreviation BTPS does not appear to have been used until November 1943, when John R. Pappenheimer coined it for a military aviation essay (100). At higher altitudes, water vapor constitutes a larger fraction of total gas pressure, making the water vapor correction in BTPS calculations much larger than at sea level. In 1952 Hermann Rahn and Daniel Hammond (116) pointed out that those reporting that vital capacity was much less at high altitude apparently had failed to make this correction. I hope that no uncorrected or miscorrected data are being published today.

In comparing this sad history of BTPS corrections with the remarkably good record for STPD corrections, I am inclined to lay the fundamental blame on Hutchinson's classic paper on spirometric measurement of vital capacity (62). Hutchinson merely wanted a useful clinical index, for which his method was adequate as long as it was used only near sea level. However, if he had looked up the then-known laws of temperature and pressure and had described his measurement of vital capacity with the corrections that would make it truly represent the volume change of the lungs, I think all subsequent authors, clinical and physiological, would have done it correctly, just as those dealing with the mass of gas did when they universally corrected to STPD following the similarly influential publication by Bunsen (14–16). Unfortunately, when incorrectly calculated data are considered to provide a standard of comparison, subsequent authors tend to calculate their data similarly in a vain attempt to make their new results comparable to the published standard. Because Hutchinson's incorrect method of calculation introduces different errors under different circumstances, precise comparability requires recalculation of Hutchinson's data.

EXTRAPOLATING FROM PAST TO FUTURE: PLEA FOR BETTER UNITS

From the ideal gas laws it is apparent that the volume occupied by any given mass of O_2 or CO_2 depends on its temperature, pressure, and humidity. Two centuries ago Lavoisier recognized that he needed to correct O_2 volume to some standard temperature and pressure to specify the mass of O_2 involved, and careful scientists have been doing that ever since. This was a logical solution to the problem in a bygone day, but it has persisted even though a better solution has long been available. The mass of other chemical reactants and solutes is commonly expressed in moles. Why should O_2 and CO_2 be expressed differently just because they are gases?

In 1971 a group of four physiologists, Johannes Piiper from Germany, Pierre Dejours from France, Pierre Haab from Switzerland, and Hermann Rahn from the United States, pointed out that it would be much more logical and convenient to abandon this anachronism and use moles to express the mass or quantity of a gas, rather than the volume STPD (110). They proposed that the standard respiratory symbols (101) adopted at the first "Respiration Dinner" in Atlantic City in 1950 be augmented to include M for the moles (or millimoles) of any gas, specifying O_2 or CO_2 by subscript as usual. The symbol $\dot{M}$ would represent the time derivative for rates of production, consumption, or transfer. The concentration of any gas in the liquid phase, already expressed by the standard symbol C, would be redefined to have the units of moles per unit volume, M/V. During the four decades since I first studied physiology, millimoles or milliequivalents per liter have replaced volumes percent for expressing CO_2 and HCO_3^- concentrations, with obvious advantages. The HCO_3^- can be directly compared with other anions and the balancing cations. Extrapolating into the future, I trust that similar advantages from expressing O_2 and hemoglobin in millimoles will be achieved. It would not be necessary to remember how many ml of O_2 STPD can be bound by each gram of hemoglobin. The O_2 capacity of hemoglobin would simply be 4 mmol/mmol. (Converting 4 mmol O_2 to milliliters STPD and 1 mmol hemoglobin to grams makes it obvious that the time-honored value of 1.34 ml/g still cited in some texts cannot be correct.)

If O_2 consumption and CO_2 production are expressed in mmol/min, their ratio, of course, still gives the same value for the respiratory exchange ratio or respiratory quotient as when both are expressed in ml/min STPD. The caloric value of O_2 would be expressed (with new numbers) in kcal/mol instead of kcal/liter STPD, making it comparable with the expressions of energy used for other chemical reactions. The extraction of O_2 from the blood could be directly related to the moles of substrate being consumed by the perfused tissue. Teachers would no longer have to explain to confused students which gas volumes should be converted to STPD, because none would be. Only actual volumes, whether in a spirometer or in the lungs, would need to be considered. Those brought up in the old-fashioned way might be tempted to convert a measured volume to ml STPD and then divide it by 22.4 ml/mmol to arrive at the number of millimoles, but it is simpler to calculate the moles directly from the observed values by using $n = PV/RT$. Care would be needed merely to distinguish the gas constant, which I have symbolized by italicizing *R* following the convention used by Dejours (29), from the respiratory exchange ratio, a nonitalicized R.

Other advantages of using moles are not so obvious. I understand from a coauthor (H. Rahn, personal communication) of the formal proposal to use moles mentioned above (110), that it was Pierre Dejours who first recognized that if CO_2 elimination in the alveolar gas equation that introduced this chapter (Eq. 1) is converted to moles per minute, the peculiar number 863 in that equation is converted to *R*T, where T is the body temperature in degrees Kelvin. This properly separates the body temperature, which really is a variable, from the physical constant, and should remind those dealing with patients that fever and hypothermia make a difference here. Moreover, Equation 1 would no longer need to be derived. It is simply a rearrangement of the ideal gas law, PV = nRT, as Dejours recognized, into the form P = (n/V)RT, where both n and V are expressed as time derivatives. The specific case, in the new symbols, becomes $P_{A_{CO_2}} = (\dot{M}_{CO_2}/\dot{V}_A)RT$. This is intuitively obvious, because the moles of CO_2 being eliminated in the alveolar ventilation each minute must indeed exert the partial pressure expressed by the ideal gas law. (Although CO_2 deviates slightly from the ideal gas law, ignoring that fact when calculating in moles introduces no more error than when calculating in ml STPD, as is presently done.)

A similar argument can be made for the use of pascals or kilopascals to replace mmHg, torr, cm of water, atmospheres, and feet of altitude, all of which are now used to express physiological pressures. I hope the historical sections of this chapter explain why a unit of length, the millimeter, has been used as a unit of pressure. The International System of Units has adopted the newton as the basic unit of force and the meter as the basic unit of length. Pressure is expressed explicitly as newtons per square meter (N/m^2). For simplicity in expression, it allows the derived unit, pascal, to be substituted for N/m^2. This is such a logical simplification that, again extrapolating history, I am tempted to predict that it will eventually be adopted in pulmonary gas exchange, as it is already being adopted in some other fields throughout the world. Of course the transition will be a nuisance for everyone used to the current practice, just as the transition from the apothecary system to the metric system for drugs was a nuisance; but future generations will be glad we made the effort. When the change has been accomplished, students will be able to see the relationships between pleural pressure, arterial pressure, and venous pressure, all in the same units. The relationship between transpulmonary pressure and the surface tension in the alveolar gas-liquid interface (in N/m) will fit obviously into the so-called law of Laplace (74), which was actually described first (22, 148) by Thomas Young (1773–1829), who was still another physician-physicist (22, 148). As a teacher, I hope that the history summarized in this chapter focuses attention on these cumbersome anachronisms and hastens their elimination from common use.

REFERENCES

1. ALLEN, W., AND W. H. PEPYS. On the changes produced in atmospheric air, and oxygen gas, by respiration. *Philos. Trans. R. Soc. Lond.* 98: 249–281, 1808.
2. AMONTONS, [G.]. Moyen de substituer commodement l'action du feu, à la force des hommes et des chevaux pour mouvoir les machines. In: *Mémoires de Mathématique et de Physique . . . de l'Académie Royale des Sciences. De l'Année 1699* (3rd ed.). Paris: Martin, Coignard, & Guerin, 1732, p. 112–126.
3. AMONTONS, [G.]. Le thermométre réduit à une mesure fixe & certaine, & le moyen d'y rapporter les observations faites avec les anciens thermométres [sic.]. In: *Mémoires de Mathématique et de Physique . . . de l'Académie Royale des Sciences. De l'Année 1703* (2nd ed.). Paris: Hochereau, 1720, p. 50–56.
4. ARNETT, J. H. The vital capacity of the lungs: early observations and instruments. *Med. Life* 43: 2–8, 1936.
5. BOHR, C. Om iltens afvigelse fra den Boyle-Mariotteske lov ved lave tryk. *K. Dan. Vidensk. Selsk. Skr. Naturvidensk. Math. Afd.* Ser. 6, 2: 401–417, 1885.
6. BOHR, C. *Experimentale Untersuchungen über die Sauerstoffaufnahme des Blutfarbstoffes.* Kopenhagen: Olsen, 1885.
7. BOHR, C. Ueber die Abweichung des Sauerstoffs von dem Boyle-Mariotte'schen Gesetze bei niedrigen Drucken. *[Wiedemann's] Ann. Phys. Chem.* Folge 3, 27: 459–479, 1886.
8. BOHR, C. Die funktionellen Änderungen in der Mittellage und Vitalkapazität der Lungen. Normales und pathologisches Emphysem. *Dtsch. Arch. Klin. Med.* 88: 385–434, 1907.
9. BORELLI, I. A. *De motu animalium.* Rome: Bernabò, 1680–1681, vol. 2, p. 162–164. (*Landmarks of Science.* New York: Readex Microprint, 1967.)
10. BOYLE, R. *New Experiments Physico-Mechanicall, Touching the Spring of the Air, and its Effects, (Made, for the most part, in a New Pneumatical Engine).* . . .Oxford: H: Hall for T: Robinson, 1660. (*Landmarks of Science.* New York: Readex Microprint, 1973.)
11. BOYLE, R. A defence of the doctrine touching the spring and weight of the air, propos'd by Mr. R. Boyle in his new physico-mechanical experiments; against the objections of Franciscus Linus. Wherewith the objector's funicular hypothesis is also examin'd. . . . In: *New Experiments Physico-Mechanical, Touching the Air. The Second Edition. Whereunto is added A Defence of the Authors Explication of the Experiments, Against the Obiections of Franciscus Linus, And, Thomas Hobbes.* Oxford: H. Hall for T: Robinson, 1662. (*Landmarks of Science.* New York: Readex Microprint, 1974.)
12. BRUNNER, C., AND G. VALENTIN. Ueber das Verhältniss der bei dem Athmen der Menschen ausgeschiedenen Kohlesäure zu dem durch jenen Process aufgenommenen Sauerstoffe. *Arch. Physiol. Heilk.* [Ser. 1], 2: 373–417, 1843.
13. BUCHWALD, J. Z. Sir William Thomas (Baron Kelvin of Largs). In: *Dictionary of Scientific Biography*, edited by C. C. Gillispie. New York: Scribner, 1976, vol. 13, p. 374–388.
14. BUNSEN, R. [W. E.]. *Gasometrische Methoden.* Braunschweig: Vieweg, 1857.
15. BUNSEN, R. [W. E.]. *Gasometry, Comprising the Leading Physical and Chemical Properties of Gases*, translated by H. E. Roscoe. London: Walton & Maberly, 1857.
16. BUNSEN, R. [W. E.]. *Méthodes gazométriques*, translated by T. Schneider. Paris: Masson, 1858.
17. CARNOT, [N. L.] S. *Réflexions sur la puissance motrice du feu et sur les machines propres à développer cette puissance.* Paris: Bachelier, 1824. (Facs. reprint. Paris: Hermann, 1903.)
18. CARNOT, [N. L.] S., É. CLAPEYRON, AND R. CLAUSIUS. *Reflections on the Motive Power of Fire, by Sadi Carnot; and Other Papers on the Second Law of Thermodynamics by É. Clapeyron and R. Clausius*, edited by E. Mendoza. New York: Dover, 1960.
19. CARPENTER, T. M. (editor). *Tables, Factors, and Formulas for Computing Respiratory Exchange and Biological Transformations of Energy.* Washington, DC: Carnegie Inst. Washington Publ. 303, 1921. (Reprint. Washington, DC: Carnegie Inst. Washington Publ., 1924, 1939, 1948.)
20. CLAPEYRON, É. Mémoire sur la puissance motrice de la chal-

eur. *J. Èc. Polytech. Paris* [Ser. 1], 14 (cahier 23): 153–190, 1834.
21. CLAUSIUS, R. Ueber die bewegende Kraft der Wärme und die Gesetze, welche sich daraus für die Wärmelehre selbst ableiten lassen. *[Poggendorff's] Ann. Phys. Chem.* Folge 2, 79: 368–397, 500–524, 1850.
22. COMROE, J. H., JR. *Retrospectroscope: Insights into Medical Discovery.* Menlo Park, CA: Von Gehr, 1977, p. 140–148.
23. CROSLAND, M. P. Joseph Louis Gay-Lussac. In: *Dictionary of Scientific Biography*, edited by C. C. Gillispie. New York: Scribner, 1972, vol. 5, p. 317–327.
24. CROSLAND, M. [P.]. *Gay-Lussac: Scientist and Bourgeois.* Cambridge: Cambridge Univ. Press, 1978.
25. DALTON, J. *Meteorological Observations and Essays.* London: Richardson, Phillips, and Pennington, 1793, p. 132–145, 200–208. (*Landmarks of Science.* New York: Readex Microprint, 1973.)
26. DALTON, J. Experimental essays on the constitution of mixed gases; on the force of steam or vapour from water and other liquids in different temperatures, both in a Torricellian vacuum and in air; on evaporation; and on the expansion of gases by heat. *Mem. Lit. Philos. Soc. Manchester* [Ser. 1], 5: 535–602, 1802.
27. DAVY, H. *Researches, Chemical and Philosophical; Chiefly Concerning Nitrous Oxide, or Dephlogisticated Nitrous Air, and its Respiration.* London: Johnson, 1800, p. 398–411.
28. DAVY, J. An account of some experiments on the blood in connexion with the theory of respiration. *Philos. Trans. R. Soc. Lond.* 128: 283–300, 1838.
29. DEJOURS, P. *Principles of Comparative Respiratory Physiology* (2nd ed.). Amsterdam: Elsevier/North-Holland, 1981.
30. DOEBEREINER, [J. W.]. Sur l'action capillaire des fissures, etc. *Ann. Chim. Phys.* Ser. 2, 24: 332–334, 1823.
31. DONDERS, F. C. Bedenken gegen die von Buys-Ballot und Fabius gegebene Formel zur Berechnung der vitalen Kapacität. *Z. Rat. Med.* Ser. 2, 4: 304–309, 1853.
32. DOUGLAS, C. G., AND J. G. PRIESTLEY. *Human Physiology: A Practical Course* (3rd ed.). Oxford: Clarendon, 1948, p. 8, 20.
33. DUCLAUX, J.-P. E. Calcul de la tension de vapeur de l'eau entre 0° et 100°C; formule donnant cette tension entre −20° et +200°. Volume de la vapeur. Chaleur de vaporisation. *C. R. Hebd. Seances Acad. Sci.* 236: 2218–2219, 1953.
34. DULONG, [P. L.], AND [A. T.] PETIT. Recherches sur les lois de dilatation des solides, des liquides et des fluides élastiques, et sur la mesure exacte des températures. *Ann. Chim. Phys.* Ser. 2, 2: 240–263, 1816.
35. DULONG, [P. L.], AND [A. T.] PETIT. Recherches sur la mesure des températures et sur les lois de la communication de la chaleur. *Ann. Chim. Phys.* Ser 2, 7: 113–154, 225–264, 337–367, 1817.
36. EXNER, F. Ueber den Durchgang der Gase durch Flüssigkeitslamellen. *[Poggendorff's] Ann. Phys. Chem.* Folge 2, 155: 321–336, 443–464, 1875.
37. FABIUS, [H.]. Neuere Beiträge zur Spirometrie. I. Spirometrische Beobachtungen. *Z. Rat. Med.* Ser. 2, 4: 281–304, 1853.
38. FICK, A. Ueber Diffusion. *[Poggendorff's] Ann. Phys. Chem.* Folge 2, 94: 59–86, 1855.
39. FINKLER, D., AND E. OERTMANN. Ueber den Einfluss der Athemmechanik auf den Stoffwechsel. *[Pfüger's] Arch. Gesamte Physiol. Menschen Tiere* 14: 38–72, 1877.
40. FOURIER, [J. B. J.]. *Théorie analytique de la chaleur.* Paris: Didot, 1822.
41. FOURIER, J. [B. J.]. *The Analytical Theory of Heat*, translated by A. Freeman. Cambridge: Cambridge Univ. Press, 1878. (Reprint. New York: Dover, 1955.)
42. FOX, R. Henri Victor Regnault. In: *Dictionary of Scientific Biography*, edited by C. C. Gillispie. New York: Scribner, 1975, vol. 11, p. 352–354.
43. GAY-LUSSAC, [J. L.]. Recherches sur la dilatation des gaz et des vapeurs. *Ann. Chim. Paris* [Ser. 1], 43: 137–175, 1802.
44. GAY-LUSSAC, [J. L.]. Mémoire sur la combinaison des substances gazeuses, les unes avec les autres. *Mem. Phys. Chim. Soc. Arcueil* 2: 207–234, 252–253, 1809.
45. GAY-LUSSAC, [J. L.]. Memoir on the combination of gaseous substances with each other. In: *Foundations of the Molecular Theory Comprising Papers and Extracts by John Dalton, Joseph-Louis Gay-Lussac, and Amadeo Avogadro (1808–1811).* Alembic Club Reprints, no. 4. Edinburgh: Livingstone, 1899. Reprinted 1950, p. 8–24.
46. GOODWYN, E. *The Connexion of Life with Respiration. . . .* London: Johnson, 1788, p. 34–37.
47. GOUGH, J. B. Jacques-Alexandre-César Charles. In: *Dictionary of Scientific Biography*, edited by C. C. Gillispie. New York: Scribner, 1971, vol. 3, p. 207–208.
48. GRAHAM, T. On the law of the diffusion of gases. *Philos. Mag.* Ser. 3, 2: 175–190, 269–276, 351–358, 1833.
49. GRAHAM, T. On the diffusion of liquids. *Philos. Trans. R. Soc. Lond.* 140: 1–46, 1850.
49a. GRAHAM, T. Supplementary observations on the diffusion of liquids. *Philos. Trans. R. Soc. Lond.* 140: 805–836, 1850.
50. GRAHAM, T. On the molecular mobility of gases. *Philos. Trans. R. Soc. Lond.* 153: 385–405, 1864.
51. GRAHAM BROWN, T., AND G. DE BEER. *The First Ascent of Mont Blanc.* London: Oxford Univ. Press, 1957, p. 52, 420–421.
52. GRÉHANT, N. Recherches physiques sur la respiration de l'homme. *[Robin's] J. Anat. Physiol. Norm. Pathol. Homme Anim.* 1: 523–555, 1864.
53. GUNTHER, R. T. *Early Science in Oxford.* Oxford: Printed for the author, 1930–1938, vols. 6–8, 10, 13.
54. HALDANE, J. [S.]. Some improved methods of gas analysis. *J. Physiol. Lond.* 22: 465–480, 1898.
55. HALDANE, J. S., AND J. G. PRIESTLEY. The regulation of the lung-ventilation. *J. Physiol. Lond.* 32: 225–266, 1905.
56. HALES, S. *Vegetable Staticks: Or, An Account of some Statical Experiments on the Sap in Vegetables: Being an Essay towards a Natural History of Vegetation. Also, a Specimen of An Attempt to Analyse the Air, By a great Variety of Chymio-Statical Experiments;. . .* London: W. & J. Innys and Woodward, 1727, p. 204–248. (Reprint. London: Scientific Book Guild, 1961, p. 117–140.)
57. HALES, S. *Statical Essays: Containing Haemastaticks; or, An Account of some Hydraulick and Hydrostatical Experiments made on the Blood and Blood-Vessels of Animals. . . .* London: Innys & Manby and Woodward, 1733. (Facs. reprint. New York: Hafner, 1964.)
58. HALL, J. A., AND C. R. BARBER. The International Temperature Scale—1948 revision. *Br. J. Appl. Physics* 1: 82–86, 1950.
59. HENRY, W. Experiments on the quantity of gases absorbed by water, at different temperatures, and under different pressures. *Philos. Trans. R. Soc. Lond.* 93: 29–42, 1803.
60. HENRY, W. C. A memoir of the life and writings of the late Dr. Henry. *Mem. Lit. Philos. Soc. Manchester* 11 [Ser. 2, vol. 6]: 99–141, 1842.
61. HERBST, E. F. G. Ueber die Capacität der Lungen für Luft, im gesunden und kranken Zustande. *[Meckel's] Arch. Anat. Physiol.* [1828]: 83–107, 1828.
62. HUTCHINSON, J. On the capacity of the lungs, and on the respiratory functions, with a view of establishing a precise and easy method of detecting disease by the spirometer. *Med.-Chir. Trans.* 29: 137–252, 1846.
63. HUTCHINSON, J. *Von der Capacität der Lungen und von den Athmungs-Functionen, mit Hinblick auf die Begründung einer genauen und leichten Methode, Krankheiten der Lungen durch das Spirometer zu entdecken*, translated by Samosch. Braunschweig: Vieweg, 1849. [Cited by Wintrich (147).]
64. INTERNATIONAL CIVIL AVIATION ORGANIZATION. *Manual of the ICAO Standard Atmosphere extended to 32 kilometres (105 000 feet)* (2nd ed.). Montreal: ICAO, 1964. (ICAO Document 7488/2.)
65. JONES, H. C., translator and editor. *The Modern Theory of Solution: Memoirs by Pfeffer, van't Hoff, Arrhenius, and Raoult.*

New York: Harper, 1899.
66. JOULE, J. P., AND W. THOMSON. On the thermal effects of fluids in motion, Part II. *Philos. Trans. R. Soc. Lond.* 144: 321–364, 1854.
67. JURIN, J. De motu aquarum fluentium. *Philos. Trans. [R. Soc. Lond.]* 30: 748–766, 1718.
68. KAUFFMAN, G. B. Thomas Graham. In: *Dictionary of Scientific Biography*, edited by C. C. Gillispie. New York: Scribner, 1972, vol. 5, p. 492–495.
69. KENTISH, E. An account of a pulmometer, by which may be known the power and capacity of the lungs to receive the atmospheric air. In: *An Account of Baths, and of a Madeira-House, at Bristol. . . .* London: Longman, Hurst, Rees, Orme, & Browne, [1814?], p. 81–117.
70. KEYES, F. G. The thermodynamic properties of water substance 0° to 150°C. *J. Chem. Phys.* 15: 602–612, 1947.
71. KROGH, A., AND M. KROGH. On the rate of diffusion of carbonic oxide into the lungs of man. *Skand. Arch. Physiol.* 23: 236–247, 1910.
72. KÜCHENMEISTER, [F.]. Ueber die Spirometrie im Allgemeinen und die Respirationsgrösse der Schwangern im Besondern. *Arch. [Ver.] [Gemein. Arb. Foerd.] Wiss. Heilkd.* 1: 504–516, 1854.
73. LA HIRE, [P.] DE. Experiences et remarques sur la dilatation de l'air par l'eau boüillante. *Mémoires de Mathématique et de Physique . . . de l'Académie Royale des Sciences. De l'Année 1708.* Paris: Compagnie des Libraires, 1730, p. 274–288.
74. LA PLACE, [P. S.] DE. Supplement to the Tenth Book. In: *Mécanique Céleste*, translated by N. Bowditch. Boston, MA: Little, Brown, 1839, vol. 4, p. 685–1018.
75. LAVOISIER, [A.-L.]. Expériences sur la respiration des animaux, et sur les changemens qui arrivent à l'air en passant par leur poumon. In: *Mémoires de Mathématique et de Physique . . . de l'Académie Royale des Sciences. Année 1777.* Paris: Imprimerie Royale, 1780, p. 185–194.
76. LAVOISIER, [A.-L.], AND [P. S.] DE LA PLACE. Mémoire sur la chaleur. In: *Mémoires de Mathématique et de Physique . . . de l'Académie Royale des Sciences. Année 1780.* Paris: Imprimerie Royale, 1784, p. 355–408.
77. LAVOISIER, [A.-L.], AND A. SÉGUIN. Second mémoire sur la respiration. *Ann. Chim. Paris* [Ser. 1], 91: 318–334, 1814.
78. LIEBIG, G. [VON]. Ueber die Respiration der Muskeln. *[Müller's] Arch. Anat. Physiol. Wiss. Med.* [1850]: 393–416, 1850.
79. LIEBIG, G. VON. Ueber das Athmen unter erhöhtem Luftdruck. *Z. Biol. Munich* [Ser. 1], 5: 1–27, 1869.
80. LIEBIG, G. [VON]. Beobachtungen über das Athmen unter dem erhöhten Luftdruck. *[Du Bois-Reymond's] Arch. Anat. Physiol. Physiol. Abt.* [1889] Suppl. Bd.: 41–90, 1889.
81. LINUS, F. *Tractatus de Corporum Inseparabilitate. . . .* London: Martin, Allestry, & Ditas, 1661.
82. LOEWY, A. *Untersuchungen über die Respiration und Circulation bei Aenderung des Druckes und des Sauerstoffgehaltes der Luft.* Berlin: Hirschwald, 1895.
83. LUNDSGAARD, C. Studies of oxygen in the venous blood. I. Technique and results on normal individuals. *J. Biol. Chem.* 33: 133–144, 1918.
84. LUNDSGAARD, C., AND D. D. VAN SLYKE. Studies of lung volume. I. Relation between thorax size and lung volume in normal adults. *J. Exp. Med.* 27: 65–86, 1918.
85. MADDISON, R. E. W. *The Life of the Honourable Robert Boyle F.R.S.* London: Taylor & Francis, 1969.
86. MAGNUS, G. Ueber die im Blute enhaltenen Gase, Sauerstoff, Stickstoff und Kohlensäure. *[Poggendorff's] Ann. Phys. Chem.* Folge 2, 40: 583–606, 1837.
87. MAGNUS, G. Ueber die Ausdehnung der Gase durch die Wärme. *[Poggendorff's] Ann. Phys. Chem.* Folge 2, 55: 1–27, 1842.
88. MAGNUS, G. Ueber die Ausdehnung der atmosphärischen Luft in höheren Temperaturen. *[Poggendorff's] Ann. Phys. Chem.* Folge 2, 57: 177–199, 1842.
89. MAGNUS, G. Sur la dilatation de l'air dans les hautes températures. *Ann. Chim. Phys.* Ser. 3, 6: 353–369, 1842.
90. MARIOTTE, [E.]. De la nature de l'air. In: *Oeuvres de Mr. Mariotte, de l'Académie Royale des Sciences.* Leiden: Pierre Vander Aa, 1717, vol. 1, p. 148–182. (See esp. p. 150–155.) (*Landmarks of Science.* New York: Readex Microprint, 1967.) (First published in 1679.)
91. MARVIN, C. F. *Barometers and the Measurement of Atmospheric Pressure* (Circular F, 7th ed.). Washington, DC: US Govt. Printing Office, 1941. (Weather Bur. no. 1010.)
92. MCKIE, D. Boyle's Law. *Endeavour* 7: 141–151, 1948.
93. MENZIES, R. *Tentamen physiologicum inaugurale, de respiratione.* Edinburgh: Creech, 1790.
94. MENZIES, R. *A Dissertation on Respiration*, translated by C. Sugrue. Edinburgh: Mudie, 1796.
95. MEYER, L. Die Gase des Blutes. *Z. rat. Med.* Ser. 2, 8: 256–316, 1857.
96. MIDDLETON, W. E. K. *The History of the Barometer.* Baltimore, MD: Johns Hopkins Press, 1964.
97. MIDDLETON, W. E. K. *A History of the Thermometer and its Use in Meteorology.* Baltimore, MD: Johns Hopkins Press, 1966.
98. MOSSO, A. *Life of Man on the High Alps*, translated by E. L. Kiesow. London: Fisher Unwin, 1898, p. 41.
99. MYERS, J. A. *Vital Capacity of the Lungs: A Handbook for Clinicians and Others Interested in the Examination of the Heart and Lungs Both in Health and Disease.* Baltimore, MD: Williams & Wilkins, 1925, p. 15–23, 120–135.
100. NATIONAL RESEARCH COUNCIL. Committee on Aviation Medicine. Subcommittee on Oxygen and Anoxia. *Handbook of Respiratory Data in Aviation.* Washington, DC, 1944, Chart R-1.
101. PAPPENHEIMER, J. R. [Chairman]. Standardization of definitions and symbols in respiratory physiology. *Federation Proc.* 9: 602–605, 1950.
102. PARTINGTON, J. R. *A History of Chemistry.* London: Macmillan, 1962, vol. 3.
103. PASCAL, [B.]. *Traitez de l'eqvilibre des liqvevrs, et de la pesantevr de la masse de l'air. . . .* Paris: Desprez, 1663.
104. PASCAL, B. *The Physical Treatises of Pascal*, translated by I. H. B. Spiers and A. G. H. Spiers. New York: Columbia Univ. Press, 1937.
105. PEABODY, F. W., AND J. A. WENTWORTH. Clinical studies of the respiration. IV. The vital capacity of the lungs and its relation to dyspnea. *Arch. Intern. Med.* 20: 443–467, 1917.
106. PEABODY, F. W., J. A. WENTWORTH, AND B. I. BARKER. Clinical studies on the respiration. V. The basal metabolism and the minute-volume of the respiration of patients with cardiac disease. *Arch. Intern. Med.* 20: 468–478, 1917.
107. PEPPER, W. The spirometer; its use in detecting disease of the lungs. *Am. J. Med. Sci.* Ser. 2, 25: 297–312, 1853.
108. PETERS, J. P., AND D. D. VAN SLYKE. *Quantitative Clinical Chemistry.* Baltimore, MD: Williams & Wilkins, 1932, vol. 2, p. 129.
109. PFLÜGER, E. [F. W.]. Ueber den Einfluss der Athemmechanik auf den Stoffwechsel. *[Pflüger's] Arch. Gesamte Physiol. Menschen Tiere* 14: 1–37, 1877.
110. PIIPER, J., P. DEJOURS, P. HAAB, AND H. RAHN. Concepts and basic quantities in gas exchange physiology. *Respir. Physiol.* 13: 292–304, 1971.
111. POISEUILLE, [J.-L.-M.]. Recherches expérimentales sur le mouvement des liquides dans les tubes de très-petits diamètres. *Mémoires présentés par divers savants à l'Académie Royale des Sciences de l'Institut de France* (Savants étrangers). 9: 433–543, 1846.
112. PRIESTLEY, J. Observations on different kinds of air. *Philos. Trans. [R. Soc. Lond.]* 62: 147–264, 1772.
113. PRINS, J. A. Johannes Diderik van der Waals. In: *Dictionary of Scientific Biography*, edited by C. C. Gillispie. New York: Scribner, 1976, vol. 14, p. 109–111.
114. RADFORD, E. P., JR. The physics of gases. In: *Handbook of Physiology. Respiration*, edited by W. O. Fenn and H. Rahn. Washington, DC: Am. Physiol. Soc., 1964, sect. 3, vol. I, chapt. 3, p. 125–152.

115. RAHN, H., AND W. O. FENN. *A Graphical Analysis of the Respiratory Gas Exchange. The O_2-CO_2 Diagram.* Washington, DC: Am. Physiol. Soc., 1955, p. 37.
116. RAHN, H., AND D. HAMMOND. Vital capacity at reduced barometric pressure. *J. Appl. Physiol.* 4: 715–724, 1952.
117. RANDALL, W. W. (translator and editor). *The Expansion of Gases by Heat. Memoirs by Dalton, Gay-Lussac, Regnault and Chappuis.* New York: Am. Book, 1902.
118. RAOULT, F.-M. Loi générale des tensions de vapeur des dissolvants. *C. R. Hebd. Seances Acad. Sci.* 104: 1430–1433, 1887.
119. REGNAULT, V. Sur le coefficient de dilatation des gaz. *C. R. Hebd. Seances Acad. Sci.* 13: 1077–1079, 1841.
120. REGNAULT, V. Recherches sur la dilatation des gaz. *Ann. Chim. Phys.* Ser. 3, 4: 5–67, 1842.
121. REGNAULT, V. Relation des expériences entreprises par ordre de monsieur le ministre des travaux publics, et sur la proposition de la commission centrale des machines à vapeur, pour déterminer les principales lois et les données numériques qui entrent dans le calcul des machines à vapeur. *Mem. Acad. R. Sci. Inst. Fr.* 21: 1–767, 1847.
122. REGNAULT, V., AND J. REISET. Recherches chimiques sur la respiration des animaux des diverses classes. *Ann. Chim. Phys.* Ser. 3, 26: 299–519, 1849.
123. ROSENTHAL, J. Die Physiologie der Athembewegungen und der Innvervation derselben. In: *Handbuch der Physiologie,* edited by L. Hermann. Leipzig: Vogel, 1882, vol. 4, pt. 2, p. 163–286.
124. ROTH, P. Modifications of apparatus and improved technic adaptable to the Benedict type of respiration apparatus. *Boston Med. Surg. J.* 186: 457–465, 491–501, 1922.
125. RUDBERG, F. Ueber die Ausdehnung der trocknen Luft zwischen 0° und 100°C. *[Poggendorff's] Ann. Phys. Chem.* Folge 2, 41: 271–293, 558–559, 1837.
126. RUDBERG, F. Zweite Reihe von Versuchen über die Ausdehnung der trocknen Luft zwischen 0° und 100°. *[Poggendorff's] Ann. Phys. Chem.* Folge 2, 44: 119–123, 1838.
127. SCHOLANDER, P. F. Analyzer for accurate estimation of respiratory gases in one-half cubic centimeter samples. *J. Biol. Chem.* 167: 235–250, 1947.
128. SCHOTT, G. *Mechanica Hydraulico-Pneumatica ... Accessit Experimentum novum Magdeburgicum, quo vacuum alij stabilire, alij evertere conantur.* Frankfurt am Main: Sumptu Heredum J. G. Schönwetterei, Excudebat H. Pigrin, 1657, p. 441–484. (*Landmarks of Science.* New York: Readex Microprint, 1975.)
129. SCHULTZ, A. W. F. Ueber die Wärmeerzeugung bei der Athmung. *[Müller's] Arch. Anat. Physiol. Wiss. Med.* [1842]: 121–144, 1842.
130. SCHUMBURG, [W. A. E. F.], AND N. ZUNTZ. Zur Kenntniss der Einwirkungen des Hochgebirges auf den menschlichen Organismus. *[Pflüger's] Arch. Gesamte Physiol. Menschen Tiere* 63: 461–494, 1896.
131. SÉGUIN, [A.], AND [A.-L.] LAVOISIER. Premier mémoire sur la respiration des animaux. *Mémoires de Mathématique et de Physique ... de l'Académie Royale des Sciences, Année 1789.* Paris: Imprimerie de du Pont, 1793, p. 566–584.
132. SEVERINGHAUS, J. W. Methods of measurement of blood and gas carbon dioxide during anesthesia. *Anesthesiology* 21: 717–726, 1960.
133. SHARLIN, H. I. *Lord Kelvin: The Dynamic Victorian.* University Park: Pennsylvania State Univ. Press, 1979.
134. THACKRAY, A. John Dalton. In: *Dictionary of Scientific Biography,* edited by C. C. Gillispie. New York: Scribner, 1971, vol. 3, p. 537–547.
135. THOMSON, W. On an absolute thermometric scale founded on Carnot's theory of the motive power of heat, and calculated from Regnault's observations. *Philos. Mag.* Ser. 3, 33: 313–317, 1848.
136. THOMSON, W. On the equilibrium of vapour at a curved surface of liquid. *Philos. Mag.* Ser. 4, 42: 448–452, 1871.
137. UOTILA, U. A. Earth, figure of. In: *The New Encyclopaedia Britannica....* (15th ed.). Chicago: Encyclopaedia Britannica, 1974, Macropaedia, vol. 6, p. 1–8.
138. VIERORDT, C. Ueber die Abhängigkeit des Kohlesäuregehaltes der ausgeathmeten Luft von der Häufigkeit der Athembewegungen: Ein Beitrag zur Experimentalphysiologie. *Arch. physiol. Heilk.* [Ser. 1], 3: 536–558, 1844.
139. VIVENOT, R. VON, JUN. Ueber die Zunahme der Lungencapacität bei therapeutischer Anwendung der verdichteten Luft. *Virchows Arch. Pathol. Anat. Physiol.* 33: 126–144, 1865.
140. WAALS, J. D. VAN DER. The continuity of the liquid and gaseous states of matter. *Physical Memoirs, Selected and Translated from Foreign Sources under the Direction of the Physical Society of London* 1 (Pt. 3): 333–496, 1890.
141. WAALS, J. D. VAN DER. Condensation of gases. In: *Encylopaedia Britannica* (11th ed.). New York: Encylopaedia Britannica, 1910, vol. 6, p. 844–849.
142. WALKER, J. E. C., R. E. WELLS, JR., AND E. W. MERRILL. Heat and water exchange in the respiratory tract. *Am. J. Med.* 30: 259–267, 1961.
143. WEAST, R. C., M. J. ASTLE, AND W. H. BEYER (editors). *CRC Handbook of Chemistry and Physics* (66th ed.). Boca Raton, FL: CRC, 1985, p. D-188–D-190, E-34–E-37, F-148–F-156.
144. WEBSTER, C. The discovery of Boyle's Law, and the concept of the elasticity of air in the seventeenth century. *Arch. Hist. Exact Sci.* 2: 441–502, 1965.
145. WEST, J. B., C. J. PIZZO, J. S. MILLEDGE, K. H. MARET, AND R. M. PETERS. Barometric pressure and alveolar gas composition on the summit of Mt. Everest (Abstract). *Federation Proc.* 41: 1109, 1982.
146. WESTFALL, R. S. Robert Hooke. *Dictionary of Scientific Biography,* edited by C. C. Gillispie. New York: Scribner, 1972, vol. 6, p. 481–488.
147. WINTRICH, M. A. Einleitung zur Darstellung der Krankheiten der Respirationsorgane. In: *Handbuch der speciellen Pathologie und Therapie,* edited by R. Virchow. Erlangen: Enke, 1854, vol. 5, pt. 1, p. 1–224.
148. YOUNG, T. An essay on the cohesion of fluids. *Philos. Trans. R. Soc. Lond.* 95: 65–87, 1805.
149. ZUPKO, R. E. *British Weights & Measures: A History From Antiquity to the Seventeenth Century.* Madison: Univ. of Wisconsin Press, 1977, p. 174.
150. ZUPKO, R. E. *French Weights and Measures Before the Revolution: A Dictionary of Provincial and Local Units.* Bloomington: Indiana Univ. Press, 1978, p. 143.

CHAPTER 3

Diffusion of gases

H. K. CHANG | *Departments of Biomedical Engineering and of Physiology and Biophysics, University of Southern California, Los Angeles, California*

CHAPTER CONTENTS

THE SUBJECT OF DIFFUSION is of great importance in biological sciences; every cell of every organism, at every moment of its existence, is dependent on the diffusion process. In studying biological gas exchange, knowledge about diffusion of gases is fundamental. As the science of physiology becomes increasingly more quantitative, the modern respiratory physiologist, whether designing an experiment, interpreting observed data, or modeling a physiological phenomenon, is in ever greater need of a firm grasp of the laws of gas diffusion.

In particular it has been convincingly demonstrated that mixing between the inspired tidal gas and the resident alveolar gas is incomplete (15) and that this incomplete mixing is not only a consequence of the geometrical and mechanical properties of the lung but also dependent on the rate of molecular diffusion in the gas phase (39). In other words, molecular diffusion in the gaseous state plays a vital role in the delivery of O_2 to, and removal of CO_2 from, the sites of gas exchange.

This chapter provides a brief outline of the essential elements in gaseous diffusion. It is written for the physiologist who has no advanced training in mathematics, physics, or engineering. Equal emphasis is placed on the physical nature of gaseous diffusion, on the practical means to estimate such quantities as diffusion coefficients, and on a mathematical framework on which a more in-depth knowledge of the diffusion phenomenon can be built.

HISTORICAL NOTE

The earliest investigators of diffusion were motivated mostly by their desire to understand the processes of biological transport. They studied diffusion of liquids, especially across membranes. In the early part of the nineteenth century, physicists and chemists who attempted to unravel the mystery of atomic and molecular forces also became interested in diffusion, principally in the gaseous state. Among this group was Thomas Graham (1805–1869). Using a glass tube that had a dense stucco plug at one end and was submerged in water at the other end, Graham measured the rate of flux of various gases through the stucco plug. Because the flux of the experimental gas does not equal the flux of air, the water level in the tube either rises or falls during diffusion. Graham correctly saw that this change in water level would lead to a pressure gradient that would in turn alter diffusion. To overcome this he continually adjusted the tube position so that the water level stayed constant. His experimental results then consisted of a volume change reflecting the diffusional property of each gas originally held in the tube. Graham showed that this volume change was inversely proportional to the square root of the density of the gas. First published in 1833, Graham's law stated (20): "The diffusion of spontaneous intermixture of two gases in contact is affected by an interchange of position of infinitely minute volumes, being, in the case of each gas, inversely proportional to the square root of the density of the gas."

Graham's experiments involved a moving frame of reference for measuring the diffusion fluxes. What was kept constant was the pressure gradient across the stucco plug, not the number of molecules exchanged between air and the experimental gas. This feature of Graham's experiments has caused considerable confusion among later workers. Furthermore the inverse square root relationship was specifically derived with air as the second gas in the diffusion process. When applied to other situations, Graham's law as it is known to today's respiratory physiologists may lead to erroneous results.

Graham later also performed some experiments on liquid diffusion, but these experiments did not lead to another important discovery. One reason for this failure was perhaps his earlier success; he looked hard for another square root relationship.

Just as one of the fundamental laws in fluid mechanics was formulated by the physician Jean Poiseuille (1799–1869), the fundamental law of diffusion was also discovered by a physician, Adolf Fick (1829–1901). Figuratively, Fick stepped out from under the roof of Graham's square root and saw the light in Fourier's heat equation.

The heat-conduction law of Joseph Fourier (1768–1830) states that the flux of heat is directly proportional to the temperature gradient that causes it. By qualitative theories, quantitative experiments, and probably a good deal of intuitive guessing, Fick (19) suggested in 1855 that "the diffusion of the dissolved material" and "the spreading of warmth in a conductor" were both "left to the influence of molecular forces basic to the same law." Hence he postulated that the concentration gradient of a substance and the resulting diffusional flux are linearly related. Namely

$$J_z = -\mathscr{D}\frac{dC}{dz} \tag{1}$$

where J_z is the mass flux and dC/dz is the concentration gradient, both in the z direction. The proportionality constant $\mathscr{D}$ is known as the diffusion coefficient. (See Table 1 for symbols and definitions used in this chapter.)

TABLE 1. *Symbols and Definitions*

A	cross-sectional area	l	smallest dimension of container in which diffusion occurs
C	molar concentration	m	molecular mass
$\mathscr{D}$	diffusion coefficient	n	number of molecules per volume, of species in multicomponent mixture, and of simultaneous equations
$\mathscr{D}_{ab}$	binary diffusion coefficient between species a and b	q	magnitude of velocity of a gas molecule
$\mathscr{D}_i$	diffusion coefficient of the ith species	r	radial axis in cylindrical coordinate system; distance of separation between two molecules
D_{ij}	multicomponent diffusion coefficient	s	standard deviation
D'_{im}	effective diffusion coefficient of species i in multicomponent mixture	s^2	variance
E_k	kinetic energy of molecule	t	time
I	an integer	u	velocity component in x direction of molecule
$\mathbf{J}$	general diffusion flux; mass diffusion flux with respect to mass average velocity	v	velocity component in y direction of molecule; mass average velocity of mixture
$\mathbf{J}_z$	diffusion flux in z direction; mass diffusion flux with respect to mass average velocity	v_i	diffusing velocity of species i in mixture
$\mathbf{J}_a^*$	molar diffusion flux of species a with respect to molar average velocity of binary mixture	v^*	molar average velocity
$\mathbf{J}_i^*$	molar diffusion flux of ith species in multicomponent mixture	w	velocity component in z direction
K	degree Kelvin	x	coordinate direction; molar fraction
L	large integer	x_i	molar fraction of ith species in mixture
M_a	molecular weight of species a	y	coordinate direction
M_b	molecular weight of species b	z	coordinate direction
$\mathbf{N}$	molar flux with respect to stationary coordinates		
$\mathbf{N}_i$	molar flux of ith species in multicomponent mixture	*Greek letters*	
$N_x(N_y, N_z)$	molar flux in $x(y, z)$ direction	Γ	frequency of molecular collision
P	pressure	$\Omega_{\mathscr{D}}$	collision integral for diffusion
P	probability	ϕ	Lennard-Jones potential energy function of single species of gas molecules
Q_0	quantity of diffusate contained in a small region	ϕ_{ab}	Lennard-Jones potential energy function of ab gas pair
R	universal gas constant	ϵ	force constant of molecules in Lennard-Jones potential
T	temperature	ϵ_{ab}	force constant of ab gas pair
V	volume	λ	mean free path
$\mathbf{V}_i$	velocity vector of ith species	η	argument of error function
X	position or small region in random walk	ξ	constant; dummy variable in error function
Lowercase letters		ρ	mass density
d	diameter of idealized spherical molecules	ρ_i	mass density of ith species
$\mathbf{i}$	unit vector in x direction	σ	collision diameter of gas molecule
$\mathbf{j}$	unit vector in y direction	σ_{ab}	averaged collision diameter of ab gas pair
$\mathbf{k}$	unit vector in z direction		

Fourier's law of heat conduction, Fick's law of diffusion, and Newton's law of viscosity (which states that the shear stress in a flowing fluid is directly proportional to the local velocity gradient) describe macroscopic phenomena. These phenomenological laws, which are similar in appearance, do not give any insight into the reasons for the behavior they describe. As was correctly foreseen by Fick, there is a molecular or microscopic basis that links these macroscopic phenomena. This link was partially unveiled by the work of Rudolf Clausius (1822–1888) and James Maxwell (1831–1879) on the kinetic theory of gases (30). In 1871 Maxwell (31) showed theoretically that the diffusion coefficient defined by Fick's law varied with the square root of the harmonic average of the densities of the two diffusing gases, thus formally establishing the molecular theory of binary diffusion.

GENERAL DESCRIPTION OF GASEOUS DIFFUSION

When a gas mixture contains two or more different kinds of molecules whose spatial distribution is nonuniform, a process termed *diffusion* occurs continuously in a way that diminishes the nonuniformity of composition. The kinetic theory of gases offers an explanation of this phenomenon.

The molecules in the gaseous state are in constant thermal motion due to their thermal energy. They collide with each other, rebound, then collide again. The motion and collisions are purely random. In homogeneous mixtures, if one considers an imaginary plane fixed in space, the net number of molecules that move across the plane, over a sufficiently long time, should be zero for molecules of the same kind. In nonhomogeneous mixtures, as a consequence of the thermal motion, more molecules of a given kind travel from regions rich in that kind to regions of scarcity than travel in the opposite direction. The process tends to smooth out the original nonuniform distribution. Obviously the net movement of each kind of molecule is likely to be in the direction in which its density decreases most rapidly, where *density* means the number of molecules of the same kind per unit volume.

The preceding description applies to a general mixture of any number of different kinds of molecules, i.e., gas species. For convenience of discussion the following description refers to binary mixtures, i.e., those mixtures containing only two kinds of gas molecules. Because each kind of molecule moves according to its own density gradient, the rate of diffusion of the two constituents generally will not be equal. For different kinds of molecules with widely different velocities of thermal motion, the difference in diffusion rates may be very large. If nothing more than the thermal motion processes were involved in the phenomenon of diffusion, a greater number of the faster-moving molecules would be transferred in one direction than of the other in the opposite direction. The gas mixture as a whole would thus move bodily toward one side. Indeed this was what Graham (20) discovered in his glass-tube experiments.

The phenomenon of bodily motion caused by diffusion requires that for a quantitative description of the diffusion process, the frame of reference be appropriately defined. The most commonly used frame of reference is the molar frame of reference, which moves with the molar average velocity, i.e., the net difference among the rates of diffusion in molar units in a mixture. Therefore, when the net flux with respect to the molar frame of reference is zero, the diffusion is termed *equimolar*. The general free diffusion with respect to a stationary frame of reference is termed *nonequimolar*.

The mathematical description of the diffusion process may be approached from either a macroscopic or a microscopic point of view. From the macroscopic point of view, diffusion is one of the transport phenomena that can be considered a direct consequence of entropy changes and whose precise form is postulated and derived in nonequilibrium thermodynamics. From the microscopic point of view, diffusion can be described by the kinetic theory of gases as a consequence of actual collisions among the gas molecules. Both approaches are valid and generally arrive at the same expressions for the diffusion phenomenon.

MOLECULAR BEHAVIOR: KINETIC THEORY OF GASES

The number of molecules per mole of a substance (Avogadro's number) is determined to be 6.023×10^{23}. From this number one can calculate that in 1 cm^3 of an ideal gas there are 2.688×10^{19} molecules. The average distance of molecular separation at atmospheric pressure is approximately the cube root of the inverse of this number, or 3.34×10^{-7} cm. The molecular diameter for a simple organic gas is in the range of $2–5 \times 10^{-8}$ cm (Table 2). Thus for the common gases the average distance of molecular separation is ~10 times the molecular diameter.

At ordinary conditions of temperature and pressure, gas molecules have speeds of the order of 10^4 cm/s (Table 2). In contrast, actual diffusion velocities are much less, ~1 cm/s. This great decrease in apparent molecular speed occurs because diffusion is dominated by collisions that deflect the molecules along tortuous paths. The collisions in turn are controlled by the forces of interaction between the molecules. Based on the formulas of kinetic theory, knowledge of these fundamental intermolecular forces can lead to predictions of the gaseous diffusion coefficients. The task of the kinetic theory of gases then is to construct a hypothetical model for the interaction between gas molecules, describe the molecular velocities and molecular collisions in a rational manner, and derive

TABLE 2. *Molecular Constants of Some Gases*

Gas	Average Velocity at 20°C, 10^2 cm	Mean Free Path at 75 cmHg, 10^{-6} cm	Collision Frequency at 20°C, 10^6 s^{-1}	Molecular Diameter, 10^{-8} cm
Air	463			
Argon	395	9.88	4,000	2.94
Carbon monoxide	471	9.73	5,100	3.12
Carbon dioxide	376	6.15	6,120	3.23
Helium	1,252	27.45	4,540	2.65
Krypton	272			3.69
Neon	557			2.66
Nitrogen	471	9.29	5,070	3.15
Nitrous oxide	392	6.10		4.66
Oxygen	440	9.93	4,430	2.92
Water vapor	587			2.88
Xenon	218			4.02

Molecular diameter computed from van der Waal's equation.

mathematically the transport coefficients and other macroscopic quantities.

The common hypotheses of all kinetic theories are that matter is composed of small discrete units known as molecules, that all molecules of a given substance are alike, and that the three states of matter differ essentially in the arrangement and state of motion of the molecules. In the kinetic theory of gases, it is further assumed that all molecules are monoatomic and all molecular collisions are binary, involving only two molecules. Three-body collisions are assumed to occur with only negligible frequency. Except at very low temperatures, pressures <100 atm are low enough to ensure the validity of this hypothesis.

The discovery of wavelike subatomic particles in modern physics has made the original hypotheses of the kinetic theory appear rather crude. Nevertheless this theory is very useful in explaining the aggregate behavior of many molecules. As a demonstration of the power of the kinetic theory of gases and also as a comparison with the more sophisticated theory to be outlined later, a very simple theory is presented first.

Simple Kinetic Theory of Gases

In this simplified theory it is assumed that gas molecules are rigid nonattracting spheres, all traveling with the same speed and only in the coordinate directions (*x, y,* and *z*); that the total number of molecules is large in a small volume; and that the conservation laws of classical mechanics apply.

Let the diameter of the gas molecules be *d*. Imagine two molecules A and B. When the centers of these two molecules are at a distance *d*, collision occurs. Thus each molecule has a "collision sphere" of radius *d*. A collision occurs whenever the center of another molecule comes within this sphere. If there are *n* molecules per unit volume and if equal numbers of molecules are traveling in each coordinate direction, then there will be $n/6$ molecules moving in the $+x$ direction, and these molecules will collide with those traveling in the $-x$ direction at a rate $(n/6)\pi d^2(2u)$, where πd^2 is the cross-sectional area of the collision sphere of each molecule and $2u$ is the relative velocity at which two molecules approach each other. The molecules moving in the $+x$ direction will collide with those moving in the $+y$, $-y$, $+z$, and $-z$ directions at a right angle and at a rate $(n/6)\pi d^2(\sqrt{2}u)$, where $\sqrt{2}u$ is the relative velocity between the colliding molecules. Because there is no collision with molecules moving in the same direction, the molecules moving in the $+x$ direction will experience

$$\Gamma = \left(\frac{n}{6}\right)\pi d^2(2u) + 4\left[\left(\frac{n}{6}\right)\pi d^2(\sqrt{2}u)\right] = 1.276\ n\pi d^2 u \qquad (2)$$

where Γ is the frequency of collisions per unit time.

An important quantity in kinetic theory is the average distance a molecule travels between collisions. This is termed the *mean free path.* The average number of collisions experienced by one molecule in unit time is given in Equation 2. In this time the molecule has traveled a distance *u*. The mean free path λ is therefore u/Γ, or

$$\lambda = \frac{1}{\xi n\pi d^2} \qquad (3)$$

where $\xi = 1.276$; for a slightly improved derivation in which the molecules are allowed to move in all directions, $\xi = \sqrt{2}$ or 1.414. Although Equation 3 is based on an ultrasimplified theory, it is qualitatively correct and yields results that are within the range of the best available data (Table 2).

Consider now the net flux of molecules in the $+z$ direction through plane 0 as shown in Figure 1. Let the number density of molecules in plane 0 be n_0. Molecules approaching 0 from below have suffered their last collision at a distance λ below plane 0. That is, they have come from plane A and have the number density n_A, which is characteristic of that location. Similarly, molecules arriving at plane 0 from above have come from plane B and possess the number density n_B, which is characteristic of that plane. As an approximation, assume a constant gradient of density dn/dz over distances of the order of magnitude of the mean free path

$$n_A = n_0 - \lambda\frac{dn}{dz}$$
$$n_B = n_0 + \lambda\frac{dn}{dz} \qquad (4)$$

The number of molecules passing through plane 0 from below is $(1/6)n_A u$ and from above is $-(1/6)n_B u$. Hence the net flux (flow of molecules per unit area)

$$J_z = -\tfrac{1}{6}(n_B - n_A)u = -\tfrac{1}{3}u\lambda\frac{dn}{dz} \qquad (5)$$

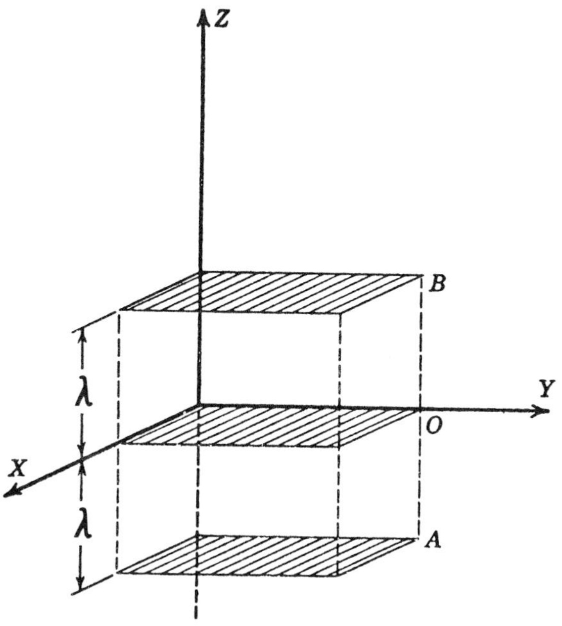

FIG. 1. Sketch of molecular flux through *plane 0* in *z* direction. *A*, *B*, planes; λ, distance; *x*, *y*, directions.

If Equation 5 is compared with Fick's law as given in Equation 1, the coefficient of self-diffusion of this kind of molecule is obtained

$$\mathcal{D} = \tfrac{1}{3}u\lambda \tag{6}$$

Thus the proportionality constant in Fick's phenomenological law is given a microscopic interpretation from this simple theory. The diffusion coefficient increases when the molecules move faster or the mean free path increases.

Rigorous Kinetic Theory of Gases

The rigorous kinetic theory of dilute gases is very complicated; no useful purpose would be served by detailing here the lengthy postulates and often tedious derivations. Those readers who are gifted in mathematical marathons and who have a propensity for mental gymnastics are referred to the highly esteemed books by Chapman and Cowling (9) and Hirschfelder et al. (23).

In this more realistic theory in which the binary collision hypothesis is still retained, three refinements are made over the simple theory presented above. First, the molecules are considered to interact according to a prescribed force field. Second, the molecules are supposed to move with a spectrum of velocities at any instant, necessitating the notion of a distribution function. Third, abstract concepts such as *n*-dimensional spaces and ensembles as well as statistical methods are used. The probability of a certain behavior then may be predicted from such a theory. Only a bare outline of these features is presented here.

LENNARD-JONES POTENTIAL. The forces acting between a pair of molecules during a collision are characterized by the potential energy of interaction ϕ. In other words, the actual intermolecular force equals $-d\phi/dr$, where r is the distance of separation between two molecules. An empirical representation of the potential energy function that has proved fairly successful is the Lennard-Jones potential model plotted in Figure 2

$$\phi(r) = 4\epsilon\left[\left(\frac{\sigma}{r}\right)^{12} - \left(\frac{\sigma}{r}\right)^{6}\right] \tag{7}$$

where σ, the collision diameter, is the value of r for which $\phi(r) = 0$ and ϵ is the maximum energy of attraction between a pair of molecules. The model exhibits weak attraction at large separations (nearly proportional to r^{-6}) and strong repulsion at small separations (nearly proportional to r^{-12}). Table 3 lists the values of σ and ϵ for various gases frequently encountered in respiratory physiology studies.

The Lennard-Jones model describes a spherically symmetrical force field and hence is intended for use with nonpolar, nearly symmetrical molecules (e.g., O_2). Molecules with appreciable dipole moments (e.g., H_2O) and those that are highly elongated interact with

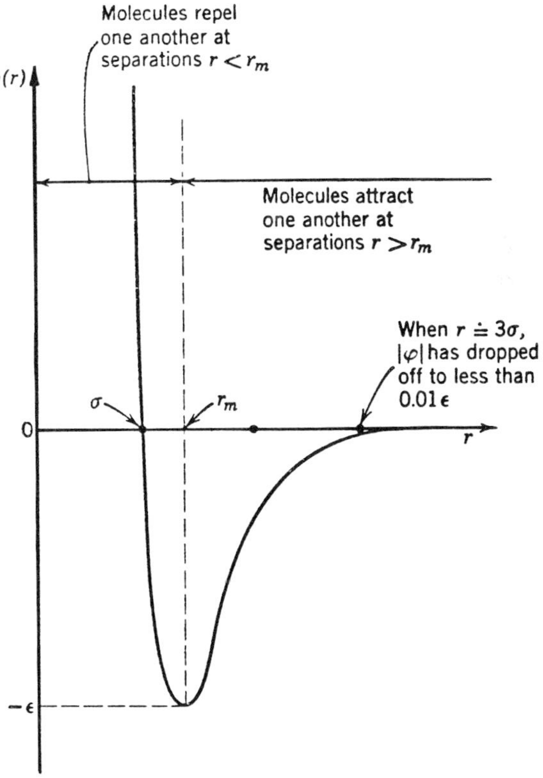

FIG. 2. Lennard-Jones potential energy function, describing interaction of 2 spherical, nonpolar molecules. r, Distance of separation between 2 molecules; r_m, separation distance where intermolecular forces change sign, i.e., repellent to attractive or vice versa; ϵ, maximum energy of attraction between pair of molecules; σ, collision diameter. [From Bird et al. (2).]

TABLE 3. *Force Constants for Lennard-Jones Potential Model*

Gas	σ, 10^{-8} cm	ϵ/k, °K
Air	3.711	79
Argon	3.542	93
Carbon monoxide	3.690	92
Carbon dioxide	3.941	195
Helium	2.551	10
Krypton	3.655	179
Neon	2.820	33
Nitrogen	3.798	71
Nitrous oxide	3.828	232
Oxygen	3.467	107
Sulfur hexafluoride	5.128	222
Water vapor	3.737	32
Xenon	4.047	231

σ, Collision diameter of gas molecules; ϵ, force constant of molecules; k, Boltzmann constant. [Data from R. A. Svehla (44).]

potentials that are angle dependent. However, for many practical purposes it is adequate to use the Lennard-Jones potential even for polar and elongated molecules.

DISTRIBUTION OF MOLECULAR VELOCITIES. In their constant motion, the molecules of a gas collide many times with one another, and these collisions provide the mechanism through which the velocities of individual molecules change continually. As a result there exists a distribution of velocities among the molecules; most have velocities far above or far below the average.

The distribution of velocities among molecules in a gas was first calculated by Maxwell (30). To present his results it is best to begin with a related problem in the theory of probability, termed the *random walk.*

Consider the case of an inebriated sailor who leaves a tavern still able to walk but unable to navigate. He is just as likely to take a step east as a step west. (The tavern happens to be located on a narrow street with an east-west orientation!) Each step has a probability of ½ of being in either direction. After he has taken L steps (L is a large number), what is the probability that he is a distance z from his starting point, if the length of each step is h?

Let $P(z, L)$ be the probability that he is at point z after L steps. It can be shown (18) that this probability is in fact the Gaussian distribution function

$$P(z, L)\Delta z = \left(\frac{1}{2\pi h^2 L}\right)^{1/2} e^{-z^2/2Lh^2}\Delta z \tag{8}$$

where Δz is a distance of a number of steps. Written in the usual manner the Gaussian distribution function is

$$P(z) = \frac{1}{(2\pi)^{1/2}s} e^{-z^2/2s^2} \tag{9}$$

where s is the standard deviation from the mean and s^2 is the variance.

To apply the random walk to the problem of molecular velocities, the wandering sailor is replaced by a gas molecule, and the displacement z by a velocity component u in the x direction. Instead of a sailor taking L steps at random under his own residual will power, we visualize a gas molecule receiving increments of velocity from random collisions with other molecules. From Equation 9, the probability that the molecule attains a velocity u is simply

$$P(u) = \frac{1}{(2\pi s^2)^{1/2}} e^{-u^2/2s^2} \tag{10}$$

From thermodynamics we know that the translational kinetic energy (E) of a gas molecule is

$$E_k = {}^3\!/_2 k\mathrm{T} \tag{11}$$

where k is the Boltzmann constant or gas constant per molecule and T is temperature. The principle of equipartition of energy holds that the kinetic energy in each of the three translational degrees of freedom is the same (25); therefore the kinetic energy in the x direction is

$$\tfrac{1}{2}m\bar{u}^2 = \tfrac{1}{2}k\mathrm{T} \ (\text{or } \bar{u}^2 = k\mathrm{T}/m) \tag{12}$$

where m is the mass of the molecule and $\bar{u}^2$ is the mean square velocity. Because the velocity can be either positive or negative, the mean value $\bar{u}$ is zero, hence

$$s^2 = \frac{1}{n}\sum_{i=1}^{n}(u_i - \bar{u})^2 = \frac{1}{n}\sum_{i=1}^{n}u_i^2 - \bar{u}^2 \tag{13}$$

By Equations 10, 12, and 13, the probability that a molecule has a velocity component between u and $u + du$ is

$$P(u)du = \left(\frac{m}{2\pi k\mathrm{T}}\right)^{1/2} e^{-mu^2/2k\mathrm{T}}du \tag{14}$$

One can show that the fraction of molecules having simultaneously a velocity component between u and $u + du$ in the x direction, v and dv in the y direction, and w and $w + dw$ in the z direction is simply the product of the three individual probabilities (25). Thus

$$\frac{dn}{n} = \left(\frac{m}{2\pi k\mathrm{T}}\right)^{3/2} e^{-(u^2 + v^2 + w^2)/2k\mathrm{T}}du\,dv\,dw \tag{15}$$

where n is the number of molecules per unit volume.

The molecules with a speed between q and $q + dq$, regardless of direction, where $q^2 = u^2 + v^2 + w^2$, have their velocity points lying within a spherical shell of thickness dq at a distance q from the origin. The volume of this shell is $4\pi q^2 dq$, and therefore the desired distribution function is

$$\frac{dn}{n} = 4\left(\frac{m}{2\pi k\mathrm{T}}\right)^{3/2} e^{-mq^2/2k\mathrm{T}}q^2 dq \tag{16}$$

Equation 16 gives the Maxwellian velocity distribution function for a system at equilibrium. Based on this distribution function, the average velocity of the molecules may be obtained

$$\bar{q} = \frac{1}{n}\int_0^\infty q dn = 4\pi\left(\frac{m}{2\pi kT}\right)^{3/2}\int_0^\infty e^{-mq^2/2kT}q^3 dq = \left(\frac{8kT}{\pi m}\right)^{1/2} \quad (17)$$

With the use of Equation 17 the molecular velocities of such gases as shown in Table 1 may be calculated.

BOLTZMANN EQUATION AND CHAPMAN-ENSKOG SOLUTION. Using the laws of classical mechanics, working with abstract concepts such as n-dimensional spaces and ensembles, and considering binary collisions, Boltzmann derived a highly complex integrodifferential equation in terms of a distribution function $f(\mathbf{r}, \boldsymbol{V}_i, t)$. This function represents the number of molecules of the ith species that at time t lie in a unit volume element about the point $\mathbf{r}$ and that have velocities within a unit range about $\boldsymbol{V}_i$. The Boltzmann equation describes a nonequilibrium system. When the system is at equilibrium, $f(\mathbf{r}, \boldsymbol{V}_i, t)$ reduces to the Maxwellian distribution given in Equation 16. Mathematically, the central task of the rigorous kinetic theory of dilute gases is to solve the Boltzmann equation and obtain the nonequilibrium distribution function.

Usually one is interested in the properties of gases that are under conditions only slightly different from equilibrium. In fact it is only under these conditions that the flux vectors (e.g., Eq. 5) are linear in the derivatives and that the usual definitions of the transport coefficients apply. In this limit the distribution function is nearly Maxwellian, and the Boltzmann equation can be solved by a successive approximation method developed independently by Chapman and Enskog (13).

The Chapman-Enskog solution of the Boltzmann equation depends on these assumptions:

Binary collisions. The Boltzmann equation itself is based on this fundamental assumption. Therefore the Chapman-Enskog theory is applicable only to dilute gases, as mentioned previously.

Small mean free paths. The Chapman-Enskog solution assumes that the dimensions of the gas container are large compared with the molecular mean free path. In gases of extremely low densities, molecules collide more frequently with the walls of the container than with each other. When molecular collisions with a container surface are significant, the theory fails.

Small perturbations. In the Chapman-Enskog theory the assumption of a small perturbation function describes small departures from the equilibrium velocity distribution functions; in other words, at conditions slightly away from equilibrium the transport property fluxes vary linearly with the gradients.

Classical mechanics. Historically, classical mechanics was used by Boltzmann, Chapman, and Enskog; however, their theory can be reformulated to account for quantum-mechanical effects.

Elastic collisions. The original Boltzmann equation and its solution by Chapman and Enskog were limited to elastic collisions between molecules interacting with central forces. Inelastic collisions occur between molecules with internal degrees of freedom, such as molecular vibration, and kinetic energy is no longer conserved, although mass and momentum are conserved. Thus diffusion and viscosity, which are dependent on molecular mass and momentum transport, are not strongly affected by the presence of internal degrees of freedom, although thermal conductivity, which depends on molecular kinetic energy transfer, is affected.

The transport properties appear finally in the Chapman-Enskog theory as solutions of infinite sets of simultaneous algebraic equations and may be expressed in terms of a set of collision integrals. These integrals explicitly involve the dynamics of molecular encounters and hence the intermolecular force law. Based on the Lennard-Jones potential model, the collision integrals $\Omega_{\mathscr{D}}$ for the diffusion coefficient are weak functions of temperature, becoming very nearly constant at high temperatures. They are tabulated in Table 4. The actual formula for diffusion coefficients is given in next section.

BINARY DIFFUSION

This section deals with some practical aspects of *binary diffusion*, a term meaning ordinary diffusion arising from a concentration gradient in a binary

TABLE 4. *Collision Integrals for Lennard-Jones Potential Model*

kT/ϵ	$\Omega_{\mathscr{D}}$	kT/ϵ	$\Omega_{\mathscr{D}}$	kT/ϵ	$\Omega_{\mathscr{D}}$	kT/ϵ	$\Omega_{\mathscr{D}}$
0.30	2.662	1.30	1.273	2.60	0.9878	4.60	0.8568
0.35	2.476	1.35	1.253	2.70	0.9770	4.70	0.8530
0.40	2.318	1.40	1.233	2.80	0.9672	4.80	0.8492
0.45	2.184	1.45	1.215	2.90	0.9576	4.90	0.8456
0.50	2.066	1.50	1.198	3.00	0.9490	5.0	0.8422
0.55	1.966	1.55	1.182	3.10	0.9406	6.0	0.8124
0.60	1.877	1.60	1.167	3.20	0.9328	7.0	0.7896
0.65	1.798	1.65	1.153	3.30	0.9256	8.0	0.7712
0.70	1.729	1.70	1.140	3.40	0.9186	9.0	0.7556
0.75	1.667	1.75	1.128	3.50	0.9120	10.0	0.7424
0.80	1.612	1.80	1.116	3.60	0.9058	20.0	0.6640
0.85	1.562	1.85	1.105	3.70	0.8998	30.0	0.6232
0.90	1.517	1.90	1.094	3.80	0.8942	40.0	0.5960
0.95	1.476	1.95	1.084	3.90	0.8888	50.0	0.5756
1.00	1.439	2.00	1.075	4.00	0.8836	60.0	0.5596
1.05	1.406	2.10	1.057	4.10	0.8788	70.0	0.5464
1.10	1.375	2.20	1.041	4.20	0.8740	80.0	0.5352
1.15	1.346	2.30	1.026	4.30	0.8694	90.0	0.5256
1.20	1.320	2.40	1.012	4.40	0.8652	100.0	0.5170
1.25	1.296	2.50	0.9996	4.50	0.8610		

k, Boltzmann constant; T, temperature; ϵ, force constant of molecules. [From Hirschfelder et al. (23).]

mixture. Mass transfer resulting from a temperature gradient or a pressure gradient is not included. Furthermore only molecular diffusion in a container whose smallest dimension l is much greater than the mean free path λ of the gas molecules is considered; diffusion in the Knudsen ($l \ll \lambda$) or transition ($l \approx \lambda$) range is not discussed. Neither of these restrictions excludes any known physiological condition.

Fick's First Law: Steady Diffusion

As given in Equation 1, Fick's law describes the relationship between the diffusional flux and the concentration gradient in steady-state diffusion. This law, sometimes also called Fick's first law (as opposed to Fick's second law; see *Fick's Second Law: Unsteady Diffusion*, p. 42), relates a concentration (C), a spatial coordinate (z), a flux (J_z), and a dimensional proportionality constant ($\mathcal{D}$). To give a precise meaning to Fick's first law of diffusion, these quantities must be clearly defined and their dimensions must be consistent.

Because diffusion in a multicomponent system is discussed in MULTICOMPONENT DIFFUSION, p. 45, the definitions that follow are not merely suitable for a binary mixture but apply equally to a mixture containing n species. The notation adopted here is one that is found in textbooks of transport phenomena (2).

CONCENTRATIONS. Mass concentration is defined as

$$\rho_i = \frac{\text{mass of the } i\text{th species (in g)}}{\text{volume of mixture (in cm}^3)}$$

and molar concentration is defined as

$$C_i = \frac{\text{moles of the } i\text{th species (in g-mol)}}{\text{volume of mixture (in cm}^3)}$$

Thus the density of the mixture is $\rho = \Sigma\rho_i$ (in g/cm^3), the total molar concentration of the mixture is $C = \Sigma C_i$ (in g-mol/cm^3), and the molar fraction is $x_i = C_i/C$.

VELOCITIES. In an n-component system, each species moves at a different velocity. The diffusion velocity of species i with respect to a stationary coordinate system is designated by v_i, which should not be mistaken as the velocity of an individual molecule but should be regarded as the average of the velocities of all the molecules of species i in the mixture. Mass average velocity is defined as

$$\boldsymbol{v} = \frac{\sum_{i=1}^{n} \rho_i \boldsymbol{v}_i}{\sum_{i=1}^{n} \rho_i} = \frac{1}{\rho}\sum_{i=1}^{n} \rho_i \boldsymbol{v}_i \qquad (18)$$

Molar average velocity can be expressed as

$$\boldsymbol{v}^* = \frac{\sum_{i=1}^{n} C_i \boldsymbol{v}_i}{\sum_{i=1}^{n} C_i} = \frac{1}{C}\sum_{i=1}^{n} C_i \boldsymbol{v}_i = \sum_{i=1}^{n} x_i \boldsymbol{v}_i \qquad (19)$$

where mass average velocity ($\boldsymbol{v}$) is the velocity of the center of mass of the system and is the hydrodynamic velocity or velocity of the mass bulk flow. Molar average velocity ($\boldsymbol{v}^*$) is the velocity of the centroid of molar concentration of the system. Thus the quantities $\boldsymbol{v}_i - \boldsymbol{v}$ and $\boldsymbol{v}_i - \boldsymbol{v}^*$ are the diffusion velocities of species i with respect to the center of mass and to the centroid of molar concentration, respectively.

FLUXES. For a pure substance, $\rho\boldsymbol{v}$ (density times velocity) gives the mass flux. In an n-component system, fluxes can be defined in various combinations of concentration and velocity according to the foregoing definitions. For simplicity, the various definitions of fluxes are given in Table 5, which is self-explanatory. For example, the most commonly used flux is $\boldsymbol{J}_i^*$, the molar flux with respect to the centroid of molar concentration. By applying Equation 19 and Table 5, one obtains

$$\begin{aligned} \boldsymbol{J}_i^* &= C_i(\boldsymbol{v}_i - \boldsymbol{v}^*) \\ &= C_i\boldsymbol{v}_i - \frac{C_i}{C}\sum_{j=1}^{n} C_j\boldsymbol{v}_j = \boldsymbol{N}_i - x_i\sum_{j=1}^{n} \boldsymbol{N}_j \end{aligned} \qquad (20)$$

From this it can be seen that the molar diffusion flux $\boldsymbol{J}_i^*$ is the difference between the molar flux with respect to a stationary coordinate system ($\boldsymbol{N}_i$) and the rate of the bodily transport of species i due to the local molar flux of the mixture. Summation of Equation 20 from $i = 1$ to $i = n$ gives

$$\sum_{i=1}^{n} \boldsymbol{J}_i^* = 0 \qquad (21)$$

which shows that the sum of molar diffusion fluxes relative to the molar velocity is zero in any mixture.

In Equation 1 the concentration gradient is given as dC/dz. This is assuming that the concentration gradient is only along the z-axis of a certain coordinate system. Generally the concentration gradients along different axes of a coordinate system are different. To generalize the concept of "gradient," the vector operator ∇, which is independent of, and therefore may be

TABLE 5. *Mass and Molar Fluxes*

	Stationary Coordinates	Center of Mass	Centroid of Molar Concentration
Velocity, cm/s	$\boldsymbol{v}_i$	$\boldsymbol{v}_i - \boldsymbol{v}$	$\boldsymbol{v}_i - \boldsymbol{v}^*$
Mass flux, g·cm^{-2}·s^{-1}	$\boldsymbol{n}_i = \rho_i\boldsymbol{v}_i$	$\boldsymbol{j}_i = \rho_i(\boldsymbol{v}_i - \boldsymbol{v})$	$\boldsymbol{j}_i^* = \rho_i(\boldsymbol{v}_i - \boldsymbol{v}^*)$
Molar flux, mol·cm^{-2}·s^{-1}	$\boldsymbol{N}_i = C_i\boldsymbol{v}_i$	$\boldsymbol{J}_i = C_i(\boldsymbol{v}_i - \boldsymbol{v})$	$\boldsymbol{J}_i^* = C_i(\boldsymbol{v}_i - \boldsymbol{v}^*)$

For definitions of symbols, see Table 1.

represented in, any given coordinate system, is used. Thus in the Cartesian system

$$\nabla C = \frac{\partial C}{\partial x}\mathbf{i} + \frac{\partial C}{\partial y}\mathbf{j} + \frac{\partial C}{\partial z}\mathbf{k} \quad (22)$$

where **i**, **j**, and **k** are the unit vectors in the x, y, and z directions, respectively. In the cylindrical system

$$\nabla C = \frac{\partial C}{\partial r}\mathbf{r} + \frac{1}{r}\frac{\partial C}{\partial \theta}\theta + \frac{\partial C}{\partial z}\mathbf{z} \quad (23)$$

where **r**, θ, and **z** are unit vectors in the r, θ, and z directions, respectively.

For a binary mixture containing species a and b, Fick's first law may be written in terms of all the fluxes in Table 5. Two forms are presented here

$$\begin{aligned} \boldsymbol{J}_a^* &= -\mathcal{D}_{ab}\nabla C_a = -C\mathcal{D}_{ab}\nabla x_a \\ \boldsymbol{J}_b^* &= -\mathcal{D}_{ba}\nabla C_b = -C\mathcal{D}_{ba}\nabla x_b \end{aligned} \quad (24)$$

$$\begin{aligned} \boldsymbol{N}_a &= x_a(\boldsymbol{N}_a + \boldsymbol{N}_b) - C\mathcal{D}_{ab}\nabla x_a \\ \boldsymbol{N}_b &= x_b(\boldsymbol{N}_a + \boldsymbol{N}_b) - C\mathcal{D}_{ba}\nabla x_b \end{aligned} \quad (25)$$

As defined in Table 5, $\boldsymbol{J}_a^*$ and $\boldsymbol{J}_b^*$ are relative to the molar average velocity and $\boldsymbol{N}_a$ and $\boldsymbol{N}_b$ are relative to stationary coordinates. These four fluxes are vectors with a component in the direction of each coordinate axis. The negative signs in Equations 24 and 25 indicate that the fluxes are positive in the direction of decreasing or negative gradients. Equation 24 is the more common form of Fick's first law; Equation 25 shows that the diffusion flux $\boldsymbol{N}_a$ relative to stationary coordinates is the resultant of two vectors, the vector $x_a(\boldsymbol{N}_a + \boldsymbol{N}_b)$, which is the molar flux of a resulting from the bulk motion of the fluid mixture, and the vector $\boldsymbol{J}_a^* = -C\mathcal{D}_{ab}\nabla x_a$, which is the molar flux of a resulting from the diffusion superimposed on the bulk flow.

From Equation 21, it is clear that

$$\boldsymbol{J}_a^* = -\boldsymbol{J}_b^* \quad (26)$$

From Equations 24–26 it is also clear that $\boldsymbol{N}_a \neq -\boldsymbol{N}_b$. By using the relation $x_a + x_b = 1$ and applying Equation 26 to Equation 24, one can easily show that

$$\mathcal{D}_{ab} = \mathcal{D}_{ba} \quad (27)$$

Thus diffusion in a binary mixture is characterized by a single diffusion coefficient.

Binary Diffusion Coefficients

Diffusion coefficients of binary mixtures of dilute gases have been comprehensively compiled, critically evaluated, and correlated by new semiempirical expressions (29). They are strongly dependent on the molecular weights of the individual gases and are generally independent of the composition of the mixture. They increase with increasing temperature and vary inversely with pressure. Table 6 gives the experimentally obtained diffusion coefficients at 1 atm of some common gas pairs.

TABLE 6. *Experimental Values of Binary Diffusion Coefficients*

Gas Pair	cm^2/s*	T, °C	Gas Pair	cm^2/s*	T, °C
Air-Ar	0.192	22	CO_2-O_2	0.153	20
Air-CO_2	0.139	0	CO_2-H_2O	0.198	34
Air-He	0.708	20	He-Kr	0.616	18
Air-Kr	0.134	0	He-Ne	1.01	20
Air-O_2	0.178	0	He-N_2	0.687	25
Air-H_2O	0.260	25	He-O_2	0.703	20
Ar-Ar	0.178	2	He-SF_6	0.4	20
Ar-CO_2	0.133	3	He-H_2O	0.902	34
Ar-He	0.729	25	He-Xe	0.518	20
Ar-Kr	0.128	15	Kr-Kr	0.101	35
Ar-Ne	0.309	20	Kr-Ne	0.233	0
Ar-N_2	0.189	20	Kr-N_2	0.159	35
Ar-SF_6	0.05	20	Kr-Xe	0.0725	18
Ar-Xe	0.107	18	Ne-Ne	0.484	20
CO-CO	0.323	100	Ne-N_2	0.315	20
CO-N_2	0.207	27	Ne-Xe	0.208	18
CO-O_2	0.211	27	N_2-N_2	0.188	0
CO_2-CO_2	0.125	40	N_2-O_2	0.208	27
CO_2-He	0.605	20	N_2-SF_6	0.1	20
CO_2-Kr	0.109	20	N_2-H_2O	0.256	34
CO_2-Ne	0.267	22	N_2O-O_2	0.096	0
CO_2-N_2	0.167	25	O_2-O_2	0.232	25
CO_2-N_2O	0.128	40	O_2-H_2O	0.282	35

* Pressure, 1 atm.

Binary diffusion coefficients of nonpolar gases may be predicted within ~5% with the formula derived from the Chapman-Enskog theory

$$\mathcal{D}_{ab} = 0.001858 \frac{T^{3/2}}{P\sigma_{ab}^2\Omega_{\mathcal{D},ab}}\left(\frac{1}{M_a} + \frac{1}{M_b}\right)^{1/2} \quad (28)$$

where T is ambient temperature in degrees Kelvin; P is ambient pressure in atm; M_a and M_b are molecular weights of gases a and b, respectively; σ_{ab} is the Lennard-Jones force constant for the binary mixture in Å (10^{-8} cm); and $\Omega_{\mathcal{D},ab}$ is the dimensionless collision integral. The Lennard-Jones potential for a binary gas mixture may be approximated by

$$\phi_{ab}(r) = 4\epsilon_{ab}\left[\left(\frac{\sigma_{ab}}{r}\right)^{12} - \left(\frac{\sigma_{ab}}{r}\right)^{6}\right] \quad (29)$$

where ϵ_{ab} and σ_{ab} are molecular force constants, as defined in the previous section. Usually for nonpolar, nonreacting molecule pairs, the force constants in Equation 29 may be estimated satisfactorily by combining the Lennard-Jones parameters of gas species a and b, namely

$$\sigma_{ab} = (\sigma_a + \sigma_b)/2 \quad (30)$$

$$\epsilon_{ab} = \sqrt{\epsilon_a\epsilon_b} \quad (31)$$

Values of σ and ϵ for some gases can be found in Table 3; values of $\Omega_{\mathcal{D},ab}$ as a function of kT/ϵ are given in Table 4. As an example of the use of the Chapman-

Enskog formula, the diffusion coefficient of the Ar-O_2 pair at 37°C and 1 atm is computed with $M_{Ar} = 39.9$ and $M_{O_2} = 32.0$. From Table 3

$$\sigma_{Ar} = 3.542\ \text{Å} \qquad \sigma_{O_2} = 3.468\ \text{Å}$$

$$\frac{\epsilon_{Ar}}{k} = 93°\text{K} \qquad \frac{\epsilon_{O_2}}{k} = 107°\text{K}$$

From Equation 30

$$\sigma_{Ar\text{-}O_2} = ½(3.542 + 3.467) = 3.505$$

From Equation 31

$$\frac{\epsilon_{Ar\text{-}O_2}}{k} = (93 \times 107)^{½} = 99.8$$

From Table 4, with T = 310°K

$$\frac{kT}{\epsilon_{Ar\text{-}O_2}} = \frac{310}{99.8} = 3.11$$

$$\Omega_{\mathcal{D},Ar\text{-}O_2}\ (3.11) = 0.9406$$

From Equation 28

$$\mathcal{D}_{Ar\text{-}O_2} = \frac{(1.858 \times 10^{-3})(310)^{1.5}(1/39.9 + 1/32.0)^{0.5}}{(1)(3.505)^2(0.9406)}$$
$$= 0.2083\ \text{cm}^2/\text{s}$$

Based on the Chapman-Enskog theory the mutual diffusion coefficients of 11 gases at 37°C and 1 atm have been calculated and are tabulated in a symmetric matrix form in Table 7.

There are many improved versions or variations of the formula given in Equation 28. Reid et al. (36) and Marrero and Mason (29) have discussed these in detail.

Fick's Second Law: Unsteady Diffusion

When unsteady or transient diffusion occurs, time must be featured as a variable in the governing equation. Thus Fick's first law, which contains no time variable, cannot be used alone; it must be combined with the principle of conservation of mass to form the unsteady diffusion equation.

To derive such an equation, consider a segment of length dz of a trumpet-shaped container whose cross-sectional area at axial position z is $A(z)$ (Fig. 3). The principle of conservation of mass can be stated as

Rate of accumulation of given substance in infinitesimal segment considered

= Rate at which this substance is brought into segment

− Rate at which this substance is removed from segment

+ Rate at which this substance is produced in segment by chemical or biological reactions

Assuming a linear variation of cross-sectional area in the infinitesimal segment between z and $z + dz$, and designating the molar concentration of the substance considered in the infinitesimal volume by C, one can write the statement before the equal sign of the above equation as

$$\frac{\partial}{\partial t}\left\{[A + (A + dA)]\,\frac{dz}{2}\,\text{C}\right\} = \frac{\partial \text{C}}{\partial t}\,Adz + \frac{\partial \text{C}}{\partial t}\cdot\frac{dAdz}{2} \approx \frac{\partial \text{C}}{\partial t}\,Adz \tag{32}$$

where the partial derivative $\partial/\partial t$ is used because C varies both with time t and with axial position z. If it is assumed that diffusion occurs only in the z direction and that no chemical reactions occur in the container, one can write the part of the equation after the equal sign for the above conservation principle as

$$AN_z - (A + dA)(N_z + dN_z) = -N_z dA - AdN_z - dAdN_z \approx -N_z dA - AdN_z \tag{33}$$

where N_z is the molar flux in the z direction relative to the stationary coordinate axis z. Combining Equations 32 and 33 yields

TABLE 7. *Binary Diffusion Coefficients Computed From Chapman-Enskog Theory*

	He	H_2O	Ne	CO	N_2	Air	O_2	Ar	CO_2	N_2O	SF_6
He	1.7790										
H_2O	0.9059	0.2039									
Ne	1.1301	0.4038	0.5349								
CO	0.7506	0.2261	0.3394	0.2163							
N_2	0.7407	0.2315	0.3363	0.2164	0.2162						
Air	0.7538	0.2313	0.3399	0.2172	0.2171	0.2180					
O_2	0.7907	0.2285	0.3491	0.2184	0.2187	0.2195	0.2204				
Ar	0.7715	0.2219	0.3319	0.2073	0.2073	0.2079	0.2083	0.1957			
CO_2	0.6345	0.1602	0.2678	0.1647	0.1663	0.1660	0.1640	0.1545	0.1191		
N_2O	0.6467	0.1584	0.2713	0.1650	0.1669	0.1665	0.1641	0.1548	0.1183	0.1173	
SF_6	0.4349	0.0992	0.1686	0.1031	0.1047	0.1037	0.1001	0.0921	0.0707	0.0698	0.0366

Diffusion coefficients in cm^2/s. Conditions: pressure, 1 atm; temperature, 37°C.

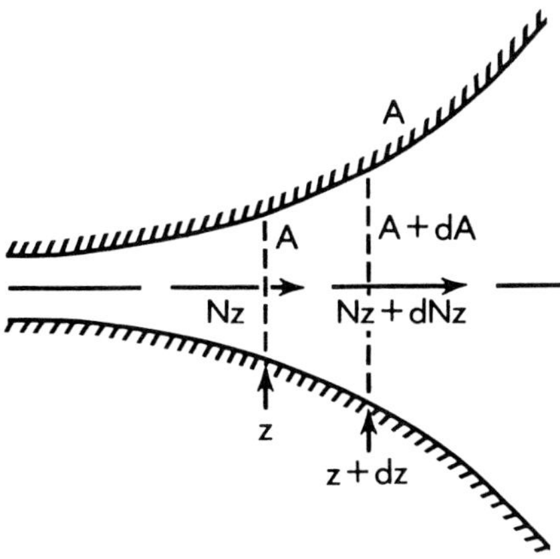

FIG. 3. Axisymmetric container segment of length dz with variable cross-sectional area (A). Diffusion takes place in this container. N, molar flux with respect to stationary frame of reference.

$$\frac{\partial C}{\partial t} Adz = -N_z dA - AdN_z \tag{34}$$

which is a general statement of unsteady-state one-dimensional mass transfer.

If there is no bulk flow through the container, from Equations 24 and 25, $J_z^* = N_z = -\mathcal{D}(\partial C/\partial z)$. Therefore Equation 34 becomes

$$\frac{\partial C}{\partial t} Adz = -\left(-\mathcal{D}\frac{\partial C}{\partial z}\right) dA - Ad\left(-\mathcal{D}\frac{\partial C}{\partial z}\right) \tag{35}$$

Recalling that $\mathcal{D}$ is a constant and dividing Equation 35 by Adz results in

$$\frac{\partial C}{\partial t} = \mathcal{D}\frac{\partial^2 C}{\partial z^2} + \frac{\mathcal{D}}{A}\frac{dA}{dz}\frac{\partial C}{\partial z} \tag{36}$$

which is the equation of the one-dimensional diffusion process in an axisymmetric container. In the limiting case in which the container becomes a cylinder, namely when $dA/dz = 0$, this equation becomes

$$\frac{\partial C}{\partial t} = \mathcal{D}\frac{\partial^2 C}{\partial z^2} \tag{37}$$

Equation 37 is the simplest form of diffusion equation and is also called Fick's second law of diffusion.

When diffusion occurs in all directions of a coordinate system, a three-dimensional equation may be derived by applying Fick's first law (Eq. 25) to a general statement of conservation of mass that may be derived in a manner similar to the derivation of Equation 34. Commonly referred to as the continuity equation, the general statement of conservation of mass can be expressed as

$$\frac{\partial C}{\partial t} + (\nabla \cdot \boldsymbol{N}) = 0 \tag{38}$$

where $\nabla \cdot$ is a vector operator termed *divergence*. In Cartesian coordinates, Equation 38 takes the form

$$\frac{\partial C}{\partial t} + \frac{\partial N_x}{\partial x} + \frac{\partial N_y}{\partial y} + \frac{\partial N_z}{\partial z} = 0 \tag{39}$$

and in cylindrical coordinates

$$\frac{\partial C}{\partial t} + \frac{1}{r}\frac{\partial}{\partial r}(rN_r) + \frac{1}{r}\frac{\partial N_\theta}{\partial \theta} + \frac{\partial N_z}{\partial z} = 0 \tag{40}$$

where r is the radial axis and θ is the azimuthal coordinate.

Applying Equation 25 to Equation 40 results in a three-dimensional diffusion equation in the cylindrical coordinates

$$\frac{\partial C}{\partial t} = \mathcal{D}\left[\frac{1}{r}\frac{\partial}{\partial r}\left(r\frac{\partial C}{\partial r}\right) + \frac{1}{r^2}\frac{\partial^2 C}{\partial \theta^2} + \frac{\partial^2 C}{\partial z^2}\right] \tag{41}$$

Equations 36, 37, and 41 are second-order parabolic-type partial differential equations. They must be solved in conjunction with an initial condition and two boundary conditions to yield the concentration throughout the container at any time (10).

Solution of Binary Diffusion Equation

Because the diffusion equation is one of the most frequently encountered partial differential equations, it has been studied extensively and solutions for various initial and boundary conditions already exist (3, 11). Four different methods of solution of the diffusion equation are outlined next.

ANALYTIC METHOD. This is the classical method. The one-dimensional diffusion equation (Eq. 37) may be solved either by separation of variables or by the Laplace transform method (3). The solutions vary, depending on the initial and boundary conditions, but they are generally in the form of convergent infinite series. Because the diffusion equation is linear, many composite solutions can be obtained by applying the superposition principle to known solutions.

As an illustration, consider diffusion in a long cylinder. Initially, half of the cylinder is filled with one substance, the other half with a second substance. At time $t = 0$, a partition in the middle of the cylinder is removed and diffusion begins. The concentration distribution of the first substance along the cylinder at all times $t > 0$ can be obtained. Letting the position of the partition be $z = 0$ and the concentration of the first substance be C results in

Initial condition	$z < 0$	$C = C_0$	(42)
$(t < 0)$	$z > 0$	$C = 0$	
Boundary conditions	$z = -\infty$	$C = C_0$	(43)
	$z = +\infty$	$C = 0$	

The solution to this problem is

$$C(z, t) = \tfrac{1}{2}C_0\left[1 - \text{erf}\left(\frac{z}{\sqrt{4t}}\right)\right] \tag{44}$$

where erf (η) is the error function, namely

$$\mathrm{erf}(\eta) = \frac{2}{\sqrt{\pi}} \int_0^{\xi} e^{-\xi^2} d\xi \qquad (45)$$

This solution gives a step concentration distribution at $z = 0$ initially, but as time goes on the step becomes more and more rounded and the concentration profile along the cylinder eventually flattens.

In modeling diffusion in the alveolar region of the lung, Rauwerda (35) and Cumming et al. (12) have used the analytic method to solve the one-dimensional diffusion equation.

FINITE-DIFFERENCE METHOD. Although useful, the analytic method of solution is restricted to simple geometries and constant diffusion coefficients throughout the domain of diffusion. For complicated geometries and boundary conditions, numerical methods are preferred and, in most cases, necessary.

A well-established numerical method for the solution of differential equations is the finite-difference method. In this method, space and time of diffusion are divided into small intervals and the derivatives are approximated by finite differences, the differences between the values of the differentiated functions at the end and at the start of the intervals. That is, a differential equation is transformed into an algebraic difference equation that can be solved numerically. The finite-difference solution of the diffusion equation is usually carried out by "marching" in time. From the known initial ($t = 0$) concentration values at all the grid points in the space domain, the values at the next time step ($t = t_1$) can be obtained. This process can be continued for $t = t_2$, $t = t_3$, etc. The amount of computational work and the accuracy of the finite-difference solution depend on the finite-difference scheme used and on the sizes of the increments chosen.

A scheme that is widely used for the diffusion equation was proposed by Crank and Nicolson (11). They replaced $\partial^2 C/\partial z^2$ by the mean of its finite-difference representation at the jth and $(j + 1)$th time steps and approximated Equation 40 by

$$\frac{C_{i,j+1} - C_{i,j}}{\Delta t} = \frac{\mathcal{D}}{2}\left[\frac{C_{i+1,j} - 2C_{i,j} + C_{i-1,j}}{(\Delta z)^2} + \frac{C_{i+1,j+1} - 2C_{i,j+1} + C_{i-1,j+1}}{(\Delta z)^2}\right] \qquad (46)$$

where the subscripts $i - 1$, i, and $i + 1$ refer to grid points in the space domain; j and $j + 1$ refer to the instants in time; Δz is the spatial increment; and Δt is the time increment. Equation 46 gives a set of n simultaneous algebraic equations with n unknowns. Thus the solution of this set of simultaneous equations is called for at each time step.

The infinite-difference method is introduced in most books on numerical methods (37); its application to the diffusion equation has been discussed by Crank (11) and Saul'yev (38). In relation to diffusion in the lung, the finite-difference method has been used by La Force and Lewis (28) in their model of diffusional transport in the human lung.

FINITE-ELEMENT METHOD. The finite-element method is a relatively new numerical scheme capable of handling certain types of differential equations over an irregularly shaped region. The region of interest is divided into many smaller regions, termed *finite elements*, and solutions are sought in each of these elements. If the finite elements are small enough, the finite-element solution can be a good approximation of the real solution of the original equation. Several approximation methods of solution are available. Zienkiewicz (54) has discussed application of the finite-element method to transient problems such as diffusion.

Advanced mathematics is required to explain the principle of this method. The general procedure, however, may be simply stated. Solution of the differential equation is achieved by a minimization scheme in which the approximate concentration values in all the finite elements are identified. In other words, concentration values that minimize a certain functional over the elements give a solution to the original differential equation. In terms of computation, the major task is to solve repeatedly a large set of algebraic equations.

In their modeling of diffusion in an alveolar sac, Chang et al. (5) solved a two-dimensional diffusion equation with the finite-element method.

RANDOM-WALK METHOD. The random-walk method has been developed since the advent of high-speed digital computers and has been found as adequate as, and sometimes superior to, the classical method for handling the diffusion problem (22, 40). It can be applied readily to systems of complicated shapes—all that is necessary is that the shape of the boundary be describable in some way. In brief, the random-walk method (using the concept introduced in MOLECULAR BEHAVIOR: KINETIC THEORY OF GASES, p. 35) ascribes a probability to the motion of each particle of the diffusate in any direction. The direction of motion at any time is independent of the previous direction. The space in which diffusion occurs is represented by a set of points, each of which is tagged by an integer X for reference. If the physical medium is continuous it must be divided into regions, each of which is associated with one of the points X. As shown in Figure 4, for each point or region X there is a set of contiguous points or regions X_1, X_2, etc., to which diffusion may occur directly from X. From any X, then, there are paths that can be tagged by integer I. Thus $I = 1$ is a path from X to X_1, $I = 2$ to X_2, etc. The diffusate is represented by particles that move from point to point in the diffusion space, always stepping from a point X to a point contiguous to X. Each particle represents a

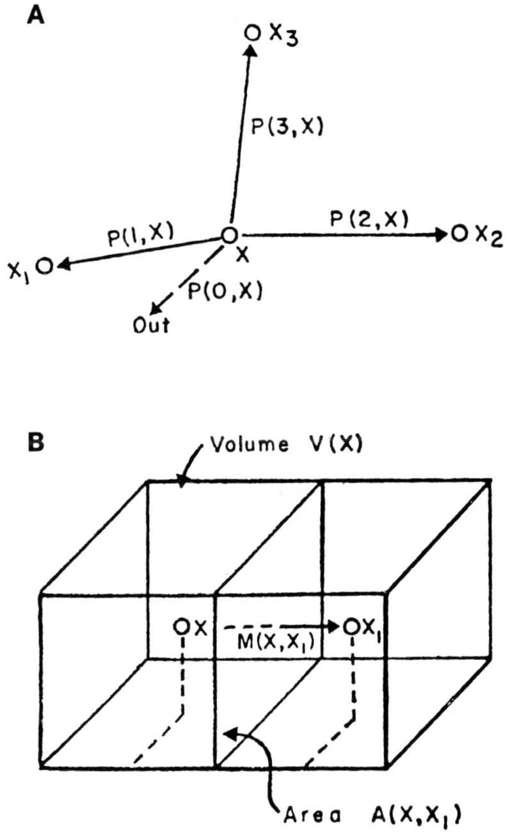

FIG. 4. Diagrams illustrating principle of random-walk method. *A*: from *point X* the "particle" in a random walk may take a step to neighboring *point* X_1, X_2, or X_3 with probabilities $P(1, X)$, $P(2, X)$, and $P(3, X)$, respectively. It may also terminate its walk with probability $P(0, X)$. *B: points* X and X_1 are surrounded by volumes $V(X)$ and $V(X_1)$ and area of contact $A(X, X_1)$ can be assigned. Particles that move through area $A(X, X_1)$ in a unit of time are named $M(X, X_1)$. [From Stibitz (42).]

finite quantity of diffusate. During its walk, each particle must keep track of a "clock time" (t) so that the time at which the particle arrives at any point X will be known. The random walk is defined by distribution functions $P(I, X, t)$, which are the probabilities that the next step from X will be I, to X_1, and by the dwell time $T(X, t)$ after which the next step will be taken.

In general, from each point X there is a possible step to a point outside the system. This fact may be stated pictorially by saying that the exterior point is contiguous to every point X in the system, and that for every point X there may be a step $I = 0$, with a probability that the walk of a particle at X will be terminated.

From these basic postulates for the model, it is intuitively evident that, in an appropriately defined system, there will at any instant t be an expected number $B(X)$ of particles at any point. Because each particle contains a quantity (Q_0) of diffusate, the expected quantity of diffusate in region X is $Q_0B(X, t)$. If one wishes to associate a volume of space, say $V(X)$, with each region or point X, then at any instant the expected concentration of diffusate at X is

$$C(X, t) = Q_0B(X, t)/V(X) \tag{47}$$

Furthermore, during any period of time, e.g., t_1 to $t_1 + \Delta t$, for any path between contiguous points, e.g., X and X_1, there is an expected number, $M(X, X_1, t)$, of particles that step from X to X_1. These particles represent a quantity $Q_0M(X, X_1, t)$ of diffusate. In the same unit period, an expected number of particles, $M(X_1, X, t)$, move from X_1 to X, and convey a quantity $Q_0M(X_1, X, t)$ from X_1 to X. The net flux of diffusate from X to X_1 then is

$$J(X, X_1, t) = Q_0[M(X, X_1, t) - M(X_1, X, t)] \tag{48}$$

A concise introduction to the random-walk method is given by Stibitz (42), who used it to consider the problem of gaseous diffusion in the lung (42, 43). The model and the solution method of Stibitz (42) and of several authors mentioned previously (12, 28, 35) have been critically reviewed by Chang and Farhi (6).

MULTICOMPONENT DIFFUSION

Exceptions to Fick's law of diffusion have been discovered frequently and continually since its formulation. The most important exceptions have to do with multicomponent systems in which more than two species are involved in the diffusion process. Under such circumstances the diffusion coefficient defined in Fick's law is often not constant but is dependent on the composition of the mixture.

As an illustration of the multicomponent effect, Figure 5 shows two connected tubes as used by Arnold and Toor (1)—one containing 50% CH_4 and 50% Ar, the other containing 50% H_2 and 50% Ar. As the partition between the two tubes is removed, although initially there is no gradient of the Ar concentration, a transient diffusion flux of Ar from the CH_4 side toward the H_2 side can be observed. This is because H_2 diffuses faster than CH_4, and, as H_2 molecules accumulate on the CH_4 side, a pressure gradient is created, causing all species on the CH_4 side, including Ar, to move to the H_2 side.

A transient pressure gradient is an inherent feature of a closed system such as the apparatus shown in Figure 5, whether the mixture is multicomponent or binary. In a binary mixture, however, the pressure gradient simply enhances the motion of the slower component and suppresses the motion of the faster component, making the net flux with respect to stationary coordinates equal. When a multicomponent mixture is contained in a closed system, the equimolar condition states

$$\sum_{i=1}^{n} \boldsymbol{N}_i = 0 \quad (49)$$

Because there are n components involved, the flux of each species becomes a function of the fluxes of the other species.

In an attempt to explore the implications of multicomponent diffusion in the lung, Chang et al. (8) made a model study of ternary equimolar diffusion. Among the cases they studied was one in which a fictitious gas film separates two gas mixtures of equal total pressure (at 710 mmHg). On one side of the film, partial pressures of O_2 (P_{O_2}), CO_2 (P_{CO_2}), and the inert gas (N_2, He, or SF_6) are 40, 46, and 624 mmHg, respectively. On the other side, P_{O_2} is 104, P_{CO_2} is allowed to vary, and the inert-gas partial pressure also varies so that the total pressure remains 710 mmHg. The resulting CO_2 fluxes as a function of P_{CO_2} difference are plotted in Figure 6. If a gas mixture obeys Fick's law, the flux should pass through the origin and the slope of the flux line will be proportional to the binary diffusion coefficient. Normal air behaves essentially like a binary mixture. The SF_6 mixture deviates from binary behavior only slightly, but the He mixture behaves very differently. In this case the flux line and the coordinate axes form a right triangle in the third quadrant. At the top of the triangle, there is a zero partial pressure gradient but a large positive flux. At the intersection of the flux line and the abscissa, the flux is zero despite a nonzero partial pressure gradient. All along the hypotenuse, the fluxes are positive when the partial pressure gradients are negative. In other

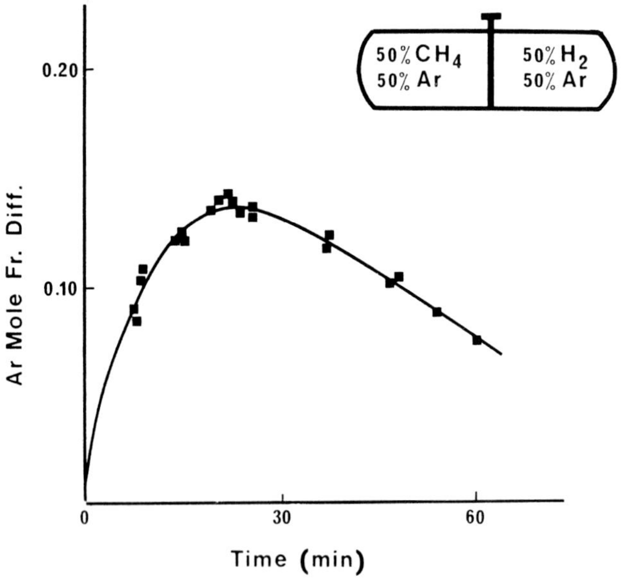

FIG. 5. Diffusion of Ar in an H_2-CH_4-Ar system. Although there is initially no gradient in Ar concentration, Ar will move transiently from CH_4 side toward H_2 side. Mole Fr. Diff., molar fractional difference. [Data from Arnold and Toor (1).]

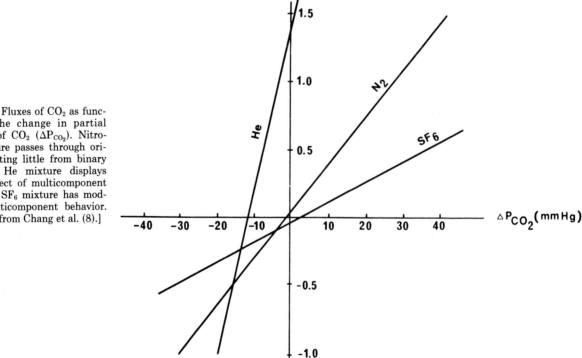

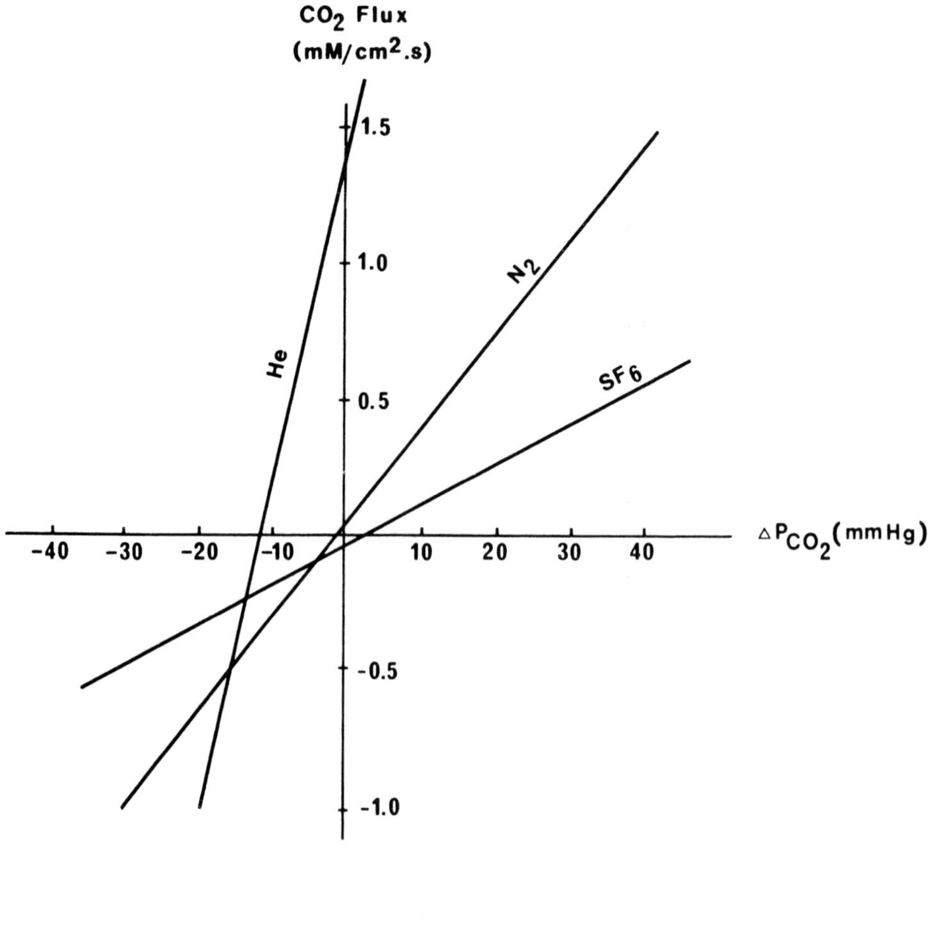

FIG. 6. Fluxes of CO_2 as function of the change in partial pressure of CO_2 (ΔP_{CO_2}). Nitrogen mixture passes through origin, deviating little from binary behavior; He mixture displays strong effect of multicomponent diffusion; SF_6 mixture has moderate multicomponent behavior. [Adapted from Chang et al. (8).]

words, CO_2 will diffuse against its own concentration gradient.

Although this model study is highly idealized, it points out the possible effects of multicomponent diffusion in the alveolar spaces (4) and other biological systems (16). Physiologists who deal with multicomponent gas mixtures therefore should be well aware of these possible effects.

The transport phenomenon of multicomponent diffusion is quite complex and often defies intuition; theoretically, it is much less well understood than is binary diffusion. Nevertheless the total knowledge about multicomponent diffusion has permitted a fair understanding of this phenomenon and provided some practical means to predict the pertinent quantities in a multicomponent system. By necessity, the treatment of this subject in this chapter is brief and is confined to ideal gas mixtures. For more thorough and systematic discussions of this topic, consult the recent reviews by Cussler (14) and Krishna and Standart (27).

Multicomponent Diffusion Equations

The equations of multicomponent diffusion can be derived either from nonequilibrium thermodynamics or from the Chapman-Enskog solution of the Boltzmann equations. For an ideal gas mixture of constant temperature and pressure, the steady-state flux equations, known as Stefan-Maxwell equations, have the form

$$\frac{\mathrm{P}}{R\mathrm{T}} \nabla x_i = \sum_{\substack{j=1 \\ j \neq i}}^{n} \frac{1}{\mathcal{D}_{ij}} (x_i \boldsymbol{N}_j - x_j \boldsymbol{N}_i) \qquad (50)$$

where P is the pressure of the mixture in atm, T is the temperature in degrees Kelvin, R is the ideal gas constant in $cm^3 \cdot atm \cdot 1°K^{-1} \cdot g\text{-}mol^{-1}$, $\boldsymbol{N}_j$ and $\boldsymbol{N}_i$ are molar fluxes in $g\text{-}mol \cdot cm^{-2} \cdot s^{-1}$ with respect to a stationary frame of reference, and $\mathcal{D}_{ij}$ is the binary diffusion coefficient of the i-j gas pair in cm^2/s. Stefan-Maxwell equations make it evident that the fluxes in a multicomponent mixture are the resultant of coupled actions of the binary gas pairs. Because total pressure is constant and $\sum x_i = 1$, there are only $n - 1$ independent equations in Equation 50.

If all the diffusion fluxes and other parameters involved are known, the concentration profiles may be obtained by integrating the $n - 1$ equations given in Equation 50. However, in most physical problems, all or at least some of the diffusion fluxes are not known. Therefore the Stefan-Maxwell equations cannot be solved easily.

An alternative form of the multicomponent flux equations has been derived by Onsager (33) from the laws of thermodynamics. These equations have the appearance of a generalized Fick's law

$$\boldsymbol{J}_i^* = -\frac{\mathrm{P}}{R\mathrm{T}} \sum_{j=1}^{n-1} D_{ij} \nabla x_j \qquad (51)$$

where $\boldsymbol{J}_i^*$ is the molar flux of the ith species with respect to the molar average velocity as already defined, and D_{ij} is the multicomponent diffusion coefficient, which is nonconstant but dependent on the composition of the mixture. It is clear from Equation 51 that the flux of any component depends on the concentration gradients of all the components in the mixture. Because the net sum of all fluxes $\boldsymbol{J}_i^*$ as well as concentration gradients ∇x_i must be zero, i.e., $\sum \boldsymbol{J}_i^* = 0$ and $\sum \nabla x_i = 0$, there are only $n - 1$ independent equations in Equation 51.

Equations 50 and 51 have been shown to be equivalent (13); each has a major disadvantage. The fluxes in the Stefan-Maxwell equations are implicitly expressed, whereas the Onsager equations require nonconstant concentration-dependent diffusion coefficients, which are difficult to measure. To solve a general multicomponent mass-transfer problem, it is more convenient to apply Equation 51 to the continuity equation. For an n-component mixture without chemical reactions the continuity equation is exactly analogous in form to Equation 38, i.e.

$$\frac{\partial \mathrm{C}_i}{\partial t} + \nabla \cdot \boldsymbol{N}_i = 0 \qquad i = 1, 2, \ldots, n - 1 \qquad (52)$$

where $\boldsymbol{N}_i = \boldsymbol{J}_i^* + \mathrm{C}_i \boldsymbol{v}^*$ (as defined in BINARY DIFFUSION, p. 39).

Combination of Equations 51 and 52 results in $n - 1$ independent equations and n unknowns. Thus an equation representing an additional physical constraint must be found. Generally three types of physical constraints have been used. The first is the consideration of a certain component (e.g., the ith component) in the mixture as stagnant, i.e., having zero rate of diffusion or $\boldsymbol{N}_i = 0$. The second is the assumption of equimolar diffusion, with Equation 49 as the needed nth equation; this means that diffusion is confined to a closed system. The third type of physical constraint specifies a certain nonzero relationship among the fluxes. For diffusion in free space

$$\sum_{i=1}^{n} \boldsymbol{N}_i M_i - 0 \qquad (53)$$

is often used, where M_i is the molecular weight of the ith component. Equation 53 implies that there is a net movement of the centroid of molar concentration of the multicomponent mixture.

The multicomponent diffusion equations are nonlinear. Toor (48, 49) and Stewart and Prober (41) independently developed a matrix method to obtain the approximate solution of the linearized equations in the equimolar diffusion case. Tai and Chang (45) extended this method to the nonequimolar case. Both the equimolar and nonequimolar solutions have been satisfactorily verified by experiment (46, 49). Using a more general matrix method, Krishna and Standart (26) developed an exact solution to the Stefan-Maxwell equations. In many cases the deviations between the fluxes estimated by the linear method and those calculated by the exact method are small (47).

Multicomponent Diffusion Coefficients

The multicomponent diffusion coefficients in Equation 51 may be determined experimentally when they are concentration independent. If they are concentration dependent, only approximate descriptions are possible (21). For mixtures of dilute gases, however, the multicomponent diffusion coefficients can be predicted from the kinetic theory, although with more difficulty than in the case of binary diffusion coefficients. Despite the complex interactions among molecules of the different species, the phenomenon of multicomponent diffusion is a result of molecular motion and binary molecular collisions. For a ternary system, Toor et al. (50) gave the $(n-1)^2 = 4$ elements of the ternary diffusion coefficient matrix as

$$D_{ii} = \mathcal{D}_{13}[(1 - x_i)\mathcal{D}_{ij} + x_i\mathcal{D}_{i3}]/S \qquad i = 1, 2;\ j = 1, 2;\ i \neq j$$

$$D_{ij} = x_i\mathcal{D}_{j3}(\mathcal{D}_{i3} - \mathcal{D}_{ij})/S \qquad i = 1, 2;\ j = 1, 2;\ i \neq j \tag{54}$$

$$S = x_1\mathcal{D}_{23} + x_2\mathcal{D}_{13} + x_3\mathcal{D}_{12}$$

The diagonal terms D_{11} and D_{22} are always positive and the off-diagonal terms D_{12} and D_{21} may be positive or negative. The off-diagonal terms may be greater or smaller than the diagonal terms. The larger the values of the off-diagonal terms, the more coupling interaction there is in the ternary system. Specifically, if D_{12}/D_{11} is much larger than unity the system has a large ternary diffusion effect. This is true when D_{12}/D_{23} is small (e.g., in the He-O_2-CO_2 mixture). Conversely, when all binary diffusion coefficients are equal or nearly equal (e.g., in the Ar-O_2-CO_2 mixture), the off-diagonal terms D_{12} and D_{21} are very small and the ternary system behaves essentially like a binary system.

A more general and straightforward predictive formula has been derived by Obermeier and Schaber (32) from elementary mean free path theory

$$D_{ik} = \frac{x_i}{(x_k/\mathcal{D}_{ik})(\mathcal{D}_{ii}/\mathcal{D}_{kk})^{1/2} + \sum(x_j/\mathcal{D}_{kj})} + \frac{(\bar{M} - M_i x_i)/M_k}{(x_i/\mathcal{D}_{ik})(\mathcal{D}_{kk}/\mathcal{D}_{ii})^{1/2} + \sum_{j\neq 1}(x_j/\mathcal{D}_{ij})} \tag{55}$$

where $\bar{M}$ is the molecular weight of the gas mixture, M_i is the molecular weight of the ith component, and $\mathcal{D}_{ii}$ and $\mathcal{D}_{ik}$ are self-diffusion and binary diffusion coefficients, respectively. This formula is satisfactory for mixtures with components of extremely different molecular weights; however, the greatest accuracy of this formula is achieved if either the molecular weights of the components do not differ strongly or if the number of components of the mixture is large.

Effective Diffusion Coefficients

As the solution of the Stefan-Maxwell equations is rather difficult, it is often advantageous to take an alternative approach, finding the effective diffusion coefficients and applying the binary form of Fick's law to obtain the diffusion fluxes. The effective diffusion coefficient is usually a function of the binary diffusion coefficients and local or boundary concentrations. With this coefficient, the flux of a certain species can be related to its own concentration gradient

$$\boldsymbol{J}_i^* = -CD'_{im}\nabla x_i \tag{56}$$

where D'_{im} denotes the effective diffusion coefficient of the ith species.

Many forms of effective diffusion coefficients have been proposed and used (14). Perhaps the simplest formula has been proposed by Wilke (51), who considered the effective diffusion coefficient of a single gas (species 1) with respect to a multicomponent mixture of stagnant gases. He obtained

$$D'_1 = \frac{1 - x_1}{x_2/\mathcal{D}_{12} + x_3/\mathcal{D}_{13} + \ldots + x_n/\mathcal{D}_{1n}} \tag{57}$$

where $x_1, x_i, \ldots, x_n$ are the molar fractions. Fairbanks and Wilke (17) tested Equation 57 experimentally and found it very satisfactory.

A more general expression has been given by Bird et al. (2), who defined D_{im} of species i in a multicomponent mixture in an analogous manner to the binary-relation Equation 25

$$\boldsymbol{N}_i = -CD'_{im}\nabla x_i + x_i \sum_{j=1}^{n} \boldsymbol{N}_j \tag{58}$$

By solving Equation 58 for ∇x_i and equating the result to x_i in the Stefan-Maxwell equations, one obtains

$$D'_{im} = \frac{\boldsymbol{N}_i - \sum_{j=1}^{n} \boldsymbol{N}_j}{\sum_{\substack{j=1\\ j\neq 1}}^{n} (1/\mathcal{D}_{ij})(x_j\boldsymbol{N}_i - x_i\boldsymbol{N}_j)} \tag{59}$$

Because x_i varies with position along the diffusion path, D'_{im} also varies. Usually the average values of x_i and x_j over the diffusion path are used with estimated fluxes to evaluate D'_{im}. For significant position dependence, linear variation of D'_{im} may be assumed, as Hsu and Bird (24) suggested.

The effective diffusion coefficients are a simple way to handle a complex problem and are preferred by

TABLE 8. *Effective Diffusion Coefficients for O_2 and CO_2 in Diffusion Between Inspired Gas and Alveolar Gas*

Mixture	Diffusing Gas	Measured at 742 mmHg, 37°C, cm^2/s*	Computed for 742 mmHg, 37°C, cm^2/s†	Computed for 713 mmHg, 37°C, cm^2/s‡
O_2-H_2 vs.	O_2	0.549	0.773	
O_2-CO_2-H_2	CO_2	0.415	0.439	
O_2-He vs.	O_2		0.620	0.530
O_2-CO_2-He	CO_2		0.440	0.438
O_2-N_2 vs.	O_2	0.240	0.251	0.240
O_2-CO_2-N_2	CO_2	0.173	0.179	0.177
O_2-SF_6 vs.	O_2	0.107	0.101	0.143
O_2-CO_2-SF_6	CO_2	0.090	0.084	0.096

Inspired gas: 21% O_2 + 79% y; alveolar gas: 14% O_2 + 6% CO_2 + 80% y; y = H_2, He, N_2, SF_6. * From Worth and Piiper (53). † From Wilke (51). ‡ From Chang and Farhi (7).

many biologist-investigators who have studied multicomponent diffusion (4, 16, 34, 52, 53). For ternary gas mixtures similar to the inspired gas and the alveolar gas, Worth and Piiper (53) have made in vitro measurements, whereas Chang and Farhi (7) have computed the effective diffusion coefficients based on the nonequimolar theory (45). The two sets of values are compared with the values computed with Equation 57 and are given in Table 8. The agreement among the three sets of values is good. When diffusion fluxes of O_2 and CO_2 in the alveolar space are computed from Fick's first law, the values in Table 8 should be used as the diffusion coefficients.

SUMMARY

The process of diffusion is fundamental to the maintenance of life in all organisms. In respiratory physiology, diffusion in the gas phase plays an important role in the delivery of O_2 to, and removal of CO_2 from, the sites of gas exchange. This is even more evident in extreme conditions such as diving and hibernation.

The macroscopic phenomenon of gaseous diffusion can be explained from a microscopic point of view with the kinetic theory of gases. The most advanced and useful version for explaining transport phenomena is that of Chapman and Enskog. In particular, it can be used to predict accurately the binary diffusion coefficients for nonpolar, nonreacting gas pairs.

Ordinary binary diffusion is well understood, and Fick's first law is a phenomenological description of steady-state diffusion caused by a concentration gradient. Mass also can be transported because of temperature or pressure gradients, but such occurrences are virtually nonexistent in biology and are therefore not discussed.

For the proper application of Fick's law, concentration as well as flux must be appropriately defined. The common definitions for concentration include mass concentration (ρ), molar concentration (C), and molar fraction (x). Fluxes may be described as mass flux or molar flux; a certain frame of reference must be specified for a proper measurement of flux, whether mass or molar.

Unsteady-state binary diffusion is characterized by the diffusion equation, the solution of which yields concentration values in the entire space domain of diffusion at all instants of time, from which fluxes and concentration profiles may be established. Four different methods—the classical analytic method, the finite-difference method, the finite-element method, and the random-walk method—are available for the solution of a given diffusion equation. The major considerations in choosing the appropriate method are the boundary and initial conditions of the diffusion problem to be solved. In terms of diffusion in the lung, all four methods have been employed.

Diffusion in multicomponent mixtures often does not obey Fick's law. The effects of multicomponent diffusion must be properly accounted for, because gas mixtures in the respiratory tract always contain more than two gases. A practical way to handle this is to use effective diffusion coefficients and to apply Fick's law or the unsteady-state diffusion equation. For alveolar gas mixtures, values of effective diffusion coefficients for O_2 and CO_2 are given.

REFERENCES

1. ARNOLD, K. R., AND H. L. TOOR. Unsteady diffusion in ternary gas mixtures. *AIChE J.* 13: 909–914, 1967.
2. BIRD, R. B., W. E. STEWART, AND E. N. LIGHTFOOT. *Transport Phenomena.* New York: Wiley, 1960.
3. CARSLAW, H. S., AND J. C. JAEGER. *Conduction of Heat in Solids.* Oxford, UK: Clarendon, 1959.
4. CHANG, H. K. Multicomponent diffusion in the lung. *Federation Proc.* 39: 2759–2764, 1980.
5. CHANG, H. K., R. T. CHENG, AND L. E. FARHI. A model study of gas diffusions in alveolar sacs. *Respir. Physiol.* 18: 386–397, 1973.
6. CHANG, H. K., AND L. E. FARHI. On mathematical analysis of gas transport in the lung. *Respir. Physiol.* 18: 370–385, 1973.
7. CHANG, H. K., AND L. E. FARHI. Ternary diffusion and effective diffusion coefficients in alveolar spaces. *Respir. Physiol.* 40: 269–279, 1980.
8. CHANG, H. K., R. C. TAI, AND L. E. FARHI. Some implications of ternary diffusion in the lung. *Respir. Physiol.* 23: 109–120, 1975.
9. CHAPMAN, S., AND T. G. COWLING. *The Mathematical Theory of Non-Uniform Gases* (3rd ed.). New York: Cambridge Univ. Press, 1970.
10. CHURCHILL, R. V. *Fourier Series and Boundary Value Problems* (2nd ed.). New York: McGraw-Hill, 1963.
11. CRANK, J. *The Mathematics of Diffusion* (2nd ed.). Oxford, UK: Clarendon, 1975.

12. Cumming, G., J. Crank, K. Horsfield, and I. Parker. Gaseous diffusion in the airways of the human lung. *Respir. Physiol.* 1: 58–74, 1966.
13. Curtiss, C. F., and J. O. Hirschfelder. Transport properties of multicomponent gas mixtures. *J. Chem. Phys.* 17: 550–555, 1949.
14. Cussler, E. L. *Multicomponent Diffusion.* Amsterdam: Elsevier, 1976.
15. Engel, L. A., and P. T. Macklem. Gas mixing and distribution in the lung. In: *Respiratory Physiology II*, edited by J. G. Widdicombe. Baltimore, MD: University Park, 1977, vol. 14, p. 37–82. (Int. Rev. Physiol. Ser.)
16. Erasmus, D., and H. Rahn. Effects of ambient pressures, He and SF_6 on O_2 and CO_2 transport in the avian egg. *Respir. Physiol.* 27: 53–64, 1976.
17. Fairbanks, D. F., and C. R. Wilke. Diffusion coefficients in multicomponent gas mixtures. *Ind. Eng. Chem.* 42: 471–475, 1950.
18. Feller, V. J. *An Introduction to Probability Theory and Its Applications* (3rd ed.). New York: Wiley, 1968, p. 50.
19. Fick, A. E. Uber die Diffusion. *Ann. Phys. Chem.* 94: 59–86, 1855.
20. Graham, T. On the law of the diffusion of gases. *Phil. Mag.* 2: 175–190, 269–276, 351–358, 1833.
21. Gupta, P. K., and A. R. Cooper, Jr. The [D] matrix for multicomponent diffusion. *Physica* 54: 39–59, 1971.
22. Haji-Sheikh, A., and E. M. Sparrow. The floating random walk and its application to Monte Carlo solutions of heat equations. *J. SIAM* 14: 370–389, 1966.
23. Hirschfelder, J. O., C. F. Curtiss, and R. B. Bird. *The Molecular Theory of Gases and Liquids.* New York: Wiley, 1954.
24. Hsu, H. W., and R. B. Bird. Multicomponent diffusion problems. *AIChE J.* 6: 516–524, 1960.
25. Jeans, J. *Introduction to the Kinetic Theory of Gases.* London: Cambridge Univ. Press, 1940.
26. Krishna, R., and G. L. Standart. A multicomponent film model incorporating an exact matrix method of solution to the Maxwell-Stefan equations. *AIChE J.* 22: 383–389, 1976.
27. Krishna, R., and G. L. Standart. Mass and energy transfer in multicomponent systems. *Chem. Eng. Commun.* 3: 201–276, 1979.
28. La Force, R. C., and B. M. Lewis. Diffusional transport in the human lung. *J. Appl. Physiol.* 28: 291–298, 1970.
29. Marrero, T. R., and E. A. Mason. Gaseous diffusion coefficients. *J. Phys. Chem. Ref. Data* 1: 1–119, 1972.
30. Maxwell, J. C. On the dynamic theory of gases. *Philos. Trans. R. Soc. Lond.* 157, 1866. (Reprint in: *Scientific Papers.* New York: Dover, 1952, vol. II, p. 26–78.)
31. Maxwell, J. C. On Loschmidt's experiments on diffusion in relation to the kinetic theory of gases. *Nature Lond.* 8: 298, 1871. (Reprint in: *Scientific Papers.* New York: Dover, 1952, vol. II, p. 343–350.
32. Obermeier, E., and A. Schaber. A simple formula for multicomponent gaseous diffusion coefficients derived from mean free path theory. *Int. J. Heat Mass Transfer* 20: 1301–1306, 1977.
33. Onsager, L. Theories and problems of liquid diffusion. *Ann. NY Acad. Sci.* 46: 241–265, 1945.
34. Paganelli, C. B., A. Ar, and H. Rahn. Multicomponent diffusion of O_2 and CO_2 across the hen's egg shell in air and helium-oxygen mixtures (Abstract). *Federation Proc.* 38: 966, 1979.
35. Rauwerda, P. E. Unequal Ventilation of Different Parts of the Lung and Determination of Cardiac Output. Gronigen, The Netherlands: Groningen State Univ., 1946. PhD thesis.
36. Reid, R. C., J. M. Prausnitz, and T. S. Sherwood. *The Properties of Gases and Liquids* (3rd ed.). New York: McGraw-Hill, 1977.
37. Salvadori, M. G., and M. C. Baron. *Numerical Methods in Engineering* (2nd ed.). Englewood Cliffs, NJ: Prentice-Hall, 1961.
38. Saul'yev, V. K. *Integration of Equations of Parabolic Type by the Methods of Nets.* New York: Macmillan, 1964.
39. Scheid, P., and J. Piiper. Intrapulmonary gas mixing and stratification. In: *Pulmonary Gas Exchange. Ventilation, Blood Flow, and Diffusion,* edited by J. B. West. New York: Academic, 1980, vol. I, p. 87–130.
40. Spitzer, F. *Principles of Random Walk.* New York: Van Nostrand Reinhold, 1964.
41. Stewart, W. E., and R. Prober. Matrix calculations of multicomponent mass transfer in isothermal systems. *Ind. Eng. Chem. Fundam.* 3: 224–235, 1964.
42. Stibitz, G. R. Calculating diffusion in biological systems by random walks with special reference to gaseous diffusion in the lung. *Respir. Physiol.* 7: 230–262, 1969.
43. Stibitz, G. R. A model of diffusion in the respiratory unit. *Respir. Physiol.* 18: 249–257, 1973.
44. Svehla, R. A. *Estimated Viscosities and Thermal Conductivities of Gases at High Temperatures.* Washington, DC: Natl. Aeronaut. and Space Admin., 1962. (NASA Tech. Rep. R-132.)
45. Tai, R. C., and H. K. Chang. A mathematical study of nonequimolar ternary gas diffusion. *Bull. Math. Biol.* 41: 591–606, 1979.
46. Tai, R. C., H. K. Chang, and L. E. Farhi. Nonequimolar counter-diffusion in ternary gas systems. *Respir. Physiol.* 40: 253–267, 1980.
47. Taylor, R., and D. R. Webb. On the relationship between the exact and linearized solutions of the Maxwell-Stefan equations for multicomponent film model. *Chem. Eng. Commun.* 7: 287–299, 1980.
48. Toor, H. L. Solution of the linearized equations of multicomponent mass transfer. I. *AIChE J.* 10: 448–455, 1964.
49. Toor, H. L. Solution of the linearized equations of multicomponent mass transfer. II. Matrix methods. *AIChE J.* 10: 460–465, 1964.
50. Toor, H. L., C. V. Seshadri, and K. R. Arnold. Diffusion and mass transfer in multicomponent mixture of ideal gases. *AIChE J.* 11: 744–755, 1965.
51. Wilke, C. R. Diffusional properties of multicomponent gases. *Chem. Eng. Prog.* 46: 95–104, 1950.
52. Worth, H., and J. Piiper. Diffusion of helium, carbon monoxide and sulfur hexafluoride in gas mixtures similar in alveolar gas. *Respir. Physiol.* 32: 155–166, 1978.
53. Worth, H., and J. Piiper. Model experiments on diffusional equilibration of oxygen and carbon dioxide between inspired and alveolar gas. *Respir. Physiol.* 35: 1–7, 1978.
54. Zienkiewicz, O. C. *The Finite Element Method in Engineering Science.* New York: McGraw-Hill, 1971.

CHAPTER 4

Diffusion and convection in intrapulmonary gas mixing

JOHANNES PIIPER | *Abteilung Physiologie, Max-Planck-Institut für experimentelle Medizin, Göttingen, Federal Republic of Germany*

PETER SCHEID | *Institut für Physiologie, Ruhr-Universität, Bochum, Federal Republic of Germany*

CHAPTER CONTENTS

BECAUSE LUNGS CONTAIN a large volume of gas at end expiration (functional residual capacity), inspired gas cannot reach the alveolar-capillary membrane by bulk flow alone (i.e., by displacement of the inspired gas/lung gas boundary toward the lung periphery); therefore other mechanisms must intervene to achieve mixing with resident gas. Thus the gas transport between the atmosphere and the alveolar-capillary membrane is provided not only by alveolar ventilation but also by intrapulmonary gas mixing. This mixing step is usually not particularly considered in analysis of pulmonary gas transport, where it is tacitly assumed that mixing in the alveolar region is virtually complete and thus does not limit gas transport. In the last decade, however, the completeness of intrapulmonary gas mixing has been questioned, mainly on the basis of experimental data obtained by refined gas-monitoring techniques.

Evidently intrapulmonary mixing is not complete, as shown by the presence of series or anatomical dead space, which diminishes with breath holding, but is never entirely suppressed. When axial (longitudinal) gas-concentration gradients in airways are designated as *stratification*, dead space undoubtedly is a manifestation of stratification. Stratification or stratified inhomogeneity (127) in the proper sense, however, means presence of gradients within the gas-exchange zone of the lungs (i.e., in the alveolar space).

Dead space and alveolar space have an anatomical background (conducting airways vs. alveolated airways) but are mainly defined functionally as non-gas-exchanging and gas-exchanging or as nonmixing and well-mixing volumes. The dead space and the alveolar space are neither anatomically nor functionally separated by a sharp boundary. This is reflected in the expirogram (plot of concentration vs. expired volume or time) by a somewhat gradual change from phase II (steep concentration change) to phase III (alveolar plateau). This transition region may be regarded as due to dead space (flattened, e.g., by distributed transit times) or to stratification in the proximal region of the alveolar space. Therefore the delimitation of changes in dead space from stratification in alveolar space may be difficult and in some cases hardly possible.

When mixing of inspired gas with lung resident gas is not complete, axial gradients for the respiratory gases will persist, with O_2 decreasing and CO_2 increasing in the direction from proximal to distal alveolar airways. This series (stratified) inhomogeneity will reduce the efficiency of gas exchange in a manner similar to the well-known parallel inhomogeneity caused by regional inequalities in the ventilation-perfusion ratio ($\dot{V}A/\dot{Q}$), as shown for corresponding two-compartment models in Figure 1. This unfavorable effect on gas exchange is the main reason for the physiological and clinical interest in intrapulmonary gas mixing. It is also evident from Figure 1 that the possibility of both parallel and series inhomogeneity is inherent to lung structure. Thus both probably occur in close association, and it can be expected that the distinction and separation of their effects may be difficult.

This chapter reviews the evidence for stratification, resulting from experiments and from model calculations. The quantitative anatomy of the airways and the physics of gas transport by convection and diffusion, which are required for analysis of experimental data and for model calculations, are also briefly examined. Various aspects of intrapulmonary gas mixing have been reviewed elsewhere (14, 21, 32, 40, 63, 111, 115, 118, 120, 133).

DIFFUSION

Because the physics of diffusion in the gas phase is more fully discussed in the chapter by Chang in this *Handbook*, we consider in this chapter only those aspects that are essential for an analysis of gas mixing and transport in the lungs.

Diffusion Laws

The basic diffusion laws are expressed in the equations of Fick. The first Fick diffusion equation

$$J = -D \cdot (dC/dx) \tag{1}$$

applies to steady-state conditions (all variables at any given site constant in time); the second Fick diffusion equation [for diffusion in one dimension (x)]

$$\partial C/\partial t = D \cdot (\partial^2 C/\partial x^2) \tag{2}$$

relates to unsteady-state conditions (concentration at

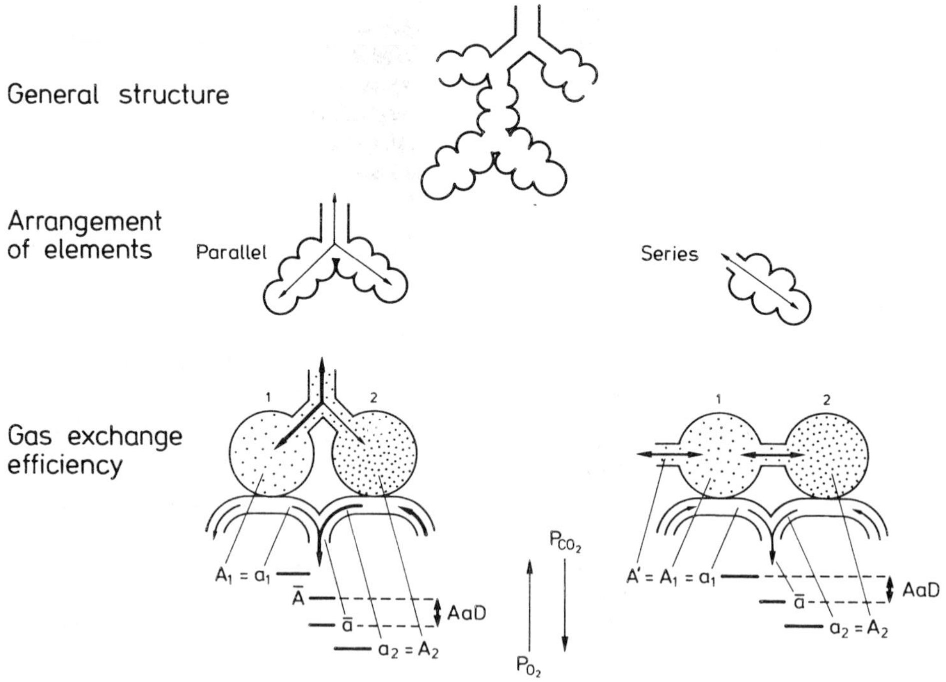

FIG. 1. Schema of lung structure shows potential for parallel [ventilation-perfusion ratio ($\dot{V}A/\dot{Q}$)] and series (stratified) inhomogeneities and their effects on efficiency of alveolar gas exchange. Levels of partial pressure of O_2 and CO_2 (P_{O_2} and P_{CO_2}) in compartments 1 and 2 [arterialized blood (a) = alveolar gas (A)] are indicated. In parallel inhomogeneity, mixed alveolar gas ($\bar{A}$) and arterial blood ($\tilde{a}$) result from ventilation-weighted and perfusion-weighted mixing, respectively. In series inhomogeneity, partial pressures in arterial blood ($\tilde{a}$) result from mixing, but values in expired alveolar gas (A′) are those of proximal compartment 1 (A_1). In both cases, there arise alveolar-arterial P_{O_2} and P_{CO_2} differences (AaD).

any site dependent on time). In these equations, J is density of diffusive flux (amount of gas × area^{-1} × time^{-1}), C is concentration (amount of gas × volume^{-1}), x is length, and t is time. The diffusion coefficient D (length^2 × time^{-1}) is dependent on the diffusing gas species and on the medium in which diffusion occurs (background gas).

It is customary to use the (dimensionless) fractional concentration of gas species y (F_y) or its partial pressure (P_y) instead of mass (or molar) concentration (C_y). They relate to each other by the equations

$$P_y = C_y/\beta_g \tag{3}$$

$$F_y = C_y/(\beta g \cdot P_T) \tag{3a}$$

where β_g (amount of gas × volume^{-1} × pressure^{-1}) is the capacitance coefficient of any ideal gas in the gas phase (116) and P_T is the total pressure, which is often equal to atmospheric pressure. Because the fractional concentration usually refers to dry gas components only, P_T in Equation 3a denotes total pressure minus water-vapor pressure; for calculation of diffusivities in humid gas mixtures, see *Diffusion in Multicomponent Systems*, this page.

In a gas phase (without local differences in P_T), the sum of partial pressures of all n components must equal P_T and the sum of fractional concentrations must equal unity

$$\sum_{y=1}^{n} P_y = P_T \tag{4}$$

$$\sum_{y=1}^{n} F_y = 1 \tag{4a}$$

This requirement introduces additional complications into the analysis of diffusion in the gas phase because it imposes a constraint on the components in a multicomponent diffusible system (see the chapter by Chang in this *Handbook*).

Binary Diffusion

An important property of binary (or mutual) diffusion, where only two gases (x and y) are present, is that the diffusion coefficient $D_{x/y}$ is (practically) independent of the fractional concentrations. Thus He in very low concentration diffuses in a sulfur hexafluoride (SF_6) medium as rapidly as SF_6 in very low concentration in an He medium.

Binary-diffusion coefficients of most gases naturally involved in gas exchange or experimentally introduced during lung function studies have been experimentally determined (4, 176). They can be predicted on the basis of empirical or theoretical relationships:

1. Graham's law is a very simple empirical approximation (for accuracy see ref. 123), which is much used in physiological literature for prediction of relative D values from the molecular mass (M) of the gases

$$D_{x/z}/D_{y/z} = (M_y/M_x)^{1/2} \tag{5}$$

where $D_{x/z}$ and $D_{y/z}$ are diffusion coefficients for the binary mixtures x with z and y with z, respectively.

2. More accurate predictions can be obtained from an equation based on the Chapman-Enskog theory of gases [(128, 133); see also the chapter by Chang in this *Handbook*]. Some important inferences can be drawn from the Chapman-Enskog equation: *a*) the diffusion coefficient D, is inversely proportional to the barometric pressure; *b*) in the range of 30°C–40°C, D increases ~0.8% when temperature is raised 1°C; and *c*) D is inversely proportional to the square root of the harmonic mean molecular mass but depends on other molecular properties as well.

Diffusion in Multicomponent Systems

Four gases are normally involved in the diffusion processes within lung airways: N_2, O_2, CO_2, and H_2O (water vapor). In lung function testing, further test gases may be introduced. For a quantitative study of diffusion problems in multicomponent gas mixtures, the Stefan-Maxwell diffusion equations have to be solved (see the chapter by Chang in this *Handbook*). This requires advanced mathematics and costly computation; therefore it is practical to examine if, and to what extent, the much simpler binary-diffusion model can be applied to studies of intrapulmonary diffusion.

In the model of Wilke, an "effective diffusion coefficient" $D'_{x/\bar{y}}$ is calculated by treating diffusion in a multicomponent gas as binary diffusion of the components "test-gas" (x) and "background-gas mixture" ($\bar{y}$) (38, 170)

$$\frac{1}{D'_{x/\bar{y}}} = \frac{1}{1 - F_x} \sum_{y=1}^{n} \frac{F_y}{D_{x/y}} \tag{6}$$

where $D_{x/y}$ is the binary diffusion coefficient for x with any component y of the background-gas mixture. This useful formula essentially means that the diffusing properties of a mixture can be approximated by the fraction-weighted harmonic mean of binary diffusion coefficients.

Experimental values for the diffusion coefficients of He, CO, and SF_6 in alveolar-like gas mixtures agreed well with the predictions from Equation 6, and the effect of water vapor corresponded to that predicted on the basis of the Wilke relationship (177). Good agreement with the Wilke prediction was also found when the diffusional equilibration of O_2 and CO_2 between inspired gas and alveolar gas (80% N_2, H_2, or SF_6) was simulated, particularly when the background was N_2 (133, 178).

It thus follows from theoretical and experimental studies that in many cases, and in most physiological and experimental conditions prevailing in lungs, the diffusion of a single-gas species may be assumed to follow closely binary-diffusion characteristics despite the presence of a multicomponent-gas mixture (133).

DIFFUSION, CONVECTION, AND THEIR INTERACTIONS

This section characterizes convection and diffusion as transport mechanisms and shows how both may interact under conditions prevailing in the airways.

The term *diffusion* may be defined as the results from the random motion of molecules due to their thermal energy. Although the motion of any given molecule is random in nature, the net mass transport by diffusion is predictable, e.g., by Fick's diffusion equations, which imply that the diffusive flux of a molecular species is proportional to its concentration (or partial pressure) gradient and to its diffusivity.

The term *convection*, on the other hand, may be defined as the results from the unidirectional displacement of a number of neighboring molecules contained in a volume element of the gas. This displacement is in general the same for all molecular species contained in the volume and is thus in particular not different for gases of different diffusivity. Convective flow occurs generally along gradients of total pressure and not along those of partial pressure, as is the case for diffusional transport. Hence gas transport is identical for all gas species when convection constitutes the limiting process, whereas a separation of two gas species of different diffusivity implies a significant limitation of the transport by diffusion.

We consider convection and diffusion as the only mechanisms of gas transport in the gas phase. Convection may be due to laminar flow, with simple or complex flow profiles, or to turbulent flow. On the other hand, diffusion (e.g., in lung airways) may be in axial or radial direction; yet its mechanism is the same, thus making the term *molecular diffusion* unnecessary. Terms such as *convective diffusion* (152), *effective diffusion* (46), *augmented diffusion* (43), and *turbulent diffusion* (15) are confusing because they are applied to particular situations where diffusion is combined with convection.

Dispersion

The term *dispersion* means flattening of concentration gradients. In lung airways, axial dispersion leads to a distribution of a thin bolus or of a sharp concentration step into a larger volume. Dispersion may be due to diffusion, to convection, or to an interaction between the two mechanisms.

DISPERSION IN LAMINAR FLOW. Figure 2*A* shows a circular tube with a fluid moving steadily under laminar-flow conditions, i.e., with parabolic velocity profile across the tube. The resulting axial dispersion of a concentration step of a nondiffusible tracer does not lead to mixing of tracer into initially tracer-free fluid. In fact, when flow is reversed with the same parabolic profile, the initial concentration front is restored. Hence, over a complete cycle in reciprocating flow, there is no net tracer transport by this reversible axial dispersion (see ref. 113).

In general, however, mixing between tracer-containing and tracer-free fluid does occur during the flow, either by diffusion or by convection (e.g., eddies when flow becomes turbulent).

In the concentration profile of Figure 2*A* there are concentration gradients at the tracer front both in radial and in axial (x) directions, leading to diffusional flux of a diffusible tracer. Figure 2*B* illustrates dispersion resulting from radial diffusion in laminar flow (148), where the effects of axial diffusion have been disregarded. By diffusion, tracer molecules move radially from the central to the peripheral region of the tube. This radial diffusion would abolish the radial concentration gradient if it were not for the flow profile that replenishes the radial gradient. This replenishment can, however, operate only in the narrow zone around the concentration front.

Radial diffusion in laminar flow results in a dispersion that is not fully reversible upon flow reversal. The amount of the remaining, irreversible dispersion increases with radial diffusivity. However, when the axial dispersion of mean concentration (averaged over the tube cross section) is considered, the effect of radial diffusion is to diminish axial dispersion (Fig. 2*B*). There exists thus a "strong tendency for ... diffusion (in radial direction) to prevent dispersion" (148). The term *Taylor dispersion* is hence not entirely appropriate.

When the mean fluid velocity is low, or the tube diameter is small, or the diffusivity of the tracer is high, the profile fails to replenish the radial concentration gradient (Fig. 2*C*). In this case, diffusion in the axial direction becomes the dominating mechanism for axial dispersion.

Taylor (148) and Aris (6) have shown that the dispersion produced by the interaction of laminar flow in a circular tube and of diffusion in radial and axial directions can be described by a differential equation that is equivalent to Fick's second diffusion equation (80, 133). The amount of axial dispersion can be measured by a dispersion coefficient (B) that corresponds to and has the same dimension as the diffusion coefficient (D)

$$B = D + 1/192\ [(\bar{u} \cdot a)^2/D] \tag{7}$$

where $\bar{u}$ is the mean fluid velocity and a is the tube diameter. Despite this equivalence of dispersion in laminar flow and diffusion, the dispersive mechanism is not diffusion alone; thus the term *Taylor diffusion* should be avoided. We shall refer to this type of dispersion as the *Taylor laminar dispersion*.

It is apparent from Equation 7 that axial dispersion is dominated by axial diffusion when $(\bar{u} \cdot a/D) \ll 10$. For respiratory gases during normal breathing, this is the case in peripheral lung airways (beyond generation 12) (171).

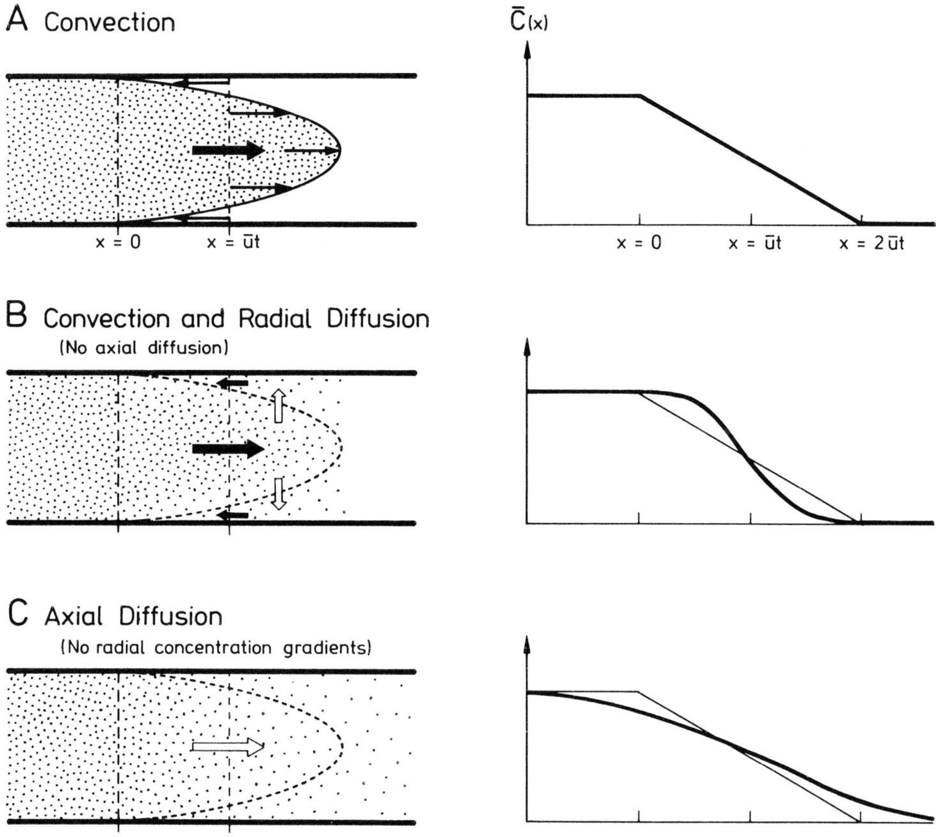

FIG. 2. Dispersion in a fluid moving steadily (mean velocity, $\bar{u}$) in circular tube under laminar-flow conditions. *Left panels*: tracer distribution [*dots*, introduced at $t = 0$ at $x = 0$ (t, time; x, length)] is displayed at $t > 0$, when imaginary plane, moving with $\bar{u}$, has moved to $x = \bar{u}t$. *Right panels*: mean tracer concentration, $\bar{C}(x)$. *A*: dispersion of nondiffusible tracer occurs only by convection (*left panel*). *Thin arrows*, radial distribution of flow relative to moving plane. *Heavy arrow*, net convective tracer transport through this plane. Axial distribution of mean concentration (*right panel*) decreases linearly in axial range from $x = 0$ to $x = 2\,\bar{u}t$. *B*: dispersion of diffusible tracer (Taylor dispersion). *Broken parabolic line* (*left panel*), denotes radial flow distribution (equal to distribution of nondiffusible tracer, see *A*). Radial diffusion (*open arrows*) leads to net convective tracer back-transport through moving plane (*closed small arrows*). Hence net convective transport through moving plane in direction of movement (*closed arrow*) is reduced and so is axial dispersion (*right panel, thin straight line* for comparison with *A*). *C*: dispersion when radial diffusion is infinitely fast and axial diffusion is significant (disregarded in *B*). Net diffusive transport through moving plane (*left panel, open arrow*) leads to axial tracer dispersion (*right panel*).

The other extreme is high flow in large tubes with low diffusivity and hence high values of $(\bar{u}\cdot a/D)$. In this case, the time spent by the fluid in the tube of finite length L may be too small for radial diffusion to establish the Taylor dispersion (171). Thus, when $(\bar{u}a^2/LD) > 10$, the dispersion coefficient of Equation 7 must be replaced by the relationship (15, 49, 153)

$$B = 0.3\bar{u}L \tag{8}$$

During normal breathing, this equation applies to the dispersion of respiratory gases in the upper lung regions (for airway generations below 8) (171).

DISPERSION IN DISTURBED FLOW. The dispersion considered so far applies to the condition of flow in straight, circular, smooth pipes with fully developed laminar-flow profile. The bronchial tubes are not straight, circular, or smooth; gas flow in them is not steady but variable with time; and the flow profiles are highly complex because of the finite length of the bronchial units and of their branching (111, 112). The laminar-dispersion theory of Taylor (148) was later extended to apply to many of these disturbing conditions (16, 42, 48–50, 163). It has been shown that under all these disturbing conditions the axial dispersion due to diffusion and convection is less than for the fully developed laminar flow (99).

Of particular interest is the dispersion observed in fully developed turbulent flow. As for laminar flow, axial dispersion in turbulent flow can be described by a differential equation of the type of Fick's second diffusion equation (149). The dispersion coefficient for turbulent flow in long straight tubes is (43, 136)

$$B = \epsilon\bar{u}a \tag{9}$$

where $\bar{u}$ is the mean fluid velocity and a is the tube diameter. The coefficient ϵ is of the order of unity and is only weakly dependent on the Reynold's number, $Re = \bar{u}a/\nu$ (ν, kinematic viscosity), at high values of Re. When ϵ is appropriately adapted, Equation 9 also may be used for turbulent flow in curved bifurcating tubes (43).

DEPENDENCE OF DISPERSION ON GAS DIFFUSIVITY. Both terms in Equation 7, the one describing axial diffusion and that corresponding to Taylor dispersion, are dependent on gas diffusivity. Whereas the first term grows with diffusivity, the second diminishes with increasing diffusivity. When both terms are of similar magnitude, dispersion is not a monotonic function of diffusivity. Thus two tracers of significantly different diffusivity may exhibit the same dispersion in a given flow, and both may disperse more than a third tracer of intermediate diffusivity. This is because the dispersion of the tracer with higher diffusivity is dominated by (axial) diffusion, whereas the Taylor mechanism prevails over dispersion of the lower-diffusivity tracer. This may be the explanation for experimental results (e.g., ref. 91) where the magnitude of dispersion does not correspond in sequence to that of the diffusivities of the tracer used. Similarly, Horsfield et al. (68) found that a heavier gas (SF_6) penetrated a hollow cast of the airways of the pig lung faster than lighter gases (Ar, He). Hogg et al. (60) found that SF_6 penetrated deeper than He into the dog lung insufflated with beads. Both author groups attributed their findings to the effects of Taylor dispersion.

At sufficiently high fluid velocity, the dispersion coefficient is independent of diffusivity and proportional to the fluid velocity. This is true both for laminar flow (Eq. 8) and turbulent flow (Eq. 9) (99, 155). This again suggests the inappropriateness of the term *Taylor diffusion.*

Attempts to Quantify Dispersion in Upper Airways

Scherer et al. (136) found the dispersion of benzene vapor in a glass model of the lung to be proportional to the mean axial velocity. The observation that the dispersion coefficient was about 3 times larger during inspiration than during expiration can be explained qualitatively by corresponding differences in the flow profiles at bifurcations (138), resulting in more radial mixing during expiration (152, 153).

It should be realized that the experimental values for the dispersion coefficient of Scherer et al. (136) apply only in the range of parameters used. For normal breathing the values should not be extrapolated to lung regions beyond generation 13 [as performed by Paiva et al. (108)].

Ultman and his colleagues (152, 153, 163) further extended the model experiments of Scherer et al. (136) and tested their results against the theoretical background of axial dispersion in laminar flow. Their experimental model comprised more generations and the flow rates covered a wider range than those of Scherer et al. (136). There was a satisfactory agreement between theory and experimental results.

Measurement of dispersion of a bolus in human airways over a complete respiratory cycle (154, 155) suggests that Taylor dispersion in fully developed laminar flow is significant during expiration only, whereas other, not diffusivity-dependent, dispersion mechanisms are important during inspiration. Similar experiments were performed by Ben Jebria et al. (8).

In conclusion, axial dispersion in the upper airways, produced by whatever mechanism, contributes very little to lung gas mixing during normal breathing, because the volume in which dispersion occurs is very small compared with the tidal volume. In particular, the Taylor mechanism is insignificant for lung gas mixing during normal breathing (11, 78, 96, 99, 174). The dominating mixing mechanism is diffusion in the axial direction (and into radially attached aveoli) in deep lung regions. Hence to omit dispersion in the upper airways from model calculations of stratification appears to be justified (see MATHEMATICAL ANALYSIS OF LUNG GAS MIXING, p. 58).

Dispersion During High-Frequency Oscillation

Dispersion in the upper airways becomes significant for gas transport, however, when tidal volumes are used far below the dead-space volume. Lunkenheimer and his colleagues (84–86) were able to maintain gas exchange in dogs by rhythmic tracheal pressure variations at high frequency. Bohn et al. (9) conducted similar experiments in dogs with tidal volumes of ~20 ml, thus substantially less than the dead-space volume. Optimal frequency for CO_2 elimination was 15 Hz. That gas exchange can be maintained with such small tidal volumes suggests that increased axial dispersion in the upper airways is significant for gas mixing between tidal and residual gas in a situation of high-frequency oscillation (HFO).

Attempts have been made to apply the theory of dispersion in the upper airways to explain the gas transport during HFO (43, 57, 134, 143, 144). All authors appear to agree that high gas-flow rates are necessary to produce sufficient axial dispersion. At these flow rates (whether flow is laminar or turbulent) the dispersion coefficient should be independent of gas diffusivity. This has indeed been confirmed experimentally in dog lungs, where no differences were observed in the washout kinetics of He and SF_6 during HFO (74).

With small tidal volume and high frequency, the breathing pattern of panting resembles the breathing pattern of HFO. It is possible that dispersion in the upper airways is an important mechanism for gas exchange during panting (9, 57).

Convective Mixing by Mechanical Action of the Heart

The mechanical action of the heartbeat evokes gas flow with relatively high frequency components in the airways of the lung. West and Hugh-Jones (168) measured in humans considerable airflows in lobar and segmental bronchi synchronous with the action of the heart. They concluded that these flows must contribute to gas mixing, as had earlier been suggested (7, 31).

Engel and Macklem (32) and their co-workers developed a technique for continuous measurement of N_2 concentration in airways of down to 2.5 mm in diameter. With this technique, Engel et al. (33) demonstrated that the reduction in dead space with breath holding in open-chest dogs was reduced after death. Similarly, the stationary concentration front (see MATHEMATICAL ANALYSIS OF LUNG GAS MIXING, p. 58) measured in a given airway with constant-flow O_2 insufflation was located more peripherally when the heart was stopped (36). Fukuchi et al. (46) extended these studies and quantified axial dispersion produced by cardiogenic oscillations to exceed axial diffusion by more than 5 times. This dispersion could effectively be reduced by filling saline into the pericardial sac, thereby reducing the tapping of the heart against the lung (44). Similar studies were performed in airway casts (69).

These studies show mixing, by the action of the heart, in the upper airways, which results in reduction in dead space. However, it may be questioned whether cardiogenic mixing occurs in the alveolar space proper and thus whether cardiogenic flow contributes to reduced stratification. Sikand et al. (141), after measuring the inspired gas/alveolar gas equilibration kinetics for He and SF_6 during breath holding in humans (see EXPERIMENTAL EVIDENCE FOR STRATIFICATION IN LUNGS, p. 62), estimated the convective (cardiogenic) conductance to exceed the diffusive conductance by ~6 times. However, the model used may have overestimated the role of convective mixing (3). Chakrabarti et al. (10), after measuring rebreathing equilibration kinetics for He and SF_6 in closed-chest and open-chest dogs, were unable to find any effect on gas mixing attributable to the heartbeat. However, the separation of He and SF_6 during washout from lungs was found to be reduced after isoproterenol infusion leading to increased heart rate (and stroke volume) in humans (82, 175), thereby suggesting a particular role for the heart action during exercise.

Slutsky (142) has attempted to treat the gas mixing produced by cardiogenic oscillations as a special case of high-frequency oscillation. With the use of Equation 7 for fully developed laminar flow and Equation 9 for fully developed turbulent flow, the dispersion predicted appeared to agree well with the experimental results (33, 36, 46). However, Slutsky (142) did not account for the possibility of developing laminar Taylor dispersion (Eq. 8); therefore his prediction of diffusivity-dependent cardiogenic mixing should be considered cautiously.

ANATOMICAL BASIS FOR MODELS OF LUNG GAS MIXING

Some morphometric details of the human airways are critical for a quantitative treatment of gas mixing (see MATHEMATICAL ANALYSIS OF LUNG GAS MIXING, p. 58). Several authors have quantitatively studied lung structure (5, 21, 54–56, 58, 61, 62, 64–67, 97, 109, 125, 126, 130, 164, 180).

Regularly Branching Lung Model

The first comprehensive account on lung morphometry was given by Weibel (164), whose symmetrical model A has been adopted by many authors as the basis for calculations. Weibel's model A constitutes a branching-tube system derived from the trachea (generation 0) by 23 orders of regular dichotomous branching. The nonalveolated part (conducting zone) extends to generation 16 (terminal bronchiole). Therefrom three generations each of respiratory bronchioles (partly alveolated, transition zone) and of alveolar ducts originate in succession; these are followed finally by the terminal structures (the alveolar sacs). The following features are of interest for lung gas mixing:

1. All paths into the $2^{23} \approx 8 \times 10^6$ alveolar sacs are identical. Because radial concentration gradients in individual bronchi can be disregarded (see MATHEMATICAL ANALYSIS OF LUNG GAS MIXING, p. 58), the walls between all bronchi of the same generation can be omitted for the purpose of gas-mixing studies; the complex lung structure can thus be approximated by a geometrically simple, solid, hollow figure representing the relationship between axial length and summed airway cross section.

2. Despite diminishing size of individual bronchi, the total airway volume per generation increases tremendously toward the lung periphery, as shown in Figure 3 for an axisymmetric solid figure with the same distribution of volume to length as the lung. When equivalent radius and length are drawn to the same scale (Fig. 3*A*), *thumbtack* (79) appears to describe this solid figure better than the conventional term *trumpet*. More than 96% of the volume is contained in the terminal 7 mm of the airways (2% of total length).

3. When a tidal volume of 500 ml is delivered to a human lung at functional residual capacity as a nonmixing bolus, its front will penetrate down to about generations 20 or 21 (first- or second-order alveolar ducts), and thus the front will be <2 mm from the distal end.

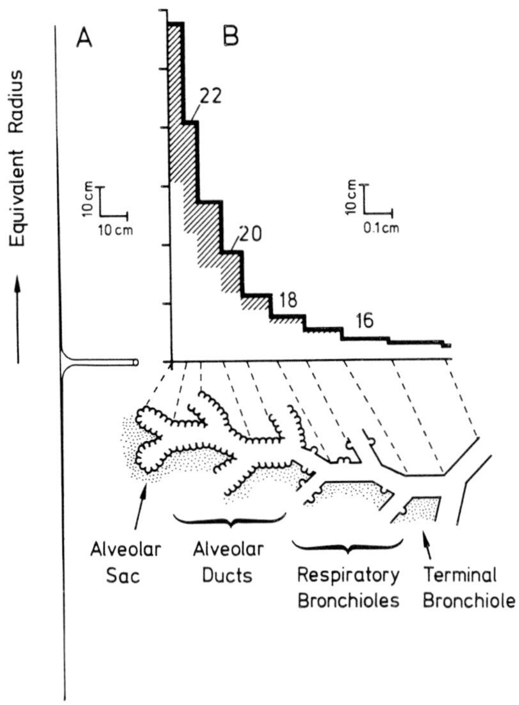

FIG. 3. Morphometric lung model according to Weibel (164). *A*: equivalent radius plotted against axial distance. Same length scale for both axes. *B*: details of terminal airways (acinus) resolved by expanding abscissa scale 100-fold, retaining ordinate scale. *Bottom schema* shows representative path in acinus, which originates from one terminal bronchiole. [From Scheid and Piiper (133).]

Irrregularly Branching Lung Model

Many investigators before and after Weibel (164) observed more irregularity and variability in the bronchial assembly, particularly in the alveolated parts, than is accounted for by the symmetrical model of Weibel (see ref. 21). Particularly useful are positive lung reconstructions used by Horsfield and Cumming and their co-workers (64, 66, 67) and by Hansen and Ampaya (54–56). The most important observation of these investigators was that the number of generations (constant at 24 in Weibel's model) could vary widely along individual paths.

Two types of models have been used to account for the branching irregularity in studies of lung gas mixing:

1. Axisymmetric solid figure. Irregularity of branching can be considered to modify the volume-to-length relationship of an otherwise axisymmetric solid figure. Thus Paiva et al. (108) represented the data of Hansen and Ampaya (54, 55) by a more rapidly widening thumbtack, whereas Horsfield (62) proposed a turnip or peg-top model to allow for some airways with extremely extended axial length. These models differ only quantitatively from the regular thumbtack of Weibel.

2. Axiasymmetric models. Because gas concentrations in corresponding generations of paths that exhibit different axial lengths generally cannot be considered identical, removal of the radial walls to represent the lung airways by an axisymmetric solid figure does not appear to be warranted. Models that quantify the irregular pattern of branching (axiasymmetric models) have been proposed (109, 146).

Conclusion

It is Weibel's distinct merit to have introduced a morphometric model that is a reasonable approximation to reality and yet is simple enough for application in mathematical analyses. However, gas-mixing studies with alternative models, which describe the lung as an axisymmetric solid figure of modified shape, have produced no qualitatively different results. When branching irregularity is introduced as an important feature for the study of lung gas mixing, Weibel's model can no longer be used. Because the irregular pattern of airway branching, even if it were described in detail, is too complex to be handled in model studies, the easiest approach is to use branched-trumpet (branched-thumbtack) models. In the simplest model (the two-trumpet model) a trumpet divides at a given generation to give rise to two trumpets. These models have recently been used in mathematical model studies of lung gas mixing (see next section).

MATHEMATICAL ANALYSIS OF LUNG GAS MIXING

Several attempts have been made to estimate the extent of stratification in lungs by simulating gas mixing in lung models. These models have increasingly been refined to more closely resemble the physiological situation with respect to lung structure and the physics of gas transport.

Models Considering Diffusive Mixing Alone

In these model calculations, the assumption is made that tidal air is inspired as a nonmixing bolus to establish an initially sharp front between tidal and resident air from which mixing proceeds by diffusion alone. Attainment of mixing is judged from persisting concentration differences in the model over a time corresponding, for example, to the respiratory period.

Rauwerda (127) performed the first calculations on a truncated cone model that was closed at both ends representing the functional terminal lung unit (acinus), which was 7 mm in length. He concluded that mixing was sufficiently rapid to abolish any concentration gradient within 1 s or less.

Cumming et al. (22) used an elongated cone to allow for gas transport across the proximal border. In their cone, which represents the terminal 13 generations in Weibel's model A, a finite concentration difference persisted after 1 s over the distal 7 mm, which amounted to 8% of the initial concentration step. The authors retained the hypothesis of Krogh and Lindhard (75) that stratification was the main reason for the sloping alveolar plateau in the single-breath N_2 test.

The elongated cone used by Cumming et al. (22) fits the thumbtack shape less than the short cone used by Rauwerda (127; cf. ref. 119). La Force and Lewis (79) have thus modeled the terminal 13 generations of Weibel's model A, represented by a solid figure resembling the thumbtack of Figure 3. The authors concluded that a concentration step, set up at generation 20, was rapidly attenuated within the volume inside the acinus.

Differences in the models chosen and differences in interpretation led to discrepancies in conclusions among the three author groups (133). The striking difference between the models resides in the distribution of volume to axial length. Concentration gradients assessed from slopes in plots against axial distance or against cumulative volume will thus differ widely among models. Particularly for a comparison with expirograms (in tests such as the single-breath N_2 test), it is appropriate to relate stratification to the concentration differences over the terminal alveolar volume rather than the terminal length corresponding to the axial length of the acinus. In general, the time course of equilibration in any (one-dimensional) system is related to both diffusion resistance (axial length) and capacitance (e.g., volume). For equilibration within the entire system (dead space plus alveolar region), the fastest time course is attained with homogeneous distribution of capacitance and resistance (e.g., in the cylinder). If, on the other hand, equilibration only in the alveolar volume (e.g., 90% of total volume) is considered, equilibration is fastest with most of the resistance in proximal and most of the capacitance in distal regions, such as in the thumbtack model (133). The model shape is therefore important for calculations of lung gas mixing, and simplified models such as cones and cylinders (104) have to be dismissed.

Models Considering Convection and Diffusion

A sharp front between tidal and resident air, assumed for the above calculations, will not be established under physiological conditions in the lung, because axial diffusion has already caused blunting and retreat of the front during inspiration. Pedley (110) and Wilson and Lin (171) have proposed equations to treat simultaneous convection and diffusion.

GAS MIXING IN AXISYMMETRIC LUNG MODELS. Cumming et al. (24), Paiva (100, 101), and Scherer et al. (135) have independently considered convection and diffusion as simultaneous gas-transport mechanisms for mixing in axisymmetric lung models, which are based on Weibel's model A.

The thumbtack or trumpet model of Paiva (102) is based on the last 13 generations. He assumed absence of dispersion in the upper airways (which thus acts merely to delay the inspiratory concentration front), assumed a flat flow profile, and disregarded radial concentration gradients both within airways and alveoli. The alveolar walls were assumed to reduce the cross section for axial diffusion and convection to that of the airways (axial diffusion and convection within the alveoli were thus disregarded).

Gas mixing in the model is thus described by the differential equation

$$\frac{\partial \mathrm{F}}{\partial t} = \frac{\mathrm{s}}{\mathrm{S}}\left[\frac{1}{\mathrm{s}}\cdot\frac{\partial}{\partial x}\left(D\cdot \mathrm{s}\cdot\frac{\partial \mathrm{F}}{\partial x}\right) - \frac{\dot{\mathrm{V}}}{\mathrm{S}}\cdot\frac{\partial \mathrm{F}}{\partial x}\right] \qquad (10)$$

where $\mathrm{F} = \mathrm{F}(x,t)$ is the concentration of the test gas at any (axial) distance x from the distal end and at any time t; S and s are the total cross section in the model with and without alveoli, and both vary with x (trumpet shape) but not with t; D is the diffusion coefficient (or, more generally, the dispersion coefficient), which may vary with x (see DIFFUSION, CONVECTION, AND THEIR INTERACTIONS, p. 54); and $\dot{\mathrm{V}} = \dot{\mathrm{V}}(t)$ is the ventilatory flow rate. This equation is similar to that proposed by Pedley (110) and used by others. The boundary conditions are determined by the trumpet shape, i.e., by the dependence of S and s on x.

Several of the simplifying assumptions underlying these calculations were later tested: *1)* Scherer et al. (135) and Davidson (27) allowed for tidal changes in the alveolar model. *2)* Davidson (25, 26) investigated the influence of gas uptake on mixing and particularly on alveolar slopes. *3)* Several studies addressed the anatomical details in the alveolated lung region and their impact on mixing (11, 13, 25, 26, 28, 103). *4)* Some studies were devoted to the influence of inspiratory mixing processes in the upper airways upon stratification (11, 35, 99).

These refined investigations confirmed qualitatively the results of the calculations of Paiva (102), which may be summarized into the following points (cf. Fig. 4):

1. During inspiration, the concentration front (i.e., axial distance at which F = 0.5) lags far behind the tidal-volume front. Whereas the latter reaches, with V_T = 500 ml, into the 22nd generation, the former stays in the 17th, a depth corresponding to only 150 ml (dead space). This shows that in the calculations of diffusive mixing alone, the assumption of an end-inspiratory concentration step at the tidal-volume front is not warranted.

2. For most of inspiration the concentration front is practically stationary, indicating that its convective advancement into the periphery is balanced by its proximal retreat due to diffusive loss of test gas into the periphery.

3. Stratification is present in the alveolar region during most of inspiration, to a considerably larger

extent than in the calculations of La Force and Lewis (79).

4. On expiration, all intrapulmonary concentration gradients are rapidly convected out of the lung, mainly because of the shape of the trumpet (or thumbtack). However, diffusion aids mixing in early expiration (compare solid and dashed lines labeled 6 and 6′ in Fig. 4). The alveolar plateau of the expirogram thus shows no significant slope. Inspiratory and expiratory flows in the calculations of Figure 4 were constant, but similar results were obtained with sinusoidally varying flow (102).

Only Scrimshire et al. (139) predicted sloping alveolar plateaus from similar calculations assuming as boundary condition that the net transport provided by (diffusive plus convective) gas fluxes at the peripheral model walls was zero. Paiva et al. (107) showed that this assumption was not warranted because at a rigid wall both diffusive and convective fluxes of an insoluble gas must individually be zero.

We conclude that calculations on lung models represented by axisymmetric solid figures show that stratification does exist in the alveolar region during most of the breath but that this stratification is unlikely to produce a measurable slope of the alveolar plateau.

GAS MIXING IN BRANCHED-TRUMPET MODELS. Anatomical studies strongly suggest (see ANATOMICAL BASIS FOR MODELS OF LUNG GAS MIXING, p. 57) that the branching pattern of the bronchial tree is not symmetric but that differences exist among individual paths in the number of airway generations, in particular within the acinus. At corresponding generations (e.g., counted from the trachea) the gas concentrations may thus differ in different paths. Mon and Ultman (93) performed calculations on lung models with inhomogeneous path lengths and suspected that observed sloping alveolar plateaus might be produced by such heterogeneity. A simple model to account for such parallel inhomogeneity is that of two parallel trumpets originating from a common stem at a branch point at variable axial levels (Fig. 5).

Paiva and Engel (105) used a branched model with two identical trumpet branches, but with each receiving different inspired volumes, to calculate gas mixing and the slope of the expired concentration curve in a single-breath test. These are the main results of their study: *1)* Only with the branch point sufficiently proximal to the (stationary) gas concentration front (outside the acinus) was the end-inspiratory concentration of a given gas in the two units 3:1, as expected from the difference in the ventilation-volume ratio ($\dot{V}/V$). When the branch point was moved to more peripheral regions, the gas concentrations within the units differed progressively less, finally becoming identical. *2)* This homogenizing effect, which is produced by diffusion, is more pronounced for He than for SF_6. Thus

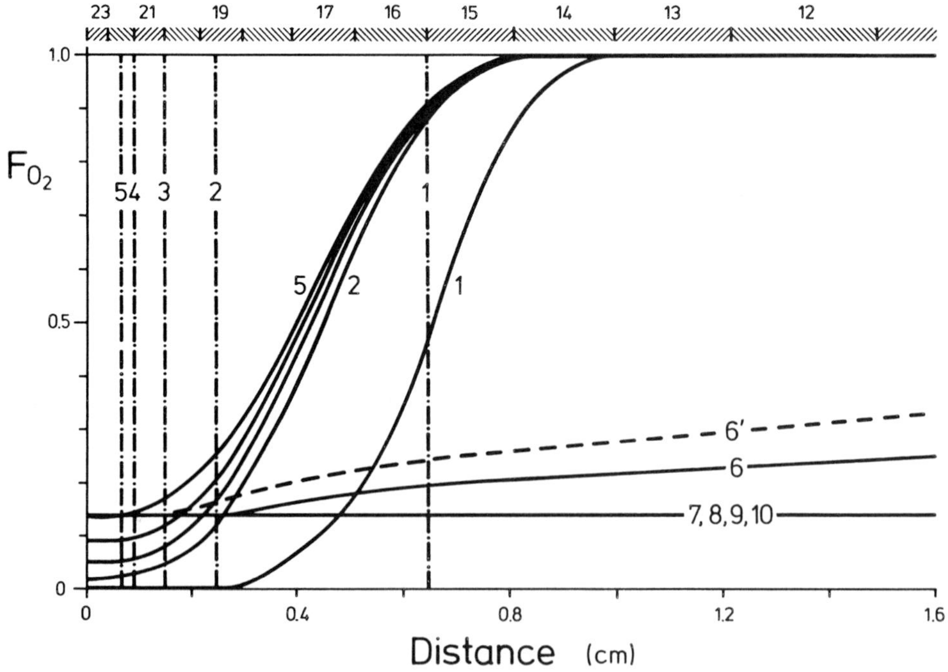

FIG. 4. Concentration profiles during respiratory cycle in trumpet model. Linear abscissa scale for axial distance from terminal end of bronchial tree. Delimitation of generations shown on *upper scale.* Ordinate: O_2 fraction (F_{O_2}). Single breath of O_2 is inhaled into, and then exhaled from, an initially O_2-free lung with constant flow. *Solid lines,* concentration profiles at successive equally timed periods during inspiration (*1–5*) and expiration (*6–10*). *Dashed-dotted lines* (*1–5*), tidal volume front (i.e., concentration front for nondiffusible tracer) during inspiration. *Dashed line* (*6′*), concentration profile calculated assuming no (axial) diffusion during expiration. [Adapted from Paiva (102).]

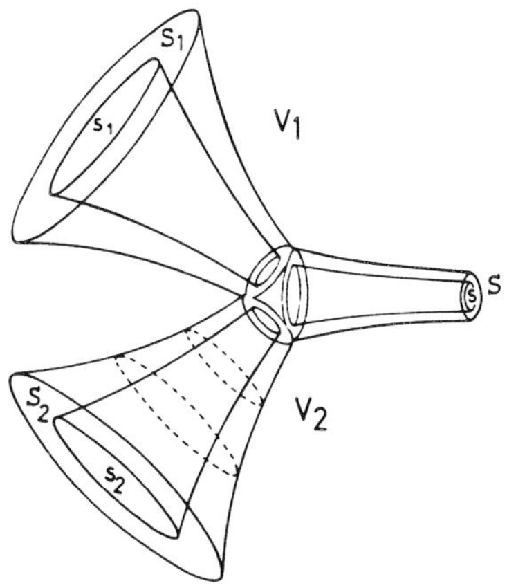

FIG. 5. Branched-trumpet model. Two trumpets branch off a common stem. By cutting off from end of second trumpet, ratio of both trumpet volumes (V_2/V_1) can be made to vary. S and s, cross-sectional area of trumpet branches with and without alveoli, respectively. [From Paiva and Engel (106).]

more He than SF_6 reaches the poorly ventilated parallel unit by the end of inspiration. *3*) On expiration this separation of He and SF_6 leads to a retention of He (relative to SF_6) within the lung, which is due to its relative accumulation in the poorly ventilated unit. *4*) In the absence of sequential emptying, the slope of the alveolar plateau is practically zero.

The inhomogeneity of volume was investigated in more detail in a later study (106) in which the volume of one trumpet branch was progressively reduced by cutting off from the peripheral end (Fig. 5).

Figure 6 shows typical calculated O_2-concentration profiles after inspiration of pure O_2 into a volume-asymmetric branched trumpet with equal $\dot{V}/V$ ratio (volume ratio is 0.12, branch point at entrance to alveolar duct region): *1*) At the end of an inspiration of pure O_2, the O_2 concentration in the smaller trumpet is significantly higher despite the same $\dot{V}/V$ ratio in both. This is due to diffusion aiding convective mass transport into the smaller trumpet, whose smaller axial dimensions favor diffusional flux, and whose smaller volume favors rapid increase in concentration. *2*) During expiration, diffusion aids convection in test gas leaving the small unit. *3*) The diffusive flux diminishes rapidly during expiration. Thus the branch-point concentration varies, resulting in a sloping alveolar plateau during phase III of the expirogram. *4*) The alveolar slope is largest for a certain volume ratio of the trumpet branches.

Also the expired profiles obtained by Fukuchi et al. (45) after test gas–bolus inhalation at various lung volumes and originally attributed merely to sequential emptying, could be qualitatively explained by this model (34).

Luijendijk et al. (83) used a similar branched-trumpet model to arrive at similar results and conclusions. They showed in particular that different slopes were obtained for He and SF_6; the branch point for producing the largest slopes was different for both gases. They also calculated the decreasing effect of breath holding on the alveolar slope.

Vries et al. (159) studied both single-breath and multibreath washout of gases of differing diffusivity in branched-trumpet models in which the branch volumes were different or in which the cross section of the entrance into one unit was reduced, thereby simulating the crossover phenomenon previously observed in experiments (95).

We conclude that branched-trumpet models, representing parallel inhomogeneity in the region of the acinus, predict both sloping alveolar plateaus and separation of gases of differing diffusivity. In these models, axial diffusion produces *1*) on inspiration, a gas distribution inhomogeneity, even without $\dot{V}/V$ inhomogeneity, which results in concentration differences between parallel units; and *2*) on expiration, a nonconstant contribution from parallel units, equivalent to sequential emptying, even with synchronous flow rates from the parallel units. It may be debated whether the axial concentration gradients, necessary for producing the sloping plateau, should be termed *stratification* (106). However, the phenomena de-

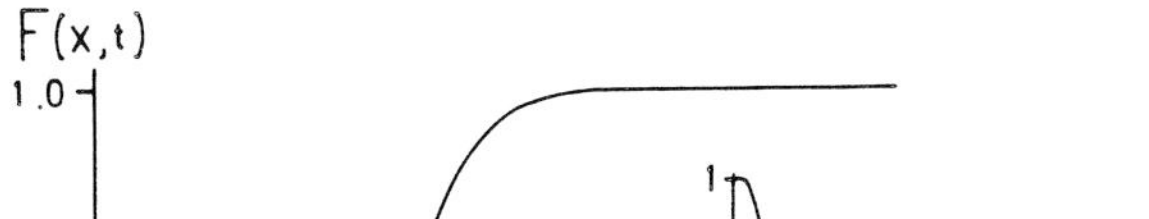

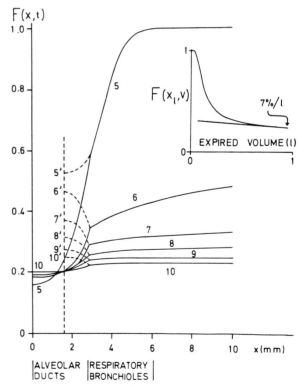

FIG. 6. Profiles of O_2 concentration during expiration, after single breath of O_2 (see Fig. 4), calculated for branched-trumpet model with uneven volume ratio ($V_2/V_1 = 0.12$). Abscissa: distance, x, from the terminal surface. Ordinate: fractional O_2 concentration, $F(x,t)$, as function of distance x (abscissa) and time t (parameter). *Dashed lines* refer to short unit; *solid lines*, long unit. Numbers *5–10*, concentration profiles at successive equally timed periods during expiration. *Inset*: expirogram. Ordinate: fractional O_2 concentration, $F(x_l v)$, at model exit (generation 13/14). [From Paiva and Engel (106).]

scribed depend on diffusion limitation; because they occur in the alveolar region, they may well be regarded as stratified inhomogeneity in lungs with parallel inhomogeneities.

EXPERIMENTAL EVIDENCE FOR STRATIFICATION IN LUNGS

Effects of Series and Parallel Inhomogeneities

Robertson et al. (129) pointed out that the multiexponential time course of insoluble gas washout from lungs can be explained by both parallel and series arrangement of compartments. Similarly, neither the measurements of differences in alveolar and arterial partial pressure of O_2 ($P_{AO_2} - Pa_{O_2}$) and CO_2 ($P_{ACO_2} - Pa_{CO_2}$) nor the clearance pattern in multiple inert gases infused intravenously (160, 162) allows a simple distinction between the presence of parallel and stratified inhomogeneities.

There are, however, some gas-exchange phenomena that are believed to be rather specific for series inhomogeneity: *1*) the sloping alveolar plateau (for O_2 and CO_2 or for insoluble and soluble inert gases) with positive slope, i.e., change of expired concentration away from the inspired value; *2*) the dependence of an inhomogeneity effect (e.g., sloping alveolar plateau) on gas diffusivity (less effect for better diffusible gas); *3*) the diminution of an inhomogeneity effect with breath-holding time; and *4*) changes of inhomogeneity effects with geometric parameters of the lung (axial distance and cross-sectional area) in the manner predicted from diffusion laws. (Criticism on the specificity for series inhomogeneity of these phenomena and criteria is presented in the next section.)

Methods and Results

SLOPING ALVEOLAR PLATEAU. In the course of an expiration, the partial pressure of O_2 (P_{O_2}) decreases and the partial pressure of CO_2 (P_{CO_2}) increases. However, these sloping alveolar plateaus do not clearly indicate the presence of stratification in lungs, because at least two alternative mechanisms may explain them as well. *1*) Continuing respiratory gas exchange exerts marked effects on alveolar P_{O_2} and P_{CO_2}, the magnitude of which depends notably on lung gas volume, blood flow, blood O_2 and CO_2 equilibrium curves, and mixed venous blood composition (29, 30). *2*) When, in a lung with parallel $\dot{V}A/\dot{Q}$ inhomogeneity, regions with low $\dot{V}A/\dot{Q}$ (and therefore low P_{O_2} and high P_{CO_2}) expire preferentially last, a positively sloping alveolar plateau for these gases results. This appears to be particularly prominent in patients with obstructive lung disease. West et al. (167) have in fact worked out a quantitative procedure for estimating $\dot{V}A/\dot{Q}$ inhomogeneity from the alveolar slopes for CO_2 and O_2.

Use of virtually insoluble inert gases (H_2, He, N_2, and Ar) obviates most of the mentioned difficulties, and the alveolar slopes of these gases (72, 76, 94, 137) seem to be better suited for detection of series inhomogeneities in alveolar gas. Unfortunately it is not possible to unequivocally attribute the measured alveolar slopes to stratification for two reasons similar to those discussed for alveolar slopes of O_2 and CO_2. *1*) Because the average gas-exchange ratio (R) is usually less than unity and diminishes further during expiration, the alveolar concentration of N_2 and other insoluble gases must rise progressively because of shrinkage of lung gas volume. This effect was excluded by Sikand et al. (140), who considered the concentration ratio of two insoluble inert gases (Ar/N_2) during expiration; this ratio definitely fell after a single inhalation of 20% O_2 in Ar. Recently the effects of continuing gas exchange have been reinvestigated (19, 20, 156). *2*) For insoluble inert gases, sloping alveolar plateaus are predicted to occur if there is an inequality of $\dot{V}A/VA$ in lungs with units of low $\dot{V}A/VA$ expiring last. This mechanism could not be excluded with certainty in the above-mentioned experiments of Sikand et al. (140; see also ref. 118).

An important improvement in the development of tests more specific for stratification was initiated by Georg et al. (47), who used multiple insoluble gases of differing diffusivity (He, Ne, and SF_6) in a single-breath maneuver. The less-diffusible gas SF_6 was preferentially found in the early expirate, whereas the highly diffusible gas He was found in the last part of the expirate, as would be expected in the presence of stratified inhomogeneity. Similar results were obtained in other studies (23, 35, 124). However, the separation of gases of different diffusivity may reflect differences in the dead space for the gases rather than the existence and diffusivity-dependence of concentration gradients within the alveolar gas (35). As expected, the diffusivity-dependent differences are particularly enhanced in hyperbaric conditions (157, 158).

SEPARATION OF INSOLUBLE GASES OF DIFFERING DIFFUSIVITY DURING WASHOUT. During washout of insoluble gases from lungs, a separation is observed between gases of differing diffusivity: the less-diffusible gas is delayed (71, 95, 98, 145, 175). Part but not all of this separation can be attributed to the fact that the dead space is larger for the less-diffusible gas (71).

Nieding et al. (95) found the He/SF_6 ratio in expired gas to be higher during early, and lower during later, parts of the washout, compared with the equilibrium value before washout. This means that there was a crossover point (He/SF_6 ratio equal to equilibrium prior to washout); this crossover point was found to be greatly delayed in patients with chronic emphysema. The delay of the crossover point could be explained by increasing airway diffusion limitation. Separation of insoluble test gases during washout is enhanced in hyperbaria (157).

ELIMINATION OF INTRAVENOUSLY INFUSED INERT GASES. The elimination of intravenously infused gases by lungs depends on their solubility in blood (39, 41). Therefore gases of identical solubility are expected to behave identically in this test, even in lungs with $\dot{V}A/\dot{Q}$ (parallel) inhomogeneity. Measurement in dog lungs of the simultaneous elimination of acetylene (C_2H_2) and Freon 22 (CHF_2Cl), which have nearly identical solubility but differing diffusivity by almost a factor of 2, showed the retention ($Pa/P\bar{v}$, where Pa is arterial partial pressure and $P\bar{v}$ is mixed venous partial pressure) for the less-diffusible Freon 22 to be higher than for acetylene, as expected in the presence of stratificational inhomogeneity (1). Knoblauch et al. (73) confirmed the results but found acetylene retention to be too high relative to that of Freon 22 when the (small but important) solubility differences between both gases are considered. In fact, in those experiments, extreme care must be devoted to the small but finite solubility differences between these gases and to their dependence on temperature (J. Piiper and P. Scheid, unpublished observations).

Truog et al. (151) used the multiple-inert-gas elimination technique (162), which is based on the model of Farhi (39), for quantifying $\dot{V}A/\dot{Q}$ inhomogeneities in anesthetized rats. The clearance of the high-molecular-weight gases (SF_6 and halothane) was found to be depressed relative to the other gases, indicating the presence of diffusion limitation in the gas phase (151). Later the theory of multiple-gas elimination from lungs was extended to accommodate the presence of both parallel and stratified inhomogeneities and was applied to experimental data (59, 132).

APPARENT SINGLE-BREATH CO DIFFUSING CAPACITY. Magnussen et al. (89) measured single-breath diffusing capacity for CO (D_{CO}) at various breath-holding times in patients with bronchial asthma. As expected on the basis of parallel inhomogeneities, D_{CO} was found to increase with decreasing breath-holding time (122). In emphysematous patients, however, D_{CO} decreased with shortening of breath-holding time, reaching negative values at shortest breath-holding times. This behavior can be attributed to stratification: CO diffuses more slowly into distal airways than He, so that its concentration in airways contributing to end-expired gas ($F_{CO,t}$) remains high; hence the initial CO concentration ($F_{CO,0}$) is underestimated when calculated from expired He concentration. If this damming up prevails over the absorption by blood, (measured) $F_{CO,t}$ may exceed (calculated) $F_{CO,0}$, and a negative value for D_{CO} is computed.

This interpretation was supported by further experiments in which SF_6 and He were used simultaneously as insoluble test gases (87, 88). Although D_{CO} in emphysematous patients was again found to decrease to negative values with decreasing breath-holding time when calculated on the basis of He dilution, it increased when calculated on the basis of SF_6 dilution.

CHANGES IN ALVEOLAR GASEOUS MEDIUM. Another technique to achieve controlled changes of diffusivity of test gases is to change the total pressure or the composition of the gaseous medium for diffusion (background gas). This approach has been used in numerous studies (51–53, 70, 77, 81, 90, 131, 150, 172, 173, 179). The measured parameters have mostly been $PA_{O_2} - Pa_{O_2}$ and $PA_{CO_2} - Pa_{CO_2}$, physiological dead space, and D_{CO}. The results are not uniform. For example, on transition from air breathing to O_2/He breathing, D_{CO} has been found to increase (173), to stay unchanged (179), to decrease (77) or to remain constant in normoxia, but to decrease in hyperoxia (53).

In most studies, however, $PA_{O_2} - Pa_{O_2}$ has been found to decrease when the denser gas (e.g., SF_6/O_2) was breathed. To explain this unexpected behavior, changes in $\dot{V}A/\dot{Q}$ distribution due to changes in airflow regime produced by changes in viscosity (179), changes in conditions for cardiogenic mixing (172), or intra-acinar stratification of blood flow (96) have been invoked. The role of the Taylor dispersion mechanism has also been postulated (70, 77), but others have denied it (96).

Attempts at Quantification

Considering the ambiguity of all experimental evidence for stratification, quantification of the effects of stratified inhomogeneities may appear to be premature. However, this section reports attempts that have been made.

LUNG MODEL. An extremely simplified lung model of the lumped-parameter type was used. In the model all resistance to intrapulmonary gas mixing is concentrated into a uniform gas-filled membrane that divides the alveolar space into a proximal and a distal compartment. The gas-transfer properties of the barrier are characterized by a mixing conductance (Gmix), which has the same dimension as the pulmonary diffusing capacity (DL), i.e., amount of gas $\times$ time^{-1} $\times$ partial pressure^{-1}.

EXPERIMENTAL RESULTS. Several methods have been used in an attempt to calculate Gmix from experimental data. Equilibration between inspired gas and lung gas was studied by inspiring a gas mixture containing He, Ar, and SF_6 and expiring after a breath hold of varied duration (141). From the decrease with breath-holding time of the concentration difference between end-expired gas and (calculated) lung resident gas a value of Gmix was obtained for each test gas. The Gmix value for O_2 obtained by interpolation averaged 78 ml·min^{-1}·Torr^{-1} in humans.

During washout of insoluble inert gases, Gmix was calculated from a comparison of the washout rate constants of He (faster) and SF_6 (slower) with the use of a modified washout equation extended by a diffusional term (71, 98). In humans, the average Gmix for O_2 was 80 ml·min^{-1}·Torr^{-1}. It follows from the design of the experiment that this value does not include contributions made by convective mixing. Introduction of the convective mixing conductance as estimated by Sikand et al. (141) increased the total Gmix for O_2 to 160 ml·min^{-1}·Torr^{-1}. Worth et al. (175) used the same method with similar results in humans.

Application of the lumped-parameter stratification model to clearance data of multiple inert gases infused intravenously in rats enabled Hlastala et al. (59) to estimate Gmix for O_2.

SIGNIFICANCE FOR LIMITATION OF ALVEOLAR GAS EXCHANGE. To evaluate the role of stratified inhomogeneity, quantitatively expressed as Gmix, in limiting alveolar-capillary gas exchange, it is appropriate to compare Gmix to DL. There is no agreement about the value of DL_{O_2} in normal resting humans (119); the estimated values range from 26 (18) to 54 ml·min^{-1}·Torr^{-1} (92). Hence the $(Gmix/DL)_{O_2}$ ratios range from 1.4 to 6.2. These ratios indicate that for alveolar O_2 transfer, stratification is somewhat less limiting than alveolar-capillary diffusion (including chemical reaction with hemoglobin) but is of the same order of magnitude. Similar conclusions were drawn from the estimated $(Gmix/DL)_{O_2}$ ratios for dog lungs (98) and for rat lungs (59).

Because the effective DL for CO_2 is much higher than for O_2 (117), whereas Gmix for CO_2 is lower than for O_2 on the basis of the diffusion coefficients, the relative importance of stratification is expected to be greater for CO_2 exchange.

CRITICAL REMARKS. Attempts to determine the quantitative role of stratification in terms of Gmix are based on a number of assumptions, many of which are critical (133). The crucial assumption is that the whole resistance to mixing (e.g., by diffusion) has been concentrated into a gas-filled membrane. The distinct advantages of this model are its simplicity and its independence of anatomical data; the important drawback is its dissimilarity to models based on morphometric data (see MATHEMATICAL ANALYSIS OF LUNG GAS MIXING, p. 58). A model study showed a further limitation of this model (3). The diffusional equilibration kinetics in a lung model was computed and therefrom Gmix was calculated on the basis of two-compartment lumped-parameter models used in the experimental studies mentioned earlier. The resulting Gmix values were shown to be time dependent and not proportional to diffusivity, in disagreement with the behavior of simple two-compartment models. The gas-membrane model can hence only be regarded as an analogue model, which when carefully analyzed may permit predictions of intrapulmonary gas mixing and of its limiting role in alveolar gas exchange.

To predict the effects of stratified inhomogeneity, as derived from insoluble-gas equilibration data, on O_2 and CO_2 exchange, the mode of blood-flow distribution must be known or assumed. Adaro and Piiper (2) assumed the model with blood flow to the distal compartment only (cf. Fig. 7). The same assumption was made by others in their analysis of multiple-inert-gas clearance data (59, 132). When part of blood flow is assumed to perfuse the proximal series compartments, the pattern of resulting $PA_{O_2} - Pa_{O_2}$ and $PA_{CO_2} - Pa_{CO_2}$ is different.

These and other uncertainties of the experimental data and their interpretations limit any attempt at quantifying the extent of stratified inhomogeneity and the resulting effects on alveolar-gas-exchange efficiency; presently the order of magnitude can only be estimated at best.

CRITICAL REMARKS AND CONCLUSIONS

Physiological Measurements Versus Morphometric Models

Trumpet models, which are based on symmetrically branching morphometric lung models, do not predict sloping alveolar plateaus that are observed experimentally. With asymmetrically branching trumpet models, this discrepancy is resolved because these models do in fact predict sloping alveolar plateaus and separation of insoluble gases of different diffusivity. Although this could and should be regarded as progress, the firm ground of morphometric data has been lost in the branched-trumpet models because all the asymmetries introduced are hypothetical, at least with respect to their quantitative extent. Hence although these models are capable of qualitatively reproducing a wide variety of results, quantitative estimates of the effects of stratified inhomogeneity can hardly be based on them.

The simplified lumped-parameter models (in which a limited number of parameters are fitted to experimental data), on the other hand, allow investigators to determine the amount of stratification. This estimate, however, is limited to the extent to which the simplified model adequately represents the physiological situation.

Dead Space Versus Stratification

It has been pointed out that the concepts of series dead space and stratification cannot easily be distinguished. Thus the diffusivity-dependence of the dead space gives rise to separation of gases even when stratification is not present. However, it can be shown that when stratification is present, it exerts a dead space–like effect that can be described as an increase in total dead space, which is beyond the series and alveolar dead space (132, 147).

Effects of Series and Parallel Inhomogeneity

Estimating the significance of stratified inhomogeneity is difficult partly because distinguishing between series and parallel inhomogeneity in lungs is virtually impossible: both types of inhomogeneity exert similar

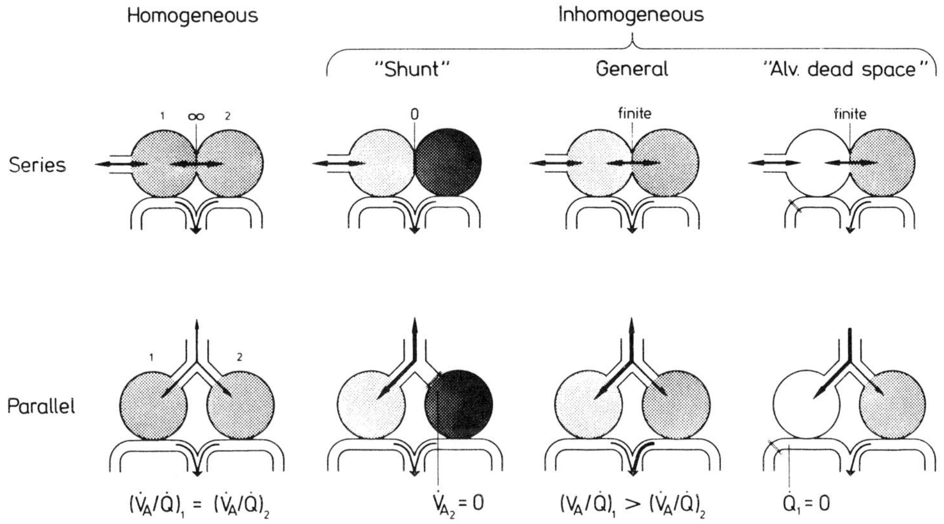

FIG. 7. Two-compartment models of series and parallel inhomogeneities. Gas-transfer conductance between compartments 1 and 2 of series model is indicated (0, finite, or ∞). Thickness of *arrows* in parallel models denotes magnitude of ventilation ($\dot{V}$A) and perfusion ($\dot{Q}$). For inhomogeneities, a general case and 2 limiting cases, shunt [giving rise to shuntlike effects, $(P_{A_{O_2}} - Pa_{O_2}) > (Pa_{CO_2} - P_{A_{CO_2}})$] and alveolar dead space [producing alveolar dead space–like effects, $(P_{A_{O_2}} - Pa_{O_2}) \approx (Pa_{CO_2} - P_{A_{CO_2}})$] are shown.

effects in global lung function tests (160, 166). This is shown in Figure 7, which illustrates inhomogeneities in simplified series and parallel models giving rise to a shuntlike effect, to an alveolar dead space–like effect, or to a mixture of both (general case).

Because the number of capillaries decreases conspicuously toward the proximal airways, the alveolar dead-space model has often been applied to analysis of gas exchange in lungs with stratified inhomogeneity. Others have used models with blood flow to the series alveolar elements, comparable to the general case shown in Figure 7 (37, 165). Experimental evidence, however, has been provided for an inhomogeneous axial distribution of blood flow favoring even proximal alveolar regions (161, 169). This would contribute a shuntlike effect to this model.

It was pointed out previously in this section that a distinction between the series and the parallel models on the basis of diffusivity-dependent effects is limited by the presence of parallel inhomogeneities on a microscale, when significant diffusion occurs between parallel compartments during the period of a breath. In fact, the branched-trumpet models constitute this type.

Mixing in Overall Pulmonary Gas Transfer

The individual processes considered in the conventional schema for the analysis of alveolar gas exchange are (alveolar) ventilation, (gas-blood) diffusion, and (pulmonary-capillary) perfusion. The functional site for the "gas mixing" is between ventilation and gas-blood diffusion.

Introduction of a Gmix allows a direct comparison of mixing with gas-blood diffusion, characterized by its conductance, which is identical with DL. The commensurate conductance values for ventilation and perfusion are proportional to alveolar ventilation ($\dot{V}$A) and pulmonary-capillary blood flow ($\dot{Q}$), respectively (119).

Because alveolar ventilation and mixing are arranged in series, their resistances R (= 1/G) can be added to obtain the total resistance to gas transfer between ambient air and the surface of the alveolar membrane. Because of the particular relationship between gas-blood diffusion and perfusion (121), its inclusion leads to a more complicated relationship for the overall conductance, $G_T = \dot{M}/(P_I - P_{\bar{v}})$, and the overall resistance, $R_T = 1/G_T$, to gas transfer between inspired gas and mixed venous blood. This model shows that the significance of stratification in overall pulmonary gas exchange can be assessed from the comparison of the resistance to mixing with both the resistance to ventilation and the resistance term describing the resistance to perfusion and the resistance to alveolar-capillary diffusion.

Parallel inhomogeneities can be included by combining this model with models for parallel inhomogeneities in terms of unequal distribution of $\dot{V}$A, DL, and $\dot{Q}$ (17, 114). Such a comprehensive model would essentially be capable of reproducing the effects obtained in branched-trumpet models (83, 105). However, because of the number of variables and their combinations, such an integrated model appears to be prohibitively complex and hardly applicable to analysis of experimental data.

REFERENCES

1. ADARO, F., AND L. E. FARHI. Effects of intralobular gas diffusion on alveolar gas exchange (Abstract). *Federation Proc.* 30: 437, 1971.
2. ADARO, F., AND J. PIIPER. Limiting role of stratification in alveolar exchange of oxygen. *Respir. Physiol.* 26: 195–206, 1976.
3. ADARO, F., AND J. PIIPER. Interpretation of simultaneous intrapulmonary equilibration of gases of differing diffusivities. *Prog. Respir. Res.* 16: 68–72, 1981.
4. ANDRUSSOW, L., AND B. SCHRAMM. Transportphänomene I (Viscosität und Diffusion). In: *Landoldt-Börnstein, Zahlenwerte und Funktionen aus Physik, Chemie, Astronomie, Geophysik und Technik*, edited by H. Borchers, H. Hausen, K.-H. Hellwege, K. Schäfer, and E. Schmidt. Berlin: Springer-Verlag, 1969.
5. ANGUS, G. E., AND W. M. THURLBECK. Number of alveoli in the human lung. *J. Appl. Physiol.* 32: 483–485, 1972.
6. ARIS, R. On the dispersion of a solute in a fluid flowing through a tube. *Proc. R. Soc. Lond. A Math. Phys. Sci.* 235: 67–77, 1956.
7. BARTELS, J., J. W. SEVERINGHAUS, R. E. FORSTER, W. A. BRISCOE, AND D. V. BATES. The respiratory dead space measured by single-breath analysis of oxygen, carbon dioxide, nitrogen or helium. *J. Clin. Invest.* 33: 41–48, 1954.
8. BEN JEBRIA, A., A. MALLET, J. L. STEIMER, J. F. BOISVIEUX, AND C. HATZFELD. Quantitative analysis of gas transport in the central airways. Computer simulations and experimental results. *Prog. Respir. Res.* 16: 96–102, 1981.
9. BOHN, D. J., K. MIYASAKA, B. E. MARCHAK, W. K. THOMPSON, A. B. FROESE, AND A. C. BRYAN. Ventilation by high-frequency oscillation. *J. Appl. Physiol.* 48: 710–716, 1980.
10. CHAKRABARTI, M. K., E. E. DAVIES, J. M. B. HUGHES, H. A. JONES, C. ORCHARD, AND M. K. SYKES. The effect of heart beat on the mixing of gases in the lungs of dogs (Abstract). *J. Physiol. Lond.* 320: 56P–57P, 1981.
11. CHANG, D. B., S. M. LEWIS, AND A. C. YOUNG. A theoretical discussion of diffusion and convection in the lung. *Math. Biosci.* 29: 331–349, 1976.
13. CHANG, H.-K., R. T. CHENG, AND L. E. FARHI. A model study of gas diffusion in alveolar sacs. *Respir. Physiol.* 18: 386–397, 1973.
14. CHANG, H.-K., AND L. E. FARHI. On mathematical analysis of gas transport in the lung. *Respir. Physiol.* 18: 370–385, 1973.
15. CHATWIN, P. C. The approach to normality of the concentration distribution of a solute in a solvent flowing along a straight pipe. *J. Fluid Mech.* 43: 321–352, 1970.
16. CHATWIN, P. C. On the longitudinal dispersion of passive contaminant in oscillatory flows in tubes. *J. Fluid Mech.* 71: 513–527, 1975.
17. CHINET, A., J. L. MICHELI, AND P. HAAB. Inhomogeneity effects on O_2 and CO pulmonary diffusing capacity estimates by steady-state methods. Theory. *Respir. Physiol.* 13: 1–22, 1971.
18. COMROE, J. H., R. E. FORSTER, A. B. DUBOIS, W. A. BRISCOE, AND E. CARLSEN. *The Lung* (2nd ed.). Chicago, IL: Yearbook, 1962.
19. CORMIER, Y., AND J. BÉLANGER. Contribution of gas exchange to slope of phase III of the single-breath nitrogen test. *J. Appl. Physiol.* 50: 1156–1160, 1981.
20. CORMIER, Y., AND J. BÉLANGER. The influence of active gas exchange on the slope of phase III at rest and after exercise. *Am. Rev. Respir. Dis.* 123: 213–216, 1981.
21. CUMMING, G. Alveolar ventilation: recent model analysis. In: *Respiratory Physiology I*, edited by J. G. Widdicombe. Baltimore, MD: University Park, 1974, vol. 2, p. 139–166. (Int. Rev. Physiol. Ser.)
22. CUMMING, G., J. CRANK, K. HORSFIELD, AND I. PARKER. Gaseous diffusion in the airways of the human lung. *Respir. Physiol.* 1: 58–74, 1966.
23. CUMMING, G., K. HORSFIELD, J. G. JONES, AND D. C. F. MUIR. The influence of gaseous diffusion on the alveolar plateau at different lung volumes. *Respir. Physiol.* 2: 386–398, 1967.
24. CUMMING, G., K. HORSFIELD, AND S. B. PRESTON. Diffusion equilibrium in the lungs examined by nodal analysis. *Respir. Physiol.* 12: 329–345, 1971.
25. DAVIDSON, M. R. Lung gas mixing during expiration following an inspiration of air. *Bull. Math. Biol.* 37: 113–126, 1975.
26. DAVIDSON, M. R. The influence of gas exchange on lung gas concentrations during air breathing. *Bull. Math. Biol.* 39: 73–86, 1977.
27. DAVIDSON, M. R. Further considerations in a theoretical description of gas transport in lung airways. *Bull. Math. Biol.* 43: 517–548, 1981.
28. DAVIDSON, M. R., AND J. M. FITZ-GERALD. Transport of O_2 along a model pathway through the respiratory region of the lung. *Bull. Math. Biol.* 36: 275–303, 1974.
29. DUBOIS, A. B. Alveolar CO_2 and O_2 during breath holding, expiration, and inspiration. *J. Appl. Physiol.* 5: 1–12, 1952.
30. DUBOIS, A. B., A. G. BRITT, AND W. O. FENN. Alveolar CO_2 during the respiratory cycle. *J. Appl. Physiol.* 4: 535–548, 1952.
31. DUBOIS, A. B., R. C. FOWLER, A. SOFFER, AND W. O. FENN. Alveolar CO_2 measured by expiration into the rapid infrared gas analyzer. *J. Appl. Physiol.* 4: 526–534, 1952.
32. ENGEL, L. A., AND P. T. MACKLEM. Gas mixing and distribution in the lung. In: *Respiratory Physiology II*, edited by J. G. Widdicombe. Baltimore, MD: University Park, 1977, vol. 14, p. 37–82. (Int. Rev. Physiol. Ser.)
33. ENGEL, L. A., H. MENKES, L. D. H. WOOD, G. UTZ, J. JOUBERT, AND P. T. MACKLEM. Gas mixing during breath holding studied by intrapulmonary gas sampling. *J. Appl. Physiol.* 35: 9–17, 1973.
34. ENGEL, L. A., AND M. PAIVA. Analyses of sequential filling and emptying of the lung. *Respir. Physiol.* 45: 309–321, 1981.
35. ENGEL, L. A., M. PAIVA, D. I. M. SIEGLER, AND Y. FUKUCHI. Dual tracer single-breath studies of gas transport in the lung. *Respir. Physiol.* 36: 103–119, 1979.
36. ENGEL, L. A., L. D. H. WOOD, G. UTZ, AND P. T. MACKLEM. Gas mixing during inspiration. *J. Appl. Physiol.* 35: 18–24, 1973.
37. EWAN, P. W., H. A. JONES, J. NOSIL, J. OBDRZALEK, AND J. M. B. HUGHES. Uneven perfusion and ventilation within lung regions studied with nitrogen-13. *Respir. Physiol.* 34: 45–59, 1978.
38. FAIRBANKS, D. F., AND C. R. WILKE. Diffusion coefficients in multicomponent gas mixtures. *Ind. Eng. Chem.* 42: 471–475, 1950.
39. FARHI, L. E. Elimination of inert gas by the lung. *Respir. Physiol.* 3: 1–11, 1967.
40. FARHI, L. E. Diffusive and convective movement of gas in the lung. In: *Circulatory and Respiratory Mass Transport*, edited by G. E. W. Wolstenholme and J. Knight. London: Churchill, 1969, p. 277–293.
41. FARHI, L. E., AND T. YOKOYAMA. Effects of ventilation-perfusion inequality on elimination of inert gases. *Respir. Physiol.* 3: 12–20, 1967.
42. FLINT, L. F., AND P. EISENKLAM. Dispersion of matter in transitional flow through straight tubes. *Proc. R. Soc. Lond. A Math. Phys. Sci.* 315: 519–533, 1970.
43. FREDBERG, J. J. Augmented diffusion in the airways can support pulmonary gas exchange. *J. Appl. Physiol.* 49: 232–238, 1980.
44. FUKUCHI, Y., M. COSIO, S. KELLY, AND L. A. ENGEL. Influence of pericardial fluid on cardiogenic gas mixing in the lung. *J. Appl. Physiol.* 42: 5–12, 1977.
45. FUKUCHI, Y., M. COSIO, B. MURPHY, AND L. A. ENGEL. Intraregional basis for sequential filling and emptying of the lung. *Respir. Physiol.* 41: 253–266, 1980.
46. FUKUCHI, Y., C. S. ROUSSOS, P. T. MACKLEM, AND L. A. ENGEL. Convection, diffusion and cardiogenic mixing of in-

spired gas in the lung: an experimental approach. *Respir. Physiol.* 26: 77–90, 1976.

47. GEORG, J., N. A. LASSEN, K. MELLEMGAARD, AND A. VINTHER. Diffusion in the gas phase of the lungs in normal and emphysematous subjects. *Clin. Sci. Lond.* 29: 525–532, 1965.
48. GILL, W. N., V. ANANTHAKRISHNAN, AND R. J. NUNGE. Dispersion in developing velocity fields. *AIChE J.* 14: 939–946, 1968.
49. GILL, W. N., AND R. SANKARASUBRAMANIAN. Exact analysis of unsteady convective diffusion. *Proc. R. Soc. Lond. A Math. Phys. Sci.* 316: 341–350, 1970.
50. GILL, W. N., AND R. SANKARASUBRAMANIAN. Dispersion of a nonuniform slug in the time-dependent flow. *Proc. R. Soc. Lond. A Math. Phys. Sci.* 322: 101–117, 1971.
51. GLEDHILL, N., A. B. FROESE, F. J. BUICK, AND A. C. BRYAN. $\dot{V}A/\dot{Q}$ inhomogeneity and $AaDO_2$ in man during exercise: effect of SF_6 breathing. *J. Appl. Physiol.* 45: 512–515, 1978.
52. GRIMRATH, U., U. SMIDT, G. VON NIEDING, AND H. KREKELER. Respiratorischer Gasaustausch bei Atmung von 20,9% Sauerstoff in verschiedenen Inertgasen. *Respiration* 35: 15–21, 1978.
53. GUÉNARD, H., M. CHAUSSAIN, AND C. LEBEAU. Respiratory gas exchange under normobaric helium-oxygen breathing at rest and during muscular exercise. *Bull. Eur. Physiopathol. Respir.* 14: 417–429, 1978.
54. HANSEN, J. E., AND E. P. AMPAYA. Lung morphometry: a fallacy in the use of the counting principle. *J. Appl. Physiol.* 37: 951–954, 1974.
55. HANSEN, J. E., AND E. P. AMPAYA. Human air space shapes, sizes, areas, and volumes. *J. Appl. Physiol.* 38: 990–995, 1975.
56. HANSEN, J. E., E. P. AMPAYA, G. H. BRYANT, AND J. J. NAVIN. Branching pattern of airways and air spaces of a single human terminal bronchiole. *J. Appl. Physiol.* 38: 983–989, 1975.
57. HASELTON, F. R., AND P. W. SCHERER. Bronchial bifurcations and respiratory mass transport. *Science Wash. DC* 208: 69–71, 1980.
58. HAYEK, H. VON. *Die menschliche Lunge* (2nd ed.). Berlin: Springer-Verlag, 1970.
59. HLASTALA, M. P., P. SCHEID, AND J. PIIPER. Interpretation of inert gas retention and excretion in the presence of stratified inhomogeneity. *Respir. Physiol.* 46: 247–259, 1981.
60. HOGG, W., J. BRUNTON, M. KRYGER, R. BROWN, AND P. MACKLEM. Gas diffusion across collateral channels. *J. Appl. Physiol.* 33: 568–575, 1972.
61. HORSFIELD, K. Some mathematical properties of branching trees with application to the respiratory system. *Bull. Math. Biol.* 38: 305–315, 1976.
62. HORSFIELD, K. Quantitative morphology and structure: functional correlations in the lung. In: *The Lung. Structure, Function and Disease*, edited by W. M. Thurlbeck. Baltimore, MD: Williams & Wilkins, 1978, p. 151–159.
63. HORSFIELD, K. Gaseous diffusion in the lungs. *Br. J. Dis. Chest* 74: 99–120, 1980.
64. HORSFIELD, K., AND G. CUMMING. Morphology of the bronchial tree in man. *J. Appl. Physiol.* 24: 373–383, 1968.
65. HORSFIELD, K., AND G. CUMMING. Functional consequences of airway morphology. *J. Appl. Physiol.* 24: 384–390, 1968.
66. HORSFIELD, K., AND G. CUMMING. Morphology of the bronchial tree in the dog. *Respir. Physiol.* 26: 173–182, 1976.
67. HORSFIELD, K., G. DART, D. E. OLSON, G. F. FILLEY, AND G. CUMMING. Models of the human bronchial tree. *J. Appl. Physiol.* 31: 207–217, 1971.
68. HORSFIELD, K., A. DAVIES, AND G. CUMMING. Role of conducting airways in partial separation of inhaled gas mixtures. *J. Appl. Physiol.* 43: 391–396, 1977.
69. HORSFIELD, K., A. DAVIES, C. MILLS, AND G. CUMMING. Effect of flow oscillations on the stationary concentration front in a hollow cast of the airways. *Lung* 157: 103–111, 1980.
70. JOHNSON, L. R., AND H. D. VAN LIEW. Use of arterial P_{O_2} to study convective and diffusive gas mixing in the lungs. *J. Appl. Physiol.* 36: 91–97, 1974.
71. KAWASHIRO, T., R. S. SIKAND, F. ADARO, H. TAKAHASHI, AND J. PIIPER. Study of intrapulmonary gas mixing in man by simultaneous wash-out of helium and sulfur hexafluoride. *Respir. Physiol.* 28: 261–275, 1976.
72. KJELLMER, I., L. SANDQVIST, AND E. BERGLUND. 'Alveolar plateau' of the single-breath nitrogen elimination curve in normal subjects. *J. Appl. Physiol.* 14: 105–108, 1959.
73. KNOBLAUCH, A., E. G. HONIG, A. SYBERT, AND G. H. GURTNER. Density-dependence of steady state airway gas transport. *Am. Rev. Respir. Dis.*, Suppl. 119: 324, 1979.
74. KNOPP, T. J., T. KAETHNER, J. KOHL, M. MEYER, AND P. SCHEID. Pulmonary washout of He and SF_6 during HFO in dogs (Abstract). *Physiologist* 24(4): 7, 1981.
75. KROGH, A., AND J. LINDHARD. On the average composition of the alveolar air and its variations during the respiratory cycle. *J. Physiol. Lond.* 47: 431–445, 1914.
76. KROGH, A., AND J. LINDHARD. The volume of the dead space in breathing and the mixing of gases in the lungs of man. *J. Physiol. Lond.* 51: 59–90, 1917.
77. KVALE, P. A., J. DAVIS, AND R. C. SCHROTER. Effect of gas density and ventilatory pattern on steady-state CO uptake by the lung. *Respir. Physiol.* 24: 385–398, 1975.
78. LACQUET, L. M., L. P. VAN DER LINDEN, AND M. PAIVA. Transport of H_2 and SF_6 in the lung. *Respir. Physiol.* 25: 157–173, 1975.
79. LA FORCE, R. C., AND B. M. LEWIS. Diffusional transport in the human lung. *J. Appl. Physiol.* 28: 291–298, 1970.
80. LEVENSPIEL, O., AND W. K. SMITH. Notes on the diffusion-type model for the longitudinal mixing of fluids in flow. *Chem. Eng. Sci.* 6: 227–233, 1957.
81. LIESE, W., K. MUYSERS, AND J. P. PICHOTKA. Die Beeinflussung der alveolär-arteriellen O_2-Druckdifferenzen durch inerte Gase. *Pfluegers Arch.* 321: 316–331, 1970.
82. LÖLLGEN, H., AND G. VON NIEDING. Use of isoproterenol infusion to study intrapulmonary gas mixing in man. *Respiration* 35: 198–203, 1978.
83. LUIJENDIJK, S. C. M., A. ZWART, W. R. DE VRIES, AND W. M. SALET. The sloping alveolar plateau at synchronous ventilation. *Pfluegers Arch.* 384: 267–277, 1980.
84. LUNKENHEIMER, P. P., I. FRANK, H. ISING, H. KELLER, AND H. H. DICKHUT. Intrapulmonaler Gaswechsel unter simulierter Apnoe durch transtrachealen, periodischen intrathorakalen Druckwechsel. *Anaesthesist* 22: 232–238, 1973.
85. LUNKENHEIMER, P. P., H. ISING, I. FRANK, M. SCHARSICH, K. WELHAM, AND H. DITTRICH. Enhancement of CO_2-elimination by intrapulmonary high frequency pressure alternation during "apnoeic oxygenation." *Adv. Exp. Med. Biol.* 94: 599–603, 1977.
86. LUNKENHEIMER, P. P., W. RAFFLENBEUL, H. KELLER, I. FRANK, H. H. DICKHUT, AND C. FUHRMANN. Application of transtracheal pressure oscillations as a modification of "diffusing respiration." *Br. J. Anaesth.* 44: 627, 1972.
87. MAGNUSSEN, H. Single breath diffusion capacity for carbon monoxide in bronchial asthma and emphysema. *Prog. Respir. Res.* 16: 147–151, 1981.
88. MAGNUSSEN, H., J. P. HOLLE, V. HARTMANN, AND M. BERRES. Measurement of single breath diffusion capacity for CO using inert gases of different diffusiveness. *Prog. Respir. Res.* 11: 297–304, 1979.
89. MAGNUSSEN, H., J. P. HOLLE, V. HARTMANN, AND J. D. SCHOENEN. D_{CO} at various breath-holding times: comparison in patients with chronic bronchial asthma and emphysema. *Respiration* 37: 177–184, 1979.
90. MARTIN, R. R., M. ZUTTER, AND N. R. ANTHONISEN. Pulmonary gas exchange in dogs breathing SF_6 at 4 Ata. *J. Appl. Physiol.* 33: 86–92, 1972.
91. MAZZONE, R. W., H. I. MODELL, AND L. E. FARHI. Interaction of convection and diffusion in pulmonary gas transport. *Respir. Physiol.* 28: 217–225, 1976.

92. MEYER, M., P. SCHEID, G. RIEPL, H.-J. WAGNER, AND J. PIIPER. Pulmonary diffusing capacities for O_2 and CO measured by a rebreathing technique. *J. Appl. Physiol.* 51: 1643–1650, 1981.
93. MON, E., AND J. S. ULTMAN. Monte Carlo simulation of simultaneous gas flow and diffusion in an asymmetric distal pulmonary airway model. *Bull. Math. Biol.* 38: 161–192, 1976.
94. MUNDT, E., W. SCHOEDEL, AND H. SCHWARZ. Über die Gleichmäßigkeit der Lungenbelüftung. *Pfluegers Arch.* 244: 99–106, 1940.
95. NIEDING, G. VON, H. LÖLLGEN, U. SMIDT, AND H. LINDE. Simultaneous washout of helium and sulfur hexafluoride in healthy subjects and patients with chronic bronchitis, bronchial asthma, and emphysema. *Am. Rev. Respir. Dis.* 116: 649–660, 1977.
96. NIXON, W., AND A. PACK. Effect of altered gas diffusivity on alveolar gas exchange—a theoretical study. *J. Appl. Physiol.* 48: 147–153, 1980.
97. OGAWA, C. The finer ramifications of the human lung. *Am. J. Anat.* 27: 315–332, 1920.
98. OKUBO, T., AND J. PIIPER. Intrapulmonary gas mixing in excised dog lung lobes studied by simultaneous wash-out of two inert gases. *Respir. Physiol.* 21: 223–239, 1974.
99. PACK, A., M. B. HOOPER, W. NIXON, AND J. C. TAYLOR. A computational model of pulmonary gas transport incorporating effective diffusion. *Respir. Physiol.* 29: 101–124, 1977.
100. PAIVA, M. Computation of the boundary conditions for diffusion in the human lung. *Comput. Biomed. Res.* 5: 585–595, 1972.
101. PAIVA, M. Méthode nouvelle de résolution de l'équation de transport de matière dans un milieu hétérogène avec diffusion (application au transport des gaz dans le poumon humain). *Biophysik* 8: 280–292, 1972.
102. PAIVA, M. Gas transport in the human lung. *J. Appl. Physiol.* 35: 401–410, 1973.
103. PAIVA, M. Gaseous diffusion in an alveolar duct simulated by a digital computer. *Comput. Biomed. Res.* 7: 533–543, 1974.
104. PAIVA, M. Boundary conditions and geometry in pulmonary gas transport models. *Comput. Biomed. Res.* 13: 271–282, 1980.
105. PAIVA, M., AND L. A. ENGEL. Pulmonary interdependence of gas transport. *J. Appl. Physiol.* 47: 296–305, 1979.
106. PAIVA, M., AND L. A. ENGEL. The anatomical basis for the sloping N_2 plateau. *Respir. Physiol.* 44: 325–337, 1981.
107. PAIVA, M., L. A. ENGEL, H. K. CHANG, AND P. SCHEID. On the boundary conditions used in calculations of gas mixing in alveolar lungs. *Respir. Physiol.* 37: 1–3, 1979.
108. PAIVA, M., L. M. LACQUET, AND L. P. VAN DER LINDEN. Gas transport in a model derived from Hansen-Ampaya anatomical data of the human lung. *J. Appl. Physiol.* 41: 115–119, 1976.
109. PARKER, H., K. HORSFIELD, AND G. CUMMING. Morphology of distal airways in the human lung. *J. Appl. Physiol.* 31: 386–391, 1971.
110. PEDLEY, T. J. A theory for gas mixing in a simple model of the lung. In: *Fluid Dynamics of Blood Circulation and Respiratory Flow. AGARD Conf. Proc.* 65: 27, 1970.
111. PEDLEY, T. J. Pulmonary fluid dynamics. *Am. Rev. Fluid Mech.* 9: 229–274, 1977.
112. PEDLEY, T. J., R. C. SCHROTER, AND M. F. SUDLOW. Gas flow and mixing in the airways. In: *Bioengineering Aspects of the Lung*, edited by J. B. West. New York: Dekker, 1977, vol. 3, p. 163–265.
113. PHILIP, J. R. Theory of flow and transport processes in pores and porous media. In: *Circulatory and Respiratory Mass Transport*, edited by G. E. W. Wolstenholme and J. Knight. London: Churchill, 1969, p. 25–44.
114. PIIPER, J. Variations of ventilation and diffusing capacity to perfusion determining the alveolar-arterial O_2 difference: theory. *J. Appl. Physiol.* 16: 507–510, 1961.
115. PIIPER, J. Series ventilation, diffusion in airways and stratified inhomogeneity. *Federation Proc.* 38: 17–21, 1979.
116. PIIPER, J., P. DEJOURS, P. HAAB, AND H. RAHN. Concepts and basic quantities in gas exchange physiology. *Respir. Physiol.* 13: 292–304, 1971.
117. PIIPER, J., M. MEYER, C. MARCONI, AND P. SCHEID. Alveolar-capillary equilibration kinetics of $^{13}CO_2$ in human lungs studied by rebreathing. *Respir. Physiol.* 42: 29–41, 1980.
118. PIIPER, J., AND P. SCHEID. Respiration: alveolar gas exchange. *Annu. Rev. Physiol.* 33: 131–154, 1971.
119. PIIPER, J., AND P. SCHEID. Blood-gas equilibration in lungs. In: *Pulmonary Gas Exchange. Ventilation, Blood Flow, and Diffusion*, edited by J. B. West. New York: Academic, 1980, vol. 1, p. 131–171.
120. PIIPER, J., AND P. SCHEID. Gas mixing and its measurement. In: *Scientific Foundations of Respiratory Medicine*, edited by J. G. Scadding, G. Cumming, and W. M. Thurlbeck. London: Heinemann, 1981, p. 129–138.
121. PIIPER, J., AND P. SCHEID. Model for capillary-alveolar equilibration with special reference to O_2 uptake in hypoxia. *Respir. Physiol.* 46: 193–208, 1981.
122. PIIPER, J., AND R. S. SIKAND. Determination of D_{CO} by the single-breath method in inhomogeneous lungs: theory. *Respir. Physiol.* 1: 75–87, 1966.
123. PIIPER, J., AND H. WORTH. Value and limits of Graham's law for prediction of diffusivities of gases in gas mixtures. *Respir. Physiol.* 41: 233–240, 1980.
124. POWER, G. G. Gaseous diffusion between airways and alveoli in the human lung. *J. Appl. Physiol.* 27: 701–709, 1969.
125. PUMP, K. K. The morphology of the finer branches of the bronchial tree of the human lung. *Dis. Chest* 46: 379–398, 1964.
126. PUMP, K. K. Morphology of the acinus of the human lung. *Dis. Chest* 56: 126–134, 1969.
127. RAUWERDA, P. E. Unequal Ventilation of Different Parts of the Lung and the Determination of Cardiac Output. Groningen, The Netherlands: State Univ. Groningen, 1946. Dissertation.
128. REID, R. C., AND T. K. SHERWOOD. *The Properties of Gases and Liquids* (2nd ed.). New York: McGraw-Hill, 1966.
129. ROBERTSON, J. S., W. E. SIRI, AND H. B. JONES. Lung ventilation patterns determined by analysis of nitrogen elimination rates; use of the mass spectrometer as a continuous gas analyzer. *J. Clin. Invest.* 29: 577–590, 1950.
130. ROSS, B. B. Influence of bronchial tree structure on ventilation in the dog's lung as inferred from measurements of a plastic cast. *J. Appl. Physiol.* 10: 1–14, 1957.
131. SALTZMAN, H. A., J. V. SALZANO, G. D. BLENKARN, AND J. A. KYLSTRA. Effects of pressure on ventilation and gas exchange in man. *J. Appl. Physiol.* 30: 443–449, 1971.
132. SCHEID, P., M. P. HLASTALA, AND J. PIIPER. Inert gas elimination from lungs with stratified inhomogeneity: theory. *Respir. Physiol.* 44: 299–309, 1981.
133. SCHEID, P., AND J. PIIPER. Intrapulmonary gas mixing and stratification. In: *Pulmonary Gas Exchange. Ventilation, Blood Flow, and Diffusion*, edited by J. B. West. New York: Academic, 1980, vol. 1, p. 87–130.
134. SCHERER, P. W., AND F. R. HASELTON. Convective exchange in oscillatory flow through bronchial tree models. *J. Appl. Physiol.* 53: 1023–1033, 1982.
135. SCHERER, P. W., L. H. SHENDALMAN, AND N. M. GREENE. Simultaneous diffusion and convection in single breath lung washout. *Bull. Math. Biophys.* 34: 393–412, 1972.
136. SCHERER, P. W., L. H. SHENDALMAN, N. M. GREENE, AND A. BOUHUYS. Measurement of axial diffusivities in a model of the bronchial airways. *J. Appl. Physiol.* 38: 719–723, 1975.
137. SCHOEDEL, W. Alveolarluft. *Ergeb. Physiol. Biol. Chem. Exp. Pharmakol.* 39: 450–488, 1937.
138. SCHROTER, R. C., AND M. F. SUDLOW. Flow patterns in models of the human bronchial airways. *Respir. Physiol.* 7: 341–355, 1969.
139. SCRIMSHIRE, D. A., R. J. LOUGHNANE, AND T. J. JONES. A reappraisal of boundary conditions assumed in pulmonary gas transport models. *Respir. Physiol.* 35: 317–334, 1978.
140. SIKAND, R., P. CERRETELLI, AND L. E. FARHI. Effects of $\dot{V}A$

and $\dot{V}A/\dot{Q}$ distribution and of time on the alveolar plateau. *J. Appl. Physiol.* 21: 1331–1337, 1966.

141. SIKAND, R. S., H. MAGNUSSEN, P. SCHEID, AND J. PIIPER. Convective and diffusive gas mixing in human lungs: experiments and model analysis. *J. Appl. Physiol.* 40: 362–371, 1976.
142. SLUTSKY, A. S. Gas mixing by cardiogenic oscillations: a theoretical quantitative analysis. *J. Appl. Physiol.* 51: 1287–1293, 1981.
143. SLUTSKY, A. S., G. G. BERDINE, AND J. M. DRAZEN. Oscillatory flow and quasi-steady behavior in a model of human central airways. *J. Appl. Physiol.* 50: 1293–1299, 1981.
144. SLUTSKY, A. S., J. M. DRAZEN, R. H. INGRAM, JR., R. D. KAMM, A. H. SHAPIRO, J. J. FREDBERG, S. H. LORING, AND J. LEHR. Effective pulmonary ventilation with small-volume oscillations at high frequency. *Science Wash. DC* 209: 609–611, 1980.
145. SMIDT, U., AND G. VON NIEDING. Experimental demonstration of stratification by simultaneous wash-in of three inert gases. *Bull. Physio-Pathol. Respir.* 9: 508–509, 1973.
146. SOONG, T. T., P. NICOLAIDES, C. P. YU, AND S. C. SOONG. A statistical description of the human tracheobronchial tree geometry. *Respir. Physiol.* 37: 161–172, 1979.
147. STRIEDER, D. J., B. A. BARNES, B. W. LEVINE, AND H. KAZEMI. Stratified dead space in excised perfused lungs. *J. Appl. Physiol.* 29: 486–492, 1970.
148. TAYLOR, G. Dispersion of soluble matter in solvent flowing slowly through a tube. *Proc. R. Soc. Lond. A Math. Phys. Sci.* 219: 186–203, 1953.
149. TAYLOR, G. The dispersion of matter in turbulent flow through a pipe. *Proc. R. Soc. Lond. A Math. Phys. Sci.* 223: 446–468, 1954.
150. THIRIET, M., D. DOUGUET, J. C. BONNET, C. CANONNE, AND C. HATZFELD. Influence du mélange He-O_2 sur la mixique dans les bronchopneumopathies obstructives chroniques. *Bull. Eur. Physiopathol. Respir.* 15: 1053–1068, 1979.
151. TRUOG, W. E., M. P. HLASTALA, T. A. STANDAERT, H. P. MCKENNA, AND W. A. HODSON. Oxygen-induced alteration of ventilation-perfusion relationships in rats. *J. Appl. Physiol.* 47: 1112–1117, 1979.
152. ULTMAN, J. S., AND H. S. BLATMAN. A compartmental dispersion model for the analysis of mixing in tube networks. *AIChE J.* 23: 169–176, 1977.
153. ULTMAN, J. S., AND H. S. BLATMAN. Longitudinal mixing in pulmonary airways. Analysis of inert gas dispersion in symmetric tube network models. *Respir. Physiol.* 30: 349–367, 1977.
154. ULTMAN, J. S., B. E. DOLL, R. SPIEGEL, AND M. W. THOMAS. Longitudinal mixing in pulmonary airways—normal subjects respiring at a constant flow. *J. Appl. Physiol.* 44: 297–303, 1978.
155. ULTMAN, J. S., AND M. W. THOMAS. Longitudinal mixing in pulmonary airways: comparison of inspiration and expiration. *J. Appl. Physiol.* 46: 799–805, 1979.
156. VAN LIEW, H. D., AND R. ARIELI. Exchanges of oxygen and carbon dioxide alter inert gas pattern in single-breath tests. *J. Appl. Physiol.* 50: 487–492, 1981.
157. VAN LIEW, H. D., E. D. THALMANN, AND D. K. SPONHOLTZ. Diffusion-dependence of pulmonary gas mixing at 5.5 and 9.5 ATA. *Undersea Biomed. Res.* 6: 251–258, 1979.
158. VAN LIEW, H. D., E. D. THALMANN, AND D. K. SPONHOLTZ. Hindrance to diffusive gas mixing in the lung in hyperbaric environments. *J. Appl. Physiol.* 51: 243–247, 1981.
159. VRIES, W. R. DE, S. C. M. LUIJENDIJK, AND A. ZWART. Helium and sulfur hexafluoride washout in asymmetric lung models. *J. Appl. Physiol.* 51: 1122–1130, 1981.
160. WAGNER, P. D., AND J. W. EVANS. Conditions for equivalence of gas exchange in series and parallel models of the lung. *Respir. Physiol.* 31: 117–138, 1977.
161. WAGNER, P., J. MCRAE, AND J. READ. Stratified distribution of blood flow in secondary lobule of the rat lung. *J. Appl. Physiol.* 22: 1115–1123, 1967.
162. WAGNER, P. D., H. A. SALTZMAN, AND J. B. WEST. Measurement of continuous distributions of ventilation-perfusion ratios: theory. *J. Appl. Physiol.* 36: 588–599, 1974.
163. WEAVER, D. W., AND J. S. ULTMAN. Axial dispersion through tube constrictions. *AIChE J.* 26: 9–15, 1980.
164. WEIBEL, E. R. *Morphometry of the Human Lung.* Berlin: Springer-Verlag, 1963.
165. WEIBEL, E. R., C. R. TAYLOR, P. GEHR, H. HOPPELER, O. MATHIEU, AND G. M. O. MALOIY. Design of the mammalian respiratory system. IX. Functional and structural limits for oxygen flow. *Respir. Physiol.* 44: 151–164, 1981.
166. WEST, J. B. Gas exchange when one lung region inspires from another. *J. Appl. Physiol.* 30: 479–487, 1971.
167. WEST, J. B., K. T. FOWLER, P. HUGH-JONES, AND T. V. O'DONNELL. Measurement of the ventilation-perfusion ratio inequality in the lung by the analysis of a single expirate. *Clin. Sci. Lond.* 16: 529–547, 1957.
168. WEST, J. B., AND P. HUGH-JONES. Pulsatile gas flow in bronchi caused by the heart beat. *J. Appl. Physiol.* 16: 697–702, 1961.
169. WEST, J. B., J. E. MALONEY, AND B. L. CASTLE. Effect of stratified inequality of blood flow on gas exchange in liquid-filled lungs. *J. Appl. Physiol.* 32: 357–361, 1972.
170. WILKE, C. R. Diffusional properties of multicomponent gases. *Chem. Eng. Prog.* 46: 95–104, 1950.
171. WILSON, T. A., AND K.-H. LIN. Convection and diffusion in the airways and the design of the bronchial tree. In: *Airway Dynamics: Physiology and Pharmacology*, edited by A. Bouhuys. Springfield, IL: Thomas, 1970, p. 5–19.
172. WOOD, L. D. H., A. C. BRYAN, S. K. BAU, T. R. WENG, AND H. LEVISON. Effect of increased gas density on pulmonary gas exchange in man. *J. Appl. Physiol.* 41: 206–210, 1976.
173. WORTH, H. Diffusionskapazität der Lunge für CO bei Atmung von Inertgasgemischen mit unterschiedlichen physikalischen Eigenschaften. *Respiration* 32: 436–444, 1975.
174. WORTH, H., F. ADARO, AND J. PIIPER. Penetration of inhaled He and SF_6 into alveolar space at low tidal volumes. *J. Appl. Physiol.* 43: 403–408, 1977.
175. WORTH, H., G. VON NIEDING, H. LÖLLGEN, AND U. SMIDT. Intrapulmonary gas mixing in man during infusion of isoproterenol studied by simultaneous wash-out of He and SF_6. *Lung* 158: 241–250, 1980.
176. WORTH, H., W. NÜSSE, AND J. PIIPER. Determination of binary diffusion coefficients of various gas species used in respiratory physiology. *Respir. Physiol.* 32: 15–26, 1978.
177. WORTH, H., AND J. PIIPER. Diffusion of helium, carbon monoxide and sulfur hexafluoride in gas mixtures similar to alveolar gas. *Respir. Physiol.* 32: 155–166, 1978.
178. WORTH, H., AND J. PIIPER. Model experiments on diffusional equilibration of oxygen and carbon dioxide between inspired and alveolar gas. *Respir. Physiol.* 35: 1–7, 1978.
179. WORTH, H., H. TAKAHASHI, H. WILLMER, AND J. PIIPER. Pulmonary gas exchange in dogs ventilated with mixtures of oxygen with various inert gases. *Respir. Physiol.* 28: 1–15, 1976.
180. YEATES, D. B., AND N. ASPIN. A mathematical description of the airways of the human lungs. *Respir. Physiol.* 32: 91–104, 1978.

CHAPTER 5

Diffusion of gases across the alveolar membrane

ROBERT E. FORSTER | *Department of Physiology, University of Pennsylvania School of Medicine, Philadelphia, Pennsylvania*

CHAPTER CONTENTS

THIS CHAPTER IS CONCERNED with the diffusion of gases across the alveolar-capillary membrane, primarily the physiology of CO and O_2 exchange between alveolar gas and pulmonary capillary blood and the diffusing capacity of the lung, taking up where the chapter on diffusion of gases in volume I of the *Handbook* section on respiration left off in 1964 (34, 35, 37). It is technically impossible to measure this step in gas exchange in the lungs without involving diffusion plus chemical reactions within the blood. Therefore some discussion of the pertinent reaction rates (CO and O_2) in blood is included. Topics covered elsewhere in this *Handbook* are not discussed, particularly CO_2 exchange and reactions in the blood and tissue (see the chapter by Klocke), diffusion of gases in the gas phase (see the chapter by Piiper and Scheid), Hb-O_2 equilibrium (see the chapter by Baumann, Bartels, and Bauer), and the effects of nonuniformity on diffusion (see the chapter by Hlastala).

Basic and important physiological questions that are considered to have been settled in the previous volume are not redefended. For example, the equilibration of chemically inert gases between alveolar air and capillary blood, which is accepted as being very rapid (i.e., complete before the blood has coursed several percent of its total path through the alveolus) is not considered here.

Investigations of gas exchange in the alveoli depend on quantitative measurement of the efficiency of the lungs in transferring gas between capillary blood and alveolar air. The measure of this transfer efficiency is the rate of flux of the gas (generally CO or O_2) between alveolar air and red cell hemoglobin divided by the mean driving pressure difference, which is termed the *pulmonary diffusing capacity* in the United States, although this exchange is not produced by diffusion alone (some chemical reaction is also included) and is not a capacity. A better term is the more general engineering expression, *transfer coefficient* or *transfer factor*, which is accepted in the United Kingdom. *Diffusing capacity* appears fairly rooted in the United States and will long remain so, judging by the speed with which the logical 200-year-old metric system is being accepted by the American public. The symbol D for diffusing capacity is used here with the symbol L for *lung*, indicating that the measurement applies to overall exchange in this organ, or the symbol m for *membrane*, referring to the transfer properties of the alveolar membrane alone. The units are milliliters of gas [standard temperature and pressure, dry (STPD)] per minute per millimeter of mercury (1 mmHg = 0.133 kP). The subscripts O_2 and CO indicate the gas in question.

The diffusing capacity of the lung (DL) is measured by one of several techniques that determine the rate of exchange of CO (or O_2) using steady-state, rebreathing, or breath-holding maneuvers and dividing by the mean pressure difference between alveolar gas and the hemoglobin in the red cells, which must be determined independently.

The DL can only be measured by CO or O_2. The permeability of the pulmonary membrane itself is so great that unless there is a large capacity, or large effective solubility, for the gas under study in the blood, it diffuses so rapidly that no measurable pressure difference remains between alveolar air and the end-capillary blood. Thus the average mean driving pressure gradient between the gas and fluid phases cannot be determined; Dm and DL cannot be measured experimentally. The membrane component (Dm) for other gases can be obtained from that of CO by multiplying by the ratio

$$\frac{\alpha_x}{\alpha_{CO}}\left(\frac{MW_{CO}}{MW_x}\right)^{1/2}$$

where α_x is the solubility of gas x and α_{CO} is the solubility of CO, both in the membrane at 37°C; MW_x and MW_{CO} are the molecular weights of x and CO, respectively. Diffusing capacity of the lung, as measured with CO, is widely used as a clinical pulmonary function test; thus there are many reports on the test itself and a large volume of experimental data on healthy subjects and patients with a variety of diseases (19, 36, 96a). Only representative articles are referenced in this chapter and only results of physiological, as opposed to clinical, pertinence are noted.

MECHANISM OF O_2 AND CO EXCHANGE IN LUNG ALVEOLI

The model of Roughton and Forster (108) has been generally accepted as describing the transport of O_2 and CO between aveolar gas and the red cells. More recent experimental data in support of this hypothesis is presented. The model is described concisely by the equation

$$1/D_L = 1/Dm + 1/\Theta Vc \qquad (1)$$

where DL is the diffusing capacity of the whole lung and Dm is the analogous diffusing capacity of the membrane alone, including alveolar epithelium, interstitium, and capillary endothelium; both indices are in milliliters per minute per millimeter of mercury. By analogy ΘVc is the diffusing capacity of the total mass of red cells in the capillary bed of the lung at any instant, where Vc is the volume of the capillary bed in milliliters and Θ is the standard rate at which 1 ml of whole blood will take up the gas, CO or O_2, in milliliters STPD per minute per millimeter of mercury of partial pressure.

In engineering terms 1/DL is the total resistance (i.e., the ratio of the driving pressure gradient to flux) between alveolar gas and hemoglobin molecules and equals the sum of the resistance across the pulmonary membrane alone, 1/Dm, and the resistance of the total volume of red cells in the alveolar capillary bed, 1/(ΘVc). In Equation 1 it is assumed that transport of gas across the pulmonary membrane (Dm) is proportional to the pressure difference across that membrane and similarly that the rate of gas uptake of red cells is proportional to the partial pressure outside red cells minus the partial pressure in equilibrium with the hemoglobin. This means that there is no active transport of O_2 or CO; no new evidence for active transport has appeared.

Ayash et al. (5), Burns et al. (12), and Mendoza et al. (82) have proposed that there is carrier-facilitated flux of O_2 and CO across the pulmonary membrane. Their candidate for this carrier is cytochrome *P*-450. The evidence presented for this facilitation is that the pulmonary diffusing capacity for CO (DL_{CO}) at very low partial pressure of CO (P_{CO}) (in the parts per million range) is greater than when alveolar P_{CO} (PA_{CO}) is ~1 mmHg. It is argued that the affinity of CO for the carrier is high; the carrier becomes saturated at partial pressures well below 1 mmHg, and the facilitated flux of CO is swamped by the ordinary diffusion flux as PA_{CO} rises further. However, other investigators using radiolabeled CO found that DL_{CO} did not increase at low PA_{CO}, certainly down to the level of 1 ppm (63, 84). Furthermore, cytochrome *P*-450 at least does not react reversibly with O_2 nor does it easily dissociate from CO; thus this pigment fails to qualify as a facilitated carrier. It seems unlikely that there is significant carrier-mediated flux of either CO or O_2 in the lung at this time.

It is easier to discuss CO diffusion in the lung, and in fact the model was developed for this gas, because it does not produce a significant change in CO saturation of the hemoglobin in one capillary transit and therefore does not produce a significant back reaction, i.e., breakdown of HbCO to form CO. Equation 2 describes the combination of CO with hemoglobin in red cells at high partial pressure of O_2 (P_{O_2})

$$CO + Hb_4(O_2)_3 \xrightarrow{l'_4} Hb_4(O_2)_3CO \qquad (2)$$

where Hb_4 indicates tetrameric hemoglobin with four binding sites for ligand (O_2 or CO) per molecule; $Hb_4(O_2)_3$ has three sites occupied by molecular O_2; $Hb_4(O_2)_3CO$ has the fourth site occupied by CO; l'_4 is the bimolecular reaction velocity constant for the binding of CO to the fourth position of the hemoglobin molecule in units of millimoles per liter per second.

The rate of $Hb_4(O_2)_3CO$ formation corresponding to Equation 2 is

$$\frac{d[Hb_4(O_2)_3CO]}{dt} = l'_4[Hb_4(O_2)_3][CO] \qquad (3)$$

where concentrations are in millimoles per liter and time is in seconds.

$$\Theta_{CO} = l'_4\alpha_{CO}\ 0.2 \times 60 \qquad (4)$$

where Θ_{CO} is the rate of CO uptake by 1 ml of normal whole blood in milliliters of CO binding per minute for a partial pressure of 1 mmHg outside the cells; α_{CO} is the solubility of CO in blood at 37°C, 0.00105 mM × $mmHg^{-1}$; 0.2 is the capacity of blood for binding CO in milliliters of gas STPD for each milliliter of blood; and 60 is the seconds in a minute.

If P_{O_2} is high (i.e., >200 mmHg) the saturation of the hemoglobin is so great that the only unsaturated species present is $Hb_4(O_2)_3$. Under this limited circumstance the equilibrium between O_2 and the incompletely saturated hemoglobin can be approximated by the equation

$$K = \frac{[Hb_4(O_2)_3][O_2]}{[Hb_4(O_2)_4]} \quad (5)$$

where K is an equilibrium constant. This O_2 equilibrium is hyperbolic, since there is only one binding site, and the concentration of the unoxygenated form can be expressed as

$$[Hb_4(O_2)_3] = \frac{K[Hb_4(O_2)_4]}{K + \alpha_{O_2}P_{O_2}} \quad (6)$$

where α_{O_2} is the solubility of O_2, which is 0.0014 mM × $mmHg^{-1}$ P_{O_2}. At high P_{O_2}, where $\alpha_{O_2} \times P_{O_2}$ is much greater than K, the concentration of unliganded hemoglobin becomes proportional to $1/P_{O_2}$.

If this approximate relationship is substituted in Equation 4

$$\Theta_{CO} \propto l_4'/P_{O_2} \quad (7)$$

To make quantitative calculations with Equation 1 (e.g., calculations of Vc and Dm) it is necessary to assume that *1)* DL and Dm are uniform along the capillary and *2)* Θ_{CO} is constant along the capillary. At normal PA_{O_2}, blood enters the lung capillary at 40 mmHg and rises to approximate the PA_{O_2}, 100 mmHg, at the end of the capillary. As blood P_{O_2} rises, the O_2 combines with the hemoglobin and reduces the concentration of unliganded hemoglobin that can react and, as indicated by Equation 7, reduces the value of Θ. Therefore the measurements of DL_{CO} must be made at a high P_{O_2} (>200 mmHg) so that PA_{O_2} equilibrates with capillary blood so early in its path that it is reasonable to assume PA_{O_2} equals mean capillary blood P_{O_2} and therefore that Θ_{CO} in the capillary can be considered constant at the value determined by PA_{O_2}. At P_{O_2} this high, CO uptake by red cells is slowed to such an extent that diffusion of CO within the red cell becomes relatively unimportant and Θ_{CO} is approximately the same in intact cells as in an equivalent concentration of hemolysate.

Probably the greatest experimental support for the validity of Equation 1 is provided by the experimental measurements of DL_{CO} in normal subjects at PA_{O_2} from <100 mmHg to >3,200 mmHg [Fig. 1; (95)]. As predicted by Equation 7, $1/DL_{CO}$ increases linearly with P_{O_2} over this entire range. This agreement between

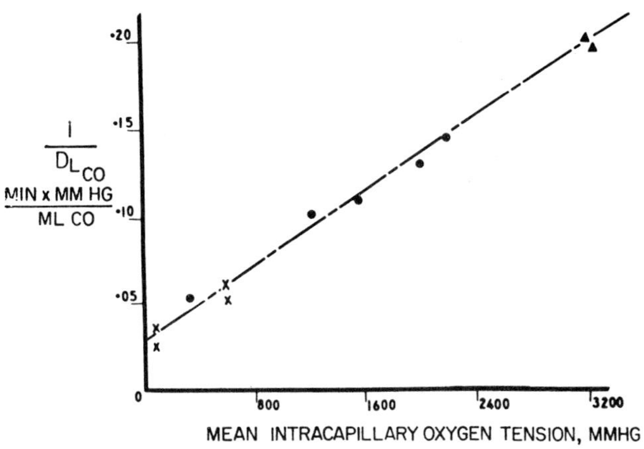

FIG. 1. Graph of $1/DL_{CO}$ (DL_{CO}, CO pulmonary diffusing capacity) versus mean intracapillary partial pressure of O_2 ($P\bar{c}_{O_2}$) at sea level (×), 3.5 atm (●), and 4.8 atm (▲), one subject. *Dashed line*, regression (r) of all points (r = 0.992). [From Nairn et al. (95).]

experiment and theory does not depend on the quantitative in vitro values of Θ_{CO}, only on the reciprocal relation between Θ and P_{O_2}. The DL_{CO} decreases to one-seventh over the whole range of P_{O_2}, and the resistance to CO uptake is almost entirely in the red cells. The diffusion resistance of the pulmonary membrane is relatively unimportant.

Another experimental finding that supports the validity of Equation 1 is that a decrease in (peripheral) hematocrit is accompanied by a decrease in DL_{CO} (9, 18, 95), and corrections for this must be made for comparisons; Θ_{CO} is the rate at which 1 ml of pulmonary capillary blood takes up CO for an extracellular P_{CO} of 1 mmHg. The rate at which individual red cells react with CO appears constant from individual to individual (some exceptions to this are discussed in MEASUREMENT OF RATES OF CO AND O_2 EXCHANGE WITH RED BLOOD CELLS (Θ), p. 77), but the number of red cells per milliliter of blood in the pulmonary capillary varies widely. It is certainly decreased in anemia, which in turn decreases ΘVc and increases the resistance of gas uptake by the blood. If CO exchange in the lung were limited by the permeability of the pulmonary membrane, a change in blood hematocrit should not affect the rate of gas exchange. The body could compensate entirely for anemia by increasing pulmonary capillary blood flow ($\dot{Q}c$) to give the same mass flow of O_2, i.e., $\dot{Q}c$ times O_2 content.

MEASUREMENT OF PULMONARY DIFFUSING CAPACITY (TRANSFER FACTOR)

Measurement of DL requires determining experimentally the flux of gas from alveolar air to capillary blood and dividing this by the mean pressure difference causing this exchange. The flux is generally easy to obtain: under steady-state conditions it is the total gas inspired minus the total gas expired; during breath holding or rebreathing it is the change in concentration times the total gas volume. The mean partial pressure difference between the alveolar gas phase and the hemoglobin molecule is much harder to obtain. Alveolar partial pressure itself can be measured by direct sampling or by calculation under steady-state conditions with experimentally measured arterial P_{CO_2} (Pa_{CO_2}) and the alveolar air equation. The partial pressure in equilibrium with the intracellular hemoglobin molecule is the most difficult measurement. In the case of O_2 it rises from 40 mmHg at the start of the capillary to ~100 mmHg at the end of the capillary when air is being breathed. The PA_{O_2} minus end-capillary P_{O_2} (Pc'_{O_2}), the end gradient, is extremely critical in defining mean PA_{O_2} minus capillary P_{O_2} (Pc_{O_2}). For this reason DL is generally measured using CO rather than the more "physiological" species O_2.

Note that CO is also a physiological gas. Approximately 0.4 ml of CO/h are produced in the normal human adult from the degradation of the porphyrin ring of heme. Each α-methene bridge carbon forms a molecule of CO (see the chapter by Coburn and Forman in this *Handbook*). Thus [HbCO] in human blood is never zero. Inhaling up to 10 times the [CO] used in a breath-holding DL_{CO} measurement does not change the mechanical properties of the human lung (59). Continuous breathing of up to 35 times this concentration (14% CO) in one lung of a dog caused no change in the pressure-volume curves and no histological alterations (32), leading to the conclusion that the levels of CO used in measuring DL_{CO} are not damaging to the lung.

When the inspired [CO] is increased to 4% from the normal level of 0.2%, DL_{CO} breath holding decreases 14% when the subject is supine and 11% when sitting (59). If $DL_{CO}/\dot{Q}c$ in any alveolus is >2.5 times the average value, the [HbCO] at the end of the capillary approaches 100% saturation and no more CO is taken up, reducing the measured DL_{CO}. Thus nonuniform distribution of $DL_{CO}/\dot{Q}c$ in the lung can explain the decrease in measured DL_{CO} at high PA_{CO} (60).

The affinity of CO for hemoglobin is so great that if PA_{CO} in the low millimeter of mercury range is used, the gas that is transported into the blood and is mopped up by the red blood cells gives a negligible arteriovenous [HbCO] difference; the capillary HbCO is effectively constant. If a large PA_{CO} were used, of course, large amounts of CO would enter the blood and the arteriovenous difference in P_{CO} ($Pa_{CO} - P\bar{v}_{CO}$) and [HbCO] would become significant. The P_{CO} in equilibrium with blood HbCO, which must be subtracted from the PA_{CO} to obtain the driving gradient for CO diffusion, can be obtained experimentally by several means. First the blood P_{CO} can be calculated from the Haldane relation

$$P_{CO} = \frac{P_{O_2} \times [\text{HbCO}]}{M \times [\text{HbO}_2]} \tag{8}$$

where M is a constant, the relative affinity of CO for hemoglobin compared with that of O_2, and is generally taken as 225. Even though HbCO is constant along the capillary, P_{O_2}/HbO_2 is not. An average P_{O_2}/HbO_2 value can be estimated with sufficient accuracy to make this calculation in most cases. Of course blood [HbCO] has to be measured directly.

A second approach is to measure PA_{CO} after a period of breath holding or rebreathing. By this time the PA_{CO} will have risen to be in equilibrium with the HbCO in the blood. This measurement can be made at a high P_{O_2} to increase the value of PA_{CO} and therefore to make its measurement more accurate, to equilibrate PA_{O_2} with capillary blood more rapidly, and to estimate P_{O_2}/HbO_2 more precisely. The measured PA_{CO} can then be reduced in proportion to the desired PA_{O_2} with the Haldane relation.

Measurement of Pulmonary Diffusing Capacity with CO

Provided PA_{CO} is ≲1%, the rate at which CO enters the capillary blood is not rapid enough to raise the blood [HbCO] significantly during lung transit and the arteriovenous [HbCO] difference is negligible. However, if there is stagnant blood in the alveolar capillaries (49, 52) or hemorrhage into the lung tissue (28), repeated inhalations of gas containing CO may increase the [HbCO] in this pigment significantly and decrease the measured DL_{CO}. Under normal circumstances there is no detectable decrease in breath-holding DL_{CO} after >10 successive measurements.

The concentration of CO in gas samples can be measured by several physical methods: infrared (Pfund) detectors, gas chromatographs, and mass spectrometers using isotopically labeled CO (^{13}CO) with a molecular weight of 29 to avoid the ubiquitous N_2 peak at mass 28.

BREATH-HOLDING METHOD. With this method, the individual makes a maximal inspiration of a gas mixture containing several 10ths percent CO and several percent He (or any other convenient chemically inert insoluble gas as a tracer), holds his breath ~10 s, and expires an alveolar gas sample that is analyzed for He and CO. Depending on the analytical instrumentation used, it is usually helpful and as convenient to measure O_2 and CO_2 in these samples as well. The equation originally developed by Krogh and Krogh (72) is used

$$DL = \frac{-VA}{\Delta t(PB - 47)} \ln\left(\frac{PI_{CO} \times \text{alveolar [He]}}{PA_{CO} \times \text{inspired [He]}}\right) \tag{9}$$

where VA is the alveolar volume STPD, Δt is the breath-holding time in seconds, PB is the barometric pressure in millimeters of mercury, and PI_{CO} is inspired P_{CO}. This modification of the Krogh equation calculates the initial P_{CO} in the expired alveolar sample at the start of the breath-holding period from the relative dilution of the inspired He. Alveolar volume needs to be determined independently. As the inspiration is

maximal, the dilution of He can be used to give a reliable measurement of VA according to the relationship

$$\text{V}_\text{A} = \text{inspired volume} \times \text{alveolar [He]/inspired [He]} \tag{10}$$

This measurement is convenient, and the He ratio is already available to calculate the initial alveolar [CO]. However, in the presence of uneven distribution of inspired gas the calculated VA will be in error.

It was originally assumed (72, 97) that inspiration and expiration of the alveolar samples could be made so rapidly that the time consumed would be negligible in comparison with the total breath-holding time and that VA could be considered constant. However, this is not always true, and different models that allow for changes in VA during inspiration and expiration have been developed to calculate $D_{L_{CO}}$ (50, 65, 94). Several widely used methods measure the breath-holding time from the midpoint in inspiration to that in expiration.

REBREATHING METHOD. In this variation of the breath-holding method the individual rebreathes from a bag containing He and CO rapidly enough to approach continuous mixing so that the bag gas concentration is considered to be the same as that in alveolar gas. The $D_{L_{CO}}$ is calculated from the Krogh equation, except that VA is replaced by VA plus gas volume in the bag plus apparatus (75). Because there is sufficient rebreathing to mix alveolar and bag gas, the dilution of the He originally in the bag gives a correct estimate of total lung VA.

STEADY-STATE METHODS. In this technique (35) the subject inspires a gas mixture containing <0.1% CO until a steady state of CO exchange has been reached (this is usually achieved in <30 s) at which point the rate of CO uptake can be calculated as inspiratory flow rate times concentration of CO inspired minus expiratory flow rate times concentration of CO expired and divided by $P_{A_{CO}}$. Alveolar P_{CO} can be obtained from an end-tidal sample, calculated from an assumed ratio of the dead-space volume to the tidal volume, or calculated from arterial P_{CO_2} (Pa_{CO_2}) and the alveolar air equation. More CO is absorbed than in the breath-holding test, so blood [HbCO] may rise significantly during the measurement. In an effort to keep the level of HbCO low, the inspired [CO] is usually made lower, which has the disadvantage of increasing the significance of the P_{CO} in equilibrium with the HbCO in the blood. Thus a correction for blood HbCO is generally made in this method. Steady-state $D_{L_{CO}}$ (end tidal) (Bates, as cited in ref. 35, p. 852) is generally about two-thirds breath-holding $D_{L_{CO}}$ in the same normal subject. If a model of CO absorption in the lung is developed with defined inspiratory and expiratory patterns, an effective breath-holding time and average DL/VA value can be calculated and a corrected $D_{L_{CO}}$ for the whole lung derived. This result agrees with the breath-holding estimate, itself corrected for finite inspiratory and expiratory times. These findings infer that the differences between the steady-state and breath-holding measurements result primarily from their peculiar errors in calculating $D_{L_{CO}}$ and that the normal lung is probably homogeneous for DL.

Measurement of Pulmonary Diffusing Capacity with O_2

Obviously if O_2 equilibrates completely between the alveolar air and the capillary blood, there will be no end gradient of P_{O_2} and $D_{L_{O_2}}$ cannot be calculated, except as a minimal value of limited use. It is generally accepted that at physiological P_{O_2} the end gradient is small or negligible, but at feasible lower $P_{A_{O_2}}$ there is a measurable end gradient. Thus using $^{16}O_2$, $D_{L_{O_2}}$ can only be measured at a $P_{A_{O_2}}$ of ~50 mmHg. However, there continue to be reports that even at this low $P_{A_{O_2}}$ the end gradient is not significant. Cohen et al. (16) reduced alveolar N_2, theoretically eliminating any effects of nonuniform alveolar ventilation/perfusion ratio ($\dot{V}A/\dot{Q}$) and were unable to find a significant $P_{A_{O_2}} - Pa_{O_2}$. They had normal subjects breathe ~100% O_2 at a reduced total barometric pressure, giving a $P_{A_{O_2}} < 60$ mmHg.

The development of P_{O_2} electrodes that permit the measurement of P_{O_2} in a very small volume of blood has probably been the major stimulus for further studies on $D_{L_{O_2}}$ over the past two decades. Prior to the availability of these instruments, obtaining measurements of blood P_{O_2} was a major part of the effort involved in the measurements.

STEADY-STATE METHODS. In the classic method for the measurement of $D_{L_{O_2}}$ (106) under steady-state conditions, the subject's O_2 and CO_2 exchange and Pa_{O_2} and Pa_{CO_2} were measured at low (55 mmHg) and high (~100 mmHg) $P_{A_{O_2}}$. The goal of the method is to analyze the alveolar-arterial P_{O_2} into that part resulting from the failure of blood P_{O_2} to reach complete equilibrium with alveolar gas [the end gradient ($P_{A_{O_2}} - Pc'_{O_2}$)] and that part resulting from venous-to-arterial shunting across the pulmonary capillary bed (venous admixture, which also includes the effect of uneven $\dot{V}A/\dot{Q}$). Alveolar P_{O_2} is calculated from the alveolar air equation, and mixed venous P_{O_2} ($P\bar{v}_{O_2}$) is estimated. On the assumption that $D_{L_{O_2}}$ and any venous-to-arterial shunt across the lung are constant at the two $P_{A_{O_2}}$ values, these values are obtained by trial and error from the two sets of experimental data, using the Bohr integration to calculate the end gradient and the shunt equation to calculate $Pc'_{O_2} - Pa_{O_2}$. The Bohr integral equation is

$$\frac{D_{L_{O_2}}}{\dot{Q}c} = \int_{[HbO_2]\bar{v}}^{[HbO_2]c'} \frac{d[HbO_2]}{P_{A_{O_2}} - Pc_{O_2}} \tag{11}$$

where $[HbO_2]\bar{v}$ and $[HbO_2]c'$ are the concentration of mixed venous and end-capillary blood, respectively, in milliliters STPD per milliliter. This equation permits calculation of an effective mean value of $P_{A_{O_2}} - Pc_{O_2}$, the diffusion gradient, from its initial and final values, without defining experimentally the shape of the capillary blood P_{O_2} or HbO_2. Arndt et al. (4) and King and Briscoe (66) have published a graphic method of solving this in combination with nonuniform distribution of $\dot{V}_A/\dot{Q}$.

At a high $P_{A_{O_2}}$, the end gradient is minimal, whereas the effect of the venous admixture on $P_{A_{O_2}} - Pa_{O_2}$ is great; the reverse is true at low $P_{A_{O_2}}$. This method is not widely used today but was a trail breaker, particularly in efforts to use it to measure $D_{L_{O_2}}$ during maximal exercise.

Although the effect of a true venous-to-arterial shunt in lowering Pa_{O_2} can be computed from the mixing of proportions of end-capillary and mixed venous blood, this is not so for the effect of uneven $\dot{V}_A/\dot{Q}$. The $Pc'_{O_2} - Pa_{O_2}$ difference produced by nonuniform $\dot{V}_A/\dot{Q}$ increases as $P_{A_{O_2}}$ increases from ~50 mmHg, reaching a maximum and then falling to minimal levels again at very high $P_{A_{O_2}}$ (such as that obtained breathing 100% O_2). Riley and Permutt (106) reexamined the effects of uneven $\dot{V}_A/\dot{Q}$ on the steady-state $D_{L_{O_2}}$ model and found that it would underestimate the value of D_L in the presence of $\dot{V}_A/\dot{Q}$ (at least for the $\dot{V}_A/\dot{Q}$ distribution used in the model).

REBREATHING AND BREATH-HOLDING METHODS. Two methods for the measurement of $D_{L_{O_2}}$ have been described: a rebreathing method and a breath-holding method. Both methods require *1*) simultaneous measurement (or nearly so) of $\dot{Q}c$ by inert-gas uptake and of O_2 uptake, *2*) a low $P_{A_{O_2}}$, approximating $P\bar{v}_{O_2}$, and *3*) subject versatility in respiratory maneuvers (or an anesthetized animal). The rebreathing method measures the uptake of the natural isotope of O_2, $^{16}O_2$; the breath-holding method measures the uptake of the stable isotope $^{18}O_2$.

In the rebreathing method (1–3, 14, 86, 100, 110) it is possible to calculate the small end gradient ($P_{A_{O_2}} - Pc'_{O_2}$) accurately because all measurements are referred to $P_{A_{O_2}}$, and the absolute partial pressure differences among $P\bar{v}_{O_2}$, $P_{A_{O_2}}$, and Pc_{O_2} are small. The technique consists of measuring P_{O_2} continuously at the mouth while the subject rebreathes from a closed-bag system. First a mixture containing N_2O, a soluble inert gas, is rebreathed to measure $\dot{Q}c$. Then a gas mixture that contains a reduced P_{O_2}, adjusted so that it is close to $P\bar{v}_{O_2}$, is rebreathed.

1. Mixed venous P_{O_2} in relation to $P_{A_{O_2}}$ is calculated by plotting the instantaneous O_2 uptake (rate of change of $P_{A_{O_2}} \times V_A$) against $P_{A_{O_2}}$ and extrapolating to zero O_2 uptake. Clearly when instantaneous O_2 uptake from alveolar gases is zero, $P\bar{v}_{O_2}$ must equal $P_{A_{O_2}}$.

2. Pulmonary blood flow is then obtained from measurements with N_2O

$$\frac{dP_{A_{N_2O}}}{dt}(V_{\text{system}} + \alpha_{ti,N_2O}Vti) = \alpha_{B,N_2O}\dot{Q}cP_{A_{N_2O}} \quad (12)$$

where $P_{A_{N_2O}}$ is the alveolar partial pressure of N_2O, V_{system} is the total volume STPD of the lungs plus rebreathing bag, α_{ti,N_2O} is the solubility of N_2O in the lung tissue of volume Vti, α_{B,N_2O} is the solubility of N_2O in blood, and $\dot{Q}c$ is the pulmonary blood flow in milliliters per second.

3. The instantaneous arterial-venous O_2 content difference ($Cc'_{O_2} - C\bar{v}_{O_2}$) is calculated from the following equation

$$Cc'_{O_2} - C\bar{v}_{O_2} = \frac{dP_{A_{O_2}}V_{\text{system}}}{dt\dot{Q}c(P_B - P_{H_2O})} \quad (13)$$

where $P_B - P_{H_2O}$ is the barometric pressure minus the pressure of water vapor.

4. Since $Cc'_{O_2} - C\bar{v}_{O_2}$ is known, the $Pc'_{O_2} - P\bar{v}_{O_2}$ can be obtained by dividing with the effective solubility of O_2 in the blood, α_{B,O_2}. This figure is taken as the slope of the Hb-O_2 equilibrium curve between the $P\bar{v}_{O_2}$ and $P_{A_{O_2}}$. At the low values of $P_{A_{O_2}}$, these O_2 tensions are close enough that this linearization produces no significant error. Having obtained $Pc'_{O_2} - P\bar{v}_{O_2}$, we add this to $P\bar{v}_{O_2}$ and obtain Pc'_{O_2}. In view of the constant effective solubility of O_2 in the blood, a Bohr integration is not necessary; the exchange of O_2 between alveolar gases and capillary blood can be described by the exponential

$$\frac{P_{A_{O_2}} - Pc'_{O_2}}{P_{A_{O_2}} - P\bar{v}_{O_2}} = \exp\left(\frac{-D_{L_{O_2}}760}{\dot{Q}c\alpha_{B,O_2}}\right) \quad (14)$$

Because $P_{A_{O_2}}$, Pc'_{O_2}, $P\bar{v}_{O_2}$, $\dot{Q}c$, and effective α_{B,O_2} are known, $D_{L_{O_2}}$ can be calculated. It may appear that there are so many calculations, all possible sources of error, that the cumulative error in the end gradient would be prohibitive. However, because the measurements are all obtained in reference to alveolar gas, most of these errors appear to cancel out. The average value for the seated human at rest was 31 $ml \cdot min^{-1} \cdot mmHg^{-1}$, which is not significantly different from the known values of single-breath $D_{L_{CO}} \times 1.23$.

In the breath-holding method for the measurement of $D_{L_{O_2}}$, O_2 uptake is measured with the stable O_2 isotope $^{18}O_2$. There are two advantages of using this labeled O_2. *1*) The partial pressure of the labeled species in mixed venous blood is negligible, therefore at least four times as much $^{18}O_2$ must diffuse into the blood from alveolar gas to reach equilibrium as $^{16}O_2$; mixed venous blood normally enters the alveolar capillaries already 75% saturated with O_2. This additional blood capacity increases $P_{A_{O_2}} - Pc'_{O_2}$ and makes this critical measurement more accurate. *2*) Because $P_{A_{O_2}}$ is set experimentally near $P\bar{v}_{O_2}$, the effective solubility of $^{18}O_2$ in capillary blood may be considered constant and equal to

$$\frac{\text{total elemental blood } O_2 \text{ content}}{\text{total elemental } P_{O_2}}$$

This means that the relation between Pc'_{O_2} and $D_{L_{O_2}}$

can be described by Equation 14 (the O_2 species becomes $^{18}O_2$).

The procedure consists of taking a single maximum inspiration of a gas mixture containing ~0.2% $^{18}O_2$, 6.5% $^{16}O_2$, 1% acetylene, 0.5% neon (as a tracer), and the remainder N_2, holding the breath for various periods of time, and expiring an alveolar sample that is then analyzed for the concentration of each of the gases (most conveniently done with mass spectrometer) (Fig. 2). Pulmonary blood flow is calculated in the same manner as for the rebreathing method. Mixed venous $P_{^{18}O_2}$ is zero.

The last datum, the $Pc_{^{18}O_2}$, can be obtained from Equation 15, which states that the instantaneous rate of $^{18}O_2$ disappearance from the alveolar gas must equal $\dot{Q}c(Cc'_{^{18}O_2} - C\bar{v}_{^{18}O_2})$. Because $P\bar{v}_{^{18}O_2}$ is zero this becomes simplified to

$$\frac{dP_{A^{18}O_2}V_A}{dt(P_B - P_{H_2O})} = \frac{-Pc'_{^{18}O_2}\alpha_{B,^{18}O_2}}{760} \quad (15)$$

Equation 14 can now be solved for DL_{O_2}. (These calculations have been simplified for exposition. The exact details can be found in refs. 57 and 60). The DL_{O_2} by this breath-holding method at a $P_{A_{O_2}}$ of 42 mmHg averaged (5 normal subjects) 33 ml·min^{-1}·mmHg^{-1} where DL_{CO} (measured simultaneously by including CO in the inspired gas mixture) was 44 ml·min^{-1}·mmHg^{-1}. This discrepancy between O_2 and CO measurements can only be explained by nonuniformity of $DL/\dot{Q}c$. Measurements were also made at a $P_{A_{O_2}}$ of 220 mmHg, in which case DL_{O_2} was 6 ml·min^{-1}·mmHg^{-1}.

Calculations of Pulmonary Diffusing Capacity From Dimensions of Alveolar-Capillary Bed

In 1964 (35) there was no method to measure the surface area of the alveolar-capillary membrane or the volume of the capillary blood, and therefore the calculations, particularly of the diffusing capacity of the pulmonary membrane (Dm), were no more accurate than those of G. Hüfner in 1897 (35). However, in the 1970s Weibel and his associates (122–124) applied histological morphometric techniques to the measurements of the dimensions of the pulmonary gas-exchange system. The necessary methods were developed largely in Weibel's laboratory and consist of a statistical calculation of the area of a structure and of its thickness from measurements of the number of intercepts on that surface by standard lines superimposed on the microscopic or electron-microscopic section. In this manner these authors calculate the total surface area of the pulmonary capillaries and of the alveolar septa. The reciprocal of Dm can be calculated as the sum of the reciprocals of the conductances of the components of the diffusion path from alveolar gas to hemoglobin molecule. This path includes the alveolar surface lining, the pulmonary membrane tissue (including epithelium, basement membrane, and endothelium), plasma, and red blood cell. Each conductance is computed as area (in centimeters) times specific permeability (in cm^2·mmHg^{-1}·min^{-1}) divided by the thickness (in centimeters). The specific permeability data are obtained from independent measurements or from the literature.

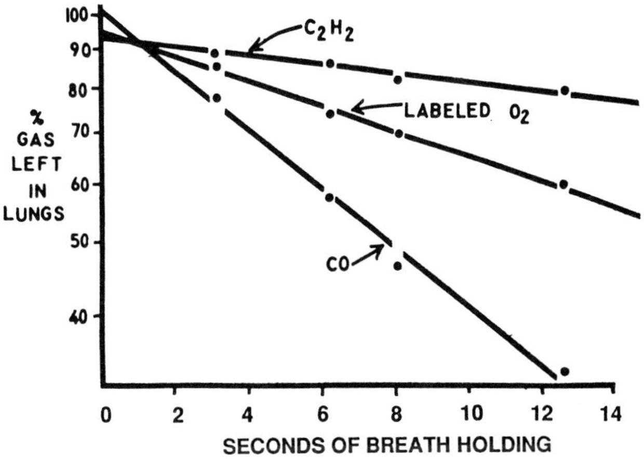

FIG. 2. Graph of logarithm of percent of C_2H_2, $^{18}O_2$, and CO left in alveolar gas (1 − fraction that has disappeared) during breath holding in one subject. Alveolar elemental P_{O_2} was 42 mmHg. Each *line* is a least-mean-squares regression. Depression of time zero intercept of *C_2H_2 curve* is caused by its solution in pulmonary tissues; depression of $^{18}O_2$ intercept is considered to be caused by initial uptake of labeled O_2 by pulmonary capillary blood. [From Hyde et al. (57).]

In general the morphometric values of DL are greater than those measured experimentally, by all techniques (22, 26, 118, 128). The Vc measured by morphometric methods (200 ml) is more than twice the value obtained by breath-holding DL_{CO} (100 ml). On the other hand, Dm_{O_2} is ~10 times greater than the comparable value of breath-holding Dm_{CO} times 1.23: 567 ml·min^{-1}·mmHg^{-1} compared with 42 ml·min^{-1}·mmHg^{-1} (128).

The Dm and DL_{O_2} increase with increasing body weight in a single species (112) and among different species (122) and increase with inflation of the lungs (41). Capillary blood volume is greater in the more dependent parts of the lung, and the relative surface area is greater in the less dependent parts of the lung (42, 130).

MEASUREMENT OF RATES OF CO AND O_2 EXCHANGE WITH RED BLOOD CELLS (Θ)

The rates at which O_2 and CO are taken up by red cells of all species are so great that their measurement must be carried out in a rapid-mixing apparatus. Only a limited number of observations have been reported and almost all on humans.

Measurement of Θ_{CO}

MEASUREMENTS OF Θ_{CO} WITH CONTINUOUS-FLOW RAPID-MIXING APPARATUS. The most useful data are those of Θ_{CO} on humans at 37°C for use in the calculation of Vc and Dm from measurements of DL_{CO} at varying P_{O_2}. The most widely used values are those Roughton and Forster (108) obtained with continuous-flow rapid-mixing instruments on blood from a limited number of normal subjects from both sides of the Atlantic with spectrophotometric and reversion spectroscopic analytical techniques.

The measurements of Θ_{CO} in 1957 (108) were made at greater than physiological extracellular pH, 7.8–8.0 rather than 7.4. Recent values of Θ_{CO} (71) obtained on blood from five normal individuals at 37°C and pH 7.4 with a continuous-flow spectrophotometric rapid-reaction apparatus are shown in Figure 3. Although the intercept of $1/\Theta$ on the ordinate is the same for all the data, at higher P_{O_2} the value of $1/\Theta$ at pH 7.4 is significantly lower. Equations 16–18 are the regression equations for these data. At pH 7.4

$$1/\Theta = 1.30 + 0.0041\ P_{O_2}\ \text{mmHg} \qquad r = 0.99 \tag{16}$$

At pH 8.2

$$1/\Theta = 1.19 + 0.0061\ P_{O_2}\ \text{mmHg} \qquad r = 0.97 \tag{17}$$

At pH 8.0 (1957 data)

$$1/\Theta = 0.7 + 0.0061\ P_{O_2}\ \text{mmHg} \tag{18}$$

When the more recent values (71) of Θ_{CO} at physiological pH are used, a larger Dm is obtained than with the 1957 data (108) and the value of Vc obtained is 15%–20% smaller. Other experimental data (71) show that Θ_{CO} decreases ~8.8% per pH unit over the physiological range. These data were obtained in fresh normal human red blood cells suspended in 0.03 M phosphate buffer in the absence of any bicarbonate. Substituting 0.0225 M $NaHCO_3$ at a P_{CO_2} of 40 mmHg and pH 7.4 gave the same value of Θ_{CO} as in the phosphate buffer. The primary variable is pH, not P_{CO_2}. Depleting red cell 2,3-diphosphoglycerate (2,3-DPG) in a limited number of experiments at high P_{O_2} had no effect on Θ_{CO}.

Roughton and Forster (35, 108) applied two theoretical corrections to their experimental values of Θ_{CO} to calculate Vc and Dm from measurements of DL_{CO} at different $P_{A_{O_2}}$. The first correction was made because P_{CO} in the in vitro rapid-mixing apparatus was ~2 orders of magnitude greater (70 mmHg) than the in vivo value in the pulmonary capillaries (<1 mmHg) in order to obtain a [CO] high enough to form adequate HbCO. The formation of HbCO at P_{O_2} from 100 to 600 mmHg, the normal physiological range, is a two-step process

$$Hb_4(O_2)_4 \rightarrow Hb_4(O_2)_3 + O_2 \tag{19a}$$

$$Hb_4(O_2)_3 + CO \rightarrow Hb_4(O_2)_3CO \tag{19b}$$

At these P_{O_2} levels there is initially little unliganded hemoglobin available to react with CO; thus the overall reaction velocity depends on the dissociation of HbO_2 to provide these unbound hemoglobin sites (Eq. 19a). The rate of the reaction of CO with unliganded hemoglobin (Eq. 19b) is proportional to the [CO]. If the [CO] is too great, this reaction consumes the unliganded hemoglobin much faster than the dissociation reaction can form it, and the overall rate of formation of HbCO, the measured end product, is limited by the rate of HbO_2 dissociation. This phenomenon has been measured in hemoglobin solution by Gibson and Roughton (44), who found that the measured value of Θ_{CO} at the higher P_{CO} is less than the value at "physiological" P_{CO} by the factor

$$\frac{1}{1 + 0.36[CO]/[O_2]} \tag{20}$$

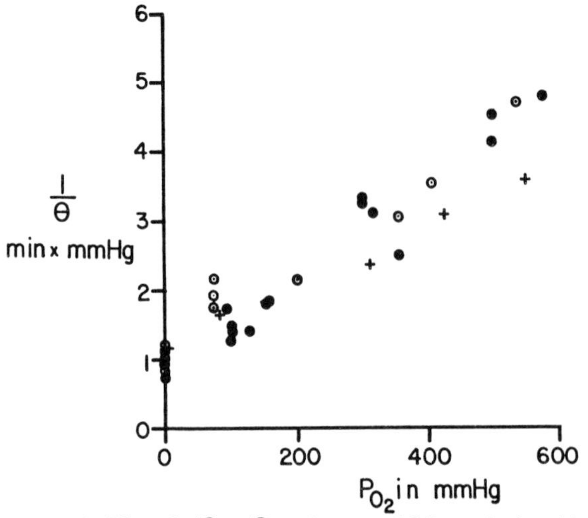

FIG. 3. Plot of $1/\Theta_{CO}$ (Θ_{CO}, the rate of CO uptake in ml/min for 1 ml of normal whole blood for a P_{CO} of 1 mmHg) against P_{O_2} in mmHg for normal human red cells at 37°C measured in a continuous-flow rapid-mixing apparatus analyzed by a split-beam spectrophotometer. ⊙, ●: Reacting solution contained 2 mM $NaHCO_3$, 2.2 mM CaCl, 2.2 mM KCl, and 145 mM NaCl; ⊙, experiments at pH 8.2 (71); ●, experiments at pH 7.8–8.0 done in 1957 (108); +, experiments in 30 mM phosphate buffer plus 112 mM NaCl at pH 7.4 (71).

The values of Θ published in 1957 (108) have been corrected by this factor. It was not technically feasible at that time to measure Θ over a wide range of P_{CO} and verify the correction. This has now been done (71) and (presumably owing to the retarding effect of simultaneous chemical reaction plus diffusion in the red cells) raising P_{CO} from 70 to 300 mmHg has no significant effect on Θ_{CO}. Therefore correcting the in vitro values of Θ_{CO} upward is not justified, and the proper values to use for the calculation of Vc and Dm are given in Figure 3 (pH 7.4) and Equation 16.

The second correction applied to the experimental data in 1957 was to allow for differences in gas permeability in the red cell plasma membrane expressed as λ, the ratio of the permeability of the membrane to the permeability of the cell interior.

There is no clear evidence that the diffusion resistance of the red cell membrane significantly limits the rate of gas uptake; there is experimental evidence against it for CO_2, whose permeability through the lipid membrane should not be strikingly different from the permeability of O_2 (111). Certainly the possible diffusion resistance of the red cell plasma membrane is far less than the resistance of the fluid stagnant layer that is concluded to exist around the red cells when the suspension is still for a millisecond or less (17, 71). In reality investigators have used the data computed for a λ of 2.5, which actually corresponds to the uncorrected experimental measurements in 1957. It seems most reasonable to accept the pH 7.4 data in Figure 3 as the best estimate for Θ for red cells in the pulmonary capillaries, acknowledging that there may be a measurably small stagnant layer about the cells in the in vitro measurements in the rapid-reaction apparatuses that are not present when the cells are in the capillaries.

MEASUREMENTS OF Θ_{CO} AND Θ_{O_2} WITH STOP-FLOW RAPID-MIXING APPARATUS. The measurement of Θ_{CO} with the continuous-flow rapid-mixing apparatus requires a relatively large amount of red cell suspension, ~1–2 ml of blood, to determine HbCO percentage at each time point, and 5–8 such time points are needed to define the time course of HbCO formation at a given P_{O_2}, which provides only one estimate of Θ_{CO} (1 point in Fig. 3). In a stop-flow rapid-mixing instrument the flowing reactants are suddenly stopped and the progress of the chemical reaction is followed by spectrophotometric methods on a cathode-ray oscilloscope. The instrument consumes <1/50 as much reactant as the continuous-flow apparatus in a single experiment, which provides the entire time course of the reaction. Thus the total gain in economy of cells is ~300- to 1,000-fold. In addition the necessity of making fewer individual runs saves time.

For all these reasons, many investigators studied the effect of physiological factors on Θ_{CO} and Θ_{O_2} with a stop-flow rapid-reaction apparatus (53, 107). Coin and Olson (17) have shown that the rates of ligand reactions with hemoglobin in intact cells in a stop-flow rapid-mixing apparatus appeared to be slowed by diffusion of the ligand through a stagnant layer of solvent at the surface of the cells. As measured by a stop-flow rapid-mixing apparatus, Θ_{CO} was as little as half the value obtained under similar conditions in a continuous-flow rapid-reaction apparatus (71). Therefore the values of Θ obtained in the continuous-flow rapid-mixing apparatus appear more correct, although we should be able to use the stop-flow data, with their greater economy of time and reactant, to estimate changes in Θ, bearing always in mind that they underestimate its absolute value.

Measurement of Θ_{O_2}

The reaction velocity constant for the combination of O_2 with hemoglobin in solution is ~30 times faster than the comparable rate for CO (35). However, Θ_{O_2} in the red cell is only approximately twice as large as Θ_{CO}, because the uptake processes within the red cell are partly rate limited by diffusion, which is the same for both gases. It is more difficult to obtain physiologically useful measurements of Θ_{O_2} than Θ_{CO}. In the body, hemoglobin is always partly saturated with O_2 at the start of the exchanging capillary, reducing the maximum change in HbO_2 that can be expected, and the exchange process goes nearly to completion by the end of the capillary transit. In the case of CO, blood normally has very little HbCO at the start of the capillary bed, and the total change in HbCO is always less than a few percent saturation. Thus a constant Θ_{CO} through the capillary bed can be assumed, but this simplifying assumption cannot be made for O_2.

Effects of Physiological Variables on Θ

CONCENTRATION OF RED BLOOD CELLS. Roughton and Forster (108) defined Θ as the rate of CO uptake in milliliters CO STPD per minute for an extracellular pressure gradient of 1 mmHg in 1 ml of blood (one could also determine the rate of CO uptake per cell and then multiply by the number of red cells per milliliter of pulmonary capillary blood). The experimental values of Θ are obtained by in vitro experiments and based on the assumption that all samples of the red cells have the same intrinsic uptake rate; the experimental data at a relatively dilute hematocrit are corrected to an assumed pulmonary capillary blood hematocrit. Thus any change in the hematocrit of pulmonary capillary blood will alter Θ. It is assumed that the hematocrit of pulmonary capillary blood is the same as that in peripheral blood samples. This may not be precisely true, but it is the best estimate that can be obtained.

FACTORS ALTERING THE GAS-UPTAKE RATE OF INDIVIDUAL RED BLOOD CELLS. *P_{O_2}*. As discussed in MEASUREMENT OF PULMONARY DIFFUSING CAPACITY (TRANSFER FACTOR), p. 73, an increase in P_{O_2} causes a decrease in Θ_{CO} (and in Θ_{O_2}).

Temperature. The Θ_{CO} increases ~2.5%/°C over the physiological range (34). This should not be an important factor, as lung temperature does not vary more than several degrees, even in fever. Hypothermic conditions during open-heart surgery lower lung temperatures significantly, but this is a highly artificial situation. Because Θ_{O_2} is faster than Θ_{CO}, the effect of temperature changes should be even less important for O_2 gradients. Temperature in the extremities is normally less than that in the body core, but even with hypothermia, exercise, and anemia, which exaggerate the P_{O_2} gradients within the blood, the effect on O_2 exchange is not important (79).

Changes in Hb-O_2 equilibrium curve. The rate of the bimolecular chemical reaction between CO and hemoglobin is proportional to the concentration of unliganded hemoglobin. As a reasonable approximation it is assumed that the reaction of O_2 with hemoglobin is essentially complete before any significant amounts of CO are taken up in the blood. Therefore the concentration of unliganded hemoglobin approximates that in red cells estimated from the Hb-O_2 equilibrium curve, and any factors that alter the O_2 half-saturation pressure of hemoglobin (P_{50}) should alter Θ_{CO}. Experimentally this has turned out to be qualitatively true. An increase in pH or decrease in P_{CO_2}, which reduces the free unliganded hemoglobin, decreases Θ_{CO} at the same P_{O_2} (34, 71). An increased red blood cell concentration of 2,3-DPG (6, 7), which increases the available unliganded hemoglobin, should increase Θ_{CO}, but in preliminary studies on intact cells no significant change in Θ_{CO} was seen.

Changes in cell size and hemoglobin concentration. There is no good evidence that changes of the mean corpuscular hemoglobin concentration, of the magnitude seen in disease, alter Θ significantly. Among different animal species, an increase in red blood cell size is accompanied by a decrease in Θ_{O_2}. This can be explained, at least semiquantitatively, by the increased diffusion distances in the larger cells (53). The possible rate limitation by stagnant layers of suspending fluid in the stop-flow rapid-mixing apparatus used may have affected the results.

The specific rate of O_2 uptake by sickle cell hemoglobin (Hb S) is about half that of normal control cells, while the dissociation rate (O_2 egress) was faster, compatible with a decreased P_{50}, possibly from the increased 2,3-DPG found in sickle cells (76, 107). These findings, combined with the fact that the P_{50} of normal hemoglobin and Hb S are the same in the same chemical environment, suggest that the rate differences are not the results of differences in the molecular hemoglobin structure. The change in Θ_{CO} should increase $D_{L_{CO}}$ by itself. However, these kinetic effects on the hemoglobin reactions are attenuated in intact cells by the simultaneous diffusion processes. No difference was detected between the O_2-uptake rates of sickled and nonsickled Hb S cells. The Θ_{O_2} for spherocytes is not remarkably different from the Θ_{O_2} for normal red blood cells (70).

Plasma membrane thickness. The diffusion resistance of the red cell membrane to O_2 and CO is probably too low to be measured (34, 73). The experimental difficulty is that the resistance to the uptake of CO and O_2 presented by simultaneous chemical reaction plus diffusion within the red cell interior can account for almost all of the rate limitation of uptake by the cells. Measurements of the kinetics of CO_2 exchange between intracellular and extracellular bicarbonate analyzed by ^{13}C nuclear magnetic resonance showed that the rate was the same in intact and lysed cells (111). This indicates that cell membrane produced no significant rate-limiting influence on the CO_2 reactions, which, in the presence of high concentrations of carbonic anhydrase, are more rapid than those of O_2 and CO intracellular hemoglobin. Certainly variations in the diffusion resistance of the red cell membrane to gas transport should not exert any influence on the value of Θ.

FACTORS INFLUENCING PULMONARY DIFFUSING CAPACITY, MEMBRANE DIFFUSING CAPACITY, AND CAPILLARY VOLUME

Introduction

If the validity of Equation 1 is accepted, we can measure $D_{L_{CO}}$ by any technique at different $P_{A_{O_2}}$, obtain the corresponding value of Θ_{CO} from the literature, and solve the equation graphically, plotting $1/D_{L_{CO}}$ versus $1/\Theta$, as in Figure 1. The slope equals 1/Vc, in this case 77 ml, and the intercept on the ordinate is 1/Dm, in this case 90 ml $\cdot$ min^{-1} $\cdot$ mmHg^{-1}. Measurements of Dm and Vc have been made in a wide range of physiological conditions and disease, and the results are reasonable. Their absolute values depend on the in vitro estimates of Θ_{CO}.

The value of DL, as a measure of the capability of the lung system as a gas-exchange organ, can be altered by changes in *1*) the diffusing characteristics of the alveolocapillary membrane (Dm) and *2*) the diffusing characteristics of the total number of red blood cells in the capillary bed (ΘVc). The important factors that alter Θ have been discussed in MEASUREMENT OF RATES OF CO AND O_2 EXCHANGE WITH RED BLOOD CELLS (Θ), p. 77, and consist of variables that change the rate of gas uptake by the individual red cells and those that change the concentration of red cells in the pulmonary capillaries. As calculated by morphometry, Dm is the effective overall transfer function of the total alveolar epithelium, basement membrane, endothelium, and plasma up to the red cell, in series. As estimated from $D_{L_{CO}}$ in different $P_{A_{O_2}}$, Dm is that fraction of the total transfer resistance, $1/D_{L_{CO}}$, that does not decrease when $P_{A_{O_2}}$ rises. The Vc is the effective volume of blood in the alveolar capillaries that take up CO. The Dm and Vc are interdependent; the alveolar-capillary surface for a capillary that contains no red cells is not included in a measurement of $D_{L_{CO}}$, although it may be in morphometric estimations. Without an alveolar-capillary membrane covering it, Vc cannot exist. Therefore the magnitude of Dm and of Vc must to some extent vary together with physiological variables. In diseased states it may be that Dm is decreased, as by thickening, without decreasing the capillary blood volume, but not in the extreme where the thickness of the capillary wall would obliterate the capillary lumen.

The diffusion coefficient (cm^2/s) for O_2 in plasma at 37°C can change ~5-fold over the range of plasma protein concentrations seen clinically (10). The "average" thickness of the layer of plasma around the red cells in the capillaries can vary from practically zero (88), if the cells are deformed against the capillary wall, to several microns if the lumen is much larger than the cells. Thus the contribution of the diffusion resistance of this plasma to $D_{L_{CO}}$ is not obvious. Weibel (128) estimates the harmonic mean of the interposed plasma thickness in humans as 0.15 μm of a total distance (air to red cell) of 0.77 μm. Because

1/Dm appears to be ~50% of the total diffusion resistance in the lung of humans under physiological circumstances, the plasma diffusion resistance should contribute <10% to the total. Thus, although it is possible that alterations in the plasma diffusion coefficient could produce measured changes in DL_{CO}, it seems unlikely to be of great importance.

Replacement of alveolar gas with fluid, as in lung lavage (74), might be considered an extreme decrease in Dm (or an exaggeration of stratified diffusion gradients in the airway). In humans CO_2 and O_2 appear to equilibrate between alveolar fluid and end-capillary blood in <30 s.

Body Size

By morphometric calculations (125, 129), DL_{O_2} increases in proportion to body mass in the same species and among species. Breath-holding DL_{CO} increase in proportion to body weight in humans (23, 35). It is eminently reasonable that resting DL_{O_2} increases with increasing body size in order that $PA_{O_2} - Pa_{O_2}$ remain approximately constant as metabolic rate increases. It has been pointed out that morphometric DL_{O_2} increases in proportion to body mass, although metabolic rate increases only as body mass to an exponent of 0.75 (128).

Alveolar Volume

With increased VA among individuals, DL_{CO} increases, since both increase with body size (73). In a single individual, DL_{CO} breath-holding increases with VA but at a rate less than proportional at rest (where most measurements are made) but nearly proportional during exercise or while supine (46, 50, 81, 87). In general DL_{CO} increases with an increase in VA because of an increase in Dm. No mechanism that is completely consistent with the experimental data is available. The effects of change in VA and of change in hemodynamic factors operating in the pulmonary capillary bed are closely related. These effects can be summarized as follows:

1. Under conditions where the alveolar capillary bed could be expected to be evenly perfused, DL increases somewhat less than proportionally to the increase in VA. These conditions would obtain during exercise and in the supine position.

2. Under conditions where the alveolar capillary bed is known to be unevenly perfused, as in the erect position or when pulmonary blood flow is reduced by the Valsalva maneuver or by positive-pressure breathing (31), the effect of an increase in VA is much less.

3. The changes in DL_{CO} with VA are similar in the breath-holding, rebreathing, and steady-state (end-tidal sample) methods, except that in the erect position at rest, an increase in VA has little effect on DL_{CO}, as measured by the rebreathing or steady-state methods, but does cause the breath-holding DL_{CO} to increase, albeit less than when the capillary bed is better filled.

It is possible that two basic mechanisms are operating. The first is that an increase in $\dot{Q}c$ and/or transmural capillary pressure increases capillary blood volume but a maximum is reached when all capillaries are open. The second is that an increase in VA per se increases Dm. When VA is increased at rest while erect, the increased hydrostatic gradients decrease capillary blood volume, at least at the apices, but increase Dm. The net effect is little change in DL_{CO}.

If breath-holding DL_{CO} is calculated from samples of the expirate, considering VA constant and taking breath-holding time from the start of inspiration to the collection of sample, gas samples from the later portions of the breath (where VA is lower) give a higher value than samples from earlier parts of the expirate. This last-gas-out should have originated largely from the apical regions of the lung where DL/VA should be low (88), so this finding is not expected. However, if corrections are made for the effective breath-holding time and the changes in DL/VA during the measurement, DL_{CO} is approximately the same in the first 90% of the expired breath (21).

Clinicians find it useful to calculate the index DL_{CO}/VA, sometimes called the Krogh constant (22, 30, 47), although since DL_{CO} does not vary in proportion to the first power of VA, this ratio would not be expected to be constant in an individual. The advantages of using the Krogh constant are *1*) it can be calculated without measuring VA independently in the breath-holding DL_{CO} technique (see Eq. 10) and *2*) it does compensate to some extent for changes in VA within an individual patient.

Pulmonary Hemodynamics and Increased Metabolic Rate

The DL provides a method to measure changes in Vc in the intact organism and to study its regulation. The DL increases with exercise; Krogh and Krogh (72) developed the CO method to demonstrate this. It appears reasonable to assume that an increase in $\dot{Q}L$ or capillary transmural pressure increases the size and uniformity of the capillary bed by straightforward hemodynamic factors. Maneuvers that would be expected to alter pulmonary blood flow or pressure generally alter DL_{CO} and DL_{O_2} (46) by all methods in the expected direction; a Valsalva maneuver decreases DL and a Müller maneuver increases it. Exceptions are noted later. The transmural pressure in the capillaries would appear to be more important than $\dot{Q}c$. If left atrial pressure is low, raising pulmonary arterial pressure causes an increase in DL_{CO} (11). If left atrial pressure is high, raising pulmonary arterial pressure has much less effect. If the capillaries are blocked by microspheres injected into the right side of the heart, the left atrial pressure becomes the determining factor in changing Vc (64). Gurtner and Fowler (48) found that all of the increase in $D_{L_{CO}}$ with exercise in the erect position could be related to the increase in V_A. However, it seems unreasonable that increasing pressure in the pulmonary circulation would have no effect on $D_{L_{CO}}$. Raising bronchial blood pressure in the perfused dog lung to 150 mmHg did not alter $D_{L_{CO}}$ (64). Inspiring against negative pressure during the breath-holding $D_{L_{CO}}$ measurement increased its value to a degree equivalent to a low level of exercise (20). The administration of epinephrine or isoproterenol or the release of a Valsalva maneuver, both while seated or supine, increased breath-holding $D_{L_{CO}}$ in proportion to the increase in $\dot{Q}c$ (77). Inhaling histamine produces a slight decrease in breath-holding $D_{L_{CO}}$ (15). Transient changes in pulmonary blood flow are associated with synchronous changes in $D_{L_{CO}}$.

Dinitrophenol produces a 600% increase in O_2 consumption in anesthetized dogs, a 150% increase in blood pulmonary flow, but only a 15% increase in breath-holding $D_{L_{CO}}$ (68, 101). Therefore O_2 metabolism itself is not a regulator of D_L. However, the lung does adapt to metabolic needs, as in hypoxia, by increasing its diffusing surface (56). An unusual finding was that exercise in a supine subject did not lead to increased breath-holding $D_{L_{CO}}$ (48), apparently because $D_{L_{CO}}$ in the supine position is already increased over its value at rest (at or above functional residual volume) and therefore cannot increase as much with increasing exercise as it does in the seated subject.

The reserve of the pulmonary capillary is large, and destruction or physiological alterations in part of the bed can be compensated for by the opening up of other areas. If the pulmonary blood can be increased enough to expand the entire bed, the D_L should give a maximum value, which would give an index of the lung exchange capabilities. However, although $D_{L_{CO}}$ has been reported to reach a maximum plateau with exercise, this apparently results from a limitation of pulmonary blood flow but not necessarily because the capillary bed is maximally expanded (3, 55, 61, 62, 114). Breath-holding $D_{L_{CO}}$ and $\dot{Q}c$, the latter measured by breath-holding acetylene disappearance, both decreased ~35% in a normal subject during exposure to 8 times normal gravity for 1 min (104). Although the decreased $\dot{Q}c$, presumably from pooling of blood in the more dependent portions of the body, may have caused the decrease in D_L directly, it is more likely that a large portion of the blood flow was diverted into nonventilated regions of the lung.

The $D_{L_{O_2}}$ increased much more than $D_{L_{CO}}$ during exercise (26). The most likely explanation is that inhomogeneity of capillary blood flow, Dm, and/or Vc decreased with the increase in $\dot{Q}c$ and increased the $D_{L_{O_2}}$ while having a minimal effect on $D_{L_{CO}}$.

Using a water-filled body plethysmograph with augmented sensitivity, Menkes et al. (83) were able to measure pulsations in soluble inert-gas uptake as well as in CO uptake. The pulsatile soluble-gas uptake represents pulsatile flow into the capillaries, with or without pulsatile changes in Vc. However, the pulsatile CO uptake is strong evidence that Vc pulses with the heartbeat. Fowler and Maloney (40) had earlier sought evidence for pulsatile Vc by measuring radioactivity at the surface of the lung after ^{51}Cr-labeled red cells had been introduced into the circulation. They were not technically able to measure rapid changes in radioactivity but ingeniously got around this by gating the radioactivity measurements to different parts of the pulse cycle. The reason they found no pulsation in Vc with the pulse is not known.

Partial Pressure of CO_2, pH, and Shifts in Hb-O_2 Equilibrium

Increasing $P_{A_{CO_2}}$ increases breath-holding $D_{L_{CO}}$ (105) in humans and in isolated cat lungs (58) perfused in the normal direction or in reverse. However, other investigators (64) have reported that breathing 10.5% CO_2 produced no change in $D_{L_{CO}}$ in isolated perfused dog lungs. Particularly because of the short duration of the measurements, it appears unlikely that these changes in the capillary bed are caused by changes in vascular dimensions; rather it is more likely that Θ_{CO} was increased by the changes in P_{CO_2} or in pH. However, the increase of Θ_{CO} with pH measured in vitro (71) does not appear great enough to explain all of the increases in $D_{L_{CO}}$ found in subjects.

Alveolar Partial Pressure of O_2

Increasing $P_{A_{O_2}}$ of course decreases Θ_{CO} because of the decreased concentration of unliganded hemoglobin reactant and therefore decreases $D_{L_{CO}}$. The Θ_{O_2} also decreases as P_{O_2} rises and for the same reason, but this is of no physiological significance since the effect only occurs after the hemoglobin has become highly saturated with O_2 (see *Measurement of Θ_{O_2}*, p. 77).

Breath-holding $D_{L_{CO}}$ decreases as $P_{A_{O_2}}$ increases in the manner shown in Figure 1. The $D_{L_{CO}}$ obtained is the same, whether the $P_{A_{O_2}}$ has been at the same value as during the breath-holding measurement for the previous 10–20 min or has been at any value from ~60 to 650 mmHg. The $P_{A_{O_2}}$ does not appear to alter Vc or Dm over this range. However, if $P_{A_{O_2}}$ is maintained at $\lesssim$50 mmHg for several minutes before the measurement, $D_{L_{CO}}$ is increased when measured at any P_{O_2} from 60 to 650 mmHg during breath holding. These results are interpreted to mean that the hemodynamic dimensions of the alveolar capillary bed are not affected by P_{O_2} over the range from 60 to 650 mmHg, but when it drops below ~50 mmHg, Vc increases, and possibly Dm, presumably as a result of hemodynamic changes. Healthy subjects in the first three days at high altitude (>14,000 ft; $P_{A_{O_2}}$ ~ 50 mmHg) showed a significant drop in $D_{L_{CO}}$ and $\dot{V}c$ sufficient to account for much of the alveolar-arterial P_{O_2} gradient seen (131).

Temperature

With decreased temperature, Θ_{O_2} decreases (see *Effects of Physiological Variables on* Θ, p. 79). However, there may be additional changes in the hemodynamics of the capillary bed, i.e., in Vc and/or Dm. The breath-holding $D_{L_{CO}}$ in isolated perfused cat lungs decreases as the temperature falls from ~37°C to 5°C, with the hemodynamic conditions maintained constant. The Q_{10} for this decrease is 1.90 and results from a fall in Dm while Vc increases, both in addition to the drop in Θ_{CO} seen in vitro (103). Single-breath $D_{L_{CO}}$ increases with age up to ~19 yr and then decreases ~2% a year (23, 43). The Vc does not fall as early as Dm (43). Insofar as possible subjects with pulmonary disease were not included, this would appear to be the result of a normal physiological aging process. Nonuniformity of the distribution of diffusing capacity, $\dot{Q}c$, and $\dot{V}A$ will alter measured $D_{L_{CO}}$, generally to decrease it (see the chapter by Hlastala in this *Handbook*).

Blood Hemoglobin Concentration

Any factor that reduces the total concentration of hemoglobin in the red cells in the alveolar capillary bed will cause the measured value of $D_{L_{CO}}$ to fall [see MEASUREMENT OF RATES OF CO AND O_2 EXCHANGE WITH RED BLOOD CELLS (Θ), p. 77].

Miscellaneous

The $D_{L_{CO}}$ decreases in diseases that have reduced dimensions of the pulmonary capillary bed, i.e., lower Dm or Vc, or a decrease in Θ_{CO}, as caused by a decreased concentration of red cells in the capillary bed (36, 96a). The physiological factors numerated in *Effects of Physiological Variables on* Θ, p. 79, can all affect $D_{L_{CO}}$. However, there has been no instance reported where Θ_{CO}, under the same physical chemical conditions, is abnormal. Nonuniformity of DL can produce changes in the measured values for the whole lung (110), but this is discussed in the chapter by Hlastala in this *Handbook* and is more of a clinical phenomenon (80).

Measurements of CO exchange in the lungs are made at low $P_{A_{CO}}$ (several mmHg or less) so that the concentration of HbCO in the capillary blood does not rise and produce a significant equilibrated P_{CO} back pressure. If there is stagnant blood in the capillaries, or hemorrhage, this hemoglobin will take up CO and increase $D_{L_{CO}}$, primarily because of an increased Vc with little change in Dm (81). Repeated measurements of breath-holding $D_{L_{CO}}$ may produce large increases in the [HbCO] in this local pool and reduce the value of experimentally determined $D_{L_{CO}}$ (28). In a normal lung, however, even a dozen rapidly repeated breath-holding measurements of CO uptake do not produce a fall in $D_{L_{CO}}$.

Values of $D_{L_{O_2}}$ calculated by morphometry (128), as shown in Figure 4, cover a wide range of body size and mammalian species. However, note that the morphometric values are 5–10 times greater than the physiological measurements. For example, Dm for a 70-kg man is 137 ml $O_2 \cdot min^{-1} \cdot mmHg^{-1}$ compared with values of 28–31 ml $O_2 \cdot min^{-1} \cdot mmHg^{-1}$ by experimental measurements with $D_{L_{CO}}$, as in Table 1. Presumably the morphometric measurement represents potential diffusion capabilities. For canids, the morphometric estimates of $D_{L_{O_2}}$ were only 2.5 times the physiological measurements (128). Rats (avg 214 g) at sea level have a $D_{L_{O_2}}$ of 0.25 $ml \cdot min^{-1} \cdot mmHg^{-1}$ calculated from the steady-state $D_{L_{CO}}$ (117) compared with 0.9 $ml \cdot min^{-1} \cdot mmHg^{-1}$ by morphometry (128). The turtle, with a simpler lung and lower metabolic rate, has a $D_{L_{CO}}$ of 0.03–0.1 $ml \cdot min^{-1} \cdot mmHg^{-1}$ (24), as compared with a value of 3.4 for a mammal of the same weight (1 kg) by morphometric estimations.

Simpler lungs, or exchange organs in other media, may have a lesser conductance, or transfer coefficient, for which they compensate by using a crosscurrent or countercurrent exchange model, rather than by diffusion from a uniform pool as in the lung (102). The catfish has an effective transfer coefficient of only 0.02 $ml \cdot min^{-1} \cdot mmHg^{-1} \cdot kg^{-1}$, but its gills have a countercurrent exchange arrangement. The blood-to-gill water thickness is ~50 times as great as the thickness of a mammalian alveolar-capillary membrane so that its diffusion resistance dominates the exchange process, and reactions within the blood are unimportant.

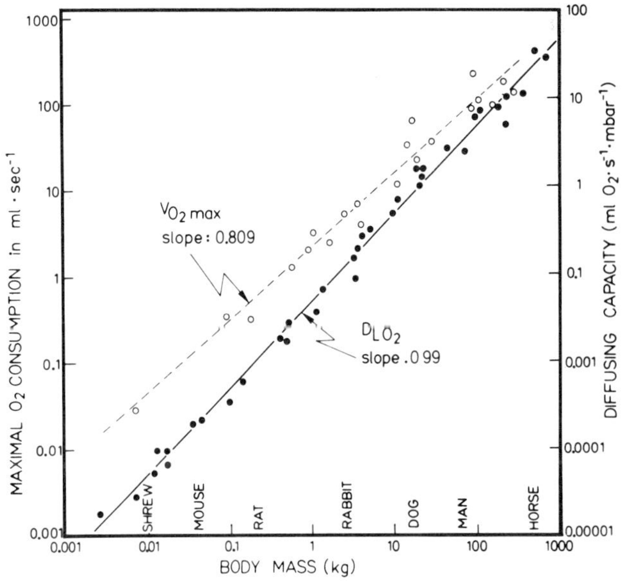

FIG. 4. Allometric plot for O_2 pulmonary diffusing capacity ($D_{L_{O_2}}$) calculated by morphometry and maximal O_2 consumption against body mass for different animal species; $D_{L_{O_2}}$ in $ml \cdot mmHg^{-1} \cdot min^{-1} = D_{L_{O_2}}$ $ml \cdot mbar^{-1} \cdot s^{-1}$ 0.0125. [From Weibel (128).]

TABLE 1. *Representative Partition of Resistance Between Alveolar-Capillary Membrane and Capillary Blood in Normal Human Lung*

DL_{CO}, ml·min^{-1}·mmHg^{-1}	Dm_{CO}, ml·min^{-1}·mmHg^{-1}	Vc, ml	R_{blood}/R_{tot}, %	Ref.
23 ($13.0 + 1.6\ \dot{Q}c$)	34 ($22.7 + 1.9\ \dot{Q}c$)	98 ($63.8 + 5.7\ \dot{Q}c$)	34	109
25 ($12 + 2.2\ \dot{Q}c$)	48 ($31 + 2.8\ \dot{Q}c$)	100 ($37 + 7\ \dot{Q}c$)	47	61

DL_{CO}, CO pulmonary diffusing capacity; Dm_{CO}, CO membrane diffusing capacity; Vc, volume of the capillary blood; R_{blood}, resistance in blood; R_{tot}, total resistance. $\dot{Q}c$, pulmonary capillary blood flow (6 liters/min). Alveolar P_{O_2} = 100 mmHg.

RESULT OF DIFFUSION: ALVEOLAR–END-CAPILLARY PARTIAL PRESSURE DIFFERENCE

The lung is such an excellent exchanger of gas between alveolar air and capillary blood that any gas that does not bind chemically to blood is equilibrated (35). The speed of the whole process is impressive. A bolus of CO injected during an inspiration can produce an alveolar CO concentration of ~0.1% and cause HbCO to appear on the surface capillaries within as little as 0.3 s (121).

In the ultimate sense O_2, and certainly CO_2, cannot be considered to have reached equilibrium between alveolar gas and capillary blood until all the complex interactions of these species with hemoglobin and movements of reactants and products across the red cell membrane have been completed. The speed of the whole process in vitro cannot be measured because the small dimensions and small diffusion distances in the lung cannot be duplicated experimentally.

How can the speed of these processes in vivo be estimated? One approach is to determine the rates of isolated segments of the overall process and assemble them into the whole with numerical calculations of a model. The Bohr shift (38, 115), Haldane shift (67), and Root shift (39) involve interactions of CO and O_2, including diffusion into the red cell, chemical reaction plus diffusion within the red cell (93), dissociation of one gas from hemoglobin, and its diffusion out of the cell. In general the total process is somewhat slower than the sum of the parts (67). These reactions can be incorporated into a model of in vivo processes (8, 29, 51, 116, 120).

Wagner and West (120) pointed out the interesting fact that although it is customarily stated that CO_2 diffuses 20 times as fast as O_2 across the alveolar-capillary membrane and therefore equilibrates completely, the effective solubility of CO_2 in blood is 10 times greater than that of O_2, which means that the time required for equilibration, an exponential process that depends on pulmonary diffusing capacity/effective solubility in blood, differs by a factor of only ~2. The major practical reason the assumption can be made that PA_{CO_2} equals Pa_{CO_2} is that the arteriovenous CO_2 difference is so small that even if equilibrium were only partially accomplished, the P_{CO_2} end gradient would be undetectable.

The rate of uptake of CO in the lungs at constant P_{O_2} and P_{CO_2} can be studied independently because, at least in the breath-holding measurement, CO-blood equilibrium is never even approached and all the significant effects of other gases are encompassed in the measurement of Θ.

The importance of the P_{O_2} gradient within the pulmonary capillary bed as compared with P_{O_2} difference across the alveolar-capillary membrane is not entirely clear. There is no experimental method by which plasma P_{O_2} can be measured; it can only be calculated by an equation for O_2 analogous to Equation 1 for CO. The Dm_{O_2} can be calculated as equal to 1.23 Dm_{CO}. The Dm_{CO} can be determined from an analysis of experimentally measured values of DL_{CO} and of Θ_{CO} at different PA_{O_2}, according to Equation 1. For a man with a pulmonary blood flow of 6 liters/min, Dm_{O_2} = 46–64 ml·min^{-1}·mmHg^{-1} and Vc = 98–100 ml.

According to Equation 1, the instantaneous P_{O_2} difference between plasma and the hemoglobin molecule in the red cell expressed as a fraction of the total P_{O_2} difference from alveolar gas to the interior of the red cell equals

$$\frac{\text{plasma } P_{O_2} - \text{red cell } P_{O_2}}{PA_{O_2} - \text{red cell } P_{O_2}} = \frac{1/\Theta Vc}{1/\Theta Vc + 1/Dm} \qquad (21)$$

As measured by a continuous-flow mixing apparatus with an O_2 electrode (113), Θ_{O_2} is 2.8 ml·min^{-1}·ml^{-1}·mmHg^{-1} from 20% to 80% HbO_2 saturation and above this level drops linearly to reach zero at 100% HbO_2. It is 2 ml·min^{-1}·ml^{-1}·mmHg^{-1} at 90% HbO_2 saturation. If values for the venous end of the capillary are used, the resistance to O_2 diffusion within the blood represents 16% of the total alveolar-to-red cell diffusion resistance. Near the arterial end of the capillary, at 90% HbO_2, this resistance rises to 22%. There are wide variations in the value of Θ_{O_2} reported in the literature (69, 89, 92). Ono and Tazawa (98) found that Θ_{O_2} is ~33% of the value reported by Staub et al. (113). If these lower values of Θ_{O_2} are used in the calculation above, the diffusion resistance within the blood becomes 38% of the total diffusion resistance at the start of the capillary and rises to 44% near the end of the capillary where the HbO_2 saturation is 90%. There seems little question that an important fraction of the resistance to O_2 uptake in the alveolar capillary lies within the blood. However, if the total PA_{O_2} − Pc'_{O_2} is small, the absolute magnitude of the P_{O_2} gradient within the blood, which is still smaller, becomes negligible.

Weibel (128) found by morphometric measurements that Dm_{O_2} should be an order of magnitude greater, ~550 ml·min^{-1}·mmHg^{-1}, than the values found experimentally. This means that the diffusion resistance of the alveolar-capillary membrane is much less than thought and increases the importance of the chemical reaction plus diffusion resistance to O_2 movement within the blood. This evidence supports the concept that a significant proportion of the total P_{O_2} gradient between alveolar gas and the hemoglobin molecule can lie within the capillary blood. In other words, the lungs are very well designed; red blood cells are exposed to alveolar gas for exchange with only a minimal amount of the structure of the lung interposed. The alveolar-capillary membrane is generally extremely thin, particularly in comparison with the thickness of the red blood cells, and it is not surprising that the diffusion resistance of the membrane, 1/Dm (Dm also includes tissue and plasma up to the red cell membrane surface), is not the major impediment to O_2 and CO exchange in the lungs. Burns and Shepard (13) perfused an isolated lung with sodium dithionite, which reacts rapidly with O_2, to increase the rate of removal of O_2 within the blood to such an extent that diffusion between the alveolar gas and the blood would become the rate-limiting step; i.e., 1/Dm would become the rate-limiting resistance. They obtained an estimate of Dm ~10 times greater than the values obtained by measuring $D_{L_{CO}}$ at different $P_{A_{O_2}}$. Thus their values approximate those of Weibel. However, this ingenious approach is limited because the rate of O_2 uptake by a cylinder of fluid containing dithionite corresponding to a capillary would not increase without limit as the concentration of the chemical increases but would reach a maximum as an advancing-front mechanism developed (34). Thus it is still possible that there were significant O_2 gradients within the dithionite solution in the capillary bed, making the Dm estimates of Burns and Shepard, as high as they were, still underestimates.

Although there is no question that the rate of CO uptake by chemical reaction plus diffusion with hemoglobin in red cells determines the value of $D_{L_{CO}}$, particularly at high P_{O_2}, the intracapillary P_{O_2} gradients are less important in limiting O_2 exchange in the lung or the peripheral capillaries for two main reasons. *1*) At the same P_{O_2}, Θ_{O_2} is about twice Θ_{CO} (34). *2*) The absolute gas-to-blood or blood-to-tissue pressure differences are much larger in the case of P_{O_2}, so the changes in HbO_2 saturation are larger and the P_{O_2} of the end-capillary blood may reach equilibrium with that in the alveolar gas or the tissue. The velocity of the O_2 reaction is still of limited importance, even under the most severe circumstances, namely in anemic peripheral blood, at a reduced temperature, during exercise (increased O_2 consumption). The P_{O_2} gradient within the blood is then still only ~13% of the total red cell–to–tissue P_{O_2} difference (78). This can be compared with the situation for CO in Table 1, where in the normal human breathing air at normal body temperature at rest, the P_{CO} gradient within blood approaches half of the total P_{CO} gradient.

REFERENCES

1. ADARO, F., P. SCHEID, J. TEICHMANN, AND J. PIIPER. A rebreathing method for estimating pulmonary D_{O_2}: theory and measurements in dog lungs. *Respir. Physiol.* 18: 43–63, 1973.
2. ADARO, F., J. TEICHMANN, A. LUDTKE-HANJERY, P. SCHEID, AND J. PIIPER. Comparison of rebreathing and steady-state pulmonary D_{L,O_2} in dogs ventilated by body respirator. *Respiration* 31: 71–84, 1974.
3. ANDREW, G. M., AND L. BAINES. Relationship of pulmonary diffusing capacity (D_L) and cardiac output ($\dot{Q}_c$) in exercise. *Eur. J. Appl. Physiol. Occup. Physiol.* 33: 127–137, 1974.
4. ARNDT, H., T. K. C. KING, AND W. A. BRISCOE. Diffusing capacities and ventilation:perfusion ratios in patients with the clinical syndrome of alveolar capillary block. *J. Clin. Invest.* 49: 408–422, 1970.
5. AYASH, R., A. SYBERT, AND G. H. GURTNER. Saturation kinetics for steady state pulmonary CO transfer in man (Abstract). *Am. Rev. Respir. Dis.* 173: 310, 1978.
6. BAUER, C., R. A. KLOCKE, AND R. E. FORSTER. A kinetic basis of the effect of 2,3-diphosphoglycerate (2,3-DPG) and pH on the oxygen affinity in hemoglobin. *Pfluegers Arch.* 319: R7, 1970.
7. BAUER, C., R. A. KLOCKE, D. KAMP, AND R. E. FORSTER. Effect of 2,3-diphosphoglycerate and H^+ on the reaction of O_2 and hemoglobin. *Am. J. Physiol.* 224: 838–847, 1973.
8. BIDANI, A., E. D. CRANDALL, AND R. E. FORSTER. Analysis of postcapillary pH changes in blood in vivo after gas exchange. *J. Appl. Physiol.* 44: 770–781, 1978.
9. BLUMENTHAL, W. S., R. F. JOHNSTON, L. A. KAUTTMAN, AND P. B. SOLNICK. The effect of anemia on pulmonary diffusing capacity with a derivation of a correction equation. *Am. Rev. Respir. Dis.* 102: 965–969, 1970.
10. BRYANT, S. C., AND R. M. NAVARI. Effect of plasma proteins on oxygen diffusion in the pulmonary capillaries. *Microvasc. Res.* 7: 120–130, 1974.
11. BURGESS, J. H., J. GILLESPIE, P. D. GRAF, AND J. A. NADEL. Effect of pulmonary vascular pressures on single-breath CO diffusing capacity in dogs. *J. Appl. Physiol.* 24: 692–696, 1968.
12. BURNS, B., Y. N. CHA, AND J. M. PURCELL. A specific carrier for O_2 and CO in the lung: effects of volatile anesthetics on gas transfer and drug metabolism. *Chest* 69: 316–320, 1976.
13. BURNS, B., AND R. H. SHEPARD. $D_{L_{O_2}}$ in exercised lungs perfused with blood containing sodium dithionite ($Na_2S_2O_4$). *J. Appl. Physiol.* 46: 100–110, 1979.
14. CERRETELLI, P., A. VEICSTEINAS, J. TEICHMANN, H. MAGNUSSEN, AND J. PIIPER. Estimation by a rebreathing method of pulmonary O_2 diffusing capacity in man. *J. Appl. Physiol.* 37: 526–532, 1974.
15. CHANDLER, C. L., D. J. CHINN, AND J. E. COTES. Effect of inhaled histamine on single breath lung transfer factor for carbon monoxide (Abstract). *J. Physiol. Lond.* 327: 51P, 1982.
16. COHEN, R., E. M. OVERFIELD, AND J. A. KYLSTRA. Diffusion component of alveolar-arterial oxygen pressure difference in man. *J. Appl. Physiol.* 31: 223–226, 1971.
17. COIN, J. T., AND J. S. OLSON. The rate of oxygen uptake by human red blood cells. *J. Biol. Chem.* 254: 1178–1190, 1979.
18. COTES, J. E., J. M. DABBS, P. C. ELWOOD, A. M. HALL, A. MCDONALD, AND M. J. SAUNDERS. Iron-deficiency anaemia: its effect on transfer factor for the lung (diffusing capacity) and ventilation and cardiac frequency during sub-maximal exercise. *Clin. Sci. Lond.* 42: 325–335, 1972.
19. COTES, J. E., AND A. M. HALL. The transfer factor of the lung: normal values in adults. In: *Normal Values in Respiratory Function in Man*, edited by P. Arcangeli. Torino, Italy: Panminerva Med., 1970, p. 327–343.

20. Cotton, D. J., J. T. Mink, and B. L. Graham. Effect of high negative inspiratory pressure on single breath CO diffusing capacity. *Respir. Physiol.* 54: 19–20, 1983.
21. Cotton, D. J., C. J. L. Newth, P. M. Portner, and J. A. Nadel. Measurement of single-breath CO diffusing capacity by continuous rapid CO analysis in man. *J. Appl. Physiol.* 46: 1149–1156, 1979.
22. Crapo, J. D., and R. O. Crapo. Comparison of total lung diffusion capacity and the membrane component of diffusion capacity as determined by physiologic and morphometric techniques. *Respir. Physiol.* 51: 181–194, 1983.
23. Crapo, R. O., and A. H. Morris. Standardized single breath normal values for carbon monoxide diffusing capacity. *Am. Rev. Respir. Dis.* 123: 185–189, 1981.
24. Crawford, E. C., Jr., R. N. Gatz, H. Magnussen, S. F. Perry, and J. Piiper. Lung volumes, pulmonary blood flow and carbon monoxide diffusing capacity of turtles. *J. Comp. Physiol.* 107: 169–178, 1976.
25. Cree, E. M., J. R. Benfield, and H. K. Rasmussen. Differential lung diffusion, capillary volume, and compliance in dogs. *J. Appl. Physiol.* 25: 186–190, 1968.
26. Cross, C. E., H. Gong, Jr., C. J. Kurpershoek, J. R. Gilliespie, and R. W. Hyde. Alterations in distribution of blood flow to the lung's diffusion surfaces during exercise. *J. Clin. Invest.* 52: 414–421, 1973.
27. Cuomo, A. J., G. M. Tisi, and K. M. Moser. Relationship of $DL_{CO(SB)}$ and K^{m-1} to lung volume and partition of pulmonary perfusion. *J. Appl. Physiol.* 35: 129–135, 1973.
28. Ewan, P. W., H. A. Jones, C. G. Rhodes, and J. M. B. Hughes. Detection of intrapulmonary hemorrhage with carbon monoxide uptake. Application in Goodpasture's syndrome. *N. Engl. J. Med.* 295: 1391–1396, 1976.
29. Filley, G. F., D. B. Bigelow, D. E. Olson, and L. M. Lacquet. Pulmonary gas transport. A mathematical model of the lung. *Am. Rev. Respir. Dis.* 98: 480–489, 1968.
30. Finley, T. N., E. P. Engelman, B. Packer, A. Aronow, and A. M. Cosentino. Use of the RC time constant for CO in measurement of diffusing capacity. *Am. Rev. Respir. Dis.* 109: 682–684, 1974.
31. Fisher, A. B., and R. W. Hyde. Decrease of diffusing capacity and pulmonary blood flow during passive lung inflation. *J. Appl. Physiol.* 27: 157–163, 1969.
32. Fisher, A. B., R. W. Hyde, A. E. Baue, J. S. Reif, and D. F. Kelly. Effect of carbon monoxide on function and structure of the lung. *J. Appl. Physiol.* 26: 4–12, 1969.
33. Fisher, T. R., R. F. Coburn, and R. E. Forster. Carbon monoxide diffusing capacity in the bullhead catfish. *J. Appl. Physiol.* 26: 161–169, 1969.
34. Forster, R. E. Rate of gas uptake by red cells. In: *Handbook of Physiology. Respiration*, edited by W. O. Fenn and H. Rahn. Washington, DC: Am. Physiol. Soc., 1964, vol. I, chapt. 32, 827–837.
35. Forster, R. E. Diffusion of gases. In: *Handbook of Physiology. Respiration*, edited by W. O. Fenn and H. Rahn. Washington, DC: Am. Physiol. Soc., 1964, vol. I, chapt. 33, p. 839–872.
36. Forster, R. E. The single-breath carbon monoxide transfer test 25 years on: a reappraisal. 1. Physiological considerations (Editorial). *Thorax* 38: 1–5, 1983.
37. Forster, R. E., and E. D. Crandall. Pulmonary gas exchange. *Annu. Rev. Physiol.* 38: 69–93, 1976.
38. Forster, R. E., and J. B. Steen. Rate limiting processes in the Bohr shift in human red cells. *J. Physiol. Lond.* 196: 541–562, 1968.
39. Forster, R. E., and J. B. Steen. The rate of the 'root shift' in eel red cells and eel hemoglobin solution. *J. Physiol. Lond.* 204: 259–282, 1969.
40. Fowler, K. T., and J. E. Maloney. A search for a pulsatile component in pulmonary capillary blood volume. *J. Appl. Physiol.* 20: 1173–1178, 1965.
41. Gehr, P., C. Hugonnaud, P. E. Burri, H. Bachofen, and E. R. Weibel. Adaption of the growing lung to increased V_{O_2}. III. The effect of exposure to cold environment in rats. *Respir. Physiol.* 32: 345–353, 1978.
42. Gehr, P., and E. R. Weibel. Morphometric estimation of regional differences in the dog lung. *J. Appl. Physiol.* 37: 648–653, 1974.
43. Georges, R., G. Saumon, and A. Loiseau. The relationship of age to pulmonary membrane conductance and capillary blood volume. *Am. Rev. Respir. Dis.* 116: 1069–1078, 1978.
44. Gibson, Q. H., and F. J. W. Roughton. The kinetics of dissociation of the first oxygen molecule from fully saturated oxyhemoglobin in sheep blood solutions. *Proc. R. Soc. Lond. B. Biol. Sci.* 143: 310–334, 1955.
45. Glass, M. L., and K. Johansen. Pulmonary oxygen diffusing capacity of the lizard *Tupinambis tequixin*. *J. Exp. Zool.* 219: 385–388, 1982.
46. Gong, H., Jr., C. J. Kurpershoek, D. H. Meyer, and C. E. Cross. Effects of cardiac output on $^{18}O_2$ lung diffusion in normal resting man. *Respir. Physiol.* 16: 313–326, 1972.
47. Graham, B. L., J. T. Mink, and D. J. Cotton. Dynamic measurements of CO diffusing capacity using discrete samples of alveolar gas. *J. Appl. Physiol.* 54: 73–79, 1983.
48. Gurtner, G. H., and W. S. Fowler. Interrelationships of factors affecting pulmonary diffusing capacity. *J. Appl. Physiol.* 30: 619–624, 1971.
49. Hallenborg, C. W., W. Holden, T. Menzel, R. Dozor, and J. A. Nadel. The clinical usefulness of a screening test to detect static pulmonary blood using a multiple-breath analysis of diffusing capacity. *Am. Rev. Respir. Dis.* 119: 349–356, 1979.
50. Hamer, N. A. J. Variations in the components of diffusing capacity as the lung expands. *Clin. Sci. Lond.* 24: 275–285, 1963.
51. Hill, E. P., G. G. Power, and L. D. Longo. Mathematical simulation of pulmonary O_2 and CO_2 exchange. *Am. J. Physiol.* 224: 904–917, 1973.
52. Holden, W. E., C. P. Hallenborg, T. E. Menzel, R. Dozor, P. D. Graf, and J. A. Nadel. Effect of static or slowly flowing blood on carbon monoxide diffusion in dog lungs. *J. Appl. Physiol.* 46: 992–997, 1979.
53. Holland, R. A. B., and R. E. Forster. The effect of size of red cells on the kinetics of their oxygen uptake. *J. Gen. Physiol.* 49: 727–742, 1966.
54. Holland, R. A. B., W. van Hezewikj, and J. Zubzanda. Velocity of oxygen uptake by partially saturated adult and fetal human red cells. *Respir. Physiol.* 29: 303–314, 1977.
55. Holmgren, A. On the variation of $D_{L_{CO}}$ with increasing oxygen uptake during exercise in healthy trained young men and women. *Acta Physiol. Scand.* 65: 207–220, 1965.
56. Hugonnaud, C., P. Gehr, E. R. Weibel, and P. H. Burri. Adaptation of the growing lung to increased oxygen consumption. II. Morphometric analysis. *Respir. Physiol.* 29: 1–10, 1977.
57. Hyde, R. W., R. E. Forster, G. G. Power, J. Nairn, and R. Rynes. Measurement of O_2 diffusing capacity of the lungs with a stable O_2 isotope. *J. Clin. Invest.* 45: 1178–1193, 1966.
58. Hyde, R. W., W. H. Lawson, and R. E. Forster. Influence of carbon dioxide on pulmonary vasculature. *J. Appl. Physiol.* 19: 734–744, 1964.
59. Hyde, R. W., M. G. Marin, R. I. Rynes, G. Karreman, and R. E. Forster. Measurement of uneven distribution of pulmonary blood flow to CO diffusing capacity. *J. Appl. Physiol.* 31: 605–612, 1971.
60. Hyde, R. W., R. Rynes, G. G. Power, and J. Nairn. Determination of distribution of diffusing capacity in relation to blood flow in the human lung. *J. Clin. Invest.* 46: 463–474, 1967.
61. Johnson, R. L., Jr., and J. M. Miller. Distribution of ventilation, blood flow, and gas transfer coefficients in the lung. *J. Appl. Physiol.* 25: 1–15, 1968.
62. Johnson, R. L., Jr., H. F. Taylor, and W. H. Lawson, Jr. Maximal diffusing capacity of the lung for carbon monoxide. *J. Clin. Invest.* 44: 349–355, 1965.

63. JONES, H. A., P. D. BUCKINGHAM, J. C. CLARK, R. E. FORSTER, J. D. HEATHER, J. M. B. HUGHES, AND C. G. RHODES. Constant rate of CO uptake with variable inspired CO concentration. *Prog. Respir. Res.* 16: 169–171, 1981.
64. KARP, R. B., P. D. GRAF, AND J. A. NADEL. Regulation of pulmonary capillary blood volume by pulmonary arterial and left atrial pressures. *Circ. Res.* 22: 1–10, 1968.
65. KINDIG, N. B., AND D. R. HAZLETT. The effects of breathing pattern in the estimation of pulmonary diffusing capacity. *Q. J. Exp. Physiol. Cogn. Med. Sci.* 59: 311–329, 1974.
66. KING, T. K. C., AND W. A. BRISCOE. Bohr integral isopleths in the study of blood gas exchange in the lung. *J. Appl. Physiol.* 22: 659–674, 1967.
67. KLOCKE, R. A. Mechanism and kinetics of the Haldane effect in human erythrocytes. *J. Appl. Physiol.* 35: 673–681, 1973.
68. KÖTTER, D., A. HUCH, H. STOTZ, AND J. PIIPER. Single breath CO diffusing capacity in anesthetized dogs with increased oxygen consumption. *Respir. Physiol.* 6: 202–208, 1969.
69. KOYAMA, T., T. FURUSE, T. ARAI, AND M. MOCHIZUKI. A study on the oxygenation velocity factor of the red blood cell by use of the rapid flow method combined with a Pt-electrode as the oxygenation detector. *Bull. Res. Inst. Appl. Electricity* 20: 144–152, 1968.
70. KOYAMA, T., T. FURUSE, AND M. MOCHIZUKI. A preliminary study on the oxygenation velocity of the spherocyte. *Bull. Res. Inst. Appl. Electricity* 20: 153–157, 1968.
71. KRAWIEC, J. A., R. E. FORSTER, T. W. GOTTLIEBSEN, AND D. FISH. Rate of CO uptake by human red blood cells (Abstract). *Federation Proc.* 42: 993, 1983.
72. KROGH, A., AND M. KROGH. Rate of diffusion of CO into the lungs of man. *Scand. Arch. Physiol.* 23: 236–247, 1909.
73. KUTCHAI, H. Role of the red cell membrane in oxygen uptake. *Respir. Physiol.* 23: 121–132, 1975.
74. KYLSTRA, J. A., W. H. SCHOENFISCH, J. M. HERRON, AND G. D. BLENKARN. Gas exchange in saline-filled lungs of man. *J. Appl. Physiol.* 35: 136–142, 1973.
75. LAWSON, W. H., JR. Rebreathing measurements of pulmonary diffusing capacity for CO during exercise. *J. Appl. Physiol.* 29: 896–900, 1970.
76. LAWSON, W. H., JR. Effect of anemia, species, and temperature on CO kinetics with red blood cells. *J. Appl. Physiol.* 31: 447–457, 1971.
77. LAWSON, W. H., JR. Effect of drugs, hypoxia, and ventilatory maneuvers on lung diffusion for CO in man. *J. Appl. Physiol.* 32: 788–794, 1972.
78. LAWSON, W. H., JR., AND R. E. FORSTER. Oxygen tension gradients in peripheral capillary blood. *J. Appl. Physiol.* 22: 970–973, 1967.
79. LAWSON, W. H., JR., R. A. B. HOLLAND, AND R. E. FORSTER. Effect of temperature on deoxygenation rate of human red cells. *J. Appl. Physiol.* 20: 912–918, 1965.
80. LEWIS, S. M., D. Z. RUBIN, AND C. MITTMAN. Distribution of ventilation and diffusing capacity in the normal and diseased lung. *J. Appl. Physiol.* 51: 1463–1470, 1981.
81. LIPSCOMB, D. J., K. PATEL, AND J. M. B. HUGHES. Interpretation of increases in the transfer coefficient for carbon monoxide (TLCO/VA or KCO). *Thorax* 33: 728–733, 1978.
82. MENDOZA, C., H. PEAVY, B. BURNS, AND G. GURTNER. Saturation kinetics for steady-state pulmonary CO transfer. *J. Appl. Physiol.* 43: 880–884, 1977.
83. MENKES, H. A., K. SERA, R. M. ROGERS, R. HYDE, R. E. FORSTER, AND A. B. DUBOIS. Pulsatile uptake of CO in the human lung. *J. Clin. Invest.* 49: 335–345, 1970.
84. MEYER, M., P. SCHEID, AND J. PIIPER. No evidence for facilitated pulmonary transfer of carbon monoxide. *Prog. Respir. Res.* 16: 168, 1981.
85. MICHAELSON, E. D., M. A. SACKNER, AND R. L. JOHNSON, JR. Vertical distributions of pulmonary diffusing capacity and capillary blood flow in man. *J. Clin. Invest.* 45: 493–500, 1966.
86. MICHELI, J. L., AND P. HAAB. Estimation de la capacité de diffusion pulmonaire pour l'oxygène chez l'homme au repos par la méthode du rebreathing hypoxique. *J. Physiol. Paris* 62, Suppl. 1: 194–195, 1970.
87. MILLER, J. M., AND R. J. JOHNSON. Effect of lung inflation on pulmonary diffusing capacity at rest and exercise. *J. Clin. Invest.* 45: 493–500, 1966.
88. MIYAMOTO, Y., AND W. MOLL. Measurements of dimensions and pathway of red cells in rapidly frozen lungs in situ. *Respir. Physiol.* 12: 141–156, 1971.
89. MOCHIZUKI, M. Study on the oxygenation velocity of the human red cell. *Jpn. J. Physiol.* 16: 635–648, 1966.
90. MOCHIZUKI, M. On the velocity of oxygen dissociation of human hemoglobin and red cell. *Jpn. J. Physiol.* 16: 649–657, 1966.
91. MOCHIZUKI, M. A theoretical study on the velocity factor of oxygenation of the red cell. *Jpn. J. Physiol.* 16: 658–666, 1966.
92. MOCHIZUKI, M. The relationship between O_2 diffusing capacity and the oxygenation velocity of the red cell. *Jpn. Circ. J.* 33: 1817–1820, 1968.
93. MOLL, W. The influence of hemoglobin diffusion on oxygen uptake and release by red cells. *Respir. Physiol.* 6: 1–15, 1969.
94. MORRIS, A. H., AND R. O. CRAPO. Standardization of computation of single-breath diffusing capacity (transfer factor). *Clin. Respir. Physiol.* In press.
95. NAIRN, J. R., G. G. POWER, R. W. HYDE, R. E. FORSTER, J. LAMBERTSEN, AND J. DICKSON. Diffusing capacity and pulmonary capillary blood flow at hyperbaric pressures. *J. Clin. Invest.* 44: 1591–1599, 1965.
96. NEWTH, C. J. L., D. J. COTTON, AND J. A. NADEL. Pulmonary diffusing capacity measured at multiple intervals during a single exhalation in man. *J. Appl. Physiol.* 43: 617–625, 1977.
96a. OGILVIE, C. The single-breath carbon monoxide transfer test 25 years on: a reappraisal. 2. Clinical observations (Editorial). *Thorax* 38: 5–9, 1983.
97. OGILVIE, C. M., R. E. FORSTER, W. S. BLAKEMORE, AND J. W. MORTON. A standardized breath holding technique for the clinical measurement of the diffusing capacity of the lung for carbon monoxide. *J. Clin. Invest.* 36: 1–17, 1957.
98. ONO, T., AND H. TAZAWA. Microphotometric method for measuring the oxygenation and deoxygenation rate in a single red blood cell. *Jpn. J. Physiol.* 25: 93–107, 1975.
99. PIIPER, J. Apparent increase of the O_2 diffusing capacity with increased O_2 uptake in inhomogenous lungs: theory. *Respir. Physiol.* 6: 209–218, 1969.
100. PIIPER, J., P. CERRETELLI, D. W. RENNIE, AND P. E. DI PRAMPERO. Estimation of the pulmonary diffusing capacity for O_2 by a rebreathing procedure. *Respir. Physiol.* 12: 157–162, 1971.
101. PIIPER, J., A. HUCH, D. KOTTER, AND R. HERBST. Pulmonary diffusing capacity at basal and increased O_2 uptake levels in anesthetized dogs. *Respir. Physiol.* 6: 219–232, 1969.
102. PIIPER, J., AND P. SCHEID. Maximum gas transfer efficacy of models for fish gills, avian lungs and mammalian lungs. *Respir. Physiol.* 14: 115–124, 1972.
103. POWER, G. G., V. S. AOKI, W. H. LAWSON, JR., AND J. B. GREGG. Diffusion characteristics of pulmonary blood-gas barrier at low temperatures. *J. Appl. Physiol.* 31: 438–446, 1971.
104. POWER, G. G., JR., R. W. HYDE, R. J. SEVER, F. G. HOPPIN, JR., AND J. R. NAIRN. Pulmonary diffusing capacity and capillary blood flow during forward acceleration. *J. Appl. Physiol.* 20: 1199–1204, 1965.
105. RANKIN, J., R. S. MCNEIL, AND R. E. FORSTER. Influence of increased alveolar CO_2 tension on pulmonary diffusing capacity for CO in man. *J. Appl. Physiol.* 15: 543–549, 1960.
106. RILEY, R. L., AND S. PERMUTT. Venous admixture component of the AaP_{O_2} gradient. *J. Appl. Physiol.* 35: 430–431, 1973.
107. ROTHMAN, H. H., R. A. KLOCKE, K. K. ANDERSON, L. D'ALECY, AND R. E. FORSTER. Kinetics of oxygenation and deoxygenation of erythrocytes containing hemoglobin S. *Respir. Physiol.* 21: 9–17, 1974.
108. ROUGHTON, F. J. W., AND R. E. FORSTER. Relative importance of diffusion and chemical reaction rates in determining

rate of exchange of gases in the human lung, with special reference to true diffusing capacity of pulmonary membrane and volume of blood in the lung capillaries. *J. Appl. Physiol.* 11: 290–302, 1957.

109. SACKNER, M. A., D. GREENELTCH, M. S. HEIMAN, L. S. EPSTEIN, AND N. ATKINS. Diffusing capacity, membrane diffusing capacity, capillary blood volume, pulmonary tissue and cardiac output measured by a rebreathing technique. *Am. Rev. Respir. Dis.* 111: 157–165, 1975.

110. SCHEID, P., F. ADARO, J. TEICHMANN, AND J. PIIPER. Rebreathing and steady state pulmonary D_{O_2} in the dog and in inhomogeneous lung models. *Respir. Physiol.* 18: 258–272, 1973.

111. SHPORER, M., R. E. FORSTER, AND M. M. CIVAN. Kinetics of CO_2 exchange in human erythrocytes analyzed by ^{13}C-NMR. *Am. J. Physiol.* 246 (*Cell Physiol.* 15): C231–C234, 1984.

112. SIEGWART, B. P., P. GEHR, J. GIL, AND E. R. WEIBEL. Morphometric estimation of pulminary diffusion capacity. IV. The normal dog lung. *Respir. Physiol.* 13: 141–159, 1971.

113. STAUB, N. C., J. M. BISHOP, AND R. E. FORSTER. Velocity of O_2 uptake by human red blood cells. *J. Appl. Physiol.* 16: 511–516, 1961.

114. STOKES, D. L., N. R. MACINTYRE, AND J. A. NADEL. Nonlinear increases in diffusing capacity during exercise by seated and supine subjects. *J. Appl. Physiol.* 51: 858–863, 1981.

115. TAZAWA, H., AND M. MOCHIZUKI. Rates of oxygenation and Bohr shift of capillary blood in chick embryos. *Nature Lond.* 261: 509–511, 1976.

116. TAZAWA, H., T. ONO, AND M. MOCHIZUKI. Oxygenation and deoxygenation velocity factors of chorioallantoic capillary blood. *J. Appl. Physiol.* 40: 399–403, 1976.

117. TUREK, Z., A. FRANS, AND F. KREUZER. Hypoxic pulmonary steady-state diffusing capacity for CO and alveolar-arterial O_2 pressure differences in growing rats after adaption to a simulated altitude of 3,500 m. *Pfluegers Arch.* 335: 1–9, 1972.

118. VREIM, C. E., AND N. C. STAUB. Indirect and direct pulmonary capillary blood volume in anesthetized open-thorax cats. *J. Appl. Physiol.* 34: 452–459, 1973.

119. WAGNER, P. D., R. W. MAZZONE, AND J. B. WEST. Diffusing capacity and anatomic dead space for carbon monoxide ($C^{18}O$). *J. Appl. Physiol.* 31: 847–852, 1971.

120. WAGNER, P. D., AND J. B. WEST. Effects of diffusion impairment on O_2 and CO_2 time courses in pulmonary capillaries. *J. Appl. Physiol.* 33: 62–71, 1972.

121. WAGNER, W. W., JR., L. P. LATHAM, P. D. BRINKMAN, AND G. F. FILLEY. Pulmonary gas transport time: larynx to alveolus. *Science Wash. DC* 163: 1210–1211, 1969.

122. WEIBEL, E. R. Morphometric estimation of pulmonary diffusion capacity. I. Model and method. *Respir. Physiol.* 11: 54–75, 1970.

123. WEIBEL, E. R. Morphometric estimation of pulmonary diffusion capacity. II. Effect of PO_2 on the growing lung. *Respir. Physiol.* 11: 247–264, 1971.

124. WEIBEL, E. R. Morphometric estimation of pulmonary diffusion capacity. III. The effect of increased oxygen consumption in Japanese waltzing mice. *Respir. Physiol.* 11: 354–366, 1971.

125. WEIBEL, E. R. Comparative analysis of mammalian lungs. *Respir. Physiol.* 14: 26–43, 1972.

126. WEIBEL, E. R. Morphological basis of alveolar-capillary gas exchange. *Physiol. Rev.* 53: 419–495, 1973.

127. WEIBEL, E. R. Oxygen demand and the size of respiratory structures in mammals. In: *Lung Biology in Health and Disease. Evolution of Respiratory Process*, edited by S. C. Wood and C. Lenfant. New York: Dekker, 1979, vol. 13, chapt. 7, p. 289–346.

128. WEIBEL, E. R. *The Pathway for Oxygen.* Cambridge, MA: Harvard Univ. Press, 1984.

129. WEIBEL, E. R., C. R. TAYLOR, J. O'NEIL, D. E. LEITH, P. GEHR, H. HOPPELER, V. LANGMAN, AND R. V. BAUDINETTE. Maximal oxygen consumption and pulmonary diffusing capacity: a direct comparison of physiologic and morphometric measurements in canids. *Respir. Physiol.* 54: 173–188, 1983.

130. WEIBEL, E. R., P. UNTERSEE, J. GIL, AND M. ZULAUT. Morphometric estimation of pulmonary diffusion capacity. VI. Effect of varying positive pressure inflation of air spaces. *Respir. Physiol.* 18: 285–308, 1973.

131. WEISKOPF, R. B., AND J. W. SEVERINGHAUS. Diffusing capacity of the lung for CO in man during acute acclimatization to 14,246 ft. *J. Appl. Physiol.* 32: 285–289, 1972.

CHAPTER 6

Facilitated diffusion of oxygen and carbon dioxide

FERDINAND KREUZER
LOUIS HOOFD | *Department of Physiology, University of Nijmegen, Nijmegen, The Netherlands*

CHAPTER CONTENTS

FACILITATED DIFFUSION of a permeant occurs under the driving force of thermal agitation (Brownian movement) just as for plain diffusion, but the transport rate is faster than expected from the nature of the substance and of the diffusion medium; i.e., the rate is higher than according to the concentration difference for plain diffusion. This enhancement may be mediated by a molecular carrier reversibly reacting with a permeant. The carrier concept originated almost a century ago and has been developed mainly to explain ion and nonelectrolyte transport, e.g., the sugar transport in red blood cells in which all sugar is transferred by a carrier (carrier transport). The facilitated transport in which the permeant is transported both in free form and combined with a carrier (as here, where the permeant is a dissolved gas) has been termed *carrier-mediated transport* (157). Such a carrier system exhibits saturation behavior due to the finite concentration of the carrier and can be inhibited by molecules structurally similar to and thus competing with the carried species.

Carrier-mediated transport is analyzed as a problem of reaction-coupled diffusion where the reversible chemical reactions between carrier and permeant must be fast compared with the carrier diffusion. Thus the permeant not only diffuses but also disappears or reappears onto or from carrier "sites"; i.e., a capacitive factor is present. If the carrier is moving, two concentration gradients (for permeant and permeant-carrier complex) contribute to transport, and the reaction rates are important for the relationship between these concentration gradients.

FACILITATED DIFFUSION OF O_2

Experimental Basis

After Roughton's (150) early suggestion of a possible contribution of HbO_2 to O_2 diffusion, Klug et al. (96) investigated the non-steady-state oxygenation of thin layers of Hb solutions and found considerable enhancement of O_2 diffusion by HbO_2, with a maximum in the middle range of Hb concentration. Independent experiments at steady state (to rule out the capacitive factor of Hb) by Wittenberg (197) and Scholander (155) firmly established the phenomenon and the basic characteristics of facilitated O_2 diffusion in Hb and Mb solutions. Total O_2 transport is the result of two additive components, plain diffusion of O_2 and specific transport mediated by the carrier Hb. Maximum enhancement occurs with full saturation of the carrier pigment on one side of the layer and full desaturation on the other side (67, 69). The gradients of O_2 and oxygenated pigment must occur across the entire layer and are not confined to the interfaces (for reviews see refs. 100 and 199). Specific O_2 transport due to an HbO_2 gradient is abolished by a certain minimum back pressure of O_2, which must probably be more than 40 Torr for Hb + O_2 (101, 109). The "dilemma" of Hemmingsen and Scholander (69)—that facilitated O_2 flux vanished at a partial pressure of O_2 (P_{O_2}) of 10 Torr where the saturation on the low-pressure side presumably was only 55%–65% [as Weigelt (192) experimentally confirmed]—may be due to an artifact, i.e., an unstirred gas layer at the low-pressure interface in these particular experiments (199). This artifact was prevented by a moist vacuum (155), by convection (131), or by directing a rapid He stream at the downstream face of the slab (198). The early as well as later steady-state experiments typically were performed on pigment solutions in a Millipore filter membrane (usually 150 μm thick) separating two gas chambers. Because of uncertainties inherent to these filters with respect to available volume and surface as well as porosity and tortuosity (78), in later experiments the solution was interposed between two plastic membranes whose diffusion resistance had to be taken into account.

The basic features of facilitated O_2 transport are visualized in Figure 1 for the system Hb + O_2. The plain diffusive O_2 flux in the solution with Hb inactivated as metHb is linearly related to P_{O_2}, as expected. The line for the total (facilitated + plain) O_2 flux rises

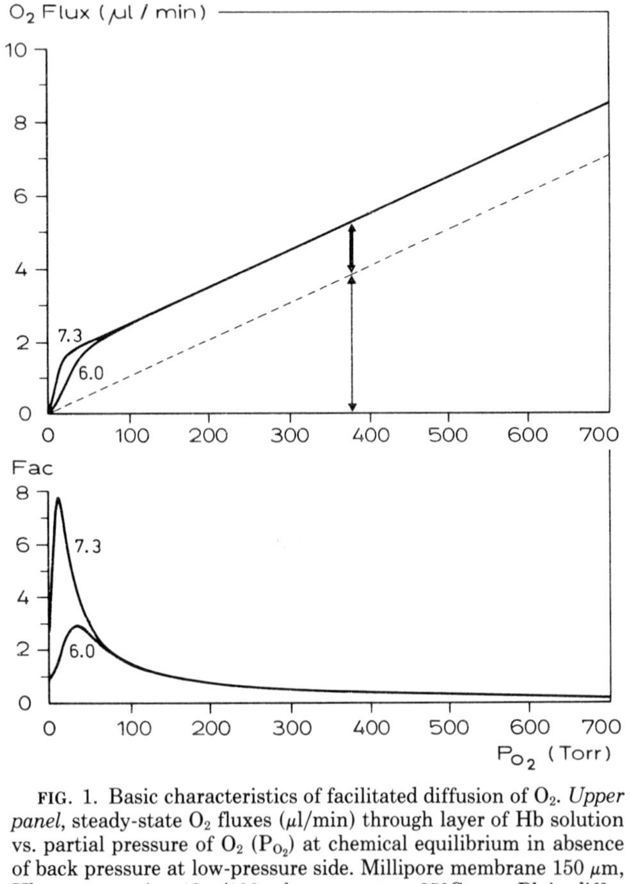

FIG. 1. Basic characteristics of facilitated diffusion of O_2. *Upper panel*, steady-state O_2 fluxes (μl/min) through layer of Hb solution vs. partial pressure of O_2 (P_{O_2}) at chemical equilibrium in absence of back pressure at low-pressure side. Millipore membrane 150 μm, Hb concentration 19 g/100 ml, temperature 25°C. ⟷, Plain diffusion component (Hb inactivated as metHb, - - - - -) of total O_2 flux (——). ⟷, Hb-augmented component. In ascending part of facilitated flux, 2 curves reflect 2 HbO_2 dissociation curves, pH 7.3 and 6.0. *Lower panel*, dimensionless relative facilitation (Fac): (total flux − plain flux)/plain flux = facilitated flux/plain flux vs. P_{O_2}. Maximum facilitation ~8 at pH 7.3 and ~3 at pH 6.0. Maximum at pH 7.3 occurs at lower P_{O_2} than at pH 6.0, due to respective position of HbO_2 dissociation curve. Two curves do not pass through origin where quotient mentioned above is 0/0 or undefined. [*Upper panel* adapted from Hemmingsen (68) and Wittenberg (198).]

from zero with increasing P_{O_2}, but its slope decreases as the point of saturation of the carrier with O_2 is reached; then the line runs parallel to that of plain diffusion with further increase of P_{O_2} (at chemical equilibrium); i.e., the enhancement becomes constant. The ascending part of the facilitated O_2 flux is a result of the prevailing O_2 dissociation curve (ODC) and thus depends on the pH. Above the point of saturation, however, the facilitated O_2 flux becomes independent of the ODC. The dimensionless relative facilitation (Fac), usually expressed as (total flux − plain flux)/plain flux = facilitated flux/plain flux, plotted against P_{O_2} starts with an undefined value (due to 0/0), reaches a maximum depending on the position of the ODC (i.e., on the pH here), and then gradually declines. Thus maximum *relative* enhancement is found with low P_{O_2} values, and the O_2 flux due to HbO_2 depends not only on the P_{O_2} difference across the layer but also on the absolute pressures at the layer boundaries. Below the point of saturation the facilitated O_2 flux depends on the position and slope of the operating range of the ODC (25, 26, 68, 71, 91, 112, 113). Higher affinity of the carrier for the permeant promotes facilitation at low pressures but also renders the system more sensitive to back pressure. Above the point of saturation, however, the facilitated O_2 flux does not increase further with rising P_{O_2}, although the HbO_2 profile steepens and moves toward the low-pressure side; this apparent paradox is resolved because the facilitation is independent of the ODC in this range. In the fully oxygenated part of the membrane the enhanced transport is carried by an increased P_{O_2} gradient, because the flux is augmented by the HbO_2 gradient near the low-pressure boundary. Thus the two gradients contribute to the total O_2 transport (equal in all planes at steady state) very differently in the upper and lower portions of the layer; plain diffusive flux is dominant near the high-pressure side and carrier-mediated flux is dominant near the low-pressure side (199).

The shape of the O_2 and the HbO_2 profiles within the layer and their mutual relationship was much discussed in the 1960s, as critically reviewed previously (100, 199). It emerged that both profiles must be nonlinear even at equilibrium. Furthermore the assumption of chemical equilibrium between Hb and O_2 was not compatible with a complete description of the two profiles (109, 201). A consistent solution for all conditions was achieved only with consideration of the reaction rates in the nonequilibrium approaches, as described in *Quantitative Interpretation*, p. 92.

Oxygenation of Hb on one side and its deoxygenation on the other side lead to a lower and higher pH respectively and thus to a pH difference across the film. The resulting countercurrent migration of H^+ and Hb ions, having different charges and mobilities, must establish a varying distribution of ions and an electric potential difference across the film. The local pH differences also affect the position and steepness of the ODC (38). Bright (7) estimated a potential difference of ≪2 mV in buffered solutions. Hoofd et al. (74) found a sharp decrease in potential difference for increasing salt concentrations, from a maximum of 4 mV at zero salt concentration to an absence of electric effects above 30 mM KCl. In the intermediate range the electric potential induced a decrease in facilitation of up to 40%.

Molecular Mechanism

Interpretation of facilitated O_2 diffusion in terms of ligand transfer, in a "bucket brigade" with fixed binding sites (155) or by molecular collision (32), was incompatible with experimental facts (100, 199). An explanation of facilitation by molecular rotation of the pigment (198) was refuted by Wyman (201), who calculated that rotation contributes only negligibly ($<5 \times 10^{-4}$ of total) to the facilitated flux because the rotational velocity of the Hb molecule is too fast (relaxation time $\sim 10^{-6}$ s is too short) and the dissociation rate of O_2 from the pigment is too slow (half-life of an O_2 molecule attached to the pigment ~0.1 s).

Translational diffusion of the carrier pigment protein as the mechanism of facilitation might at first seem unlikely because the protein molecule diffuses so much more slowly than the O_2 molecules [e.g., at high protein concentrations the diffusion coefficient of Hb (D_{Hb}) is ~100 times lower than the diffusion coefficient of O_2 (D_{O_2})]. However, even a slow movement of the pigment can contribute substantially to O_2 transport because under many experimental and physiological conditions the amount of O_2 combined with the pigment is much larger (~100 times for Hb) than that in free solution (100, 199, 201). Because the flux is proportional to the product of the diffusion coefficient and concentration difference, the contribution of plain O_2 diffusion and oxygenated pigment diffusion may easily be of similar order of magnitude.

Three lines of evidence support translational diffusion of a mobile carrier pigment as a mechanism.

1. Influence of membrane thickness. The fact that both facilitated and diffusive fluxes through Hb solutions in layers 25–300 μm thick are inversely proportional to the path length L points to a translational diffusion process within the body of the solution (198). Below 25 μm the $1/L$ behavior breaks down due to deviation from chemical equilibrium (109). However, the true diffusion path length may not be identical to the layer thickness, particularly in Millipore membranes (80, 102, 136, 152, 198).

2. Influence of temperature. The relative insensitivity to temperature above saturation of the carrier was taken as evidence for a diffusive rather than chemical nature of the process (68, 69).

3. Influence of molecular size and mobility of the pigment. There is an inverse relationship between flux augmentation and molecular weight (MW) of the pigment when comparing various individual pigments (198). Oxygen flux that is facilitated by a pigment of increasing concentration first increases up to a maximum at a concentration of ~15 g/100 ml for Hb or Mb and then decreases due to increasing viscosity reducing molecular motion (68, 155, 198). Facilitated flux is a linear function of the product of protein concentration and diffusion coefficient, according to Wittenberg (199). The line for Hb is steeper than the line for Mb, which suggests that the saturation difference between the boundaries is greater for Hb (0.8) than for Mb (0.45). Because at equilibrium the saturation difference should be unity, this points to a disequilibrium, particularly for Mb. For the same reason this relationship cannot be strictly linear (152). Comparing Hb and Mb is important because Mb is smaller and therefore more mobile, has only one site for O_2 binding, and shows much higher O_2 affinity. In view of these differences it is surprising that the facilitations by Hb and Mb per mole heme (not per mole protein) are the same [Wittenberg paradox; (198, 199)]. This seems to be a fortuitous result of counteracting parameters, Mb having a larger diffusion coefficient but a smaller dissociation rate constant (152, 198, 199). Furthermore facilitation by Mb may be underestimated due to stronger oxidation to metMb (152). Final proof for the necessity of protein mobility was provided by Colton et al. (21), who showed that an Hb solution lost its facilitation on immobilization of Hb by sorption in a swollen collodion film at steady state, although the Hb retained its capacity for reversible binding of O_2.

The rate of combination is unlikely to be limiting (198, 199), although a fall of this rate with decreasing P_{O_2} eventually may lead to disequilibrium and hence to lower flux (7). The rate of dissociation, however, must be rate limiting because pigments of appropriate molecular size (ascaris body wall Hb and succinyl ascaris perienteric fluid Hb), but with very low rate of O_2 dissociation, showed no facilitation of O_2 diffusion (198). According to Wittenberg (198), the O_2 affinity is of secondary importance, because Hb H and ascaris body wall Hb with similar affinities show very different facilitations, whereas Hb H and Hb A with very different affinities exhibit similar facilitations. However, varying affinity will not affect the facilitated flux above the point of saturation, as pertains in these experiments (Fig. 1), and other properties—such as dissociation rate, deviation from equilibrium, and sensitivity to back pressure—may explain differences in facilitation between various pigments. At nonequilibrium the reaction velocity constants k′ (forward) and k (backward; K = k′/k) must be of different importance at the high and low boundaries: k′ is more important on the high-pressure side and k is more important on the low-pressure side (109). The recurring problems of chemical equilibrium encountered here call for a detailed quantitative examination of facilitated O_2 diffusion in terms of equilibrium versus nonequilibrium, as is outlined next.

Quantitative Interpretation

Carrier-mediated transport due to translational carrier diffusion and reversible permeant-carrier reaction throughout the membrane (distributed parameter model) is a classic diffusion-reaction problem with a bimolecular chemical reaction between the carrier **C** and the permeant substrate **S** to form a carrier-substrate complex **CS**

$$\mathbf{C} + \mathbf{S} \underset{k}{\overset{k'}{\rightleftharpoons}} \mathbf{CS} \tag{1}$$

This reaction scheme implies a one-step reaction, whereas actually the reactions of O_2 and CO with Hb are more complicated, e.g., according to a four-step reaction scheme. The one-step reaction can often be a satisfactory approximation, though not always.

The usual model is based on one-dimensional diffusion across an infinitely extended flat layer of a homogeneous liquid membrane interposed between two gas chambers. This layer is supposed to contain a homogeneous globally nonreactive (passive, i.e., no net reaction in membrane) medium at steady state (concentration gradients independent of time; total flux independent of position x in the layer).

For this model, differential equations can be derived for situations in the absence of electric, convective, and coupled diffusive effects. Local material balance (conservation of species) provides at steady state

$$D_S \frac{d^2C_S}{dx^2} = D_C \frac{d^2C_C}{dx^2} = -D_{CS} \frac{d^2C_{CS}}{dx^2} = -\theta = k'C_CC_S - kC_{CS} \tag{2}$$

where D is the respective diffusion coefficient, C is the respective concentration, and θ is the reaction rate. The situation where $\theta = 0$ is chemical equilibrium.

The boundary conditions for both boundaries include Henry's law (possibly corrected for interfacial effects) and the fact that the boundaries are impervious to **C** and **CS**; i.e., the species **C** and **CS** are confined to the layer, whereas species **S** can enter and leave the layer. The boundary concentrations of **S** are under direct experimental control, whereas those of **C** and **CS** are not. Application of all the boundary conditions and constraints leads to a set of equations of the same number as the unknown quantities.

Equations 3 and 4 are solutions with constant diffusion coefficients for total **C**

$$D_CC_C + D_{CS}C_{CS} = H \tag{3}$$

and total **S**

$$\frac{d}{dx}(D_SC_S + D_{CS}C_{CS}) = -J \tag{4}$$

where H and J are integration constants and J is the total flux of **S**.

The assumptions that all values of D are independent of the substrate concentration and $D_C = D_{CS}$ (differences of ±20% in D_C vs. D_{CS} have no great effect on the calculated fluxes) lead to the constraint that the total carrier concentration $C_C + C_{CS} = C_T$ is constant everywhere in the layer. Because one of the concentrations C_C or C_{CS} is redundant, the number of boundary conditions is reduced from 6 to 4.

Integration of Equation 4 between $x = 0$ (high-concentration side) and $x = L$ (low-concentration side) provides an exact relationship between the flux and the boundary concentrations of **S** and **CS**

$$D_S(C_{S_{x=0}} - C_{S_{x=L}}) + D_{CS}(C_{CS_{x=0}} - C_{CS_{x=L}}) = JL \tag{5}$$

where the first expression is free diffusion of **S** and the second expression is facilitated diffusion of **S** by **CS**.

Even after this partial solution, Equation 2 is a system of nonlinear (due to bimolecular kinetics with saturation behavior) second-order differential equations to describe the concentration field in the layer, which cannot be solved analytically. However, at chemical equilibrium (due to infinite reaction rates) the reaction terms in Equation 2 become undefined, and a solution is found using the equilibrium relationship between **CS** and **S** (ODC). Thus the number of boundary conditions reduces from 4 to 2, and Equation 5 provides a direct solution. Whenever the reaction rates are finite, however, specific numerical solutions or analytic approximations must be developed.

Numerical solutions (109, 134, 203) have the advantage of being applicable also to nonlinearities in the equations and of providing solutions of any desirable accuracy in principle. However, they are not generally applicable, provide no information about mechanisms, require a priori specification of parameters, and can involve excessive computer time (44).

When trying to account for reaction-rate limitations one is confronted with problems involving "stiff" differential equations (for situations including steep local gradients) of the boundary-layer or singular-perturbation variety (44). To appreciate the possibilities and limitations of approximate analytic solutions it may be useful to inspect Figure 2, which schematically shows the regions where approximate analytic solutions may be obtained (for one reaction and one permeant **S**), depending on the concentration difference **ΔS**, the equilibrium constant K, and a Damköhler number γ (see below). Over the entire range shown, an analytic treatment with linearized kinetics is possible when **ΔS** becomes very small (small driving force), as shown by Friedlander and Keller (39). Increasing K (increasing affinity) decreases the region of validity for any analytic solution, particularly concerning **ΔS**.

Approximate analytic solutions may be particularly useful for the two extreme asymptotic regimes (see Fig. 2, hatched areas), the near-diffusion regime (Fig.

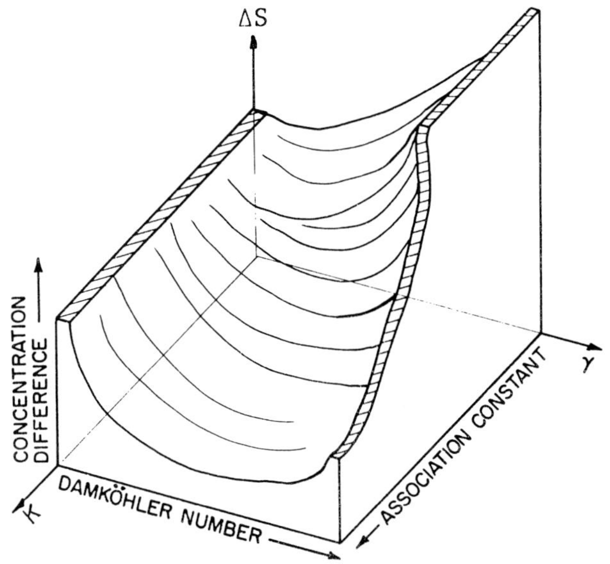

FIG. 2. Regions where approximate analytic solutions can be obtained (for one reaction and one permeant **S**), depending on concentration difference Δ**S**, equilibrium (association) constant K, and Damköhler number γ. Two extreme asymptotic regimes are hatched (*left*, near-diffusion regime; *right*, near-equilibrium regime). [From Schultz et al. (157).]

2, *left*) and the near-equilibrium regime (Fig. 2, *right*). These regimes are characterized by the Damköhler number γ (for a single homogeneous reaction), which is the ratio of characteristic or relaxation times of diffusion (τ_D) and reaction (τ_R)

$$\gamma = \frac{\tau_D}{\tau_R} = \frac{\theta L^2}{CD} = \left(\frac{L}{\lambda}\right)^2 \qquad (6)$$

where θ is a typical reaction rate, and system length $\lambda = \sqrt{CD/\theta}$ is a characteristic reaction-diffusion (reaction-layer) length scale [Friedlander and Keller (39)]; thus $\sqrt{\gamma} \equiv L/\lambda$. A typical value of λ for Hb is 0.1 μm at 25°C.

A large Damköhler number characterizes the near-equilibrium regime where the chemical reaction is so predominant that it determines the course of events and the facilitated flux approaches its maximum corresponding to chemical equilibrium. A small Damköhler number characterizes the near-diffusion regime. Here the residence time of reacting species in the layer may be so short as to preclude an appreciable chemical reaction, so that diffusion prevails over chemical reaction. In this regime, facilitation is much smaller than its maximum possible, although it may be substantial as compared with free diffusion. In the limit of $\gamma \rightarrow 0$ the near-diffusion regime provides the nonreactive (passive) physical permeability for **S** (181).

As shown above, assumption of chemical equilibrium as a limiting case ($\gamma \rightarrow \infty$) permits an analytic solution (144). Indeed, the first mathematical descriptions of facilitated O_2 diffusion [reviewed by Kreuzer (100) and Wittenberg (199)] neglected these boundary effects and were based on the assumption of chemical equilibrium according to the ODC. Because these solutions were compared with experimental results obtained on relatively thick layers (typically on Millipore membranes 150 μm thick), the assumption of chemical equilibrium was a useful approximation.

Equation 5 for Hb + O_2 at chemical equilibrium becomes

$$P_{O_2}\Delta P_{O_2}\left(1 + \frac{D_{Hb}C_T}{P_{O_2}}\frac{\Delta S_{O_2}}{\Delta P_{O_2}}\right) = JL \qquad (7)$$

where P_{O_2} = O_2 permeability = $\alpha_{O_2}D_{O_2}$ (α_{O_2} = O_2 solubility), C_T is total heme concentration, and $\Delta S_{O_2}/\Delta P_{O_2}$ is the slope of ODC. A calculation for the experimental situation shown in Figure 1 provided a plain flux of O_2 of 3 μl/min at a P_{O_2} difference of 300 Torr and a facilitated flux (above the point of saturation) of 1.5 μl/min, both in good agreement with the experimental values. The calculated values of D_{Hb}/D_{O_2} also agreed well with values obtained independently [(164); see also Fig. 5].

However, it was realized that the facilitated O_2 flux often was overestimated, as compared with the experimental data, when assuming chemical equilibrium. In numerical calculations Kutchai et al. (109) found the deviation from chemical equilibrium to be more marked at the low-pressure side where the HbO_2 concentration increases above the equilibrium value as L decreases, accompanied by a decrease of facilitation. This deviation was reduced on increases in k′, k, or K.

Departure from chemical equilibrium can be calculated with singular-perturbation methods. Perturbations originate at the boundaries where the boundary conditions are not compatible with chemical equilibrium (39, 184). Because **S** can cross the boundaries, whereas **C** and **CS** cannot, there must always be an association of **S** with **C** at the high-pressure side and a dissociation of **S** from **CS** at the low-pressure side; a finite reaction rate intuitively implies nonequilibrium near the boundaries (109). Thus three parts of the layer can be distinguished: two boundary zones with thicknesses determined by the penetration depth λ and a middle core (as shown in Fig. 3 for carrier Mb and substrate O_2). At the boundaries the gradient of **S** or P_{O_2} carries the total flux (no gradient in **CS** or saturation) and is equal on both sides at steady state (Fig. 3, solid lines). This excludes solutions with asymptotic profiles of **S** at the low-pressure side, as constructed by Wyman (201), Murray (136), and others. The boundary zones can be analyzed under these conditions and interpreted as boundary-layer resistances (43), but a full solution is obtained only by matching them to the middle core. The choice of the ODC is important; a one-step reaction scheme with a hyperbolic ODC for HbO_2 overestimates corrections at the low-pressure side because of its steeper course;

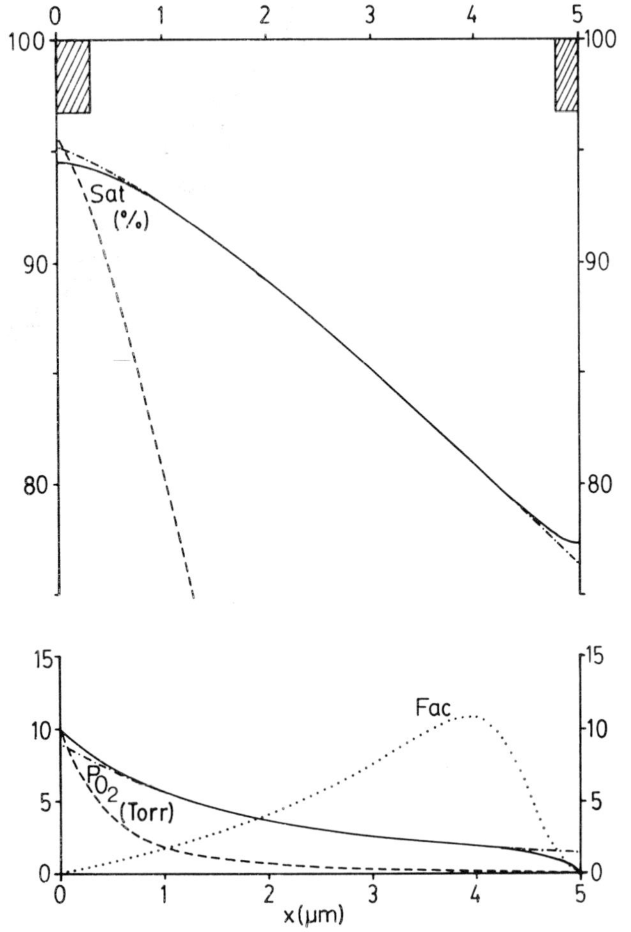

FIG. 3. Profiles of O_2 pressure (P_{O_2}, *bottom*), O_2 saturation (Sat, *top*), and nonequilibrium facilitation (Fac, ·····) plotted against distance (x) in 5-μm-thick layer of 15 g/100 ml Mb solution at steady state, exposed to P_{O_2} of 10 (*left*) and 0 (*right*) Torr. *Curves* are scaled for same flux contribution. Saturation scale only covers range from 75% to 100%. ——, Calculated profiles for nonequilibrium (76, 102); at boundaries, P_{O_2} slopes are equal (steady state) and slopes of MbO_2 saturation are 0 (no flux). —·—·—, Equilibrium core extensions. - - - - -, Profiles for equilibrium presumed throughout layer. *Top*, - - - - -: saturation starts at equilibrium value of <100% because a P_{O_2} of 10 Torr is not sufficient for complete saturation and would continue to 0 on *right side*. ▨, Penetration depth λ for nonequilibrium (39); although this penetration depth is smaller at low-pressure boundary, its effect of raising the MbO_2 saturation is enormous (from 0% at equilibrium to 77% at nonequilibrium) due to steep course of MbO_2 dissociation curve in this range.

an Adair four-step scheme would be more adequate (43) with diffusion paths longer than 4 μm (49).

Two different approaches have been discerned and identified: a weak-boundary-layer and a strong-boundary-layer method (47, 157).

In the weak-boundary-layer solution the assumption of chemical equilibrium throughout the layer ($\gamma \to \infty$; Fig. 3, broken lines) is a zero-order approximation. Deviations from chemical equilibrium are calculated in terms of a small parameter defining the dimensionless thickness of the perturbed layer relative to the total thickness (λ/L), which essentially is $\gamma^{-1/2}$ and is called ϵ (46) or $\epsilon^{1/2}$ (64, 98, 130, 136, 152). The method is straightforward, works well as long as the deviations are small ($\epsilon \ll 1$), and produces explicit formulas for calculation of profiles and facilitation. First- and higher-order terms can be calculated (46, 152) but do not necessarily lead to better approximations. Mitchell and Murray (130, 136) applied this technique to zero order only (called first order by these authors) and thus essentially reduced the problem to the equilibrium approach. Instead of calculating higher orders they used the experimentally measured flux (198) to formally prescribe the saturation on the low-pressure side. This saturation deviates from equilibrium and thus might imply an interface resistance at the low-pressure boundary. Therefore Jacquez et al. (80) numerically solved the equations by quasi linearization for the possibility of an interface resistance (back pressure) and concluded that Murray's analysis is not adequate for a description of the results of Wittenberg (198), even at thicknesses of 25 and 64 μm, but is good only for very thick membranes essentially at equilibrium throughout the layer.

Equilibrium in the core is a strong constraint in strong-boundary-layer (or shock-layer) techniques (101), also in first-order solution (161), but consequently such an equilibrium profile no longer can meet the boundary conditions. Therefore the equilibrium is uncoupled from the boundaries and is coupled to the boundary-zone solutions; extension of the core solution provides virtual values of P_{O_2} and saturation (Fig. 3, dashed-dotted lines). The virtual P_{O_2} is lower at the upstream boundary and higher at the downstream boundary, as compared with the actual values; the corresponding virtual saturations differ in the same way from the values predicted by these actual P_{O_2} values according to the ODC. Because the ODC is steeper at low P_{O_2} in general, the deviation is much more important at the downstream boundary; i.e., small changes in P_{O_2} will induce larger changes in saturation (e.g., from 0% to 77% for Mb in Fig. 3). The resulting formulas are now implicit and must be solved by iterative procedures, but the technique can be applied to much smaller values of γ.

The various strong-boundary-layer methods differ in the solution for the boundary zones. Kreuzer and Hoofd (101) constructed a solution by assuming that the reduced Hb concentration is constant in the boundary zones (strictly correct only for $P_{O_2} = 0$). The facilitated fluxes of O_2 in Hb solutions agreed well with the experimental data of Wittenberg (198). This solution was improved (102) by solving for all the boundary-layer profiles as small deviations from their equilibrium core extensions, which were assumed to be nearly constant. It was found that the system Hb + O_2 is not far from equilibrium down to $L = 200$ μm, whereas the system Mb + O_2 is not at equilibrium at $L < 1{,}000$ μm. In the latter case, equilibrium would lead to a facilitation almost double the experimental values of Wittenberg (198), but nonequilibrium provides better agreement. Increasing P_{O_2} on the high-pressure side reduces the facilitated flux; i.e., high P_{O_2} removes the system from equilibrium, the more so as the system tends to nonequilibrium (e.g., Mb + O_2), as Rubinow and Dembo (152) confirmed. The nonequilibrium profiles calculated for HbO_2 and O_2 were ascertained experimentally (192) by microcryophotometric determination of the HbO_2 saturation profiles in Millipore membranes 150 μm thick.

Smith et al. (161) developed separate approximate analytic solutions for thick and for thin layers. For thick layers a strong-boundary zone was solved with a first-order ($1/L$) or a second-order ($1/L^2$) approximation. Comparison with the numerical results of Kutchai et al. (109) for Hb + O_2 or Hb + CO and with their own numerical calculations provided excellent agreement.

Solutions for the near-diffusion regime ($\gamma \rightarrow 0$, due to slow reaction or thin layer) are based on the gradients of **C** and **CS** being small. No gradient in **CS** ($\gamma = 0$) means no facilitation. For constant **C** and **CS**, Equation 2 can be solved directly for **S** [slow-reaction solution of Ward (189)]. With γ as a small parameter in thin layers, first- and higher-order terms can be calculated for the near-diffusion regime (161).

The near-equilibrium and near-diffusion regimes were combined by Hoofd and Kreuzer (75, 76), who developed a solution for the substrate concentration consisting of the sum of two terms to be solved for small and large γ. Although the method originated from the shock-layer model, it no longer depends on the existence of a middle core and therefore is applicable to any situation.

Yung and Probstein (203) and Smith and Quinn (160) combined the two asymptotic solutions for the flux and derived approximate equations for flux prediction over the entire range of regimes.

Nedelman and Rubinow (140) constructed a solution for small facilitation (small **CS** gradient for Mb + O_2 and Hb + CO) ensuing from the large affinity of carrier for permeant and/or high pressures. In this case the permeant profile is approximately linear and therefore linearization is applicable. The authors obtained a solution in terms of Airy (Bessel) functions. Their calculations agree with those obtained by Hoofd and Kreuzer (76), but the numerical results are dubious because of questionable parameters chosen for experimental situations (131, 198).

Figure 4 is a comparison of the performance of the various quantitative interpretations of facilitated O_2 diffusion, as described above, for the entire range of Damköhler numbers.

In summary, the most useful analytic methods are, in the order of increasing complexity and applicability [modified from Goddard et al. (47)], *1)* classic chemical equilibrium approximation ($\epsilon = 0$ for $\gamma = \infty$); *2)* minor deviations from a limiting regime, permitting linearization of kinetics ($\Delta\mathbf{S} \rightarrow 0$, $KP_{O_2} \rightarrow \infty$, $\epsilon \rightarrow 0$ for $\gamma \rightarrow \infty$ or $\epsilon \gg 1$ for $\gamma \ll 1$); *3)* weak-boundary-layer analysis

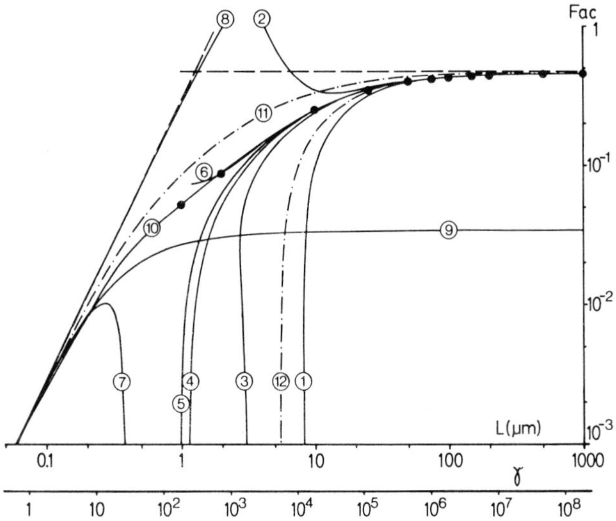

FIG. 4. Comparison of various approximate analytic approaches to describe facilitated diffusion in plot of facilitation (Fac) against layer thickness L and Damköhler number γ. Calculations for Hb solution of 15 g/100 ml and P_{O_2} difference of 200 vs. 2 Torr to compare with numerical results (●) of Kutchai et al. (109). -----, Asymptotes; near-diffusion asymptote (*left*) coincides with thin-layer first-order solution (161) and near-equilibrium asymptote (*top*) corresponds with thick-layer zero-order solutions (maximum facilitation). *Lines* and -·-·- (approximate formulas) indicate the solutions: *1*, weak boundary layer, first order (46, 130); *2*, weak boundary layer, second order (46, 152); *3*, strong boundary layer (101); *4*, strong boundary layer (102); *5*, thick layer, first order (161); *6*, thick layer, second order (161); *7*, thin layer, second order (161); *8*, slow reaction (189); *9*, single-point linearization (39, 46); *10*, wide range, improved for flat layers (76); *11*, interpolation formula, modified for nonzero back pressure (203); see ref. 160 for similar solution; *12*, approximation for sufficiently thick layers (161).

for definite but small deviations from chemical equilibrium, with singular-perturbation methods near equilibrium ($\epsilon \ll 1$ for $\gamma \gg 1$); *4)* strong-boundary-layer analysis with separate treatment of the boundary-layer effects and matching with equilibrium core solution ($\epsilon < 1$ for $\gamma > 1$); and *5)* combined Damköhler number solution applicable to any regime. Recent reviews with particular emphasis on mathematical treatment were published by Way et al. (191) and Jacquez (79).

Two groups have studied the dependence of optimum facilitation on the value of the equilibrium binding constant K. Schultz et al. (157) derived an expression for the equilibrium facilitation factor, showing that this factor goes through a maximum as the equilibrium binding constant K goes from zero to infinity. This optimum facilitation moves to lower values of K when the back pressure at the downstream boundary is increased according to optimum $K = 1/(C_{S_0}C_{S_L})^{1/2}$, where C_{S_0} is the permeant concentration at the upstream boundary and C_{S_L} is the permeant concentration at the downstream boundary. With no back pressure the curve of facilitation factor versus K reaches a plateau at high values of K. Noble and co-workers (93, 143) analyzed the possibility of optimizing the choice of parameters and regimes for O_2 facilitation and of evaluating the extent of deviation from the optimum in a given situation. They extended the analysis of Schultz et al. (157) to nonequilibrium and again found optimum facilitation at an intermediate value of K, depending on γ, of course. A kinetic efficiency factor η for diffusion and reaction in parallel, defined as the ratio of actual facilitation and equilibrium facilitation, declines with decreasing γ, as expected, the more so, paradoxically, as the mobility of the carrier increases, because with increasing mobility, equilibrium facilitation increases more than actual facilitation. The value of $1/\eta$ was found to be a qualitative measure of the time necessary to reach steady state.

Kemp and Noble (94) calculated that imposition of a temperature gradient across the diffusion membrane can significantly increase or decrease the facilitated flux and in extreme cases even reverse the direction of the facilitated flux.

Recently the attention paid to the shape factors affecting facilitated O_2 diffusion has increased. Noble (141, 142) and Folkner and Noble (37) developed analytic solutions for steady-state and transient response of facilitated transport for planar, cylindrical, and spherical geometries under the two extreme regimes of large and small Damköhler numbers γ. A shape factor was derived that permits evaluation of the performance of any of these geometries from the performance of another geometry on the basis of experimental data. Hoofd and Kreuzer (77) found good agreement of their analytic combined Damköhler number technique (76) with numerical calculations for spheres with a membrane, planar layers, and O_2 uptake by muscle cylinders. Stroeve and Eagle (174) calculated that nonequilibrium facilitation is maximal in planar geometry, followed by cylindrical and spherical geometries, whereas equilibrium facilitation is independent of configuration. Stroeve et al. (177) applied the combined Damköhler number technique of Hoofd and Kreuzer (76) to a sphere with a central core as a sink and a peripheral shell or membrane with reversible carrier reaction. Their analytic solutions agreed well with the numerical results of Folkner and Noble (37). Internal and external resistances decrease the flux of both freely diffusing permeant and facilitated component. Internal resistance in the membrane reduces facilitated flux more than does external resistance in the surrounding continuous phase.

Diffusion Coefficients of O_2 and Hemoglobin

Calculations of facilitated O_2 diffusion crucially depend on the assumed physical parameters, particularly the diffusion coefficients of O_2 (D_{O_2}) and the pigment protein (D_{pr}). Conversely D_{O_2} and D_{pr} may be estimated from the measured plain and facilitated fluxes of O_2 respectively. The diffusion coefficients decrease with increasing protein concentration due to the obstruction effect by the large protein molecules in solution, where an envelope of hydration water around the protein molecules has to be taken into account (170). A plot of D_{O_2} against Hb concentration (Fig. 5, *top*), with values of various authors, provided a smooth curve (48, 100, 102); a plot of D_{O_2} against the concentration of plasma or serum proteins resulted in a similar though not quite identical regression line (100, 102). In an Hb solution of a concentration equivalent to that in the red blood cells (RBC) (~35 g/100 ml), D_{O_2} is about one-third of the value in water or saline.

The D_{pr} is inversely related to the molecular weight

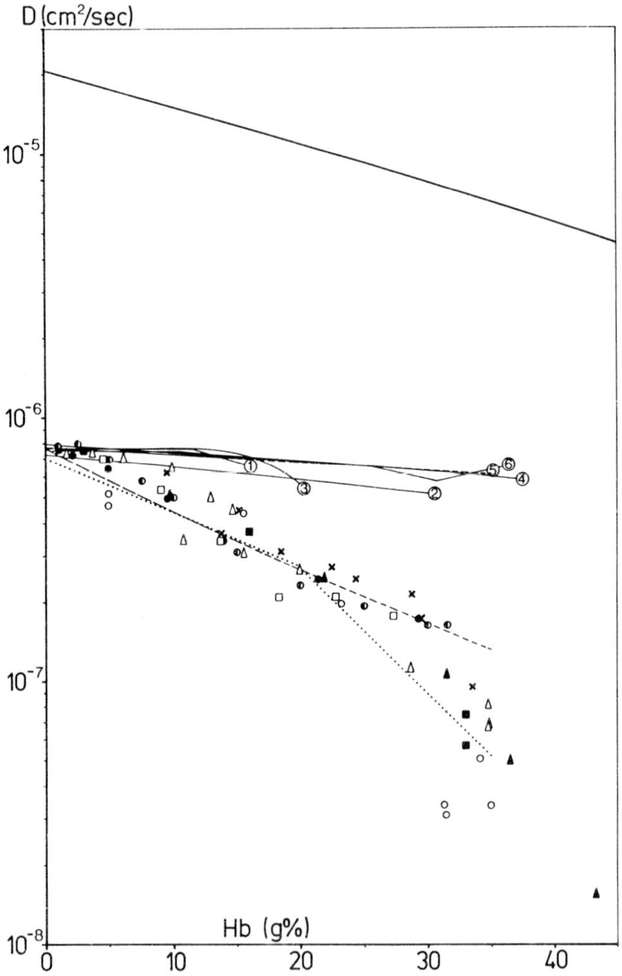

FIG. 5. Curve of diffusion coefficient of O_2 (D_{O_2}, *top*) from Goldstick and Fatt (48) and Kreuzer (100) and values of D_{Hb} obtained by various authors as a function of Hb concentration at 25°C. Symbols, tracer D_{Hb} (D_t, except ●): □, Keller and Friedlander (92), pH 7.4; ■, Moll (132); ○, Adams and Fatt (1); ●, Keller et al. (90), mutual D_m, pH 7.3; ◐, Keller et al. (90), tracer D_t, pH 7.3; △, Riveros-Moreno and Wittenberg (149), pH 7.3; ▲, Gros (51), pH 7.2, ionic strength I = 150 mM; ×, Spaan et al. (164). Numbered lines, mutual D_{Hb} (D_m): *1*, Wilson et al. (193), pH 7.0; *2*, Alpert and Banks (2), pH 7.0, I = 100 mM; *3*, Veldkamp and Votano (185), pH 7.2, I = 125 mM; *4*, Jones et al. (81), pH 6.9 = isoelectric point IP, I = 100 mM; *5*, Hall et al. (63), pH 6.7 = IP of deoxy Hb, I = 200 mM; *6*, LaGattuta et al. (115), pH 6.9, I = 150 mM; - - - - -, D_t calculated from D_m according to Hall et al. (63) up to 16 g/100 ml; --------, D_t calculated from D_m (63) extrapolated up to 35 g/100 ml; ·····, D_t calculated from Stokes-Einstein equation according to Equation 8 in Young et al. (202) with values of viscosity coefficient obtained by Kreuzer (99).

and to the viscosity of the solution, and the decrease of the self-diffusion coefficients with concentration is related to the volume fraction of the solution occupied by the protein (199).

The D_{pr} may be obtained in two ways. The mutual diffusion coefficient (D_m) is measured from diffusion due to a difference in total protein concentration, e.g., on opposite sides of a porous diaphragm. To measure the tracer or self-diffusion coefficient (D_t), protein solutions of equal concentrations are placed on each side of the membrane and labeled protein is present on one side; i.e., the total protein concentration is constant everywhere.

The D_t equals kT/f (where k is the Boltzmann constant, T is absolute temperature, and f is a frictional factor), whereas D_m equals D_t (1 + d log a/dlog C) (1 − ϕ) (where a is the activity coefficient, C is concentration, and ϕ is the volume fraction of solute); the dependence of activity a on C can be calculated (62, 90); the term (1 − ϕ) may have to be omitted (6). Thus D_t equals D_m only in very dilute ideal solution (2, 63, 95, 147, 185), but at finite protein concentration D_m is larger than D_t by the terms given above and the values of D_m and D_t are interconvertible according to the relationship shown. It is surprising therefore and remains unexplained that Keller et al. (90) did not find any difference between D_m and D_t for Hb. There seems to be agreement now that the photon correlation spectroscopy (laser) method provides reliable values of D_m, whereas the classic diaphragm diffusion cell method is able to provide D_t (63) but is not reliable to measure D_m because it is beset with difficulties when applied to proteins (62).

The concentration dependence of D_m and D_t (as found by many authors) is plotted for Hb in Figure 5 (*bottom*). The discrepancy between the values of D_m and D_t becomes more marked as the Hb concentration increases. The dependence of D_m on Hb concentration is linear throughout or over a wide range, contrary to D_t, which shows considerable scattering, particularly at higher Hb concentrations. For our purpose it is important that in the presence of a constant total Hb concentration (as pertains in typical measurements of facilitated O_2 diffusion) the interdiffusion of HbO_2 and Hb is given by D_t (e.g., ref. 164), which is reduced to ~10% at the Hb concentration in the RBC as compared to diluted solutions.

At higher concentrations there will be molecular interactions between the diffusing particles, reflecting in nonideal osmotic behavior (81, 149, 185). At low ionic strength, electrostatic interactions ensue (61). Most important is the possibility of a structural change of the Hb molecule by tetramer dissociation (promoted by decrease in concentration, increase in pH, or oxygenation), which has not been considered sufficiently (2, 61, 81, 185). Tetramers and dimers differ not only in molecular weight and thus mobility (153) but also in electric charge; this must affect the movement and electrostatic interaction of the particles, depending on the pH by way of the hydration (which is increasing with pH), particularly in solutions of low ionic strength (16, 115, 147). On the other hand there may also be intertetrameric aggregation (115) as well as conformational changes (186).

Facilitated Diffusion of CO

Theoretically one should expect a facilitation of CO diffusion in a film of Hb or Mb solution even greater than that of O_2 diffusion, due to the much higher CO affinity that results in large HbCO concentration gradients in the presence of very low concentrations of dissolved CO. There was some enhancing effect, though small and inconclusive, in dilute Hb solutions in non-steady-state thin-layer experiments (97). At steady state Mochizuki and Forster (131) found, with partial pressure of CO (P_{CO}) up to 10 Torr, a facilitation very much greater than that of O_2 with Hb but still only 1/10 the value to be expected at chemical equilibrium. Facilitation of CO diffusion increased in the presence of raised O_2 concentrations, which was ascribed to an increased rate of dissociation of CO from HbCO by O_2; at equilibrium the HbCO concentration difference should fall in this case. Thus reaction rates were limiting and placed this system far from chemical equilibrium at the boundaries. There is an O_2 diffusion countercurrent to CO diffusion in the absence of or even against a P_{O_2} gradient (103, 111, 114, 131).

Wittenberg (198), however, found no facilitated CO diffusion in various pigment solutions at high P_{CO} values (70–750 Torr), not even in the presence of O_2, whereas CO in even small amounts markedly reduced facilitated O_2 diffusion (8, 197, 198). The absence of facilitated CO diffusion was explained primarily by the extreme sensitivity of the CO system to even minute back pressures due to its high affinity and the experimental difficulty of adequate stirring to prevent back pressure (139, 201).

However, Kutchai et al. (109) challenged this explanation and emphasized the importance of marked chemical nonequilibrium due to the slow dissociation of CO from HbCO downstream, extant even in layers 500 μm thick. Suchdeo et al. (179) explained the absence of facilitated CO diffusion in the experiments of Wittenberg (198) as a result of the high P_{CO} values applied, moving the system toward the near-diffusion regime. Their calculated facilitated CO fluxes without O_2 were even much higher than those reported by Mochizuki and Forster (131). Hoofd and Kreuzer (75, 103) computed that CO fluxes facilitated by Mb reach a maximum at L ~ 30 μm with a P_{CO} ~ 2 Torr. However, with the often-used layer thickness of 150 μm this flux maximum is only 8% of the equilibrium value and thus much further removed from equilibrium than a corresponding O_2 system. When the reaction rates were carefully considered, there was satisfactory agreement with the experiments of Mochizuki and Forster (131). With low P_{CO} the facilitated CO flux was much greater than the free CO flux for both Hb and Mb, whereas it was reduced to a few percent of the total CO flux (75) in the presence of a P_{CO} of 100 Torr, as used by Wittenberg (198) and Murray and Wyman (139). This means that the absence of facilitated CO diffusion suggested by these authors pertains to a physiologically abnormal situation of high P_{CO} only and implies no general solution of the problem of facilitated CO diffusion.

Facilitated O_2 Diffusion in Non-Steady-State Oxygenation

Most of the analyses presented so far concern experiments at steady state to rule out the capacitive factor of Hb or Mb, which interferes with facilitation. Because the gas-exchange processes in the body, however, are non-steady-state phenomena, the question arises as to what extent non-steady-state oxygenation of Hb solutions is affected by facilitation.

At chemical equilibrium the half time of O_2 saturation of a layer should be proportional to L^2. In an Hb solution of 32.25 g/100 ml at pH 7.4 and 37°C, this relationship was obeyed when $L > 1.6$ μm, whereas below this limit the chemical reaction rates were intervening. The effect of O_2 facilitation was zero at 0.25 μm and increased with L up to its maximum at $L \geq$ 10 μm. This maximum facilitation was reached at lower L than in steady state and amounted to a 35% shortening of the saturation half time, which is less than the facilitating effect at steady state in layers of the same thickness (106).

Kutchai (108) found that numerical solutions that use the unmodified advancing front theory (i.e., neglecting HbO_2 diffusion) were able to describe the O_2 uptake by layers 1.8–20 μm thick for saturations from 30% to 90%. He confirmed his conclusion of a negligible role of HbO_2 diffusion (107) when he compared his numerical calculations with the experimental data of Klug et al. (96). However, from a similar comparison Spaan (162), using the advancing front theory corrected for the physically dissolved O_2, concluded that HbO_2 diffusion cannot be neglected and suggested a simultaneous determination of D_{O_2} and D_{Hb} from non-steady-state oxygenation experiments.

Spaan and co-workers (163, 164) calculated the oxygenation of layers of Hb solutions thick enough to ensure chemical equilibrium between Hb and O_2. Plots of the oxygenation times against $1/P_{O_2}$ (where P_{O_2} = O_2 driving pressure) in any particular Hb solution permitted the simultaneous derivation of the O_2 permeability (or, knowing O_2 solubility, of D_{O_2}) and of D_{Hb}. The experimental oxygenation times were measured spectrophotometrically in Hb solutions of 10–34 g/100 ml in layers 50–250 μm thick with O_2 driving pressures between 35 and 700 Torr at 25°C. The values of the oxygenation times agreed well with similar previous data (99): those of the O_2 permeability agreed well with data of Stroeve et al. (173) at steady state, and those of D_{O_2} agreed well with a previous curve (100). The D_{Hb} values are plotted in Figure 5.

Non-steady-state O_2 facilitation was numerically calculated during the deoxygenation of layers of Hb solution also under the conditions of tissue microcirculation. There was no chemical equilibrium in these thin layers of 1.6 and 6 μm (deviations up to 40%), and the reaction kinetics should be accounted for to be compatible with the actual ODC. The resistance to O_2 transport in blood was not constant but depended on the wall O_2 flux and the position (time) along the capillary (159).

Physiological Significance of Facilitated O_2 Diffusion

OXYGEN DIFFUSION FACILITATED BY HEMOGLOBIN IN RED BLOOD CELLS. The RBC interior can be considered as equivalent to a highly concentrated (~35 g/100 ml) but true, though not ideal, solution of Hb whose tracer D_{Hb} (D_t) is ~10^{-7} cm²/s or ~100 times smaller than D_{O_2} (Fig. 5). Despite the absence of an intracellular structure, the physicochemical situation in the RBC is complex because of the influence of effectors on the function of Hb (pH, CO_2, organic phosphates, small anions), ionic exchanges, and a potential across the membrane.

In experiments on RBC, hemolysis results in a spurious increase of facilitated O_2 diffusion (110, 176), particularly in Millipore membranes. Marked enhancement, though less than in Hb solutions, was demonstrated (135, 155), particularly even when hemolysis was minor (68, 110). This facilitation often was similar to the free diffusion of O_2 but must be below its equilibrium maximum for the dimensions of the RBC where deviations from equilibrium can be expected (39, 91, 109). The HbO_2 diffusion markedly accelerates the rate of deoxygenation of the RBC in traversing the capillaries; the Nusselt number as a measure of the O_2 flux may be increased by a factor of two to three by HbO_2 diffusion when varying D_{Hb} from 0 to 6.5×10^{-8} cm²/s in a 6-μm layer of Hb solution after 0.75 s (159). Gonzalez-Fernandez and Atta (49), who numerically investigated the O_2 transport in solutions of Hb (and Mb) at steady state, were concerned with the contribution of O_2 facilitation in capillaries at an Hb concentration equivalent to that in the RBC. For a diffusion path of 0.75–1 μm, they calculated for physiologically possible P_{O_2} differences in hypoxia a contribution of O_2 facilitation of 56%–69% of the total O_2 flux. Antonini et al. (3) found by microspectrophotometry on single RBC that combination of Hb with O_2 was 10 times faster than combination with CO; because this difference could not be explained by plain diffusion of these gases, they suspected the presence of facilitated diffusion in the case of O_2 combination.

Because there is mounting evidence that the diffusive resistance of the RBC membrane for O_2 is negligible (105, 110, 167), each RBC can be considered a homogeneous particle with a D_{O_2} and D_{Hb} according to its Hb concentration. A heterogeneous media theory can be applied to a suspension of RBC (dispersed phase) in plasma (continuous phase) to predict an effective D_{O_2} (encompassing facilitation) from the diffusion properties of the two phases. The heterogeneous media theories of Maxwell and Fricke were applied to flowing blood (165) and to stagnant blood (173, 176). There was substantial facilitation, though well below its value at equilibrium. Under physiological conditions (hematocrit 45, driving pressure difference from 95 to 40 Torr P_{O_2}, 37°C), however, equilibrium may be presumed with a maximum facilitation of 15% (173, 176); facilitation would be considerably larger at hypoxia. Goddard (45) calculated that the peripheral mass transfer resistance of quasi spheres in a suspension can become dominant even at near equilibrium and that therefore the reactive enhancement of mass transfer can be much smaller in dispersions than in homogeneous solutions; he gave a theoretical limit for the transport rate in heterogeneous dispersions. Stroeve (172) reviewed the field of diffusion with chemical reaction in two-phase heterogeneous media.

In non-steady-state systems in vivo both the P_{O_2} and the HbO_2 gradients change continuously during oxygenation and deoxygenation, and deviations from chemical equilibrium may be more marked here (39). Moll (134), assuming chemical equilibrium and neglecting any resistance of the RBC membrane, has shown by numerical calculations for layers 1.6 and 3.6 μm thick that Hb diffusion speeded up only the last two-thirds of saturation change by ~30% of the time; the acceleration of the O_2 uptake by Hb diffusion was more marked in the presence of lower P_{O_2}. Kutchai (106, 107) calculated, based on the nonequilibrium approach, that for a 32.25 g/100 ml Hb solution 1.6 μm thick at 37°C and pH 7.4, the non-steady-state initial rate of O_2 uptake (first 10% only) is influenced in decreasing importance by k′, D_{O_2}, D_{Hb}, and k.

In flowing blood any effect on HbO_2 diffusion may be overridden by shear-induced effective mixing of the contents of the RBC, which helps loading and unloading of O_2 (25, 204). Clark et al. (15) theoretically analyzed a possible effect of tank-treading motion and kneading motion of the RBC on O_2 transport. They estimated that cell rotation does not have a significant effect, whereas distortion of the RBC with mixing of its contents might be significant.

OXYGEN DIFFUSION FACILITATED BY MYOGLOBIN IN MUSCLE. The situation is more complicated for Mb than for Hb, because not only the Mb concentration in the tissue but also the characteristics of the highly structured cellular medium (total protein concentration ~20 g/100 ml and a corresponding viscosity) and the condition of Mb in relation to its environment are important. Distribution and mobility of Mb in the cell remain controversial issues. Histochemical studies seemed to suggest that Mb may be preferentially located near the cell membrane, at fibrillar structures possibly related to an internal cell membrane system, at the myofibrils mainly in the A band (except in the H zone), and also at the Z line, but methodological difficulties preclude a definitive conclusion concerning facilitation [reviewed by Kreuzer (100) and Wittenberg (199)]. In aqueous solutions Riveros-Moreno and Wittenberg (149) determined the tracer D_{Mb} as a function of the Mb concentration up to 27 g/100 ml and found D_{Mb} to be roughly twice D_{Hb} above 10 g/100 ml. In muscle homogenates Moll (133) found a D_{Mb} of 2.7×10^{-7} cm²/s at 37°C or about one-third of the value in an Mb solution of the same Mb concentration. Livingston et al. (116) who recently used the proton nuclear magnetic resonance (NMR) technique in bovine heart muscle at 25°C, suggest that intracellular Mb diffusion at an Mb concentration of 0.2 mM occurs at nearly half the rate observed in dilute aqueous solution (0.5 mM).

The requirements for physiological facilitation of O_2 transport by Mb in the muscle are *1)* Mb must be present in sufficiently high concentration; *2)* Mb must be mobile, at least partially; and *3)* there must be partial (preferably marked) desaturation along a P_{O_2} gradient in the muscle at low P_{O_2} in view of the high affinity of Mb for O_2. The transport of O_2 in respiring muscle includes three basic processes: free diffusion of O_2, diffusion of MbO_2 coupled with reversible reaction between Mb and O_2 (facilitated O_2 diffusion), and the irreversible reaction of O_2 consumption in the mitochondria.

Of three possible Mb functions—O_2 transport, catalysis, and O_2 storage—Millikan (129) found evidence only for storage and argued that Mb acts as a short-time O_2 store to tide the muscle over from one contraction to the next, covering a few seconds. Later in vitro experiments, however, provided evidence for an O_2 transport function of Mb (155, 197). During intermittent muscular activity there is fast (within 1 s) deoxygenation and reoxygenation of Mb, and during sustained muscular contraction there is a steady level of partial desaturation (129); therefore an MbO_2 gradient is possible. Thus it appears that the conditions for facilitation in vivo are met with the exception of the unknown mobility of Mb in the muscle.

According to Wittenberg (199), who reviewed the experimental evidence on the function of Mb in muscle and heart from 1939 [Millikan (129)] up to 1970, the steady state of Mb oxygenation and of mitochondrial oxidation-reduction in the beating heart does not support the view that Mb primarily serves as a short-term O_2 store; instead, because Mb in the beating heart is only partially oxygenated, gradients of MbO_2 may be present to favor a function of Mb in terms of facilitation of O_2 diffusion. Fletcher (36) noted that a small MbO_2 disequilibrium can induce deoxygenation and thus O_2 unloading, even when the local MbO_2

fraction is near the saturation value. The MbO_2 can also readily respond to small local pressure variations within the tissue. The mitochondria may produce small local regions with high P_{O_2} gradients, which are seen only as average gradients across these regions. In such a case the local MbO_2 could direct O_2 into these higher consumption regions by its ability to transfer O_2 over the smaller MbO_2 gradients outside these regions (36).

Calculated estimates of the facilitation of O_2 diffusion by Mb in vivo suggested an enhancement possibly similar to plain O_2 diffusion at low P_{O_2} in the muscle [reviewed by Kreuzer (100) and Wittenberg (199)]. Facilitation was calculated to occur, when assuming chemical equilibrium, with O_2 consumption of zero order or according to Michaelis-Menten kinetics (137, 138, 183), but deviation from equilibrium as well as the presence of cell boundaries reduces the facilitating effect (45, 184a). Application of Maxwell's heterogeneous media theory to a muscle with cells of radius 3.5 μm showed that facilitation is about the same as inert O_2 permeability and that it is 85% of its maximum equilibrium value (171, 175), in agreement with experimental results (23); i.e., the assumption of chemical equilibrium is an acceptable approximation. The facilitation factor can be influenced by an irreversible reaction (consumption). For larger cell radii, irreversible reaction decreases concentration of the diffusing species and therefore increases facilitation [(175); see also Fig. 1]. In tissue, the O_2 penetration depth into tissue was calculated to reach farther in the presence of a subcritical linear dependency of the cellular O_2 consumption on P_{O_2} than with zero-order kinetics of the O_2 consumption, which may be important in hypoxia (104, 187).

Wittenberg et al. (196) measured the steady-state O_2 uptake of fiber bundles from resting pigeon breast muscle in a chamber perfused with a succinate-containing Krebs-Ringer solution at 37°C. The O_2 consumption with P_{O_2} values below 150 Torr was reduced by inactivation of Mb (e.g., by nitrite, supposedly not affecting the O_2 uptake of isolated mitochondria in the presence of Mb) to about half the value found with active Mb, leading to the conclusion that Mb in the intact muscle facilitates the O_2 transport to the mitochondria. However, a mathematical treatment was impossible, and therefore no quantitative data in terms of diffusional parameters were presented. Later the same group (20) failed to demonstrate any difference in O_2 uptake with and without nitrite below a P_{O_2} of 400 Torr, when an isolated dog heart preparation with intact microcirculation was perfused with a fluorocarbon suspension at 28°C. The authors suspected that a heterogeneous distribution of the P_{O_2} gradients in the myocardium with predominant regions of high and near-zero P_{O_2} might have concealed any facilitation. In view of these difficulties, Wittenberg and Wittenberg (200) isolated fresh cells from adult rat ventricles, providing better controlled experimental conditions. Steady-state O_2 uptake of this preparation was O_2 limited only at very low P_{O_2}, near 0.1 Torr, which, however, still is much higher than that of the mitochondria, suggesting steep intracellular O_2 gradients. Wittenberg and Robinson (195) and Wittenberg and Monahan (194), however, concluded that their half-maximum P_{O_2} of 0.15 Torr in adult rat heart myocytes differed little from that of isolated skeletal muscle mitochondria (0.02–0.05 Torr); they concluded that the intracellular impediment to O_2 diffusion is minimal and that therefore a major part of the resistance to O_2 flux in Mb-containing heart muscle cells should be sought outside the cells. Katz et al. (87), using monoamine oxidase as an intracellular probe of P_{O_2} in isolated cardiac myocytes, found the P_{O_2} gradient from outside the cell to the outer mitochondrial membrane to be at most 2 Torr, even with strong respiration; i.e., the large P_{O_2} difference (~20 Torr) between capillary lumen and mitochondria of the working heart must be extracellular.

Cole et al. (19) studied the effect of Mb on O_2 consumption and ATP production in isolated mitochondria of rat skeletal muscle in steady state at 25°C. The half-maximum P_{O_2} was 0.02–0.05 Torr for both O_2 consumption and ATP production with and without functional Mb. Thus Mb had no direct influence on the O_2 transport immediately around the isolated mitochondria. The Mb did, however, enhance the O_2 flux across the stagnant layer at the gas-liquid interface. The authors warned, though, against extrapolating these results to muscle tissue in vivo.

Cole (17, 18) perfused the canine isolated working gastrocnemius-plantaris muscle in situ with blood equilibrated with 10% O_2 at 37°C. Reversible inactivation of Mb by H_2O_2 reduced the O_2 consumption during stimulation by 35% and the twitch-tension amplitude by ~45% without the muscle being hypoxic; there was no change in O_2 consumption at rest. The decrease in O_2 consumption correlated best with a decrease in O_2 extraction; there was no change in flow. Cole concluded that Mb is important for maintaining isometric exercise in hypoxia.

De Koning et al. (23) studied the possible significance of facilitated O_2 diffusion in thin layers (300–700 μm) of respiring chicken gizzard smooth muscle at steady state and 37°C. Oxygen flux measurements at high P_{O_2} yielded maximum O_2 consumption and inert O_2 permeability, whereas a mathematical analysis of O_2 uptake from measurements at lower (subcritical) P_{O_2} provided values of q_{50} (the P_{O_2} for half-maximum O_2 consumption) and facilitation. It appeared that in this situation the effects of P_{O_2}-dependent O_2 consumption and facilitation counteract one another, whereas both enhance O_2 consumption into the tissue (104). Zero facilitation was defined as that obtained in the presence of 1% CO; maximum possible facilitation was calculated from the prevailing

Mb concentration, assuming full mobility of Mb. Facilitation without CO was 50%–100% of the theoretical maximum, i.e., in the same range as the 85% facilitation calculated by Stroeve and Eagle (175). Microcryophotometric measurements of the MbO_2 gradients in this resting muscle suggested that at most 40% of the O_2 transport could be mediated by Mb (158). The average value of 2 Torr for q_{50} is much higher than the mitochondrial Michaelis-Menten constant K_m and thus is an apparent K_m accounting for diffusion resistances in the tissue (30, 104).

Driedzic and co-workers (28, 29) compared the isolated perfused heart preparations of two fish species, one rich in Mb (sea raven, *Hemitripterus americanus*) and the other poor in Mb (ocean pout, *Macrozoarces americanus*). Both hearts have no coronary arteries and are metabolically quite similar. The power output during electric pacing and perfusion with blood equilibrated with 5% O_2 in the presence of iodoacetate and pyruvate declined faster with time when Mb was inactivated by hydroxylamine only in the Mb-rich heart of the sea raven. Thus Mb was important for maintaining cardiac activity during hypoxia in this species, possibly because of O_2 facilitation.

Stevens and Carey (169) investigated why warmth enhances muscular performance. Tunas are warm-blooded fish with high O_2 consumption, an extraordinary capacity to maintain high cruising speeds for a long time, and much red muscle rich in Mb. Elevated temperature increases the mobility of Mb and thus favors O_2 facilitation by MbO_2; it also shifts the MbO_2 dissociation curve to the right, which promotes the occurrence of MbO_2 concentration gradients in the cell at low P_{O_2}. To prove this, Stevens (168) measured the rate of O_2 diffusion across rat Hb solutions in Millipore filters. The value of Q_{10} of the experimental diffusion rate constant plotted against Hb concentration first increased about threefold up to a maximum at an Hb concentration of 21 g/dl and then decreased at high Hb concentrations of up to 40 g/dl. This behavior is remarkably similar to that in a Wittenberg (198) curve for the facilitated O_2 flux as a function of Hb and Mb concentration.

The important problem of the O_2 gradients in tissue must be examined. Where these gradients are located and whether they enable MbO_2-mediated facilitated O_2 diffusion are physiologically relevant questions.

In the isolated, Hb-free perfused rat heart, there may be sharp intracellular O_2 gradients between cytosol containing Mb and mitochondrial inner membrane (182). Such gradients were also suggested for isolated hepatocytes (84, 85) and for resting isolated rat cardiac myocytes near steady state (83). In the hepatocytes, the O_2 gradients were thought to be located in proximity to the mitochondria within a distance of 1 μm where the intracellular D_{O_2} was calculated to be only ~1/100 of the extracellular value and to be a function of mitochondrial respiration. Jones (82) detected this O_2 gradient at the outer mitochondrial membrane of isolated hepatocytes by the use of monoamine oxidase activity as a sensor for O_2 concentration and the respiratory rate of the mitochondria. In the myocytes, the half-maximum value of MbO_2 saturation depended on the O_2 consumption; it was 8.9 μM O_2 in the resting controls, 2.2 μM O_2 for isolated Mb with zero O_2 consumption, and ~25 μM O_2 with stimulated O_2 consumption (83). Inactivation of Mb by H_2O_2 had no effect on the O_2 dependency of cytochrome *aa*$_3$ oxidation (half-maximum value = 5.8 μM O_2) and thus showed that the presence of active Mb does not alter the O_2 supply to mitochondria under these O_2-limiting conditions (83). Some of these measurements can be criticized because O_2 concentration was measured in the suspension fluid, thus neglecting the diffusion resistance in the boundary layer around the myocytes (22).

Gayeski and Honig (41) found a uniformly high MbO_2 saturation (>70%) in resting dog gracilis muscle at 37°C and concluded that this was not compatible with facilitation. The MbO_2 saturation did not decrease during the first seconds of twitch contraction when stimulating at moderate frequencies of 1/s or 4/s (22). However, a study of steadily working skeletal muscle or of a continuously working muscle such as that of the heart might be more revealing than the situation in resting skeletal muscle, because facilitation is supposed to be beneficial particularly in situations of high O_2 demand and/or low P_{O_2}.

The results concerning myocardial variations of MbO_2 saturation are conflicting. Tamura et al. (182) found in the isolated, Hb-free perfused rat heart that Mb is more oxygenated during systole and diastole and deoxygenated in the resting period, whereas cytochrome *aa*$_3$ is more reduced in systole and diastole and oxidized in the resting state. During perfusion with 95% O_2-saturated Krebs-Ringer-HCO_3^- buffer at 25°C, there were fluctuations with only 5%–10% of the Mb being in the deoxygenated form, which is not thought to be enough to elicit facilitation. Hassinen et al. (65) detected a considerable myocardial (subepicardial) O_2 gradient in the rat heart and found that the oxygenation level of Mb oscillated in pace with the contraction-relaxation cycle of the heart, with deoxygenation occurring during systole. This oscillation was not increased when the perfusate O_2 concentration was lowered. Makino et al. (121), however, did not see any variation of myocardial MbO_2 saturation during the cardiac cycle in aerobic and anaerobic steady state in the isolated perfused rat heart. Figulla et al. (35) found in the blood-free perfused guinea pig heart an MbO_2 saturation of 93% and a cytochrome *aa*$_3$ oxidation of 91%, from which they concluded a partial anoxia of 9%. Araki et al. (4) found in the isolated, Hb-free perfused rat heart that Mb was deoxygenated >50% even during normoxia. Barlow et al. (5) induced ischemia by coronary artery ligation in the isolated, Hb-free perfused rabbit heart. There was a sharp interface between fully reduced and normoxic tissue, but the width of this border zone was not affected by oxidation of the intracellular Mb by nitrite, suggesting that Mb did not exert any facilitatory effect for O_2 diffusion across this zone. Gonzalez-Fernandez and Atta (50) numerically calculated that the presence of membranes in the diffusion path lowers O_2 facilitation. The extent of this decrease depends on the location and number of membranes; the mechanism is based on the cumulative effect of jump discontinuities in the concentration of MbO_2 at the membranes.

Some of these studies, particularly those of Tamura et al. (182), Jones and Mason (85), and Jones and Kennedy (83, 84), are subject to some doubt because they did not measure O_2 gradients directly but imputed them from optical signals in heterogeneous tissue populations. If cytochrome aa_3 is reduced in some (anoxic) mitochondria and oxidized in others, no conclusions can be drawn about gradients around an individual mitochondrion. Both values of O_2 half-saturation pressure (P_{50}) of Mb and of the critical P_{O_2} are similar in vivo and in vitro (C. Honig, unpublished observations). In heterogeneous tissue, interpretation of results averaged over a certain tissue volume is difficult in terms of gradients and the resolution of the methods is not sufficient to measure the postulated steep gradients directly (13).

For the above reasons, Honig et al. (73) measured MbO_2 saturation at many sites in dog gracilis muscle that was freeze clamped during tetanic contraction and calculated the corresponding P_{O_2} values from the MbO_2 dissociation curve. The O_2 distribution within this working muscle cell is remarkably uniform; the largest intracellular gradient found was only 14% MbO_2 saturation, corresponding to a P_{O_2} of 1.2 Torr, and the gradients were irregular in terms of intracellular pattern. Federspiel (34) also computed an intracellular P_{O_2} gradient of only 1–3 Torr in the presence of a sufficiently high Mb concentration and concluded that this gradient was enough to account for the measured O_2 flux. These flat gradients are incompatible with the assumption of the Krogh tissue model that the major resistance to O_2 diffusion resides within the tissue.

Furthermore the tissue is not homogeneous; there may be steep intercellular gradients in the extracellular medium where the capillaries are located. Because, in the working muscle, some fibers are working and others are resting, the capillary distribution is not homogeneous; the individual diffusion fields interact and an O_2 exchange between adjacent fields may occur, leading to redistribution of O_2 by even small driving forces, where Mb might be involved. Thus Mb, together with intracellular convection (42), might contribute to buffering the tissue P_{O_2} at a low and uniform level and thus minimize heterogeneity of O_2 concentration in exercise without compromising O_2 consumption. This would increase the P_{O_2} difference between capillary and tissue cells, enhance the O_2 release from the RBC, and inhibit the diffusional shunting between capillaries. In this way the small MbO_2 saturation gradients in working skeletal muscle would not be thought of as the missing cause (41) but rather as the consequence of Mb-mediated O_2 facilitation (40). Such a mechanism is similar to a function that is assigned to legume Hb (Leg Hb or Lb) in N_2 fixation (200). Performance of all these functions is greatly enhanced if there is significant desaturation of Mb in exercise. Because the turnover of cytochrome aa_3 does not become O_2 limited until Mb is almost fully desaturated, the large fall in MbO_2 saturation and tissue P_{O_2} in exercise does not signify hypoxia; instead it is an essential adaptation to high O_2 demand. This concept would call for a thorough revision of the Krogh tissue model.

Where is most of the resistance to O_2 diffusion between the capillaries and the tissue cells located? Whereas in the Krogh tissue model the resistance to O_2 diffusion by the capillary wall and the blood is neglected, Honig et al. (73) postulated a carrier-free layer, consisting of plasma, endothelium, and extracellular fluid between RBC and muscle cell, that would throttle the O_2 release. This layer and the high O_2 flux density at the capillary would result in a region of disequilibrium between Hb and O_2 in the RBC interior adjacent to the RBC membrane (16). This O_2 gradient between RBC and sarcolemma may represent ~50% of the total resistance to O_2 diffusion (66) or may be at least an order of magnitude larger than that between sarcolemma and mitochondria (73); i.e., the bottleneck would be at the capillary. Indeed, gradients from Hb to Mb on the order of 10–15 Torr/μm, acting over a distance of <6 μm, have been observed in working dog gracilis muscle, and P_{O_2} in equilibrium with Mb is less than venous P_{O_2} at almost all locations. Furthermore the combined surface area of the mitochondria exceeds the effective capillary surface area by a factor of 200 or more. Therefore the O_2 flux density near a mitochondrion is ~1/200 of that near a capillary. The P_{O_2} gradient around a mitochondrion was calculated to be no greater than 0.03 Torr at maximum O_2 consumption; i.e., there are no observable "O_2 wells" around the mitochondria (14; C. Honig, unpublished observations).

Furthermore, in exercise, blood flow increases and in an increasing number of capillaries the RBC transit time, as compared with the O_2 release time, is too short to allow equilibration between blood and tissue (72). This increased heterogeneity results in a functional convective arteriovenous O_2 shunt with, on one hand, a paradoxically increased venous O_2 saturation and P_{O_2} and, on the other hand, a decreased tissue P_{O_2}. Myoglobin might mitigate this effect by buffering tissue P_{O_2} way below capillary P_{O_2} and thus enhance O_2 release from the blood, compensating for short

RBC transit times. Buffering is most effective near the P_{50} of Mb (40). Thus Mb balances discrepancies between O_2 delivery and O_2 consumption in exercise.

Whether convection by stirring in the muscle cells, particularly during contraction, might be more effective in promoting O_2 transport within the muscle than Mb-facilitated O_2 diffusion needs to be examined.

FACILITATED O_2 DIFFUSION IN TISSUES OTHER THAN MUSCLE. Longmuir and McCabe (119) found that the respiration rate of various tissues (particularly liver and kidney) behaved according to Michaelis-Menten kinetics rather than according to zero-order O_2 consumption, which is assumed in the classic diffusion model (188). Longmuir et al. (118) suggested cytochrome *P*-450 as a carrier; this however, was discounted recently (I. Longmuir, unpublished observations).

Facilitated O_2 and CO transport has been suggested for the sheep placenta (58) and for the lungs of sheep and dogs (10), again invoking cytochrome *P*-450 as a carrier. However, this contention could not be confirmed for the placenta, because the data were shown to be not good enough for a conclusive proof (120). Application of the dithionite technique yielded very high values of the lung membrane diffusing capacity ($D_{M_{O_2}}$) and thus excluded any membrane diffusion limitation (11). Five pieces of evidence exclude the facilitation hypothesis and thus cytochrome *P*-450 as a carrier (12; B. Burns, unpublished observations). *1)* Because P_{50} of pulmonary cytochrome *P*-450 is nearly equal for O_2 and CO and very low (0.26 Torr), the carrier would always be saturated and CO binding would be impossible even at a P_{O_2} as low as 10 Torr. *2)* Cytochrome *P*-450 occurs in the wrong place, in the bronchial epithelial Clara cells rather than in the alveolar septum. *3)* Temperature dependence of $D_{M_{O_2}}$ is of diffusional rather than chemical magnitude. *4)* There are no drug effects on $D_{M_{O_2}}$; earlier inhibition results are explicable by variation in the blood diffusing capacity (possibly altering Hb-mediated facilitation of O_2 diffusion in the RBC) or by the action of Hb as a drug-metabolizing enzyme. *5)* The enormous values of $D_{M_{O_2}}$ render a carrier both unnecessary and undetectable by conventional methods. Gurtner and Peavy (59) maintained that the steady-state methods of measuring pulmonary diffusing capacity for O_2 and CO assess the true gas-to-blood transport and support the carrier hypothesis. They explained the discrepancy between the two groups by systematic differences in experimental design and suggested that the values of $D_{M_{O_2}}$ obtained by Burns and Shepard (11) might be much too high artifactually, because dithionite enters freely into the extravascular space and lowers markedly, by this shunt, the alveolar-capillary diffusion resistance.

Recent experimental evidence obtained by other workers (86, 88, 128, 148, 151) does not support the contentions of the groups of Longmuir (118, 119) and Gurtner (10, 58, 59).

FACILITATED DIFFUSION OF CO_2

Theory

Facilitation of CO_2 transport is mediated basically by HCO_3^-, which, however, is interfered with by other ions in complex systems. Although HCO_3^- is not a carrier of CO_2 in the sense defined thus far but rather a special chemical form of CO_2, it has become customary to speak of facilitated transport nonetheless; this transport is chemically enhanced, rather than carrier mediated, to a rate greater than can be accounted for by diffusion of physically dissolved CO_2 alone. The CO_2 dissolved in an aqueous medium is first hydrated to form carbonic acid or HCO_3^- at a slow rate when uncatalyzed. The carbonic acid is rapidly ionized to HCO_3^- and H^+ (proton); H^+ is possibly buffered. In the range of physiological pH, which will be considered exclusively here, HCO_3^- is ~20 times more abundant than the nonionic form (mainly CO_2); the second ionization to carbonate and the direct combination of CO_2 with proteins to form carbamate may be neglected; thus HCO_3^- largely prevails in the transport of CO_2. Because facilitation depends on the HCO_3^- gradient, which is maximum at chemical equilibrium, the acceleration of HCO_3^- formation by catalysis [carbonic anhydrase (CA)], favoring the attainment of equilibrium, is crucial. The uncatalyzed CO_2 system is more apt to be far from chemical equilibrium than systems involving O_2, because a typical value of λ is 100 μm or three orders of magnitude higher than for Hb + O_2 (see *Quantitative Interpretation*, p. 92); sufficient catalysis, however, reduces λ by possibly two to three orders of magnitude.

The extent of HCO_3^- formation is limited by the buildup of protons. Hence more-alkaline solutions are better CO_2 transporters, and buffers consuming protons also increase HCO_3^- concentration and therefore diffusion. The buffer, however, must be diffusible (57); an immobilized buffer eradicates HCO_3^--facilitated CO_2 diffusion despite an HCO_3^- concentration gradient, because of the electric diffusion potential caused by the difference in mobility between buffer and HCO_3^-.

The migration of HCO_3^- due to a concentration gradient must be met by an equal charge of positive ions in the same direction or of other negative ions in the opposite direction to implement the constraint of zero electric current. If the mobilities of these ions are different, an electric potential ensues to ensure zero electric current. This potential, the steady-state concentrations of the ions, and the total CO_2 flux in the presence of a CO_2 difference in a flat layer of an ionic solution can be obtained by solving the local material balance (continuity equation) for all species together with the Nernst-Planck equation (24, 122, 124, 127, 178), which is

$$J_j = -D_j \frac{dC_j}{dx} - D_j z_j C_j \frac{F}{RT}\frac{dU}{dx} \quad (8)$$

where the first expression on the right-hand side of the equation is the Fick term and the second expression is the electric potential term; J_j is flux, D_j is diffusion coefficient, C_j is concentration, and z_j is charge of species j; U is electric potential; F is the Faraday constant; R is universal gas constant; T is absolute temperature; and x is distance.

Solution of these equations is subject to the boundary conditions at the two boundaries and to the constraints of zero electric current (charge conservation in an electrically floating system) and of local electroneutrality. These two constraints can only be made consistent if either all diffusion coefficients are equal or the potential gradient dU/dx is not zero.

Substitution of the Nernst-Planck equation and of local electroneutrality into the equation of zero electric current (for the important ions involved, including proteins) provides an expression for the local electric field or potential gradient (24, 122)

$$\frac{dU}{dx} = \frac{RT}{F} \cdot \frac{D_{HCO_3^-} - D_{pr}}{D_{HCO_3^-}C_{HCO_3^-} + D_{pr}(\overline{z_{pr}^2}C_{pr} + \sum z_i^2 C_i)} \frac{dC_{HCO_3^-}}{dx} \quad (9)$$

where pr is protein, $\overline{z_{pr}^2}$ is local average squared protein charge, z_i is charge of inert ions, and C_i is concentration of inert ions. Because the charges of proteins and inert ions are squared, the respective terms hold for both anions and cations; the inert-ion term is related to ionic strength. Equation 9 neglects carbonate, carbamate, H^+, and OH^-, which, however, may become important at more-alkaline pH values; also the effects of possible binding of Cl^- and O_2 to protein are neglected.

Equation 9 shows that the potential mainly is a consequence of the difference in the $D_{HCO_3^-}$ and D_{pr} values. Diffusion potentials are smaller in simple salt solutions but are greater in the presence of proteins because the D_{pr} is much less than the $D_{HCO_3^-}$. With a given $D_{HCO_3^-}$, any increase in D_{pr} leads to a decrease of the potential and vice versa. Furthermore the potential gradient is proportional to the HCO_3^- concentration gradient (and hence to the P_{CO_2} gradient) and inversely proportional to HCO_3^- concentration and thus P_{CO_2}, average squared protein charge, and ionic strength. Average squared protein charge is related to the average protein charge $\overline{z}_{pr}$, according to the Linderstrøm-Lang equation, $\overline{z_{pr}^2} = \overline{z}_{pr}^2 + \beta/2.3$, where β is the buffer capacity. Therefore the electric potential gradient is maximum at the isoelectric point (IP), where $z_{pr} = 0$ and $\overline{z_{pr}^2} = \beta/2.3$ = minimum. The inert ions are distributed passively in response to the potential.

Equation 9 cannot be solved by a straightforward procedure, even when assuming local chemical reaction equilibrium in the presence of CA. However, its denominator usually is found to be only weakly dependent on x and therefore may be taken as constant. Then the diffusion potential is simply proportional to the product of the difference between the $D_{HCO_3^-}$ and D_{pr} values and the HCO_3^- concentration difference across the layer.

The total CO_2 flux (the sum of the fluxes of CO_2 and HCO_3^-) is obtained by application of the continuity equation for total carbon. A facilitation (Fac) is the ratio of the facilitated and free fluxes of CO_2 or Fac = $(J_{CO_2} - J_{CO_2}^{inert})/J_{CO_2}^{inert}$; an effective CO_2 permeability is $Pe_{CO_2} = P_{CO_2}^{inert}(1 + \text{Fac})$, where $P_{CO_2}^{inert}$ is permeability of free CO_2. The total CO_2 flux, J_{CO_2}, emerges as

$$J_{CO_2} = Pe_{CO_2} \frac{(P_{CO_2}^0 - P_{CO_2}^L)}{L} \quad (10)$$

where $P_{CO_2}^0$ is upstream P_{CO_2}, $P_{CO_2}^L$ is downstream P_{CO_2}, and L is thickness of the layer.

A comparison of the profiles with and without diffusion potential exposes the effects of a potential, as shown in Figure 6 (122, 166, 178). The potential primarily redistributes electric charge—positive charge (Na^+) against and negative charge (inert Cl^-) with the potential gradient—leading to new equilibria. A charge deficit at the upper boundary (Fig. 6, *left*) lowers HCO_3^- concentration and pH and raises mean protein charge (z_{Hb}), whereas a charge surplus at the lower boundary (Fig. 6, *right*) has an opposite effect. In the presence of unequal mobilities of HCO_3^- and protein, a potential gradient ensues that depresses the HCO_3^- gradient (and flux) and steepens the protein charge gradient to maintain zero electric current. Furthermore the electric potential term in Equation 8 also is counter to the HCO_3^- gradient. Thus the potential gradient decreases facilitation. Note how marked this effect can be: a potential as small as −1.3 mV lowers the facilitation by about one order of magnitude. This detrimental effect is strengthened by protein immobilization, where $D_{HCO_3^-} - D_{pr}$ and therefore the potential gradient are maximum (Eq. 9). Increased inert-ion (e.g., Na^+) concentration decreases the potential gradient (Eq. 9) and therefore increases CO_2 permeability.

Experimental Studies

BICARBONATE SOLUTIONS. The first evidence for CO_2 facilitation due to HCO_3^- diffusion promoted by CA was obtained in RBC and in the lung by Enns (33), who also stressed the possibility of CO_2 transport by the enzyme alone acting as a CO_2 carrier. The apparent (effective) D_{CO_2} (117) and the CO_2 permeability (9,

190) are increased by CA. The extent of facilitation depends on the concentration of HCO_3^- and on the approach to equilibrium, as influenced by the concentration of CA and the film thickness (27, 145, 180, 181). The theoretical studies neglected the electric field effects and therefore must have overestimated CO_2 facilitation, possibly by as much as 30% (126).

WEAK ACIDS, BUFFERS. Enhancement of CO_2 transport by buffers was suggested by Gutknecht and Tosteson (60) and Gros and Moll (56). Meldon et al. (125) found that buffering by salts of weak acids can play a role at least as important as that of hydration catalysts. The effect of noncatalytic buffers maximizes when the weak acid pK (negative logarithm of dissociation constant) is in the range of the pH value prevailing in solution, i.e., when buffering is maximal. Engasser and Horvath (31) proposed that buffers might act as carriers for H^+. In phosphate buffer solutions with sufficient CA the necessary proton transport can be provided only by phosphate-diffusion-facilitated proton transfer where the mobility of the buffer is indispensable (57). There was good agreement between theory and experiment when accounting for the effect of electric potential. Meldon (123) objected to the notion of buffer-facilitated proton transport used by Gros et al. (57), because there is appreciable facilitation of CO_2 transport in simple carbonate-HCO_3^- solutions without any buffer, and CO_2 is the only species with a net transport. The transport of charge (proton, carbonate, or buffer) to maintain zero current in the presence of an HCO_3^- flux, e.g., by a reverse weak-acid anion flux (125), is important.

PROTEIN SOLUTIONS. Facilitation of CO_2 diffusion in bovine RBC and Hb solutions occurred only at low P_{CO_2} and amounted to a 60% enhancement of CO_2 transport (55). It could not be fully explained by the conventional mechanisms, but later rotational diffusion was demonstrated for transport enhancement in earthworm Hb solutions (MW 3.7×10^6) over a concentration range of up to 26 g/100 ml (53, 54). Here the conditions for a rotational diffusion effect are more favorable than for Hb and O_2 because the rate of protonation is greater than that of oxygenation by several orders of magnitude and the speed of rotation of earthworm Hb is much smaller than that of Hb.

Experimental studies in Hb solutions (24, 124) demonstrated the electric potentials induced by CO_2 gradients (38 vs. 2 Torr) in the presence of sufficient CA. With increasing Hb concentration the potential rose almost linearly, mainly due to an increase in the HCO_3^- concentration gradient by buffering. Without CA the potential also increased with L; reaction equi-

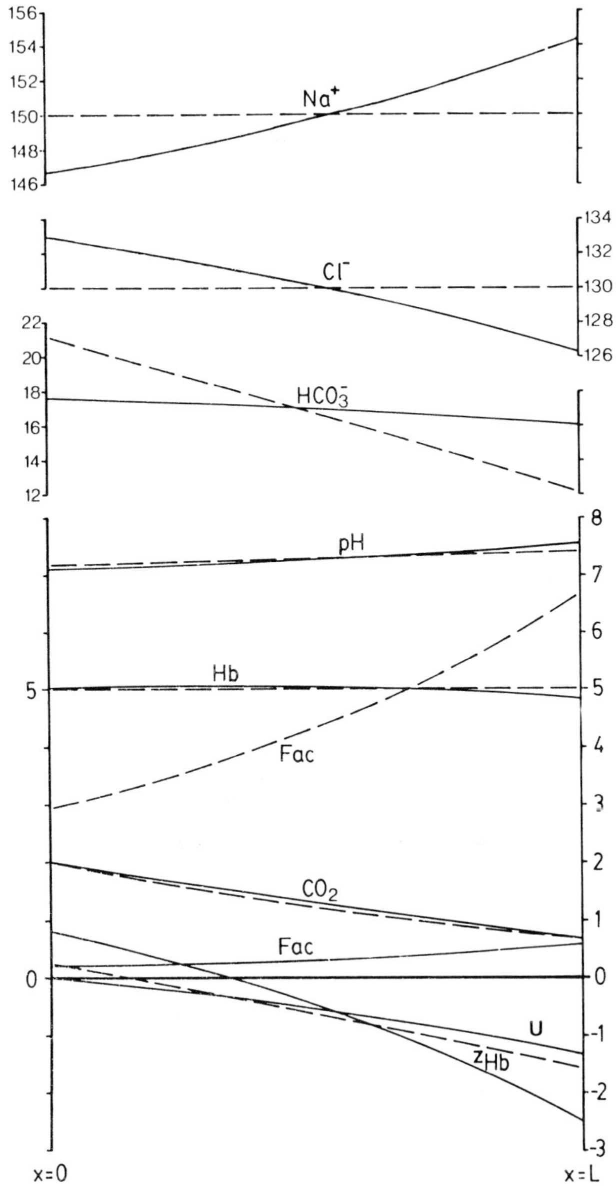

FIG. 6. Schematic profiles of species important in facilitated CO_2 diffusion across a layer. Conditions assumed [according to De Koning et al. (24)]: P_{CO_2} difference from 45 Torr ($x = 0$) to 15 Torr ($x = L$); mean concentrations: $Na^+ = 150$ mM, $Cl^- = 130$ mM (not bound to Hb), Hb = 5 mM. Temperature, 21°C. Values at upper ($x = 0$) vs. lower ($x = L$) boundary. ——, With potential; - - - -, without potential.

Parameter	With Potential		Without Potential	
	P_{CO_2} 45 Torr	P_{CO_2} 15 Torr	P_{CO_2} 45 Torr	P_{CO_2} 15 Torr
Na^+, mM	146.6	154.4	150	150
Cl^-, mM	133.0	126.3	130	130
HCO_3^-, mM	17.7	16.1	21.1	12.2
CO_3^{2-}, mM*	0.03	0.07	0.04	0.04
pH	7.09	7.53	7.17	7.41
Hb, mM	5.02	4.82	5	5
Facilitation (Fac)	0.32†		4.3†	
CO_2, mM	2.00	0.67	2.00	0.67
Charge of Hb (z_{Hb})	+0.8	−2.5	+0.2	−1.6
Potential (U), mV	0	−1.3	0	

* Not shown on figure. † Mean values over the whole layer.

librium was reached only at $L \rightarrow \infty$, which again points to the importance of a catalysis by CA. There was satisfactory agreement between experiments and theory including a potential. Stroeve and Ziegler (178) confirmed these results concerning the potential, using experimental CO_2-flux data from bovine Hb solutions, and found that interfacial potentials were not significant.

A 30 g/100 ml albumin solution at low P_{CO_2} also showed facilitation with a maximum of 90% in the presence of CA at pH 7.2 (56). The electric potential was assumed to be small (0.05 mV) and was calculated to have no appreciable effect on the fluxes of HCO_3^- and albumin because the CO_2 and HCO_3^- gradients were small and the albumin charge was highly negative at a pH far from the IP of 5.2 (122).

Experimental data from bovine serum albumin solutions showed reasonable agreement with the theoretical treatment of Stroeve and Ziegler (178) when taking into account the diffusion potential (166). These albumin results were qualitatively similar to those of Hb (178), but facilitation was smaller than with Hb, because pH and HCO_3^- concentration were lower due to the lower IP of albumin. The change in aggregation of a protein (formation of dimers in albumin solutions or dissociation of tetrameric Hb in Hb solutions) might have to be taken into account because it affects the D_{pr}, but this factor has been neglected.

Physiological Significance

Most of the conditions in the in vitro model experiments and calculations deviate widely from the situations in vivo and therefore do not provide any solid basis for extrapolation to the very complex and diverse physiological milieux in cells and extracellular spaces. There have been only a few speculations derived from principles established in model studies and even fewer experimental physiological investigations in muscle, which yielded no more than suggestive and semiquantitative evidence for facilitation.

Calculations for the RBC based on model experiments suggested a much smaller potential (by almost two orders of magnitude) and yet an only threefold reduction of CO_2 facilitation (24, 124). However, in these model experiments the P_{CO_2} difference was seven times larger and the Na^+ concentration four times smaller than in the physiological situation. Reduced protein mobility (as may occur in cells) was calculated to increase the potential difference only moderately but to decrease facilitation by about one order of magnitude in model systems. Apart from the diffusion potential inherent to the HCO_3^--mediated CO_2 transport in solutions containing proteins, there are, in many cells, in vivo potential differences from other sources, which may be much greater than the diffusion potentials considered here, but nothing is known about this possible interference (122, 178).

Facilitation of CO_2 transport was demonstrated within the RBC and in RBC ghosts as well as in lung tissue of isolated canine lung lobes where the CO_2 diffusing capacity was halved by acetazolamide (70).

Kawashiro and Scheid (89), studying CO_2 transport in thin layers of intact rat skeletal muscle at 37°C, concluded that CO_2 diffusion is facilitated in the presence of sufficiently low P_{CO_2} values (<100 Torr). They calculated that facilitation resulted in a 25%–35% reduction of the P_{CO_2} gradient between a single muscle fiber and blood (fraction of 1 Torr at rest and ~2 Torr in heavy muscular activity), but a real physiological effect still needs direct experimental confirmation. Although the magnitude of CO_2 facilitation diminishes with decreasing path length of HCO_3^- diffusion (181), Scheid et al. (154) believe that the path length to be considered is the diameter of the muscle fiber rather than the entire layer thickness. Gros et al. (53) contend that for diffusion paths as short as the diameter of a muscle fiber a facilitation of CO_2 diffusion is possible only in the presence of CA, which has been demonstrated in skeletal muscle (205). The CA is most effective in promoting facilitated CO_2 transport if it is uniformly dispersed; therefore tissues with a spatial distribution of CA may have a decreased facilitated flux (156). Gros et al. (52) experimentally found a facilitation of CO_2 transport by 60% due to the presence of Ca III in intact, partially red, muscle layers from abdominal muscles of the rat.

Much more experimental work is needed to assess the physiological role of facilitated CO_2 diffusion.

We thank Drs. Jerome S. Schultz, Pieter Stroeve, Hendrik J. van Ouwerkerk, Henricus M. Fijnaut, Peter M. Breepoel, Zdenek Turek, and Carl R. Honig for their reading of the manuscript and their suggestions.

We are grateful to Ted Hendriksen for helping with the collection of the literature, to Uschi Lubowski for typing, and to Christa Kreuzer-Paustian for correcting the manuscript.

REFERENCES

1. ADAMS, L. R., AND I. FATT. The diffusion coefficient of human hemoglobin at high concentrations. *Respir. Physiol.* 2: 293–301, 1967.
2. ALPERT, S. S., AND G. BANKS. The concentration dependence of the hemoglobin mutual diffusion coefficient. *Biophys. Chem.* 4: 287–296, 1976.
3. ANTONINI, E., M. BRUNORI, B. GIARDINA, P. A. BENEDETTI, AND N. PINTUS. Kinetics of oxygen reactions within single erythrocytes. Observation by microspectrophotometry. In: *Hemoglobin and Oxygen Binding*, edited by C. Ho. New York: Elsevier/North-Holland, 1982, p. 449–452.
4. ARAKI, R., M. TAMURA, AND I. YAMAZAKI. The effect of intracellular oxygen concentration on lactate release, pyridine nucleotide reduction and respiration rate in the rat cardiac tissue. *Circ. Res.* 53: 448–455, 1983.
5. BARLOW, C. H., B. CHANCE, W. HARDEN III, M. B. SIMSON,

AND A. H. HARKEN. Spectroscopic mapping of oxygen supply-demand in heart. In: *Biochemical and Clinical Aspects of Oxygen*, edited by W. S. Caughey. New York: Academic, 1979, p. 845–856.

6. BATCHELOR, G. K. Brownian diffusion of particles with hydrodynamic interaction. *J. Fluid Mech.* 74: 1–29, 1976.
7. BRIGHT, P. B. The basic flow equations of electrophysiology in the presence of chemical reactions. II. A practical application concerning the pH and voltage effects accompanying the diffusion of O_2 through hemoglobin solution. *Bull. Math. Biophys.* 29: 123–138, 1967.
8. BRITTON, N. F., AND J. D. MURRAY. The effect of carbon monoxide on haem-facilitated oxygen diffusion. *Biophys. Chem.* 7: 159–167, 1977.
9. BROUN, G., E. SELEGNY, C. TRAN MINH, AND D. THOMAS. Facilitated transport of CO_2 across a membrane bearing carbonic anhydrase. *FEBS Lett.* 7: 223–226, 1970.
10. BURNS, B., AND G. H. GURTNER. A specific carrier for oxygen and carbon monoxide in the lung and placenta. *Drug Metab. Dispos.* 1: 374–379, 1973.
11. BURNS, B., AND R. H. SHEPARD. DL_{O_2} in excised lungs perfused with blood containing sodium dithionite ($Na_2S_2O_4$). *J. Appl. Physiol.* 46: 100–110, 1979.
12. BURNS, B., AND R. H. SHEPARD. Membrane diffusion. Comparison between dithionite DO_2 and DL_{CO}. *Prog. Respir. Res.* 16: 130–141, 1981.
13. CHANCE, B., AND B. QUISTORFF. Study of tissue oxygen gradients by single and multiple indicators. *Adv. Exp. Med. Biol.* 94: 331–338, 1978.
14. CLARK, A., JR., AND P. A. A. CLARK. Local oxygen gradients near mitochondria in tissue. *Microvasc. Res.* 29: 212–213, 1985.
15. CLARK, A., JR., G. R. COKELET, AND W. J. FEDERSPIEL. Erythrocyte motion and oxygen transport. *Bibl. Anat.* 20: 385–388, 1981.
16. CLARK, A., JR., W. J. FEDERSPIEL, P. A. A. CLARK, AND G. R. COKELET. Oxygen delivery from red cells. *Biophys. J.* 47: 171–181, 1985.
17. COLE, R. P. Myoglobin function in exercising skeletal muscle. *Science Wash. DC* 216: 523–525, 1982.
18. COLE, R. P. Skeletal muscle function in hypoxia. Effect of alteration of intracellular myoglobin. *Respir. Physiol.* 53: 1–14, 1983.
19. COLE, R. P., P. C. SUKANEK, J. B. WITTENBERG, AND B. A. WITTENBERG. Mitochondrial function in the presence of myoglobin. *J. Appl. Physiol.* 53: 1116–1124, 1982.
20. COLE, R. P., B. A. WITTENBERG, AND P. R. B. CALDWELL. Myoglobin function in the isolated fluorocarbon-perfused dog heart. *Am. J. Physiol.* 234 (*Heart Circ. Physiol.* 3): H567–H572, 1978.
21. COLTON, C. K., P. STROEVE, AND J. G. ZAHKA. Mechanism of oxygen transport augmentation by hemoglobin. *J. Appl. Physiol.* 35: 307–309, 1973.
22. CONNETT, R. J., T. E. J. GAYESKI, AND C. R. HONIG. Lactate accumulation in fully aerobic, working, dog gracilis muscle. *Am. J. Physiol.* 246 (*Heart Circ. Physiol.* 15): H120–H128, 1984.
23. DE KONING, J., L. J. C. HOOFD, AND F. KREUZER. Oxygen transport and the function of myoglobin. Theoretical model and experiments in chicken gizzard smooth muscle. *Pfluegers Arch.* 389: 211–217, 1981.
24. DE KONING, J., P. STROEVE, AND J. H. MELDON. Electrical potentials during carbon dioxide transport in hemoglobin solutions. *Adv. Exp. Med. Biol.* 94: 183–188, 1978.
25. DILLER, T. E., AND B. B. MIKIC. Modeling the oxygen diffusion effects of red cell motions in flowing blood. In: *Advances in Bioengineering*, edited by V. C. Mow. New York: Am. Soc. Mech. Eng., 1980, p. 177–180.
26. DILLER, T. E., AND I. A. PATTANTYUS. Analytical modeling of facilitated transport in flowing hemoglobin solutions. In: *Advances in Bioengineering*, edited by D. L. Bartel. New York: Am. Soc. Mech. Eng., 1983, p. 7–8.
27. DONALDSON, T. T., AND J. A. QUINN. Kinetic constants determined from membrane transport measurements. Carbonic anhydrase activity at high concentrations. *Proc. Natl. Acad. Sci. USA* 71: 4995–4999, 1974.
28. DRIEDZIC, W. R. The fish heart as a model system for the study of myoglobin. *Comp. Biochem. Physiol. A Comp. Physiol.* 76: 487–493, 1983.
29. DRIEDZIC, W. R., J. M. STEWART, AND D. L. SCOTT. The protective effect of myoglobin during hypoxic perfusion of isolated fish hearts. *J. Mol. Cell. Cardiol.* 14: 673–677, 1982.
30. ENGASSER, J.-M. A fast evaluation of diffusion effects on bound enzyme activity. *Biochim. Biophys. Acta* 526: 301–310, 1978.
31. ENGASSER, J.-M., AND C. HORVATH. Buffer-facilitated proton transport. pH Profile of bound enzymes. *Biochim. Biophys. Acta* 358: 178–192, 1974.
32. ENNS, T. Molecular collision-exchange transport of oxygen by hemoglobin. *Proc. Natl. Acad. Sci. USA* 51: 247–252, 1964.
33. ENNS, T. Carbonic anhydrase facilitated transport of CO_2 (Abstract). *Federation Proc.* 24: 397, 1965.
34. FEDERSPIEL, W. J. The effect of myoglobin concentration on muscle cell PO_2 gradients. *Adv. Exp. Med. Biol.* 180: 539–543, 1984.
35. FIGULLA, H. R., J. HOFFMANN, AND D. W. LÜBBERS. Coronary conductivity and tissue oxygenation as measured by the myoglobin O_2 saturation and the cytochrome aa_3 redox state in the Langendorff guinea pig heart preparation. *Adv. Exp. Med. Biol.* 159: 579–585, 1983.
36. FLETCHER, J. E. On facilitated oxygen diffusion in muscle tissue. *Biophys. J.* 29: 437–458, 1980.
37. FOLKNER, C. A., AND R. D. NOBLE. Transient response of facilitated transport membranes. *J. Membr. Sci.* 12: 289–301, 1983.
38. FOX, M. A., AND H. D. LANDAHL. Theory of hemoglobin facilitated oxygen transport. *Bull. Math. Biophys.* 27: 183–190, 1965.
39. FRIEDLANDER, S. K., AND K. H. KELLER. Mass transfer in reacting systems near equilibrium. Use of the affinity function. *Chem. Eng. Sci.* 20: 121–129, 1965.
40. GAYESKI, T. E. J., R. J. CONNETT, AND C. R. HONIG. Oxygen transport in the rest-work transition illustrates new functions for myoglobin. *Am. J. Physiol.* 248 (*Heart Circ. Physiol.* 17): H914–H921, 1985.
41. GAYESKI, T. E. J., AND C. R. HONIG. Myoglobin saturation and calculated PO_2 in single cells of resting gracilis muscles. *Adv. Exp. Med. Biol.* 94: 77–84, 1978.
42. GAYESKI, T. E. J., AND C. R. HONIG. Direct measurement of intracellular O_2 gradients; role of convection and myoglobin. *Adv. Exp. Med. Biol.* 159: 613–621, 1983.
43. GIJSBERS, G. H., AND H. J. VAN OUWERKERK. Boundary layer resistance of steady-state oxygen diffusion facilitated by a four-step chemical reaction with hemoglobin in solution. *Pfluegers Arch.* 365: 231–241, 1976.
44. GODDARD, J. D. Further applications of carrier-mediated transport theory—a survey. *Chem. Eng. Sci.* 32: 795–809, 1977.
45. GODDARD, J. D. A model of facilitated transport in concentrated two-phase dispersions. *Chem. Eng. Commun.* 9: 345–361, 1981.
46. GODDARD, J. D., J. S. SCHULTZ, AND R. J. BASSETT. On membrane diffusion with near-equilibrium reaction. *Chem. Eng. Sci.* 25: 665–683, 1970.
47. GODDARD, J. D., J. S. SCHULTZ, AND S. R. SUCHDEO. Facilitated transport via carrier-mediated diffusion in membranes. Pt. III. Mathematical aspects and analyses. *AIChE J.* 20: 625–645, 1974.
48. GOLDSTICK, T. K., AND I. FATT. Diffusion of oxygen in solutions of blood proteins. *Chem. Eng. Prog. Symp. Series* 66: 101–113, 1970.
49. GONZALEZ-FERNANDEZ, J. M., AND S. E. ATTA. Transport of

oxygen in solutions of hemoglobin and myoglobin. *Math. Biosci.* 54: 265–290, 1981.
50. GONZALEZ-FERNANDEZ, J. M., AND S. E. ATTA. Facilitated transport of oxygen in the presence of membranes in the diffusion path. *Biophys. J.* 38: 133–141, 1982.
51. GROS, G. Concentration dependence of the self-diffusion of human and *Lumbricus terrestris* hemoglobin. *Biophys. J.* 22: 453–468, 1978.
52. GROS, G., F. GANGHOFF, P. SCHEID, W. SIFFERT, W. TESKE, AND D. KRÜGER. Concentration, properties, and functional significance of skeletal muscle carbonic anhydrase III. *Pfluegers Arch.* 400, Suppl.: R58, 1984.
53. GROS, G., H. GROS, D. LAVALETTE, B. AMAND, AND F. POCHON. Mechanisms of facilitated CO_2 and H^+ diffusion in protein solutions. In: *Biophysics and Physiology of Carbon Dioxide*, edited by C. Bauer, G. Gros, and H. Bartels. Berlin: Springer-Verlag, 1980, p. 36–48. (Symp. Univ. Regensburg, April 17–20, 1979.)
54. GROS, G., D. LAVALETTE, W. MOLL, H. GROS, B. AMAND, AND F. POCHON. Evidence for rotational contribution to protein-facilitated proton transport. *Proc. Natl. Acad. Sci. USA* 81: 1710–1714, 1984.
55. GROS, G., AND W. MOLL. The diffusion of carbon dioxide in erythrocytes and hemoglobin solutions. *Pfluegers Arch.* 324: 249–266, 1971.
56. GROS, G., AND W. MOLL. Facilitated diffusion of CO_2 across albumin solutions. *J. Gen. Physiol.* 64: 356–371, 1974.
57. GROS, G., W. MOLL, H. HOPPE, AND H. GROS. Proton transport by phosphate diffusion—a mechanism of facilitated CO_2 transfer. *J. Gen. Physiol.* 67: 773–790, 1976.
58. GURTNER, G. H., AND B. BURNS. Possible facilitated transport of oxygen across the placenta. *Nature Lond.* 240: 473–475, 1972.
59. GURTNER, G. H., AND H. H. PEAVY. Evidence for facilitated transport of O_2 and CO in the lungs. *Prog. Respir. Res.* 16: 161–165, 1981.
60. GUTKNECHT, J., AND D. C. TOSTESON. Diffusion of weak acids across lipid bilayer membranes: effects of chemical reactions in the unstirred layers. *Science Wash. DC* 182: 1258–1261, 1973.
61. HAAS, D. D., AND B. R. WARE. Electrophoretic mobilities and diffusion coefficients of hemoglobin at high pH. *Biochemistry* 17: 4946–4950, 1978.
62. HALL, R. S., AND C. S. JOHNSON, JR. Experimental evidence that mutual and tracer diffusion coefficients for hemoglobin are not equal. *J. Chem. Phys.* 72: 4251–4253, 1980.
63. HALL, R. S., Y. S. OH, AND C. S. JOHNSON, JR. Photon correlation spectroscopy in strongly absorbing and concentrated samples with applications to unliganded hemoglobin. *J. Phys. Chem.* 84: 756–767, 1980.
64. HANNA, R. E., AND J. B. GARNER. An analysis of facilitated-diffusion problems. *Math. Biosci.* 63: 9–20, 1983.
65. HASSINEN, I. E., J. K. HILTUNEN, AND T. E. S. TAKALA. Reflectance spectrophotometric monitoring of the isolated perfused heart as a method of measuring the oxidation-reduction state of cytochromes and oxygenation of myoglobin. *Cardiovasc. Res.* 15: 86–91, 1981.
66. HELLUMS, J. D. The resistance to oxygen transport in the capillaries relative to that in the surrounding tissue. *Microvasc. Res.* 13: 131–136, 1977.
67. HEMMINGSEN, E. A. Enhancement of oxygen transport by myoglobin. *Comp. Biochem. Physiol.* 10: 239–244, 1963.
68. HEMMINGSEN, E. A. Accelerated transfer of oxygen through solutions of heme pigments. *Acta Physiol. Scand. Suppl.* 246: 1–53, 1965.
69. HEMMINGSEN, E., AND P. F. SCHOLANDER. Specific transport of oxygen through hemoglobin solutions. *Science Wash. DC* 132: 1379–1381, 1960.
70. HILL, E. P., AND T. ENNS. CO_2 diffusing capacity in isolated lungs. *Prog. Respir. Res.* 16: 172–176, 1981.
71. HILLS, B. A. Chemical facilitation of gas transfer liquids. *Br. Chem. Eng.* 16: 175–177, 1971.
72. HONIG, C. R., M. L. FELDSTEIN, AND J. L. FRIERSON. Capillary lengths, anastomoses, and estimated capillary transit times in skeletal muscle. *Am. J. Physiol.* 233 (*Heart Circ. Physiol.* 2): H122–H129, 1977.
73. HONIG, C. R., T. E. J. GAYESKI, W. FEDERSPIEL, A. CLARK, JR., AND P. CLARK. Muscle O_2 gradients from hemoglobin to cytochrome: new concepts, new complexities. *Adv. Exp. Med. Biol.* 169: 23–38, 1984.
74. HOOFD, L., P. BREEPOEL, AND F. KREUZER. Facilitated diffusion and electrical potentials in protein solutions with ionic species. *Adv. Exp. Med. Biol.* 169: 133–143, 1984.
75. HOOFD, L., AND F. KREUZER. Calculation of the facilitation of O_2 or CO transport by Hb or Mb by means of a new method for solving the carrier-diffusion problem. *Adv. Exp. Med. Biol.* 94: 163–168, 1978.
76. HOOFD, L., AND F. KREUZER. A new mathematical approach for solving carrier-facilitated steady-state diffusion problems. *J. Math. Biol.* 8: 1–13, 1979.
77. HOOFD, L., AND F. KREUZER. The mathematical treatment of steady state diffusion of reacting species. *AIChE Symp. Ser.* 77: 123–129, 1981.
78. HOOFD, L., AND A. LAMBOO. Oxygen permeability of methemoglobin solutions soaked in Millipore filters. *Adv. Exp. Med. Biol.* 191: 565–570, 1985.
79. JACQUEZ, J. A. The physiological role of myoglobin: more than a problem in reaction-diffusion kinetics. *Math. Biosci.* 68: 57–97, 1984.
80. JACQUEZ, J. A., H. KUTCHAI, AND E. DANIELS. Hemoglobin-facilitated diffusion of oxygen: interfacial and thickness effects. *Respir. Physiol.* 15: 166–181, 1972.
81. JONES, C. R., C. S. JOHNSON, JR., AND J. T. PENNISTON. Photon correlation spectroscopy of hemoglobin: diffusion of oxy-HbA and oxy-HbS. *Biopolymers* 17: 1581–1593, 1978.
82. JONES, D. P. Intracellular O_2 gradients—detection at the outer mitochondrial membrane by monoamine oxidase activity (Abstract). *Federation Proc.* 42: 994, 1983.
83. JONES, D. P., AND F. G. KENNEDY. Intracellular O_2 gradients in cardiac myocytes. Lack of a role for myoglobin in facilitation of intracellular O_2 diffusion. *Biochem. Biophys. Res. Commun.* 105: 419–424, 1982.
84. JONES, D. P., AND F. G. KENNEDY. Intracellular oxygen supply during hypoxia. *Am. J. Physiol.* 243 (*Cell Physiol.* 12): C247–C253, 1982.
85. JONES, D. P., AND H. S. MASON. Gradients of O_2 concentration in hepatocytes. *J. Biol. Chem.* 253: 4874–4880, 1978.
86. JONES, H. A., P. D. BUCKINGHAM, J. C. CLARK, R. E. FORSTER, J. D. HEATHER, J. M. B. HUGHES, AND C. G. RHODES. Constant rate of CO uptake with variable inspired CO concentration. *Prog. Respir. Res.* 16: 169–171, 1981.
87. KATZ, I. R., J. B. WITTENBERG, AND B. A. WITTENBERG. Monoamine oxidase, an intracellular probe of oxygen pressure in isolated cardiac myocytes. *J. Biol. Chem.* 259: 7504–7509, 1984.
88. KAWASHIRO, T., J. PIIPER, AND P. SCHEID. Dependence of O_2 uptake on surface P_{O_2} in intact, excised skeletal muscle of the rat: validity of the Warburg model (Abstract). *J. Physiol. Lond.* 284: 45P–46P, 1978.
89. KAWASHIRO, T., AND P. SCHEID. Measurement of Krogh's diffusion constant of CO_2 in respiring muscle at various CO_2 levels: evidence for facilitated diffusion. *Pfluegers Arch.* 362: 127–133, 1976.
90. KELLER, K. H., E. R. CANALES, AND S. I. YUM. Tracer and mutual diffusion coefficients of proteins. *J. Phys. Chem.* 75: 379–387, 1971.
91. KELLER, K. H., AND S. K. FRIEDLANDER. The steady-state transport of oxygen through hemoglobin solutions. *J. Gen. Physiol.* 49: 663–679, 1966.
92. KELLER, K. H., AND S. K. FRIEDLANDER. Diffusivity measurements of human methemoglobin. *J. Gen. Physiol.* 49: 681–687, 1966.

93. KEMENA, L. L., R. D. NOBLE, AND N. J. KEMP. Optimal regimes of facilitated transport. *J. Membr. Sci.* 15: 259–274, 1983.
94. KEMP, N. J., AND R. D. NOBLE. Heat transfer effects in facilitated transport liquid membranes. *Sep. Sci. Technol.* 18: 1147–1165, 1983.
95. KITCHEN, R. G., B. N. PRESTON, AND J. D. WELLS. Diffusion and sedimentation of serum albumin in concentrated solutions. *J. Polym. Sci. Polym. Symp.* 55: 39–49, 1976.
96. KLUG, A., F. KREUZER, AND F. J. W. ROUGHTON. The diffusion of oxygen in concentrated haemoglobin solutions. *Helv. Physiol. Pharmacol. Acta* 14: 121–128, 1956.
97. KLUG, A., F. KREUZER, AND F. J. W. ROUGHTON. Simultaneous diffusion and chemical reaction in thin layers of haemoglobin solution. *Proc. R. Soc. Lond. B Biol. Sci.* 145: 452–472, 1956.
98. KOLKKA, R. W., AND E. P. SALATHÉ. A mathematical analysis of carrier-facilitated diffusion. *Math. Biosci.* 71: 147–180, 1984.
99. KREUZER, F. Modellversuche zum Problem der Sauerstoffdiffusion in den Lungen. *Helv. Physiol. Pharmacol. Acta* 11, Suppl. 9: 1–99, 1953.
100. KREUZER, F. Facilitated diffusion of oxygen and its possible significance; a review. *Respir. Physiol.* 9: 1–30, 1970.
101. KREUZER, F., AND L. J. C. HOOFD. Facilitated diffusion of oxygen in the presence of hemoglobin. *Respir. Physiol.* 8: 280–302, 1970.
102. KREUZER, F., AND L. J. C. HOOFD. Factors influencing facilitated diffusion of oxygen in the presence of hemoglobin and myoglobin. *Respir. Physiol.* 15: 104–124, 1972.
103. KREUZER, F., AND L. J. C. HOOFD. Facilitated diffusion of CO and oxygen in the presence of hemoglobin or myoglobin. *Adv. Exp. Med. Biol.* 75: 207–215, 1976.
104. KREUZER, F., AND L. HOOFD. Facilitated diffusion of oxygen: possible significance in blood and muscle. *Adv. Exp. Med. Biol.* 169: 3–21, 1984.
105. KREUZER, F., AND W. Z. YAHR. Influence of red cell membrane on diffusion of oxygen. *J. Appl. Physiol.* 15: 1117–1122, 1960.
106. KUTCHAI, H. Numerical study of oxygen uptake by layers of hemoglobin solution. *Respir. Physiol.* 10: 273–284, 1970.
107. KUTCHAI, H. O_2 uptake by 100 μ layers of hemoglobin solution. Theory vs. experiment. *Respir. Physiol.* 11: 378–383, 1971.
108. KUTCHAI, H. Wider applicability for Hill's advancing front theory of oxygen uptake. *J. Appl. Physiol.* 31: 302–304, 1971.
109. KUTCHAI, H., J. A. JACQUEZ, AND F. J. MATHER. Nonequilibrium facilitated oxygen transport in hemoglobin solution. *Biophys. J.* 10: 38–54, 1970.
110. KUTCHAI, H., AND N. C. STAUB. Steady-state, hemoglobin-facilitated O_2 transport in human erythrocytes. *J. Gen. Physiol.* 53: 576–589, 1969.
111. LA FORCE, R. C. Steady-state diffusion in the carbon monoxide + oxygen + hemoglobin system. *Trans. Faraday Soc.* 62: 1458–1468, 1966.
112. LA FORCE, R. C., AND I. FATT. Steady-state diffusion of oxygen through whole blood. *Trans. Faraday Soc.* 58: 1451–1464, 1962.
113. LA FORCE, R. C., AND I. FATT. Steady-state gas transport through hemoglobin solutions. *Biopolym. Symp.* 1: 555–562, 1964.
114. LA FORCE, R. C., AND I. FATT. Conditions for countergradient diffusion of oxygen through a hemoglobin barrier. In: *Chemical Engineering in Medicine and Biology*, edited by D. Hershey. New York: Plenum, 1967, p. 107–115.
115. LAGATTUTA, K. J., V. S. SHARMA, D. F. NICOLI, AND B. K. KOTHARI. Diffusion coefficients of hemoglobin by intensity fluctuation spectroscopy. Effects of varying pH and ionic strength. *Biophys. J.* 33: 63–79, 1981.
116. LIVINGSTON, D. J., G. N. LA MAR, AND W. D. BROWN. Myoglobin diffusion in bovine heart muscle. *Science Wash. DC* 220: 71–73, 1983.
117. LONGMUIR, I. S., R. E. FORSTER, AND C.-Y. WOO. Diffusion of carbon dioxide through thin layers of solution. *Nature Lond.* 209: 393–394, 1966.
118. LONGMUIR, I. S., D. C. MARTIN, H. J. GOLD, AND S. SUN. Nonclassical respiratory activity of tissue slices. *Microvasc. Res.* 3: 125–141, 1971.
119. LONGMUIR, I. S., AND M. G. P. MCCABE. Evidence for an oxygen carrier in tissue. *J. Polarogr. Soc.* 10: 45–48, 1964.
120. LONGO, L. D. Placental diffusing capacity for carbon monoxide (Letter to the editor). *J. Appl. Physiol.* 45: 155, 1978.
121. MAKINO, N., H. KANAIDE, R. YOSHIMURA, AND M. NAKAMURA. Myoglobin oxygenation remains constant during the cardiac cycle. *Am. J. Physiol.* 245 (*Heart Circ. Physiol.* 14): H237–H243, 1983.
122. MELDON, J. H. The theoretical effect of diffusion potential on carbon dioxide transport in protein solutions. *Int. Biophys. Congr., 5th, Copenhagen, 1975*, Abstract 413.
123. MELDON, J. H. The effect of diffusion potentials on facilitated CO_2 diffusion. In: *Biophysics and Physiology of Carbon Dioxide*, edited by C. Bauer, G. Gros, and H. Bartels. Berlin: Springer-Verlag, 1980, p. 49–57. (Symp. Univ. Regensburg, April 17–20, 1979.)
124. MELDON, J. H., J. DE KONING, AND P. STROEVE. Electrical potentials induced by CO_2 gradients in protein solutions and their role in CO_2 transport. *Bioelectrochem. Bioenerg.* 5: 77–87, 1978.
125. MELDON, J. H., K. A. SMITH, AND C. K. COLTON. The effect of weak acids upon the transport of carbon dioxide in alkaline solutions. *Chem. Eng. Sci.* 32: 939–950, 1977.
126. MELDON, J. H., K. A. SMITH, AND C. K. COLTON. An analysis of electrical effects induced by carbon dioxide transport in alkaline solutions. *Recent Developments in Separation Science*, edited by N. N. Li. Boca Raton, FL: CRC, 1979, vol. 5, p. 1–10.
127. MELDON, J. H., P. STROEVE, AND C. E. GREGOIRE. Facilitated transport of carbon dioxide: a review. *Chem. Eng. Commun.* 16: 263–300, 1982.
128. MEYER, M., W. LESSNER, P. SCHEID, AND J. PIIPER. Pulmonary diffusing capacity for CO independent of alveolar CO concentration. *J. Appl. Physiol.* 51: 571–576, 1981.
129. MILLIKAN, G. A. Muscle hemoglobin. *Physiol. Rev.* 19: 503–523, 1939.
130. MITCHELL, P. J., AND J. D. MURRAY. Facilitated diffusion: the problem of boundary conditions. *Biophysik* 9: 177–190, 1973.
131. MOCHIZUKI, M., AND R. E. FORSTER. Diffusion of carbon monoxide through thin layers of hemoglobin solution. *Science Wash. DC* 138: 897–898, 1962.
132. MOLL, W. The diffusion coefficient of haemoglobin. *Respir. Physiol.* 1: 357–365, 1966.
133. MOLL, W. The diffusion coefficient of myoglobin in muscle homogenate. *Pfluegers Arch.* 299: 247–251, 1968.
134. MOLL, W. The influence of hemoglobin diffusion on oxygen uptake and release by red cells. *Respir. Physiol.* 6: 1–15, 1968.
135. MOLL, W. Measurements of facilitated diffusion of oxygen in red blood cells at 37°C. *Pfluegers Arch.* 305: 269–278, 1969.
136. MURRAY, J. D. On the molecular mechanism of facilitated oxygen diffusion by haemoglobin and myoglobin. *Proc. R. Soc. Lond. B Biol. Sci.* 178: 95–110, 1971.
137. MURRAY, J. D. On the role of myoglobin in muscle respiration. *J. Theor. Biol.* 47: 115–126, 1974.
138. MURRAY, J. D. On the functional role of myoglobin in skeletal muscle. In: *Myoglobin: Colloq. on Myoglobin, Brussels, May 22, 1976*, p. 179–201.
139. MURRAY, J. D., AND J. WYMAN. Facilitated diffusion. The case of carbon monoxide. *J. Biol. Chem.* 246: 5903–5906, 1971.
140. NEDELMAN, J., AND S. I. RUBINOW. Facilitated diffusion of oxygen and carbon monoxide in the large affinity regime. *J. Math. Biol.* 12: 73–90, 1981.
141. NOBLE, R. D. Shape factors in facilitated transport through membranes. *Ind. Eng. Chem. Fundam.* 22: 139–144, 1983.
142. NOBLE, R. D. Two-dimensional permeate transport with facilitated transport membranes. *Sep. Sci. Technol.* 19: 469–478, 1984.

143. NOBLE, R. D. Kinetic efficiency factors for facilitated transport membranes. *Sep. Sci. Technol.* 20: 577–585, 1985.
144. OLANDER, D. R. Simultaneous mass transfer and equilibrium chemical reaction. *AIChE J.* 6: 233–239, 1960.
145. OTTO, N. C., AND J. A. QUINN. The facilitated transport of carbon dioxide through bicarbonate solutions. *Chem. Eng. Sci.* 26: 949–961, 1971.
147. PHILLIES, G. D. J., G. B. BENEDEK, AND N. A. MAZER. Diffusion in protein solutions at high concentrations: a study by quasielastic light scattering spectroscopy. *J. Chem. Phys.* 65: 1883–1892, 1976.
148. POWER, G. G., AND W. C. BRADFORD. Measurement of pulmonary diffusing capacity during blood-to-gas exchange in humans. *J. Appl. Physiol.* 27: 61–66, 1969.
149. RIVEROS-MORENO, V., AND J. B. WITTENBERG. The self-diffusion coefficients of myoglobin and hemoglobin in concentrated solutions. *J. Biol. Chem.* 247: 895–901, 1972.
150. ROUGHTON, F. J. W. Diffusion and chemical reaction velocity as joint factors in determining the rate of uptake of oxygen and carbon monoxide by the red blood corpuscle. *Proc. R. Soc. Lond. B Biol. Sci.* 111: 1–36, 1932.
151. RUBIN, D. Z., D. FUJINO, C. MITTMAN, AND S. M. LEWIS. Competitive inhibition of carbon monoxide transport: evidence against a carrier. *J. Appl. Physiol.* 50: 1061–1064, 1981.
152. RUBINOW, S. I., AND M. DEMBO. The facilitated diffusion of oxygen by hemoglobin and myoglobin. *Biophys. J.* 18: 29–42, 1977.
153. SANDERS, A. H., D. L. PURICH, AND D. S. CANNELL. Oxygenation of hemoglobin. Correspondence of crystal and solution properties using diffusion coefficient measurements. *J. Mol. Biol.* 147: 583–595, 1981.
154. SCHEID, P., T. KAWASHIRO, AND J. PIIPER. Evidence for facilitated transport of CO_2 in muscle tissue. In: *Biophysics and Physiology of Carbon Dioxide*, edited by C. Bauer, G. Gros, and H. Bartels. Berlin: Springer-Verlag, 1980, p. 58–63. (Symp. Univ. Regensburg, April 17–20, 1979.)
155. SCHOLANDER, P. F. Oxygen transport through hemoglobin solutions. *Science Wash. DC* 131: 585–590, 1960.
156. SCHULTZ, J. S. Facilitation of CO_2 through layers with a spatial distribution of carbonic anhydrase. In: *Biophysics and Physiology of Carbon Dioxide*, edited by C. Bauer, G. Gros, and H. Bartels. Berlin: Springer-Verlag, 1980, p. 15–22. (Symp. Univ. Regensburg, April 17–20, 1979.)
157. SCHULTZ, J. S., J. D. GODDARD, AND S. R. SUCHDEO. Facilitated transport via carrier-mediated diffusion in membranes. I. Mechanistic aspects, experimental systems and characteristic regimes. *AIChE J.* 20: 417–445, 1974.
158. SCHWARZMANN, V., AND W. A. GRUNEWALD. Myoglobin-O_2-saturation profiles in muscle sections of chicken gizzard and the facilitated O_2 transport by Mb. *Adv. Exp. Med. Biol.* 94: 301–310, 1978.
159. SHETH, B. V., AND J. D. HELLUMS. Transient oxygen transport in hemoglobin layers under conditions of the microcirculation. *Ann. Biomed. Eng.* 8: 183–196, 1980.
160. SMITH, D. R., AND J. A. QUINN. The prediction of facilitation factors for reaction augmented membrane transport. *AIChE J.* 25: 197–200, 1979.
161. SMITH, K. A., J. H. MELDON, AND C. K. COLTON. An analysis of carrier-facilitated transport. *AIChE J.* 19: 102–111, 1973.
162. SPAAN, J. A. E. Transfer of oxygen into haemoglobin solution. *Pfluegers Arch.* 342: 289–306, 1973.
163. SPAAN, J. A. E., F. KREUZER, AND L. HOOFD. A theoretical analysis of nonsteady-state oxygen transfer in layers of hemoglobin solution. *Pfluegers Arch.* 384: 231–239, 1980.
164. SPAAN, J. A. E., F. KREUZER, AND F. K. VAN WELY. Diffusion coefficients of oxygen and hemoglobin as obtained simultaneously from photometric determination of the oxygenation of layers of hemoglobin solutions. *Pfluegers Arch.* 384: 241–251, 1980.
165. SPAETH, E. E., AND S. K. FRIEDLANDER. The diffusion of oxygen, carbon dioxide, and inert gas in flowing blood. *Biophys. J.* 7: 827–851, 1967.
166. SPAVINS, J. C. Interplay of Diffusion, Chemical Reactions and Electrical Potentials in Thin Liquid Films. Buffalo: State Univ. of New York, 1980. Master's thesis.
167. STEIN, T. R., J. C. MARTIN, AND K. H. KELLER. Steady-state oxygen transport through red blood cell suspensions. *J. Appl. Physiol.* 31: 397–402, 1971.
168. STEVENS, E. D. The effect of temperature on facilitated oxygen diffusion and its relation to warm tuna muscle. *Can. J. Zool.* 60: 1148–1152, 1982.
169. STEVENS, E. D., AND F. G. CAREY. One why of the warmth of warm-bodied fish. *Am. J. Physiol.* 240 (*Regulatory Integrative Comp. Physiol.* 9): R151–R155, 1981.
170. STROEVE, P. On the diffusion of gases in protein solutions. *Ind. Eng. Chem. Fundam.* 14: 140–141, 1975.
171. STROEVE, P. Myoglobin-facilitated oxygen transport in heterogeneous red muscle tissue. *Ann. Biomed. Eng.* 10: 49–70, 1982.
172. STROEVE, P. Diffusion with chemical reaction in two-phase heterogeneous media. In: *Advances in Transport Processes*, edited by E. F. Mujumbar and R. A. Mashelkar. New Delhi: Wiley, 1984, vol. 3, p. 361–386.
173. STROEVE, P., C. K. COLTON, AND K. A. SMITH. Steady state diffusion of oxygen in red blood cell and model suspensions. *AIChE J.* 22: 1133–1142, 1976.
174. STROEVE, P., AND K. EAGLE. An analysis of diffusion in a medium containing dispersed reactive cylinders. *Chem. Eng. Commun.* 3: 189–198, 1979.
175. STROEVE, P., AND K. EAGLE. Myoglobin-facilitated oxygen transport in heterogeneous red muscle tissue. In: *Advances in Bioengineering*, edited by V. C. Mow. New York: Am. Soc. Mech. Eng., 1980, p. 341–344.
176. STROEVE, P., K. A. SMITH, AND C. K. COLTON. An analysis of carrier facilitated transport in heterogeneous media. *AIChE J.* 22: 1125–1132, 1976.
177. STROEVE, P., P. P. VARANASI, AND L. J. C. HOOFD. Facilitated transport in spherical shells: application of the combined Damköhler number technique. *J. Membr. Sci.* 19: 155–171, 1984.
178. STROEVE, P., AND E. ZIEGLER. The transport of carbon dioxide in high molecular weight buffer solutions. *Chem. Eng. Commun.* 6: 81–103, 1980.
179. SUCHDEO, S. R., J. D. GODDARD, AND J. S. SCHULTZ. An analysis of the competitive diffusion of O_2 and CO through hemoglobin solutions. *Adv. Exp. Med. Biol.* 37B: 951–961, 1973.
180. SUCHDEO, S. R., AND J. S. SCHULTZ. Mass transfer of CO_2 across membranes: facilitation in the presence of bicarbonate ion and the enzyme carbonic anhydrase. *Biochim. Biophys. Acta* 352: 412–440, 1974.
181. SUCHDEO, S. R., AND J. S. SCHULTZ. The permeability of gases through reacting solutions: the carbon dioxide-bicarbonate membrane system. *Chem. Eng. Sci.* 29: 13–23, 1974.
182. TAMURA, M., N. OSHINO, B. CHANCE, AND I. A. SILVER. Optical measurements of intracellular oxygen concentration of rat heart in vitro. *Arch. Biochem. Biophys.* 191: 8–22, 1978.
183. TAYLOR, B. A., AND J. D. MURRAY. Effect of the rate of oxygen consumption on muscle respiration. *J. Math. Biol.* 4: 1–20, 1977.
184. ULANOWICZ, R. E., AND G. C. FRAZIER, JR. The transport of oxygen and carbon dioxide in hemoglobin systems. *Math. Biosci.* 7: 111–129, 1970.
184a. VAN OUWERKERK, H. J. Facilitated diffusion in a tissue cylinder with an anoxic region. *Pfluegers Arch.* 372: 221–230, 1977.
185. VELDKAMP, W. B., AND J. R. VOTANO. Effects of intermolecular interaction on protein diffusion in solution. *J. Phys. Chem.* 80: 2794–2801, 1976.
186. VELDKAMP, W. B., AND J. R. VOTANO. Temperature dependence of macromolecular interactions in dilute and concentrated hemoglobin solutions. *Biopolymers* 19: 111–124, 1980.
187. VENKATARAMAN, K., T. WANG, AND P. STROEVE. Oxygen diffusion into heterogeneous tissue with combined oxygen

consumption kinetics. *Ann. Biomed. Eng.* 8: 17–27, 1970.

188. WARBURG, O. Versuche an überlebendem Carcinomgewebe (Methoden). *Biochem. Z.* 142: 317–333, 1923.
189. WARD, W. J., III. Analytical and experimental studies of facilitated transport. *AIChE J.* 16: 405–410, 1970.
190. WARD, W. J., III, AND W. L. ROBB. Carbon dioxide-oxygen separation: facilitated transport of carbon dioxide across a liquid film. *Science Wash. DC* 156: 1481–1484, 1967.
191. WAY, J. D., R. D. NOBLE, T. M. FLYNN, AND E. D. SLOAN. Liquid membrane transport: a survey. *J. Membr. Sci.* 12: 239–259, 1982.
192. WEIGELT, C. Mikrokryophotometrische Messungen zur Untersuchung des erleichterten Sauerstofftransports in Gegenwart von Hämoglobin. Bochum, FGR: Bochum Univ., 1975. Dissertation.
193. WILSON, W. W., M. R. LUZZANA, J. T. PENNISTON, AND C. S. JOHNSON, JR. Pregelation aggregation of sickle cell hemoglobin. *Proc. Natl. Acad. Sci. USA* 71: 1260–1263, 1974.
194. WITTENBERG, B. A., AND M. J. MONAHAN. Intracellular oxygen gradients in isolated cardiac cells during controlled steady state hypoxia (Abstract). *J. Mol. Cell. Cardiol.* 14, Suppl. 1: 69, 1982.
195. WITTENBERG, B. A., AND T. F. ROBINSON. Oxygen requirements, morphology, cell coat and membrane permeability of calcium-tolerant myocytes from hearts of adult rats. *Cell Tissue Res.* 216: 231–251, 1981.
196. WITTENBERG, B. A., J. B. WITTENBERG, AND P. R. B. CALDWELL. Role of myoglobin in the oxygen supply to red skeletal muscle. *J. Biol. Chem.* 250: 9038–9043, 1975.
197. WITTENBERG, J. B. Oxygen transport—a new function proposed for myoglobin. *Biol. Bull. Woods Hole* 117: 402–403, 1959.
198. WITTENBERG, J. B. The molecular mechanism of hemoglobin-facilitated oxygen diffusion. *J. Biol. Chem.* 241: 104–114, 1966.
199. WITTENBERG, J. B. Myoglobin-facilitated oxygen diffusion: role of myoglobin in oxygen entry into muscle. *Physiol. Rev.* 50: 559–636, 1970.
200. WITTENBERG, J. B., AND B. A. WITTENBERG. Facilitated oxygen diffusion by oxygen carriers. In: *Oxygen and Living Processes: An Interdisciplinary Approach*, edited by D. L. Gilbert. New York: Springer-Verlag, 1981, p. 177–199.
201. WYMAN, J. Facilitated diffusion and the possible role of myoglobin as a transport mechanism. *J. Biol. Chem.* 241: 115–121, 1966.
202. YOUNG, M. E., P. A. CARROAD, AND R. L. BELL. Estimation of diffusion coefficients of proteins. *Biotechnol. Bioeng.* 22: 947–955, 1980.
203. YUNG, D., AND R. F. PROBSTEIN. Similarity considerations in facilitated transport. *J. Phys. Chem.* 77: 2201–2205, 1973.
204. ZANDER, R., AND H. SCHMID-SCHÖNBEIN. Influence of intracellular convection on the oxygen release by human erythrocytes. *Pfluegers Arch.* 335: 58–73, 1972.
205. ZBOROWSKA-SLUIS, D. T., A. L'ABBATE, AND G. A. KLASSEN. Evidence of carbonic anhydrase activity in skeletal muscle: a role for facilitative carbon dioxide transport. *Respir. Physiol.* 21: 341–350, 1974.

CHAPTER 7

Ventilation: total, alveolar, and dead space

N. R. ANTHONISEN | *General Hospital, Health Sciences Centre, Winnipeg, Manitoba, Canada*

J. A. FLEETHAM | *Department of Medicine, Health Sciences Centre Hospital, University of British Columbia, Vancouver, British Columbia, Canada*

CHAPTER CONTENTS

THE GAS-CONTAINING LUNG may be regarded as composed of two parts: alveoli, small saccular structures in which gas exchange occurs, and conducting airways, which connect the alveoli to the environment and in which no gas exchange occurs. In the human there are approximately 16 generations of conducting airways between the mouth and the alveoli (144). Because of the length and relatively small cross-sectional area of the airways, gas transport by diffusion between alveoli and environment is impractical, and mass movement or convection of environmental gas into proximity with alveoli is essential for gas exchange. This mass movement of gas is qualitatively termed *ventilation* and is accomplished by breathing. Breathing is cyclical: gas is inspired and then expired. The volume of gas inspired or expired per unit time (usually per minute) is defined as *ventilation* when the term is used quantitatively. Ventilation therefore equals mean tidal volume (volume of each breath) times breathing frequency. Inspired minute ventilation ($\dot{V}_I$) equals expired minute ventilation ($\dot{V}_E$) only when the volume of O_2 taken up ($\dot{V}_{O_2}$) in the alveoli equals the volume of CO_2 excreted ($\dot{V}_{CO_2}$), which is not usually the case; the term *ventilation*, unless otherwise specified, usually refers to $\dot{V}_E$. Differences between $\dot{V}_I$ and $\dot{V}_E$ are usually small, however.

The $\dot{V}_E$ may be considered as consisting of two components, one that has undergone gas exchange in the alveoli [alveolar ventilation ($\dot{V}_A$)] and another that has been expired from the conducting airways or dead space and has not undergone gas exchange. In a system as complicated as the mammalian lung, in which small conducting airways contain gas that has undergone exchange with blood and in which the number of conducting airways serving different alveolated structures may vary greatly, separation of the alveolar and dead-space components of the expirate is extremely difficult. In this chapter we consider the approaches that have been used to define each of these components and the known physiological determinants of dead space and $\dot{V}_A$ for each approach. Conventional symbols are used (104).

ALVEOLAR VENTILATION AND ALVEOLAR GAS COMPOSITION

Alveolar and Dead-Space Ventilation

During air breathing, $\dot{V}_A$ is usually defined in terms of CO_2 exchange. Production of CO_2 ($\dot{V}_{CO_2}$) equals $\dot{V}_E$ times the fractional concentration of CO_2 expired ($F_{E_{CO_2}}$) minus $\dot{V}_I$ times the fractional concentration of CO_2 inspired ($F_{I_{CO_2}}$)

$$\dot{V}_E F_{E_{CO_2}} - \dot{V}_I F_{I_{CO_2}} = \dot{V}_{CO_2} \tag{1}$$

When the inspired gas is air, $F_{I_{CO_2}} = 0$ and

$$F_{E_{CO_2}} \dot{V}_E = \dot{V}_{CO_2} \tag{2}$$

Because all gas exchange occurs in the alveoli, $\dot{V}_{CO_2}$ also equals the amount of CO_2 expired from alveoli

$$F_{A_{CO_2}} \dot{V}_A = \dot{V}_{CO_2} = F_{E_{CO_2}} \dot{V}_E \tag{3}$$

where $F_{A_{CO_2}}$ is the fractional concentration of CO_2 in alveolar gas. Thus $\dot{V}_A$ may be computed given $\dot{V}_{CO_2}$ and $F_{A_{CO_2}}$. Quantities of gas can occupy different volumes, depending on their temperature and pressure. It is customary to report $\dot{V}_{O_2}$ and $\dot{V}_{CO_2}$ in terms of standard temperature (0°C) and pressure, dry (STPD). Ventilation, however, is usually reported in terms of body temperature and pressure, saturated (BTPS). In equations relating ventilation to $\dot{V}_{O_2}$ or $\dot{V}_{CO_2}$ (see Eqs. 3 and 4), all these volumes and gas concentrations refer to gas at the same temperature, pressure, and water saturation. In normal subjects, under normal conditions, alveolar gas is reasonably homogeneous (see MEAN AND IDEAL ALVEOLAR GAS, p. 117) and this computation is meaningful; under other circumstances, mean alveolar concentration may be extremely difficult to measure and $\dot{V}_A$ is defined in terms of arterial CO_2 tension (Pa_{CO_2})

$$\frac{Pa_{CO_2}\dot{V}_A}{(P_B - 47)} = \dot{V}_{CO_2} \tag{4}$$

where P_B is barometric pressure. Equation 4 defines $\dot{V}_A$ as the minute volume of gas that, when in CO_2 equilibrium with arterial blood, must be expired to maintain $\dot{V}_{CO_2}$. The $\dot{V}_A$ therefore equals the minute volume of gas expired from alveolar structures only when all these structures have a mean P_{CO_2} that equals Pa_{CO_2}. Relationships between arterial and alveolar CO_2 are discussed in ALVEOLAR-ARTERIAL DIFFERENCES IN PARTIAL PRESSURE OF CARBON DIOXIDE, p. 117.

When $\dot{V}_A$ is defined in terms of $\dot{V}_{CO_2}$, dead-space ventilation ($\dot{V}_{DS}$) is also defined (15)

$$\dot{V}_E = \dot{V}_A + \dot{V}_{DS} \tag{5}$$

Combining Equations 2 and 3 and substituting Equation 5

$$F_{E_{CO_2}}\dot{V}_E = F_{A_{CO_2}}(\dot{V}_E - \dot{V}_{DS}) \tag{6}$$

$$\dot{V}_{DS} = \frac{(F_{A_{CO_2}} - F_{E_{CO_2}})\dot{V}_E}{F_{A_{CO_2}}} \tag{7}$$

Dividing both sides by breathing frequency

$$V_{DS} = \frac{(F_{A_{CO_2}} - F_{E_{CO_2}})V_T}{F_{A_{CO_2}}} \tag{8}$$

where V_{DS} is dead-space volume and V_T is tidal volume.

This type of equation, first derived by Bohr (15), may be applied to other inhaled gases, provided account is taken of the inspired concentration of gas in question. For example

$$F_{A_{O_2}}(\dot{V}_E - \dot{V}_{DS}) + F_{I_{O_2}}\dot{V}_{DS} = F_{E_{O_2}}\dot{V}_E \tag{9}$$

Alveolar Gas Equation and Alveolar Gas Composition

Alveolar gas composition was simply and quantitatively described during World War II by a number of authors (see ref. 99), but Fenn and Rahn (34, 112) made the most definitive presentation of these relationships. In this chapter we derive the most widely used version of the alveolar gas equation and indicate how it can be applied to assess overall gas exchange.

DERIVATION. As noted in Equation 1, $\dot{V}_{CO_2}$ equals the amount of CO_2 expired minus the amount inspired. Similarly for $\dot{V}_{O_2}$

$$\dot{V}_I F_{I_{O_2}} - \dot{V}_E F_{E_{O_2}} = \dot{V}_{O_2} \tag{10}$$

The ratio of $\dot{V}_{CO_2}$ to $\dot{V}_{O_2}$ is defined as the respiratory exchange ratio R

$$R = \frac{\dot{V}_{CO_2}}{\dot{V}_{O_2}} = \frac{\dot{V}_E F_{E_{CO_2}} - \dot{V}_I F_{I_{CO_2}}}{\dot{V}_I F_{I_{O_2}} - \dot{V}_E F_{E_{O_2}}} \tag{11}$$

In the steady state, the body takes up and releases essentially no N_2. Thus

$$\dot{V}_I F_{I_{N_2}} = \dot{V}_E F_{E_{N_2}} \tag{12}$$

and

$$\dot{V}_I = \frac{\dot{V}_E F_{E_{N_2}}}{F_{I_{N_2}}} \tag{13}$$

Under steady-state conditions, and only under steady-state conditions, Equation 13 may be substituted into Equation 11

$$R = \frac{F_{E_{CO_2}} - F_{I_{CO_2}}(F_{E_{N_2}}/F_{I_{N_2}})}{F_{I_{O_2}}(F_{E_{N_2}}/F_{I_{N_2}}) - F_{E_{O_2}}} \tag{14}$$

Equation 14 allows calculation of R without knowledge of ventilation. The usefulness of this is limited, however, by difficulties in assessing N_2 concentrations. Therefore

$$F_{I_{N_2}} = 1 - F_{I_{O_2}} - F_{I_{CO_2}} \tag{15}$$

and

$$F_{E_{N_2}} = 1 - F_{E_{N_2}} - F_{E_{CO_2}} \tag{16}$$

are substituted into Equation 14

$$R = \frac{(1 - F_{I_{O_2}})F_{E_{CO_2}} - (1 - F_{E_{O_2}})F_{I_{CO_2}}}{(1 - F_{E_{CO_2}})F_{I_{O_2}} - (1 - F_{I_{CO_2}})F_{E_{O_2}}} \tag{17}$$

During air breathing $F_{I_{CO_2}} = 0$ and

$$R = \frac{(1 - F_{I_{O_2}})F_{E_{CO_2}}}{(1 - F_{E_{CO_2}})F_{I_{O_2}} - F_{E_{O_2}}} \tag{18}$$

If expired gas is contaminated by the addition of inspired gas, there is no change in R, as computed from Equations 17 or 18. A volume V′ of inspired gas is added to a volume V of expired gas

$$F'_{E_{O_2}} = \frac{F_{E_{O_2}}V + F_{I_{O_2}}V'}{V + V'}$$

$$F'_{E_{CO_2}} = \frac{F_{E_{CO_2}}V + F_{I_{O_2}}V'}{V + V'}$$

These expressions are substituted into Equation 17

$$R = \frac{(1 - F_{I_{O_2}}) \dfrac{F_{E_{CO_2}}V + F_{I_{CO_2}}V'}{V + V'} - \left[1 - \left(\dfrac{F_{E_{O_2}}V + F_{I_{O_2}}V'}{V + V'}\right)\right]F_{I_{CO_2}}}{\left[1 - \left(\dfrac{F_{E_{CO_2}}V + F_{I_{CO_2}}V'}{V + V'}\right)\right]F_{I_{O_2}} - (1 - F_{I_{CO_2}}) \dfrac{F_{E_{O_2}}V + F_{I_{O_2}}V'}{V + V'}} = \frac{(1 - F_{I_{O_2}})F_{E_{CO_2}} - (1 - F_{E_{O_2}})F_{I_{CO_2}}}{(1 - F_{E_{CO_2}})F_{I_{O_2}} - (1 - F_{I_{CO_2}})F_{E_{O_2}}}$$

which is identical to Equation 17.

Alveolar gas differs from expired gas because expired gas is "contaminated" with inspired gas; thus Equations 17 and 18 apply equally well to alveolar gas

$$R = \frac{(1 - F_{I_{O_2}})F_{A_{CO_2}} - (1 - F_{A_{O_2}})F_{I_{CO_2}}}{(1 - F_{A_{CO_2}})F_{I_{O_2}} - (1 - F_{I_{CO_2}})F_{A_{O_2}}} \quad (19)$$

When $F_{I_{CO_2}} = 0$

$$R = \frac{(1 - F_{I_{O_2}})F_{A_{CO_2}}}{(1 - F_{A_{CO_2}})F_{I_{O_2}} - F_{A_{O_2}}} \quad (20)$$

Solving Equation 20 for $F_{A_{O_2}}$ and collecting terms containing $F_{A_{CO_2}}$

$$F_{A_{O_2}} = F_{I_{O_2}} - F_{A_{CO_2}}\left[F_{I_{O_2}} + \frac{(1 - F_{I_{O_2}})}{R}\right] \quad (21)$$

Multiplying both sides of the equation by $P_B - 47$ converts it to partial pressures

$$P_{A_{O_2}} = P_{I_{O_2}} - P_{A_{CO_2}}\left[F_{I_{O_2}} + \frac{(1 - F_{I_{O_2}})}{R}\right] \quad (22)$$

where $P_{A_{O_2}}$ is the alveolar partial pressure of O_2 and $P_{I_{O_2}}$ is the inspired partial pressure of O_2. Similar solutions may be derived for instances in which $F_{I_{CO_2}}$ is not zero (Eq. 19), but this is not illustrated here because assessment of alveolar gas composition during the steady-state inhalation of CO_2 is uncommon.

INTERPRETATION. Equations 18 and 22 are the most commonly used of the alveolar gas equations. They state that, for a given inspirate, expired or alveolar O_2 and CO_2 concentrations are related to one another and to the respiratory exchange ratio. If two are defined, only one value for the third can exist; e.g., for a given inspirate, R, and $P_{A_{CO_2}}$, only one $P_{A_{O_2}}$ is possible. This is intuitively reasonable, because R defines the relationship between $\dot{V}_{O_2}$ and $\dot{V}_{CO_2}$ (Eq. 11) and $P_{A_{CO_2}}$ defines the relationship between $\dot{V}_A$ and $\dot{V}_{CO_2}$ (Eq. 4). Thus $P_{A_{CO_2}}$ is dependent on ventilation and $\dot{V}_{CO_2}$: if other things are equal and $\dot{V}_{CO_2}$ is large in relation to $\dot{V}_A$, $P_{A_{CO_2}}$ rises; if $\dot{V}_{CO_2}$ is small in relation to $\dot{V}_A$, $P_{A_{CO_2}}$ falls. For both gases, $\dot{V}_A$ is the same, and $\dot{V}_{CO_2}$ and R define $\dot{V}_{O_2}$; for a given $\dot{V}_A$, $P_{A_{O_2}}$ is reciprocally related to $\dot{V}_{O_2}$. Alveolar $\dot{V}_{O_2}$ and $\dot{V}_{CO_2}$ depend on blood flow; thus alveolar gas composition depends on the alveolar ventilation-perfusion ratio $\dot{V}_A/\dot{Q}$.

The use of the above equations is not limited to the assessment of alveolar gas composition. In subjects inhaling mixtures other than 100% O_2, $\dot{V}_{O_2}$ is usually calculated by measuring $\dot{V}_{CO_2}$ (Eq. 1 or 2) and R in the mixed expired gas (Eq. 19 or 20).

There are certain restrictions for the use of these equations. Equations 12 and 13 apply only to steady-state conditions: when inspired gas composition, $\dot{V}_{O_2}$, $\dot{V}_{CO_2}$, and R do not vary with time. Because the subsequent equations depend on Equations 12 and 13, they also apply only to the steady state. Equations 20 and 22 are frequently applied to overall pulmonary gas exchange (see below). In so doing, the overall R, $P_{A_{O_2}}$, and $P_{A_{CO_2}}$ are defined. It is important to recognize that such overall values do not apply to all alveoli, even in normal subjects under ideal conditions, and that as conditions become less ideal, overall values calculated with these equations may not coincide with those present in any single alveolus. However, the alveolar gas equations were derived without anatomical reference and apply to single gas-exchange units as well as they do to the whole lung. Thus, if the appropriate information were available, $P_{A_{O_2}}$, $P_{A_{CO_2}}$, and R could be computed for every alveolus in a lung with these equations.

Finally, the composition of the inspirate is usually considered to be that of the gaseous environment. This overlooks the fact that alveoli reinspire gas from the dead space, which is an important problem. We consider it briefly here [see the classic paper by Ross and Farhi (120)].

The best and simplest way to summarize the relationships among $P_{A_{O_2}}$, $P_{A_{CO_2}}$, and R is graphically. Equation 22 states that when CO_2 is absent from the inspirate, $P_{A_{O_2}}$ is a linear function of $P_{A_{CO_2}}$ (the slope of the relationship varies with R). An example of such a plot is shown in Figure 1; the inspirate here is atmospheric air ($P_{I_{O_2}}$ = 149 mmHg). The R isopleths are plotted on P_{O_2}-P_{CO_2} coordinates. The values of P_{O_2} and P_{CO_2} on each isopleth indicate all the possible gas compositions that, given the inspirate, are compatible with that particular R value.

When R = 1 the slope ($\Delta P_{A_{CO_2}}/\Delta P_{A_{O_2}}$) of the line of Figure 1 is −1; when R is less, the slope is less. When R = 0 the slope is zero; it is also independent of $F_{I_{O_2}}$. However, as $F_{I_{O_2}}$ increases, changes in R influence the slope of the P_{O_2}-P_{CO_2} relationship less (Eq. 22) and the R isopleths become closer to each other. When 100% O_2 is breathed ($F_{I_{O_2}}$ = 1.0), $P_{A_{O_2}}$ = 1 − $P_{A_{CO_2}}$ and, because N_2 is absent, Equations 12 and 13 do not apply; thus R cannot be computed from these equations.

The problem of reinspired dead-space gas may be approached graphically (120). Figure 2*A* shows, on the P_{O_2}-P_{CO_2} coordinates of Figure 1, a line representing gas composition when O_2 and CO_2 exchange at R = 0.8. A point (A) representing a typical alveolus is indicated on the line. Mixed expired gas from this

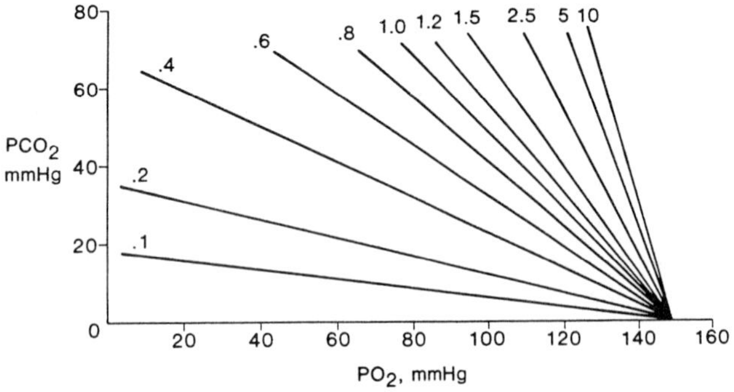

FIG. 1. Graphic representation of Equation 22. Relationship between alveolar P_{O_2} and alveolar P_{CO_2} when inspired gas (P_{O_2} = 149 mmHg; P_{CO_2} = 0 mmHg) exchanges at a variety of respiratory exchange ratio (R) values. *Isopleths,* gas compositions applying to gas exchanged at indicated R value. [Adapted from Rahn and Fenn (112).]

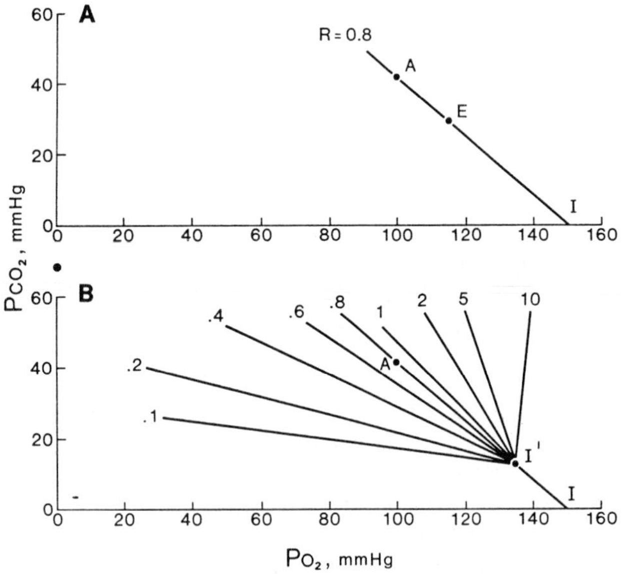

FIG. 2. Dead-space effects on alveolar gas composition. *A: isopleth,* gas compositions given R = 0.8 (R, gas-exchange ratio) and inspired gas of composition I (room air). *Alveolar point (A)* is indicated. Expired gas from this alveolus or lung must lie on same *R isopleth;* its location (*E*) depends on ratio of dead space to tidal volume (VDS/VT). *Length AE/length AI* equals VDS/VT. *B:* lung with R = 0.8 in which all dead space is common to all alveoli and VDS/VT is constant among alveoli. I′, composition of inspired gas, which is mean of gas of composition I weighted by VT − VDS and gas of composition A weighted by VDS. *R isopleths* for inspired gas of composition I′ are shown. [Adapted from Ross and Farhi (120).]

alveolus must also lie on this line (Eqs. 18–20); its precise composition depends on the degree of dilution of alveolar gas by inspired or dead-space gas. Indeed, the ratio of the length of line A–E to the length of line A–I equals the ratio of the dead-space volume to tidal volume (VDS/VT) (Fig. 2*A*). In an alveolus such as the one shown in Figure 2*A*, reinspiration of dead-space gas, which is simply gas from that alveolus mixed with inspired gas, has no influence on gas exchange as formulated above. The inspirate may be thought of as a combination of dead-space gas, which has the same composition as alveolar gas and therefore cannot exchange, and the conventional inspirate, which exchanges according to the equations summarized by Figure 1.

Unfortunately Figure 2*A* is an oversimplification because it implies that the dead space of each alveolus is peculiar to that alveolus. In the lung a substantial amount of the dead space—main-stem bronchi, trachea, and upper airway—is common to all alveoli. If all the dead space is common to all alveoli and if the distribution of reinspired gas from the dead space is the same as the distribution of ventilation (i.e., if VDS/VT is constant), alveolar gas composition may be assessed with no loss of accuracy, as in Figure 2*B*. In this figure the inspirate (point I), instead of room air, is composed of room air plus an amount of mixed alveolar gas (point A) appropriate to VDS/VT. This new inspired point (point I′) necessarily lies on the same R line as the mixed alveolar point; therefore for the lung as a whole or for alveoli with R = 0.8, the situation is the same as depicted in Figure 2*A*. For alveoli with other exchange ratios, appropriate isopleths may be calculated with gas of composition I′ as the inspirate.

Figures 2*A* and 2*B* are extreme solutions to the problem of reinspired dead-space gas: in Figure 2*A* all dead space is peculiar to the alveolus to which it is connected, and in Figure 2*B* all dead space is common to all alveoli. Neither situation applies in a real lung; some dead space is common to all alveoli, some common to some alveoli, and probably very little serves only alveoli with uniform gas composition. Furthermore, the distribution of VDS/VT is most unlikely to be constant throughout the lung, so that both the composition and the amount of reinspired dead-space gas are unknown. Ross and Farhi (120) and more recently Fortune and Wagner (39) discussed the importance of this problem in the study of gas exchange.

Assessment of Alveolar Gas Composition

INHOMOGENEITY OF ALVEOLAR GAS. As implied in INTERPRETATION, p. 115, alveolar gas composition may vary from alveolus to alveolus. Indeed, given normal biological variation, there must be extreme differences among the 300 million alveoli that make up a normal human lung. Details of this variation are considered elsewhere in this *Handbook* section on the respiratory system. Our concern is the estimation of overall alveolar gas composition in a system with wide variation. Under the best of circumstances such an estimate is a mean, with the contribution of each alveolus weighted according to its ventilation.

Note also that in a given alveolus, gas composition must vary as a function of time, because alveolar volume changes with the breathing cycle and because pulmonary capillary flow and volume, which relate to instantaneous $\dot{V}_{CO_2}$ and $\dot{V}_{O_2}$, are pulsatile. Several time variations of alveolar gas composition have been modeled (26, 35, 60, 86, 98, 100), most recently in a very sophisticated way. Figure 3 shows the respiratory oscillations of P_{O_2} and P_{CO_2} from the model of Hlastala (60). One respiratory cycle is shown; minor fluctuations of gas tensions that occur throughout the breath are the result of capillary pulsations. The exchange ratio (not shown) also varies throughout the breathing cycle. Throughout expiration, P_{O_2} decreases and P_{CO_2} increases as gas exchanges with a progressively decreasing alveolar volume. These changes persist early in inspiration as gas from the dead space is inspired. Then, as the alveolar gas is diluted by inspired air, P_{O_2} rises and P_{CO_2} falls, reaching their respective maximum and minimum values at end inspiration. The mean P_{O_2} and P_{CO_2} values appear to occur slightly more than half way through both inspiration and expiration; these mean values need not occur simultaneously. If time is allowed for the transit of gas from alveoli to mouth, Figure 3 suggests that the end-tidal gas (i.e., gas exhaled during the last 20% of the expiration) would adequately represent a mean value with respect to time, as Rahn (110) suggested on the basis of the original model of time-dependent alveolar gas composition proposed by DuBois (26).

MEAN AND IDEAL ALVEOLAR GAS. Rahn (110) defined mean alveolar gas as gas from all ventilated alveoli mixed so that its exchange ratio was the same as that of mixed expired gas. He showed that in resting young normal subjects, end-tidal gas fulfilled this criterion. In such subjects, when expired gas tensions are measured by rapid gas analyzers, little change is observed over the latter part of expiration; thus end-tidal gas concentrations are reproducible and easy to measure (110).

In normals at exercise and in patients with lung disease, large changes in expired gas tensions occur during single tidal expirations; end-tidal values are difficult to define and may not be representative of mean alveolar gas. A number of alternate approaches have been employed. With the Bohr equation (Eqs. 8 and 9), mean alveolar gas composition can be computed from measurements of mixed expired gas and either a measured or predicted dead space. Measuring the dead space does not obviate the problem of the mean alveolar sample, and using predicted normal values for dead space adds another source of error to the determination. Mean alveolar gas has been estimated by continuously recording expired P_{O_2} and P_{CO_2} and plotting them against each other on the coordinates shown in Figure 1. Mean alveolar gas tensions are those that fall on the appropriate R isopleth, as determined by analysis of mixed expired gases (5). Luft et al. (87) systematically compared those methods with that of end-tidal sampling in a large group of patients with abnormal lungs. They found that the end-tidal R was very close to mixed expired R and that end-tidal P_{CO_2} showed less variation than $P_{A_{CO_2}}$ derived by either of the other two methods.

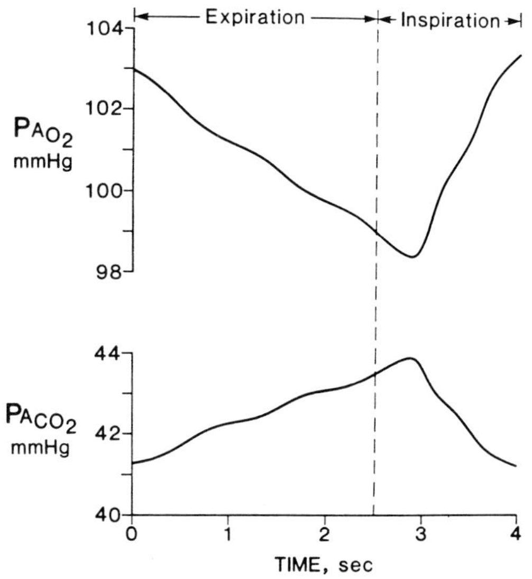

FIG. 3. Variations of $P_{A_{O_2}}$ and $P_{A_{CO_2}}$ with time. One complete respiratory cycle is shown, with phases indicated at *top*. "Ripples" on *traces* are due to pulsatile changes of capillary flow and volume. [From Hlastala (60).]

The most widely used method of assessing alveolar gas composition is to sidestep the issue of mean alveolar gas and estimate "ideal" alveolar gas tensions, an approach Riley et al. (114) pioneered. They measured Pa_{CO_2} and substituted it for $P_{A_{CO_2}}$ in the alveolar air equation (Eq. 22). When Riley et al. measured R in mixed expired gas, they calculated "ideal" $P_{A_{O_2}}$, which is the $P_{A_{O_2}}$ that would be present in a lung exchanging gas at the measured R and with $P_{A_{CO_2}} = Pa_{CO_2}$. In resting normal supine subjects, Pa_{CO_2} and end-tidal P_{CO_2} agree closely (13), but this may not be true in erect resting normals or in patients with disease. In these subjects, Pa_{CO_2} is higher than end-tidal P_{CO_2}, reflecting contributions to the latter by units with high $\dot{V}_A/\dot{Q}$ values. By analogy, end-tidal P_{O_2} should be higher than ideal $P_{A_{O_2}}$ for the same reason. Differences between ideal $P_{A_{O_2}}$ and measured Pa_{O_2} chiefly reflect the contributions of low $\dot{V}_A/\dot{Q}$ units to the latter. This approach enjoys widespread popularity, which is well deserved because it is a simple and sensitive way to assess the efficiency of pulmonary O_2 exchange. At the bedside, Pa_{CO_2} is relatively easy to determine but R is not; thus values ranging from 0.8–1.0 are frequently assumed and ideal $P_{A_{O_2}}$ is calculated by a simplified equation

$$P_{A_{O_2}} = P_{I_{O_2}} - Pa_{CO_2}/R \qquad (23)$$

Errors inherent in the simplification and the assumption of a value for R may be assessed by comparing Equation 23 with Equation 22.

ALVEOLAR-ARTERIAL DIFFERENCES IN PARTIAL PRESSURE OF CARBON DIOXIDE. As noted above, Pa_{CO_2}

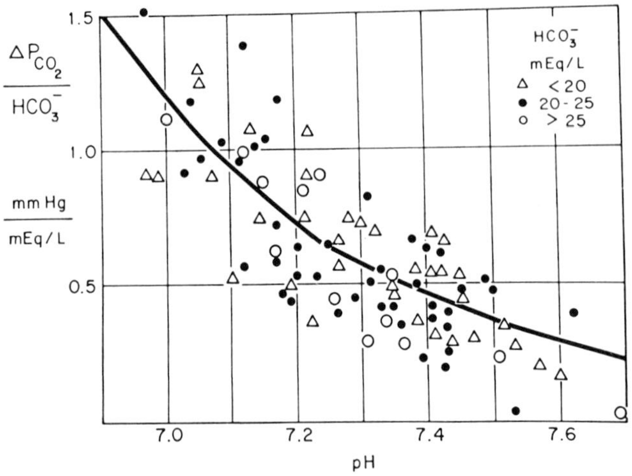

FIG. 4. Alveolar-arterial CO_2 differences in rebreathing dogs. Ordinate: P_{CO_2} ($P_{A_{CO_2}} - Pa_{CO_2}$) normalized for HCO_3^- concentration. Abscissa: arterial pH. ○, △, ●, Ranges of HCO_3^- concentrations. In these experiments, $P_{A_{CO_2}}$ exceeded Pa_{CO_2} substantially. [From Gurtner et al. (52).]

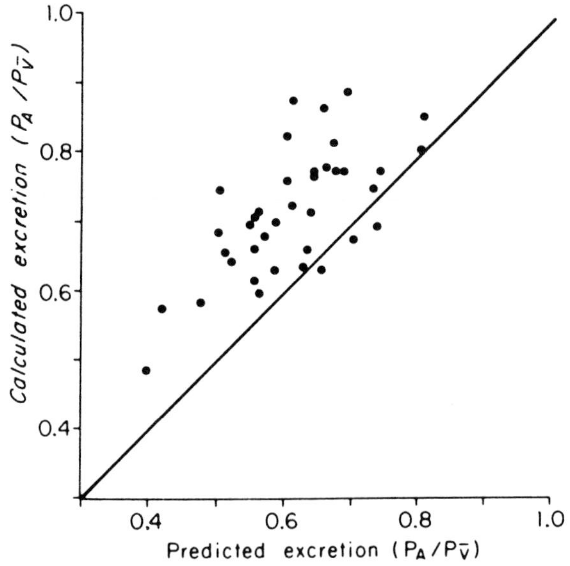

FIG. 5. Excretion of CO_2 (ordinate) compared to predicted excretion of an inert gas of similar solubility (abscissa). More-efficient CO_2 excretion suggests that it differs from that of inert gases. PA, alveolar partial pressure; P$\bar{v}$, mixed venous partial pressure. [From Robertson and Hlastala (115).]

exceeds end-tidal P_{CO_2} in lungs in which units with high $\dot{V}A/\dot{Q}$ contribute to end-tidal gas. In diseased lungs, this difference may be as large as 15 mmHg. This is considered in DEAD SPACE (see next section), but note that the calculation of ideal alveolar gas composition does not assume that Pa_{CO_2} equals mean $P_{A_{CO_2}}$ but describes a lung exchanging as if this were the case.

The classic concepts of gas exchange are based on the assumption of alveolocapillary equilibration of CO_2 within gas-exchange units. This proposition has recently been challenged by the finding that in some circumstances mean $P_{A_{CO_2}}$ exceeded Pa_{CO_2} (52, 68, 70, 135). Differences of this kind had been observed before (24) but discounted as due to errors in estimating mean $P_{A_{CO_2}}$. Such errors are not present in more recent experiments. Jones et al. (70) noted that in normal humans during rebreathing, which minimized CO_2 exchange, $P_{A_{CO_2}}$ regularly exceeded Pa_{CO_2}, whether O_2 exchange was occurring or not. Gurtner et al. (52) hypothesized that the increased $P_{A_{CO_2}}$ was due to a transient disequilibrium of H^+ and HCO_3^- within the capillary, with production of CO_2 near the capillary wall. Polyelectrolytes such as proteins dissociate when exposed to an electrical field (the Wien effect), and Gurtner proposed that negative charges on the wall of the pulmonary capillary induced such dissociation. The resulting free H^+ migrated to the capillary wall and reacted with HCO_3^- to produce CO_2, with the high CO_2 near the capillary wall equilibrating with alveolar gas so that $P_{A_{CO_2}}$ was greater than mean capillary P_{CO_2}. The increased difference between $P_{A_{CO_2}}$ and Pa_{CO_2} with increases of H^+ and HCO_3^- (Fig. 4) is compatible with this hypothesis, as were subsequent experiments conducted by Gurtner and Traystman (53).

However, both Gurtner's experimental findings and his interpretation are subjects of controversy (37, 51). Guyatt et al. (54) duplicated Gurtner's findings in a similar preparation, but Scheid et al. (122) and Scheid and Piiper (121) have been unable to do so, finding that $P_{A_{CO_2}} = Pa_{CO_2}$ in rebreathing dogs. Robertson and Hlastala (115) measured the excretion of intravenously infused inert gases and found that $\dot{V}_{CO_2}$ exceeded that predicted on the basis of CO_2 solubility (Fig. 5), supporting Gurtner's findings by suggesting that $\dot{V}_{CO_2}$ was accomplished by a mechanism that did not apply to inert gases. This provocative experiment has not been repeated. The results might be explained by the fact that the inert gases used had substantially higher molecular weights than CO_2; thus their excretion might have been limited by diffusion in lung gas [(62); see also the chapter by Hlastala in this *Handbook*]. The mechanism (Wien effect) proposed by Gurtner has been criticized because it would require significant separation of charged ions over most of the capillary length and for most of the blood transit time (37). Furthermore it has been argued that to maintain intracapillary P_{CO_2} gradients of the size postulated by Gurtner et al. (52) would require more free energy than could be supplied by the pulmonary circulation (27).

Forster (37) has suggested that an alternative mechanism is responsible for the difference between $P_{A_{CO_2}}$ and Pa_{CO_2} observed by Jones et al. (70) and Gurtner et al. (52). Equilibration of CO_2, H^+, and HCO_3^- within capillary blood is rate-limited by the uncatalyzed hydration of CO_2 in the plasma. In systemic capillaries this limitation is such that plasma CO_2 may be elevated so that during rebreathing, if nonequilibrated plasma enters the pulmonary capillary and equilibrates with the gas phase, $P_{A_{CO_2}}$ may be higher than Pa_{CO_2}, which is measured in blood samples some minutes after pulmonary capillary transit, when full CO_2 equilibrium has been established. Recent work has indicated that this is unlikely. Predictions of the differences between $P_{A_{CO_2}}$ and $P_{a_{CO_2}}$ that could result from delayed equilibration yielded results that were substantially smaller than those observed (38, 59). Furthermore several investigators (21, 28, 55, 72, 73) have shown that the pulmonary capillary endothelial surface has carbonic anhydrase activity, which would assure rapid equilibration of CO_2, H^+, and HCO_3^- in pulmonary capillary blood.

In summary, there is evidence (which has been contested) that CO_2 transfer in the lung is more complicated than previously assumed by respiratory physiologists. Because the assumption of alveolar-capillary CO_2 equilibrium underlies several classic physiological concepts, resolution of this controversy is urgently needed.

DEAD SPACE

General Considerations: Gas Mixing in Airways

At end inspiration, upper airways are filled with inspired gas that has undergone no gas exchange, and alveolar units contain gas that approximates pulmonary capillary blood in composition. Between these two sites, in intrapulmonary airways, gas composition must vary between these two extremes, approaching or equaling inspired composition in central airways and alveolar composition in peripheral airways. The dead space is conceptualized as the volume of distribution of gas of inspired composition, i.e., the volume occupied by the inspirate if there were a sharp, all-or-nothing transition between it and gas of alveolar composition. The size of this virtual volume obviously depends on the degree of mixing of inspired and alveolar gas in the airways, which has been the subject of much recent investigation. This is reviewed here as it pertains to the dead space; a more general consideration of gas mixing in the lung may be found in the chapter by Piiper and Scheid in this *Handbook*.

During inspiration, because of the rapid increase in airway cross-sectional diameter, linear velocities of gas flow are much smaller in peripheral airways than in central airways. At some point in the peripheral airways, transport of inspired gas to the periphery by convection is so small that it equals diffusion of gas from the periphery to more-central airways (29, 30, 50, 101, 103). At this point the front between inspired and alveolar gas becomes stationary, although inspiration continues. Thus, because of diffusion, the volume or distance that the front of inspired gas penetrates into the lung is less than predicted on the basis of the volume of inspiration. The position and characteristics of this front are important in determining the size of the dead space. Although the front is stationary, transport of inspired gas to the periphery continues, balanced by diffusion of residual gas in the opposite direction. Gas transport may be summarized for inspired gas (29, 30)

$$\dot{V}_I = \dot{V}F_I - DA(\partial F_I/\partial X) \qquad (24)$$

and for residual gas

$$\dot{V}F_R = DA(\partial F_R/\partial X) \qquad (25)$$

where $\dot{V}$ is inspiratory flow, $\dot{V}_I$ is peripheral transport of inspired gas, F_I is the concentration of inspired gas, F_R is the concentration of residual gas, D is the diffusion coefficient for the gas considered, A is the cross-sectional area of the airways at the stationary front, and $\partial F/\partial X$ is the axial concentration gradient at the front. In mathematical models (101, 103) employing physiological inspiratory flow rates, the best available models of lung anatomy, and neglecting nondiffusive forms of mixing, the stationary front appears to establish itself in respiratory bronchioles: airway generations 17–20 (Fig. 6). These models have characteristically considered two molecular species and have applied principles of binary diffusion to them. In real life, when there are more than two molecular species, laws of ternary diffusion should apply (18, 137), but under nonextreme circumstances, differences in gas transport in binary and ternary systems are small (39, 149).

Equation 25 allows predictions of dead-space size that qualitatively agree with experimental results (see below), despite the fact that the equation applies only for steady inspiratory flow and does not consider events during expiration, when gas composition in the periphery of symmetrical lung models becomes uniform (Fig. 5) and during which further diffusion mixing must decrease the dead space. Increasing inspira-

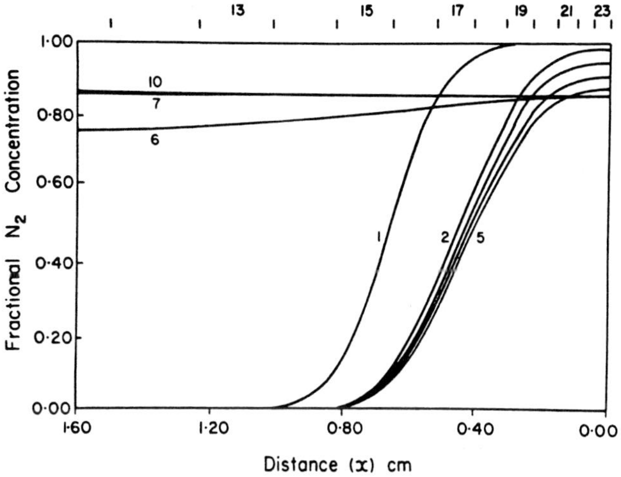

FIG. 6. Nitrogen concentration in peripheral airways as function of airway generation (*top* abscissa) and linear distance (*bottom* abscissa) during a breath of 100% O_2 at constant flow. *Lines*, N_2 concentration at successive intervals of 0.4 s. During inspiration (*lines 2–5*), large N_2 differences are present in airways, but position of front changes little with time. During expiration (*lines 6–10*), N_2 differences disappear. [Adapted from Paiva (101).]

tory flow increases convective gas transport and moves the stationary front toward the periphery to the point that the resulting increase in cross-sectional area allows a similar increase in diffusive transport. Decreases in inspiratory flow should have the opposite effect, and when inspiratory flow is zero, as in breath holding, diffusive transport is unopposed and the front should move centrally. Changes in lung volume influence the cross-sectional area of the airways ($A \propto V^{2/3}$) so that increases in volume should displace the front centrally. Finally, gas diffusivity should have a major influence on the front: diffusive transport is decreased when the gases involved have a low diffusion coefficient and the position of the front is more peripheral. Because of diffusive mixing in peripheral airways, increases in the volume of these airways influence the dead space much less than similar increases of the volume of central airways (3).

To the extent that nondiffusive mixing occurs in airways, the dead space should be affected. One type of convective mixing, Taylor dispersion (138), has been examined extensively as it applies to the lung. Taylor noted that in laminar flow, axial mixing of a tracer fluid occurs by virtue of its parabolic profile and that this axial mixing is inversely related to molecular diffusion because radial diffusion of the tracer blunts its concentration profile. Axial mixing of tracer fluid can be quantitated in terms of an effective diffusion coefficient (30, 146). Wilson and Lin (146) examined the effects of Taylor dispersion in a lung model assuming laminar flow and concluded that it was an important form of gas transport in airway generations 8–12; Scherer et al. (123) showed that in a large airway model, Taylor dispersion could be an important mechanism of gas transport, greater in inspiration than in expiration. Subsequent and more-complete model studies have indicated that Taylor dispersion is not important in mixing the inspirate with residual gas (96, 100), probably because the effect is maximum in large airways, in which little mixing occurs because they are normally filled with inspirate very early in inspiration. Spread of the front of inspired gas is small between central and peripheral airways, indicating little convective mixing (29), and only 15% of inhaled aerosols, which have a molecular diffusion coefficient of zero and therefore mix entirely by convection, are not recovered on the subsequent tidal expiration (93).

Due chiefly to the work of Engel and co-workers (29–32, 47), it has been established that gas mixing in airways is substantially increased by the mechanical impulses imposed on the lung by the heartbeat. When 100% O_2 is inspired and N_2 is sampled by catheters in airways, rhythmic increases in F_{N_2} are observed that coincide with the heartbeat, are absent in the absence of a heartbeat, and present if the heart is oscillated manually. The stationary front between inspired and residual gas extends to airways that are much more central than predicted in model studies, and when compared to lungs not agitated by the heart the position of the front is displaced by an amount equivalent to a fivefold increase in the gas diffusion coefficient of Equation 25. This enhancement of airway mixing applied during breath holding promotes central movement of the front between inspired and residual gas. Although gas mixing in airways is unquestionably promoted by cardiogenic mixing, studies of the mixing of gas in alveolar regions have failed to show a major influence due to the heartbeat (65, 69).

Beyond the fact that cardiogenic mixing depends on the motion of the heart itself and not on transmitted vascular pressure pulses (31), little is known about its mechanism. In a symmetrical lung model, oscillatory flows such as might be induced by the heartbeat produce relatively little mixing on the basis of molecular diffusion, as long as the velocity profiles of oscillatory flows are blunt (29). If velocity profiles are not blunt, Taylor dispersion (138) may produce mixing similar to that observed in the dog, as shown by the model experiments of Slutsky (130). On the other hand, in a more realistic asymmetrical lung model, small flow oscillations could produce the requisite amount of mixing in the absence of Taylor dispersion, because gas is exchanged between airways and acini of differing size and path length by molecular diffusion (102). Thus it is not clear that Taylor dispersion plays a role in cardiogenic gas mixing. Not surprisingly, the effectiveness of cardiac mixing varies with the location considered (47); it is greatest in canine middle lobes and least in upper lobes.

HIGH-FREQUENCY VENTILATION. It has recently been demonstrated that adequate pulmonary gas exchange can be maintained in animals (14) and humans (49) by artificial ventilation employing high frequency (>2 Hz) and tidal volumes that are smaller than the volume of the conducting airways. Obviously this is achieved by mixing inspired and alveolar gas in large airways and has excited a great deal of interest. We consider here only this aspect of high-frequency ventilation (for recent reviews see refs. 17, 25, 46, and 133). Briscoe, Forster, and Comroe (16) anticipated this literature to some extent; they noted that when normal subjects inhaled volumes of tracer gas that were smaller than the anatomical dead space, tracer mixed with alveolar gas. As Drazen et al. (25) have pointed out, the degree of mixing observed was compatible with subsequent high-frequency ventilation experiments.

Results of experiments involving high-frequency ventilation often depend on the techniques used; it is useful to review them briefly. Inspirate has been delivered in two general ways. High-speed piston pumps, which both push gas into the lung and actively withdraw it, have been used; this generates sinusoidal volume and flow waves. High-speed interrupter valves have also been employed. These valves are connected to a high-pressure source and open intermittently;

expiration is passive. Interrupters have been used with "jets" in which the inspirate is delivered through a small tube near the carina and with the valve connected to the whole cross section of the trachea.

Whatever the method of delivery of inspired gas, expired gas must be removed from the system. Jet ventilators leave the trachea open, and gas flows out during periods between inspiratory jets. How much of the delivered jet actually flows into the lungs with this configuration is not clear, however. Interrupter valves that are connected to the whole airway usually are open to the atmosphere during the exhalation phase. Oscillator pumps are employed with a continuous or bias flow into and out of the trachea, so that the expirate is cleared. The presence of a bias flow may influence the amount of gas delivered to the lungs, because the oscillator may entrain inspirate, and may pump gas into the tracheal vent. The result is that the performance of the ventilator is likely to vary with the configuration of the system, frequency, and tidal volume. These problems can be obviated in large part by employing a very high-impedence bias flow, delivered across a small orifice from a high-pressure source and removed from the trachea via a small orifice connected to a vacuum (132, 134). Alternatively the bias-flow system may be closed, that is, consist of a blower with CO_2 absorber, with O_2 supplied across a small orifice to maintain a constant system volume—or mean tracheal pressure (95).

Finally, there is evidence that oscillatory pressure applied to the pleural surface or chest wall can maintain gas exchange (143, 152).

Many mechanisms are potentially important in high-frequency ventilation. Alveoli are not equidistant from the airway opening (63, 119), so it is possible that some are ventilated conventionally with relatively small tidal volumes. If this mechanism contributes to gas exchange during high-frequency ventilation, ventilatory efficiency should decrease sharply at very low tidal volumes. There is some evidence that this is the case (17).

Given the high frequencies employed and the inhomogeneity of the mechanical properties of lung units, one would expect volume and pressure phase differences among peripheral units and perhaps between airway and peripheral units. Pendelluft (flow from one peripheral unit to another) has been observed with high-frequency oscillation of isolated lungs (81) and intact animals (124). Out-of-phase flows between airways and peripheral units could be a very important form of mixing during high-frequency oscillation (67). Pendelluft probably contributes to gas exchange during high-frequency ventilation, at least by homogenizing gas concentrations in regional conducting airways (17).

In a branching diverging system such as the airways, oscillatory flow produces velocity profiles that are less symmetrical or more skewed during inspiration than during expiration; thus dispersion or axial mixing occurs during inspiration that is not reversed during expiration (58). This mixing can occur in the absence of an axial concentration gradient and almost certainly must occur in large and medium airways during high-frequency ventilation.

Taylor-type mixing (138, 139) has been regarded as a likely mechanism for gas mixing in the airways during high-frequency ventilation. This occurs when there is an axial concentration gradient of gas that, due to convection, has a nonuniform concentration across the tube. Lateral mixing occurs by diffusion in laminar flows and by convective eddies in turbulent flows. In both cases mixing in tubes is much greater than would be predicted on the basis of molecular diffusion. Mathematical evaluations of Taylor mixing are complicated and difficult to apply to the lung (see ref. 129 for a recent review). It is very likely that turbulent Taylor mixing occurs in major airways during high-frequency ventilation but less clear that laminar Taylor dispersion is an important mechanism in smaller airways (17).

Many models have been formulated that theoretically are able to explain high-frequency ventilation. Typically these models assume that the pulmonary airways have a certain geometry and impedance and that these airways are rigid. A particular gas-mixing regime is applied to the model; results are analyzed in terms of conductance, i.e., the rate of washout of an alveolar gas divided by the difference in pressure from the alveoli to airway opening for that gas. This expression for conductance assumes that convective transport of alveolar gas, as in conventional ventilation, is negligible.

Fredberg (44) modeled high-frequency ventilation on the basis of turbulent Taylor mixing in major airways and showed that adequate gas-transport rates could be achieved. He further predicted that gas transport would be related to the product of tidal volume and frequency and independent of lung volume if impedence did not change with volume.

Slutsky et al. (131) modified the Fredberg model by arguing that significant gas transport (by Taylor mechanisms) could occur in airways with laminar flows. In addition, the model of Slutsky et al. included zero resistances to gas transport in the alveolar zone—well mixed by molecular diffusion—and at the airway opening where the bias flow convectively removed expired gas. The effects of the bias flow and tidal volume interacted so that gas transport depended more on tidal volume than frequency. At a given tidal volume, transport increased linearly with frequency, but the slope of this relationship increased as tidal volume increased. Again transport was independent of lung volume, as long as volume changes did not change mechanical impedence.

Permutt et al. (106) introduced a model that did not specify a mechanism of gas mixing. The airways were modeled as a series of compartments with differing transit times. Under these circumstances gas transport would be proportional to the product of frequency and the square of tidal volume but would also depend on the particular distribution of transit times.

Although the models cited above allow prediction of changes in gas transport with changes in tidal volume, frequency, and lung volume, it would be premature to regard congruent experimental data as validating one or another model, because of the multiple assumptions involved in the models. There is much experimental data on high-frequency ventilation; we briefly review studies that bear on the physiological mechanisms involved but do not review the many considerations of high-frequency ventilation as a therapeutic modality.

Studies of the effect of tidal volume and frequency on gas transport are complicated by the fact that the delivered tidal volume may be very difficult to determine, particularly in systems in which the tidal volume interacts with the bias flow. Such interactions are common with a low-impedance bias-flow system and may account for gas-transport optima at certain frequencies when frequency is increased with a "fixed" tidal volume (14, 150). When high-impedance bias-flow systems are used, increasing frequency at a given tidal volume results in a linear increase in gas transport in both humans and dogs (49, 134). If tidal volume is increased, the increase in gas transport is greater than if the frequency–tidal volume product is increased a similar amount by an increase in frequency. In both dogs and humans ventilated with a fixed tidal volume and varying frequency, gas transport becomes nearly independent of frequency at high frequencies: 5 Hz in humans and 25 Hz in dogs (49, 134). This occurs at lower frequencies in dogs with peripheral bronchoconstriction and probably indicates that at high frequencies the tidal volume is not delivered beyond the central airway, either because of gas compression or nonrigid behavior of the central airway. The latter has been observed in dogs with bronchoconstriction (48). Clearly, both compression and oscillation of central airway volume would increase as peripheral mechanical impedance increases (as in bronchoconstriction); humans have higher impedance per unit lung volume than dogs. An alternative explanation for the failure of gas transport to increase at very high frequencies is that whatever the mechanism of alveolar gas transport, it does not go to "completeness" during a very short cycle (25).

In humans, gas transport increases as lung volume increases (49), but apparently this is not true in dogs (134); this may relate to species differences in the relationship between lung volume and mechanical lung impedance.

Several studies of gas mixing during high-frequency ventilation have been published. Schmid et al. (124) noted that there was appreciable mixing between topographially separated lung regions; the degree could be explained on the basis of mixing between alveolar and dead-space gas. Gas transport during high-frequency ventilation has been shown to be largely independent of the molecular diffusivity of the gas being transported (71, 84), although diffusivity-related concentration differences may exist in alveolar gas (71). Thus, although peripheral transport is diffusion-limited, this limitation is small when compared to non-diffusion-related limitation of gas transport in central airways, including attached equipment such as the endotracheal tube.

Because high-frequency ventilation is a relatively new topic in respiratory physiology and is currently under intense investigation, an accurate summary is not possible. Whether this technique will be useful in medicine or give insights applicable to physiology under less-extreme circumstances is not clear.

Measurement of Dead Space

MORPHOLOGICAL ESTIMATES OF AIRWAY VOLUME. Although the dead space is usually defined in physiological terms, it must have some relation to the volume of conducting airways that has been measured by many investigators for nearly a century. The difficulty in equating such measurements with the dead space as measured by physiological techniques is that the physiological boundary between inspired and alveolar gas need not coincide with the morphological boundary between conducting airways and alveoli.

In 1894 Loewy (83) made a plaster-of-paris cast of bronchi in collapsed human lungs and found a volume of 144 ml. Rohrer (117) measured airway dimensions in collapsed human lungs down to branches 1 mm in diameter and found a volume of 162 ml. Allowing for a change in airway volume with lung expansion, he calculated that in life, airway volume varies between 180 ml and 260 ml, depending on lung inflation, and that ~50% of this volume is in extrathoracic airways. Nunn et al. (97) filled cadaver airways with water, obtained a mean volume of 138 ml, and noted that this was markedly influenced by jaw position. They too found that ~50% of their volume was in extrathoracic airways. More recently Weibel (144) and Horsfield and Cumming (63) have made resin casts of bronchi in single human inflated lungs and found the volume of the first 10 generations of airways to be 60 ml and 71 ml respectively.

SINGLE-BREATH MEASUREMENTS. These are usually carried out by measuring N_2 or CO_2 at the mouth with a rapid-response analyzer and, after the subject inhales a gas mixture devoid of indicator, plotting indicator gas concentration against expired gas volume. The resulting plot (Fig. 7) shows three clear-cut phases. In phase I, no indicator gas is evident; the expired gas is the same composition as the inspirate. In phase II, the indicator gas concentration rises rapidly, as a mix of dead space and alveolar gas is exhaled. In phase III, there is a slower, more-or-less linear increase in gas concentration, which is thought to represent alveolar gas. Such curves are analyzed by

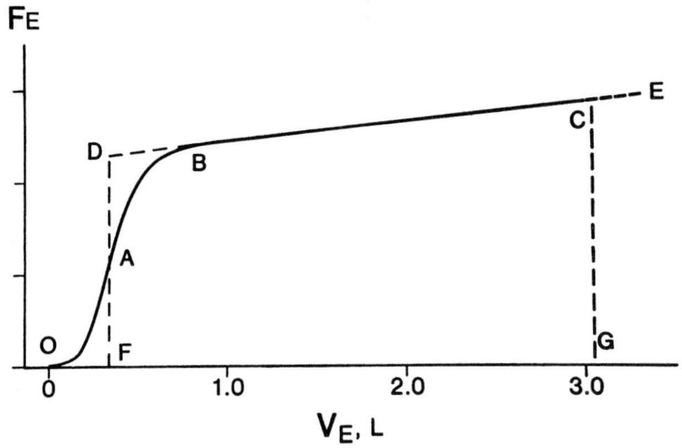

FIG. 7. Tracing of expired gas concentration (FE) from rapid analyzer as function of volume expired (VE,L) during single expiration after inspiration of mixture devoid of gas being analyzed. Alveolar plateau (*line BC*) has been extrapolated (*line DE*). [Adapted from Aitken and Clark-Kennedy (1).]

rectifying phase II and measuring the volume preceding the resulting square front. This was originally done by integrating the curve (area OABCG, Fig. 7) and constructing a trapezoid (DCGF, Fig. 7) containing an equal amount of the tracer gas (1). The dead space was then the volume expired to point F. Subsequent workers, most notably Fowler (40), rectified phase II by equating area OAF with area ADB. Using O_2 as the inspirate and N_2 as his indicator gas, Fowler found an average dead space of 156 ml in 45 healthy humans. When the same technique is used with foreign gases to measure dead space (94), expired concentration decreases from 100% of that inspired and the same three phases are evident in the concentration-volume plot. If the same method of analysis is used, dead-space volumes are similar for a variety of indicator gases (6), at least as long as their diffusivities are similar (77). A simplified method was introduced by Young (151), who used CO_2 as his indicator and designated the dead space as the volume equivalent to the point during phase II at which the expired CO_2 was 50% of the back-extrapolated alveolar CO_2 (Fig. 7). Results of this procedure were comparable to those of the Fowler technique. Single-breath measurements are widely used and are the source of most data on "anatomical" dead space.

The major difficulty with this technique is defining the junction of phases II and III. The analysis outlined above assumes that this junction demarcates the end of dead-space washout: phase II contains a mixture of dead-space and alveolar gas, whereas phase III contains only alveolar gas. Allowance is made for the slope of phase III (which is thought to be due to continuing gas exchange and sequential emptying of alveolar units) by back extrapolating this slope to the volume of interest (Fig. 7). In normal subjects the junction of phases II and III is fairly clear-cut and corresponds to the departure of the curve from a linear extrapolation of phase III. In patients with airway disease, phase III is steeper and may be less linear; the junction between phases II and III may be more difficult to detect. Fowler (41) suggested a number of modifications of his technique to render the junctions of phases II and III more clear in patients with airway disease, but the physiological significance of the results is not clear.

In a lung consisting of alveolar units that are equidistant from the mouth and that contribute equal amounts to the expirate, phase II would be a measure of the washout characteristics of airways containing inspired gas. This of course is not the case: pathway lengths from alveolus to trachea vary, and it is possible that units with the same path length differ in their contribution to a given aliquot of the total expirate. Ross (119) found that in the dog lung, path length from alveolus to carina varied from 2 to 14 cm; in a human lung at 75% total lung capacity, Weibel (144) found path lengths varying from 22 to 40 cm. Cumming et al. (22) emphasized that phase II represented not only the washout characteristics of the upper airways but also the distribution of gas transit times from the lung periphery; these transit times were related to asymmetrical path lengths and regional flow rates.

ISOSATURATION METHOD. This method was introduced by Pappenheimer et al. (105), who rearranged the Bohr equation (Eq. 9)

$$\frac{V_{DS}}{V_T} = \left(\frac{1}{P_I - P_A}\right) P_E - \left(\frac{1}{P_I - P_A}\right) P_A \quad (26)$$

where P_E is expired gas pressure and P_I is inspired gas pressure. If alveolar gas pressure (P_A) were considered equal to arterial gas pressures and kept constant while V_T was varied and P_E was measured, and if V_{DS} were constant, P_E and $1/V_T$ would be linearly related; when extrapolated to $1/V_T = 0$, $P_E = P_A$, and when extrapolated to $P_E = P_I$, $1/V_T = 1/V_{DS}$. Pappenheimer et al. found that there was a linear relationship between $1/V_T$ and both $P_{E_{O_2}}$ and $P_{E_{CO_2}}$ and that the derived dead spaces were the same. However, the extrapolated P_A differed from arterial values in a way that suggested that V_{DS} was not a constant but increased linearly with V_T (36). More recent workers have used somewhat similar approaches (19), again developing data compatible with an increase in V_{DS} as V_T increases.

MULTIPLE-BREATH MEASUREMENTS. The speed of washout or washin of multiple-breath inert gas is affected by the dead space; the gas is washed out or in by the alveolar tidal volume ($V_T - V_{DS}$), and if the speed of washout and tidal volume are known, dead space may be calculated. Open-circuit N_2 washout is measured by observing the rate of decrease in N_2 concentration in successive breaths after the subject begins to breathe 100% O_2. In the simplest case (23)

$$F_{A_n} = F_{A_0} \omega^n \quad (27)$$

where F_{A_n} is N_2 concentration at breath n, F_{A_0} is initial N_2 concentration, and ω is the alveolar dilution ratio FRC/(FRC + $V_T - V_{DS}$) (FRC, functional residual capacity), the amount lung N_2 is diluted by each successive breath of O_2. If mean expired concentration is measured

$$F_E = F_A\left(\frac{V_T - V_{DS}}{V_T}\right)$$

and

$$F_E = F_{A_0}\omega^n\left(\frac{V_T - V_{DS}}{V_T}\right)$$

If F_E is plotted logarithmically against n, a straight line results with slope ω, and if F_{A_0} and V_T are known, V_{DS} may be calculated (8, 40). Closed-circuit rebreathing washin of He may be analyzed similarly (9).

These analyses assume that washin or washout may be described as a single exponential function; i.e., all units have the same alveolar dilution ratio. This is not true in most lungs (43), and when it is not the resulting dead space is too large (8, 9). More complex washouts may be analyzed by treating them as the sum of a series of exponentials, each with its own alveolar dilution ratio. Fowler et al. (43) compared these to an ideal alveolar dilution ratio, which described washout from lungs with the same volume and the same total ventilation ($V_T - V_{DS}$) as the sum of the compartments defined by the differing exponentials. From this ideal ratio the dead space could be calculated. Although they obtained reasonable values for dead space, Fowler et al. regarded this approach as inferior to the single-breath technique, because it was very sensitive to the value of the alveolar dilution ratio assigned to the rapid-washout exponential.

More recently, Martin and colleagues (84, 88) developed a technique for assessing dead space during multiple-breath N_2 washout. By computer they analyzed the curve as the sum of four exponentials; one of them, the dead space, with an alveolar dilution ratio of zero, was a compartment that completely filled and emptied with each breath. This dead space was substantially larger than simultaneously measured single-breath dead space and larger in disease than in health. Martin and co-workers suggested that this was because the dead space contributed to portions of the expirate previously thought to contain only alveolar gas, but it is not clear whether the additional volume measured by their technique was in fact dead space (as defined in terms of gas exchange) or simply units with small alveolar dilution ratios.

PHYSIOLOGICAL DEAD SPACE. In the steady state the dead space may be estimated with the Bohr equation (Eq. 8), usually with CO_2 the indicator gas. In normal subjects at rest, use of end-tidal CO_2 as $P_{A_{CO_2}}$ results in values for the dead space approximating those from single-breath methods (2, 76). However, when end-tidal gas is sampled during exercise (2) or after a forced expiration (23), the resulting dead space is too large. The validity of end-tidal sampling is also questionable in the presence of lung disease. For these reasons Pa_{CO_2} is frequently substituted for $P_{A_{CO_2}}$ in the Bohr equation and the result is termed *physiological dead space.* Enghoff (33) introduced this procedure, which is widely used to assess gas exchange. Assuming alveolar-capillary equilibrium for CO_2, Pa_{CO_2} represents a blood flow–weighted mean of the various $P_{A_{CO_2}}$ values in the lung, whereas true mean $P_{A_{CO_2}}$ represents a ventilation-weighted mean of $P_{A_{CO_2}}$ values. Because the venoarterial P_{CO_2} difference is small, venoarterial shunting and units with low $\dot{V}_A/\dot{Q}$ contribute little to differences between Pa_{CO_2} and mean $P_{A_{CO_2}}$. Units with high $\dot{V}_A/\dot{Q}$ may have low P_{CO_2}, however, so the presence of such units creates a difference between Pa_{CO_2} and mean $P_{A_{CO_2}}$; the physiological dead space will be larger than that measured by end-tidal sampling (the anatomical or series dead space), and the difference has been termed the *alveolar* or *parallel dead space* (126).

In theory, physiological and alveolar dead space could be calculated with appropriate data for any gas exchanging in the lung. However, alveolar-arterial gas tension differences and therefore the alveolar dead space depend not only on $\dot{V}_A/\dot{Q}$ distribution within the lung but also on the solubility of the gas considered (61). Generally, for a given $\dot{V}_A/\dot{Q}$ distribution, the more insoluble the gas, the larger the physiological dead space resulting from the application of the Enghoff-Bohr equation. This phenomenon is discussed in detail in the chapters by Hlastala and Farhi in this *Handbook*; an example of its effect is the increase in physiological dead space when high concentrations of O_2 are inhaled (7). Blood CO_2 solubility decreases as O_2 saturation increases (Haldane effect); thus, without other changes, alveolar and therefore physiological dead space would be expected to increase. It is probable that the actual increase observed is too large to be fully explained by the Haldane effect (82).

Calculation of the alveolar dead space appears to estimate the fraction of the ventilation distributed to peripheral lung units with a P_{CO_2} of zero. The solubility of CO_2 is such that the alveolar dead space reflects units with high $\dot{V}_A/\dot{Q}$, but within such units the relationship between $P_{A_{CO_2}}$ and $\dot{V}_A/\dot{Q}$ is not linear; $\dot{V}_A/\dot{Q}$ must be increased 5- to 10-fold from the normal value of unity to halve $P_{A_{CO_2}}$. Thus measurements of alveolar dead space underestimate the amount of lung with high $\dot{V}_A/\dot{Q}$. Furthermore, implicit in the calculation of alveolar dead space is the assumption that if a unit is unperfused, its P_{CO_2} is zero. This neglects gas reinspired from the common dead space, so that measurements of alveolar dead space underestimate the fraction of the tidal volume entering unperfused units. This is probably why increases in anatomical or series dead space, which increase reinspired dead-space gas, are not accompanied by similar increases in physiological dead space (129, 136).

In summary, the physiological dead space for CO_2 (as calculated by the Enghoff-Bohr equation) includes the series or anatomical dead space, a true alveolar or parallel dead space that is underestimated, and a contribution from units with high $\dot{V}_A/\dot{Q}$, which varies with the particular $\dot{V}_A/\dot{Q}$ distribution. Despite these difficulties, physiological dead space is a readily available measure of "wasted" ventilation, and measurements of physiological and alveolar dead space have shed light on factors affecting lung perfusion distribution. An alveolar dead space has been found to develop in normal humans when tilted from the supine to erect positions (13), presumably because of underperfusion of the lung apex in erect subjects. Other workers (4, 79) have failed to confirm this, however. Positive-pressure breathing is also associated with a measurable alveolar dead space (12, 36), because increases of airway pressure create underperfused lung regions. In patients with obstructive lung disease, Pa_{CO_2} is regularly greater than end-tidal P_{CO_2} (82, 87), and physiological dead space may increase substantially with O_2 breathing (80). This change was attributed to increased $\dot{V}_A/\dot{Q}$ inhomogeneity consequent to relief of hypoxic vasoconstriction (80), a hypothesis that has not yet been confirmed.

Other estimates of physiological dead space have been obtained by applying the Enghoff-Bohr equation to measurements obtained during the infusion of inert gases with very high solubilities (61, 107). The excretion of such gases is little affected by $\dot{V}_A/\dot{Q}$ in units that receive any blood flow, so their physiological dead space essentially reflects units with no perfusion. Depending on $\dot{V}_A/\dot{Q}$ distribution, this inert-gas dead space may be smaller than that calculated with CO_2 as the indicator gas, because the CO_2 dead space includes units with high but finite $\dot{V}_A/\dot{Q}$. The inert-gas physiological dead space has been separated into series and parallel components, but there is a tendency to underestimate both because of reinspired dead-space gas (107). However, the inert-gas dead space is insensitive to changes in $\dot{V}_A/\dot{Q}$ distribution and is affected only slightly by nonextreme changes in the distribution of reinspired dead-space gas.

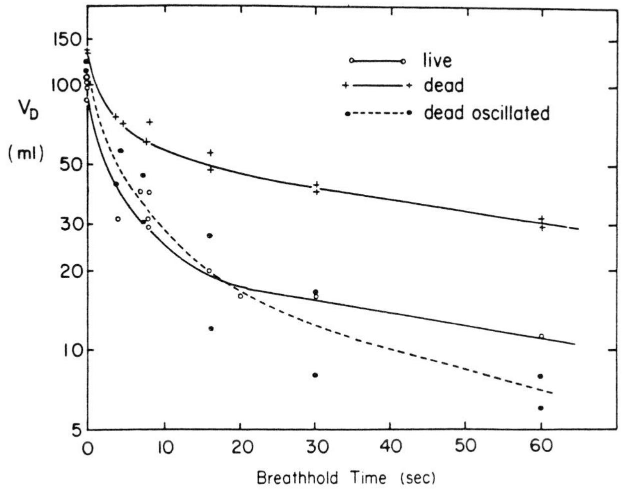

FIG. 8. Single-breath dead space (VD) in dog lungs as function of breath-holding time (abscissa). In animals with a heartbeat, dead space falls more rapidly than in dead animals; this fall can be duplicated by manually oscillating the heart of dead animals. [Adapted from Engel et al. (31).]

Factors Affecting Dead Space

Except where otherwise noted, all data reviewed below derive from single-breath measurements of "anatomical" dead space.

SPECIES. Morphological estimates of conducting airway volume are available in a variety of mammalian species, with values of 150 ml in the dog (119), 380 ml in the cow (119), and 150–300 liters in the whale (125). Tenney and Bartlett (140, 141) measured tracheal dimensions in a wide variety of mammals and found that tracheal volume, which presumably related to dead space, was proportional to body mass to the 1.05 power. Because FRC increases with body mass by approximately the same amount, VDS/FRC is approximately constant among species. Interestingly, the trachea is relatively small in newborn animals. The VDS/FRC is also smaller in newborns than in adults but appears to vary little among newborns of differing species (92). For obvious reasons the giraffe has held a particular fascination for students of the dead space. Recent studies compared single-breath dead space in the giraffe with that of other mammals and found that the giraffe's VDS/VT was not unusual (66, 78, 116). Although long, the giraffe's trachea is apparently also relatively narrow.

AGE, SEX, AND BODY SIZE. In adults, dead space clearly increases with body size, probably accounting for the fact that dead space is greater in males than in females (40). Although the dead space has been related to height (56) and body surface area (147), the most commonly used normative index is that of Radford (109), who noted that in nonobese adults the dead space in milliliters approximated the body weight in pounds. In infants the ratio of physiological dead space to tidal volume is similar to that in adults (19). In elderly people both single-breath (41) and physiological (142) dead space increase, but this may be due to an age-related increase in FRC (see next section), because age has no effect on dead space measured at full inflation. Detailed prediction formulas have been developed for physiological dead space in normals (57): normal values depended on the age, height, tidal volume, and breathing frequency of the subject. In supine normals, physiological dead space is smaller than in erect normals (13, 113); the difference is too large to explain on the basis of changes in lung volume (113).

LUNG VOLUME. Although increases in lung volume should, in the presence of a constant inspiratory flow, displace centrally the front between inspired and alveolar gas, measured dead space increases as a function of end-inspiratory lung volume (10, 127), because intrapulmonary airways are not rigid and their volume increases as inflation increases their transmural pressure. The relationship between dead space and end-inspiratory volume is alinear but approximates 2–3 ml/0.1-liter change in lung volume (10). Dead space has been found to relate linearly to end-inspiratory transpulmonary pressure (127). The relationship between end-inspiratory volume and dead space accounts for changes in single-breath dead space observed with chest compression (90) and changes in tidal volume (127). Dead-space volume also depends on lung volume history (45). At the same end-inspiratory volume, dead space was smaller after a series of deflations than after a series of inflations, implying that the dead space had greater pressure-volume hysteresis than did the pulmonary parenchyma.

BREATHING PATTERN AND GAS DIFFUSIVITY. During breath holding, dead space decreases (6, 91, 118, 127), rapidly at first and then slowly. The magnitude of the decrease is such that it has been estimated that the front between alveolar and inspired gas must migrate to the main stem or lobar bronchi, too great a distance for molecular diffusion (6, 64). Engel et al. (31) showed conclusively that cardiogenic mixing was a major cause of the reduction in dead space with breath holding (Fig. 8). In the same lungs, dead space decreased more when the heart was beating than when it was not, and the effect of the spontaneous heartbeat could be duplicated by manually oscillating the heart (Fig. 8).

As breathing frequency is increased, dead space [both anatomic (77, 118) and physiological (85)] is increased, probably because high inspiratory-flow rates peripherally displace the front between inspired and residual gas. In experiments where inspiratory- and expiratory-flow rates were independently controlled, the volume of dead space increased with inspiratory-flow rate (148). Single-breath dead space is smaller during forced expirations from total lung capacity than it is during slow expirations; this was ascribed to different emptying sequences (7), but no change in dead space with expiratory-flow rate was observed when expiration was initiated from less-extreme lung volumes (148).

Gas-density effects have been best studied by comparing the effects of low-density gas (H_2 or He) with those of a high-density gas. Dead space tended to be greater when measured with dense gas (77, 108, 128, 148), as would be predicted on the basis of better diffusive mixing of the lighter gas. With breath holding the difference between the two dead spaces decreases (108, 128). This suggests that mixing during breath holding is convective and therefore favors the denser gas (30, 128) but is also compatible with the denser gas diffusing more rapidly toward the mouth because the cross-sectional area available for its diffusion is larger than that for the lighter gas, which has a more centrally placed front at the beginning of breath holding. When, in the steady state, dense gas is substituted for N_2, physiological dead space increases (89), which also implies impaired diffusional gas mixing in the airways.

DRUGS AND SURGERY. Bronchodilator drugs tend to increase dead space and bronchoconstrictor drugs tend to decrease it (145), but these changes are relatively small and inconsistent, probably because the agents used affect major central airways only slightly. Dead space is decreased after pneumonectomy (42) and reduced 30%–50% by tracheostomy (11).

REFERENCES

1. AITKEN, R. S., AND A. E. CLARK-KENNEDY. On the fluctuation in the composition of the alveolar air during the respiratory cycle in muscular exercise. *J. Physiol. Lond.* 65: 389–411, 1928.
2. ASMUSSEN, E., AND M. NIELSEN. Physiological dead space and alveolar gas pressures at rest and during muscular exercise. *Acta Physiol. Scand.* 38: 1–21, 1956.
3. BAKER, L. G., J. S. ULTMAN, AND R. A. RHODES. Simultaneous gas flow and diffusion in a symmetric airway system: a mathematical model. *Respir. Physiol.* 21: 119–138, 1974.
4. BANZETT, R., K. STROHL, B. GEFFROY, AND J. MEAD. Effect of transrespiratory pressure on $P_{ET_{CO_2}} - Pa_{CO_2}$ and ventilatory reflexes in humans. *J. Appl. Physiol.* 51: 660–664, 1981.
5. BARGETON, D. Analysis of the capnogram and oxygram in man. *Bull. Physio-Pathol. Respir.* 3: 503–526, 1967.
6. BARTELS, J., J. W. SEVERINGHAUS, R. E. FORSTER, W. A. BRISCOE, AND D. V. BATES. The respiratory dead space measured by single breath analysis of oxygen, carbon dioxide, nitrogen or helium. *J. Clin. Invest.* 33: 41–48, 1954.
7. BASHOFF, M. A., R. H. INGRAM, JR., AND D. P. SCHILDER. Effect of expiratory flow rate on the nitrogen concentration vs. volume relationship. *J. Appl. Physiol.* 23: 895–901, 1967.
8. BATEMAN, J. B. Studies of lung volume and intrapulmonary mixing. Nitrogen clearance curves: apparent respiratory dead space and its significance. *J. Appl. Physiol.* 3: 143–160, 1950.
9. BIRATH, G. Lung volume and ventilation efficiency. Changes in collapse treated and non-collapse-treated pulmonary tuberculosis and in pulmonectomy and lobectomy. *Acta Med. Scand. Suppl.* 154: 1–166, 1944.
10. BIRATH, G. Respiratory dead space measurements in a model lung and healthy human subjects according to the single breath method. *J. Appl. Physiol.* 14: 517–520, 1959.
11. BIRATH, G., R. MALMBERG, M. BECK, AND N. P. BERGH. The airway dead space in tracheotomized patients (Abstract). *Acta Chir. Scand. Suppl.* 245: 51, 1959.
12. BITTER, H. S., AND H. RAHN. *Redistribution of Alveolar Blood Flow With Passive Lung Distention.* Washington, DC: U.S. Dept. Commerce, Off. Tech. Serv., 1956, p. 1–20. (WADC Tech. Rep. 56-466.)
13. BJURSTEDT, H., C. M. HESSER, G. LILJESTRAND, AND G. MATELL. Effects of posture on alveolar-arterial CO_2 and O_2 differences and on alveolar dead space in man. *Acta Physiol. Scand.* 54: 65–82, 1962.
14. BOHN, D. J., K. MIYASAKA, B. E. MARCHAK, W. K. THOMPSON, A. B. FROESE, AND A. C. BRYAN. Ventilation by high-

frequency oscillation. *J. Appl. Physiol.* 48: 710–716, 1980.

15. BOHR, C. Ueber die Lungenathmung. *Skand. Arch. Physiol.* 2: 236–268, 1891.
16. BRISCOE, W. A., R. E. FORSTER, AND J. H. COMROE, JR. Alveolar ventilation at very low tidal volumes. *J. Appl. Physiol.* 7: 27–30, 1954.
17. CHANG, H. K. Mechanisms of gas transport during ventilation by high-frequency oscillation. *J. Appl. Physiol.* 56: 553–563, 1984.
18. CHANG, H. K., AND L. E. FARHI. Ternary diffusion coefficients in alveolar spaces. *Respir. Physiol.* 40: 269–279, 1980.
19. COOK, C. D., R. B. CHERRY, D. O'BRIEN, P. KARLBERG, AND C. A. SMITH. Studies of respiratory physiology in the newborn infant. I. Observations on normal premature and full-term infants. *J. Clin. Invest.* 34: 975–982, 1955.
20. COON, R. L., E. J. ZUPERKU, AND J. P. KAMPINE. Measurement of dead space ventilation using a pH_a servo-controlled ventilator. *J. Appl. Physiol.* 51: 154–159, 1981.
21. CRANDALL, E. C., AND J. E. O'BRASKY. Direct evidence for participation of rat lung carbonic anhydase in CO_2 reactions. *J. Clin. Invest.* 62: 618–622, 1978.
22. CUMMING, G., J. G. JONES, AND K. HORSFIELD. Inhaled argon boluses in man. *J. Appl. Physiol.* 27: 447–451, 1969.
23. DARLING, R. C., A. COURNAND, AND D. W. RICHARDS, JR. Studies on the intrapulmonary mixing of gases. V. Forms of inadequate ventilation in normal and emphysematous lungs analyzed by means of breathing pure oxygen. *J. Clin. Invest.* 23: 55–67, 1944.
24. DOUGLAS, C. G., AND J. S. HALDANE. The capacity of the air passages under varying physiological conditions. *J. Physiol. Lond.* 45: 235–238, 1912.
25. DRAZEN, J. M., R. D. KAMM, AND A. S. SLUTSKY. High-frequency ventilation. *Physiol. Rev.* 64: 505–543, 1984.
26. DUBOIS, A. B. Alveolar CO_2 and O_2 during breath holding, expiration, and inspiration. *J. Appl. Physiol.* 5: 1–12, 1952.
27. EFFROS, R. M. Pulmonary capillary carbon dioxide gradients and the Wien effect. *J. Appl. Physiol.* 32: 221–222, 1972.
28. EFFROS, R. M., R. S. Y. CHANG, AND P. SILVERMAN. Acceleration of plasma bicarbonate conversion to carbon dioxide by pulmonary carbonic anhydrase. *Science Wash. DC* 199: 427–429, 1978.
29. ENGEL, L. A. Gas mixing within the acinus of the lung. *J. Appl. Physiol.* 54: 609–618, 1983.
30. ENGEL, L. A., AND P. T. MACKLEM. Gas mixing and distribution in the lung. In: *Respiratory Physiology II*, edited by J. G. Widdicombe. Baltimore, MD: University Park, 1977, vol. 14, chapt. 2, p. 37–82. (Int. Rev. Physiol. Ser.)
31. ENGEL, L. A., H. MENKES, L. D. H. WOOD, G. UTZ, J. JOUBERT, AND P. T. MACKLEM. Gas mixing during breath holding studied by intrapulmonary gas sampling. *J. Appl. Physiol.* 35: 9–17, 1973.
32. ENGEL, L. A., L. D. H. WOOD, G. UTZ, AND P. T. MACKLEM. Gas mixing during inspiration. *J. Appl. Physiol.* 35: 18–24, 1973.
33. ENGHOFF, H. Volumen inefficax. Bemerkungen zur Frage des schadlichen Raumes. *Uppsala Läkarefoeren. Förh.* 44: 191–218, 1938.
34. FENN, W. O., H. RAHN, AND A. B. OTIS. A theoretical study of the composition of the alveolar air at altitude. *Am. J. Physiol.* 146: 637–653, 1946.
35. FLUMERFELT, R. W., AND E. D. CRANDALL. An analysis of external respiration in man. *Math. Biosci.* 3: 205–230, 1968.
36. FOLKOW, B., AND J. R. PAPPENHEIMER. Components of the respiratory dead space and their variation with pressure breathing and with bronchoactive drugs. *J. Appl. Physiol.* 8: 102–110, 1955.
37. FORSTER, R. E. Can alveolar P_{CO_2} exceed pulmonary end-capillary CO_2? No. *J. Appl. Physiol.* 42: 323–328, 1977.
38. FORSTER, R. E., AND E. D. CRANDALL. Time course of exchanges between red cells and extracellular fluid during CO_2 uptake. *J. Appl. Physiol.* 38: 710–718, 1975.
39. FORTUNE, J. B., AND P. D. WAGNER. Effects of common dead space on inert gas exchange in mathematical models of the lung. *J. Appl. Physiol.* 47: 896–906, 1979.
40. FOWLER, W. S. Lung function studies. II. The respiratory dead space. *Am. J. Physiol.* 154: 405–416, 1948.
41. FOWLER, W. S. Lung function studies. V. Respiratory dead space in old age and in pulmonary emphysema. *J. Clin. Invest.* 28: 1439–1444, 1950.
42. FOWLER, W. S., AND W. S. BLAKEMORE. Lung function studies. VII. The effect of pneumonectomy on respiratory dead space. *J. Thorac. Surg.* 21: 433–437, 1951.
43. FOWLER, W. S., E. R. CORNISH, AND S. M. KETY. Lung function studies. VIII. Analysis of alveolar ventilation by pulmonary N_2 clearance curves. *J. Clin. Invest.* 31: 40–50, 1952.
44. FREDBERG, J. J. Augmented diffusion in the airways can support pulmonary gas exchange. *J. Appl. Physiol.* 49: 232–238, 1980.
45. FROEB, H. F., AND J. MEAD. Relative hysteresis of the dead space and lung in vivo. *J. Appl. Physiol.* 25: 244–248, 1968.
46. FROESE, A. B., AND A. C. BRYAN. High frequency ventilation. *Am. Rev. Respir. Dis.* 123: 249–250, 1981.
47. FUKUCHI, Y., C. S. ROUSSOS, P. T. MACKLEM, AND L. A. ENGEL. Convection, diffusion and cardiogenic mixing of inspired gas in the lung: an experimental approach. *Respir. Physiol.* 26: 77–90, 1976.
48. GAVRIELY, N., J. SOLWAY, S. LORING, R. H. INGRAM, JR., R. BROWN, A. SLUTSKY, AND J. DRAZEN. Airway dynamics during high frequency ventilation (HFV): a cineradiographic study (Abstract). *Physiologist* 25: 282, 1982.
49. GOLDSTEIN, D., A. S. SLUTSKY, R. H. INGRAM, JR., P. WESTERMAN, J. VENEGAS, AND J. DRAZEN. CO_2 elimination by high frequency ventilation (4 to 10 Hz) in normal subjects. *Am. Rev. Respir. Dis.* 123: 251–255, 1981.
50. GOMEZ, D. M. A physico-mathematical study of lung function in normal subjects and in patients with obstructive pulmonary disease. *Med. Thorac.* 22: 275–294, 1965.
51. GURTNER, G. H. Can alveolar P_{CO_2} exceed pulmonary end-capillary CO_2? Yes. *J. Appl. Physiol.* 42: 323–328, 1977.
52. GURTNER, G. H., S. H. SONG, AND L. E. FARHI. Alveolar to mixed venous P_{CO_2} difference under conditions of no gas exchange. *Respir. Physiol.* 7: 173–187, 1969.
53. GURTNER, G. H., AND R. J. TRAYSTMAN. Gas-to-blood P_{CO_2} differences during severe hypercapnia. *J. Appl. Physiol.* 47: 67–71, 1979.
54. GUYATT, A. R., C. J. YU, B. LUTHERER, AND A. B. OTIS. Studies on alveolar-mixed venous CO_2 and O_2 gradients in the rebreathing dog lung. *Respir. Physiol.* 17: 178–194, 1973.
55. HANSON, M. A., P. C. G. NYE, AND R. W. TORRANCE. Studies on the localization of pulmonary carbonic anhydrase in the cat. *J. Physiol. Lond.* 319: 93–109, 1981.
56. HARRIS, E. A., E. R. SEELYE, AND M. L. WHITLOCK. Revised standards for normal resting dead space volume and venous admixture in men and women. *Clin. Sci. Mol. Med.* 55: 125–128, 1978.
57. HART, M. C., M. M. ORZALESI, AND C. D. COOK. Relation between anatomic respiratory dead space and body size and lung volume. *J. Appl. Physiol.* 18: 519–522, 1963.
58. HASELTON, F. R., AND P. W. SCHERER. Bronchial bifurcations and respiratory mass transport. *Science Wash. DC* 208: 69–71, 1980.
59. HILL, E. P., G. G. POWER, AND L. D. LONGO. Mathematical simulation of pulmonary O_2 and CO_2 exchange. *Am. J. Physiol.* 224: 904–917, 1973.
60. HLASTALA, M. P. A model of fluctuating alveolar gas exchange during the respiratory cycle. *Respir. Physiol.* 15: 214–232, 1972.
61. HLASTALA, M. P., AND H. T. ROBERTSON. Inert gas elimination characteristics of the normal and abnormal lung. *J. Appl. Physiol.* 44: 258–266, 1978.
62. HLASTALA, M. P., P. SCHEID, AND J. PIIPER. Interpretation of inert gas retention and excretion in the presence of stratified inhomogeneity. *Respir. Physiol.* 46: 247–259, 1981.
63. HORSFIELD, K., AND G. CUMMING. Morphology of the bron-

chial tree in man. *J. Appl. Physiol.* 24: 373–383, 1968.

64. HORSFIELD, K., AND G. CUMMING. Functional consequences of airway morphology. *J. Appl. Physiol.* 24: 384–390, 1968.
65. HORSFIELD, K., I. GABE, C. MILLS, M. BUCKMAN, AND G. CUMMING. Effect of heart rate and stroke volume on gas mixing in dog lung. *J. Appl. Physiol.* 53: 1603–1607, 1982.
66. HUGH-JONES, P., C. E. BARTER, J. M. HIME, AND M. M. RUSBRIDGE. Dead space and tidal volume of the giraffe compared with some other mammals. *Respir. Physiol.* 35: 53–58, 1978.
67. ISABEY, D., A. HARF, AND H. K. CHANG. Alveolar ventilation during high-frequency oscillation: core dead space concept. *J. Appl. Physiol.* 56: 700–707, 1984.
68. JENNINGS, D. B., AND C. C. CHEN. Negative arterial-mixed expired P_{CO_2} gradient during acute and chronic hypercapnia. *J. Appl. Physiol.* 38: 382–388, 1975.
69. JONES, H. A., M. K. CHAKRABARTI, E. E. DAVIS, J. M. B. HUGHES, AND M. K. SYKES. The contribution of heart beat to gas mixing in the lungs of dogs. *Respir. Physiol.* 50: 177–185, 1982.
70. JONES, N. L., E. J. M. CAMPBELL, G. J. R. MCHARDY, B. E. HIGGS, AND M. CLODE. The estimation of carbon dioxide pressure in mixed venous blood during exercise. *Clin. Sci.* 32: 311–327, 1967.
71. KAETHNER, T., J. KOHL, AND P. SCHEID. Gas concentration profiles along airways of dog lungs during high-frequency ventilation. *J. Appl. Physiol.* 56: 1491–1499, 1984.
72. KLOCKE, R. A. Catalysis of CO_2 reactions by lung carbonic anhydrase. *J. Appl. Physiol.* 44: 882–888, 1978.
73. KLOCKE, R. A. Equilibrium of CO_2 reactions in the pulmonary capillary. *J. Appl. Physiol.* 48: 972–976, 1980.
74. KNOPP, T. J., T. KAETHNER, M. MEYER, K. REHDER, AND P. SCHEID. Gas mixing in the airways of dog lungs during high-frequency ventilation. *J. Appl. Physiol.* 55: 1141–1146, 1983.
75. KROGH, A. On the mechanism of gas exchange in the lungs. *Skand. Arch. Physiol.* 23: 248–278, 1910.
76. KROGH, A., AND J. LINDHARD. The volume of the dead space in breathing and the mixing of gases in the lungs of man. *J. Physiol. Lond.* 51: 59–90, 1917.
77. LACQUET, L. M., L. P. VAN DER LINDEN, AND M. PAIVA. Transport of H_2 and SF_6 in the lung. *Respir. Physiol.* 25: 157–173, 1975.
78. LANGMAN, V. A., O. S. BAMFORD, AND G. M. O. MALOIY. Respiration and metabolism in the giraffe. *Respir. Physiol.* 50: 141–152, 1982.
79. LARSON, C. P., JR., AND J. W. SEVERINGHAUS. Postural variations in dead space and CO_2 gradients breathing air and O_2. *J. Appl. Physiol.* 17: 417–420, 1962.
80. LEE, J., AND J. READ. Effect of oxygen breathing on distribution of pulmonary blood flow in chronic obstructive lung disease. *Am. Rev. Respir. Dis.* 96: 1173–1180, 1967.
81. LEHR, J., J. M. DRAZEN, P. A. WESTERMAN, AND S. C. ZATZ. Regional expansion of excised dog lungs during high frequency ventilation (Abstract). *Federation Proc.* 41: 1747, 1982.
82. LENFANT, C. Arterial-alveolar difference in P_{CO_2} during air and oxygen breathing. *J. Appl. Physiol.* 21: 1356–1362, 1966.
83. LOEWY, A. Ueber die Bestimmung der Grosse des "Schadlichen Luftraumes" im Thorax und der alveolaren Sauerstoffspannung. *Pfluegers Arch. Gesamte Physiol. Menschen Tiere* 58: 416–427, 1894.
84. LEWIS, S., AND C. J. MARTIN. Characteristics of the washout dead space. *Respir. Physiol.* 36: 51–63, 1979.
85. LIFSHAY, A., C. W. FAST, AND J. B. GLAZIER. Effects of changes in respiratory pattern on physiological dead space. *J. Appl. Physiol.* 31: 478–483, 1971.
86. LIN, K. H., AND G. CUMMING. A time varying model of gas exchange in the human lung during a respiratory cycle at rest. *Respir. Physiol.* 17: 93–112, 1973.
87. LUFT, U. C., J. A. LOEPPKY, AND E. M. MOSTYN. Mean alveolar gases and alveolar-arterial gradients in pulmonary patients. *J. Appl. Physiol.* 46: 534–540, 1979.
88. MARTIN, C. J., S. DAS, AND A. C. YOUNG. Measurements of the dead space volume. *J. Appl. Physiol.* 47: 319–324, 1979.
89. MARTIN, R. R., M. ZUTTER, AND N. R. ANTHONISEN. Pulmonary gas exchange in dogs breathing SF_6 at 4 Ata. *J. Appl. Physiol.* 33: 86–92, 1972.
90. MCILROY, M. B., J. BUTLER, AND T. N. FINLEY. Effects of chest compression on reflex ventilatory drive and pulmonary function. *J. Appl. Physiol.* 17: 701–705, 1962.
91. MILLS, R. J., AND P. HARRIS. Factors influencing the concentrations of expired nitrogen after a breath of oxygen. *J. Appl. Physiol.* 20: 103–109, 1965.
92. MORTOLA, J. P. Dysanaptic lung growth: an experimental and allometric approach. *J. Appl. Physiol.* 54: 1236–1241, 1983.
93. MUIR, D. C. F. Distribution of aerosol particles in exhaled air. *J. Appl. Physiol.* 23: 210–214, 1967.
94. MUNDT, E., W. SCHOEDEL, AND H. SCHWARZ. Über den effektiven schädlichen Raum der Atmung. *Pfluegers Arch. Gesamte Physiol. Menschen Tiere* 244: 107–119, 1941.
95. NGEOW, Y. K., AND W. MITZNER. A new system for ventilating with high-frequency oscillation. *J. Appl. Physiol.* 53: 1638–1642, 1982.
96. NIXON, W., AND A. PACK. Effect of altered gas diffusivity on alveolar gas exchange—a theoretical study. *J. Appl. Physiol.* 48: 147–153, 1980.
97. NUNN, J. F., E. J. M. CAMPBELL, AND B. W. PECKETT. Anatomical subdivisions of the volume of respiratory dead space and effect of position of the jaw. *J. Appl. Physiol.* 14: 174–176, 1959.
98. NYE, R. E. Influence of the cyclical pattern of ventilatory flow on pulmonary gas exchange. *Respir. Physiol.* 10: 321–337, 1970.
99. OTIS, A. B. Quantitative relationships in steady-state gas exchange. In: *Handbook of Physiology. Respiration*, edited by W. O. Fenn and H. Rahn. Washington, DC: Am. Physiol. Soc., 1964, sect. 3, vol. I, chapt. 27, p. 681–698.
100. PACK, A., M. B. HOOPER, W. NIXON, AND J. C. TAYLOR. A computational model of pulmonary gas transport incorporating effective diffusion. *Respir. Physiol.* 29: 101–124, 1977.
101. PAIVA, M. Gas transport in the human lung. *J. Appl. Physiol.* 35: 401–410, 1973.
102. PAIVA, M., AND L. A. ENGEL. Influence of bronchial asymmetry on cardiogenic gas mixing in the lung. *Respir. Physiol.* 49: 325–338, 1982.
103. PAIVA, M., L. M. LACQUET, AND L. P. VAN DER LINDEN. Gas transport in a model derived from Hansen-Ampaya anatomical data of the human lung. *J. Appl. Physiol.* 41: 115–119, 1976.
104. PAPPENHEIMER, J. R. Standardization of definitions and symbols in respiratory physiology. *Federation Proc.* 9: 602–605, 1950.
105. PAPPENHEIMER, J. R., A. P. FISHMAN, AND L. M. BORRERO. New experimental methods for determination of effective alveolar gas composition and respiratory dead space, in the anesthetized dog and in man. *J. Appl. Physiol.* 4: 855–867, 1952.
106. PERMUTT, S., W. MITZNER, AND G. WEINMANN. Model of gas transport during high-frequency ventilation. *J. Appl. Physiol.* 58: 1956–1970, 1985.
107. PETRINI, M. F., H. T. ROBERTSON, AND M. P. HLASTALA. Interaction of series and parallel dead space in the lung. *Respir. Physiol.* 54: 121–136, 1983.
108. POWER, G. G. Gaseous diffusion between airways and alveoli in the human lung. *J. Appl. Physiol.* 27: 701–709, 1969.
109. RADFORD, E. P., JR. Ventilation standards for use in artificial respiration. *J. Appl. Physiol.* 7: 451–460, 1955.
110. RAHN, H. A concept of mean aveolar air and the ventilation-bloodflow relationships during pulmonary gas exchange. *Am. J. Physiol.* 158: 21–30, 1949.
111. RAHN, H., AND L. E. FARHI. Ventilation, perfusion, and gas exchange—the $\dot{V}A/\dot{Q}$ concept. In *Handbook of Physiology. Respiration*, edited by W. O. Fenn and H. Rahn. Washington, DC: Am. Physiol. Soc., 1964, sect. 3, vol. I, chapt. 30, p. 735–766.
112. RAHN, H., AND W. O. FENN. *A Graphical Analysis of the*

Respiratory Gas Exchange. Washington, DC: Am. Physiol. Soc., 1955, 38 p.

113. Rea, H. H., S. J. Withy, E. R. Seelye, and E. A. Harris. The effect of posture on venous admixture and respiratory dead space in health. *Am. Rev. Respir. Dis.* 115: 571–580, 1977.
114. Riley, R. L., J. L. Lilienthal, Jr., D. D. Proemmel, and R. E. Franke. On the determination of the physiologically effective pressures of oxygen and carbon dioxide in alveolar air. *Am. J. Physiol.* 147: 191–198, 1946.
115. Robertson, H. T., and M. P. Hlastala. Elevated alveolar P_{CO_2} relative to predicted values during normal gas exchange. *J. Appl. Physiol.* 43: 357–364, 1977.
116. Robin, E. D., J. M. Corson, and G. J. Dammin. The respiratory dead space of the giraffe. *Nature Lond.* 186: 24–26, 1960.
117. Rohrer, F. Der Strömungswiderstand in den menschlichen Atemwegen und der Einfluss der unregelmässigen Verzweigung des Bronchialsystems auf den Atmungsverlauf in verschiedenen Lungenbezirken. *Pfluegers Arch. Gesamte Physiol. Menschen Tiere* 162: 225–299, 1915.
118. Roos, A., H. Dahlstrom, and J. P. Murphy. Distribution of inspired air in the lungs. *J. Appl. Physiol.* 7: 645–659, 1955.
119. Ross, B. B. Influence of bronchial tree structure on ventilation in the dog's lung as inferred from measurements of a plastic cast. *J. Appl. Physiol.* 10: 1–14, 1957.
120. Ross, B. B., and L. E. Farhi. Dead-space ventilation as a determinant in the ventilation-perfusion concept. *J. Appl. Physiol.* 15: 363–371, 1960.
121. Scheid, P., and J. Piiper. Blood/gas equilibrium of carbon dioxide in lungs. A critical review. *Respir. Physiol.* 39: 1–31, 1980.
122. Scheid, P., J. Teichmann, F. Adaro, and J. Piiper. Gas-blood CO_2 equilibration in dog lungs during rebreathing. *J. Appl. Physiol.* 33: 582–588, 1972.
123. Scherer, P. W., L. H. Shendalman, N. M. Greene, and A. Bouhuys. Measurement of axial diffusivities in a model of the bronchial airways. *J. Appl. Physiol.* 38: 719–723, 1975.
124. Schmid, E. R., T. J. Knopp, and K. Rehder. Intrapulmonary gas transport and perfusion during high-frequency oscillation. *J. Appl. Physiol.* 51: 1507–1514, 1981.
125. Scholander, P. F. Experimental investigations on the respiration in diving mammals and birds. *Hvabaadets. Skr. Nr. Nor. Vidensk. Akad.* 22: 1–131, 1940.
126. Severinghaus, J. W., and M. Stupfel. Alveolar dead space as an index of distribution of blood flow in pulmonary capillaries. *J. Appl. Physiol.* 10: 335–348, 1957.
127. Shepard, R. H., E. J. M. Campbell, H. B. Martin, and T. Enns. Factors affecting the pulmonary dead space as determined by single breath analysis. *J. Appl. Physiol.* 11: 241–244, 1957.
128. Sikand, R. S., H. Magnussen, P. Scheid, and J. Piiper. Convective and diffusive gas mixing in human lungs: experiments and model analysis. *J. Appl. Physiol.* 40: 362–371, 1976.
129. Singleton, G. J., C. R. Olsen, and R. L. Smith. Correction for mechanical dead space in the calculation of physiological dead space. *J. Clin. Invest.* 51: 2769–2772, 1972.
130. Slutsky, A. S. Gas mixing by cardiogenic oscillations: a theoretical quantitative analysis. *J. Appl. Physiol.* 51: 1287–1293, 1981.
131. Slutsky, A. S., G. G. Berdine, and J. M. Drazen. Oscillatory flow and quasi-steady behavior in a model of human central airways. *J. Appl. Physiol.* 50: 1293–1299, 1981.
132. Slutsky, A. S., J. M. Drazen, R. H. Ingram, Jr., R. D. Kamm, A. H. Shapiro, J. J. Fredberg, S. H. Loring, and J. Lehr. Effective pulmonary ventilation with small-volume oscillation at high frequency. *Science Wash. DC* 209: 609–611, 1980.
133. Slutsky, A. S., R. D. Kamm, and J. M. Drazen. Alveolar ventilation at high frequencies using tidal volumes smaller than the anatomical dead space. In: *Lung Biology in Health and Disease. Gas Mixing and Distribution in the Lung*, edited by L. A. Engel and M. Pavia. New York: Dekker, 1985, vol. 25, chapt. 4, p. 137–176.
134. Slutsky, A. S., R. D. Kamm, T. H. Rossing, S. H. Loring, J. Lehr, A. H. Shapiro, R. H. Ingram, Jr., and J. M. Drazen. Effects of frequency, tidal volume, and lung volume on CO_2 elimination in dogs by high frequency (2–30 Hz), low tidal volume ventilation. *J. Clin. Invest.* 68: 1475–1484, 1981.
135. Steinbrook, R. A., V. Fencl, R. A. Gabel, D. E. Leith, and S. E. Weinberger. Reversal of arterial-to-expired CO_2 partial pressure differences during rebreathing in goats. *J. Appl. Physiol.* 55: 736–741, 1983.
136. Suwa, K., and H. H. Bendixen. Change in Pa_{CO_2} with mechanical dead space during artificial ventilation. *J. Appl. Physiol.* 24: 556–562, 1968.
137. Tai, R. C., H. K. Chang, and L. E. Farhi. Non-equimolar counter-diffusion in ternary gas systems. *Respir. Physiol.* 40: 253–267, 1980.
138. Taylor, G. I. Dispersion of soluble matter in solvent flowing slowly through a tube. *Proc. R. Soc. Lond. A Math. Phys. Sci.* 219: 186–203, 1953.
139. Taylor, G. I. The dispersion of matter in turbulent flow through a pipe. *Proc. R. Soc. Lond. A Math. Phys. Sci.* 223: 446, 1954.
140. Tenney, S. M. Some aspects of the comparative physiology of muscular exercise in mammals. *Circ. Res.* 20/21: 1–7, 1967.
141. Tenney, S. M., and D. Bartlett, Jr. Comparative quantitative morphology of the mammalian lung: trachea. *Respir. Physiol.* 3: 130–135, 1967.
142. Tenney, S. M., and R. M. Miller. Dead space ventilation in old age. *J. Appl. Physiol.* 9: 321–327, 1956.
143. Ward, H. E., J. T. Power, and T. E. Nicholas. High-frequency oscillations via the pleural surface: an alternative mode of ventilation? *J. Appl. Physiol.* 54: 427–433, 1983.
144. Weibel, R. R. *Morphometry of the Human Lung.* Berlin: Springer-Verlag, 1963.
145. Widdicombe, J. G. The regulation of bronchial caliber. In: *Advances in Respiratory Physiology*, edited by C. G. Caro. Baltimore, MD: Williams & Wilkins, 1966, p. 48–82.
146. Wilson, T. A., and K. H. Lin. Convection and diffusion in the airways and the design of the bronchial tree. In: *Airway Dynamics: Physiology and Pharmacology*, edited by A. Bouhuys. Springfield, IL: Thomas, 1970, p. 5–19.
147. Wood, L. D. H., S. Prichard, T. R. Weng, K. Kruger, A. C. Bryan, and H. Levison. Relationship between anatomic dead space and body size in health, asthma, and cystic fibrosis. *Am. Rev. Respir. Dis.* 104: 215–222, 1971.
148. Worth, H., F. Adaro, and J. Piiper. Penetration of inhaled He and SF_6 into alveolar space at low tidal volumes. *J. Appl. Physiol.* 43: 403–408, 1977.
149. Worth, H., and J. Piiper. Model experiments on diffusional equilibration of oxygen and carbon dioxide between inspired and alveolar gas. *Respir. Physiol.* 35: 1–7, 1978.
150. Wright, K., R. K. Lyrene, W. E. Truog, T. A. Standaert, J. Murphy, and D. E. Woodrum. Ventilation by high-frequency oscillation in rabbits with oleic acid lung disease. *J. Appl. Physiol.*, 50: 1056–1060, 1981.
151. Young, A. C. Dead space at rest and during exercise. *J. Appl. Physiol.* 8: 91–94, 1955.
152. Zidulka, A., D. Gross, H. Minami, V. Vartian, and H. K. Chang. Ventilation by high frequency chest wall compression in dogs with normal lungs. *Am. Rev. Respir. Dis.* 127: 709–713, 1983.

CHAPTER 8

Phylogeny of the gas-exchange system: red cell function

STEPHEN C. WOOD | *Department of Physiology, University of New Mexico, School of Medicine, Albuquerque, New Mexico*

CLAUDE LENFANT | *National Heart, Lung, and Blood Institute, National Institutes of Health, Bethesda, Maryland*

CHAPTER CONTENTS

THIS CHAPTER ATTEMPTS to place the basic concepts of gas transport from environment to cell and of blood O_2 transport in mammals into a phylogenetic context. This requires what some may view as an unacceptable amount of speculation. However, the only available approach, or at least the one we have chosen, is to examine modern species of different groups of vertebrates. The premise is that the respiratory adaptations of modern species to their mode of breathing (water or air) and environmental variables (temperature and O_2 availability) provide insights into the phylogeny of respiratory processes.

EVOLUTION OF HEMOGLOBIN MOLECULE

Recent technological developments for determining gene structure have provided major breakthroughs in the study of molecular evolution. In 1977 the primary base sequence was determined for genes coding for hemoglobin (Hb). A number of workers have since suggested that ancestral Hb was synthesized by gene segments (exons) rather than by a continuous strand of operable DNA (23). Gilbert (43) suggests that the presence of exons and intervening nonfunctional gene segments could speed the rate of evolution because novel proteins (e.g., Hb) could be produced by recombination of gene segments rather than by substitution of single nucleotides.

The phylogenetic emergence of Hb probably occurred ~450 million years ago (46), with myoglobin (Mb) as the prototype structure. Although aggregation of this monomeric Hb to form homotetramers is likely, it would not have resulted in cooperativity in O_2 binding and other properties needed by an effective O_2 transport pigment. Homotetrameric Hb does not undergo a conformational change when oxygenated, and such a change is clearly necessary for allosteric phenomena like the Bohr effect and the organic phosphate effect, as well as for cooperativity in O_2 binding (37).

Hemoglobin in modern species conforms to the general model for allosteric effects in proteins; i.e., it exists in two distinct conformational states. Deoxygenated Hb (tense conformation) has a low O_2 affinity, whereas oxygenated Hb (relaxed conformation) has a high O_2 affinity. Goodman et al. (46) have shown that the mutations in Hb structure that improved function (by providing for cooperativity and allosteric interactions) occurred early in Hb evolution. They have also suggested that residue positions in Hb necessary for cooperativity changed more rapidly than other sites. They conclude that this is more consistent with Darwinian-type evolution: i.e., positive selection for improved function rather than evolution based on random, neutral mutations.

Eaton (35) suggests that the primitive Hb gene duplicated ~400 million years ago and segregated to different chromosomes where further duplication occurred. The result was the development of heterodimers (e.g., $\alpha\beta$-dimers) with the important functional advantage of subunit cooperativity and the resulting sigmoid O_2 dissociation curve. The only modern example of this type of Hb is found in certain primitive fishes; e.g., lamprey Hb is a monomer when oxygenated, but it aggregates to form a homodimer in the deoxy state. Subsequent evolution of $\alpha\beta$-Hb produced the heterotetramer characteristic of most modern species. Figure 1 shows a simplified phylogenetic tree illustrating Hb evolution and the cofactors regulating Hb function.

During the evolution of heterotetrameric Hb (~450 million to 300 million years ago) the environment, particularly the composition of the atmosphere and climate, changed dramatically. When Hb evolved in the first fishes, the partial pressure of O_2 (P_{O_2}) was probably as low as 15 Torr; the present value of ~155 Torr was not reached until 300 million years ago, when the first reptiles appeared (29). Consequently when the first lungfishes appeared ~420 million years ago, the air they began to breathe had a P_{O_2} of only 20 Torr.

Nothing is known about the O_2 dissociation curves of these early forms of Hb. However, to function as a transport pigment and still provide some O_2 reserves in the blood, the O_2 affinity of the blood must have been quite high, e.g., with an O_2 half-saturation pressure of Hb (P_{50}) half that of the environmental P_{O_2}. It is intriguing that these early forms, like their modern counterparts, are thought to have had ATP as a major intracellular regulator of O_2 affinity (Fig. 1). Thus they may have had low red cell ATP with a resulting high O_2 affinity, like the response of modern fish species to hypoxia.

Modern lungfishes could not have easily tolerated that primitive environment because their O_2 dissociation curves are positioned to function at higher environmental and blood P_{O_2} values (78). As Riggs (98) suggests, it seems reasonable to suppose that evolution of Hb, rather than being neutral, occurred in response to the selective pressures of dramatic environmental changes. Additionally, the evolution of the function of whole blood would have been tempered by the changes in the metabolism of red cells, particularly that of organic phosphates, in response to the increasing availability of O_2.

In summary it seems clear that the genetic engineering of Hb has permitted tremendous plasticity in the primary structure and therefore the intrinsic O_2-binding properties. However, this provided adaptability to environmental changes only over spans of time measured in generations. For the individual animal, Hb function must be adaptable to changing environmental conditions over shorter periods (days, seasons). Therefore it was essential that Hb function be controllable by regulation of its intracellular milieu.

HEMOGLOBIN FUNCTION INSIDE RED CELLS

The need to have Hb packaged inside cells has been questioned. Indeed, in some invertebrates, Hb is not intracellular but circulates in free solution as high-molecular-weight polymers. However, in vertebrates (except icefishes and certain eel larvae that have no red cells) Hb is universally found only inside red cells.

Two main arguments have been used to rationalize the intracellular packaging of Hb. First, a solution of free Hb with the same O_2 capacity as whole blood would have a much higher viscosity and thus increase cardiac work (82). Second, a low molecular weight (compared with invertebrate Hb) may be essential to a high O_2 capacity; if so, packaging in red cells is essential to avoid Hb loss by renal filtration (110). Low-molecular-weight Hb, if present in solution, would greatly elevate colloid osmotic pressure, which would then require a comparable increase in hydrostatic pressure to maintain normal Starling forces, again elevating cardiac work (103).

Schmidt-Nielsen and Taylor (105) tested the first argument for the advantage of red cells. They found, in contrast to the putative viscosity-reducing effect of red cells, that hemolysis of blood reduced viscosity.

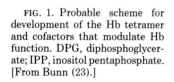

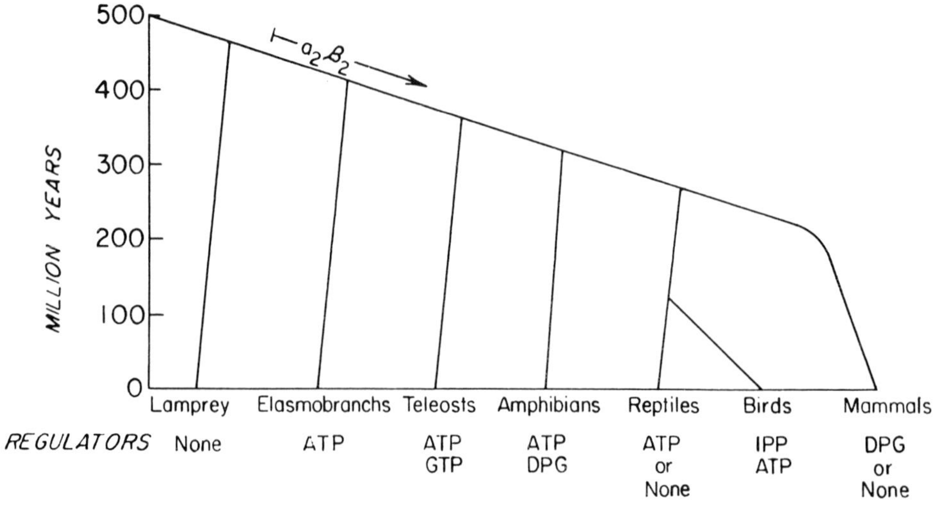

FIG. 1. Probable scheme for development of the Hb tetramer and cofactors that modulate Hb function. DPG, diphosphoglycerate; IPP, inositol pentaphosphate. [From Bunn (23).]

However, later experiments that measured viscosity in tubes with diameters approaching those of the resistance vessels in vivo revealed that red cells did reduce viscosity (109). The different results attest to the non-Newtonian nature of blood as a fluid (the Fahraeus-Lindqvist phenomenon). The net effect of confining Hb to red cells is a slight reduction of total viscosity. For example, a 40-mmHg increase in arterial pressure is needed to achieve the same flow in dog blood after hemolysis (109).

Ambersom et al. (2) tested the colloid osmotic effect of low-molecular-weight Hb by infusing Hb-saline solutions into mammals. At a relatively low (5%) Hb concentration, renal filtration was not a particular problem and the osmotic pressure was only slightly greater than that of normal plasma. However, this amount of Hb was not adequate for O_2 transport. More concentrated solutions of Hb would be rapidly diluted by the transfer of extravascular fluid into the general circulation (31).

Other recent arguments for packaging Hb in red cells were prompted by the realization that the red cell, once considered to be merely a bag of Hb, actually has very important metabolic functions. For example, the glycolytic system of red cells provides hydride ions. These are necessary to reduce the iron atoms, which yield nonfunctional MetHb when spontaneously oxidized (42). The red cell membrane also protects Hb from the proteolytic and oxidative denaturation of proteins that occurs in plasma. Consequently the turnover of Hb is only ~1% a day compared with 5%–40% for some plasma proteins. Furthermore the separation of Hb from plasma by a membrane permits the evolution of a metabolically controlled, allosteric regulation of Hb. This permits metabolic control of the microenvironment of Hb and fine-tuning of the intrinsic respiratory properties imparted by the primary structure of the molecule.

Red Cell Metabolism

Mammalian red cells are unique among plant and animal cells in losing their nucleus by a physiological process during maturation. That process apparently did not occur prior to the evolution of mammals. The red cells of fish, amphibians, reptiles, and birds are, with rare exceptions (52), nucleated. The red cells of most nonmammalian vertebrates are also characterized by the presence of mitochondria, aerobic metabolism, and oxidative phosphorylation. Predictably this produces some profound differences in the intracellular milieu and allosteric control of Hb (106).

Nucleated red cells, in contrast to the red cells of mammals, generally consume a considerable amount of the molecule they are supposed to transport. For example, the O_2 uptake of human red cells at 37°C is ~0.085 $\mu l \cdot min^{-1} \cdot ml^{-1}$ cells (76). The O_2 uptake of pigeon red cells is 10 times higher (80). In trout red cells, the O_2 demand is even greater, ~2.5 $\mu l \cdot mm^{-1} \cdot ml^{-1}$ cells (36). Incredibly, this accounts for 5% of the total O_2 uptake of the trout, whereas the work of the heart accounts for only 1% (70). In humans and most other mammals the relative roles of red cell and heart metabolism are reversed, with values of ~1% and 10% of total O_2 uptake, respectively (42). Because the relatively high rate of O_2 uptake in nucleated red cells must be satisfied by diffusion, it is appropriate to consider an important variable of diffusion, red cell size.

The diversity of red cell size among vertebrate groups is even greater than the diversity of red cell contents and metabolism. This was pointed out by Gulliver (50) in 1875 in a treatise that showed red cells ranging from 2 μm in diameter in the mouse deer to 63 μm by 40 μm in the salamander (*Amphiuma*). This is equivalent to the difference between a grape and a watermelon. There is some evidence that the small ratio of surface area to volume in amphibian red cells limits O_2 uptake, resulting in lower rates of oxidative metabolism in the larger red cells (45).

The most important effect of the different metabolism of nucleated versus mammalian red cells on O_2 transport properties is the difference in the O_2 dependence of organic phosphate production. As discussed in the next section, the virtual loss of oxidative phosphorylation and the disappearance of ATP as a major red cell organic phosphate in mammalian red cells resulted in a fundamental change in the control of Hb function.

Allosteric Controllers of Hemoglobin Function

Since the late 1960s the role of organic phosphates as allosteric regulators of Hb function has become well known. In 1925 an initial hint appeared in a report on a high concentration of organic phosphates in pig red cells (48). A stronger hint emerged in 1964 in a study showing that organic phosphates would bind to Hb (25). Then, in 1967, two papers reported that by binding preferentially to deoxygenated Hb, organic phosphates decreased the O_2 affinity of Hb, resulting in a right shift of the O_2 dissociation curve (17, 26). These papers also showed that Hb in free solution has a much higher O_2 affinity than whole blood. This was later shown to be due to the pH gradient across the red cell membrane (see next section) as well as the allosteric effect of intracellular organic phosphates. The basic finding of an effect of organic phosphates on Hb function stimulated a great deal of research on the physiological significance of this potential control mechanism in mammals, particularly for hypoxia adaptation. These papers are amply reviewed elsewhere (23, 27, 42). Subsequent studies with nucleated red cells revealed major differences with respect to hypoxia response and adaptation.

The evolutionary significance (or even presence) of organic phosphates as controllers of Hb function is speculative (Fig. 1). However, the presence and the importance of organic phosphates in red cells of extant vertebrates are now well documented. The types of organic phosphates in vertebrate red cells was first described in 1941 by Rappoport and Guest (95) and largely verified by later studies (11). The allosteric control of Hb function in lower vertebrates was first described in 1971 for fish (44) and amphibians (121). Subsequent studies have, with one exception, demonstrated an allosteric role of organic phosphates in red cells of all vertebrate groups including primitive species, e.g., the coelacanth and lungfishes (66, 127). The exception is a report that crocodile Hb is unaffected by organic phosphates but is strongly influenced by molecular CO_2 (14). The molecular basis of this has not yet been explained, but the mild antagonism between O_2 and CO_2 binding, which probably appeared very early in the evolution of Hb, is intensified about sixfold in the crocodile. As suggested by Bauer and Jelkmann (14), this could be adaptive to the typical behavior pattern of crocodiles: i.e., short-term bursts of activity. The rapid release of CO_2 stores in tissues would greatly facilitate O_2 delivery.

A fundamental difference between mammalian red cells and those of other vertebrates is the role of O_2 in organic phosphate metabolism. The aerobic metabolism of nucleated red cells results in a predominance of ATP or some other organic phosphate (e.g., GTP) that depends directly or indirectly on O_2 for its synthesis. In contrast, the dominant organic phosphate of mammalian red cells is 2,3-diphosphoglycerate (2,3-DPG), which is produced anaerobically in the glycolytic pathway. How the red cell responds to hypoxia in mammals versus other vertebrates is greatly affected by this basic difference. Despite the largely opposite control mechanisms and responses of red cells to hypoxia, both mammals and other vertebrates have adaptive responses of Hb function during hypoxia.

The mechanisms controlling Hb function in mammals and other vertebrates are compared in Figures 2 and 3. In mammals (Fig. 2) the initial effect of hypoxia is an increase in plasma and red cell pH. This results from hyperventilation and desaturation of Hb (a weaker acid than oxygenated Hb). The increase in red cell pH stimulates enzymatic production of 2,3-DPG. The negative-feedback control of 2,3-DPG production is provided by its effect on the Donnan distribution of H^+ across the red cell membrane. As 2,3-DPG production is increased, the red cell pH is reduced, inhibiting further 2,3-DPG production. The initial elevation of red cell pH and subsequent production of 2,3-DPG have offsetting effects on the O_2 affinity of blood that provide a stabilizing influence on the O_2 dissociation curve, particularly during acute exposure to high altitude. For instance, although the O_2 dissociation curve of human blood under standard conditions (pH 7.4, 37°C) is right-shifted after acute altitude exposure, the in vivo curve may be unchanged from that at sea level.

The negative-feedback control of organic phosphates just described for mammalian red cells does not occur in nucleated red cells, at least for most species in which ATP is the principal red cell organic phosphate. Furthermore the offsetting effects of pH changes on O_2 affinity (Bohr effect vs. organic phosphate effect) do not occur. The acid-base and organic phosphate changes induced by hypoxia have complementary effects on O_2 affinity (Fig. 3), i.e., a left shift of the O_2 dissociation curve. There are species, especially fish, in which GTP is the major allosteric controller of Hb (119). This compound, synthesized in the citric acid cycle, may have control systems independent of ATP production, but it still has been shown to be depleted during hypoxia (126).

Red Cell pH

Organic phosphates have two effects on Hb that work in concert to alter the O_2 affinity. The direct, or allosteric, effect is a result of the stabilization by

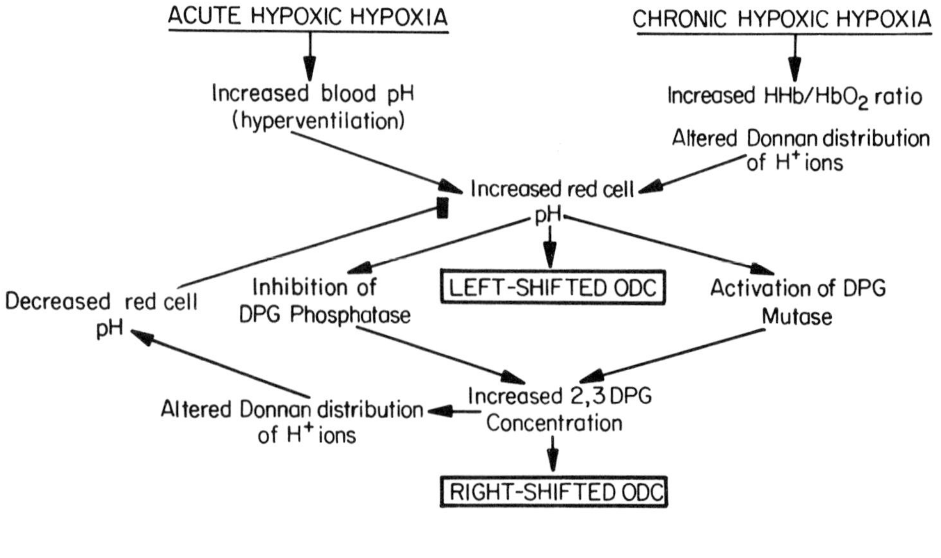

FIG. 2. Mechanisms controlling 2,3-diphosphoglycerate (2,3-DPG) metabolism and Hb-O_2 affinity of human red blood cells during hypoxia. ODC, O_2 dissociation curve. [Adapted from Gerlach and Duhm (42a).]

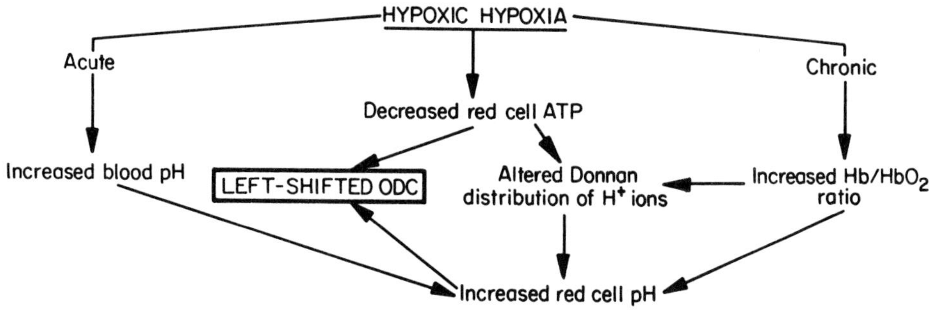

FIG. 3. Mechanisms controlling O_2 affinity and intracellular pH of nucleated red blood cells. [From Wood and Lenfant (129), by courtesy of Marcel Dekker, Inc.]

organic phosphates of Hb in the deoxygenated form. As polymeric anions, organic phosphates also have an indirect effect (via the Bohr effect) on O_2 affinity. An increase in red cell organic phosphate concentration favors a Donnan redistribution of H^+ to the inside of the red cell, decreasing intracellular pH and right-shifting the O_2 dissociation curve with no change in extracellular (plasma) pH (33). A comparison of the O_2 affinity of blood from different species at constant plasma pH can therefore be misleading if this phenomenon is not considered.

The relative importance of the indirect and direct effects of organic phosphates on O_2 affinity has been examined in only a few studies. For human blood the indirect effect is more important than the allosteric effect (33). This is consistent with the findings that the dose-response curve of 2,3-DPG on O_2 affinity flattens out at normal 2,3-DPG levels, but elevation to supranormal levels further lowers O_2 affinity (33). The indirect effect becomes increasingly important as pH increases because the allosteric interaction becomes weak or absent at higher red cell pH values (33). This is particularly relevant to ectothermic vertebrates at cooler body temperatures because blood pH is usually inversely related to body temperature (94). For example, in eels the normal blood pH is ~7.8 at 14°C. Exposure to hypoxia results in a large shift to the left of the O_2 dissociation curve that is 85% due to the indirect effect of ATP and GTP depletion on intracellular pH (122).

OXYGEN CAPACITY OF BLOOD

The O_2 capacity of blood is defined as the amount of O_2 contained in blood when the Hb is fully saturated. A few addenda to this definition are needed when dealing with the blood of ectothermic vertebrates.

1. The O_2 capacity should be corrected for dissolved O_2 (P_{O_2} × solubility coefficient). Although not too important in bloods with high Hb concentrations, this correction is significant in relatively anemic bloods, particularly at lower temperatures where the solubility is high. Icefish get along entirely on dissolved O_2 (55).

2. The O_2 capacity may be a function of blood pH in fish having blood with a Root effect. This appears to reflect an extreme pH dependency of O_2 affinity; at low pH it is impossible to fully saturate Hb even at high levels of P_{O_2} (21). This was first described by Root (99), who later showed that it did not occur in hemolysates but, rather, required intact red cells (100). The intracellular factor necessary for the extreme pH dependence has yet to be identified, but ATP has been ruled out, at least for some species (21).

3. The O_2 capacity should be measured, not calculated from total Hb concentration. Again this is not so critical for mammalian and avian red cells in which a significant amount of nonfunctional Hb is unusual, because enzymatic reductase systems reverse the ongoing oxidation of heme iron. This normally keeps MetHb levels at <1%. However, in some ectothermic vertebrates, this is not the case. Otherwise healthy turtles have been found with 90% MetHb levels (113).

4. The O_2 capacity, at least in reptiles, appears to be a function of temperature even when measured in vitro (89). The mechanism of this is not yet known. It is interesting that the temperature corresponding to maximum O_2 capacity is within the range of preferred body temperature. More study is required to explain this unusual phenomenon.

The relative anemia of many ectotherms, the numerous reports of significant amounts of MetHb in reptiles (128), and the ability of some ectotherms to survive the complete loss of their red cells (39) suggest that the role of the red cell in metabolic homeostasis is apparently much less important in ectotherms than in homeotherms.

It is tempting to conclude that the relatively sloppy control of red cell mass and function in many ectotherms is undoubtedly due largely to their O_2 demand, which is lower by orders of magnitude. Consequently, there is a relative lack of selective pressure for synthesis of much Hb and more finely tuned Hb function. This is particularly evident in the more sluggish species of ectotherms. However, the relationship of the blood flow required for a given O_2 uptake to blood O_2 capacity clearly contradicts this conclusion (30). As Figure 4 shows, the blood convection requirement becomes very pronounced at low Hb concentrations, with the icefish at the extreme. The relationship shown in Figure 4 is based on the Fick principle [$\dot{Q}/\dot{V}_{O_2} = 1/(Ca_{O_2} - C\bar{v}_{O_2})$, where $\dot{Q}$ is blood flow, $\dot{V}_{O_2}$ is O_2 uptake and $Ca_{O_2} - C\bar{v}_{O_2}$ is the arteriovenous O_2 concentration difference]. Oxygen capacity is included

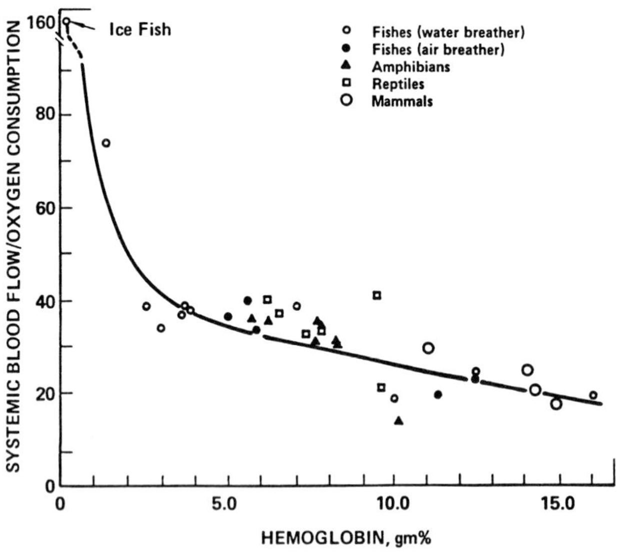

FIG. 4. Effect of Hb concentration on blood flow/O_2 uptake ratio (blood convection requirement) in different vertebrates. [From Lenfant et al. (78a).]

only as a factor limiting maximum Ca_{O_2}. This leaves as important variables the $C\bar{v}_{O_2}$ and (for amphibians and most reptiles) the degree of central vascular or intracardiac shunt that often lowers Ca_{O_2} to values well below O_2 capacity.

It seems likely that red cell mass and other components of the O_2 transport system (e.g., diffusing capacity and cardiac output) have evolved to be well matched to the metabolic machinery and O_2 demand. The higher blood flows required with smaller blood O_2 capacity may or may not be energetically more costly, depending on the hemodynamic effects of reduced viscosity and subsequent cardiac work.

HEMATOPOIESIS IN ECTOTHERMIC VERTEBRATES

The hematopoietic response to hypoxia seen in mammals is often absent in ectothermic vertebrates. This could also be viewed as evidence for reduced importance of red cells in metabolic homeostasis (57). However, some studies on this topic may have been biased in that altitude exposure was accompanied by a decreased air temperature, body temperature, and metabolic rate. Also, recent data show that ectothermic animals exposed to hypoxia in a temperature gradient respond by behaviorally lowering their normal (preferred) body temperature (125).

There is evidence for a true hematopoietic response (not dehydration) in lizards exposed to simulated altitude (118), but there appears to be no correlation between O_2 capacity and altitude in natural populations of lizards (28). Likewise there is no compelling evidence for amphibians that habitat altitude influences O_2 capacity in frogs (61) or salamanders (60).

Three compensatory mechanisms available to ectotherms may account for the relatively minor role of hematopoiesis in compensating for hypoxia. *1*) Most ectotherms have a relatively high potential for anaerobic metabolism. This has been reported for frogs and toads during anoxia (3, 69). *2*) Ectotherms may respond to hypoxic stress by a general lowering of metabolism (at a constant body temperature) or by cardiovascular adjustments (62, 120). An interesting example is the resident frog of Lake Titicaca (3,812-m altitude), which has, among other adaptations, the lowest metabolic rate of any frog (61). *3*) A potent compensation for hypoxia that is available to ectotherms is a reduction of body temperature by behavioral and physiological means.

In an evolutionary (or teleological) view, the lack of regulation of red cell quantity and subsequent compensatory mechanisms are energy-saving devices that avoid the cost of red cell production. The role of the qualities of the red cells in metabolic homeostasis is considered next.

OXYGEN DISSOCIATION CURVE AND THE ENVIRONMENT

The tradition of correlating O_2 affinity with the environment dates back to 1919 (73) and is a frequent topic of articles and reviews of Hb function (7, 27, 29, 41, 64, 67, 77, 92, 129). The dominant environmental factors in the phylogeny of vertebrates were the availability of water, O_2 concentration, and temperature. These remain dominant factors in the ontogeny as well as the daily life of modern ectotherms. Consequently these factors have been the independent variables of numerous studies on the physiology of ectotherms, including the adaptability of red cells to the environment. These investigators invariably concluded something about the adaptive significance of an observed change in O_2 affinity of blood or the appropriateness of a given O_2 dissociation curve to environmental conditions: e.g., left-shifted curve in water breathers versus right-shifted curve in air breathers.

A well-founded conclusion about the appropriateness of a given O_2 dissociation curve must be based on more than just the environmental conditions. The best and ultimate test of the physiological significance of a particular dissociation curve or shift of that curve is the effect on arterial partial pressure of O_2 (Pa_{O_2}) and mixed venous partial pressure of O_2 ($P\bar{v}_{O_2}$). As suggested in an earlier review (128), to draw physiological inferences from data on O_2 dissociation, the following criteria should be met. *1*) Whole blood, not Hb solutions, must be studied. *2*) The O_2 dissociation curve must pertain to temperatures and pH values that are ecologically realistic (many curves in the older literature were reported only at pH 7.4, whereas pH 7.8 is normal for 20°C). *3*) Acclimation history, season, sex, and age must be known. *4*) Concentration of MetHb should be measured because its presence alters the O_2 affinity of normal Hb. *5*) In vivo values of Pa_{O_2}, $P\bar{v}_{O_2}$, partial pressure of CO_2 (P_{CO_2}), pH, and O_2 content should be measured in unanesthetized, unrestrained animals. *6*) The O_2 dissociation curve should be measured by a method that accounts for, or is unaffected by, the O_2 uptake of red cells. *7*) In addition, as pointed out in a recent study (83), the possibility of multiple forms of Hb and their effect on nonstandard curve shapes must be considered.

Studies that meet these criteria and can apply the dissociation curve to the Fick principle, $\dot{V}_{O_2} = \dot{Q}(Ca_{O_2} - C\bar{v}_{O_2})$, are the exception, not the rule. Unfortunately, meeting these criteria is necessary for a critical assessment of the role of the O_2 dissociation curve. Other factors complicate a physiological assessment of the O_2 dissociation curves of ectotherms as well as homeotherms. One factor is the tremendous reserve for other components of the O_2 transport system, e.g., autoregulation of flow, to compensate for altered O_2 affinity of blood. Even in mammals the position of the O_2 dissociation curve seems to have little influence on O_2 uptake by exercising muscle or maximum O_2 uptake. In contrast some organs (heart, brain, liver) have O_2-consuming processes that are much more dependent on a higher P_{O_2} and therefore on the affinity of blood for O_2 (130). Chronic changes in O_2 affinity of human blood due to mutant Hb are compensated for by changes in Hb concentration (112). As a result, blood P_{50} values ranging from 12 to 70 Torr can provide roughly the same O_2 delivery ($Ca_{O_2} - C\bar{v}_{O_2}$) at similar $P\bar{v}_{O_2}$ values and cause no problems in otherwise healthy individuals (86).

The O_2 dissociation curve is much more labile in ectotherms than homeotherms due to the large daily fluctuations of temperature and pH. This further complicates efforts to assess the significance of the curve position. Among amphibians the range of blood P_{50} is similar to the range reported for human Hb mutants, 12 to 70 Torr. Similar large ranges in P_{50} exist for fish and reptiles. Although the trend for correlations between P_{50} and environmental variables is present, accessory data are still too scarce to allow any sweeping generalizations. Some of the available data for salamander blood illustrates a common problem in interpreting interspecies differences in O_2 affinity (Fig. 5). Not only are the O_2 affinities of different species very widely scattered but the differences are pH dependent. Both the magnitude and the direction of the Bohr effect are variable. Thus how much (or even whether) one species has a higher O_2 affinity than another depends on the pH selected for comparison.

Despite the above caveats, some consideration of environmental adaptations of the O_2 dissociation curve is worthwhile. Although much of the following discussion is speculative, the ideas are testable and may, we hope, provide some impetus for further study.

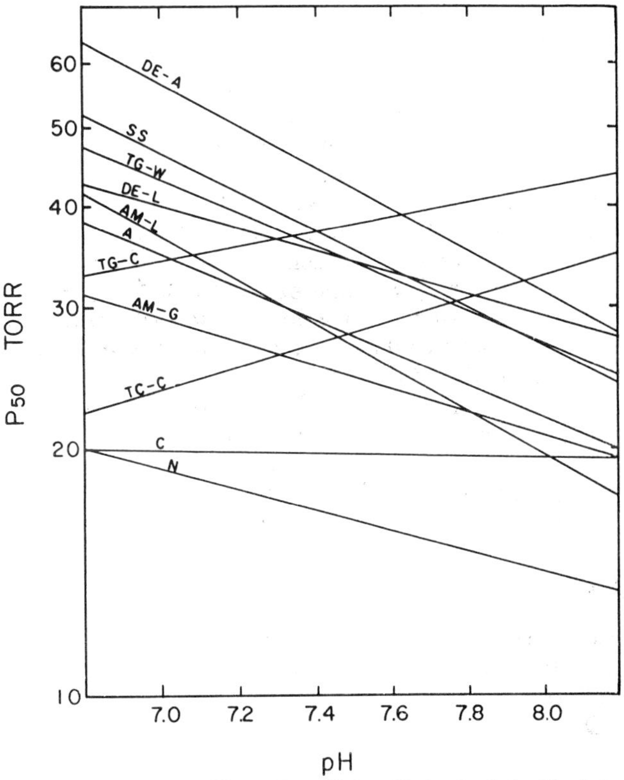

FIG. 5. Effect of pH on O_2 affinity (P_{50}) of whole blood in salamanders. DE-A, *Dicamptodon ensatus*, adult; DE-L, *D. ensatus*, larvae; TG-W, *Taricha granulosa*, warm acclimated; TG-C, *T. granulosa*, cold acclimated (121; S. C. Wood, unpublished observations). SS, *Salamandra salamandra*; AM-L, *Ambystoma mexicanum*, lung form; AM-G, *A. mexicanum*, gill form (41a). TC-C, *Triton cristatus*, cold acclimated (84a). A, *Amphiuma means*; N, *Necturus maculosa* (77). C, *Cryptobranchus* (113a).

Adaptations to Temperature

Body temperature has been an independent variable in an enormous number of comparative studies, in part because it is easy to vary and it affects almost everything. A more important reason, however, is that change in body temperature is the primary variable to which ectotherms must adapt. The mechanisms and patterns of adaptation are diverse, but the end results are similar. In Barcroft's words (4):

> Nature has learned so to exploit the biochemical situation as to escape from the tyranny of a single application of the Arrhenius equation. She can manipulate living processes in such a way as to rule and not be ruled by, the obvious chemical situation.

How does this "escape from the tyranny of the Arrhenius equation" apply to red cell function? When the temperature of a solution of Hb and O_2 is increased, the O_2 affinity is decreased. How much the curve shifts to the right depends on the heat of the combination of O_2 with Hb [apparent enthalpy (ΔH)]. The equation describing this relationship (derived from the Arrhenius equation for general chemical reactions) is

$$d(\log P_{50})/d(1/T) = \Delta H/2.303R$$

where T is temperature and R is the gas constant (1.987 cal·°K^{-1}·mol^{-1}). The nature of the bond between heme iron and O_2 is such that little or no interspecies variation is expected (71), and the apparent enthalpy of the bound O_2 should be ca. −9 kcal/mol. Although this is generally true for mammals ($\Delta H = -9$ to -14 kcal/mol), there are numerous cases of very low temperature sensitivity of Hb in ectotherms. Before citing some examples and suggesting possible mechanisms, it is appropriate to consider the selective pressures that may have favored evolution of blood with a low ΔH.

At first glance it seems that a normal temperature sensitivity would clearly be adaptive; e.g., increased temperature results in increased O_2 demand while simultaneously right-shifting the O_2 dissociation curve to promote increased O_2 delivery. This has been the classic rationale for mammals during exercise-induced hyperthermia, and it is supported by experimental data (42). The same rationale can be applied to the much wider range of excursions in body temperature and O_2 demand of ectotherms. Why then would a reduced ΔH be favorable?

One possibility for a selective pressure favoring reduced ΔH of ectotherm blood is related to the dual effect of temperature on O_2 affinity. The direct effect just described is complemented in most species by the temperature-induced change in blood pH [d(pH)/dT]. The magnitude of this effect varies but prototypically is ca. −0.016 (94). Thus an ectotherm with a normal blood pH of 7.8 at 15°C will have a normal blood pH of 7.48 when warmed to 35°C. If both the temperature effect and the Bohr effect of blood in ectotherms had normal (i.e., mammalian) values, the O_2 dissociation curve could be excessively shifted when temperature changes. That potential problem may be ameliorated by a reduction in either the temperature effect or the Bohr effect. Alternatively, O_2 affinity of blood may show temperature acclimation analogous to that seen in the metabolic rate. These strategies of adaptation and their mechanisms are described next.

There are, at least mathematically, three possible ways to reduce the effects of changing body temperature on blood O_2 affinity: i.e., via a reduction in magnitude of the three coefficients involved in this phenomenon.

1. The coefficient $d(\log P_{50})/dT$, normally ca. −0.024 in mammalian blood (19, 42), is a function of ΔH and may be reduced per se or show apparent reduction over long-term temperature acclimation. Hemoglobins showing a reduced ΔH are fairly common among ectotherms, with values ranging from 0 to −7 for fishes (122), amphibians (41, 65), and reptiles (122). An interesting example and suggestion for adaptiveness of a low ΔH involves tuna. Hochachka and Somero (56) suggested that the low ΔH (−1.8) of Hb in the bluefin tuna (*Thunnus thynnus*) could serve to prevent too rapid an unloading (and possible O_2 emboli) when cool peripheral blood entered the countercurrent heat exchanger of deep muscles [this species may have a 21°C temperature gradient from core to periphery (24a)]. Carey (24a) has recently shown that the ΔH of *Thunnus* Hb is not only low, as previously reported, but actually reversed in sign; i.e., O_2 binds less tightly as temperature decreases.

Another species with a reported positive ΔH value (mean value close to zero) is an African tree frog (*Chiromantis petersi*). Figure 6 illustrates the dual effects of temperature on O_2 affinity in this species (65). This animal may start a typical day at a body temperature of 25°C with a corresponding blood pH of 7.65. Its blood, even more so than most amphibians, has a relatively low O_2 affinity under these conditions (P_{50} = 48 Torr). The lower portion of Figure 6 shows what actually happens to P_{50} when this species warms to 40°C during the day. With a mean ΔH value close to zero, there is no effect of temperature per se on P_{50}. However, during warming the blood [assuming a coefficient of d(pH)/dT = −0.016] would be acidified to a pH of ~7.4. The Bohr effect in this species [$d(\log P_{50})/d(pH) = -0.3$] would then increase P_{50} to ~59 Torr, which is a high value but still not too high to allow saturation of Hb in the pulmonary capillaries. The upper portion of Figure 6 shows the potential effects of warming to 40°C if this species had a normal temperature sensitivity ($\Delta H = -8.2$). The dual effects of temperature would increase P_{50} to ~123 Torr, limiting saturation of Hb in the lungs to a maximum of ~50%. Similar quantitative arguments for a low ΔH have been developed for other ectotherms (122), and this seems to be the most common strategy.

Another strategy for long-term temperature exposure is acclimation of O_2 affinity. As illustrated in Figure 7, animals acclimated to either a cold or a warm temperature have blood with normal and equal tem-

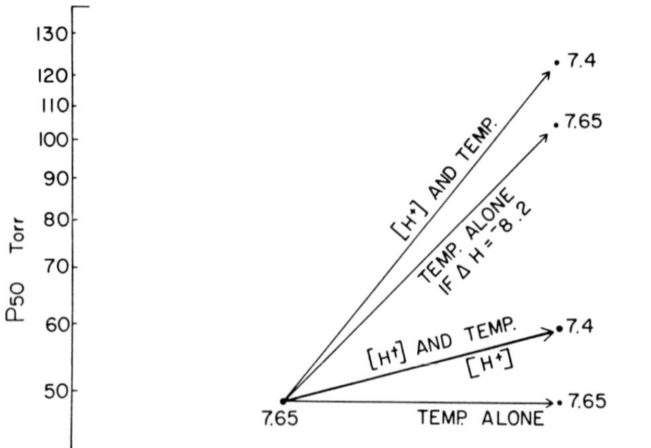

FIG. 6. Dual effect of temperature (direct and pH-mediated) on the O_2 affinity of blood in the African tree frog, *Chiromantis petersi*. ΔH, apparent enthalpy. [Data from Johansen et al. (65).]

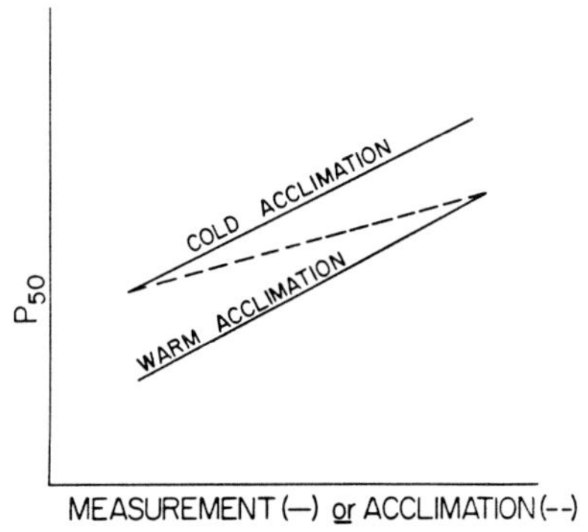

FIG. 7. Pattern of thermal acclimation of Hb function seen in some fishes and amphibians. Acutely measured temperature coefficient does not change (*solid lines*), but long-term coefficient is reduced (*dashed line*).

perature coefficients. However, at a given temperature the O_2 affinity of blood in warm-acclimated animals is relatively high. Consequently, acclimation results in a relative homeostasis of O_2 affinity; the long-term temperature coefficient may be half that of the acutely measured one. This pattern of O_2-affinity acclimation has been reported for fish, amphibians, and reptiles and is mediated, at least in one case, by a reduction in red cell organic phosphates after warm acclimation (122).

2. A reduction in the magnitude of the Bohr effect, d(log P_{50})/d(pH), could also reduce the dual effects of temperature on O_2 affinity. However, this is uncommon. Many ectotherms have mammalian-sized or larger Bohr coefficients, suggesting that selective pressures have favored retention of this interaction between CO_2 and O_2 transport. Only among urodele amphibians is a small (or in some cases reversed) Bohr effect quite common (see Fig. 5).

3. The coefficient d(pH)/dT, while quite variable, is significantly less than zero in most ectotherms. In some cases, both in the intra- and extracellular compartment, its value is close to the d(pH)/dT of neutral water, i.e., −0.017 (94). The biological significance of this effect of temperature has been related to the maintenance of a constant net charge (alphastat) on proteins, regardless of body temperature (96). However, a recent compilation of available data (53a) for all ectotherms shows that only rarely does the (d)pH/dT = 0.017 and satisfy the alphastat hypothesis. Rather, the average (d)pH/dT is ca. −0.011.

In summary, it appears that a direct reduction in ΔH is the major adaptation of ectotherms in stabilizing O_2 affinity in the face of large temperature cycles. The mechanism of reducing ΔH is not entirely clear. Organic phosphates play a major role simply because their own binding to Hb, like that of O_2, is exothermic. Therefore when O_2 binds to Hb, organic phosphates are displaced and the resulting absorption of heat is subtracted from the release of heat due to O_2 binding. In human blood ΔH is reduced from −10.7 kcal/mol with no 2,3-DPG present to −7.3 kcal/mol with 2,3-DPG present (19).

Thus the very low ΔH of tuna blood and other bloods could result from interaction between Hb and some allosteric effector, such as ATP or GTP, that is bound with a ΔH close to that of O_2. Evidence consistent with this speculation was reported by Powers et al. (92), who found that interspecific differences in the ΔH of blood do not persist when purified Hb is studied. However, there is at least one report of an intrinsically low ΔH in the purified form of a component of trout Hb (6).

Adaptations to Hypoxia

The role of O_2 affinity in hypoxia adaptation, particularly when high altitude is the cause, has been debated recently (34). The center of these debates has been whether a right shift or a left shift of the O_2 dissociation curve is better suited to life at high altitude. Both ontogenetic and interspecific differences in the response to hypoxia have sparked these debates. Earlier studies on humans as sojourners to altitude showed that both 2,3-DPG levels and the standard P_{50} were increased (79). In contrast, mammals in utero and mammals native to high altitude (e.g., llama) have bloods with higher O_2 affinity than adults or their sea-level counterparts (7, 8).

It is now fairly clear that the important factor to consider is the degree of hypoxia (116, 124). A right-shifted dissociation curve for humans is advantageous (unloading is increased more than loading is reduced) up to an altitude of ~4,300 m (108). There is convincing experimental evidence that a left-shifted dissociation curve is adaptive during more severe hypoxia; i.e., only those animals with a (pharmacologically) left-shifted dissociation curve survived (34).

Aquatic ectotherms, even at sea level, often encounter levels of hypoxia equivalent to those found at altitudes >4,300 m. Furthermore, water P_{O_2} may have daily cycles (due to photosynthesis and other factors) with values ranging from 10 to 300 Torr (131). Fishes living in certain midwater pelagic regions of the ocean encounter similar large ranges of water P_{O_2}, from ~1 Torr at a 300-m depth to 150 Torr during their daily migration to the surface (32). Longer-term changes in O_2 levels are experienced by those species that migrate between the ocean and rivers, e.g., salmon and eels. A more dramatic change, in terms of total O_2 available, occurs during the transition from aquatic to aerial respiration during amphibian metamorphosis and in facultative air-breathing fishes (see next section).

The comparative data on red cell function during hypoxia are quite consistent. Except for the fishes that inhabit the O_2-minimum zones of the ocean, the consistent finding in fish exposed to hypoxia is a left-shifted dissociation curve due to decreased red cell organic phosphates (e.g., 81, 91, 111, 126). The major compensation in fishes in the O_2-minimum zone, like that of some amphibians, seems to be a reduced metabolic rate (32). An intriguing metabolic compensation to hypoxia is found in goldfish. Like the tissues of other vertebrates, goldfish tissues respond to O_2 deprivation by switching to anaerobic metabolism. However, instead of producing lactate, an acidifying end product, this species produces ethanol, which leaves the fish by diffusion (108a, 116a).

Transition From Water Breathing to Air Breathing

Does ontogeny recapitulate phylogeny? In the case of red cell function, this is obviously an open question and one that has received its share of study and comment. The putative sequence of water breathing giving rise to air breathing in vertebrate evolution has modern parallels of two types: interspecific and ontogenetic. There are pronounced interspecific differences in the dependence on air breathing among lungfish (78) and amphibians (77). These studies (77, 78), as well as other interspecific comparisons, have shown a clear correlation between blood O_2 affinity and dependence on air breathing (cf. 64, 67). As first suggested by Krogh and Leitch (73), the O_2 dissociation curve is progressively right-shifted as the dependence on air breathing increases. Such interspecific comparisons may be interesting and provocative, but their utility as a basis for evolutionary concepts is limited by genetic diversity as well as allometric and morphological variables. These problems are partially solved by studying the transition from aquatic to aerial respiration that occurs within a species, i.e., the ontogeny of O_2 transport.

Developmental changes in Hb function have been studied in all classes of vertebrates. With rare exception the characteristic fetal-maternal shift of placental mammals has been found to accompany the development of other vertebrates (8). In many species the increase in P_{50} that occurs with birth, hatching, or metamorphosis is associated with the synthesis of a new Hb. However, that is not necessarily the cause of the change in O_2 affinity. For human Hb, the increase in P_{50} is due to a greater sensitivity of adult Hb than fetal Hb to 2,3-DPG (13). For amphibians, the increase in P_{50} at metamorphosis (or birth in the case of a viviparous species) is due to an increase in the amount of red cell ATP (114, 121). These studies support the generalization based on interspecific differences; i.e., the right shift of the O_2 dissociation curve during development is invariably associated with a switch to (or increased dependence on) air breathing. The lower O_2 affinity is argued to be adaptive to the 40- to 70-fold increase in O_2 availability as well as the increased cost of locomotion on land (67, 129). Although appealing, this argument remains to be critically evaluated by the criteria described earlier for dissociation-curve data.

ORGANISMIC ADAPTATIONS

Oxygen Uptake and Metabolic Machinery

We suggested earlier in this chapter that a smaller premium is placed on the red cells of ectotherms in terms of maintaining metabolic homeostasis. Why does a level of anemia that would be lethal for a homeotherm have little or no effect on a frog? Why is there such a huge variation in the O_2 affinities of blood, even within the same group of ectotherms? Why don't many ectotherms show a hematopoietic response to altitude or other hypoxic stresses? At least some of the answers to these questions can be derived by examining the differences between ectotherms and homeotherms at the tissue and cell level, i.e., the metabolic machinery.

The extent to which an increase in metabolic demand accompanied the evolution of homeothermy can only be inferred by comparing modern species. When data for all kinds of ectotherms are considered, the resting metabolic rate for homeotherms is ~30 times that for ectotherms (54). A 100-g bird at rest expends ~10 times as many calories as a 100-g lizard at the same body temperature (10). This is equivalent to an O_2 uptake that is 48-fold higher. The total drop in P_{O_2} from air to cells is probably about the same in these animals. Consequently the O_2 conductance ($\dot{V}_{O_2}/\Delta P_{O_2}$) must be ~30 times higher in birds. The increased demand this places on the O_2 transport system of homeotherms is reflected in all components: lung structure, complete separation of systemic and pulmonary circulation, increased perfusion pressures, cardiac performance, and red cell properties. The hematologic correlates of homeothermy include increased O_2 capacity, increased buffer capacity, and carefully regulated O_2 affinity.

What mechanisms account for the significant increase in the "cost of living" for birds and mammals? After almost a century of considerable speculation, the answers are only now beginning to emerge. One recent study shows that at least some of the extra heat in homeotherms comes from an increase in mitochondrial activity and relative organ size (38).

The argument that the lower cost of living reduces the importance of the red cell for O_2 delivery in ectotherms applies only to animals at rest, the condition under which the metabolic rates previously discussed were measured. However, the role of the red cell during activity is of greater physiological interest. Much less is known about the cost of active living and how ectotherms compare with homeotherms. Clearly there are tremendous behavioral differences in activity levels among both ectotherms and homeotherms. However, calculations by Hemmingsen (54) of maximum sustainable metabolic rate suggested that the ratio of homeotherms to poikilotherms approached unity. A recent review of data for maximum burst metabolic rate also suggested little difference between homeotherms and at least some poikilotherms (93). Data for maximum O_2 uptake in animals ranging in size from a 31-mg blowfly to a 100-ton blue whale fell on a single regression line with a slope of 0.75. Perhaps the evolution of homeothermy did not increase the maximum metabolic capacity but simply boosted the resting metabolic rate to a higher fraction of the maximum.

Allometry

One difficulty in comparing the physiological parameters of different species is the effect (often exponential) of body size, i.e., allometric influence. This carries over into attempts to draw conclusions relevant to the phylogeny of a physiological parameter like red cell function.

Numerous cardiopulmonary parameters have been related to body mass in vertebrates. The O_2 capacity of blood has been correlated with body mass in turtles and other vertebrate classes (24). The higher O_2 capacity in smaller species was suggested to be adaptive to the higher weight-specific metabolic rate. The O_2 affinity has also been reported to vary with body mass in mammals (104) and reptiles (128). The trend for lower O_2 affinity in smaller species was also regarded as an adaptation to the higher O_2 demand.

Several recent studies have cast some doubt on these allometric arguments. Most basic is a study showing that smaller mammals do not have a higher weight-specific O_2 uptake if the measurements are made in their thermoneutral zones (115). Because of the high ratio of surface area to volume in small mammals, the thermoneutral range of temperature is much smaller than previous investigators realized. Consequently some earlier studies mistakenly attributed to small body size what were probably thermoregulator increases in metabolic rate. In addition, the clear trend for lower O_2 affinity in smaller species is present only under constant conditions of P_{CO_2}, pH, and temperature. When O_2 affinities are compared under in vivo blood conditions, the trend largely disappears (74).

Circulatory Shunts

A significant contributing factor in the evolution of homeothermy was undoubtedly the development of a four-chambered heart allowing complete separation of pulmonary and systemic circulations (63). The elimination of intracardiac and central vascular shunts (e.g., Panizzae's foramen in crocodilian reptiles) permitted two significant changes that were highly adaptive to increased metabolism. First, the saturation of systemic arterial blood was increased by the vast reduction in venous admixture. Second, the systemic perfusion pressure could be increased now that the pulmonary circulation was shielded from left ventricular pressure. These features of cardiovascular function in mammals and birds greatly enhance O_2 transport potential by increasing delivered O_2, cardiac output, and the capacity for redistribution of blood flow. Among lower vertebrates only varanid lizards possess similar circulatory attributes (63).

Central vascular or intracardiac shunts affect O_2 transport in ectotherms in obvious and not so obvious ways. Clearly a right-to-left shunt will lower arterial saturation and, unless total flow increases, lower the maximum O_2 deliverable to tissues (i.e., cardiac output $\times$ Ca_{O_2}). However, the effect of a shunt on the P_{O_2} of systemic arterial blood is not so obvious because P_{O_2} becomes a dependent variable of O_2 content. Thus P_{O_2} can be quite high if the O_2 affinity is low. This in vivo phenomenon is analogous to the mixing method, an in vitro technique used to measure the P_{50} of blood (51). With this method, known ratios of saturated and desaturated blood are mixed anaerobically to produce 50% (or any other percent) saturation. The P_{O_2} of this mixture is then measured, providing one point on an O_2 dissociation curve. Any factor that right-shifts the dissociation curve will, for a given saturation, increase the measured P_{O_2}. The same principle applies when shunting occurs in normal (e.g., amphibians and reptiles) and abnormal (e.g., cyanotic heart disease) circulations. Figure 8 illustrates a two-compartment model where the mixing of bloods from the perfect compartment and the shunt compartment determines the O_2 content of the systemic arterial blood. In this model the shunt compartment also includes any blood that does not equilibrate with lung P_{O_2} for reasons other than anatomical shunt, i.e., ventilation-perfusion ($\dot{V}/\dot{Q}$) mismatch or impaired diffusion (101). The important point is that the saturation of blood in the perfect compartment is a function of P_{O_2} and O_2 affinity; thus

$$Sp_{O_2} = f(Pp_{O_2}, P_{50})$$

where Sp_{O_2} is O_2 saturation in perfect blood and Pp_{O_2} is O_2 pressure in perfect blood. The Pp_{O_2} is equal to the lung P_{O_2} and is therefore a function (f) of inspired P_{O_2}, lung P_{CO_2}, and the respiratory exchange ratio. The O_2 content of this blood (Cp_{O_2}) is a function of saturation and Hb concentration; thus

$$Cp_{O_2} = f(Sp_{O_2}, Hb)$$

However, in the systemic arterial blood, the O_2 content is a function of the shunt fraction ($\dot{Q}s/\dot{Q}_T$) and the O_2 contents of mixed venous and perfect blood; consequently

$$Ca_{O_2} = (\dot{Q}s/\dot{Q}_T)(C\bar{v}_{O_2}) + (\dot{Q}_{NS}/\dot{Q}_T)(Cp_{O_2})$$

where Ca_{O_2} is O_2 content, $\dot{Q}_{NS}/\dot{Q}_T$ is the non-shunt fraction, and $C\bar{v}_{O_2}$ is mixed venous O_2 content. Saturation of systemic arterial blood is a function of Ca_{O_2} and Hb concentration. Systemic Pa_{O_2} becomes a dependent variable of arterial saturation of O_2 (Sa_{O_2}) and P_{50}; thus

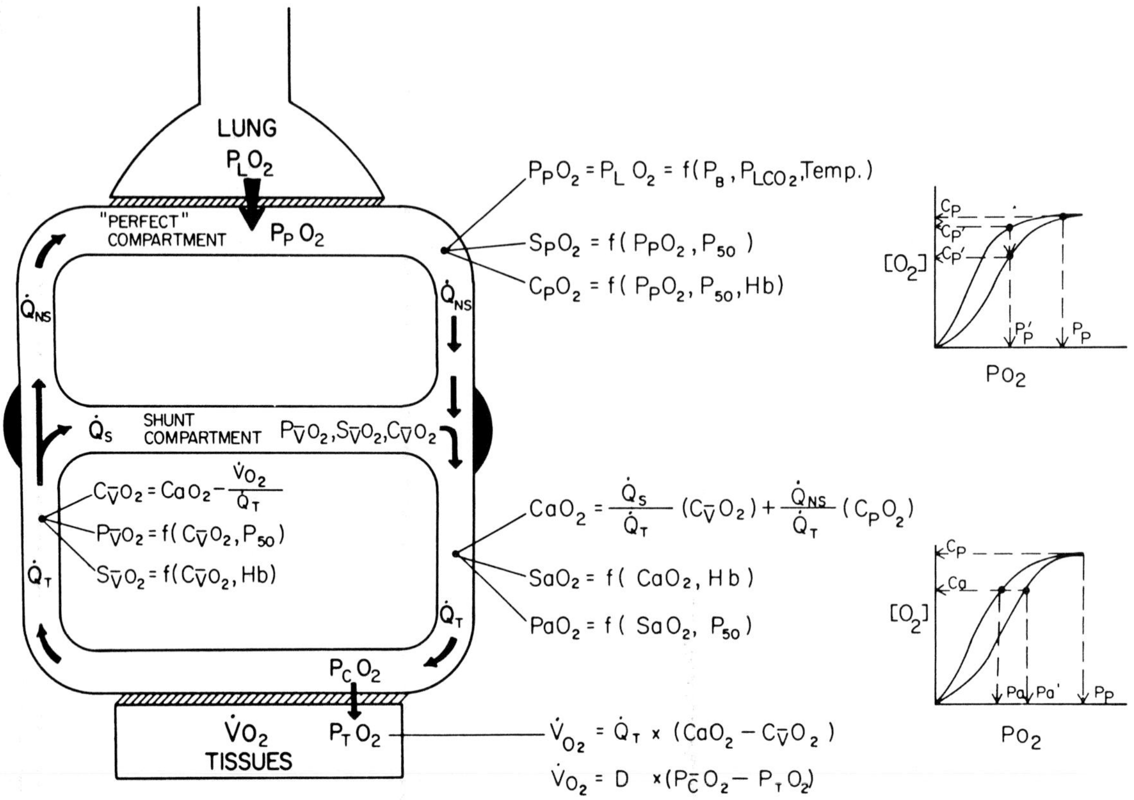

FIG. 8. Two-compartment model of O_2 transport applicable to animals with central vascular or intracardiac shunts. [From Wood (124).]

$$Pa_{O_2} = f(Sa_{O_2}, P_{50})$$

Thus, for a given saturation, Pa_{O_2} will be higher in bloods with lower O_2 affinities.

Models of gas exchange in mammals predict this phenomenon (higher Pa_{O_2} with lower O_2 affinity) in physiological shunts ($\dot{V}/\dot{Q}$ mismatch) and anatomical shunts (101, 116). Experimental data have verified this model in dogs with physiological or artificial shunts (40, 123) and in amphibians and reptiles with naturally occurring central shunts (123).

The physiological significance of this dependence of Pa_{O_2} and O_2 affinity remains to be tested. Animals with a large right-to-left shunt would clearly benefit from blood with a high P_{50} as long as the blood in the perfect compartment could become fully saturated, i.e., as long as the dissociation curve were not shifted too far to the right for the existing lung P_{O_2}. There are indeed many species of reptiles, particularly lizards, that have blood with very low O_2 affinity compared with mammals and birds (128). Also hypoxemia due to shunt differs in a fundamental way from hypoxemia due to low lung P_{O_2}. When lung P_{O_2} is reduced, the degree of hypoxia determines whether a right or left shift of the dissociation curve is adaptive. However, when a shunt is present, a right shift of the curve is generally adaptive within physiological limits of P_{50}; i.e., both Pa_{O_2} and $P\bar{v}_{O_2}$ are increased. For ectotherms, a typical factor inducing a right shift of the dissociation curve is elevated body temperature. This also increases O_2 uptake, which would undoubtedly be facilitated by the higher capillary P_{O_2} if shunt fraction were fairly stable. Further research is necessary to determine the influence, if any, of O_2 affinity on O_2 uptake in animals with shunts.

One situation in which a right-shifted curve and high body temperature may be deleterious is hypoxia. If the curve is right-shifted due to a relatively high preferred body temperature, there is little reserve for hypoxia in the upper, flat portion of the curve. Therefore, during hypoxia, blood leaving the pulmonary compartment may not be fully saturated, further reducing systemic arterial saturation. The behavioral compensation for hypoxia (voluntary hypothermia) also alleviates this potential problem by left-shifting the dissociation curve and increasing O_2 loading in the lungs.

CONCLUSION

The structure-function relationships of Hb are a fascinating area of study in modern species. The complexity of these relationships is increased by the fine-tuning of Hb function that occurs by allosteric controllers inside the red cell. Understanding the biochemistry of Hb function leads to the challenge of understanding the physiological significance. For modern species this is not always easy. Many generalizations have been made about the physiological significance of certain respiratory properties of blood, particularly O_2 affinity. Some have not survived when subjected to experimental verification. As only one link in the pathway for O_2, the red cell is protected from having paramount importance by the voluminous reserves in the other steps. This seems particularly evident in lower vertebrates, but even then the quantity and quality of red cells seems matched to the metabolic demand for O_2.

When the function of red cells is considered in a phylogenetic perspective it is possible to produce generalizations that are protected from experimental scrutiny. This is a frustrating situation to the laboratory scientist but inherent to paleophysiology, the study of the evolutionary basis of animal function.

We thank Dr. R. K. Dupre for helpful comments on the manuscript.

The work of S. C. Wood was supported by a grant from the National Science Foundation (PCM 8300476).

REFERENCES

1. Adamson, J. W., and C. Finch. Hemoglobin function, oxygen affinity, and erythropoietin. *Annu. Rev. Physiol.* 37: 351–369, 1975.
2. Ambersom, W. R., J. Flexner, and F. R. Steggerada. On the use of Ringer-Locke solutions containing hemoglobin as a substitute for normal blood in mammals. *J. Cell. Comp. Physiol.* 5: 359–364, 1934.
3. Armentrout, D., and F. L. Rose. Some physiological responses to anoxia in the great plains toad, *Bufo cognatus*. *Comp. Biochem. Physiol. A Comp. Physiol.* 39: 447–455, 1971.
4. Barcroft, J. *Features in the Architecture of Physiological Function.* London: Cambridge Univ. Press, 1934, p. 40.
5. Barnikol, W. K. R., and O. Burkhard. The fine structure of O_2 binding in animals: *Rana esculenta* (Abstract). *Pfluegers Arch.* 379: R27, 1979.
6. Barra, D. F., F. Bossa, J. Bonaventura, and M. Brunori. Hemoglobin components from trout (*Salmo irideus*): determination of the carboxyl and amino terminal sequences and their functional implications. *FEBS Lett.* 35: 151–154, 1973.
7. Bartels, H. Comparative physiology of oxygen transport in mammals. *Lancet* 2: 599–604, 1964.
8. Bartels, H. (editor). *Prenatal Respiration.* Amsterdam: North-Holland, 1970, p. 50. (Frontiers Biol. Ser. 17.)
9. Bartels, H., and C. Bauer. Relation between oxygen dissociation curve and tissue oxygenation. *Forsvarsmedicin* 5: 227–233, 1969.
10. Bartholomew, G. A. Body temperature and energy metabolism. In: *Animal Physiology: Principles and Adaptations* (4th ed.), edited by M. S. Gordon. New York: Macmillan, 1972, p. 298–368.
11. Bartlett, G. R. Phosphate compounds in red cells of reptiles, amphibians, and fish. *Comp. Biochem. Physiol. A Comp. Physiol.* 55: 211–214, 1976.
12. Battaglia, F. C., H. McGaughey, E. L. Makowski, and G. Meschia. Postnatal changes in oxygen affinity of sheep red cells: a dual role of diphosphoglyceric acid. *Am. J. Physiol.* 219: 217–221, 1970.
13. Bauer, C. On the respiratory function of haemoglobin. *Rev. Physiol. Biochem. Pharmacol.* 70: 1–31, 1974.
14. Bauer, C., and W. Jelkmann. Carbon dioxide governs the oxygen affinity of crocodile blood. *Nature Lond.* 269: 825–827, 1977.
15. Bauer, C., I. Ludwig, and M. Ludwig. Different effects of 2,3-diphosphoglycerate and adenosine triphosphate on the oxygen affinity of adult and foetal human haemoglobin. *Life Sci.* 7: 1339–1343, 1968.
16. Benesch, R., and R. E. Benesch. The chemistry of the Bohr effect. I. The reaction of *N*-ethylmaleimide with the oxygen-linked acid groups of hemoglobin. *J. Biol. Chem.* 236: 405–410, 1961.
17. Benesch, R., and R. E. Benesch. The effect of organic phosphates from the human erythrocyte on the allosteric properties of hemoglobin. *Biochem. Biophys. Res. Commun.* 26: 162–167, 1967.
18. Benesch, R., and R. E. Benesch. Homos and heteros among the hemos. *Science Wash. DC* 185: 905–908, 1974.
19. Benesch, R. E., R. Benesch, and C. I. Yu. The oxygenation of hemoglobin in the presence of 2,3-diphosphoglycerate. Effect of temperature, pH, ionic strength, and hemoglobin concentration. *Biochemistry* 8: 2567–2571, 1969.
20. Bennett, A. F., and J. Ruben. High altitude adaptation and anaerobiosis in sceloporine lizards. *Comp. Biochem. Physiol. A Comp. Physiol.* 50: 105–108, 1975.
21. Bonaventura, J., C. Bonaventura, and B. Sullivan. Hemoglobins and hemocyanins: comparative aspects of structure and function. *J. Exp. Zool.* 194: 155–174, 1975.
22. Bonaventura, J., and S. C. Wood. Respiratory pigments: overview. *Am. Zool.* 20: 5–6, 1980.
23. Bunn, H. F. Evolution of mammalian hemoglobin function. *Blood* 58: 189–197, 1981.
24. Burke, J. D. Vertebrate blood oxygen capacity and body weight. *Nature Lond.* 212: 46–48, 1966.
24a. Carey, F. H. Warm fish. In: *A Companion to Animal Physiology*, edited by C. R. Taylor, K. Johansen, and L. Bolis. Cambridge, UK: Cambridge Univ. Press, 1982, p. 216–223.
25. Chanutin, A., and R. R. Curnish. Factors influencing the electrophoretic patterns of red cell hemolysates analyzed in cacodylate buffers. *Arch. Biochem. Biophys.* 106: 433–439, 1964.
26. Chanutin, A., and R. R. Curnish. Effect of organic and inorganic phosphates on the oxygen equilibrium of human erythrocytes. *Arch. Biochem. Biophys.* 121: 96–102, 1967.
27. Coates, M. L. Hemoglobin function in the vertebrates: an evolutionary model. *J. Mol. Evol.* 6: 285–307, 1975.
28. Dawson, W. R., and T. L. Poulson. Oxygen capacity of lizard blood. *Am. Midl. Nat.* 68: 154–163, 1962.
29. Dejours, P. (editor). *Principles of Comparative Respiratory Physiology.* Amsterdam: North-Holland, 1975.
30. Dejours, P., W. F. Garey, and H. Rahn. Comparison of ventilatory and circulatory flow rates between animals in various physiological conditions. *Respir. Physiol.* 9: 108–117, 1970.
31. DeVenuto, F., H. I. Friedman, J. R. Neville, and C. C. Peck. Appraisal of hemoglobin solution as a blood substitute. *Surg. Gynecol. Obstet.* 149: 417–436, 1979.
32. Douglas, E. L., W. A. Friedl, and G. V. Pickwell. Fishes in oxygen-minimum zones: blood oxygenation characteristics. *Science Wash. DC* 191: 957–959, 1976.
33. Duhm, J. The effect of 2,3-DPG and other organic phosphates on the Donnan equilibrium and the oxygen affinity of human blood. In: *Oxygen Affinity of Hemoglobin and Red Cell Acid-Base Status*, edited by M. Rørth and P. Astrup. Copenhagen: Munksgaard, 1972, p. 583–598. (Alfred Benzon Symp., 4th, 1971.)
34. Eaton, J. W., T. D. Skelton, and E. Berger. Survival at extreme altitude: protective effect of increased hemoglobin-oxygen affinity. *Science Wash. DC* 183: 743–744, 1974.
35. Eaton, W. A. The relationship between coding sequences and

function in haemoglobin. *Nature Lond.* 284: 183–185, 1980.

36. EDDY, F. B. Oxygen uptake by rainbow trout blood. *Salmo gairdneri. J. Fish Biol.* 10: 87–90, 1977.
37. EDSALL, J. T. Hemoglobin and the origins of the concept of allosterism. *Federation Proc.* 39: 226–235, 1980.
38. ELSE, P. L., AND A. J. HULBERT. Comparison of the "mammal machine" and the "reptile machine": energy production. *Am. J. Physiol.* 240 (*Regulatory Integrative Comp. Physiol.* 9): R3–R9, 1981.
39. FLORES, G., AND E. FRIEDEN. Induction and survival of hemoglobin-less and erythrocyte-less tadpoles and young bullfrogs. *Science Wash. DC* 159: 101–103, 1968.
40. FRANS, A., Z. TUREK, H. YOKOTA, AND F. KREUZER. Effect of variations in blood hydrogen ion concentration on pulmonary gas exchange of artificially ventilated dogs. *Pfluegers Arch.* 380: 35–39, 1979.
41. GAHLENBECK, H., AND H. BARTELS. Temperaturadaptation der Sauerstoffaffinitat des Blutes von *Rana esculenta* L. *Z. Vgl. Physiol.* 59: 232–240, 1968.

41a. GAHLENBECK, H., AND H. BARTELS. Blood gas transport properties in gill and lung forms of the axolotl (*Ambystoma mexicanum*). *Respir. Physiol.* 9: 175–182, 1970.

42. GARBY, L., AND J. H. MELDON (editors). *The Respiratory Functions of Blood.* New York: Plenum, 1977, p. 282.

42a. GERLACH, E., AND J. DUHM. 2,3-DPG metabolism of red cells: regulation and adaptive changes during hypoxia. In: *Oxygen Affinity of Hemoglobin and Red Cell Acid-Base Status*, edited by M. Rørth and P. Astrup. Copenhagen: Munksgaard, 1972, p. 552–569. (Alfred Benzon Symp., 4th, 1971.)

43. GILBERT, W. Why genes in pieces? *Nature Lond.* 271: 501, 1978.
44. GILLEN, R. G., AND A. RIGGS. The haemoglobins of a freshwater teleost, *Cichlasoma cyanoguttatum* (Baird and Girard). I. The effects of phosphorylated organic compounds upon the oxygen equilibria. *Comp. Biochem. Physiol. B Comp. Biochem.* 38: 585–595, 1971.
45. GONIAKOWSKA, L. The respiration of erythrocytes of some amphibia in vitro. *Bull. Acad. Pol. Sci. Ser. Sci. Biol.* 18: 793–797, 1970.
46. GOODMAN, M. G., W. MOORE, AND G. MATSUDA. Darwinian evolution in the genealogy of haemoglobin. *Nature Lond.* 253: 603–608, 1975.
47. GRATZER, W. B., AND A. C. ALLISON. Multiple haemoglobins. *Biol. Rev. Camb. Philos. Soc.* 35: 459–503, 1960.
48. GREENWALD, I. A new type of phosphoric acid compound isolated from blood with some remarks on the effect of substitution on the notation of *l*-glyceric acid. *J. Biol. Chem.* 63: 339–349, 1925.
49. GRIGG, G. Temperature-induced changes in the oxygen equilibrium curve of the blood of the brown bullhead, *Ictalurus nebulosus. Comp. Biochem. Physiol.* 29: 1203–1223, 1969.
50. GULLIVER, G. On red blood corpuscles. *Proc. Zool. Soc. Lond.* p. 474–495, 1875.
51. HAAB, P. E., J. PIIPER, AND H. RAHN. Simple method for rapid determination of an O_2 dissociation curve of the blood. *J. Appl. Physiol.* 15: 1148–1149, 1960.
52. HANSEN, V. K., AND K. G. WINGSTRAND. Further studies on the non-nucleated erythrocytes of *Maurolicus mulleri*, and comparison with the red cells of related fishes. *Dana-Rep. Carlsberg Found.* 54: 3–14, 1960.
53. HASHIMOTO, K., Y. YAMAGUCHI, AND F. MATSURA. Comparative studies on the two hemoglobins of salmon. IV. Oxygen dissociation curve. *Bull. Jpn. Soc. Sci. Fish.* 26: 827–830, 1960.

53a. HEISLER, N. Comparative aspects of acid-base regulation. In: *Acid-Base Regulation in Animals*, edited by N. Heisler. Amsterdam: Elsevier, in press.

54. HEMMINGSEN, A. M. Energy metabolism as related to body size and respiratory surfaces and its evolution. *Rep. Steno. Mem. Hosp. Nord. Insulinlab.* 9: 1–110, 1960.
55. HEMMINGSEN, E. A., AND E. L. DOUGLAS. Respiratory characteristics of the haemoglobin-free fish. *Chaenocephalus aceratus. Comp. Biochem. Physiol.* 33: 733–744, 1970.
56. HOCHACHKA, P. W., AND G. N. SOMERO. *Strategies of Biochemical Adaptation.* Philadelphia, PA: Saunders, 1973, p. 841–842.
57. HOCK, R. J. Animals in high altitudes: reptiles and amphibians. In: *Handbook of Physiology. Adaptation to the Environment*, edited by D. B. Dill and E. F. Adolph. Washington, DC: Am. Physiol. Soc., 1964, sect. 4, chapt. 53, p. 841–842.
58. HOLLE, J. P., M. MEYER, AND P. SCHEID. Oxygen affinity of duck blood determined by in vivo and in vitro technique. *Respir. Physiol.* 29: 355–361, 1977.
59. HOUSTON, A. H., AND D. CYR. Thermoacclimatory variation in the haemoglobin systems of goldfish. (*Carassius auratus*) and rainbow trout (*Salmo gairdneri*). *J. Exp. Biol.* 61: 455–461, 1974.
60. HOYT, R. W. Respiratory Function in Tiger Salamanders: Effects of Metamorphosis and Hypoxia. Albuquerque: Univ. of New Mexico, 1981. PhD Thesis.
61. HUTCHISON, V. H., H. B. HAINES, AND G. ENGBRETSON. Aquatic life at high altitude: respiratory adaptations in the Lake Titicaca frog, *Telmatobius culeus. Respir. Physiol.* 27: 115–129, 1976.
62. JACKSON, D. C., AND K. SCHMIDT-NIELSEN. Heat production during diving in the fresh water turtle, *Pseudemys scripta. J. Cell. Physiol.* 67: 225–231, 1966.
63. JOHANSEN, K. Cardiovascular support of metabolic functions in vertebrates. In: *Lung Biology in Health and Disease. Evolution of Respiratory Processes: A Comparative Approach*, edited by S. C. Wood and C. Lenfant. New York: Dekker, 1979, vol. 13, p. 107–192.
64. JOHANSEN, K., AND C. LENFANT. A comparative approach to the adaptability of O_2-Hb affinity. In: *Oxygen Affinity of Hemoglobin and Red Cell Acid-Base Status*, edited by M. Rørth and P. Astrup. Copenhagen: Munksgaard, 1972, p. 750–780. (Alfred Benzon Symp., 4th, 1971.)
65. JOHANSEN, K., G. LYKKEBOE, S. KORNERUP, AND G. M. O. MALOIY. Temperature insensitive O_2 binding in blood of the tree frog, *Chiromantis petersi. J. Comp. Physiol.* 136: 71–76, 1980.
66. JOHANSEN, K., G. LYKKEBOE, R. E. WEBER, AND G. M. O. MALOIY. Respiratory properties of blood in awake and estivating lungfish, *Protopterus amphibius. Respir. Physiol.* 27: 335–345, 1976.
67. JOHANSEN, K., AND R. E. WEBER. On the adaptability of haemoglobin function to environmental conditions. In: *Perspectives in Experimental Biology. Zoology and Botany*, edited by P. Spencer Davis and N. Sunderland. New York: Pergamon, 1976, vol. 1, p. 219–234.
69. JONES, D. R. Oxygen consumption and heart rate of several species of anurans and amphibians during submergence. *Comp. Biochem. Physiol.* 20: 691–707, 1967.
70. JONES, D. R. Theoretical analysis of factors which may limit the maximum oxygen uptake of fish: the oxygen cost of the cardiac and branchial pumps. *J. Theor. Biol.* 32: 341–349, 1971.
71. KLOTZ, I. M., AND T. A. KLOTZ. Oxygen carrying proteins: a comparison of the oxygenation reaction in hemocyanin with that in hemoglobin. *Science Wash. DC* 121: 477–480, 1955.
72. KROGH, A. *Comparative Physiology of Respiratory Mechanisms.* Philadelphia: Univ. of Pennsylvania Press, 1941.
73. KROGH, A., AND I. LEITCH. The respiratory functions of the blood in fishes. *J. Physiol. Lond.* 52: 288–297, 1919.
74. LAHIRI, S. Blood oxygen affinity and alveolar ventilation in relation to body weight in mammals. *Am. J. Physiol.* 229: 529–536, 1975.
75. LEFTWICH, F. B., AND J. D. BURKE. Blood oxygen capacity in Ranid frogs. *Am. Midl. Nat.* 72: 241–248, 1964.
76. LENFANT, C., AND C. AUCUTT. Oxygen uptake and change in carbon dioxide tension in human blood stored at 37 C. *J. Appl. Physiol.* 20: 503–508, 1965.
77. LENFANT, C., AND K. JOHANSEN. Respiratory adaptations in selected amphibians. *Respir. Physiol.* 2: 247–260, 1967.

78. Lenfant, C., K. Johansen, and G. C. Grigg. Respiratory properties of blood and pattern of gas exchange in the lungfish *Neoceratodus forsteri. Respir. Physiol.* 2: 1–21, 1966.
78a. Lenfant, C., K. Johansen, and D. Hanson. Bimodal gas exchange and ventilation-perfusion relationship in lower vertebrates. *Federation Proc.* 29: 1124–1129, 1970.
79. Lenfant, C., J. Torrance, E. English, C. A. Finch, C. Reynafarje, C. Ramos, and J. Faura. Effect of altitude on oxygen finding by hemoglobin and on organic phosphate levels. *J. Clin. Invest.* 47: 2652–2656, 1968.
80. Lutz, P. L., I. S. Longmuir, J. V. Tuttle, and K. Schmidt-Nielsen. Dissociation curve of bird blood and effect of red cell oxygen consumption. *Respir. Physiol.* 17: 269–275, 1973.
81. Lykkeboe, G., and R. E. Weber. Changes in the respiratory properties of the blood in the carp, *Cyprinus carpio*, induced by diurnal variation in ambient oxygen tension. *J. Comp. Physiol.* 128: 117–125, 1978.
82. MacFarlane, H. T., and A. H. T. Robb-Smith (editors). *Functions of the Blood.* New York: Academic, 1961.
83. Maginniss, L. A., Y. K. Song, and R. B. Reeves. Oxygen equilibria of ectotherm blood containing multiple hemoglobins. *Respir. Physiol.* 42: 329–343, 1980.
84. McCutcheon, F. J., and F. G. Hall. Hemoglobin in the amphibia. *J. Cell Comp. Physiol.* 9: 191–197, 1937.
84a. Morpurgo, G., P. A. Battaglia, and T. Leggio. Negative Bohr effect in newt haemolysates and its regulation. *Nature Lond.* 225: 76–77, 1970.
85. Morse, M. D., D. E. Cassals, and M. Holder. The position of the oxygen dissociation curve of the blood in cyanotic congenital heart disease. *J. Clin. Invest.* 29: 1098–1103, 1950.
86. Parer, J. T. Oxygen transport in human subjects with hemoglobin variants having altered oxygen affinity. *Respir. Physiol.* 9: 43–49, 1970.
87. Perutz, M. F. Stereochemistry of cooperative effects in haemoglobin. *Nature Lond.* 228: 726–739, 1970.
88. Perutz, M. F. Nature of haem-haem interaction. *Nature Lond.* 237: 495–499, 1970.
89. Pough, F. H. The effect of temperature on oxygen capacity of reptile blood. *Physiol. Zool.* 49: 141–151, 1976.
90. Pough, F. H. Ontogenetic change in molecular and functional properties of blood of garter snakes, *Thamnophis sirtalis. J. Exp. Zool.* 201: 47–55, 1977.
91. Powers, D. A. Molecular ecology of teleost fish hemoglobins: strategies for adaptation to changing environments. *Am. Zool.* 20: 139–162, 1980.
92. Powers, D. A., J. P. Martin, R. L. Garlick, and H. J. Fyhn. The effect of temperature on the oxygen equilibrium of fish haemoglobin in relation to environmental thermal variability. *Comp. Biochem. Physiol. A Comp. Physiol.* 62: 82–94, 1979.
93. Prothero, J. W. Maximal oxygen consumption in various animals and plants. *Comp. Biochem. Physiol. A Comp. Physiol.* 64: 463–466, 1979.
94. Rahn, H. Evolution of the gas transport system in vertebrates. *Proc. R. Soc. Med.* 59: 493–494, 1966.
95. Rappoport, S., and G. M. Guest. Distribution of acid-soluble phosphorus in the blood cells of various vertebrates. *J. Biol. Chem.* 138: 269–282, 1941.
96. Reeves, R. B., and H. Rahn. Patterns in vertebrate acid-base regulation. In: *Lung Biology in Health and Disease. Evolution of Respiratory Processes: A Comparative Approach*, edited by S. C. Wood and C. Lenfant. New York: Dekker, 1979, vol. 13, p. 225–252.
97. Riggs, A. The nature and significance of the Bohr effect in mammalian hemoglobin. *J. Gen. Physiol.* 4: 737–752, 1960.
98. Riggs, A. Factors in the evolution of hemoglobin function. *Federation Proc.* 35: 2115–2118, 1976.
99. Root, R. W. The respiratory function of blood of marine fishes. *Biol. Bull. Woods Hole* 61: 427–456, 1931.
100. Root, R. W., L. Irving, and E. C. Black. The effect of hemolysis upon the combination of oxygen with the blood of some marine fishes. *J. Cell. Comp. Physiol.* 13: 303–313, 1939.
101. Rossoff, L., R. Zeldin, E. Hew, and A. Aberman. Changes in blood P_{50}. Effects on oxygen delivery when arterial hypoxemia is due to shunting. *Chest* 77: 142–146, 1980.
102. Scheid, P., and T. Kawashiro. Metabolic changes in avian blood and their effects on determination of blood gases and pH. *Respir. Physiol.* 23: 291–300, 1975.
103. Schmidt-Nielsen, K. *Animal Physiology.* Cambridge, UK: Cambridge Univ. Press, 1978.
104. Schmidt-Nielsen, K., and J. L. Larimer. Oxygen dissociation curves of mammalian blood in relation to body size. *Am. J. Physiol.* 195: 424–428, 1958.
105. Schmidt-Nielsen, K., and C. R. Taylor. Red blood cells: why or why not? *Science Wash. DC* 162: 274–275, 1968.
106. Schweiger, H. G. Pathways of metabolism in nucleate and anucleate erythrocytes. *Int. Rev. Cytol.* 13: 135–201, 1962.
107. Scott, A. F., H. F. Bunn, and A. H. Brush. Functional aspects of hemoglobin evolution in the mammals. *J. Mol. Evol.* 8: 311–316, 1976.
108. Shappell, S. D., and C. Lenfant. Physiological role of the oxyhemoglobin dissociation curve. In: *The Red Blood Cell* (2nd ed.), edited by D. M. Surgenor. New York: Academic, 1974, p. 842–873.
108a. Shoubridge, E. A., and P. W. Hochachka. Ethanol: novel end product of vertebrate anaerobic metabolism. *Science Wash. DC* 209: 308–309, 1980.
109. Snyder, G. K. Erythrocyte evolution: the significance of the Fahraeus-Lindqvist phenomenon. *Respir. Physiol.* 19: 271–278, 1973.
110. Snyder, G. K. Blood corpuscles and blood hemoglobins: a possible example of coevolution. *Science Wash. DC* 195: 412–413, 1977.
111. Soivio, A., M. Nikinmaa, and K. Westman. The blood oxygen binding properties of hypoxic *Salmo gairdneri. J. Comp. Physiol.* 136: 83–87, 1980.
112. Stamatoyannopoulos, G., A. J. Bellingham, and C. Lenfant. Abnormal hemoglobins with high and low oxygen affinity. *Annu. Rev. Med.* 22: 221–234, 1971.
113. Sullivan, B., and A. Riggs. Haemoglobin: reversal of oxidation and polymerization in turtle red cells. *Nature Lond.* 204: 1098–1099, 1964.
113a. Taketa, F., and M. A. Nickerson. Hemoglobin of the aquatic salamander, *Cryptobranchus. Comp. Biochem. Physiol. A Comp. Physiol.* 46: 583–591, 1973.
114. Toews, D., and D. MacIntyre. Blood respiratory properties of a viviparous amphibian. *Nature Lond.* 266: 464–465, 1977.
115. Tracy, C. R. Minimum size of mammalian homeotherms: role of the thermal environment. *Science Wash. DC* 198: 1034–1035, 1977.
116. Turek, Z., and F. Kreuzer. Effects of shifts of the O_2 dissociation curve upon alveolar-arterial O_2 gradients in computer models of the lung with ventilation-perfusion mismatching. *Respir. Physiol.* 45: 133–139, 1972.
116a. Van Den Thillart, G. Adaptations of fish energy metabolism to hypoxia and anoxia. *Mol. Physiol.* 2: 49–61, 1982.
117. Vinegar, A., and S. D. Hillyard. The effects of altitude on oxygen-binding parameters of the blood of the iguanid lizards, *Sceloporus jarrovi* and *Sceloporus occidentalis. Comp. Biochem. Physiol. A Comp. Physiol.* 43: 317–320, 1972.
118. Weathers, W. W., and J. J. McGrath. Acclimation to simulated altitude in the lizard, *Dipsosaurus dorsalis. Comp. Biochem. Physiol. A Comp. Physiol.* 42: 263–268, 1977.
119. Weber, R. E., S. C. Wood, and J. P. Lomholt. Temperature acclimation and oxygen binding properties of blood and multiple haemoglobins of rainbow trout. *J. Exp. Biol.* 65: 333–345, 1976.
120. White, F. N., and G. Ross. Circulatory changes during experimental diving in the turtle. *Am. J. Physiol.* 211: 15–18, 1966.
121. Wood, S. C. Effect of metamorphosis on blood respiratory properties and erythrocyte adenosine triphosphate level of the

salamander, *Dicamptodon ensatus. Respir. Physiol.* 12: 53–65, 1971.
122. WOOD, S. C. Adaptation of red blood cell function to hypoxia and temperature in ectothermic vertebrates. *Am. Zool.* 20: 163–172, 1980.
123. WOOD, S. C. Effect of O_2 affinity on arterial P_{O_2} in animals with central vascular shunts. *J. Appl. Physiol.* 53: 1360–1364, 1982.
124. WOOD, S. C. Cardiovascular shunts and oxygen transport in lower vertebrates. *Am. J. Physiol.* 247 (*Regulatory Integrative Comp. Physiol.* 16): R3–R14, 1984.
125. WOOD, S. C., J. W. HICKS, AND R. K. DUPRE. Hypoxic reptiles: hearts, heat, and hemoglobin. *Am. Zool.* In press.
126. WOOD, S. C., AND K. JOHANSEN. Adaptation to hypoxia by increased HbO_2 affinity and decreased red cell ATP concentration. *Nature New Biol.* 237: 278–279, 1972.
127. WOOD, S. C., K. JOHANSEN, AND R. E. WEBER. Haemoglobin in the coelacanth. *Nature Lond.* 239: 283–285, 1972.
128. WOOD, S. C., AND C. LENFANT. Respiration: mechanics, control, and gas exchange. In: *Biology of the Reptilia*, edited by C. Gans and W. R. Dawson. New York: Academic, 1976, vol. 5, p. 225–274.
129. WOOD, S. C., AND C. LENFANT. Oxygen transport and oxygen delivery. In: *Lung Biology in Health and Disease. Evolution of Respiratory Processes: A Comparative Approach*, edited by S. C. Wood and C. Lenfant. New York: Dekker, 1979, vol. 13, p. 193–223.
130. WOODSON, R. D. Physiological significance of oxygen dissociation curve shifts. *Crit. Care Med.* 7: 368–373, 1979.
131. ZAAIJER, J. P., AND P. WOLVEKAMP. Some experiments on the hemoglobin oxygen affinity in the blood of the ramshorn (*Planorbis corneus* L.). *Acta Physiol. Pharmacol. Neerl.* 7: 56–77, 1958.

CHAPTER 9

Blood oxygen transport

ROSEMARIE BAUMANN
HEINZ BARTELS
Zentrum Physiologie, Medizinische Hochschule Hannover, Hannover, Federal Republic of Germany

CHRISTIAN BAUER
Institut für Physiologie, Universität Regensburg, Regensburg, Federal Republic of Germany

CHAPTER CONTENTS

ONE OF THE MAJOR FUNCTIONS of blood in vertebrates is the transport of O_2. The physical solubility of O_2 in aqueous media is low, however. Therefore the efficiency of gas transport relies on the presence of specific O_2 carriers; one of the most widely distributed is hemoglobin (Hb), the O_2 transport protein of all vertebrates, which is present inside the red blood cell (RBC).

An often-asked question is why vertebrates transport Hb inside the RBC. There are two major functional aspects: *1*) a high O_2-carrying capacity is desirable and *2*) O_2 uptake and release must occur at O_2 pressures compatible with environmental and physiological conditions inside the organism, respectively. A high O_2-carrying capacity requires the presence of high concentrations of Hb in the circulation, which in many mammals is ~150 g/liter blood, carrying a maximum of 200 ml O_2/liter blood. Freely circulating Hb would result in an unduly high oncotic pressure, whereas an Hb of higher molecular weight present at the same concentration would drastically increase viscosity. The second aspect requires that the functional properties of Hb, i.e., its O_2 affinity, must be adaptable. Vertebrate Hb is largely regulated by constituents of the RBC that are subject to metabolic control.

In this chapter we discuss in greater detail the properties of Hb with respect to its O_2 transport function and regulation. The scope of the article is limited to a discussion of predominantly mammalian Hb. Extensive reviews of human Hb structure and function are found in references 15, 16, and 64.

ANATOMY OF THE HEMOGLOBIN MOLECULE

Hemoglobin is a tetrameric protein (mol wt ~64,500) due to combination of two pairs of nonidentical chains ($\alpha_2\beta_2$): the α-chain (141 amino acids) and the β-chain (146 amino acids). Heme, the prosthetic O_2-binding group, is attached to each globin chain. Its center has a bivalent iron atom that reversibly binds O_2. Analysis of the Hb pattern of many species shows that multiple forms are present very

TABLE 1. *Hemoglobin Pattern of Adult Human Blood*

Hemoglobin Type	Molecular Structure	Percentage of Total
Hb A	$\alpha_2\beta_2$	90
Hb A_2	$\alpha_2\delta_2$	2.5
Hb F	$\alpha_2\gamma_2$	0.5
Hb A_1	$\alpha_2\beta_2{}^{NH_2\text{-}R}$	1.6
Hb A_{1b}	$\alpha_2\beta_2{}^{NH_2\text{-}R}$	0.8
Hb A_{1c}	$\alpha_2\beta_2{}^{NH_2\text{-glucosamine}}$	4

often; likewise, Hb polymorphism due to the presence of alleles is often found.

In addition to genetic heterogeneity of the Hb pattern (Table 1), there are possible posttranslational modifications of the Hb, e.g., by nonenzymatic glycosylation as found in the human Hb variants Hb A_{1a}, Hb A_{1b}, and Hb A_{1c} or by acetylation (cf. ref. 64). Because of the presence of multiple forms of Hb, or Hb polymorphism, the functional properties assessed for individual species in whole blood often represent the sum of the properties of various Hb species.

It has been proposed that Hb multiplicity might help to achieve the very high solubility necessary for Hb inside the RBCs (cf. ref. 208). In most cases the intracellular Hb concentration ranges between 5 and 6 mmol/liter RBCs. The major reason for the high solubility of Hb is that hydrophobic side chains are oriented toward the interior of the molecule, whereas charged residues are oriented toward the surface. Because of the large volume of the Hb molecule the intermolecular distances shorten considerably under physiological conditions, thus increasing the chance for possible intramolecular interactions. Riggs (208) has suggested that the high solubility probably imposes evolutionary constraints on the development of the Hb molecule. The amino acid sequence (primary structure) of the α- and β-chains has been established for several types of vertebrate Hb, which allows the construction of phylogenetic trees (76, 106). The comparison of the sequence data indicates that the ancestral Hb was a monomer that diverged from myoglobin (Mb) 450–500 million years ago. Subsequent gene duplication (~400 million years ago) established the β-chain and the possibility for cooperative heterotetramers. Goodman et al. (106) concluded that after this event substitutions leading to allosteric functions occurred at an accelerated rate, which they interpreted as an indication that positive selection has played a dominant role in the evolution of Hb function (106).

The three-dimensional structure of crystalline deoxygenated Hb and carboxyhemoglobin (HbCO) has been clarified through X-ray structural analysis by Baldwin (15), Fermi (90), Muirhead and Greer (169), and Perutz et al. (193). Whereas the structure of deoxygenated Hb could be determined directly, it has not yet been possible to determine the structure of oxyhemoglobin (HbO_2) because of the rapid formation of methemoglobin (MetHb). However, to all intents the HbCO structure that has been elucidated is isomorphous with the structure of HbO_2.

All globin chains show a high degree (~80%) of α-helix content. The helical segments are denoted starting from the α-amino end with the letters A to H. Nonhelical segments are characterized through the adjoining helical segments, e.g., FG. Despite large differences in the primary structure of the α- and β-chains, the tertiary structures, i.e., the spatial folding of the α- and β-chains, show a large degree of similarity.

Between the α- and β-chains there are two main contact regions, the $\alpha_1\beta_1$ and the $\alpha_1\beta_2$. The $\alpha_1\beta_2$-contact region shows large structural changes with ligand binding (188), and substitutions in this region have been shown to lead in most cases to a large reduction of cooperativity of O_2 binding (191).

The tertiary and the quaternary structure (i.e., the relative alignment of the chains toward each other) are largely the result of a multitude of hydrophobic interactions between the chains. In addition there are a number of hydrogen bonds that play a smaller but not negligible role (90).

The heme group, which consists of a protoporphyrin ring system, is in a hydrophobic pocket between the helical segments F and G in the α- and β-chains, respectively. The hydrophobic environment apparently protects the iron atom from oxidation, which rapidly occurs when the heme group is exposed to a polar medium. Under physiological conditions there is a continuous autoxidation of the bivalent iron; however, the MetHb reductase systems present in the RBC instantaneously reduce the iron. Because of this the MetHb content of the RBC is <1%.

Between the heme group and the globin chain are ~80 contacts (188), most of them noncovalent. The iron atom is covalently bound to the four nitrogen atoms of the protoporphyrin ring with one coordination site toward FG8 His of the corresponding globin chain. The sixth coordination site is free for the binding of other ligands such as H_2O or O_2. With ligand binding the most pronounced changes occur in the FG nonhelical part of each chain, which is in the immediate vicinity of the heme group.

MOLECULAR BASIS FOR COOPERATIVE OXYGEN BINDING

The most important step in the evolution of vertebrate Hb was probably the acquisition of *cooperative ligand binding*; this term means that the ligand affinity of a protein depends on the degree of saturation with ligand.

Hemoglobin is a protein with positive cooperativity, hence the affinity for O_2 increases with increasing O_2 saturation, which is reflected in the sigmoid shape of the O_2 equilibrium curve (Fig. 1), which was first

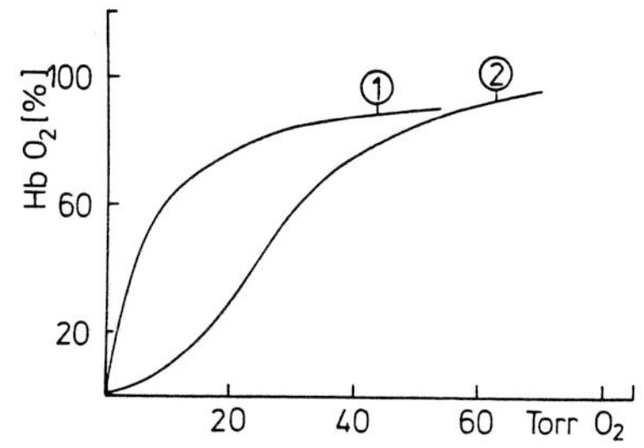

FIG. 1. Oxygen-binding curves of human Mb (*1*) and Hb (*2*) under physiological conditions (whole blood, plasma pH = 7.4, 37°C).

determined by Bohr (52). The physiological benefit of this type of binding is that in the steep part of the curve it allows large changes in O_2 saturation with only small changes in O_2 pressure. Cooperativity requires that a protein can assume different conformational states, which are characterized by different affinities for the ligand.

The fact that different structures have been demonstrated for crystalline liganded Hb and deoxygenated Hb (188) has created the possibility to look for structural characteristics that correspond to specific functional properties of the Hb molecule. However, it should be clear that deoxygenated Hb and HbCO, as representatives of the ligand form, represent only two of several possible species, because there is no information available about the dynamics of the structural changes in the protein during ligand binding. The differences observed between HbO_2 and deoxygenated Hb in crystalline conformation are also found in solution. These include changes in the reactivity of the SH groups of β93 Cys (206) and differences in the dimer-tetramer dissociation constants (142, 143) and in the UV spectrum (58).

The analysis of the cooperativity of Hb is often carried out in terms of the allosteric model of Monod, Wyman, and Changeux [MWC model (166)]. The allosteric protein is composed of identical subunits that are arranged symmetrically and can exist in two different quaternary structures. The T state (T for tense, indicating quaternary constraints) has a low affinity for ligands, and the R state (R for relaxed) has a high affinity. Deoxygenated Hb corresponds to the T state and liganded Hb to the R state. The binding of ligand shifts the conformational equilibrium, which in the absence of ligand favors the T state, progressively toward the R state with corresponding changes in affinity. Allosteric effector molecules are bound preferentially to one conformation; hence in their presence the conformational equilibrium is shifted and with it the ligand affinity.

It has been shown that the O_2 affinity of fully oxygenated Hb is even slightly higher than that of the isolated chains (130), which as monomers cannot be subjected to quaternary constraints. A main effort has been directed toward explaining the low affinity of deoxygenated Hb. Perutz (188, 189) suggested that the quaternary deoxystructure imposes strains on the heme, which oppose the change in spin state of the iron atom that occurs on ligand binding. However, a structural reason for this was not found.

Recent work of Gelin and Karplus (99) suggests that the low affinity of deoxygenated Hb is caused by steric repulsion between the proximal F8 His and the heme porphyrin, which arises when the ligand tries to bind to the heme in deoxygenated Hb. In the absence of ligand the deoxygenated heme is not subject to strain (16, 99). The strain cannot be relaxed unless there is a change in the relative position of the F helix toward the heme. Thus the liganded quaternary deoxystructure is less stable, which promotes the transition toward the liganded quaternary structure, allowing a subsequent readjustment of the F helix and F8 His, thereby removing the strain on the heme group. A detailed description of these structural events is given by Baldwin and Chothia (16).

Because the distance between the heme groups is large (~30 Å), the structural perturbation induced on ligand binding to deoxygenated Hb cannot be directly transmitted. Compared with the distance between the heme groups, the distance from the heme toward the next $\alpha_1\beta_2$-intersubunit contact region is ~10–12 Å. The main impact of the stereochemical changes of the heme group that occur on ligand binding is thus transmitted from the heme group to the $\alpha_1\beta_2$-intersubunit contact regions, thereby inducing changes in the packaging of the chains relative to each other (16), which in turn alter the geometry of the heme environment in the neighboring subunit and thus its O_2 affinity.

ALLOSTERIC MODIFICATION OF OXYGEN BINDING

The functional properties of most Hb as determined under physiological conditions are largely dependent on the presence of allosteric heterotropic molecules. For mammalian Hb and most other Hb of higher vertebrates the unifying feature of all known physiological effector molecules is their capacity to reduce the O_2 affinity of the Hb. Irrespective of the detailed molecular mechanism the basis for this behavior is that all allosteric effectors are bound preferentially to deoxygenated Hb, thereby shifting the conformational equilibrium in favor of the low-affinity form.

There is no investigated mammalian Hb that has an intrinsic O_2 affinity that does not need modulation by effectors for adaptation to physiological conditions. The major regulators of O_2 affinity are protons (which cause the pH dependence of O_2 binding known as the Bohr effect), organic phosphates, CO_2, and Cl^-. The following sections describe in greater detail the molecular mechanism of their action.

Protons

The pH dependence of Hb-O_2 affinity was first observed by Bohr et al. (53), who found that with increasing partial pressure of CO_2 (P_{CO_2}) the O_2 affinity decreased. For human Hb this decrease is observed between pH 6 and 9, the "alkaline Bohr effect." Below pH 6 one finds an increase of the O_2 affinity with increasing proton concentration, the "acid Bohr effect."

The physiological importance of the Bohr effect is twofold. *1*) The O_2-linked proton release results in an improved buffer capacity of deoxygenated Hb for CO_2 uptake in the systemic capillaries [see the chapter by Klocke in this *Handbook*; (72)]. *2*) The pH dependence of the O_2 affinity helps to facilitate O_2 release to the tissue because the pH of blood passing through the capillaries drops continuously due to uptake of CO_2 and other acids. Thus the Bohr effect is particularly important under conditions of heavy muscular exercise (236). During development the Bohr effect augments the O_2 transfer from maternal to fetal blood in placentas, because the maternal blood is continuously acidified during passage through the placenta, whereas the reverse is true for fetal blood (18).

On a molecular level the Bohr effect is caused by the O_2-linked release or uptake of protons from the Hb molecule. Whereas it was long thought that the Bohr effect presents primarily an intrinsic phenomenon, i.e., the Bohr protons come from ionizable groups in the Hb molecule that alter their pK with changes in quaternary or tertiary structure, it is now clear that a major part of the Bohr effect of Hb is caused through the binding of allosteric effectors, notably Cl^- and organic phosphates.

A thermodynamic linkage of the pH-induced changes in affinity and the number of protons that are released with binding of O_2 was first developed by Wyman (256)

$$\left|\frac{\Delta \log P_{O_2}}{\Delta pH}\right| S_{O_2} = \left|\frac{\Delta H^+}{\Delta HbO_2}\right| pH$$

where P_{O_2} is the partial pressure of O_2 and S_{O_2} is O_2 saturation. This relationship allows the calculation of the release of protons from the change in O_2 affinity with pH. The term ($\Delta \log P_{O_2}$)/ΔpH is conventionally referred to as the Bohr coefficient and $\Delta H^+/\Delta HbO_2$ as the Haldane coefficient. However, the relationship holds only under certain conditions: *1*) the activity of all other allosteric effectors except protons remains constant during ligand binding and *2*) the cooperativity of O_2 binding is pH independent.

The application of Wyman's formula implies a uniform change with pH of the O_2 equilibrium over the entire saturation range and a noncooperative binding of protons. Kinetic investigations by Antonini et al. (5) and Gray (107) demonstrated a linearity of O_2 binding and proton release in human Hb solutions that contained only neutral salts, and differential titration studies carried out under similar experimental conditions showed that there was a sufficient agreement between the Bohr and Haldane coefficients, proving the validity of Wyman's concept.

An important consequence of the results was that proton release occurs as a consequence of ligand-induced changes in the tertiary structure and that the contribution of the α- and β-chains must be more or less identical. However, Imai and Yonetani (132) showed a nonuniform change of the equilibrium constants K_1 to K_4. Although they observed a pH invariance for K_4 and a different pH dependence for K_1 to K_3 in each case, they still obtained a good agreement between the Haldane and Bohr coefficients. This result is to be expected when the intermediary structures HbO_2 to $Hb(O_2)_3$ occur only in small stationary concentrations in comparison with Hb and $Hb(O_2)_4$, respectively. Under these conditions the population of $Hb(O_2)_4$ increases proportionally to the O_2 saturation and a linear relationship between proton release and ligand binding is found.

Furthermore binding of anions such as Cl^- or 2,3-diphosphoglycerate (2,3-DPG) also leads to a proton uptake (13, 77, 210, 245). This makes it difficult in a given experimental situation, when several types of allosteric effectors are present, to decide whether the nonlinearity of proton release or uptake is caused by interactions of Hb with anions or represents a property of the intrinsic Bohr effect. Irrespective of all models, a linear relationship between proton binding and O_2 release during gas exchange is physiologically desirable, because an effective coupling of O_2 and CO_2 transport by Hb is achieved only in this way.

BINDING SITES FOR BOHR PROTONS. The elucidation of the residues participating in the alkaline Bohr effect has been completed for human Hb only recently. Crystallographic studies showed that in deoxygenated Hb the COOH-terminal histidine is linked with a salt bridge to the COOH group of β94 Asp (188). This salt bridge between the imidazole group of β146 His and the COOH group of β94 Asp raises the pK of the imidazole group. This was shown by Kilmartin et al. (145), who studied the COOH-terminal histidine with nuclear magnetic resonance (NMR) titration and found that the pK of the imidazole group was 7.2 in HbCO and 8.1 in deoxygenated Hb. Thus this group causes ~50% of the alkaline Bohr effect of human Hb at physiological pH. From NMR titration studies, α122 His, α20 His, and α89 His have also been suggested as intrinsic Bohr groups (178, 182), but these results are not unequivocally accepted.

The remaining part of the Bohr effect (in the absence of organic phosphates) is due to O_2-linked binding of Cl^-. A direct effect of Cl^- on the O_2-linked proton release of Hb was first demonstrated by Rollema et al. (210). About 25% of the Bohr effect, measured at a physiological Cl^- concentration of 0.1 mol, has to be attributed to O_2-linked Cl^- binding.

Much work has been directed toward the identification of the binding sites for inorganic anions. Results of these studies have led to the identification of the NH_2-terminal α-amino group of the α-chain as the principal site responsible for the contribution of O_2-linked Cl^- binding to the Bohr effect (8, 175, 181). Arnone et al. (8) found that at the NH_2-terminal of the α-chain there are 2–3 potential anion-binding sites. Van Beek et al. (244, 245) determined the pK value for the α-chain NH_2-terminal α-amino group at different Cl^- concentrations. Whereas the pK value of the β-chain NH_2-terminal α-amino group is independent of the Cl^- concentration, there is a marked increase of the pK of the NH_2-terminal α-amino group of the deoxy α-chain from 7.4 to 8.0 when the Cl^- concentration is raised from 10 to 100 mM. These results are in agreement with the studies of O'Donnell et al. (181), who titrated specifically carbamylated Hb and found that blockage of the α-chain NH_2-terminal abolished the effect of Cl^- in the Bohr effect. Note, however, that the binding of Cl^- to the α-chain NH_2-terminal is mainly responsible for the augmentation of the Bohr effect, whereas much of its action on the O_2 affinity is caused through binding at other sites (54, 56, 177, 181).

Because binding of 2,3-DPG to Hb also leads to a proton uptake (13, 77), whereas binding of CO_2 has the reverse effect (215), the physiological Bohr effect measured in whole blood is an expression of the interaction of Hb with various cofactors and only partly the expression of the intrinsic Bohr effect. In principal the studies on human Hb show that the alkaline Bohr effect is caused through two different processes: *1*) ligand binding induces intramolecular conformational changes, which cause the formation or the solvation of salt bridges between groups that ionize in the physiological pH region, and *2*) O_2-linked anion binding at α-amino or imidazole groups causes a shift in the ionization of these groups with resulting proton uptake.

A comparison of the amino acid sequences of mammalian Hb shows that β146 His and β94 Asp are invariant amino acids. Thus one can assume that these groups participate in the Bohr effect in all these types of Hb. The Bohr coefficient, (Δlog P_{50})/ΔpH, measured in the blood of mammalian or avian species is generally in the region between −0.40 and −0.65, when the change in P_{50} (O_2 half-saturation pressure of Hb) is related to the plasma pH. If the relationship between plasma and RBC pH is known, the intracellular Bohr coefficient can then be calculated according to the equation

$$(\Delta pH_e/\Delta pH_i)BF_e = BF_i$$

where BF_e is the Bohr coefficient related to plasma pH (pH_e) and BF_i is the Bohr coefficient related to RBC pH (pH_i). The variation of pH in the determination of the Bohr effect of whole blood is achieved either by changes in P_{CO_2}, which correspond more closely to the physiological conditions, or through addition of fixed acid at constant P_{CO_2}. The Bohr effect measured this way is called the fixed-acid Bohr effect. The fixed-acid Bohr effect and the Bohr effect induced by changes in P_{CO_2} are identical only under the condition that there is no O_2-linked carbamate formation. This has been found in some avian species where O_2-linked carbamate formation is completely suppressed due to competitive action of organic phosphates (31, 163, 211). Where O_2-linked carbamate is formed (even a relatively small quantity) the CO_2 and fixed-acid Bohr effects are different from each other (227, 255).

Because of the interaction of Hb with organic phosphates and CO_2 the Bohr and the Haldane coefficients can be different at physiological conditions. The interaction of Hb with these cofactors under physiological conditions and the pH dependence of their binding constants can result in a dependence of the Bohr coefficient on the saturation.

Organic Phosphates

The presence of high concentrations of organic phosphates, notably 2,3-DPG, in mammalian and other vertebrate RBCs was established long before an understanding of their function in the RBC (108, 201), which came through the work of Chanutin and Curnish (67) and Benesch and Benesch (42). They demonstrated that the O_2 affinity of human Hb could be drastically reduced in the presence of 2,3-DPG. This finding was subsequently shown to hold for many types of vertebrate Hb of different vertebrate classes; however, knowledge about the mechanism of interaction with Hb is most precise for mammalian, especially human, Hb. Whereas 2,3-DPG is the major organic phosphate for most mammalian Hb, birds use predominantly inositol pentaphosphate (IPP) and inositol tetraphosphate (ITP), whereas amphibians use ATP and fish use GTP and ATP. A survey of the distribution of organic phosphates among the various vertebrate classes is given by Bartlett (22).

METABOLIC REGULATION OF 2,3-DIPHOSPHOGLYCERATE IN MAMMALIAN RED BLOOD CELLS. The organic phosphate 2,3-DPG is a metabolite of the glycolytic pathway, formed from 1,3-diphosphoglycerate (1,3-DPG) by the action of bisphosphoglycerate mutase (202), and is an essential cofactor for the phosphoglycerate mutase reaction that converts 3-phosphoglycerate (3-PG) into 2-phosphoglycerate (2-PG). The 2,3-DPG concentrations in most mammalian RBCs are, however, about two orders of magnitude larger than necessary for the maximum velocity of the phosphoglycerate mutase reaction.

In their survey of many mammalian species, Scott et al. (222, 223) found 4.2–12 mmol 2,3-DPG/liter RBC, which corresponds to a stoichiometric ratio of ~0.8–2.6 mol 2,3-DPG/mol Hb, not including the

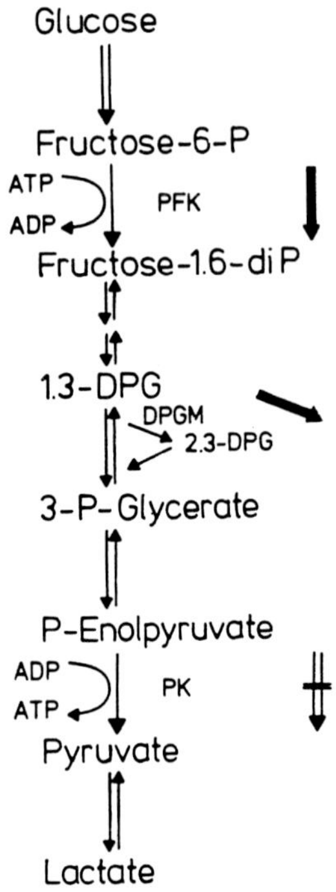

FIG. 2. Scheme of RBC glycolysis. The 2,3-diphosphoglycerate (2,3-DPG) accumulates with an increased activity of phosphofructokinase (PFK) and bisphosphoglycerate mutase [diphosphoglycerate mutase (DPGM)] (*solid arrows*) and decreased activity of pyruvate kinase (PK) (*broken arrow*). [Adapted from Jelkmann and Bauer (137).]

RBCs of felines and ruminants such as sheep, goats, and cattle, which contain only traces of 2,3-DPG. The concentration of 2,3-DPG in the RBC mainly depends on three factors: *1*) the overall glycolytic rate, *2*) the rate of conversion from 1,3-DPG to 2,3-DPG, and *3*) the rate of the glycolytic pathway below the formation of 3-PG (Fig. 2). The principal enzymes involved in the regulation are 6-phosphofructokinase (PFK), which has a decisive influence on the overall glycolytic rate, bisphosphoglycerate mutase, which catalyzes the conversion from 1,3-DPG to 2,3-DPG, and pyruvate kinase (PK), which determines the rate in the lower part of glycolysis. A comprehensive review is given by Jacobasch et al. (133). Comparative studies on several mammalian species have shown that those species that as adults possess low concentrations of 2,3-DPG in their RBCs have a very low activity of bisphosphoglycerate mutase (114). Likewise a low concentration of 2,3-DPG has been demonstrated in humans with inherited bisphosphoglycerate mutase defects (195, 213), with an inherited low activity of PFK (69), and with inherited elevation of PK activity (258).

Because the PFK activity is strongly pH dependent (maximum pH ~8), the intracellular RBC pH decisively influences the concentration of 2,3-DPG. An increase of RBC pH is associated with an overall increase in glycolytic rate and hence 2,3-DPG formation. This pH dependence of the 2,3-DPG concentration is important especially with regard to the increase observed with exposure to hypoxic hypoxia as seen at high altitude, because Duhm and Gerlach (82) showed that on prevention of the accompanying respiratory alkalosis there was no net increase of the 2,3-DPG concentration.

BINDING OF ORGANIC PHOSPHATE TO HEMOGLOBIN. At physiological ionic strength (I) of 0.1, organic phosphates are bound in a ratio of 1 mol organic phosphate/1 mol deoxygenated Hb (43). Investigations of substituted or chemically modified human Hb (45, 63) as well as X-ray structural analysis of the deoxygenated Hb–2,3-DPG (6) and deoxygenated Hb–inositol hexaphosphate (IHP) (9) complexes have led to identification of those residues that participate in the binding of 2,3-DPG and other organic phosphates in deoxygenated Hb. Organic phosphates are bound to the central cavity of deoxygenated Hb to a number of positively charged β-chain residues (Fig. 3). The binding is electrostatic and in human Hb includes the NH_2-terminal α-amino group of the β-chain, the imidazole groups of β143 His and β2 His, and the ϵ-amino group of β82 Lys (6, 9). Of prime importance for the stability of the phosphate-Hb complex are the NH_2-terminal α-amino groups and the imidazole group of β2 His.

A substitution or deletion of one or more of the residues involved in the binding of 2,3-DPG to Hb has been found in all types of mammalian Hb that show a low O_2 affinity in the absence of organic phosphates and whose function in vivo is not regulated through 2,3-DPG. These include ruminant (36, 91) and feline (61, 234) Hb. All of these hemoglobins lack β2 His, which is deleted in ruminant Hb. This deletion also precludes the participation of the NH_2-terminal α-amino groups of the β-chain in the binding of 2,3-DPG, because it increases the distance between the two NH_2-terminal α-amino groups so that electrostatic binding with the corresponding phosphate groups of 2,3-DPG is no longer possible. In cat Hb, β2 His is substituted by phenylalanine, and in addition the β-chain NH_2-terminal is blocked in one of the two major Hb fractions (234).

Because of the participation of the α-amino and the imidazole groups, the association constants for 2,3-DPG to human Hb are strongly dependent on pH in the physiological pH range, and the association of 2,3-DPG to Hb decreases rapidly with increasing pH (46). Although it has been shown that 2,3-DPG is also bound to HbO_2 (77, 100) in a stoichiometric ratio of 1:1, which suggests the central cavity as a binding site, it is still not clear which sites are participating in the binding of 2,3-DPG to HbO_2, because X-ray studies show that the central cavity in the liganded forms of Hb is too small to accommodate 2,3-DPG in the same way as in deoxygenated Hb. The association constants for the binding of 2,3-DPG to human HbO_2 and deoxygenated Hb under simulated physiological conditions have been determined (100, 243).

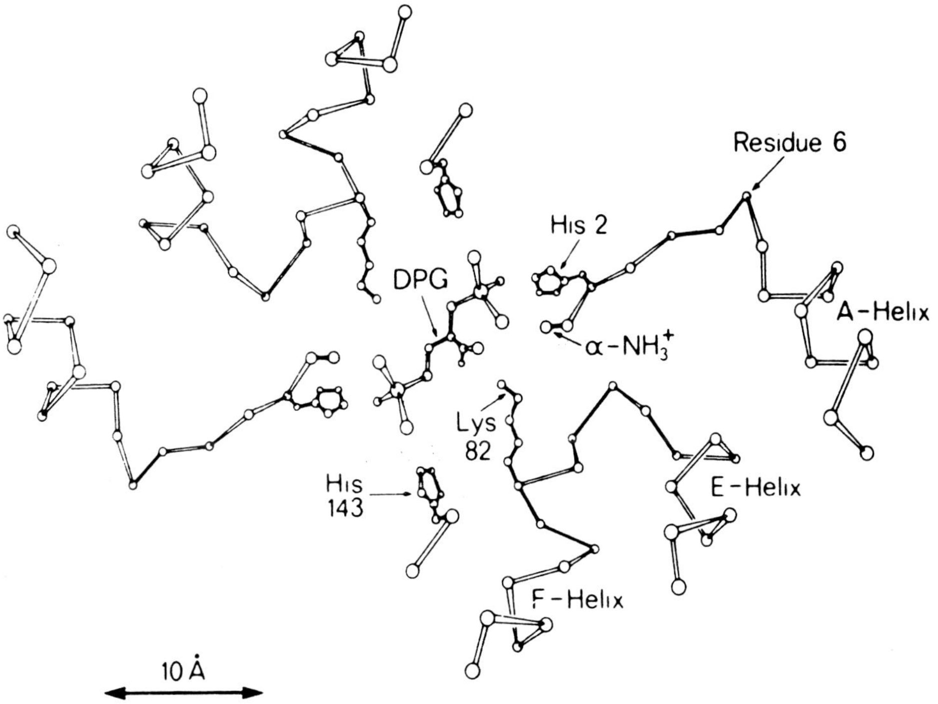

FIG. 3. Binding site for 2,3-DPG in human deoxygenated Hb. [From Arnone (6). Reprinted by permission from *Nature*, copyright 1972, Macmillan Journals Limited.]

Using the approach developed by Baldwin (14) and Szabo and Karplus (232), one can determine the association constants from experiments where the change in P_{50} in dependence of 2,3-DPG or other organic phosphates is measured according to the equation

$$\log P_{50}^{+DPG} = \log P_{50}^{-DPG} + 1/4 \left(\frac{1 + vK_D}{1 + vK_O}\right)$$

where the P_{50}^{+DPG} and P_{50}^{-DPG} are the O_2 half-saturation pressures of Hb in the presence and absence of organic phosphates, respectively, K_D and K_O are the association constants for deoxygenated Hb and HbO_2, respectively, and v is the concentration of free 2,3-DPG at P_{50}. The estimated binding constants and those obtained from direct measurements show good agreement. A comparison of several association constants for various mammalian species, some showing substitutions at the 2,3-DPG–binding site, is given in Table 2.

Inositol pentaphosphate, the major allosteric effector of avian Hb, is the most powerful organic phosphate. In addition to the residues that were shown to participate in the binding of 2,3-DPG to human Hb, the binding site for IPP of avian Hb contains two other residues, β135 Arg and β139 His. The residue β143 His is substituted by arginine (9). Consequently the binding of IPP to bird Hb is much stronger than that of 2,3-DPG to human Hb and it shows much less pH dependence of binding (60). Rollema and Bauer (209) determined the binding constants for IPP of two species of geese Hb under nearly physiological conditions. A comparison with the association constants obtained for the 2,3-DPG–human Hb complex shows

TABLE 2. *Association Constants for Binding of 2,3-Diphosphoglycerate to Hemoglobin*

Hemoglobin Type	K_{deoxy}, mol^{-1}	K_{oxy}, mol^{-1}	Ref.
Human Hb A	3.5×10^4	4.1×10^2	244
	5.0×10^3	2.5×10^2	100
	1.2×10^4	1.3×10^2	29
Human fetal Hb*	2.1×10^3	16	29
Llama Hb†	5.1×10^3	3.4×10^2	29
Camel Hb	1.6×10^3	4.6×10^2	29

Experimental conditions: pH 7.2, 37°C, 0.1 mol Cl$^-$. * β143 His → Ser. † β2 His → Asp.

TABLE 3. *Association Constants for Binding of Inositol Pentaphosphate and Inositol Hexaphosphate to Hemoglobin*

	K_{deoxy}, mol^{-1}	K_{oxy}, mol^{-1}	Ref.
Inositol pentaphosphate			
Bar-headed goose*	1×10^9	2.3×10^5	210
Greylag goose*	9×10^8	1.5×10^5	210
Inositol hexaphosphate			
Human Hb A†	1×10^6	2.5×10^3	86, 257

* Experimental conditions: pH 7.2, 37°C, 0.1 mol Cl$^-$. † Experimental conditions: pH 7.3, 20°C, 0.1 mol Cl$^-$.

that the binding of IPP to HbO_2 or deoxygenated Hb of birds is about several orders of magnitude larger at physiological pH (Table 3). Qualitatively similar results have been obtained with IHP, whose association constants for the binding to human Hb were determined by Edalji et al. (86).

The binding of 2,3-DPG or IPP to Hb causes extensive changes in the quaternary and tertiary structures of deoxygenated Hb (6, 9), which are regarded as stabilizing forces for the deoxystructure. Because deoxygenated Hb preferentially binds organic phosphates, there is a shift in the conformational equilibrium between the oxy- and deoxyconformation in the presence of organic phosphate, which is thought to cause the observed changes in O_2 affinity. Furthermore it is conceivable that the O_2 affinity of the deoxygenated Hb–phosphate complex is different from that of the phosphate-free deoxygenated Hb. Experimental results that support such a possibility have been reported by Bonaventura et al. (55), who observed that the binding of IHP to Hb H (β_4) induces cooperative O_2 binding and a decrease of the O_2 affinity.

PHYSIOLOGICAL IMPORTANCE OF ORGANIC PHOSPHATES. Since the finding that organic phosphates are major allosteric regulators of Hb, it has become increasingly clear that the intrinsic O_2 affinity of many types of mammalian and nonmammalian Hb in the absence of allosteric effectors is very high; indeed it may be as high or even higher than that of Mb. Therefore the principal action of organic phosphates and of other allosteric effectors is to shift the O_2 affinity of the cooperative Hb tetramer into a region that is compatible with the physiological demands. Thus human Hb in the absence of organic phosphate has a P_{50} of 13.2 Torr at pH 7.2 and 37°C, which is shifted to 24 Torr in the presence of physiological concentrations of 2,3-DPG. That birds use a more powerful allosteric effector, i.e., IPP or ITP, correlates with the observation that generally the intrinsic O_2 affinity of avian Hb is even higher than that of mammalian Hb, which requires a correspondingly greater decrease of O_2 affinity to match the physiological demands (Table 4).

Compared with this major role of organic phosphates the possibility of inducing adaptive changes in O_2 affinity through metabolic variation of the 2,3-DPG content in mammalian RBCs is clearly of secondary importance. Because the binding of O_2 to the α- and β-subunits of Hb is preferentially to the α-subunits in the presence of organic phosphates (11, 140) and because there is also a nonlinear release of 2,3-DPG during ligand binding to Hb (127), the binding of organic phosphates may also cause changes in the cooperativity of O_2 binding.

TABLE 4. *Major Red Blood Cell Organic Phosphates and P_{50} for Whole Blood and Purified Hemoglobin Solution of Several Mammalian and Avian Species*

	P_{50} Hb Solution, Torr*	P_{50} Whole Blood, Torr†	P_{50} Whole Blood/ P_{50} Hb Solution	Organic Phosphate as Cofactor	Ref.
Sheep B	33.2	41.8	1.25		35
Musk shrew	17.4	33.5	1.92	2,3-DPG	19
Human	13.2	27.0	2.04	2,3-DPG	74
Etruscan shrew	13.1	35.2	2.68	2,3-DPG	19
Mouse BALB/c	13.0	41.0	3.15	2,3-DPG	196
Rabbit	10.2	30.0	2.94	2,3-DPG	135
Chicken	7.4	48.3	6.52	IPP	31
Greylag goose	6.0	39.5	6.58	IPP	197
Bar-headed goose	4.6	29.7	6.46	IPP	197

P_{50}, O_2 half-saturation of Hb. 2,3-DPG, 2,3-diphosphoglycerate. IPP, inositol pentaphosphate. * Experimental conditions: 37°C, pH 7.2, 0.15 mol Cl^-. † Experimental conditions: 37°C, pH 7.4, partial pressure of CO_2 (P_{CO_2}) = 40 Torr.

INTERACTIONS BETWEEN ORGANIC PHOSPHATES AND CHLORIDE. It has long been known that inorganic anions decrease Hb-O_2 affinity (226). Of physiological significance in this respect is Cl^-, because its concentration inside the RBC is high enough to overcome the relatively low affinity of Hb for inorganic anions as compared with organic phosphates.

Benesch et al. (46) observed that the effect of 2,3-DPG on Hb was reduced and finally abolished with increasing Cl^- concentrations. This result was taken to indicate that 2,3-DPG and Cl^- had identical binding sites in the deoxygenated Hb molecule and that the major difference between both types of effectors was the much lower affinity of Cl^- for the binding site in deoxygenated Hb compared with 2,3-DPG. However, investigations carried out during recent years have shown that inorganic anions like Cl^- are also bound at sites not shared with organic phosphates. Chiancone et al. (70, 71) and Nigen et al. (175, 176) showed that Cl^- was also bound to the α-chain of human Hb. As indicated by X-ray analysis (181), inorganic anion-binding sites are located at the α-chain NH_2-terminal, and functional studies make it plausible that the binding of Cl^- to the α-chain NH_2-terminal is partly responsible for the observed dependence of the Bohr effect on Cl^- (181, 210).

However, blocking the α-chain NH_2-terminal and thereby removing the binding site for Cl^- does not completely abolish the effect of Cl^- on the O_2 affinity (181). Thus other sites located on the β-chains contribute to the effect of Cl^- on O_2 affinity. One identified site is β82 Lys, which is substituted in human Hb mutants Providence and Rahere (cf. ref. 54). The effect of Cl^- on O_2 affinity is reduced in both types of Hb (54, 56). Nigen et al. (177) finally prepared Hb carbamylated at the α-chain NH_2-terminal and showing substitutions at β82 Lys, thereby removing two of the potential Cl^--binding sites. However, even in Hb prepared this way, there is still a residual activity of Cl^- concerning the O_2 affinity so that one has to conclude that at least in human Hb there are three O_2-linked binding sites for Cl^- (α1 Val, β82 Lys, and an unknown site), only one of which is shared with organic phosphates (β82 Lys). Thus the action of Cl^- and organic phosphates on Hb can in some way be seen as complementary. Conversely the splitting of binding sites for organic and inorganic anions means that large substitutions or changes in the primary structure of the organic phosphate–binding site do not necessarily abolish the action of Cl^- on the respective Hb.

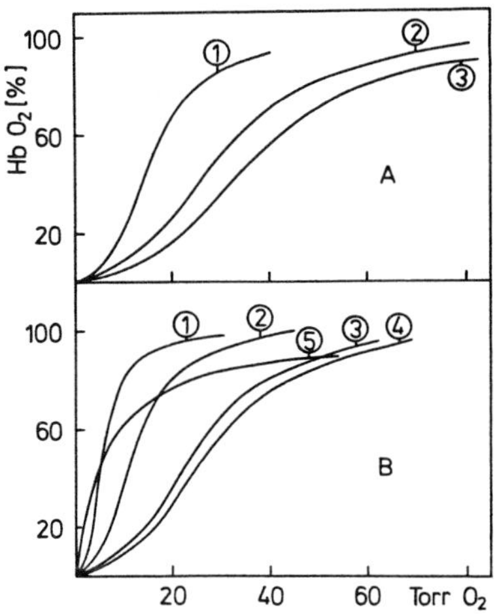

FIG. 4. Comparison of intrinsic O_2 affinity and effect of allosteric effectors on cat Hb A and human Hb. *A*: cat Hb. ① 10 mmol Cl^-, O_2 half-saturation pressure of Hb (P_{50}) = 15.6 Torr; ② 100 mmol Cl^-, P_{50} = 29.2 Torr; ③ partial pressure of CO_2 (P_{CO_2}) = 40 Torr, P_{50} = 36.7 Torr. *B*: human Hb. ① 10 mmol Cl^-, P_{50} = 5.6 Torr; ② 100 mmol Cl^-, P_{50} = 11.5 Torr; ③ 1 mol 2,3-DPG/mol Hb, P_{50} = 24 Torr; ④ P_{CO_2} = 40 Torr, P_{50} = 27 Torr; ⑤ human Mb. Experimental conditions for all data: pH 7.2 and 37°C.

This finding is important because even those types of mammalian Hb that lack a substantial effect of 2,3-DPG on their O_2 affinity and are not regulated by 2,3-DPG under physiological conditions need allosteric modification to have an O_2 affinity compatible with physiological demands. Because their intrinsic affinity is lower than that of other types of mammalian Hb they need a correspondingly smaller amplification of their P_{50}. This is illustrated in Figure 4, which shows the comparison of human and cat Hb at various concentrations of Cl^- and 2,3-DPG. Whereas human Hb in the absence of organic phosphate and with only 10 mmol Cl^- has (under physiological conditions of pH and temperature) an O_2 affinity (P_{50} = 5.6 Torr) similar to Mb, the O_2 affinity of cat Hb A under the same conditions is about threefold lower. However, the resulting P_{50} (15 Torr) is still not high enough for physiological conditions. With physiological concentrations of Cl^- and the addition of CO_2, P_{50} increases by ~21 Torr to 36 Torr, which corresponds to the P_{50} value measured in whole blood (20).

In human Hb, on the other hand, the combined action of CO_2, 2,3-DPG, and Cl^- shifts the P_{50} from 5 to ~27 Torr. Thus in absolute terms the shift in P_{50} achieved by the weak effectors in the case of cat Hb and the more powerful allosteric effectors in the case of human Hb is about the same. This illustrates that the action of weak allosteric effectors such as Cl^- and CO_2 cannot be neglected, even in the case of those types of Hb that have a relatively low intrinsic O_2 affinity.

INFLUENCE OF ORGANIC PHOSPHATES ON THE BOHR EFFECT. Aside from the change in O_2 affinity caused by the binding of 2,3-DPG it was observed early that combination of Hb with 2,3-DPG also changes the pH dependence of the O_2 affinity, i.e., the Bohr effect (207), due to the pH dependence of the binding constants of 2,3-DPG to HbO_2 and deoxygenated Hb. De Bruin and Janssen (77) showed that the binding of 2,3-DPG to HbO_2 or deoxygenated Hb is accompanied by proton absorption. Above pH 6.7, the proton absorption for human deoxygenated Hb exceeds that observed for HbO_2; therefore in the presence of 2,3-DPG one observes an increased O_2-linked proton release (13, 77). The proton uptake of Hb with binding of 2,3-DPG is the sum of two processes. *1*) When 2,3-DPG is bound to Hb the p*K* of the phosphate groups of 2,3-DPG is decreased, which leads to a proton release from the corresponding groups. *2*) The p*K* of the imidazole groups of β2 His and β143 His and the α-amino group of β1 Val is increased, which leads to an additional proton uptake. Because a net proton uptake is observed for both HbO_2 and deoxygenated Hb, one must conclude that the second process dominates. The determination of the additional proton absorption has been used as an excellent method to determine the stoichiometry and the association constants for organic phosphate binding to Hb (60, 86, 243, 257).

In the discussion of the Bohr effect it was noted that $(\Delta \log P_{O_2})/\Delta pH$ and $\Delta H^+/\Delta HbO_2$ are equal only when the activity of other components interacting with Hb does not change with ligand binding. Because under physiological conditions the concentration of 2,3-DPG is about equimolar to that of Hb, the free concentration of 2,3-DPG will change with oxygenation; hence $(\Delta \log P_{O_2})/\Delta pH \neq \Delta H^+/\Delta HbO_2$, which has been confirmed by experiment (47, 48).

The influence of 2,3-DPG on the pH dependence of the O_2 affinity is most pronounced at low-to-intermediate concentrations of 2,3-DPG, where the pH dependence of the association constants exercises the strongest effect. It disappears, however, when experiments are carried out under conditions where the concentration of 2,3-DPG is high enough to give complete saturation of the binding site (46).

The important point with respect to physiological conditions is that one commonly tries to estimate the O_2-linked proton release via measurement of the pH dependence of the O_2 affinity. However, because the linked function relation developed by Wyman (256) is not applicable under such conditions, each characteristic has to be determined independently.

REGULATION OF RED BLOOD CELL PH THROUGH HEMOGLOBIN AND ORGANIC PHOSPHATES. The plasma pH of mammalian or avian arterialized blood under physiological conditions is usually between 7.4 and 7.5 at rest, and corresponding values for the RBC pH are between 7.1 and 7.25. Because of the pH dependence of the O_2 affinity of Hb and of the cofactor binding, the regulation of RBC pH is important.

The distribution of monovalent anions and H^+ in mammalian RBCs follows the Donnan equilibrium (95, 247) and is characterized by the distribution ratio r such that

$$r = \frac{(Cl^-)_i}{(Cl^-)_e} = \frac{(OH^-)_i}{(OH^-)_e} = \frac{(\alpha H^+)_e}{(\alpha H^+)_i}$$

where i is intraerythrocytic concentration or activity and e is plasma concentration. Thus there is a direct dependence of the intracellular on the extracellular pH, which allows the Bohr effect to gain physiological significance.

In order to obtain $r < 1$ (i.e., a lower intracellular pH), the concentration of impermeable anions in the RBC must be higher than that in plasma. The main nondiffusible anions are Hb and organic phosphates. In human RBCs, Hb accounts for ~60% of the impermeable anion equivalent, whereas organic phosphates contribute ~40% (81). Rapoport and Guest (200) were the first to draw attention to this role of organic phosphates. Similar relations must hold for all other mammalian species with comparable organic phosphate concentrations in the RBC.

On the other hand, those species where 2,3-DPG does not regulate Hb-O_2 affinity and where the organic phosphate concentration is low rely entirely on the Hb net charge for the maintenance of RBC pH. Thus the isoelectric point and buffer capacity of Hb, which determine the net charge carried at physiological pH, must be important criteria for selection, and apparently mammalian Hb has already been positively selected in this respect.

There is only a small variation in RBC pH between mammalian species with high and low 2,3-DPG concentrations. The mouse has 7.5 mmol 2,3-DPG/liter RBC and an intracellular pH (pH_c) of 7.18 at an extracellular pH (pH_e) of 7.4 (197), compared with pH_c 7.23 in the sheep (35), which has <0.1 mmol 2,3-DPG/liter RBC. It follows that the sum of impermeable anions is regulated within narrow bounds and consequently the contributions of Hb and organic phosphates must be complementary; i.e., an increase in organic phosphate concentration compensates a low Hb net charge. This might explain the observation of Scott et al. (223) that RBCs of several mammalian species (e.g., rodents) contain far more 2,3-DPG (i.e., up to 12 mmol/liter RBC) than is necessary for its allosteric action. Duhm (81) has shown that above a concentration of 6 mmol 2,3-DPG/liter RBC the changes in O_2 affinity of human blood are entirely due to the decrease of RBC pH caused by 2,3-DPG (Fig. 5).

Because of the Bohr effect an increase in organic phosphate concentration will cause a lowering of Hb-O_2 affinity irrespective of any specific interaction between the phosphate and Hb. This mechanism plays an important role in the pre- and postnatal changes of O_2 affinity in a number of mammalian species (79, 83).

Interaction Between Hemoglobin and Carbon Dioxide

The direct combination of CO_2 with Hb was first described by Henriques (121). The unequivocal demonstration of carbamate compounds of Hb and the O_2-linked nature of carbamate formation was achieved through the work of Rossi-Bernardi and Roughton (215). The authors showed that at constant pH and P_{CO_2}, human deoxygenated Hb binds more CO_2 than HbO_2. This difference is the equivalent of the O_2-

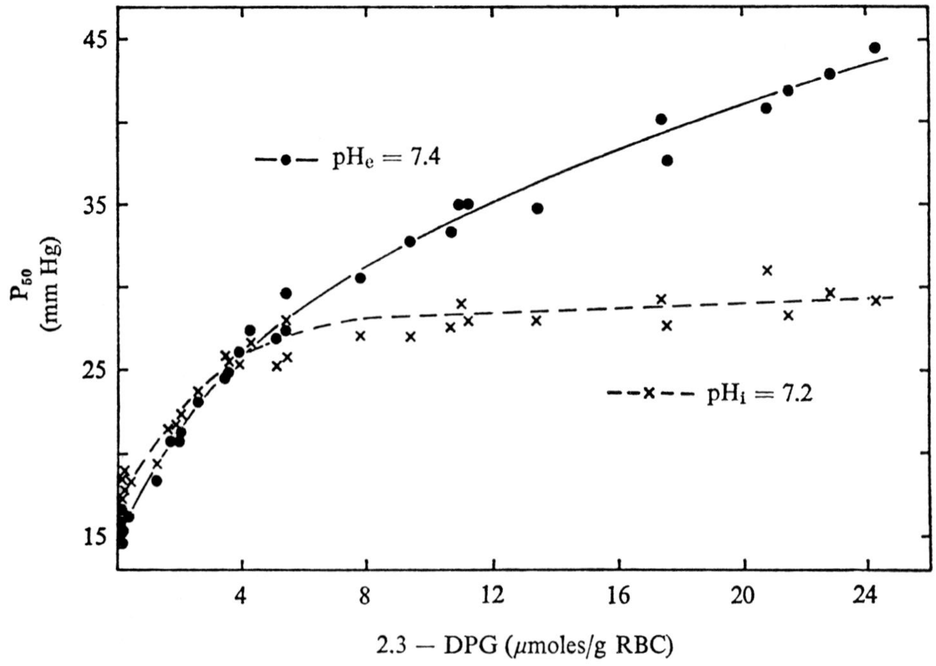

FIG. 5. Relationship between P_{50} of whole blood (37°C, P_{CO_2} = 40 Torr) and 2,3-DPG concentration of human RBCs. *Solid line,* P_{50} determined at plasma pH (pH_e) of 7.4. *Broken line,* P_{50} corrected to intracellular pH (pH_i) of 7.2. [From Duhm (81).]

linked carbamate. The reaction between CO_2 and Hb is characterized by the reaction scheme

$$RNH_3 \rightleftharpoons RNH_2 + H^+ \qquad K_z \qquad (1)$$

$$RNH(COOH) \rightleftharpoons RNH_2 + CO_2 \qquad K \qquad (2)$$

$$RNH(COO^-) + H^+ \rightleftharpoons RNHCOOH \qquad K_x \qquad (3)$$

When K and K_x are combined to give K_c

$$RNH(COO^-) + H^+ \rightleftharpoons RNH_2 + CO_2 \qquad K_c = K_x \cdot K$$

where K_z is the equilibrium constant for the amino group, K is the equilibrium constant for the carbamate reaction, K_x is the dissociation constant for carbamic acid, and K_c, the combined equilibrium constant for the carbamate reaction, contains the dissociation constant for the carbamic acid. However, this approach is justified, because at physiological pH the carbamino groups are nearly completely ionized because the ionization constant pK_x is ~5.2.

Because the carbamate reaction occurs preferentially with unprotonized amino groups, one long suspected the NH_2-terminal α-amino groups of the α- and β-chains to be the binding sites for CO_2 in the physiological pH region. The experimental verification came through the work of Kilmartin and Rossi-Bernardi (147), who worked with horse Hb that had been specifically blocked with cyanate at the NH_2-terminal α-amino groups. The selective blockage of the α- and β-chain NH_2-terminal amino groups as well as the investigation of human Hb variants that are partially blocked at the NH_2-terminal allowed the clarification of the question to what extent the α- and β-chains of human Hb participate in the O_2-linked carbamate formation (25, 146). Thus, in agreement with results obtained by indirect determinations of O_2-linked carbamate (25, 146), when the effect of CO_2 on the O_2 affinity was used, it was found that the β-chains of human Hb are the principal site for the formation of O_2-linked carbamate (109, 159, 186, 187).

The main reason for the difference in the O_2-linked carbamate formation between the α- and β-chain NH_2-terminals are the different ionization constants of the NH_2-terminal α-amino groups. The pK value of the α-chain NH_2-terminal increases with deoxygenation from 7 to 7.8 (98), whereas the pK value for the β chain NH_2 terminal amino groups remains unchanged. The decrease of the carbamate formation at the β-chains with oxygenation is exclusively due to an increase in pK_c (159). The main reason for the low values of pK and pK_c at the β-chain NH_2-terminal in deoxygenated Hb lies in the large number of positively charged groups that are found in the direct neighborhood of the β-chain NH_2-terminals, which can directly influence pK_z and through a stabilization of the carbamate anion also affect pK_x and therefore pK_c. This implies that the tertiary structure in the NH_2-terminal region of the β-chain decisively influences the carbamate formation.

Crystallographic results demonstrating the presence of CO_2 at the NH_2-terminals of β-chains (7) also showed that CO_2 binding to deoxygenated Hb does not lead to changes in the tertiary or quaternary structure that can be resolved through crystallography. Arnone (7) proposed that the formation of a salt bridge between the carbamate anion of the β-chain NH_2-terminal and the ϵ-amino group of β82 Lys acts as a stabilizing force on the β-chain tertiary deoxy-structure. Changes in the tertiary structure of the β-chains with CO_2 binding are indicated by alterations of the reactivity of the SH groups at position β93 of various types of Hb in the presence of CO_2 (32).

INFLUENCE OF CARBON DIOXIDE BINDING ON HEMOGLOBIN FUNCTION. Carbon dioxide is bound preferentially to deoxygenated Hb, and therefore the O_2 affinity of Hb decreases. Under the assumption that CO_2 binding to the NH_2-terminals is not cooperative but independent, it is possible to use the change in O_2 affinity as a measure for the O_2-linked carbamate formation (25, 146). The O_2-linked carbamate formation results in a release of protons from deoxygenated Hb; therefore in the presence of CO_2 the Bohr effect is decreased (Fig. 6).

The physiological importance of CO_2 as an allosteric regulator of Hb-O_2 affinity is largely determined through the interactions between CO_2 and organic phosphate. Because organic phosphates and CO_2 share the same binding site at the NH_2-terminal α-amino groups of the β-chains in deoxygenated Hb there is a direct competition between both types of effectors (24). Thus in the presence of organic phosphates there is a pronounced reduction of O_2-linked carbamate

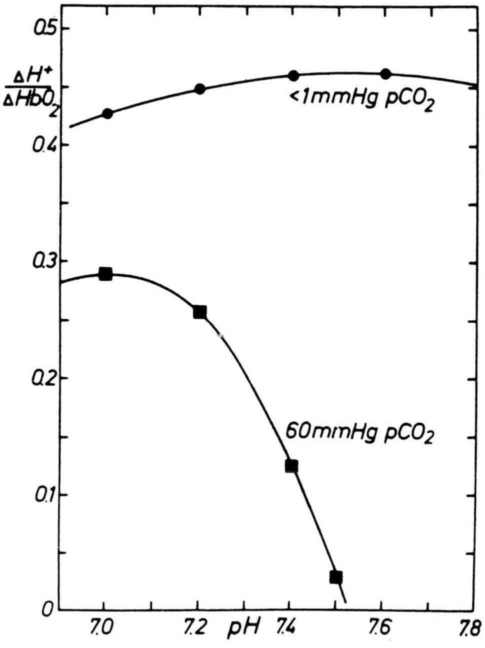

FIG. 6. Effect of P_{CO_2} on Bohr effect of sheep Hb B at 37°C and ionic strength of 0.16. [From Baumann, Bauer, and Haller (35).]

formation, which was first shown for human Hb (24).

Investigations about the influence of CO_2 on the O_2 affinity have been nearly exclusively conducted on mammalian Hb and on a few types of bird Hb (31, 35, 66, 74). In most types of Hb, especially mammalian and avian, the O_2-linked CO_2 binding plays a minor role in the regulation of O_2 affinity when organic phosphates are the principal allosteric regulators because CO_2 binding to the β-chains will be reduced or abolished. However, in those mammalian species (e.g., felines and ruminants) where control of Hb function is not coupled to organic phosphates, O_2-linked carbamate formation has an important role in the regulation of in vivo O_2 affinity (33, 35, 37).

OXYGEN-HEMOGLOBIN EQUILIBRIUM CURVE

General Aspects

The physiological function of Hb is best assessed through the measurement of the O_2-Hb equilibrium curve. Two methods are used to express O_2-binding data. The first was devised by Hill (122), who arrived at the empirical expression

$$y = k(P_{O_2})^n/1 + k(P_{O_2})^n$$

where y is the fractional saturation and k is the dissociation constant. The exponent n was thought to represent the maximum number of subunits in the polymer, which requires maximum cooperativity. The linearized form of the equation

$$\log \frac{y}{1 - y} = \log k + n(\log P_{O_2})$$

holds for the saturation range between ~20%–80% and permits the evaluation of P_{50}. The slope n is used as an empirical index of cooperativity.

For mammalian hemoglobins, n value is in the range between 2.6 and 3.0 at physiological pH. It is decreased when the conformational transition with ligand binding is impaired, as in many types of pathological human Hb, and reaches the minimum value of 1 in the absence of conformational transition, as, for example, in human Hb H (β_4), which consists only of β-chains, behaves functionally like a monomer, and shows no structural transition on ligand binding (192).

A mathematically sufficient form of treatment for the O_2 equilibrium curve was devised by Adair (2). He assumed that each subunit of the tetrameric Hb molecule has individual association, dissociation, and equilibrium constants according to the equations

$$Hb_4 + O_2 \underset{k_1}{\overset{k_1'}{\rightleftharpoons}} Hb_4O_2 \qquad K_1 = k_1'/k_1$$

to

$$Hb_4(O_2)_3 + O_2 \underset{k_4}{\overset{k_4'}{\rightleftharpoons}} Hb_4(O_2)_4 \qquad K_4 = k_4'/k_4$$

that give the fractional saturation (y) of the Hb molecule such that

$$y = \frac{K_1p + 2K_1K_2p^2 + 3K_1K_2K_3p^3 + 4K_1K_2K_3K_4p^4}{4(1 + K_1p + K_1K_2p^2 + K_1K_2K_3p^3 + K_1K_2K_3K_4p^4)}$$

where p is P_{O_2}.

Of the four equilibrium constants, only K_1 and K_4 can be determined directly, which in either case necessitates extremely precise measurements of O_2 equilibrium either in the very low or very high saturation range. With K_1 and K_4 determined, K_2 and K_3 can subsequently be calculated. Measurements of K_1 to K_4 under physiological conditions (217) show that the affinity of the Hb molecule increases ~500-fold between the binding of the first to the fourth ligand (217), whereas at low salt concentrations and in the absence of organic phosphates there is only a 35-fold increase in O_2 affinity (135).

Another point of interest with respect to the O_2 equilibrium curve is the question whether O_2 is bound statistically to the α- and β-chains or if there is a preferential binding order. This question was investigated by Johnson and Ho (140), who first reported that in the presence of organic phosphates, O_2 is bound preferentially to the α-chains of human Hb; recent work of Viggiano and Ho (248) and Asakura and Lau (10) has confirmed and extended these findings. On the other hand, in the presence of buffer and Cl^- but without organic phosphate, there is no preferential binding order to either the α- or β-chain. Thus the consequence of O_2 binding to Hb largely depends on the composition of the milieu in which the Hb is tested. The reaction of Hb with O_2 is exothermic with an apparent heat of oxygenation (ΔH) of −11 to −14 kcal/mol for mammalian Hb (4). The apparent heat of oxygenation contains the heat of solution of O_2 and the heat of ionization of O_2-linked proton- or anion-binding groups (4) in addition to the intrinsic heat of oxygenation.

Due to the exothermic nature of O_2 binding to Hb the O_2 affinity decreases with increasing temperature. This is described in the temperature coefficient $(\Delta \log P_{50})/\Delta T$, which for human blood is ~0.02 (10). Physiologically the temperature dependence in warm-blooded animals is unimportant, except under conditions of heavy muscular exercise, where the temperature-dependent decrease of O_2 affinity in conjunction with the Bohr effect allows a better utilization of the O_2 supply (236).

Methodological Aspects

PREPARATION OF HEMOGLOBIN SOLUTIONS FOR MEASUREMENTS OF OXYGEN-HEMOGLOBIN EQUILIBRIUM CURVES. The preceding discussion on the influence of various allosteric effector molecules on the properties of Hb has made it clear that to get meaningful results it is necessary to conduct measurements of the O_2-Hb equilibrium curve in Hb solutions under carefully controlled conditions with respect to pH, ionic strength, and the concentration of various cofactors. Because organic phosphates are bound with high affinity to most types of Hb, care must be taken to completely remove these cofactors. Procedures have been devised to assure this, usually using column chromatography (cf. ref. 134). Starting with these cofactor-free Hb solutions, which are often referred to as stripped Hb, one can investigate the effect of the various effector molecules under controlled conditions.

Another problem is a tendency to form MetHb, which changes the O_2 affinity. This can be minimized by adding enzymatic mixtures that reduce MetHb to the Hb solution (117) and by trying to keep the MetHb production as low as possible during the preparation of the Hb solution. This includes carrying out most or all preparatory steps in the cold.

Furthermore it is important to select the Hb-concentration range in which the O_2-binding curve is measured. Although in the physiological range of Hb concentration no concentration-dependent effects on human Hb-O_2 affinity are observed (109), this is not true for measurements carried out at very low Hb concentrations (in the micromolar range). Under these conditions substantial dissociation of tetrameric Hb into dimers is observed with consequent effect on the O_2 dissociation curve (1). An increased dissociation and hence greater dependence of O_2 binding on the Hb concentration has been found in some pathological Hb (12).

The results obtained in O_2 equilibrium studies of Hb solutions that are a mixture of several types of Hb cannot be analyzed straightforwardly, unless the properties of each component are known and no interaction occurs among the various Hb components. Physically meaningful data are only obtained if purified Hb solutions containing only one fraction are used.

PREPARATION OF SAMPLES FOR WHOLE-BLOOD MEASUREMENTS. Although the analysis of O_2-binding properties of isolated Hb components gives insight into their molecular properties and regulation, the physiologist is more often interested in the properties of whole blood with respect to O_2 uptake and release and therefore in the construction of O_2-binding curves of whole blood.

The methodological difficulties and precautions that have to be taken are different from those that occur when one works with Hb solutions. First, it is important to define physiologically meaningful conditions of temperature, CO_2 concentration, and pH, if these measurements are used to extrapolate on the properties of blood in the living animal. Very often, P_{50} measurements of mammalian blood are related to a standard state (pH 7.4, 37°C, $P_{CO_2} = 40$ Torr), which corresponds to the resting state. However, in the assessment of adaptive processes, e.g., to hypoxia, the data are only meaningful when related to the actual acid-base state of the subject. Because Hb-O_2 affinity is often regulated by organic phosphates that are actively metabolized, it is important to keep the time lapse between the actual withdrawal of a blood specimen and the analysis as short as possible (<2 h) and to store the blood in the cold during transfer.

The RBC population present in the circulation represents various subpopulations of different ages, which differ with respect to the concentration of organic phosphate and, in the case of human blood, also with respect to the concentration of minor components that are blocked at the NH_2-terminal. In addition there might be variation in intracellular pH within the various subpopulations that cannot be accounted for. This implies that again the measurements of the O_2 dissociation curve of whole blood do not represent an assessment of the physical functions of the individual Hb but rather the contributions coming from the individual subpopulations. Thus the P_{50} or the n values determined from the Hill plot are phenomenological data rather than straightforward physicochemical data. Measurements of whole-blood O_2 affinity should be complemented by determinations of the concentrations of organic phosphates inside the RBC to be able to assess their importance for the regulation of Hb-O_2 affinity.

Because the pH of the RBC interior is different from that of whole blood or plasma, one should also try to measure intracellular pH if possible to be able to relate the observed properties of Hb to the correct pH. Although there is little variation in intracellular pH of adult mammalian or avian RBCs, variations in intracellular pH can occur during ontogeny, where they are accompanied by concomitant changes in organic phosphates (see *Postnatal Period*, p. 162).

TECHNIQUES FOR MEASUREMENT OF THE OXYGEN-HEMOGLOBIN EQUILIBRIUM CURVE. In order to construct O_2-Hb equilibrium curves, different methods are applied. Primarily, samples of blood or Hb solutions are equilibrated at body temperature with gas mixtures of various O_2 pressures and O_2 saturation is measured. A great deal of the knowledge on Hb-O_2 binding is based on results of gasometric methods, mainly the manometric version (194). These methods required very skillful handling and several milliliters of blood for one curve. They were time consuming but unsurpassed in their accuracy until the present. A further advantage was that the CO_2 concentration could be measured in the same sample, thus allowing a reliable pH calculation by applying the Henderson-Hasselbalch equation with appropriate solubility factors for CO_2. A modification of the manometric method for small samples (246) gave satisfactory results with 1 ml yielding a curve with four to six points. Other manometric micromethods have also been described (124, 171). A volumetric micromethod was accurate and widely used (218). The accuracy of gasometric methods decreases with decreasing Hb concentration, as is true for the mixing technique (see later in this section).

Spectrophotometric methods can be applied with reasonable accuracy at low concentrations of the pigment (≤1 g/100 ml). They are rapid but pH must be measured, except with RBC suspensions or Hb in buffered solutions. Two approaches have been used to measure O_2 dissociation curves. Either the saturation is determined in samples equilibrated to a known P_{O_2} or the sample is deoxygenated in a tonometer-cuvette combination and then is oxygenated stepwise and the saturation measured after each addition of O_2 (44). Dynamic methods allow rapid recording of whole O_2-Hb equilibrium curves (174, 203, 225). In a drop of blood, RBC suspension, or Hb solution (10 μl) of zero O_2 saturation, full saturation is reached within 5–10 min by time-controlled diffusion of O_2 into the measuring cell. Specially constructed optical cells allow the measurement of O_2 equilibrium in a very concentrated Hb solution (80).

Electrolytic cell analysis (Lex-O_2-Con) has replaced gasometric methods almost completely, although there is not unanimous agreement on its accuracy and reproducibility (150, 224). Small sample volumes (20 μl), rapid analysis (5 min), and simple handling are the advantages. An equilibrium curve consisting of five points, including one analysis of O_2 capacity and one pH measurement in the five samples requires ~150 μl blood.

The mixing technique consists of mixing of two blood samples of given O_2 saturation in a predetermined volume ratio. A calculable S_{O_2} of the mixture and its measured P_{O_2} yield a point of an O_2 equilibrium curve. After its first application (111), others have proved the reliability of the method and given more methodological advice (87, 154, 237). A careful evaluation of accuracy and reliability showed that exact adjustment of S_{O_2} to a predetermined value is the prominent advantage of the method, thus facilitating P_{50} and Bohr effect measurements (221). Errors are mainly based on inaccuracies of volume determination. Small blood volumes and low Hb (pigment) concentration limit the applicability of the method.

More or less automatic devices mainly for clinical laboratories were developed recently and commercially produced. Three of them use spectral absorbance changes versus P_{O_2} (91, 131, 144); others use O_2 uptake of a deoxygenated sample (84, 215). They measure the change of spectral absorbance versus the change in P_{O_2}, which is monitored by an O_2 electrode attached to the cuvette. Of critical importance are the properties of the O_2 electrode, which must have a small lag phase and a linear response over the entire P_{O_2} range.

OXYGEN TRANSPORT OF HEMOGLOBIN DURING DEVELOPMENT

During the intrauterine and postnatal development of mammals there is a timely coordinated production of different populations of RBCs. These cells differ with respect to their morphology, enzyme and Hb composition, and O_2-binding properties. In the embryo the earliest Hb-containing cells are produced in the yolk sac blood islands. These erythroid cells are nucleated and mature in a relatively synchronized manner. Later in the development, erythropoiesis shifts to the liver and spleen. Fetal RBCs are anucleated and carry either fetal or adult Hb. In the latter case there is a distinct fetal pattern of glycolytic enzymes leading to alterations in the concentration of organic phosphates, compared with adult RBCs. In the late fetal period, blood formation gradually ceases in the liver and erythropoiesis in the bone marrow is initiated proportionally. The ontogenetic variations of RBC functional characteristics (covering the embryonic, fetal, and postnatal period) are considered next.

Embryonic Period

The embryonic period covers the stages of organogenesis and early organ differentiation. The end of this so-called metamorphosis is around day 60 after conception in humans and around day 14 in rabbits, day 16 in rats, and day 32 in sheep (18). The erythroid cells, which are produced by the yolk sac, synthesize embryonic Hb, which is specific for this stage of development. The types of embryonic Hb most extensively studied on a structural level are those of humans, mice, and rabbits (cf. ref. 89). In human embryos, three types of embryonic Hb have been identified: Hb Portland, Hb Gower 1, and Hb Gower 2. The structures of Hb Portland and Hb Gower 2 are $\zeta_2\gamma_2$ and $\alpha_2\epsilon_2$, respectively (97, 125, 126). Hemoglobin Gower 1 was originally thought to be a homotetramer consisting of ε-chains (ϵ_4) but was later shown to have the structure $\zeta_2\epsilon_2$ (97, 125).

Both the α-like and the β-like globin chains of the family of human embryonic, fetal, and adult Hb are encoded by a small family of genes whose organization parallels the ontogenetic sequence of gene expression. The human α-like globin gene cluster is located on chromosome 16 and has the development $5'$-ζ_2-ζ_1-Ψ_{α_2}-α_2-α_1-$3'$ (152). Because the direction of transcription starts at the 5′ side, the 5′-to-3′ organization of the genes reflects their order of expression during development. The functional globin genes coding for the embryonic α-type (ζ) globin with α_1-α_2 being their adult counterparts are ζ_1 and ζ_2; Ψ_{α_2} is an apparently nonfunctional α-like pseudogene (52). The same development-related arrangement is found with the β-like globin genes on chromosome 11 ($5'$-ϵ-γ^G-γ^A-δ-β-$3'$) (94).

The ε-gene codes for the embryonic β-type (ε) globins, which are found in Hb Gower 1 and Hb Gower 2 (97). The γ-chains of human fetal Hb are encoded by two different structural genes differing only in the presence of glycine or alanine at position 136. Shortly before birth the γ-globin chains are gradually replaced by the adult β- and δ-globin polypeptides. Whether the developmentally correlated gene arrangement plays a role in the sequential activation of globin genes is not known at present, but certain models have been developed that indicate that this particular arrangement is more than the simple consequence of gene duplication events (cf. refs. 158, 199, 249, and 252).

The erythroid cells of mouse and rabbit embryos also contain several types of embryonic Hb. They are tetramers that consist either of embryonic α- and β-type chains or of adult α- and embryonic β-type globin chains (88, 89, 162, 231).

The functional properties of human embryonic Hb Portland 1 and of mouse and rabbit embryonic Hb exhibit remarkable similarities (30, 136, 239). They have a higher O_2 affinity and a smaller Bohr effect than either human fetal Hb or the respective adult Hb (Table 5). These functional characteristics are related to the embryonic α-type chains, at least in the rabbit (136), which appear to have a much older evolutionary age than the embryonic β-type chains (162). However, studies on the O_2-binding properties of intact nucleated erythroblasts have given different results. Rabbit and rat embryonic cells have about the same low O_2 affinity as adult RBCs, which coincides with high concentrations of 2,3-DPG and ATP in these cells [Fig. 7; (104, 135)].

Conflicting results were obtained for embryonic mouse blood, where Wells (251) reported the O_2 affinity of embryonic blood to be higher than that of maternal blood, whereas Popp et al. (198) found a lower O_2 affinity in embryonic blood. Embryonic RBCs from human embryos that contained ~40% embryonic Hb and ~60% fetal Hb have the same O_2 affinity as human fetal RBCs (126).

In summary it must be said that due to the difficulties in obtaining sufficient amounts of material, the knowledge about the O_2-binding properties of blood from the earlier stages of embryonic development is scarce. The clearest results were obtained with rabbit and rat embryonic blood (Fig. 7). If any generalized deduction can be made from these studies it seems that the first O_2-transporting corpuscles that appear in the circulation of mammalian embryos have O_2-binding characteristics that would favor the unloading of O_2 from the blood.

TABLE 5. *Oxygen-Binding Parameters of Adult and Embryonic Hemoglobins*

Hemoglobin Type	P_{50}, Torr	$(\Delta \log P_{50})/\Delta pH$	Ref.
Adult human*	13.8	−0.62	239
Embryonic human (Portland)*	5.4	−0.31	239
Adult mouse	18.2	−0.48	30
Embryonic mouse	11.0	−0.36	30
Adult rabbit	10.0	−0.50	136
Embryonic rabbit (E_{I-III})	6.0	−0.25	136
Embryonic rabbit (L_{I-III})	9.1	−0.50	136

Experimental conditions: pH 7.2 and 37°C. * Values were corrected from 25°C to 37°C using a temperature coefficient of $\Delta \log P_{50}/\Delta T = 0.02$.

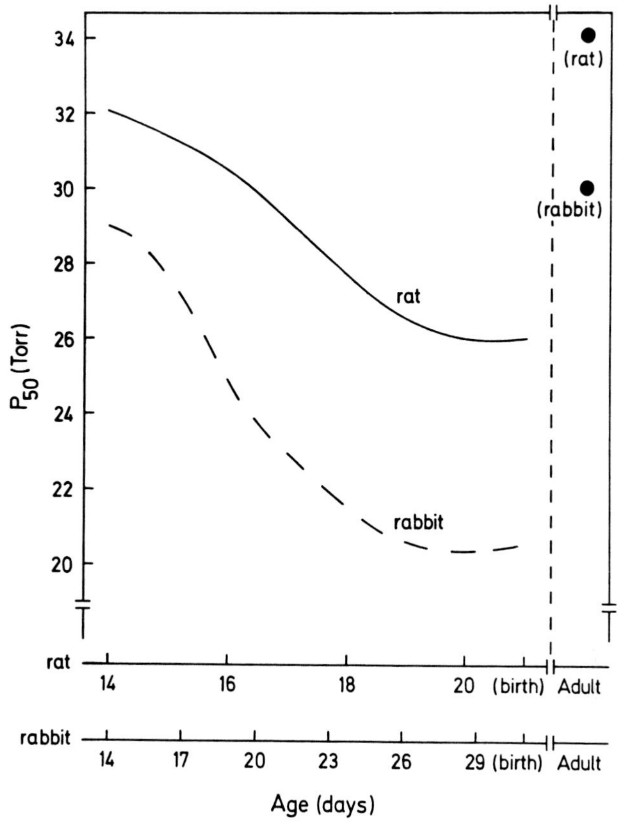

FIG. 7. Change of P_{50} of RBCs (pH 7.4, 37°C) during development of rabbit and rat embryos and fetuses. *Closed circles*, P_{50} values of adult animals. [Adapted from Jelkmann and Bauer (135) and Gilman (104).]

Fetal Period

The fetal period begins with the end of the metamorphosis and terminates with the birth of the individual. During the last third of gestation, RBCs have a higher O_2 affinity than maternal RBCs in virtually all mammalian species, although the degree of difference varies widely (18). In humans, for example, the difference in P_{50} between maternal and fetal blood is ~5 Torr. In other mammals, including ruminants and small rodents, there is a larger difference of 10–20 Torr, whereas in the domestic cat there is almost none. The higher O_2 affinity of fetal blood can be attained by three different mechanisms, two of which involve a specific fetal Hb, which has a specific β-like chain, the γ-chain, and therefore the general structure $\alpha_2\gamma_2$.

In primates and ruminants the higher O_2 affinity of fetal RBCs is related to the synthesis of a specific fetal Hb that is produced during fetal life. In the postnatal period, erythropoiesis switches from the liver and spleen to the bone marrow and the fetal Hb is gradually replaced by the adult pigment. This gradual replacement of fetal Hb by adult Hb is independent of the site of erythropoiesis (253, 254); i.e., the relative amounts of fetal and adult Hb synthesized at different stages of gestation are very similar in liver, spleen, and bone marrow. The molecular and cellular mechanisms that are involved in the process of Hb switching appear to be interrelated (cf. ref. 252), but the exact nature of the biological clock controlling the regulation of the switch has not yet been identified (173, 252). The mammalian species that possess a fetal Hb can be divided into two groups with regard to the mechanisms by which fetal blood has a high O_2 affinity. In ruminants, fetal Hb has a high intrinsic O_2 affinity and, like the adult pigment, is completely unresponsive toward 2,3-DPG (36, 51, 229). In the case of bovine fetal Hb, the high intrinsic O_2 affinity may be related to the replacement of the amino acid A12β Trp by A12γ Phe, which may lower the stability of the tertiary deoxystructure (190) and therefore increase the O_2 affinity of fetal Hb in ruminants.

On the other hand, in primates there is little difference in the intrinsic O_2 affinity of the purified fetal and adult Hb, and the higher affinity of fetal and maternal RBCs results from the decreased interaction of fetal Hb with 2,3-DPG (28, 63, 233, 242). In human fetal Hb, for example, the association constant of 2,3-DPG is smaller by a factor of 6 compared with the adult pigment (29). The reduced binding of 2,3-DPG in human fetal Hb can be explained by the replacement of a positively charged amino acid by a neutral one [β143(H21)His$\rightarrow\gamma$Ser] and furthermore by structural alterations of the binding site of 2,3-DPG in fetal Hb, which result in a poorer fit of the phosphate molecule (93).

In many mammalian species there is a direct switch from the synthesis of embryonic Hb to adult Hb; i.e., no fetal Hb is synthesized during the fetal period (148). The fetal cells of these species achieve a higher O_2 affinity by a reduced concentration of 2,3-DPG. Examples of this kind include rabbits, small rodents, dogs, horses, and pigs (cf. refs. 137 and 138). In rabbits, in four species of small rodents, and in dogs, the low concentration of 2,3-DPG in fetal RBCs was found to be secondary to a high activity of the glycolytic enzyme PK in comparison with RBCs from adult animals (50, 137, 138). In addition, rat fetal RBCs are characterized by very low activities of the enzyme bisphosphoglycerate mutase, which converts 1,3-DPG to 2,3-DPG (105, 138).

PHYSIOLOGICAL SIGNIFICANCE OF HIGH OXYGEN AFFINITY OF FETAL BLOOD. While the molecular mechanisms leading to a high O_2 affinity of fetal blood are fairly well understood, the physiological significance of the difference in O_2 affinity between maternal and fetal blood is less clear. From studies on families with hemoglobinopathies leading to a high O_2 affinity of maternal blood (68) or to human pregnancies with a low O_2 affinity of fetal blood (179) it became apparent that intrauterine survival of the fetus is not affected in such cases. What do these results indicate? Obviously the O_2 supply to the fetus is well buffered and not critically dependent on just one variable, the difference in O_2 affinity between the maternal and fetal blood. Therefore fetal survival in utero must be regarded as too crude a measure to obtain information on the biological significance that may be attached to the high O_2 affinity of fetal compared with maternal blood. It seems more promising to examine pregnancies in carriers of high-affinity Hb regarding certain physical or biochemical stigmata at birth, such as reduced weight, polycythemia, or cardiomegaly, and also placental alterations such as hypervascularity (68). In fact, two independent studies have shown that an experimentally induced increase of O_2 affinity of pregnant rats leads to a significant reduction of the fetal birth weight and also to fetal polycythemia (26, 118). These data support the findings obtained in sheep fetuses where replacement of fetal blood by adult blood led to fetal hypoxia, as indicated by an increased reticulocyte count (23). In view of these results it is to be expected that an abolishment of the fetal-maternal O_2-affinity difference is associated with a significant decrease of birth weight in human newborns and changes in other important parameters.

Postnatal Period

In most mammals the O_2 affinity of blood decreases rapidly after birth (cf. ref. 18). In those species where fetal Hb is synthesized the decrease of the percentage of fetal Hb after birth is correlated with an increase in P_{50}. Such an inverse relationship between the percentage of fetal Hb in the RBC and P_{50} after birth has been described for humans (39, 78), goats (51, 184), and sheep (36, 51). The molecular and cellular events that may be associated with the switch in synthesis from fetal to adult Hb have been recently reviewed by Wood and Jones (252). In species without fetal Hb the decrease in blood O_2 affinity is secondary to an increase in the concentration of 2,3-DPG. This has been found in horses (65), pigs (38), dogs (79, 168), mice (196), and rabbits (135). In two of these species, rabbits (135) and dogs (50), the low concentrations of 2,3-DPG are secondary to a fall in PK activity. In RBCs from rats an additional increase in bisphosphoglycerate mutase activity has been found to occur postnatally (105, 138). Evidence was presented in these studies to show that there is a changeover from a fetal RBC type to an adult RBC type that is characterized by high concentrations of 2,3-DPG, high activity of bisphosphoglycerate mutase, and low PK activity (105, 138). This change is therefore similar to the switch in biosynthesis of fetal Hb to adult Hb that occurs in humans and certain other mammals.

EFFECTS OF HYPOXIC HYPOXIA

Animals Residing at High Altitude

Since 1936 it has been known that the blood O_2 affinity of animals residing at high altitude is generally higher than that of lowland species of similar size (113). This pattern has been observed in amphibians, mammals, and birds (21, 113, 128, 197). The molecular mechanism that leads to the high O_2 affinity of animals normally living under conditions of high altitude has been investigated in the llama (*Lama glama*) and the bar-headed goose (*Anser indicus*). Under standard conditions (pH 7.4, 37°C) llama blood has a P_{50} of ~22 Torr compared with 27 Torr in human blood. This difference is due to a reduced interaction of the allosteric cofactor 2,3-DPG with llama Hb compared with human Hb, which in turn is related to an amino acid exchange at the 2,3-DPG binding site in llama Hb, where β_2 His is replaced by asparagine (29).

A completely different molecular strategy is found in the bar-headed goose (*Anser indicus*), which breeds in the highlands of Central Asia at ~4,000 m. Its blood O_2 affinity is much higher than that of its lowland relatives, the greylag goose (*Anser anser*) and the Canada goose (*Branta canadensis*). At pH 7.4 the blood P_{50} of the bar-headed goose is 12–14 Torr less than that of the greylag and Canada goose (49, 197). It is noteworthy that the intraerythrocytic concentration of the major phosphate compound (IPP) in avian RBCs is quite similar in all three species (197). A detailed analysis of the functional properties of Hb from the bar-headed and greylag goose in the absence and presence of IPP revealed that its binding constant to the respective Hb is very similar in magnitude (209). There is a small difference in P_{50} of phosphate-free Hb from the bar-headed and greylag goose amounting to 1.3 Torr. Because the interaction between IPP and Hb is virtually identical in the two species, addition of IPP leads to a similar increase in P_{50} so that in the presence of IPP the P_{50} of the Hb from the bar-headed goose is 13 Torr less than that of the Hb from the greylag goose (209). This figure is in good agreement with that obtained with whole blood (49, 197).

The physiological significance of a high O_2 affinity in the tolerance of severe hypoxic hypoxia has been established by several investigators. Llamas, for example, can tolerate a reduction of barometric pressure to 335 Torr without any sign of discomfort, whereas sheep with a P_{50} of ~40 Torr show marked cyanosis and hyperventilation at the same barometric pressure (17).

Similarly, rodents with a left-shifted O_2-binding curve have been shown to survive much longer at severe hypoxia than those with a normally positioned O_2-binding curve (85, 112, 185). This increased tolerance toward hypoxic hypoxia in animals with a high blood O_2 affinity is probably related to the fact that they can maintain a high cardiac output even at very low P_{O_2} (75, 241). Under such conditions the P_{O_2} in the tissue of the cardiac muscle may be so low that the position of the O_2-binding curve no longer determines the unloading capacity of the blood. Instead it must be the higher arterial O_2 content of the blood in animals with a high O_2 affinity (17, 49, 75, 240) that limits the O_2 supply to the cardiac muscle. It is interesting to note that humans with a high blood O_2 affinity due to an abnormal Hb showed no significant decrement in maximum O_2 consumption compared with normal controls with elevation to 3,100 m (119). Therefore this result indicates that a left-shifted O_2-binding curve may confer an advantage even at moderately high altitude in humans.

Natives at High Altitude

The ancestors of South American Indians and Sherpas in Tibet and Nepal may have been living for centuries or even millenia at altitudes of 4,000–5,000 m. In Indian natives a P_{50} of ~30 Torr was repeatedly reported (156, 157, 238). The lower O_2 affinity of the blood from Indian natives relative to sea-level dwellers appears to be secondary to an increase in the intraerythrocytic concentration of 2,3-DPG, which amounts to ~6 mmol 2,3-DPG/liter RBC in Indian natives as compared with 5 mmol 2,3-DPG/liter RBC found in sea-level residents. In Sherpas from Nepal permanently living at elevations of ~4,000 m, a very high blood O_2 affinity has been reported (167). However, later studies in which the time lapse between blood sampling and analysis of the O_2-binding properties of the blood was kept reasonably short did not show any significant difference in P_{50} between acclimatized lowlanders and Sherpas living at high altitude (220). It should be pointed out in this connection that all P_{50} values measured by the various investigators are related to standard conditions, i.e., pH 7.4, P_{CO_2} = 40 Torr, and 37°C. Under conditions of high altitude, however, hypocapnia and an incompletely compensated respiratory alkalosis have to be considered. These two effects counteract the influence of the increased concentration of 2,3-DPG. Therefore under in vivo conditions the blood O_2 affinity of humans living permanently at high altitude would not be expected to differ significantly from that found at sea level.

Sojourners at High Altitude

The necessity of considering the in vivo conditions of the blood with respect to pH and P_{CO_2} becomes particularly important during the acute phase of adaptation to high altitude. Rørth et al. (212) have shown that during the first 24 h of exposure to a lowered P_{O_2}, the P_{50}, when related to the actual pH and P_{CO_2}, is decreased; i.e., there is an increase in the RBC affinity for O_2 in vivo. At the end of the 24-h period after exposure to low P_{O_2}, the in vivo P_{50} is normalized, despite an increase in pH and a decrease in P_{CO_2}. This change in O_2 affinity is due to a gradual accumulation of 2,3-DPG in RBCs, which others have also observed (155, 156, 170). Note that the degree of muscular exercise appears to influence the rise in 2,3-DPG concentration, possibly by an increased influx of oxidants, such as pyruvate, in the RBC (212). With the assumption that the degree of muscular activity determines the availability of pyruvate to the human RBC and therefore the accumulation of 2,3-DPG, it seems possible that the lack of influence of high altitude on P_{50} in humans, which Weiskopf and Severinghaus (250) reported, is due to this phenomenon. If rats and guinea pigs are exposed to acute and chronic hypoxic hypoxia, there is an increase in both P_{50} and the concentration of 2,3-DPG that is more pronounced during the acute phase of adaptation (34). The fall of the 2,3-DPG concentration in the chronic experiments may be due to a compensation of the respiratory alkalosis, which in turn will decrease the net synthesis of 2,3-DPG (84, 212).

KINETICS OF OXYGEN BINDING AND DISSOCIATION

The Adair model (2) can be used to illustrate the reaction of Hb with O_2, with four equilibrium steps that have four "on" and four "off" reactions.

$$Hb_4 + O_2 \underset{k_1}{\overset{k_1'}{\rightleftharpoons}} Hb_4O_2 \qquad K_1 = k_1'/k_1$$

$$Hb_4O_2 + O_2 \underset{k_2}{\overset{k_2'}{\rightleftharpoons}} Hb_4(O_2)_2 \qquad K_2 = k_2'/k_2$$

$$Hb_4(O_2)_2 + O_2 \underset{k_3}{\overset{k_3'}{\rightleftharpoons}} Hb_4(O_2)_3 \qquad K_3 = k_3'/k_3$$

$$Hb_4(O_2)_3 + O_2 \underset{k_4}{\overset{k_4'}{\rightleftharpoons}} Hb_4(O_2)_4 \qquad K_4 = k_4'/k_4$$

This model might not be considered adequate because it does not allow for possible differences between the functional properties of α- and β-chains nor does it carry any structural information. However, from a phenomenological point of view it is useful as a framework for a discussion of the essential features of the Hb reaction.

Combination and Dissociation Velocity of the First and Last Oxygen-Binding Step

The binding of the first O_2 molecule to deoxygenated Hb appears to be a very rapid process. In fact, the apparent combination rate constant (k_1') is 4×10^7 $mol^{-1} \cdot s^{-1}$ (129), which is ~10 times larger than the apparent rate constant of overall O_2 binding. Therefore the low O_2 affinity of deoxygenated human Hb (190) must be due to a very high dissociation rate of O_2 of the singly liganded tetramer. The values for k_1 that have been determined experimentally are ~1,000 s^{-1} (101, 129). This high value for k_1 was attributed to only one pair of chains, provisionally identified as the β-chains (102). However, α- and β-chains appear to have very similar O_2 affinities, at least in the absence of organic phosphates (151), so that a chain heterogeneity with respect to k_1 should be associated with a similar heterogeneity with respect to k_1'.

The last O_2-binding step also has a high recombination rate constant (k_4') of 3–5 $\times 10^7$ $mol^{-1} \cdot s^{-1}$ (59, 101, 129, 160), which is therefore similar in magnitude to the first O_2-binding step, k_1'. Because the rate of dissociation of the first O_2 molecule from fully liganded Hb, k_4, is smaller by a factor of 50–100 (101, 129, 161) compared with k_1, ranging from 10 to 20 s^{-1}, it can easily be seen that the very high O_2 affinity of fully liganded Hb is due to a dramatic reduction of the dissociation velocity constant if the Hb molecule assumes the oxystructure. It is interesting that k_4 of human Hb is much less affected by pH (183) and 2,3-DPG (219) than are k_1, k_2, and k_3. This implies that these allosteric modifiers are probably released from Hb after binding of the third O_2 molecule.

Overall Rates of Oxygen Association and Dissociation in Hemoglobin Solutions

As mentioned in the previous section, the overall association rate is ~10 times smaller than the combination rate of the first and last O_2 molecules that bind to tetrameric Hb. Therefore the rate-determining step in the O_2-binding reaction must be attributed to intermediate O_2-binding steps (129). One question that has attracted the attention of several workers involves the kinetic basis for the effects of organic phosphates, notably 2,3-DPG, and H^+ on the O_2 affinity of Hb. In the first papers that dealt with the reactions of O_2 and Hb, Hartridge and Roughton (115, 116) stated that it is mainly the overall dissociation velocity that increases with increasing acidity. However, later it was demonstrated that an increase in H^+ activity not only increases the overall dissociation rate but also decreases the overall association rate (27). Likewise the effect of 2,3-DPG on the O_2 affinity of Hb is due to effects on both the association and the dissociation velocity (27), which is not true for inorganic phosphates, where only k_1, k_2, and k_3 are affected (101) but not the corresponding association rate constants.

Comparison of Oxygen Combination and Dissociation Velocity in Hemoglobin Solutions and Red Blood Cells

Of particular interest is the comparison of the rate of O_2 uptake of Hb in solution and in the RBC under physiological conditions, i.e., 37°C and pH 7.1–7.2. Gibson and co-workers (103) measured the overall rate of O_2 uptake under these conditions and found a mean value of ~3.2 $\times 10^6$ $mol^{-1} \cdot s^{-1}$ in a dilute Hb solution. These authors and later Roughton (216) and Sirs and Roughton (228) also noted that the initial rate of the combination of O_2 with deoxygenated RBCs is ~30 times smaller than the association reaction measured in a dilute Hb solution. Three possibilities may be considered that could explain this large difference between the combination velocity of RBCs and dilute Hb solutions. *1*) The O_2-binding properties of Hb are altered by the presence of intraerythrocytic cofactors such as 2,3-DPG. *2*) The RBC membrane offers an appreciable diffusion resistance. *3*) There is an unstirred layer of solvent adjacent to the RBC surface that acts as a diffusion barrier.

The first possibility can be safely excluded as a cause for the observed difference because even high concentrations of 2,3-DPG decrease the overall velocity constant only by a factor of 2 (27). The same conclusion has been reached by Coin and Olson (73), who positively demonstrated that a slow chemical reaction cannot account for the low rate of O_2 uptake observed experimentally. The second possibility can be excluded because the RBC membrane seems to offer little or no resistance to O_2 diffusion (149). Furthermore, if the diffusion of Hb inside the RBC is taken into account, Moll (165) was able to simulate closely the experimentally determined time course of the deoxygenation reaction of oxygenated RBCs in the presence of sodium dithionite (153). Under these experimental conditions the O_2 concentration at the surface of the RBC is virtually zero. Therefore the result of the computations performed by Moll (165) also argues against a membrane resistance for the release of O_2 from RBCs. Note, however, that this interpretation is only valid if it is assumed that the RBC membrane is impermeable to the dithionite anion. Coin and Olson (73) have actually shown that this is not the case but instead found that the rate of diffusion of dithionite through the RBC membrane is much too slow to influence the time course of the O_2 efflux. Regarding the third possibility, when the appropriate diffusion coefficients for Hb and O_2 in the RBC interior are employed, the calculated half time for the rate of combination of O_2 with deoxygenated RBCs is still ~3–5 times smaller than that observed with rapid-mixing experiments (73, 92, 172, 216). This discrepancy is in all likelihood due to the presence of an unstirred layer of solvent adjacent to the RBC surface (76).

Unstirred layers form within 2–3 ms after mixing, thus creating an external diffusion barrier that is 2–4 μm thick, depending on the experimental conditions (73, 96, 207, 235). This external diffusion resistance is large enough to quantitatively account for the time course of the O_2 uptake by deoxygenated RBCs measured in rapid-mixing experiments. Plasma layers ~2 μm thick have been observed by Miyamoto and Moll (164) in the capillaries of rapidly frozen lungs in situ. Therefore it seems reasonable to conclude that such solvent layers may slow gas exchange significantly not only in the rapid-mixing apparatus but also in the living organism.

PATHOLOGICAL HEMOGLOBINS

More than 200 variants of human Hb have been found that show changes in their primary structure (cf. ref. 64). The large majority of these show a substitution only at one site, due to a point mutation. From a physiological point of view those Hb variants with changes in their O_2 affinity are the most interesting, because they allow an estimate of the limits within which Hb-O_2 affinity can be altered without the need for compensatory mechanisms.

Hemoglobins With Altered Oxygen Affinity

Surveys of the existing literature show that ~90 types of abnormal Hb have been identified with changes in their O_2-binding characteristics (41, 64, 141). The majority of these are high-affinity variants. They show substitutions either in intersubunit contact regions or in those regions that are important for the binding of allosteric effectors, such as the central cavity.

The lowest P_{50} value that has been recorded in human whole blood is ~11 Torr (139), which is comparable to the P_{50} value for normal human Hb in the absence of 2,3-DPG and CO_2. The increase in O_2 capacity observed in the carriers of high-affinity Hb obviously fully compensates for the loss in O_2 release capacity due to the shift in O_2 affinity (41, 141).

It should be noted that in almost any case of high-affinity Hb the cooperativity of O_2 binding is drastically reduced (64, 141). Thus Hb Syracuse, for which the P_{50} value of 11 Torr has been reported (139), has an *n* value of 1.1; i.e., the cooperativity of O_2 binding is nearly abolished. Similar observations have been made for the high-affinity variants, Hb Rainier and Hb Bethesda (3, 62). Bellingham (40) has pointed out that the large decrease of cooperativity observed with many types of high-affinity Hb obviously presents an advantage, because with a low cooperativity, O_2 unloading occurs more rapidly than with normal cooperativity.

Because of the reduced cooperativity the increase in circulating Hb is less than would be necessary for high-affinity mutants with normal cooperativity. The Hb values recorded for high-affinity variants are in the range of 17–23 g/100 ml blood and the hematocrit values recorded do not exceed 60%.

Clinical studies show that carriers of the high-affinity Hb are apparently not hindered in their normal physical activity, although they are probably reduced in their maximum work capacity (182). This finding corroborates the notion that the combination of low cooperativity and high O_2 capacity results in practically normal O_2 delivery at physiological arterial and venous O_2 tensions.

Out of the small number of low-affinity variants observed, the most extensively investigated is probably Hb Kansas (57, 204). Here the O_2 affinity (P_{50} ~

70 Torr) is so low that at the normal arterial O_2 pressure the blood is only saturated to ~75%, which gives rise to clinically visible cyanosis. Under these conditions a normal O_2 capacity has to be kept to provide sufficient tissue oxygenation at rest. In other low-affinity variants with less pronounced decreases in O_2 affinity, a mild anemia has been observed, which is explained by the improved O_2-delivery properties of the system, which in turn, through a feedback loop, effect the release of the erythropoietin from the kidney (230). Thus Hb Seattle (P_{50} = 40.5) only has an O_2 capacity of 13.2 ml O_2/100 ml blood (230). However, because some types of low-affinity Hb are also slightly more unstable than normal human Hb, anemia might also result as the consequence of the molecular instability rather than of the low O_2 affinity.

The fact that fewer low-affinity than high-affinity variants have been reported is probably associated with the absence of clinical symptoms in the latter case. Whereas in the high-affinity variants the increase in circulating RBC mass is the leading symptom, low-affinity variants associated with no further instability are only characterized by a slightly decreased Hb concentration that could be diagnosed as mild anemia.

The study of abnormal Hb has added quite substantially to the understanding of Hb function, because in many cases the results of a single substitution dramatically alter the functional characteristics of the molecule. One of the many interesting results is that the cooperativity of O_2 binding and the Bohr effect are relatively independent of each other. Thus in many high-affinity variants that are characterized by a nearly absent cooperativity the alkaline Bohr effect has been reported to be normal or only slightly reduced (41, 64, 141). This illustrates the point made in the discussion of the Bohr effect (see *Protons*, p. 150) that the release of protons during ligand binding must largely be associated with tertiary structure alterations rather than with quaternary transition.

Another fact that emerges from the study of high-affinity Hb is that the normal cooperativity found in mammalian Hb apparently is beneficial only under conditions where the O_2 affinity is shifted into the physiological region. On the other hand, because it has been shown that in the absence of allosteric effectors the O_2 affinity of many types of Hb with normal cooperativity is very high, it follows that the development of cooperativity and the binding sites for the various allosteric effectors must have occurred more or less simultaneously, because otherwise the physiological advantage of such an Hb would have been questionable.

Christian Bauer's present address is Physiologisches Institut Universität, Zurich, Switzerland.

REFERENCES

1. ACKERS, G. K., M. L. JOHNSON, F. C. MILLS, R. HALVORSEN, AND S. SHAPIRO. The linkage between oxygenation and subunit dissociation in human hemoglobin. Consequences for the analysis of oxygenation curves. *Biochemistry* 14: 5128–5134, 1975.
2. ADAIR, G. S. The hemoglobin system. VI. The oxygen dissociation curve of hemoglobin. *J. Biol. Chem.* 63: 529–545, 1925.
3. ADAMSON, J. W., J. T. PARER, AND G. STAMATOYANNOPOULOS. Erythrocytosis associated with hemoglobin Rainier: oxygen equilibria and marrow regulation. *J. Clin. Invest.* 48: 1376–1386, 1969.
4. ANTONINI, E., AND M. BRUNORI. *Hemoglobin and Myoglobin in Their Reactions With Ligands.* Amsterdam: North-Holland, 1971.
5. ANTONINI, E., T. M. SCHUSTER, M. BRUNORI, AND J. WYMAN. The kinetics of the Bohr effect in the reaction of human hemoglobin with carbon monoxide. *J. Biol. Chem.* 240: 2262–2264, 1965.
6. ARNONE, A. X-ray diffraction study of binding of 2,3-diphosphoglycerate to human deoxyhaemoglobin. *Nature Lond.* 237: 146–149, 1972.
7. ARNONE, A. X-ray studies of the interaction of CO_2 with human deoxyhaemoglobin. *Nature Lond.* 247: 143–144, 1974.
8. ARNONE, A., R. E. BENESCH, AND R. BENESCH. Structure of human deoxyhemoglobin specifically modified from pyridoxal compounds. *J. Mol. Biol.* 115: 627–642, 1977.
9. ARNONE, A., AND M. F. PERUTZ. Structure of inositol hexaphosphate–human deoxyhemoglobin complex. *Nature Lond.* 249: 34–36, 1974.
10. ASAKURA, T., AND P.-W. LAU. Sequence of oxygen binding by hemoglobin. *Proc. Natl. Acad. Sci. USA* 75: 5462–5465, 1978.
11. ASTRUP, P., K. ENGEL, J. W. SEVERINGHAUS, AND E. MUNSON. The influence of temperature and pH on the dissociation curve of oxyhemoglobin of human blood. *Scand. J. Clin. Lab. Invest.* 17: 515–523, 1965.
12. ATHA, D. H., M. L. JOHNSON, AND A. F. RIGGS. The linkage between oxygenation and subunit association in human hemoglobin Kansas. Concentration dependence of the oxygen binding equilibria. *J. Biol. Chem.* 254: 12390–12398, 1979.
13. BAILEY, J. E., J. G. BEETLESTONE, AND D. H. IRVINE. Reactivity differences between hemoglobins. XVII. The variability of the Bohr effect between species and the effect of 2,3-diphosphoglyceric acid on the Bohr effect. *J. Chem. Soc. A* 5: 756–762, 1970.
14. BALDWIN, J. M. Structure and function of haemoglobin. *Prog. Biophys. Mol. Biol.* 29: 225–320, 1975.
15. BALDWIN, J. M. The structure of human carbonmonoxy hemoglobin at 2.7 Å resolution. *J. Mol. Biol.* 136: 103–128, 1980.
16. BALDWIN, J. M., AND C. CHOTHIA. Hemoglobin: the structural changes related to ligand binding and its allosteric mechanism. *J. Mol. Biol.* 129: 175–220, 1979.
17. BANCHERO, N., AND R. F. GROVER. Effect of different levels of simulated altitude on O_2 transport in llama and sheep. *Am. J. Physiol.* 222: 1239–1245, 1972.
18. BARTELS, H. *Prenatal Respiration.* Amsterdam: North-Holland, 1970.
19. BARTELS, H., R. BARTELS, R. BAUMANN, R. FONS, K.-D. JÜRGENS, AND P. WRIGHT. Blood oxygen transport and organ weights of two shrew species (*S. etruscus* and *C. russula*). *Am. J. Physiol.* 236 (*Regulatory Integrative Comp. Physiol.* 5): R221–R224, 1979.
20. BARTELS, H., AND H. HARMS. Sauerstoffdissociationskurven des Blutes von Säugetieren. *Pfluegers Arch.* 268: 334–365, 1959.
21. BARTELS, H., P. HILPERT, K. BARBEY, K. BETKE, K. RIEGEL, E. M. LANG, AND J. METCALFE. Respiratory functions of blood of the yak, llama, camel, Dybowski deer, and African elephant.

Am. J. Physiol. 205: 331–336, 1963.

22. Bartlett, G. R. Phosphate compounds in red cells of reptiles, amphibians and fish. *Comp. Biochem. Physiol. A Comp. Physiol.* 55: 211–214, 1976.
23. Battaglia, F. C., W. Bowes, H. R. McGaughey, E. L. Makowski, and G. Meschia. The effect of fetal exchange transfusions with adult blood upon fetal oxygenation. *Pediatr. Res.* 3: 60–65, 1969.
24. Bauer, C. Reduction of the carbon dioxide affinity of human haemoglobin solutions by 2,3-diphosphoglycerate. *Respir. Physiol.* 10: 10–19, 1970.
25. Bauer, C., R. Baumann, U. Engels, and B. Pacyna. The carbon dioxide affinity of various human hemoglobins. *J. Biol. Chem.* 250: 2173–2176, 1975.
26. Bauer, C., W. Jelkmann, and W. Moll. High oxygen affinity of maternal blood reduces fetal weight in rats. *Respir. Physiol.* 43: 169–178, 1981.
27. Bauer, C., R. A. Klocke, D. Kamp, and R. E. Forster. Effect of 2,3-diphosphoglycerate and H^+ on the reaction of O_2 and hemoglobin. *Am. J. Physiol.* 224: 838–847, 1973.
28. Bauer, C., I. Ludwig, and M. Ludwig. Different effects of 2,3-diphosphoglycerate and adenosine triphosphate on the oxygen affinity of adult and foetal haemoglobin. *Life Sci.* 7: 1339–1343, 1968.
29. Bauer, C., H. S. Rollema, H. W. Till, and G. Braunitzer. Phosphate binding by llama and camel hemoglobin. *J. Comp. Physiol.* 136: 67–70, 1980.
30. Bauer, C., R. Tamm, D. Petschow, R. Bartels, and H. Bartels. Oxygen affinity and allosteric effects of embryonic mouse haemoglobins. *Nature Lond.* 257: 333–334, 1975.
31. Baumann, F. H., and R. Baumann. A comparative study of the respiratory properties of bird blood. *Respir. Physiol.* 31: 333–343, 1977.
32. Baumann, R. Effect of CO_2 binding to hemoglobin on the reactivity of the SH groups at position β93. *Biochem. Biophys. Res. Commun.* 61: 845–851, 1974.
33. Baumann, R. Interaction between hemoglobins, CO_2 and anions. In: *Biophysics and Physiology of Carbon Dioxide*, edited by C. Bauer, G. Gros, and H. Bartels. Berlin: Springer-Verlag, 1980, p. 114–121.
34. Baumann, R., C. Bauer, and H. Bartels. Influence of chronic and acute hypoxia on oxygen affinity and red cell 2,3-diphosphoglycerate of rats and guinea pigs. *Respir. Physiol.* 11: 135–144, 1971.
35. Baumann, R., C. Bauer, and E. A. Haller. Oxygen-linked CO_2 transport in sheep blood. *Am. J. Physiol.* 229: 334–339, 1975.
36. Baumann, R., C. Bauer, and A. M. Rathschlag-Schaefer. Causes of the postnatal decrease of blood oxygen affinity in lambs. *Respir. Physiol.* 15: 151–158, 1972.
37. Baumann, R., and E. A. Haller. Cat hemoglobin A and B: differences in the interaction with Cl^-, phosphate, and CO_2. *Biochem. Biophys. Res. Commun.* 65: 220–227, 1975.
38. Baumann, R., F. Teischel, R. Zoch, and H. Bartels. Changes in red cell 2,3-diphosphoglycerate concentration as cause of the postnatal decrease of pig blood oxygen affinity. *Respir. Physiol.* 19: 153–161, 1973.
39. Beer, R., E. Doll, and J. Wenner. Die Verschiebung der Sauerstoffdissoziationskurve des Blutes von Säuglingen während der ersten Lebensmonate. *Pfluegers Arch.* 265: 526–540, 1958.
40. Bellingham, A. J. The physiological significance of the Hill parameter "n." *Scand. J. Haematol.* 9: 552–556, 1972.
41. Bellingham, A. J. Haemoglobins with altered oxygen affinity. *Br. Med. Bull.* 32: 234–238, 1976.
42. Benesch, R., and R. E. Benesch. The effect of organic phosphates from the human erythrocyte on the allosteric properties of human hemoglobin. *Biochem. Biophys. Res. Commun.* 26: 162–167, 1967.
43. Benesch, R., R. E. Benesch, and C. I. Yu. Reciprocal binding of oxygen and diphosphoglycerate by human hemoglobin. *Proc. Natl. Acad. Sci. USA* 59: 526–532, 1968.
44. Benesch, R., G. MacDuff, and R. E. Benesch. Determination of oxygen equilibria with a versatile new tonometer. *Anal. Biochem.* 11: 81–87, 1965.
45. Benesch, R. E., R. Benesch, R. D. Renthal, and N. Maeda. Affinity labeling of the polyphosphate binding site of hemoglobin. *Biochemistry* 11: 3576–3582, 1972.
46. Benesch, R. E., R. Benesch, and C. I. Yu. The oxygenation of hemoglobin in the presence of 2,3-diphosphoglycerate. Effect of temperature, pH, ionic strength, and hemoglobin concentration. *Biochemistry* 8: 2567–2571, 1969.
47. Benesch, R. E., R. Edalji, and R. Benesch. Reciprocal interaction of hemoglobin with oxygen and protons. The influence of allosteric polyanions. *Biochemistry* 16: 2594–2597, 1977.
48. Benesch, R. E., and H. Rubin. Interaction of hemoglobin with three ligands: organic phosphates and the Bohr effect. *Proc. Natl. Acad. Sci. USA* 72: 2465–2467, 1975.
49. Black, C. P., and S. M. Tenney. Oxygen transport during progressive hypoxia in high-altitude and sea-level waterfowl. *Respir. Physiol.* 39: 217–239, 1980.
50. Black, J. A., and P. A. Mueggler. Molecular changes which contribute to canine postnatal anemia. *Acta Biol. Med. Ger.* 40: 645–651, 1981.
51. Blunt, M. H., J. L. Kitchens, S. M. Mayson, and T. H. Huisman. Red cell 2,3-diphosphoglycerate and oxygen affinity in newborn goats and sheep. *Proc. Soc. Exp. Biol. Med.* 138: 800–803, 1971.
52. Bohr, C. Theoretische Behandlung der quantitativen Verhältnisse bei der Sauerstoffaufnahme der Hemoglobins. *Zentralbl. Physiol.* 17: 682–691, 1903.
53. Bohr, C., K. Hasselbalch, and A. Krogh. Über einen in biologischer Beziehung wichtigen Einfluβ, den die Kohlensäurespannung des Blutes auf dessen Sauerstoffspannung ausübt. *Scand. Arch. Physiol.* 16: 402–412, 1904.
54. Bonaventura, C., and J. Bonaventura. Competition in oxygen-linked anion binding to normal and variant human hemoglobins. *Hemoglobin* 4: 275–289, 1980.
55. Bonaventura, J., C. Bonaventura, G. Amiconi, L. Tentori, M. Brunori, and E. Antonini. Allosteric interactions in non-alpha chains isolated from normal human hemoglobin, fetal hemoglobin, and hemoglobin Abbruzzo. *J. Biol. Chem.* 250: 6278–6281, 1975.
56. Bonaventura, J., C. Bonaventura, B. Sullivan, G. Ferruzzi, P. R. McCurdy, J. Fox, and W. F. Moo-Penn. Hemoglobin Providence. Functional consequences of two alterations of the 2,3-diphosphoglycerate binding site at position β82. *J. Biol. Chem.* 251: 7563–7571, 1976.
57. Bonaventura, J., and A. Riggs. Hemoglobin Kansas, a human hemoglobin with a neutral amino acid substitution and an abnormal oxygen equilibrium. *J. Biol. Chem.* 243: 980–981, 1968.
58. Briehl, R., and J. F. Hobbs. Ultraviolet difference spectra in hemoglobin. I. Difference spectra in hemoglobin A and their relation to the function of hemoglobin. *J. Biol. Chem.* 245: 544–554, 1970.
59. Brunori, M., and E. Antonini. Kinetics of the reaction with oxygen of mixtures of oxy- and carbon monoxide hemoglobin. *J. Biol. Chem.* 247: 4305–4308, 1972.
60. Brygier, J., S. H. De Bruin, M. K. B. Peter, and H. S. Rollema. The interaction of organic phosphates with human and chicken hemoglobin. *Eur. J. Biochem.* 60: 379–383, 1975.
61. Bunn, H. F. Differences in the interaction of 2,3-diphosphoglycerate with certain mammalian hemoglobins. *Science Wash. DC* 172: 1049–1050, 1971.
62. Bunn, H. F., T. B. Bradley, W. E. Davis, J. W. Drysdale, J. F. Burke, W. S. Beck, and M. B. Laver. Structural and functional studies on hemoglobin Bethesda ($\alpha_2\beta_2^{145\ His}$), a variant associated with compensatory erythrocytosis. *J. Clin. Invest.* 51: 2299–2309, 1972.
63. Bunn, H. F., and R. W. Briehl. The interaction of 2,3-

diphosphoglycerate with various human hemoglobins. *J. Clin. Invest.* 49: 1088–1095, 1970.
64. BUNN, H. F., B. G. FORGET, AND H. M. RANNEY. *Human Hemoglobins.* Philadelphia, PA: Saunders, 1977.
65. BUNN, H. F., AND H. KITCHEN. Hemoglobin function in the horse: the role of 2,3-diphosphoglycerate in modifying the oxygen affinity of maternal and fetal blood. *Blood* 42: 471–479, 1973.
66. BURSAUX, E., A. FREMINET, AND C. POYART. Effects of CO_2 and diphosphoglycerate on foetal blood affinity for oxygen. *Respir. Physiol.* 20: 181–189, 1974.
67. CHANUTIN, A., AND R. R. CURNISH. Effect of organic and inorganic phosphate on the oxygen equilibrium of human erythrocytes. *Arch. Biochem. Biophys.* 121: 96–102, 1967.
68. CHARACHE, S., AND E. A. MURPHY. Is placental oxygen transport normal in carriers of high affinity hemoglobins? In: *Molecular Interactions of Hemoglobin,* edited by D. Labie, C. Poyart, and J. Rosa. Paris: INSERM, 1978, p. 285–294.
69. CHASSIN, S. L., W. C. KRUCKEBERG, AND G. J. BREWER. Thermal inactivation differences of phosphofructokinase in erythrocytes from genetically selected high and low DPG rat strains. *Biochem. Biophys. Res. Commun.* 83: 1306–1311, 1978.
70. CHIANCONE, E., J.-E. NORNE, S. FORSÉN, J. BONAVENTURA, M. BRUNORI, E. ANTONINI, AND J. WYMAN. Identification of chloride-binding sites in hemoglobin by nuclear-magnetic-resonance quadrupole-relaxation studies of hemoglobin digests. *Eur. J. Biochem.* 55: 385–390, 1975.
71. CHIANCONE, E., J.-E. NORNE, S. FORSÉN, A. MANSOURI, AND K. H. WINTERHALTER. Anion binding to proteins. NMR quadrupole relaxation study of chloride binding to various human hemoglobins. *FEBS Lett.* 63: 309–312, 1976.
72. CHRISTIANSEN, J., C. G. DOUGLAS, AND J. S. HALDANE. The absorption and dissociation of carbon dioxide by human blood. *J. Physiol. Lond.* 48: 244–271, 1914.
73. COIN, J. T., AND J. S. OLSON. The rate of oxygen uptake by human red blood cells. *J. Biol. Chem.* 254: 1178–1190, 1979.
74. DAHMS, T., S. M. HORVATH, M. LUZZANA, L. ROSSI-BERNARDI, F. J. W. ROUGHTON, AND G. STELLA. The regulation of oxygen affinity of human haemoglobin (Abstract). *J. Physiol. Lond.* 223: 29P–31P, 1972.
75. DAWSON, T. J., AND J. V. EVANS. Effect of hypoxia on oxygen transport in sheep with different hemoglobin types. *Am. J. Physiol.* 210: 1021–1025, 1966.
76. DAYHOFF, M. O. *Atlas of Protein Sequence and Structure.* Washington, DC: Natl. Biomed. Res. Found., 1975.
77. DE BRUIN, S. H., AND L. H. M. JANSSEN. The interaction of 2,3-diphosphoglycerate with human hemoglobin. Effects on the alkaline and acid Bohr effect. *J. Biol. Chem.* 248: 2774–2777, 1973.
78. DELIVORIA-PAPADOPOULOS, M., N. P. RONCEVIC, AND F. A. OSKI. Postnatal changes in oxygen transport of term, premature and sick infants. The role of red cell 2,3-diphosphoglycerate and adult hemoglobin. *Pediatr. Res.* 5: 235–245, 1971.
79. DHINDSA, D. S., A. S. HOVERSLAND, AND J. W. TEMPLETON. Postnatal changes in oxygen affinity and concentrations of 2,3-diphosphoglycerate in dog blood. *Biol. Neonat.* 20: 226–235, 1972.
80. DOLMAN, D., AND S. J. GILL. Membrane-covered thin-layer optical cell for gas-reaction studies of hemoglobin. *Anal. Biochem.* 87: 127–134, 1978.
81. DUHM, J. Effects of 2,3-diphosphoglycerate and other organic phosphate compounds on oxygen affinity and intracellular pH of human erythrocytes. *Pfluegers Arch.* 326: 341–356, 1971.
82. DUHM, J., AND E. GERLACH. On the mechanisms of the hypoxia-induced increase of 2,3-diphosphoglycerate in erythrocytes. Studies on rat erythrocytes in vivo and on human erythrocytes in vitro. *Pfluegers Arch.* 326: 254–269, 1971.
83. DUHM, J., AND H. D. KIM. Effect of the rapid postnatal increase of 2,3-diphosphoglycerate concentration in erythrocytes on the oxygen affinity of pig blood. In: *Erythrocytes, Thrombocytes, Leukocytes. Recent Advances in Membrane and Metabolic Research,* edited by E. Gerlach, K. Moser, E. Deutsch, and W. Williams. Stuttgart, FRG: Thieme, 1973, p. 164–167. (2nd Int. Symp., Vienna.)
84. DUVELLEROY, M. A., R. G. BUCKLES, S. ROSENKAIMER, C. TUNG, AND M. B. LAVER. An oxyhemoglobin dissociation analyzer. *J. Appl. Physiol.* 28: 227–233, 1970.
85. EATON, J. W., T. D. SKELTON, AND E. BERGER. Survival at extreme altitude: protective effect of increased hemoglobin-oxygen affinity. *Science Wash. DC* 183: 743–744, 1974.
86. EDALJI, R., R. E. BENESCH, AND R. BENESCH. Binding of inositol hexaphosphate to deoxyhemoglobin. *J. Biol. Chem.* 251: 7720–7721, 1976.
87. EDWARDS, M. J., AND R. J. MARTIN. Mixing technique for the oxygen-hemoglobin equilibrium and Bohr effect. *J. Appl. Physiol.* 21: 1898–1902, 1966.
88. FANTONI, A., A. BANK, AND P. A. MARKS. Globin composition and synthesis of hemoglobins in developing fetal mice erythroid cells. *Science Wash. DC* 157: 1327–1329, 1967.
89. FANTONI, A., M. G. FARACE, AND R. GAMBARI. Embryonic hemoglobins in man and other mammals. *Blood* 57: 623–633, 1981.
90. FERMI, G. Three-dimensional fourier synthesis of human deoxyhaemoglobin at 2–5 Å resolution: refinement of the atomic model. *J. Mol. Biol.* 97: 237–256, 1975.
91. FESTA, R. S., AND T. ASAKURA. The use of an oxygen dissociation curve analyzer in transfusion therapy. *Transfusion Phila.* 19: 107–113, 1979.
92. FORSTER, R. E. Rate of gas uptake by red cells. In: *Handbook of Physiology. Respiration,* edited by W. O. Fenn and H. Rahn. Washington, DC: Am. Physiol. Soc., 1964, sect. 3, vol. I, chapt. 32, p. 827–837.
93. FRIER, J. A., AND M. F. PERUTZ. Structure of human foetal deoxyhaemoglobin. *J. Mol. Biol.* 112: 97–112, 1977.
94. FRITSCH, E. F., R. M. LAWN, AND T. MANIATIS. Molecular cloning and characterization of the human β-like globin gene cluster. *Cell* 19: 959–972, 1980.
95. FUNDER, J., AND J. O. WIETH. Chloride and hydrogen ion distribution between human red cells and plasma. *Acta Physiol. Scand.* 68: 234–245, 1966.
96. GAD-EL-HAK, M., J. B. MORTON, AND H. KUTCHAI. Turbulent flow of red cells in dilute suspensions. *Biophys. J.* 18: 289–300, 1977.
97. GALE, R. E., J. B. CLEGG, AND E. R. HUEHNS. Human embryonic haemoglobin Gower 1 and Gower 2. *Nature Lond.* 280: 162–164, 1979.
98. GARNER, M. H., R. A. BOGARDT, JR., AND F. R. N. GURD. Determination of the p*K* values for the α-amino groups of human hemoglobin. *J. Biol. Chem.* 250: 4398–4404, 1975.
99. GELIN, B. R., AND M. KARPLUS. Mechanism of tertiary structural change in hemoglobin. *Proc. Natl. Acad. Sci. USA* 74: 801–805, 1977.
100. GERBER, G., H. BERGER, G. R. JÄNIG, AND S. M. RAPOPORT. Interaction of haemoglobin with ions. Quantitative description of the state of magnesium adenosine-5′-triphosphate, 2,3-bisphosphoglycerate, and human haemoglobin under simulated intracellular conditions. *Eur. J. Biochem.* 38: 563–571, 1973.
101. GIBSON, Q. H. The reaction of oxygen with hemoglobin and the kinetic basis of the effect of salt on binding of oxygen. *J. Biol. Chem.* 245: 3285–3288, 1970.
102. GIBSON, Q. H. The contribution of the α- and β-chains to the kinetics of oxygen binding to and dissociation from hemoglobin. *Proc. Natl. Acad. Sci. USA* 70: 1–4, 1973.
103. GIBSON, Q. H., F. KREUZER, E. MEDA, AND F. J. W. ROUGHTON. The kinetics of human haemoglobin in solution and the red cell at 37°C. *J. Physiol. Lond.* 129: 65–89, 1955.
104. GILMAN, J. G. Rat embryonic and foetal erythrocytes. *Biochem. J.* 192: 355–359, 1980.
105. GILMAN, J. G. Red cells of newborn rats have low bisphosphoglyceromutase and high pyruvate kinase activities in association with low 2,3-bisphosphoglycerate. *Biochem. Biophys.*

Res. Commun. 98: 1057–1062, 1981.

106. GOODMAN, M., G. W. MOORE, AND G. MATSUDA. Darwinian evolution in the genealogy of haemoglobin. *Nature Lond.* 253: 603–608, 1975.
107. GRAY, R. D. The kinetics of the alkaline Bohr effect of human hemoglobin. *J. Biol. Chem.* 245: 2914–2921, 1970.
108. GREENWALD, I. New type of phosphoric acid isolated from blood; effect of substitution on rotation of α-glyceric acid. *J. Biol. Chem.* 63: 339–349, 1925.
109. GROS, G., H. S. ROLLEMA, AND R. E. FORSTER. The carbamate equilibrium of α- and ϵ-amino groups of human hemoglobin at 37°C. *J. Biol. Chem.* 256: 5471–5480, 1981.
110. GROS, G., H. S. ROLLEMA, W. JELKMANN, H. GROS, C. BAUER, AND W. MOLL. Net charge and oxygen affinity of human hemoglobin are independent of hemoglobin concentratin. *J. Gen. Physiol.* 72: 765–773, 1978.
111. HAAB, P. E., J. PIIPER, AND H. RAHN. Simple method for rapid determination of an O_2 dissociation curve of the blood. *J. Appl. Physiol.* 15: 1148–1149, 1960.
112. HALL, F. G. Minimal utilizable oxygen and the oxygen dissociation curve of rodents. *J. Appl. Physiol.* 21: 375–378, 1966.
113. HALL, F. G., D. B. DILL, AND I. S. GUZMAN BARRON. Comparative physiology in high altitudes. *J. Cell. Comp. Physiol.* 8: 301–313, 1936.
114. HARKNESS, D. R., J. PONCE, AND V. GRAYSON. A comparative study on the phosphoglyceric acid cycle in mammalian erythrocytes. *Comp. Biochem. Physiol.* 28: 129–138, 1969.
115. HARTRIDGE, H., AND F. J. W. ROUGHTON. The kinetics of haemoglobin. II. The velocity with which oxygen dissociates from its combination with haemoglobin. *Proc. R. Soc. Lond. Ser. A Math. Phys. Sci.* 104: 395–430, 1923.
116. HARTRIDGE, H., AND F. J. W. ROUGHTON. The kinetics of haemoglobin. III. The velocity with which oxygen combines with reduced haemoglobin. *Proc. R. Soc. Lond. Ser. A Math. Phys. Sci.* 107: 654–683, 1925.
117. HAYASHI, A., T. SUZUKI, AND M. SHIN. An enzymatic reduction system for metmyoglobin and methemoglobin, and its application to functional studies. *Biochim. Biophys. Acta* 310: 309–316, 1973.
118. HEBBEL, R. P., E. M. BERGER, AND J. W. EATON. Effect of increased maternal hemoglobin oxygen affinity on fetal growth in the rat. *Blood* 55: 969–974, 1980.
119. HEBBEL, R. P., J. W. EATON, R. S. KRONENBERG, E. D. ZANJANI, L. G. MOORE, AND E. M. BERGER. Human llamas: adaptation to altitude in subjects with high hemoglobin oxygen affinity. *J. Clin. Invest.* 62: 593–600, 1978.
120. HEIDNER, E. J., R. C. LADNER, AND M. F. PERUTZ. Structure of horse carbonmonoxyhaemoglobin. *J. Mol. Biol.* 104: 707–722, 1976.
121. HENRIQUES, O. M. Über Carbhämoglobin. *Ergeb. Physiol. Biol. Chem. Exp. Pharmakol.* 28: 625–689, 1929.
122. HILL, A. V. The possible effects of aggregation of the molecules of haemoglobin on its dissociation curve. *J. Physiol. Lond.* 40: iv–vii, 1910.
123. HILPERT, P., R. G. FLEISCHMANN, D. KEMPE, AND H. BARTELS. The Bohr effect related to blood and erythrocyte pH. *Am. J. Physiol.* 205: 337–340, 1963.
124. HOLADAY, D. A., AND M. VEROSKY. Improved micromanometric methods for the analysis of respiratory gases in plasma and whole blood. *J. Lab. Clin. Med.* 47: 634–644, 1956.
125. HUEHNS, E. R., N. DANCE, G. H. BEAVEN, J. V. KEIL, F. HECHT, AND A. G. MOTULSKY. Human embryonic haemoglobins. *Nature Lond.* 201: 1095–1097, 1964.
126. HUEHNS, E. R., AND A. M. FAROOQUI. Oxygen dissociation properties of human embryonic red cells. *Nature Lond.* 254: 335–337, 1975.
127. HUESTIS, W. H., AND M. A. RAFTERY. ^{19}F-NMR studies of oxygen binding to hemoglobin. *Biochem. Biophys. Res. Commun.* 49: 1358–1365, 1972.
128. HUTCHISON, V. H., H. B. HAINES, AND G. ENGBRETSON. Aquatic life at high altitude: respiratory adaptations in the Lake Titicaca frog, *Telematobius culeus*. *Respir. Physiol.* 27: 115–129, 1976.
129. ILGENFRITZ, G., AND T. M. SCHUSTER. Kinetics of oxygen binding to human hemoglobin. Temperature jump relaxation studies. *J. Biol. Chem.* 249: 2959–2973, 1974.
130. IMAI, K. Analyses of oxygen equilibria of native and chemically modified human adult hemoglobin on the basis of Adair's stepwise oxygenation theory and the allosteric model of Monod, Wyman, and Changeux. *Biochemistry* 12: 798–807, 1973.
131. IMAI, K., H. MORIMOTO, M. KOTANI, H. WATARI, W. HIRATA, AND M. KURODA. Studies on the function of abnormal hemoglobins. I. An improved method for automatic measurement of the oxygen equilibrium curve of hemoglobin. *Biochim. Biophys. Acta* 200: 189–196, 1970.
132. IMAI, K., AND T. YONETANI. pH dependence of the Adair constants of human hemoglobin. Nonuniform contribution of successive oxygen bindings to the alkaline Bohr effect. *J. Biol. Chem.* 250: 2227–2231, 1975.
133. JACOBASCH, G., S. MINAKAMI, AND S. M. RAPOPORT. Glycolysis of the erythrocyte. In: *Cellular and Molecular Biology of Erythrocytes*, edited by H. Yoshikawa and S. M. Rapoport. Munich, FRG: Urban & Schwarzenberg, 1974.
134. JELKMANN, W., AND C. BAUER.What is the best method to remove 2,3-diphosphoglycerate from hemoglobin? *Anal. Biochem.* 75: 382–388, 1976.
135. JELKMANN, W., AND C. BAUER. Oxygen affinity and phosphate compounds of red cells during intrauterine development of rabbits. *Pfluegers Arch.* 372: 149–156, 1977.
136. JELKMANN, W., AND C. BAUER. Embryonic hemoglobins: dependency of functional characteristics on tetramer composition. *Pfluegers Arch.* 377: 75–80, 1978.
137. JELKMANN, W., AND C. BAUER. High pyruvate kinase activity causes low concentration of 2,3-diphosphoglycerate in fetal rabbit red cells. *Pfluegers Arch.* 375: 189–195, 1978.
138. JELKMANN, W., AND C. BAUER. 2,3-DPG levels in relation to red cell enzyme activities in rat fetuses and hypoxic newborns. *Pfluegers Arch.* 389: 61–68, 1980.
139. JENSEN, M., F. A. OSKI, D. G. NATHAN, AND H. F. BUNN. Hemoglobin Syracuse ($\alpha_2\beta_2$-143(H21)His $\rightarrow$ Pro), a new high-affinity variant detected by special electrophoretic methods. Observations on the auto-oxidation of normal and variant hemoglobins. *J. Clin. Invest.* 55: 469–477, 1975.
140. JOHNSON, M. E., AND C. HO. Effects of ligands and organic phosphates on functional properties of human adult hemoglobin. *Biochemistry* 13: 3655–3661, 1974.
141. JONES, R. T., AND T. B. SHIH. Hemoglobin variants with altered oxygen affinity. *Hemoglobin* 4: 243–261, 1980.
142. KELLETT, G. L. Dissociation of haemoglobin into subunits. Ligand-linked dissociation at neutral pH. *J. Mol. Biol.* 59: 401–424, 1971.
143. KELLETT, G. L., AND H. GUTFREUND. Reactions of haemoglobin dimers after ligand dissociation. *Nature Lond.* 227: 921–926, 1970.
144. KIESOW, L. A., J. B. SHELTON, AND J. W. BLESS. The determination of O_2-dissociation curves in hemoglobin solutions with a liquid fluorocarbon O_2-transport system. *Anal. Biochem.* 58: 14–24, 1974.
145. KILMARTIN, J. V., J. J. BREEN, G. C. K. ROBERTS, AND C. HO. Direct measurement of the p*K* values of an alkaline Bohr group in human hemoglobin. *Proc. Natl. Acad. Sci. USA* 70: 1246–1249, 1973.
146. KILMARTIN, J. V., J. FOGG, M. LUZZANA, AND L. ROSSI-BERNARDI. Role of the α-amino groups of the α- and β-chains of human hemoglobin in oxygen-linked binding of carbon dioxide. *J. Biol. Chem.* 248: 7039–7043, 1973.
147. KILMARTIN, J. V., AND L. ROSSI-BERNARDI. Inhibition of CO_2 combination and reduction of the Bohr effect in haemoglobin chemically modified at its α-amino groups. *Nature Lond.* 222: 1243–1246, 1969.
148. KITCHEN, H., AND I. BRETT. Embryonic and fetal hemoglobin

in animals. *Ann. NY Acad. Sci.* 241: 653–671, 1974.

149. KREUZER, F., AND W. Z. YAHR. Influence of red cell membrane on diffusion of oxygen. *J. Appl. Physiol.* 15: 1117–1122, 1960.
150. KUSUMI, F., W. C. BUTTS, AND W. L. RUFF. Superior analytical performance by electrolytic cell analysis of blood oxygen content. *J. Appl. Physiol.* 35: 299–300, 1973.
151. LAU, P. W., AND T. ASAKURA. Comparative study of oxygen and carbon monoxide binding by hemoglobin. *J. Biol. Chem.* 255: 1617–1622, 1980.
152. LAUER, J., C.-K. SHEN, AND T. MANIATIS. The chromosomal arrangement of human α-like globin genes: sequence homology and α-globin gene deletions. *Cell* 20: 119–130, 1980.
153. LAWSON, W. H., JR., R. A. B. HOLLAND, AND R. E. FORSTER. Effect of temperature on deoxygenation rate of human red cells. *J. Appl. Physiol.* 20: 912–918, 1965.
154. LENFANT, C., AND K. JOHANSEN. Gas transport by hemocyanin-containing blood of the Cephalopod *Octopus dofleini*. *Am. J. Physiol.* 209: 991–998, 1965.
155. LENFANT, C., J. D. TORRANCE, E. ENGLISH, C. A. FINCH, C. REYNAFARJE, J. RAMOS, AND J. FAURA. Effect of altitude on oxygen binding by hemoglobin and on organic phosphate levels. *J. Clin. Invest.* 47: 2652–2656, 1968.
156. LENFANT, C., J. D. TORRANCE, AND C. REYNAFARJE. Shift of the O_2-Hb dissociation curve at altitude: mechanism and effect. *J. Appl. Physiol.* 30: 625–631, 1971.
157. LENFANT, C., P. WAYS, C. AUCUTT, AND J. CRUZ. Effect of chronic hypoxia on the O_2-Hb dissociation curve and respiratory gas transport in man. *Respir. Physiol.* 7: 7–29, 1969.
158. MANIATIS, T., E. F. FRITSCH, J. LAUER, AND R. M. LAWN. The molecular genetics of human hemoglobin. *Annu. Rev. Genet.* 14: 145–178, 1980.
159. MATTHEW, J. B., J. S. MORROW, R. J. WITTEBORT, AND F. R. N. GURD. Quantitative determination of carbamino adducts of α- and β-chains in human adult hemoglobin in presence and absence of carbon monoxide and 2,3-diphosphoglycerate. *J. Biol. Chem.* 252: 2234–2244, 1977.
160. MCCRAY, J. A. Oxygen recombination kinetics following laser photolysis of oxyhemoglobin. *Biochem. Biophys. Res. Commun.* 47: 187–193, 1972.
161. MCDONALD, M. J., AND R. W. NOBLE. The effect of pH on the rates of ligand replacement reactions of human adult and fetal hemoglobins and their subunits. *J. Biol. Chem.* 247: 4282–4287, 1972.
162. MELDERIS, H., G. STEINHEIDER, AND W. OSTERTAG. Evidence for a unique kind of α-type globin chain in early mammalian embryos. *Nature Lond.* 250: 774–776, 1974.
163. MEYER, M., J. P. HOLLE, AND P. SCHEID. Respiratory and metabolic Bohr effect in duck blood (Abstract). *Pfluegers Arch.* 365: R18, 1976.
164. MIYAMOTO, Y., AND W. MOLL. Measurements of dimensions and pathway of red cells in rapidly frozen lungs in situ. *Respir. Physiol.* 12: 141–156, 1971.
165. MOLL, W. The influence of hemoglobin diffusion on oxygen uptake and release by red cells. *Respir. Physiol.* 6: 1–15, 1968.
166. MONOD, J., J. WYMAN, AND J. P. CHANGEUX. On the nature of allosteric transitions: a plausible model. *J. Mol. Biol.* 12: 88–118, 1965.
167. MORPURGO, G., P. ARESE, A. BOSIA, G. P. PESCARMONA, M. LUZANA, G. MODIANO, AND S. KRISHNA RANJIT. Sherpas living permanently at high altitude: a new pattern of adaptation. *Proc. Natl. Acad. Sci. USA* 73: 747–751, 1976.
168. MUEGGLER, P. A., G. JONES, J. S. PETERSON, J. M. BISSONNETTE, R. D. KOLER, J. METCALFE, R. T. JONES, AND J. A. BLACK. Postnatal regulation of canine oxygen delivery: erythrocyte components affecting Hb function. *Am. J. Physiol.* 238 (*Heart Circ. Physiol.* 7): H73–H79, 1980.
169. MUIRHEAD, H., AND J. GREER. Three-dimensional Fourier synthesis of human deoxyhaemoglobin at 3.5 Å units. *Nature Lond.* 228: 516–519, 1970.
170. MULHAUSEN, R. O., P. ASTRUP, AND K. MELLEMGAARD. Oxygen affinity and acid-base status of human blood during exposure to hypoxia and carbon monoxide. *Scand. J. Clin. Lab. Invest. Suppl.* 103: 9–15, 1968.
171. NATELSON, S. Routine use of ultra micro methods on the clinical laboratory. *Am. J. Clin. Pathol.* 21: 1153–1172, 1951.
172. NICOLSON, P., AND F. J. W. ROUGHTON. A theoretical study on the influence of diffusion and chemical reaction velocity on the rate of exchange of carbon monoxide and oxygen between the red blood corpuscle and surrounding fluid. *Proc. R. Soc. Lond. B Biol. Sci.* 138: 241–264, 1951.
173. NIENHUIS, A. W., AND G. STAMATOYANNOPOULOS. Hemoglobin switching. *Cell* 15: 307–315, 1978.
174. NIESEL, W., AND G. THEWS. Ein neues Verfahren zur schnellen und genauen Aufnahme der Sauerstoffbindungskurve des Blutes und konzentrierter Hämoproteinlösungen. *Pfluegers Arch.* 273: 380–395, 1961.
175. NIGEN, A. M., B. D. BASS, AND J. M. MANNING. Reactivity of cyanate with valine-1 (α) of hemoglobin. A probe of conformational change and anion binding. *J. Biol. Chem.* 251: 7638–7643, 1976.
176. NIGEN, A. M., AND J. M. MANNING. The interaction of anions with hemoglobin carbamylated on specific NH_2-terminal residues. *J. Biol. Chem.* 250: 8248–8250, 1975.
177. NIGEN, A. M., J. M. MANNING, AND J. O. ALBEN. Oxygen-linked binding sites for inorganic anions to hemoglobin. *J. Biol. Chem.* 255: 5525–5529, 1980.
178. NISHIKURA, K. Identification of histidine-122α in human haemoglobin as one of the unknown alkaline Bohr groups by hydrogen-tritium exchange. *Biochem. J.* 173: 651–657, 1978.
179. NOVY, M. J. Alterations in blood oxygen affinity during fetal and neonatal life. In: *Oxygen Affinity of Hemoglobin and Red Cell Acid Base Status*, edited by M. Rørth and P. Astrup. Copenhagen: Munksgaard, 1972, p. 696–712. (Alfred Benzon Symp., 4th, 1971.)
180. NOVY, M. J., M. J. EDWARDS, AND J. METCALFE. Hemoglobin Yakima. II. High blood oxygen affinity associated with compensatory erythrocytosis and normal hemodynamics. *J. Clin. Invest.* 46: 1848–1854, 1967.
181. O'DONNELL, S., R. MANDARO, T. M. SCHUSTER, AND A. ARNONE. X-ray diffraction and solution studies of specifically carbamylated human hemoglobin A. Evidence for the location of a proton- and oxygen-linked chloride binding site at valine 1α. *J. Biol. Chem.* 254: 12204–12208, 1979.
182. OHE, M., AND A. KAJITA. Changes in pK_a values of individual histidine residues of human hemoglobin upon reaction with carbon monoxide. *Biochemistry* 19: 4443–4450, 1980.
183. OLSON, J. S., M. E. ANDERSEN, AND Q. H. GIBSON. The dissociation of the first oxygen molecule from some mammalian oxyhemoglobins. *J. Biol. Chem.* 246: 5919–5923, 1971.
184. PARER, J. T., A. S. HOVERSLAND, AND J. METCALFE. Some respiratory characteristics of the blood of the adult and young African pygmy goat. *J. Appl. Physiol.* 22: 756–759, 1967.
185. PENNEY, D., AND M. THOMAS. Hematological alterations and response to acute hypobaric stress. *J. Appl. Physiol.* 39: 1034–1037, 1975.
186. PERELLA, M., G. GUGLIELMO, AND A. MOSCA. Determination of the equilibrium constants for oxygen-linked CO_2 binding to human hemoglobin. *FEBS Lett.* 78: 287–290, 1977.
187. PERELLA, M., J. V. KILMARTIN, J. FOGG, AND L. ROSSI-BERNARDI. Identification of the high and low affinity CO_2 binding sites of human haemoglobin. *Nature Lond.* 256: 759–761, 1975.
188. PERUTZ, M. F. Stereochemistry of cooperative effects in haemoglobin. *Nature Lond.* 228: 726–739, 1970.
189. PERUTZ, M. F. Nature of haem-haem interaction. *Nature Lond.* 237: 495–499, 1972.
190. PERUTZ, M. F., AND K. IMAI. Regulation of oxygen affinity of mammalian haemoglobins. *J. Mol. Biol.* 136: 183–191, 1980.
191. PERUTZ, M. F., AND H. LEHMANN. Molecular pathology of human haemoglobin. *Nature Lond.* 219: 902–909, 1968.
192. PERUTZ, M. F., AND L. MAZZARELLA. A preliminary X-ray analysis of haemoglobin H. *Nature Lond.* 199: 639, 1963.

193. PERUTZ, M. F., H. MUIRHEAD, J. M. COX, AND L. C. G. GOAMAN. Three-dimensional Fourier synthesis of horse oxy-haemoglobin at 2.89 Å resolution: the atomic model. *Nature Lond.* 219: 131–139, 1968.
194. PETERS, J. P., AND D. D. VAN SLYKE. *Quantitative Clinical Chemistry.* Baltimore, MD: Williams & Wilkins, 1932, Vol. 2, p. 981. (Reprinted 1958.)
195. PETERSON, L. L. Red cell diphosphoglycerate mutase. Immunochemical studies in vertebrate cells, including a human variant lacking 2,3-DPG. *Blood* 52: 953–958, 1978.
196. PETSCHOW, D., I. WÜRDINGER, R. BAUMANN, J. DUHM, G. BRAUNITZER, AND C. BAUER. Causes of high blood O_2 affinity of animals living at high altitude. *J. Appl. Physiol.* 42: 139–143, 1977.
197. PETSCHOW, R., D. PETSCHOW, R. BARTELS, R. BAUMANN, AND H. BARTELS. Regulation of oxygen affinity in blood of fetal, newborn and adult mouse. *Respir. Physiol.* 35: 271–282, 1978.
198. POPP, R. A., C. L. MARSH, AND L. C. SKOW. Expression of embryonic hemoglobin genes in mice heterozygous for α-thalassemia or β-duplication traits and in mice heterozygous for both traits. *Dev. Biol.* 85: 123–128, 1981.
199. PROUDFOOT, N. J., M. H. M. SHANDER, J. L. MANLEY, M. L. GEFTER, AND T. MANIATIS. Structure and in vitro transcription of human globin genes. *Science Wash. DC* 209: 1329–1336, 1980.
200. RAPOPORT, S., AND G. M. GUEST. The role of diphosphoglyceric acid in the electrolyte equilibrium of blood cells. Studies of pyloric obstruction in dogs. *J. Biol. Chem.* 131: 675–689, 1939.
201. RAPOPORT, S., AND G. M. GUEST. Distribution of acid soluble phosphorus in the blood cells of various species. *J. Biol. Chem.* 138: 269–282, 1941.
202. RAPOPORT, S., AND J. LUEBERING. The formation of 2,3-diphosphoglycerate in rabbit erythrocytes: the existence of diphosphoglycerate mutase. *J. Biol. Chem.* 183: 507–516, 1950.
203. REEVES, R. B. A rapid micro method for obtaining oxygen equilibrium curves on whole blood. *Respir. Physiol.* 42: 299–315, 1980.
204. REISSMAN, K. R., W. E. RUTH, AND T. NAMARA. A human hemoglobin with lowered oxygen affinity and impaired heme-heme interactions. *J. Clin. Invest.* 40: 1826–1833, 1971.
205. RICE, S. A. Hydrodynamic and diffusion considerations of rapid-mix experiments with red blood cells. *Biophys. J.* 29: 65–77, 1980.
206. RIGGS, A. The binding of *N*-ethyl maleimide by human hemoglobin and its effect upon the oxygen equilibrium. *J. Biol. Chem.* 236: 1948–1954, 1961.
207. RIGGS, A. Mechanism of the enhancement of the Bohr effect in mammalian hemoglobins by diphosphoglycerate. *Proc. Natl. Acad. Sci. USA* 68: 2062–2065, 1971.
208. RIGGS, A. Factors in the evolution of hemoglobin function. *Federation Proc.* 35: 2115–2118, 1976.
209. ROLLEMA, H. S., AND C. BAUER. The interaction of inositol pentaphosphate with the hemoglobins of highland and lowland geese. *J. Biol. Chem.* 254: 12038–12043, 1979.
210. ROLLEMA, H. S., S. H. DE BRUIN, L. H. M. JANSSEN, AND G. A. J. VAN OS. The effect of potassium chloride on the Bohr effect of human hemoglobin. *J. Biol. Chem.* 250: 1333–1339, 1975.
211. ROLLEMA, H., J. WEINGARTEN, C. BAUER, AND P. SCHEID. Interactions among H^+, CO_2, and inositolhexaphosphate in binding to chicken hemoglobin (Abstract). *Pfluegers Arch.* 373: R44, 1978.
212. RØRTH, M., S. F. NYGAARD, AND H. H. PARVING. Red cell metabolism and oxygen affinity of healthy individuals during exposure to high altitude. *Adv. Exp. Med. Biol.* 28: 361–372, 1972.
213. ROSA, R., M.-O. PREHU, Y. BEUZARD, AND J. ROSA. The first case of a complete deficiency of diphosphoglycerate mutase in human erythrocytes. *J. Clin. Invest.* 62: 907–915, 1978.
214. ROSSI-BERNARDI, L., M. LUZZANA, M. SAMAJA, M. DAVI, D. DARIVA-RICCI, J. MINOLI, B. SEATON, AND R. L. BERGER. Continuous determination of the oxygen dissociation curve for whole blood. *Clin. Chem.* 21: 1747–1753, 1975.
215. ROSSI-BERNARDI, L., AND F. J. W. ROUGHTON. The specific influence of carbon dioxide and carbamate compounds on the buffer power and Bohr effects in human haemoglobin solutions. *J. Physiol. Lond.* 189: 1–29, 1967.
216. ROUGHTON, F. J. W. Diffusion and simultaneous chemical reaction velocity in haemoglobin solutions and red cell suspensions. *Prog. Biophys. Biophys. Chem.* 9: 56–104, 1959.
217. ROUGHTON, F. J. W., E. C. DELAND, J. C. KERNOHAN, AND J. W. SEVERINGHAUS. Some recent studies of the oxyhemoglobin dissociation curve of human blood under physiological conditions and the fitting of the Adair equation to the standard curve. In: *Oxygen Affinity of Hemoglobin and Red Cell Acid-Base Status*, edited by M. Rørth and P. Astrup. Copenhagen: Munksgaard, 1972, p. 73–82. (Alfred Benzon Symp., 4th, 1971.)
218. ROUGHTON, F. J. W., AND P. F. SCHOLANDER. Micro gasometric estimation of the blood gases. I. Oxygen. *J. Biol. Chem.* 148: 541–550, 1943.
219. SALHANY, J. M., D. H. MATHERS, AND R. S. ELIOT. The deoxygenation kinetics of hemoglobin partially saturated with carbon monoxide. Effect of 2,3-diphosphoglycerate. *J. Biol. Chem.* 247: 6985–6990, 1972.
220. SAMAJA, M., A. VEICSTEINAS, AND P. CERRETELLI. Oxygen affinity of blood in altitude Sherpas. *J. Appl. Physiol.* 47: 337–341, 1979.
221. SCHEID, P., AND M. MEYER. Mixing technique for study of oxygen-hemoglobin equilibrium: a critical evaluation. *J. Appl. Physiol.* 45: 818–822, 1978.
222. SCOTT, A. F., H. F. BUNN, AND A. H. BRUSH. Functional aspects of hemoglobin evolution in mammals. *J. Mol. Evol.* 8: 311–316, 1976.
223. SCOTT, A. F., H. F. BUNN, AND A. H. BRUSH. The phylogenetic distribution of red cell 2,3-diphosphoglycerate and its interaction with mammalian hemoglobins. *J. Exp. Zool.* 201: 269–288, 1977.
224. SELMAN, B. J., Y. S. WHITE, AND A. R. TAIT. An evaluation of the Lex-O_2-Con oxygen analyser. *Anaesthesia* 30: 206–211, 1975.
225. SICK, H., AND K. GERSONDE. Methods for continuous registration of O_2-binding curves of hemoproteins by means of a diffusion chamber. *Anal. Biochem.* 32: 362–376, 1969.
226. SIDWELL, A. E., R. H. MUNCH, E. S. GUZMAN-BARRON, AND T. R. HOGNESS. The salt effect on the hemoglobin-oxygen equilibrium. *J. Biol. Chem.* 123: 335–350, 1938.
227. SIGGAARD-ANDERSEN, O. Oxygen-linked hydrogen binding of human hemoglobin. Effects of carbon dioxide and 2,3-diphosphoglycerate. I. Studies on erythrolysate. *Scand. Clin. Lab. Invest.* 27: 351–360, 1971.
228. SIRS, J. A., AND F. J. W. ROUGHTON. Stopped-flow measurements of CO and O_2 uptake by hemoglobin in sheep erythrocytes. *J. Appl. Physiol.* 18: 158–165, 1963.
229. SMITH, R. C., G. J. GARBUTT, R. E. ISAACKS, AND D. R. HARKNESS. Oxygen binding of fetal and adult bovine hemoglobin in the presence of organic phosphate and uric acid riboside. *Hemoglobin* 3: 47–55, 1979.
230. STAMATOYANNOPOULOS, G., J. T. PARER, AND C. A. FINCH. Physiological implications of a hemoglobin with decreased oxygen affinity (Hemoglobin Seattle). *N. Engl. J. Med.* 281: 916–919, 1969.
231. STEINHEIDER, G., H. MELDERIS, AND W. OSTERTAG. Embryonic ϵ-chains of mice and rabbits. *Nature Lond.* 257: 714–716, 1975.
232. SZABO, A., AND M. KARPLUS. Analysis of the interaction of organic phosphates with hemoglobin. *Biochemistry* 15: 2869–2877, 1976.
233. TAKENAKA, O., AND H. MORIMOTO. Oxygen equilibrium characteristics of adult and fetal hemoglobin of Japanese monkey (*Macaca fuscata*). *Biochim. Biophys. Acta* 446: 457–462, 1976.

234. TAKETA, F. Organic phosphates and hemoglobin structure-function relationships in the feline. *Ann. NY Acad. Sci.* 241: 524–537, 1974.
235. THEWS, G. Untersuchung der Sauerstoffaufnahme und -abgabe sehr dünner Blutlamellen. *Pfluegers Arch.* 268: 308–317, 1959.
236. THOMSON, J. M., J. A. DEMPSEY, L. W. CHOSY, N. T. SHAHIDI, AND W. G. REDDAN. Oxygen transport and oxyhemoglobin dissociation during prolonged muscular work. *J. Appl. Physiol.* 37: 658–664, 1974.
237. TORRANCE, J. D., AND C. LENFANT. Methods for determination of O_2 dissociation curves, including Bohr effect. *Respir. Physiol.* 8: 127–136, 1969.
238. TORRANCE, J. D., C. LENFANT, J. CRUZ, AND E. MARTICORENA. Oxygen transport mechanisms in residents at high altitude. *Respir. Physiol.* 11: 1–15, 1970/71.
239. TUCHINDA, S., K. NAGAI, AND H. LEHMANN. Oxygen dissociation curve of haemoglobin Portland. *FEBS Lett.* 49: 390–391, 1975.
240. TUREK, Z., F. KREUZER, AND B. E. M. RINGNALDA. Blood gases at several levels of oxygenation in rats with a left-shifted blood oxygen dissociation curve. *Pfluegers Arch.* 376: 7–13, 1978.
241. TUREK, Z., F. KREUZER, M. TUREK-MAISCHNEIDER, AND B. E. M. RINGNALDA. Blood O_2 content, cardiac output, and flow to organs at several levels of oxygenation in rats with a left-shifted blood oxygen dissociation curve. *Pfluegers Arch.* 376: 201–207, 1978.
242. TYUMA, I., AND K. SHIMIZU. Different response to organic phosphates of human fetal and adult hemoglobins. *Arch. Biochem. Biophys.* 129: 404–405, 1969.
243. VAN BEEK, G. G. M., AND S. H. DE BRUIN. The pH dependence of the binding of D-glycerate 2,3-bisphosphate to deoxyhemoglobin and oxyhemoglobin. *Eur. J. Biochem.* 100: 497–502, 1979.
244. VAN BEEK, G. G. M., AND S. H. DE BRUIN. Identification of the residues involved in the oxygen-linked chloride-ion binding sites in human deoxyhemoglobin and oxyhemoglobin. *Eur. J. Biochem.* 105: 353–360, 1980.
245. VAN BEEK, G. G. M., E. R. P. ZUIDERWEG, AND S. H. DE BRUIN. The binding of chloride ions to ligated and unligated human hemoglobin and its influence on the Bohr effect. *Eur. J. Biochem.* 99: 379–383, 1979.
246. VAN SLYKE, D. D., AND J. PLAZIN. *Micrometric Analyses.* Baltimore, MD: Williams & Wilkins, 1961.
247. VAN SLYKE, D. D., H. WU, AND F. L. MCLEAN. Studies of gas and electrolyte equilibria in the blood. V. Factors controlling the electrolyte and water distribution in the blood. *J. Biol. Chem.* 56: 765–849, 1923.
248. VIGGIANO, G., AND C. HO. Proton nuclear magnetic resonance investigation of structural changes associated with cooperative oxygenation of human adult hemoglobin. *Proc. Natl. Acad. Sci. USA* 76: 3673–3677, 1979.
249. WEATHERALL, D. J., AND J. B. CLEGG. Recent developments in the molecular genetics of human hemoglobin. *Cell* 16: 467–479, 1979.
250. WEISKOPF, R. B., AND J. W. SEVERINGHAUS. Lack of effect of high altitude on hemoglobin oxygen affinity. *J. Appl. Physiol.* 33: 276–277, 1972.
251. WELLS, R. M. G. Hemoglobin oxygen affinity in developing embryonic erythroid cells of the mouse. *J. Comp. Physiol.* 129: 333–338, 1979.
252. WOOD, W. G., AND R. W. JONES. Erythropoiesis and hemoglobin production: a unifying model involving sequential gene activation. In: *Hemoglobins in Development and Differentiation*, edited by G. Stamatoyannopoulos and A. W. Nienhuis. New York: Liss, 1981.
253. WOOD, W. G., J. NASH, D. J. WEATHERALL, J. S. ROBINSON, AND F. A. HARRISON. The sheep as an animal model for the switch from fetal to adult hemoglobins. In: *Cellular and Molecular Regulation of Hemoglobin Switching*, edited by G. Stamatoyannopoulos and A. W. Nienhuis. New York: Grune & Stratton, 1979, p. 153–165.
254. WOOD, W. G., AND D. J. WEATHERALL. Haemoglobin synthesis during human foetal development. *Nature Lond.* 244: 162–165, 1973.
255. WRANNE, B., R. D. WOODSON, AND J. C. DETTER. Bohr effect: interaction between H^+, CO_2, and 2,3-DPG in fresh and stored blood. *J. Appl. Physiol.* 32: 749–754, 1972.
256. WYMAN, J. Heme proteins. *Adv. Protein Chem.* 4: 407–531, 1948.
257. ZUIDERWEG, E. R. P., L. F. HAMERS, S. H. DE BRUIN, AND C. W. HILBERS. Equilibrium aspects of the binding of myo-inositol hexakisphosphate to human hemoglobin as studied by ^{31}P NMR and pH-stat techniques. *Eur. J. Biochem.* 118: 85–94, 1981.
258. ZÜRCHER, C. J., A. LOOS, AND H. K. PRINS. Hereditary high ATP content of human erythrocytes. *Bibl. Haematol.* 23: 549–556, 1965.

Carbon dioxide transport

ROBERT A. KLOCKE | *Departments of Medicine and Physiology, State University of New York at Buffalo, Buffalo, New York*

CHAPTER CONTENTS

CARBON DIOXIDE EXCRETION is a passive phenomenon, and CO_2 transfer proceeds down an electrochemical gradient from the site of production to the environment. This process is uncomplicated in single-cell organisms; CO_2 diffuses directly from the cell into the environment. Cellular partial pressure of CO_2 (P_{CO_2}) is only slightly greater than the surrounding P_{CO_2}, and there is no need for elaborate transport and buffering systems. Excretion via this mechanism is not feasible in more complex organisms because of the length of diffusion pathways between the sites of metabolism and the body surface. Convective movement is necessary to transport CO_2 from the tissue to the interface with the environment.

The efficiency of a transport system is a function of convection (blood flow) and capacity of the carrier (blood content). Fortunately, large quantities of CO_2 can be carried in blood, thus reducing flow requirements. This large capacity creates an additional problem, because CO_2 hydrates to form carbonic acid, a moderately strong acid. Accordingly, blood must possess potent buffering systems to prevent large changes in acidity associated with CO_2 transport.

CARBON DIOXIDE CONTENT OF BLOOD

Carbon dioxide is only moderately soluble in aqueous media, and transport of CO_2 in physical solution alone is not adequate to keep pace with metabolic production. Fortunately CO_2 can be transported in other forms in blood. Most CO_2 is carried as HCO_3^-, the conjugate base of carbonic acid. Smaller amounts of CO_2 exist in blood as carbamates, compounds formed by binding of CO_2 to amino groups of proteins. Carbamates are present in relatively small concentration but are physiologically important because of the influence of oxygenation on CO_2 binding to Hb.

The transformation of CO_2 to HCO_3^- and carbamate compounds greatly increases the CO_2 capacity of blood. No other chemical forms of CO_2 contribute significantly to this capacity. In the 1964 edition of the *Handbook* section on respiration, Roughton (129) summarized evidence that suggested the presence of "y-bound" CO_2, a small portion of blood CO_2 content that could not be accounted for by calculations of dissolved CO_2, HCO_3^-, and carbamate concentrations. There is no evidence for the existence of y-bound CO_2. Most likely the inability to account for all CO_2 measured in blood was the result of imprecise experimental data.

Dissolved CO_2

Under normal circumstances, ~5% of the total CO_2 content of blood exists as dissolved CO_2. If all dissolved CO_2 were removed from blood during transit through the lung, only 60% of basal CO_2 production could be excreted. This would also require maintenance of alveolar P_{CO_2} close to zero, thereby imposing immense ventilatory requirements on the organism.

Excretion of dissolved CO_2 also increases in direct

proportion to an increase in cardiac output. However, there is no feasible combination of increased ventilation and perfusion that would permit adequate transport of CO_2 in physical solution even under resting conditions. Despite its relatively low capacitance in blood, dissolved CO_2 has a critical role in gas transport. Only dissolved CO_2 can rapidly cross the vascular endothelium; all other forms of CO_2 must be converted to free CO_2 to enter or leave blood.

Carbon dioxide is considerably more soluble in lipids than aqueous media, enhancing its ability to cross membrane barriers. This diffusive movement is so rapid that the pulmonary diffusing capacity for CO_2 cannot be measured under physiological circumstances, and only approximate limits have been estimated in vivo (75).

Bicarbonate Ion

Carbonic acid and CO_2 are linked through the hydration-dehydration reaction

$$CO_2 + H_2O \rightleftharpoons H_2CO_3 \tag{1}$$

The equilibrium constant of this hydration-dehydration reaction, K_h, is usually expressed as a constant that incorporates the water term of Equation 1 so that $[H_2CO_3]/[CO_2] = K_h$. At the pH of most physiological fluids, carbonic acid instantly dissociates into H^+ and HCO_3^-

$$H_2CO_3 \overset{K_1}{\rightleftharpoons} H^+ + HCO_3^- \tag{2}$$

where K_1 is the first acidic dissociation constant of carbonic acid. Bicarbonate can further dissociate into carbonate ion with liberation of a proton

$$HCO_3^- \overset{K_2}{\rightleftharpoons} H^+ + CO_3^{2-} \tag{3}$$

where K_2 is the second acidic dissociation constant of carbonic acid. The concentration of carbonate ion in blood is miniscule because $pK_2 > 10.0$ (38). For this reason, carbonate ion is usually ignored when considering CO_2 transport in blood.

Carbonic acid is often viewed as a weak acid but in reality is a moderately strong acid ($pK_1 \sim 3.8$). By comparison, it is as strong an acid as formic or lactic acids. This impression results from combining the hydration and ionization processes (Equations 1 and 2), thereby treating the sum of CO_2 and H_2CO_3 as the undissociated acid. This common practice is pragmatic because carbonic acid and CO_2 cannot be distinguished from each other by chemical analysis. Thus

$$[H^+][HCO_3^-]/([CO_2] + [H_2CO_3]) = K_a \tag{4}$$

where K_a, the apparent dissociation constant for the reaction, is related to the hydration and ionization constants by

$$K_a = K_1K_h/(1 + K_h) \approx K_1K_h \tag{5}$$

because $1 \gg K_h$. Carbon dioxide is present in far greater concentration than carbonic acid, so the hydration constant K_h is numerically quite small. Compared to K_1, the product of K_h and K_1 (which equals K_a) is substantially smaller, which suggests that carbonic acid is a weak acid. The logarithmic form of Equation 4 is the well-known Henderson-Hasselbalch equation (94), which describes the relationship between pH, HCO_3^-, and dissolved CO_2

$$pH = pK_a' + \log \frac{[HCO_3^-]}{S \cdot P_{CO_2}} \tag{6}$$

where S is the solubility coefficient of CO_2 and equals 0.0307 mM/Torr at 37°C in human plasma (8). The pK_a' incorporates activity coefficients and has a normal value of 6.10 in humans but varies slightly depending on the physiological circumstances (124).

HYDRATION-DEHYDRATION KINETICS. Previously, only the reactions in Equations 1 and 2 were thought to be involved in hydration of CO_2 (129), but Eigen et al. (43) suggested an alternate pathway

$$CO_2 + H_2O \rightleftharpoons H^+ + HCO_3^- \tag{7}$$

whereby CO_2 and H_2O react directly to form H^+ and HCO_3^-. Equations 1, 2, and 7 are interrelated according to the scheme depicted in Figure 1 (38, 94). The ratio of the rate constants k_2/k_2' equals K_1, the first acidic dissociation constant of H_2CO_3. The rate constants k_2 and k_2' are much larger than the other rate constants in Figure 1; thus HCO_3^- and carbonic acid can be considered as always in equilibrium (38). In contrast, reactions utilizing the k_1-k_1' and k_3-k_3' pathways are much slower. In 1935 Roughton (128) estimated that changes in plasma CO_2 concentration would have a half time of 1.5 min if the hydration-dehydration process occurred in vivo at its natural uncatalyzed rate. This simple calculation avoided complex buffering reactions, and more recent computer simulations have revised this estimate to 30 s (57). Nevertheless this approach was sufficiently accurate to prompt Henriques (68) to speculate five years before the discovery of carbonic anhydrase (carbonic dehydratase, E.C. 4.2.1.1) (103, 140) that CO_2 reactions were catalyzed in vivo.

The rate of uncatalyzed formation of CO_2 is

$$d[CO_2]/dt = k_1'[H_2CO_3] + k_3'[H^+][HCO_3^-] - k_1[CO_2] - k_3[CO_2] \tag{8}$$

Substituting the equilibrium relationship for Equation 2 and rearranging

$$d[CO_2]/dt = k_{H_2CO_3}[H_2CO_3] - k_{CO_2}[CO_2] \tag{9}$$

where $k_{H_2CO_3} = k_1' + k_3'K_1$ and $k_{CO_2} = k_1 + k_3$. The relative contributions of the k_1-k_1' and k_3-k_3' pathways have not been determined, but the composite description of the two permits calculation of the rates of the uncatalyzed hydration and dehydration. The variation

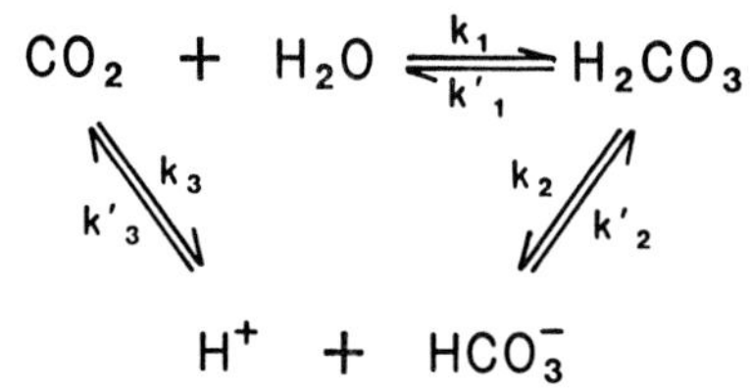

FIG. 1. Pathways for hydration-dehydration reaction. The k_2-k_2' reaction is much faster than other two reactions, which are rate limiting for the process.

of these kinetic constants with temperature is shown in Figure 2. Both $k_{H_2CO_3}$ and k_{CO_2} are fairly temperature sensitive (activation energies 15.3 and 18.3 kcal/mol, respectively), but the ratio of the two rate constants, K_h, varies relatively little with temperature. Between 0°C and 40°C the ratio of $[CO_2]$ to $[H_2CO_3]$ varies only from 883 to 434, a factor of ~2. The first acidic dissociation constant of carbonic acid under similar conditions of ionic strength and temperature can be calculated from K_h and Equation 5 if K_a is known.

Basic constituents of numerous buffering systems can catalyze the hydration-dehydration reaction

$$d[CO_2]/dt = (k_{H_2CO_3}[H_2CO_3] - k_{CO_2}[CO_2])(1 + k_B[B]) \tag{10}$$

where k_B is the catalytic factor of the conjugate base and [B] is the concentration of the conjugate base (129). Conjugate acids, unless possessing a negative charge, cannot catalyze CO_2 reactions (34). The range of catalytic factors can be quite large, e.g., from 50,000 for the hypochlorite ion to 10 for the dibasic phosphate ion. Physiologically, basic catalysis is unimportant because of the low values of k_B and concentrations of potential catalysts that are present in vivo. For example, the concentration of phosphate ion in plasma is <0.002 M and $k_B[B]$ is so small that it has no appreciable effect on the rate of change in $[CO_2]$ in Equation 10.

Interconversion of HCO_3^- and CO_2 can be achieved by a pathway not shown in Figure 1. Hydroxyl ion can combine directly with CO_2 to form HCO_3^-.

$$CO_2 + OH^- \rightleftharpoons HCO_3^- \tag{11}$$

This reaction becomes more significant with increasing pH because of the greater OH^- concentration (94). Hence the rate of formation of CO_2 is

$$d[CO_2]/dt = k_{H_2CO_3}[H_2CO_3] + k_{HCO_3^-}[HCO_3^-] - k_{CO_2}[CO_2] - k_{OH^-}[CO_2] \tag{12}$$

where $k_{HCO_3^-}$ and k_{OH^-} are the rate constants for Equation 11. Rearranging and substituting the equilibrium relationship for Equation 2

$$d[CO_2]/dt = (k_{H_2CO_3}[H^+]/K_1 + k_{HCO_3^-})[HCO_3^-] - (k_{CO_2} + k_{OH^-}[OH^-])[CO_2] \tag{13}$$

The relative importance of the hydration-dehydration reaction and hydroxyl pathway can be ascertained by comparing the two terms in either set of parentheses in Equation 13

$$\frac{\text{hydration-dehydration}}{\text{hydroxyl pathway}} = \frac{k_{H_2CO_3}[H^+]}{K_1 k_{HCO_3^-}} = \frac{k_{CO_2}}{k_{OH^-}[OH^-]} \tag{14}$$

At pH 7.4 and 37°C, only 9% of reaction product is formed via the hydroxyl pathway. This is somewhat less than the calculation of Roughton (129), principally because of the unusually high value of the ionization constant of water used in his calculation. At pH 7.2 and 7.6, this fraction becomes 6% and 14%, respectively.

The effect of temperature on k_{OH^-} is shown in Figure 2, based on the data of Sirs (138) and Pinsent et al. (118). The activation energy (13.7 kcal/mol) is quite similar to that of $k_{H_2CO_3}$ and k_{CO_2}. As a result the importance of the OH^- pathway is primarily a function of pH rather than temperature. The rate constant $k_{HCO_3^-}$ can be computed from

$$k_{HCO_3^-} = (k_{OH^-} K_w)/K_a \tag{15}$$

where K_w is the dissociation constant of water.

The uncatalyzed reactions of CO_2 proceed too slowly to permit adequate CO_2 exchange. Fortunately carbonic anhydrase is a potent catalyst and its action greatly facilitates excretion of CO_2. However, the uncatalyzed reactions undoubtedly have physiological

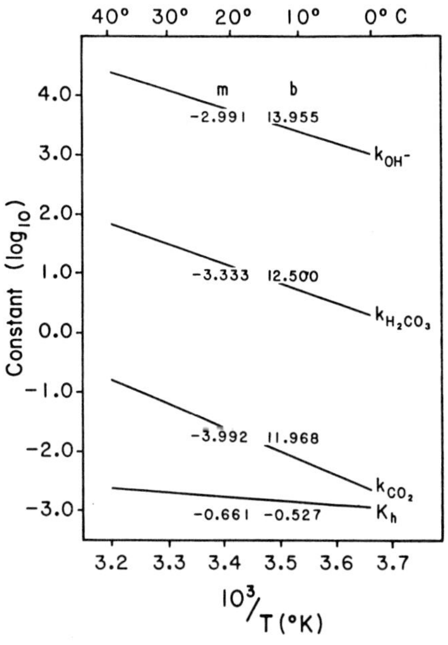

FIG. 2. Arrhenius plot illustrating effect of temperature on constants involved in CO_2 reactions. Straight lines fitted to experimental data are given by Constant ($\log_{10}$) = $m[10^3/T(°K)] + b$; m and b values for each process are listed in figure. [Data for k_{OH^-} from Pinsent et al. (118) and Sirs (138). Data for $k_{H_2CO_3}$ from Edsall (38). Data for k_{CO_2} from Roughton (129). Hydration constant K_h computed from $k_{H_2CO_3}$ and k_{CO_2}.]

importance because some body tissues do not contain carbonic anhydrase (99).

CARBONIC ANHYDRASE. The enzyme carbonic anhydrase is widely distributed throughout nature, including mammals, fish, invertebrates, and plants. Carbonic anhydrase is thought to be important in the transfer of H^+ and HCO_3^- in organs such as the pancreas, stomach, eye, kidney, and ovarian shell gland (24). Most forms of the enzyme have a molecular weight (MW) of ~30,000. The plant enzyme (MW 160,000) is an exception; this enzyme is composed of six subunits, which appear to be similar to the mammalian enzyme (121). These monomers may be held together by cysteine residues. Each molecule of mammalian carbonic anhydrase has a single zinc atom, which is essential for enzyme activity (78). Binding of the unsubstituted -SO_2NH_2 group of aromatic sulfonamides directly to the zinc ion renders the enzyme incapable of catalyzing CO_2 reactions (97). Acetazolamide is the prototype of this group of inhibitors.

Human erythrocytes contain two isoenzymes—a low-activity isoenzyme [carbonic anhydrase I (CA I)] and a high-activity isoenzyme (CA II); CA I and CA II were formerly designated CA B and CA C, respectively. A third isoenzyme, CA A, has been described but is identical in composition and activity to CA I (121); the separate designation is no longer used. Human CA II has 259 amino acid residues (67). Although similar in size, CA I has only 59% of its residues common to those of CA II (3). Erythrocytes of most mammalian species contain both low- and high-activity forms (121). The ox, cow, sheep, and dog are exceptions to this rule; their erythrocytes contain only a high-activity form similar to human CA II (24).

The X-ray crystallographic studies of human CA II reveal that the active zinc site is located in a cavity 15 Å deep. The zinc atom is liganded to the protein through three histidine groups (97). A fourth position on the zinc atom is occupied by either a water molecule or OH^-. Hydrophobic and hydrophilic amino acids in the cavity are distributed so that the cavity is divided into polar and nonpolar halves. Generally the side chains of the molecule are arranged with hydrophobic groups turned inward into the molecule and hydrophilic groups outward toward the solvent (121). Although the amino acid sequence of CA I is substantially different, its structure is quite similar to the high-activity isoenzyme.

Recently a third isoenzyme, designated CA III, has been described. Holmes (73, 74) noted carbonic anhydrase activity associated with several tissues, particularly muscles. The enzyme was absent in chicken breast, which is composed of white fast-twitch muscle fibers, but was abundant in the red slow-twitch fibers of leg muscle. The enzyme is distributed in many tissues of various species in different patterns. However, skeletal muscle, especially red muscle composed of slow-twitch fibers, is a common source of CA III. Interestingly, cardiac muscle is conspicuous for the absence of the isoenzyme (77). This confirms the indirect findings of Zborowska-Sluis et al. (147, 148), which support this distribution of carbonic anhydrase. These authors observed a volume of distribution of labeled HCO_3^- in skeletal muscle that was greater than the water space, implying interconversion of HCO_3^- and CO_2 with subsequent trapping of the label in the tissues. After administration of acetazolamide, the HCO_3^- label remained in the vascular space. In cardiac muscle, HCO_3^- space was similar to the vascular space, even in the absence of acetazolamide. Histochemical evidence indicates that the enzyme may be localized in the capillary endothelium (123), but its function remains speculative.

Koester et al. (95) have characterized CA III as a protein (MW ~ 30,000) that has one zinc atom per molecule. Thus it is similar to the other two isoenzymes but still is immunochemically distinct. In addition, Koester et al. demonstrated that CA III has only 20% and 3% of the hydratase catalytic activity of CA I and CA II, respectively. Another dissimilarity is its resistance to inhibition by sulfonamide inhibitors. The I_{50} of acetazolamide (the concentration of inhibitor needed to reduce enzyme activity to 50% of its native value) is three orders of magnitude greater than the I_{50} of the other two isoenzymes.

The catalytic activity of carbonic anhydrase appears to follow simple Michaelis-Menten kinetics (121). The initial velocity (v) of substrate conversion when the reaction is far from equilibrium is

$$v = \frac{-d[S]}{dt} = k_{cat}[E_0]\left(\frac{[S]}{[S] + K_m}\right) \tag{16}$$

where [S] is the substrate concentration, $[E_0]$ is the total enzyme concentration, k_{cat} is the turnover number, and K_m is the apparent Michaelis binding constant of the enzyme-substrate complex. Khalifah (81) has studied the catalysis of the hydration reaction at 25°C by purified preparations of human CA I and CA II. The K_m values averaged 4 mM and 9 mM, respectively, and were independent of pH (Fig. 3). In contrast, k_{cat} was markedly pH dependent for both isoenzymes, increasing with increasing pH. The k_{cat} of human CA II reaches a plateau at pH ~ 8.0, consistent with a single active acidic group with a pK ~ 7.0. The variation of k_{cat} of CA I with pH did not appear to be consistent with the titration of a single ionizing group. These data indicate closer similarity of the two isoenzymes than previously thought (99). The K_m values of the two isoenzymes differ by less than threefold, and the maximum difference in k_{cat} was no greater than a factor of 7 (81).

Pocker and Bjorkquist (120) have extensively studied the kinetic behavior of bovine carbonic anhydrase, a high-activity isoenzyme with properties almost identical to human CA II. With enzyme-catalyzed hydration of CO_2, K_m was independent of pH and had a

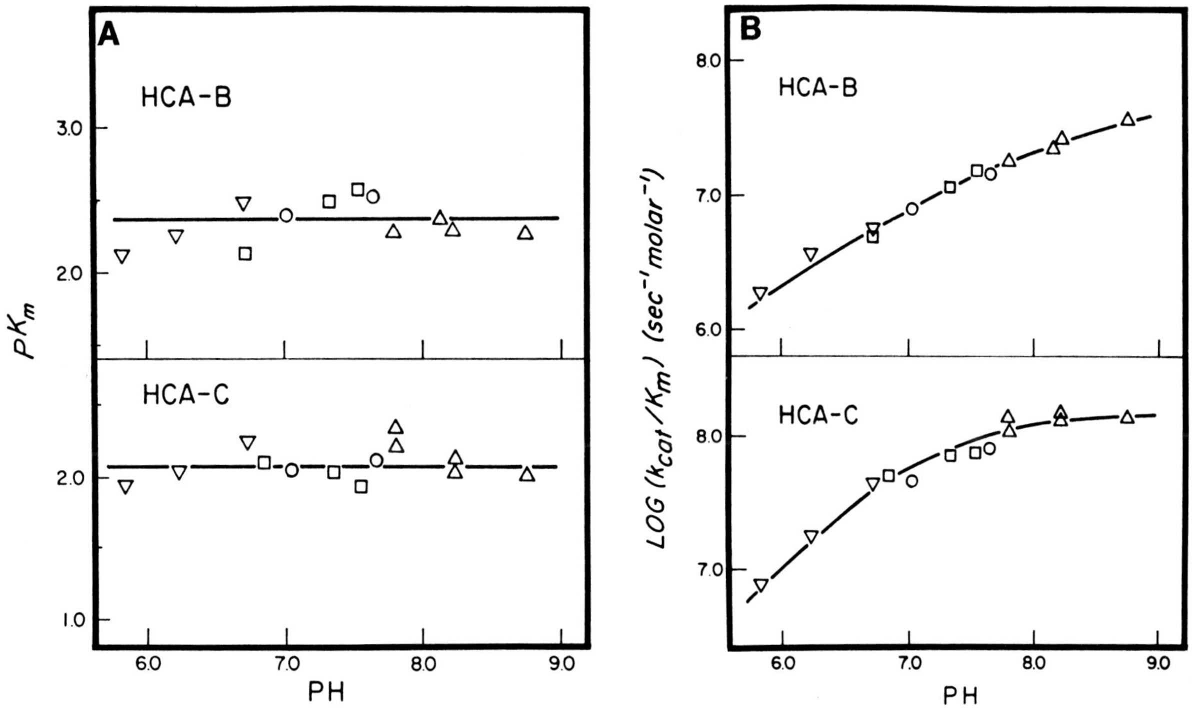

FIG. 3. Effect of pH on Michaelis constant (K_m; *A*) and turnover number (k_{cat}; *B*) of human carbonic anhydrase I (HCA-B) and II (HCA-C) at 25°C and 0.2 M ionic strength. The pH variation of k_{cat}/K_m is result of changes in k_{cat} because K_m is constant over this pH range. The following buffers were used in the experiments: ▽, 3,5-lutidine; ○, imidazole; □, *N*-methylimidazole; △, 1,2-dimethylimidazole. [From Khalifah (81).]

value of 15 mM at 25°C, close to that reported by Khalifah (81) for purified human CA II. Similarly, they found a pH-dependent increase in k_{cat} that leveled off above pH 8.0 at a k_{cat} of close to 10^6.

Pocker and Bjorkquist (120) also studied the catalysis of the dehydration reaction. Again, K_m (22 mM) was independent of pH but k_{cat} was markedly influenced by pH. The enzyme was most active at acidic pH with k_{cat} having a maximum value of 3.8×10^5/s. As pH rose, k_{cat} decreased, consistent with the titration of an active site with a p$K \sim 6.9$.

These observations led to the concept that the active site of the enzyme involves a single ionizing group with a p$K \sim 7.0$. The basic uncharged form is necessary for hydration of CO_2, and the protonated acidic form is required for catalysis of the dehydration reaction. The closeness of the pK of the active site to physiological pH is fortuitous, because this ensures a maximum cumulative activity for both the hydration and dehydration reactions. The very high turnover numbers associated with the reactions suggest that carbonic acid is not the substrate of the dehydration reaction. DeVoe and Kristiakowsky (35) calculated the rate of diffusion of carbonic acid from the surrounding solution to the active enzyme site during the dehydration reaction. Because the concentration of H_2CO_3 is so low, diffusion of the acid is not sufficient to maintain the observed rate of catalysis. This has led to the conclusion that HCO_3^- serves as the substrate with transfer of OH^- to form CO_2 (121)

$$HCO_3^- \rightleftharpoons OH^- + CO_2 \qquad (17)$$

This seems feasible because HCO_3^- is abundant in the reacting media. Furthermore it is consistent with the binding of this anion to the positively charged acidic conformation of the active site.

The hypothesis that HCO_3^-, rather than carbonic acid, is the product and substrate of the hydration and dehydration reactions carries a similar limitation. Khalifah (82) argued that if HCO_3^- were the substrate and product, the active enzyme site must change its state of ionization during catalysis and transfer of OH^- occurs via the reaction in Equation 17. Because the turnover of substrate approaches 10^6/s, this would require a rate of diffusion of OH^- or H^+ that is orders of magnitude greater than that observed experimentally. He postulated that this limiting step could be overcome if buffers participated in the proton transfer. Even in poorly buffered solutions, the concentration of buffer-bound H^+ is far greater than the concentration of free protons. The importance of this buffer-mediated facilitation of proton diffusion was confirmed when Silverman and Tu (135) demonstrated that enzyme catalysis increased substantially as buffer was added up to a concentration of 10 mM.

Despite extensive studies of carbonic anhydrase, its

behavior in vivo is still not completely clear. The data of Maren et al. (100) indicate that human CA I activity is inhibited by anions. The I_{50} for Cl^- is only 6 mM for the hydration reaction. Thus it appears that CA I is almost completely inhibited in the normal erythrocyte milieu. This has led Maren et al. (100) to speculate that CA I has a function completely separate from catalysis of CO_2 reactions. In contrast, CA II is markedly resistant to anion inhibition, with an I_{50} of 200 mM for the hydration reaction, and is postulated to be the major determinant of erythrocytic CO_2 kinetics.

Unfortunately it has not been possible to study carbonic anhydrase under conditions similar to those occurring in vivo. Investigations of enzyme activity utilizing the usual kinetic techniques have been conducted in dilute solutions because the reaction proceeds too rapidly when enzyme concentration is at its usual level. Kernohan et al. (79) observed linear catalysis of CO_2 reactions with increasing concentrations of carbonic anhydrase. In these experiments an enzyme concentration equal to 10% of the physiological level was reached. Extrapolation of their data to intracellular conditions indicated that the native human enzyme could be expected to catalyze CO_2 reactions 13,000-fold. Their experiments were conducted in the presence of 80 mM Cl^-, thus including the effect of Cl^- inhibition.

Donaldson and Quinn (37) have developed an ingenious method of characterizing chemical kinetics that depends on the rate of facilitated diffusion of isotopic CO_2 in a setting of chemical equilibrium. Under appropriate experimental conditions, transfer of CO_2 across a thin fluid layer depends on the rate of CO_2-HCO_3^- reactions. Under these conditions Donaldson and Quinn have demonstrated a linear increase in CO_2 kinetics with increasing concentration of bovine carbonic anhydrase even up to levels of 4 g/liter, the normal physiological concentration. This verifies extrapolations of measurements of enzyme kinetics in dilute solutions to physiological circumstances.

Carbamate Compounds

Uncharged amino groups of proteins can reversibly bind both protons and CO_2 (130). The relationship with H^+ is

$$\text{R-NH}_3^+ \overset{K_z}{\rightleftharpoons} \text{R-NH}_2 + \text{H}^+ \tag{18}$$

where R is the protein moiety and K_z is the acidic dissociation constant of the amino group. The uncharged amino group is also able to form a carbamic acid by binding CO_2

$$\text{R-NH}_2 + \text{CO}_2 \underset{k}{\overset{k'}{\rightleftharpoons}} \text{R-NHCOOH} \tag{19}$$

where k' is the association rate constant and k is the dissociation rate constant. Both CO_2 and H^+ compete for the uncharged amino binding site, thereby influencing binding of each other. The pK values of the carbamic acids thus formed are ~4.0–5.0 (126). As a result the acid completely dissociates at physiological pH to form carbamate with the release of a proton

$$\text{R-NHCOOH} \overset{K_x}{\rightleftharpoons} \text{R-NHCOO}^- + \text{H}^+ \tag{20}$$

where K_x is the acidic dissociation constant of the carbamic acid. Faurholt (44) treated Equations 19 and 20 as a single step because of the complete ionization of the carbamic acid and described the equilibriums involved in carbamate formation

$$\frac{[\text{R-NH}_2][\text{H}^+]}{[\text{R-NH}_3^+]} = K_z \tag{21}$$

$$\frac{[R\text{-}NHCOO^-][H^+]}{[R\text{-}NH_2][CO_2]} = \frac{K_x k'}{k} = K_c \tag{22}$$

where K_c is the effective equilibrium constant for the formation and dissociation of the carbamic acid. This approach is only valid as long as the carbamic acid dissociates completely.

Inspection of Equations 21 and 22 reveals that H^+ is involved in both reactions. A proton is released with ionization of the carbamic acid formed by combination of CO_2 with the uncharged amino group in Equation 22. Carbon dioxide binding decreases the concentration of uncharged amino groups, thereby shifting the equilibrium of Equation 21. The formation of new uncharged amino groups through this reaction is accompanied by further release of H^+. Hence binding of a single molecule of CO_2 leads to the release of more than one proton. The actual number varies between one and two, depending on the values of K_c and K_z.

Blood proteins transport CO_2 by direct binding of the molecule. The quantity of carbamates formed depends on pH, P_{CO_2}, the number of amino groups, and the values of K_z and K_c of these groups. An α-amino group is present at one end of each protein chain. This end-terminal amino group may not be available for carbamate formation because amino groups can be involved in a variety of chemical reactions that preclude carbamate formation (19, 59). In contrast to the maximum of one available α-amino group per protein chain, numerous ϵ-amino groups, principally located on lysine residues, are available. Previous work discounted the participation of the ϵ-amino groups in carbamate formation (129), but more recent data indicate that these amino groups can bind significant quantities of CO_2 if appropriate acid-base circumstances prevail (60, 62).

Estimation of the physiological role of carbamates has been hampered by the paucity of reliable data (129). Separation of protein-bound CO_2 from HCO_3^- in aqueous solutions was first accomplished with a difficult barium precipitation technique (47). More recent estimations of carbamate formation based on kinetic measurements of changes in P_{CO_2} (51) or separation by column chromatography (112) are more accurate but complex, thereby limiting the volume of

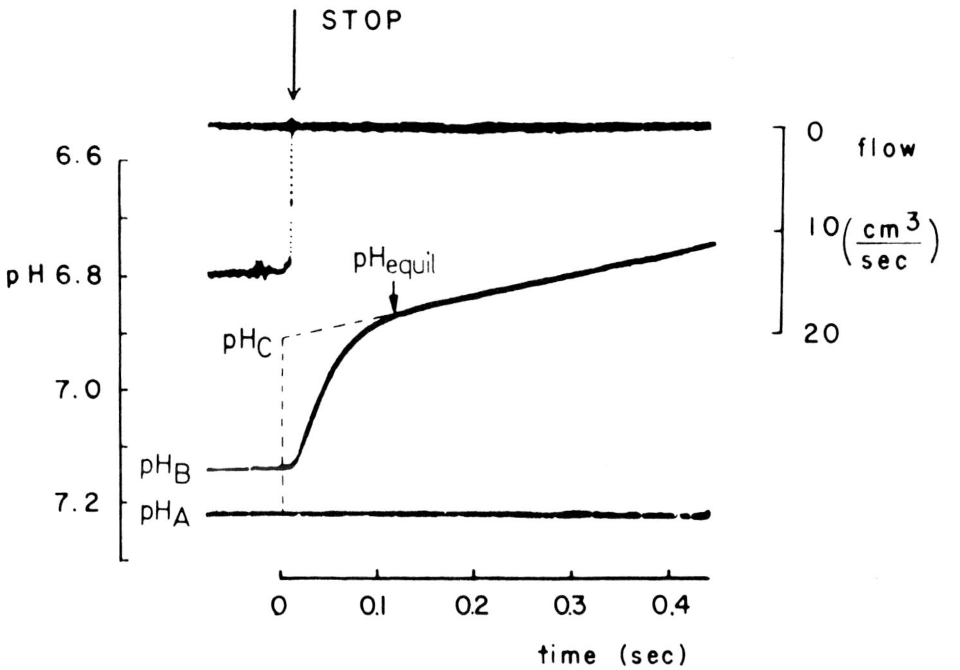

FIG. 4. Oscilloscopic tracing of change in pH after rapid mixing (STOP) of solution containing CO_2 with 4 mM glycylglycine at 37°C. pH_A, pH of glycylglycine solution prior to mixing. pH_B, pH of mixture after mixing but prior to reaction. pH_{equil}, carbamate equilibrium; subsequent pH change is due to continuing uncatalyzed hydration of CO_2. pH_C, extrapolation of pH to time of mixing; this pH would occur as result of carbamate formation alone. [From Gros et al. (60).]

data obtained. Perrella et al. (109) isolated carbamate compounds with a kinetic ion-exchange technique that has provided significant new information concerning the reactions of CO_2 with component chains of Hb (111). Gros et al. (60) developed a kinetic pH method that has been applied to both plasma proteins and Hb. Solutions of protein containing a carbonic anhydrase inhibitor are mixed in a pH stopped-flow apparatus with unbuffered solutions equilibrated with known P_{CO_2}. The pH changes rapidly with formation of carbamates and then more slowly as the uncatalyzed hydration of CO_2 takes place (Fig. 4). Carbamate formation is calculated from the initial rapid change in pH and the buffering capacity of the mixture.

CARBAMATE FORMATION IN PLASMA. In the only extensive investigation of CO_2 binding to plasma proteins, Gros et al. (60) demonstrated the release of more than two protons per protein molecule, the maximum possible number associated with carbamate formation at NH_2-terminal amino groups. With increases in both pH and P_{CO_2} the number of ions released increased exponentially, reaching values as great as 10 H^+ per protein molecule. The only plausible explanation of these data is participation of ε-amino groups in carbamate formation. The authors were unable to reconcile their data with single values of K_z, K_c, and the number (n) of participating amino groups per protein molecule. They postulated two types (α and ϵ) of amino groups able to bind CO_2 and calculated the values of the corresponding constants that fit the data with the least residual sum of squares (Table 1). The number of α-amino groups per protein molecule is within the expected theoretical range, although somewhat less than the maximum value of 1.0 expected with albumin. The value of 5.92 ε-amino groups is well below the 59 ε-amino groups of the albumin molecule. Gros et al. (60) speculated that only a portion of ε-amino groups was accessible for carbamate formation under the experimental conditions. The model utilized to calculate the constants of the carbamate reactions, as the authors acknowledged, underestimates the complexity of carbamate formation in plasma. A uniform molecular weight of 69,000 was chosen for plasma proteins, and all proteins were assumed to behave similarly as to the number of available amino groups and their equilibrium constants. Despite these drawbacks, this work provides clear insight into the role of plasma carbamates in CO_2 transport. As expected, the pK_c values of both α- and ε-amino groups are quite low and similar. Conversely the pK_z values differ significantly. The lower pK_z of the α-amino groups increases the likelihood of their participation in CO_2 transport, but the 10-fold greater number of participating ε-amino groups negates the effect of this difference in pK_z to a large extent. Total carbamate concentration resulting from both α- and ε-contributions can be calculated (60)

$$[\text{R-NHCOO}^-] = \frac{n_\alpha[\text{protein}][CO_2]}{[CO_2] + [H^+]/K_{c_\alpha} + [H^+]^2/K_{c_\alpha}K_{z_\alpha}} + \frac{n_\epsilon[\text{protein}][CO_2]}{[CO_2] + [H^+]/K_{c_\epsilon} + [H^+]^2/K_{c_\epsilon}K_{z_\epsilon}} \quad (23)$$

TABLE 1. *Equilibrium Constants Describing Carbamate Formation in Plasma and Hemoglobin Solutions*

Protein and Amino Group	n	pK_c	pK_z	Ref.
Plasma				60
α-Amino	0.55	4.20	7.00	
ϵ-Amino	5.92	4.26	9.03	
Reduced Hb				62
α-Amino, type 1	2.0*	5.19	7.05	
α-Amino, type 2	2.0*	4.36	6.13	
ϵ-Amino	14.5	4.99	9.82	
Oxygenated Hb				62
α-Amino	2.0*	4.73	7.16	
ϵ-Amino	15.4	4.71	10.18	

Solutions in absence of 2,3-diphosphoglycerate and at 37°C. n, Number of reacting sites per molecule; pK_c, negative logarithm of equilibrium constant K_c; pK_z, negative logarithm of equilibrium constant K_z. * Held invariant at 2.0 in the data analysis.

where n is the number of reacting sites per molecule. The two terms on the right side of Equation 23 describe the relative contributions of α- and ϵ-amino groups. At pH 7.40 and P_{CO_2} 40 Torr, ϵ-amino groups are responsible for 40% of plasma carbamate concentration. Gros et al. (60) have constructed carbamate dissociation curves for human plasma based on the constants extracted from their data (Fig. 5). The curves are relatively horizontal, indicating that carbamate formation is more sensitive to changes in pH than P_{CO_2}. Because the differences in plasma pH and P_{CO_2} between arterial and venous blood are small, the arterial-venous difference in carbamate concentration is only 0.002 mM. Plasma carbamate concentration is normally 0.6 mM, but the lack of significant change in concentration during capillary transit dictates that these compounds have no importance in CO_2 exchange.

HEMOGLOBIN CARBAMATES. Carbon dioxide also binds to both α- and ϵ-amino groups of Hb. Gros et al. (62) used the kinetic pH method to document progressive carbamate formation with increasing pH or P_{CO_2}. However, the ϵ-amino groups of Hb have a higher pK_z than plasma proteins (Table 1), precluding any contribution to CO_2 binding under physiological circumstances. The authors confirmed this conclusion by reacting the α-amino groups with cyanate to render them incapable of binding CO_2 (62). This carbamylation of the end-terminal α-amino groups of the α- and β-chains of Hb was associated with a complete lack of carbamate formation below pH 7.5, even though the ϵ-amino groups were not inactivated. At higher pH, ϵ-amino participation occurs but is inconsequential in vivo because this intraerythrocytic pH is present only when plasma pH > 8.0.

Oxylabile carbamate. Hemoglobin carbamates are involved in CO_2 excretion despite a relatively low concentration in blood (~1.0 mM). Ferguson and Roughton (47) demonstrated that reduced Hb forms substantially more carbamate than the oxygenated protein. The difference between bound CO_2 in the two states, termed *oxylabile carbamate,* causes increased CO_2 excretion in the lung as Hb is oxygenated. Conversely, reduction of Hb in peripheral tissues permits increased transport of CO_2. Rossi-Bernardi and Roughton (126) compared total CO_2 contents of oxygenated and reduced Hb solutions having identical pH and P_{CO_2}. Because these two variables were held constant, both solutions had the same concentrations of dissolved CO_2 and HCO_3^-. They reasoned that any difference between CO_2 contents must be due to the presence of oxylabile carbamate, and their data indicated an arterial-venous difference of 0.58 mM of oxylabile carbamate. Rossi-Bernardi and Roughton (126) calculated that this arterial-venous difference accounted for 27% of the CO_2 excreted by the lung. According to these computations, carbamate has a significant role in CO_2 exchange despite a relatively low absolute concentration.

Prior to the observation in 1967 of binding of 2,3-diphosphoglycerate (2,3-DPG) to the Hb molecule (13, 25), studies of Hb carbamate formation were performed with dialyzed Hb solutions, which were free of organic phosphate. Bauer (9, 10) repeated the earlier work of Rossi-Bernardi and Roughton (126) but added 2,3-DPG to some of the Hb preparations. Under conditions of constant P_{CO_2}, the total CO_2 content of reduced Hb at any pH is clearly less in the presence of 2,3-DPG (Fig. 6), implying inhibition of carbamate formation by the organic phosphate. Comparison of CO_2 contents of reduced and oxygenated Hb solutions in the presence of 2,3-DPG indicated that 2,3-DPG substantially decreased the amount of oxylabile carbamate. Direct determinations of the quantity of CO_2 formed from carbamate compounds during oxygenation confirmed the substantial reduction of oxylabile carbamate in the presence of 2,3-DPG (85, 86). Figure 7 illustrates that oxylabile carbamate decreases with

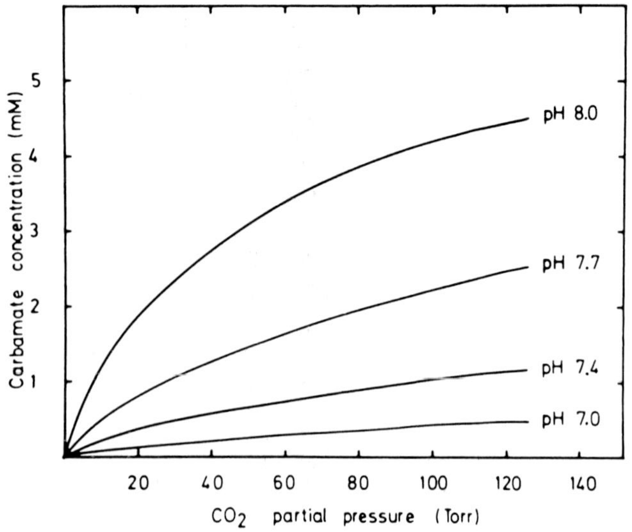

FIG. 5. Carbamate dissociation curves of human plasma at 37°C. [From Gros et al. (60).]

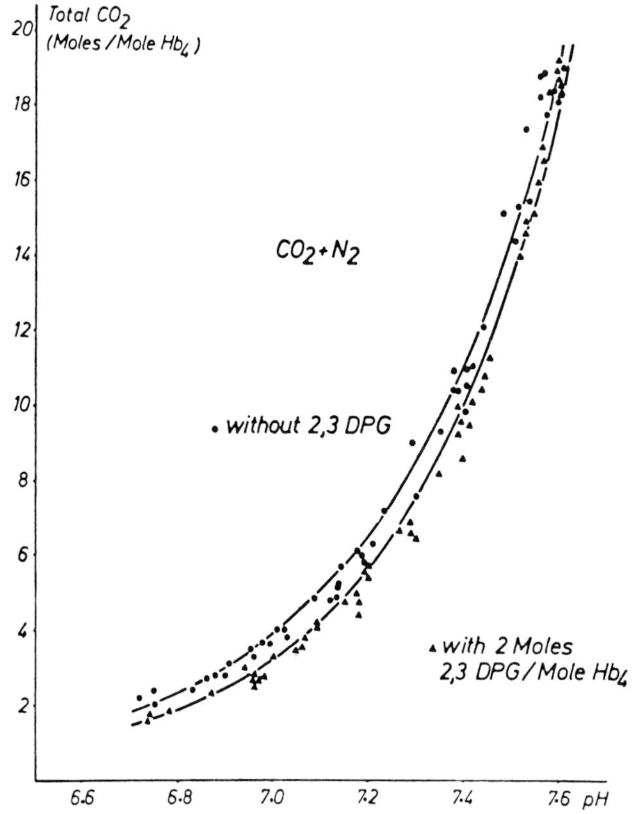

FIG. 6. Carbon dioxide content of deoxygenated solutions of human Hb at constant partial pressure of CO_2 (P_{CO_2}, 40 Torr). *Upper curve* obtained in absence of 2,3-DPG; *lower curve* obtained after addition of 2 mol 2,3-DPG/mol Hb tetramer. [From Bauer (10).]

increasing concentration of 2,3-DPG but is clearly present under physiological circumstances and has a role in CO_2 exchange, albeit much less than earlier estimates (129, 130).

The mechanism of the antagonism between CO_2 and 2,3-DPG binding to Hb was established by Bunn and Briehl (19). They utilized naturally occurring variants of Hb to demonstrate that the end-terminal valines of the β-chain are two of the principal amino acid residues involved in binding of 2,3-DPG. Electrostatic binding of this negatively charged molecule induces ionization of these two end-terminal α-amino groups, inhibiting binding of the uncharged CO_2 molecule. The end-terminal amino groups of the α-chains of Hb are not involved in binding of 2,3-DPG, and their ability to form carbamates is unaffected by organic phosphate (111).

Properties of α-amino binding sites. Attempts to describe all the α-amino groups reacting with CO_2 by a single set of values of K_c and K_z were only partially successful (51, 126, 130). As more reliable data became available, it was clear that α-amino groups had to be separated into at least two groups. All recent reports have assumed dissimilar behavior of amino groups associated with the α- and β-chains of Hb but still have met with limited success in defining the pK values of the reacting sites in question.

Perrella et al. (111) initially were unable to calculate the appropriate equilibrium constants of both α- and β-chains. However, they utilized further measurements of their own and data from the literature to later obtain a set of eight constants describing the ionization of the amino groups of both chains in oxygenated and deoxygenated Hb at 37°C (110). They concluded that changes of K_c with deoxygenation were more important than variation in K_z for oxylabile carbamate formation. Gros et al. (62) measured carbamate formation by the kinetic pH method at 37°C over a wide range of experimental conditions. The large variation in pH in their data provided more leverage in the calculation of dissociation constants but also required inclusion of the effects of ϵ-amino carbamate formation. In reduced Hb solution they were able to characterize two types of α-amino groups, each having two reactive sites, but their data best fit a model of only one type α-amino group with two reactive sites in the oxygenated state (Table 1). Matthew et al. (101) were also unable to fit constants to the β-chain amino groups in the oxygenated state. There has been little consistency in these reports. In some circumstances not only has the quantitative agreement been poor but reported changes in pK

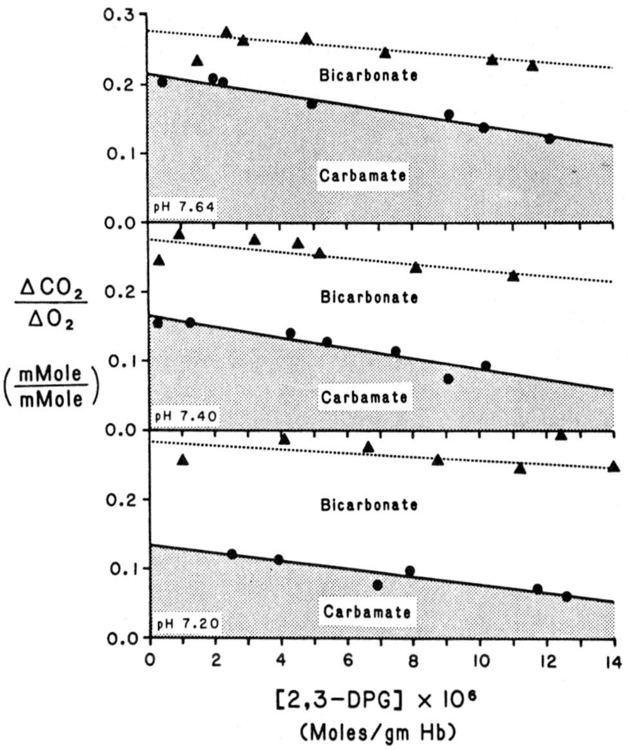

FIG. 7. Influence of 2,3-diphosphoglycerate (2,3-DPG) on Haldane effect in erythrocytes. ●, Data obtained with carbonic anhydrase inhibition. ▲, Data obtained without carbonic anhydrase inhibition. Relative contributions of HCO_3^- (*clear areas*) and carbamate (*shaded areas*) to total Haldane effect are labeled. [Adapted from Klocke (86).]

values with oxygenation have been opposite in algebraic sign. This difficulty in determining values of K_c and K_z may be the result of errors in the determination of the small quantities of carbamate formed (111), unpredicted alteration in the behavior of the β-chain amino groups with oxygenation (62), or perhaps the choice of an incorrect model. Physiologically, even if accurate these models are of limited value because all were obtained in the absence of 2,3-DPG. No investigator has successfully computed K_c and K_z in the presence of organic phosphates.

The inability to fit data to a model of oxylabile carbamate involving both α- and β-chains does not indicate that only one type of chain forms oxylabile carbamate. Arnone et al. (6) have provided crystallographic evidence of oxylabile formation by the α-amino groups of both α- and β-chains, despite an earlier report from the same laboratory that described only β-chain involvement (5). Studies of the O_2 dissociation curve (11, 83, 84), direct carbamino determination (111), and nuclear magnetic resonance studies (101, 104) strongly support oxylabile carbamate formation on both Hb chains.

In the original description of the use of carbamylated Hb to study behavior of the individual chains of the protein, Kilmartin and Rossi-Bernardi (84) concluded that the NH_2-terminal groups of both α- and β-chains were equally involved in carbamate formation in dialyzed Hb. Later work by Kilmartin et al. (83) on the O_2 half-saturation pressure of Hb (P_{50}) of carbamylated derivatives indicated that the β-chain was involved to a much greater extent in carbamate formation in the absence of 2,3-DPG. Bauer et al. (11) also concluded that the β-chain was responsible for 70%–80% of oxylabile carbamate in similar experiments with Hb variants. Nuclear magnetic resonance studies with $^{13}CO_2$ also indicated greater β-chain participation in the absence of 2,3-DPG (101, 104).

In the presence of 2,3-DPG the contribution of the β-chain is markedly reduced and both chains contribute equally to oxylabile carbamate formation. This is supported by studies of O_2-Hb affinity (83), nuclear magnetic resonance (101), and direct determination of carbamate (111). In the latter work, Perrella et al. (111) studied Hb that was selectively carbamylated at the end-terminal α-amino groups of either α- or β-chains. Carbamylation with cyanate at these sites prevents CO_2 binding and permits delineation of the relative participation of each chain in carbamate formation. The number of CO_2 molecules bound to noncarbamylated α-chains is illustrated in Figure 8*B*. Carbamate formation is substantially increased in deoxygenated Hb but is unaffected in either the liganded or reduced state by 2,3-DPG. It is apparent from Figure 8*A* that 2,3-DPG has no effect on CO_2 binding to the NH_2-terminals of β-chains in the liganded circumstance. In contrast, 2,3-DPG markedly inhibits CO_2 binding to β-chains in reduced Hb solution. At physiological P_{CO_2} in the absence of organic

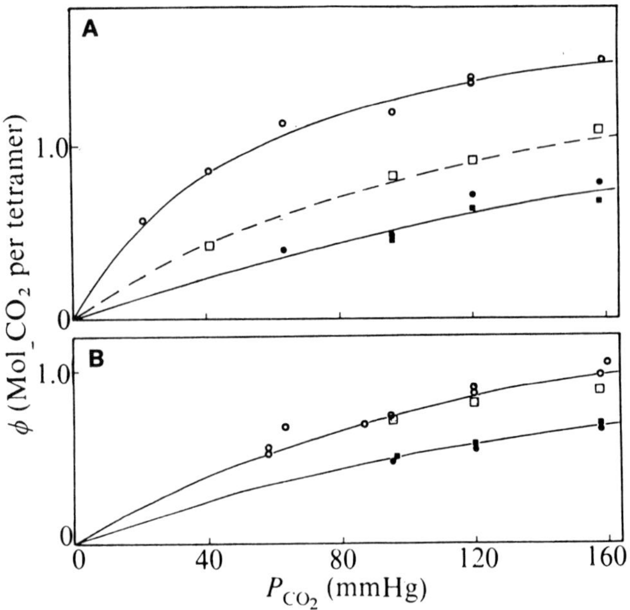

FIG. 8. Carbon dioxide bound to β-chain (*A*) and α-chain (*B*) of Hb selectively carbamylated at NH_2-terminal amino groups. ○, □, Deoxygenated solutions. ●, ■, Solutions of Hb liganded with CO. ○, ●, Solutions free of 2,3-DPG. □, ■, Data obtained in presence of 2 mol 2,3-DPG/mol Hb tetramer. [From Perrella et al. (111). Reprinted by permission from *Nature*, copyright 1975, MacMillan Journals Limited.]

phosphate, oxylabile carbamate associated with the β-chains is more than three times as great as that of the α-chains. However, 2,3-DPG reduces this β-chain involvement to approximately the same level as α-chains. As a result, total oxylabile carbamate decreases by 50% in the presence of large quantities of organic phosphate.

Role of carbamate in CO_2 excretion. Previous estimates of the importance of carbamate in CO_2 excretion (126, 129) must be revised in view of the effect of 2,3-DPG on oxylabile carbamate (9, 10, 86). Bauer and Schröder (12) observed a difference of 0.081 mmol in bound CO_2/mmol Hb (monomer) between reduced and oxygenated human blood, <40% of the value measured by Rossi-Bernardi and Roughton (126) in the absence of 2,3-DPG. Using this data, they calculated that only 10.5% of total CO_2 excreted in lungs in resting humans was transported as oxylabile carbamate. Even this reduced estimate of oxylabile carbamate has been challenged (7). The specific effect of CO_2 on the O_2 dissociation curve, $\Delta \log P_{O_2}/\Delta \log P_{CO_2}$, decreases with increasing O_2 saturation of blood (7, 54, 71). According to the linked-function theory (145), oxylabile carbamate should be similarly reduced at higher O_2 saturations. Arturson et al. (7) have calculated that this should result in a reduction of oxylabile carbamate to 3%–5% of total CO_2 excretion under normal circumstances. Unfortunately the application of the linked-function theory to oxylabile carbamate formation has not been verified. The only information available is from a single experiment by

Ferguson (46), who used the cumbersome barium precipitation technique. These data show a constant increase in carbamate formation with increasing O_2 saturation in contrast to the linked-function prediction of less carbamate formation at high O_2 saturation. A conclusive answer to this discrepancy awaits more precise experimental work employing more modern techniques.

Bauer and Schröder (12) found that oxylabile carbamate formation is 44% greater in fetal than adult human blood. This increase is the result of the presence of a glycine residue at the NH_2-terminal of the γ-chain of fetal Hb. The pK_z of this amino group is greater than that of the NH_2-terminal valine of the corresponding β-chain of adult Hb (59). The higher pK_z leads to a greater chance of the group being uncharged at physiological pH and to decreased binding to the negatively charged 2,3-DPG molecule. Both conditions favor carbamate formation. On this basis, Bauer and Schröder estimated that 19% of CO_2 excretion in the fetus occurred via the oxylabile carbamate pathway. Bursaux et al. (20), because of the influence of CO_2 on the fetal O_2 dissociation curve, have used the linked-function theory to revise this figure to 9%. This estimate also needs direct experimental confirmation.

CARBON DIOXIDE DISSOCIATION CURVE

In 1914 Christiansen, Douglas, and Haldane (27) provided the first accurate description of the CO_2 dissociation curve and its relationship to oxygenation. This classic investigation was prompted by their calculation that venous P_{CO_2} had to be substantially greater than arterial P_{CO_2} if CO_2 contents of both specimens were plotted on the same dissociation curve. Using 3- to 4-ml samples of fresh defibrinated blood obtained from finger punctures, they meticulously constructed CO_2 dissociation curves of both reduced and oxygenated blood (Fig. 9*A*). These data indicated that a substantial decrement in blood CO_2 content was associated with oxygenation at any given P_{CO_2}. Experiments with different O_2 and carbon monoxide mixtures demonstrated that the difference in CO_2 content was a linear function of binding of ligands to the heme moiety. This phenomenon is usually referred to as the Haldane effect; the names of the first two authors are omitted in favor of the more well-known Haldane.

A flurry of work followed this report in the 1920s. Peters (114) made the empirical observation that the CO_2 dissociation curve was linear when plotted on logarithmic axes (Fig. 9*B*). He and his colleagues (115) documented that the slope of the dissociation curve was a function of the Hb concentration of blood. This permits complete description of an individual CO_2 dissociation curve with the experimental determinations of a single point on the curve and the Hb concentration of blood (116). At least one experimental point on the curve is required because alterations

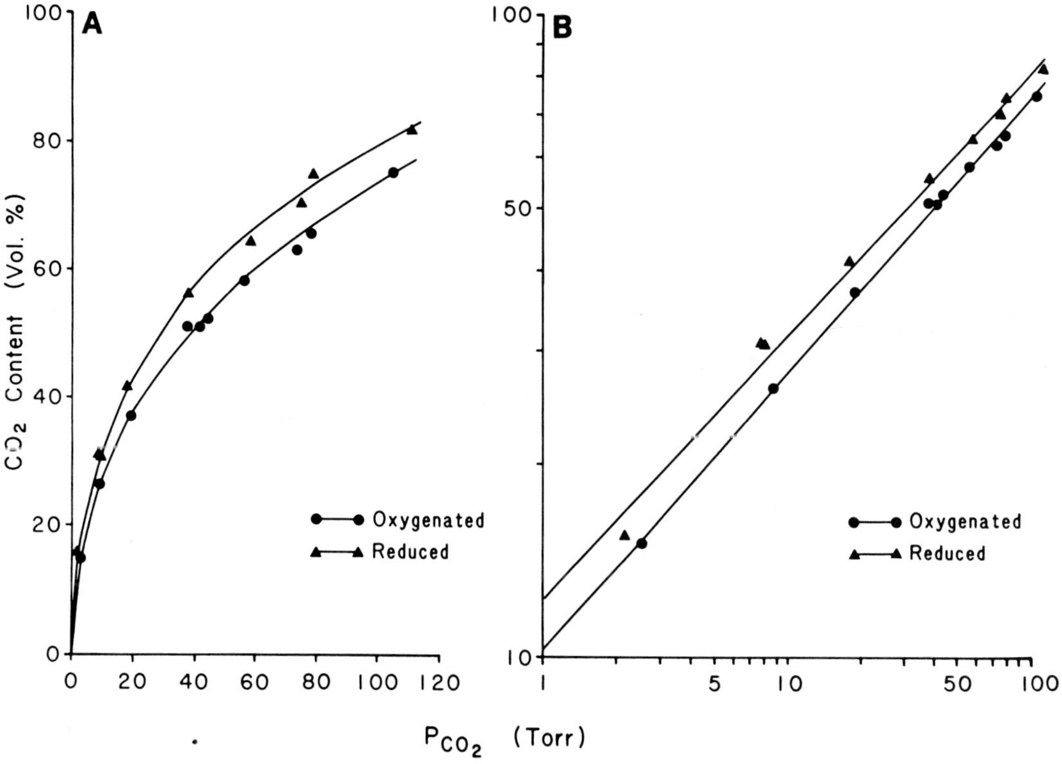

FIG. 9. Carbon dioxide dissociation curve of human blood plotted on linear (*A*) and logarithmic (*B*) axes. [Data from Christiansen et al. (27).]

in acid-base status can shift the vertical position of the dissociation curve. Christiansen, Douglas, and Haldane (27) observed that "violent exertion" led to "an enormous temporary alteration in the absorption curve." They correctly surmised that this was the result of transient lactic acidosis with buffering that is accompanied by reduction in blood HCO_3^-.

Most subsequent investigators have not even measured total CO_2 content to obtain a point on the dissociation curve but have calculated blood CO_2 content from Hb concentration, O_2 saturation, and plasma pH with an empirical relationship such as that described by Visser (142). This approach has been successful because interest has focused on changes in CO_2 content associated with gas exchange rather than the absolute CO_2 content of blood. McHardy (102) has demonstrated that the slope of the dissociation curve, and therefore the arterial-venous content difference for a given change in P_{CO_2}, is constant over a wide range of conditions as long as non-HCO_3^- buffering power of blood is considered. Hemoglobin is responsible for most of this buffering and appears to be the only factor necessary to consider, although plasma protein concentration will affect the buffering power of separated plasma (125). The effect of other blood constituents that may affect carbamate formation, such as 2,3-DPG, is unknown. However, in their original description, Christiansen et al. (27) emphasized the importance of using fresh blood to construct the curves. As a result, 2,3-DPG concentration would not have changed and the standard dissociation curves in the literature (2) can be applied to in vivo circumstances without apparent error.

Buffering of CO_2

Addition of CO_2 to blood generates significant quantities of H^+, which must be buffered by non-HCO_3^- compounds to prevent large changes in pH. Carbon dioxide in aqueous solutions is in equilibrium with carbonic acid, which in turn dissociates into H^+ and HCO_3^-. In the absence of buffers, H^+ lowers solution pH, thereby limiting the increment in HCO_3^- concentration and total CO_2 content. The non-HCO_3^- buffering power of physiological solutions is expressed in slykes $\{d[HCO_3^-]/d(pH)\}$ with HCO_3^- concentration expressed as millimoles per liter. Addition of buffers to a solution improves buffering capacity and therefore the increment in HCO_3^- concentration with any given change in pH. This is illustrated in Table 2. With increasing concentration, the buffering power of a phosphate solution improves and more CO_2 can be absorbed and converted into HCO_3^-.

TABLE 2. *Slope of In Vitro CO_2 Dissociation Curve*

Substance	β	Ref.
Phosphate buffer		
2.5 mM	1.0	
10.0 mM	4.0	
25.0 mM	10.0	
Separated plasma, dog		125
Protein 0.0 g/100 ml	0.7	
Protein 8.2 g/100 ml	6.0	
Protein 13.9 g/100 ml	9.6	
"True" plasma, human		1
Hb 0.0 g/100 ml	7.5	
Hb 5.0 g/100 ml	15.1	
Hb 10.0 g/100 ml	23.1	
Hb 15.0 g/100 ml	32.3	
Hb 20.0 g/100 ml	40.9	
Erythrocytes, human	47.9	2
Whole blood, human	34.4	2

β, Buffering power, corrected for water content and expressed as millimoles per liter of water per pH unit at pH 7.4.

TABLE 3. *Slope of In Vivo CO_2 Dissociation Curve of "True" Plasma*

Duration of CO_2 Exposure, h	β
0.5	18.4
1	32.9
3	38.0
5	37.2
7	46.3
15	42.0
24	58.0
48	90.0

β, Buffering power, calculated as millimoles per liter of plasma per pH unit (1) from data of Nichols (105) obtained in rats.

Plasma separated from erythrocytes and then equilibrated with CO_2 has the ability to absorb CO_2 because of the buffering provided by plasma proteins. This capacity is proportional to protein concentration (Table 2). However, this is substantially less than the apparent buffering power of "true" plasma—plasma that has been separated from erythrocytes after equilibration with CO_2. Plasma CO_2 content then reflects not only plasma buffering but also buffering provided by intracellular Hb. Bicarbonate formed due to buffering of CO_2 inside the cell exchanges for plasma Cl^-, thereby increasing plasma HCO_3^- more than could be achieved by plasma buffering alone. Erythrocyte buffering power, corrected for intracellular water content, is greater than that of plasma. Whole blood, a mixture of plasma and erythrocytes, has an intermediate value. The buffering powers of "true" plasma, erythrocytes, and whole blood are predominantly a function of Hb concentration. These buffering powers all pertain to solutions equilibrated in vitro.

Blood buffering in vivo differs because buffering is not confined to the intracellular compartment (88). This was first pointed out by Shaw and Messer (133) in 1932 and more recently emphasized by Brown and Clancy (18). In fact, CO_2 entering the body gradually distributes throughout the entire body and is even buffered by bone. Renal generation of HCO_3^-, though not true buffering in a chemical sense, also influences the whole-body buffering value. Thus the slope of the CO_2 dissociation curve determined in the intact organism changes temporally as more mechanisms come into play (Table 3). These changes are quite significant from an acid-base standpoint. However, the in vitro dissociation curve is the relationship of interest when considering gas exchange. Most lung tissue equilibrates with CO_2 in a few seconds, but tissue volume and buffering power are so small that the CO_2 dissociation curve in the pulmonary capillary is identical to the in vitro curve (19).

Distribution of CO_2 Content Between Cells and Plasma

Regardless of the form in which CO_2 is carried in blood, all components of the total CO_2 content originally enter blood as molecular CO_2. Only free CO_2 can readily traverse the capillary endothelium during the short time blood remains in a capillary. The P_{CO_2} quickly becomes uniform in blood because of its substantial diffusivity. The content of free CO_2 in cells and plasma is proportional to blood P_{CO_2} and the water contents of each compartment. Carbamate formation in both plasma and the erythrocyte is a function of four variables: P_{CO_2}, local pH, the number of amino groups that bind CO_2, and the dissociation constants of these groups. At equilibrium, blood and plasma HCO_3^- concentrations depend only on P_{CO_2} and local pH. As CO_2 is entering or leaving blood, the concentration of HCO_3^- also depends on the amount of available carbonic anhydrase because the uncatalyzed reaction between HCO_3^- and CO_2 is much too slow to reach equilibrium in the capillary.

ERYTHROCYTES. When blood is exposed to alveolar gas in the pulmonary capillaries, molecular CO_2 rapidly diffuses from both cells and plasma (Fig. 10). This volume of CO_2 is small because the gas is relatively insoluble and there is little difference between mixed venous and alveolar P_{CO_2}. However, as molecular CO_2 leaves the blood, the resulting chemical disequilibrium leads to generation of more free CO_2 from the HCO_3^- and carbamate pathways. Over 90% of CO_2 excreted in alveolar gas originally entered the lung in the form of HCO_3^- or carbamate. Sufficient carbonic anhydrase is present inside the erythrocyte to accelerate the dehydration reaction by a factor of 13,000 (79). As quickly as CO_2 is generated from this reaction, it leaves the cell and diffuses through plasma and the alveolar-capillary membrane into the alveolar gas. The dehydration reaction slows as intracellular stores of HCO_3^- are depleted. These stores are significantly less than those of plasma. The volume of intracellular fluid space is less than plasma and therefore can hold less HCO_3^-. Furthermore, confinement of the negatively charged Hb molecule to the cell interior leads to a Donnan distribution of freely exchangeable ions such as HCO_3^-, Cl^-, and H^+. Accordingly, erythrocyte HCO_3^- concentration is approximately two-thirds of the plasma concentration at pH 7.4 and 37°C (122). Intracellular HCO_3^- stores are partially repleted by diffusion of plasma HCO_3^- into the cell after disruption of the Donnan distribution (Fig. 10). Extracellular

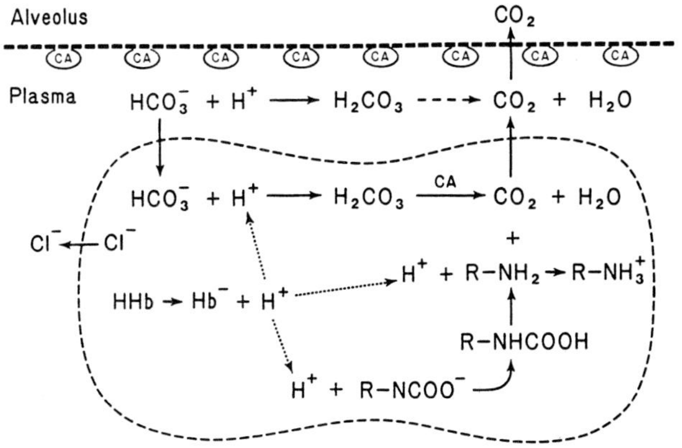

FIG. 10. Reactions of CO_2 in pulmonary capillary. CA, carbonic anhydrase, either free inside cell or bound to capillary endothelium. --›, Dehydration reaction proceeds much more slowly in plasma than erythrocyte. ⟶, Processes that proceed rapidly. •••›, Participation of H^+ associated with Hb buffering.

HCO_3^- is exchanged for intracellular Cl^- to maintain electroneutrality. This "chloride shift," also known as the "Hamburger shift" (66), provides plasma HCO_3^- access to the large quantities of intracellular carbonic anhydrase necessary for catalysis of the dehydration reaction.

After the initial rapid decrease in intracellular P_{CO_2}, molecular CO_2 is also generated from carbamate compounds. This requires association of an H^+ with the carbamate ion, followed by dissociation of the CO_2 molecule from the amino group. The small changes in pH and P_{CO_2} occurring in blood during gas exchange are not sufficient to produce any measurable release of CO_2 bound as carbamate. However, as described previously, the dissociation constants of Equations 21 and 22 change with oxygenation of Hb, leading to the release of significant quantities of CO_2.

Generation of free CO_2 via the carbamate and dehydration reactions consumes H^+. Conversion of HCO_3^- to CO_2 requires an equal number of protons. Release of CO_2 from carbamate utilizes even more H^+. The formation of carbamic acid from the carbamate ion (Fig. 10) consumes a single proton. As CO_2 is released from the carbamic acid, the concentration of uncharged amino groups increases. A portion of these groups ionize, consuming more H^+. Generation of CO_2 by the carbamate pathway requires more than a single proton, the exact number depending on the values of K_z and K_c and their change with oxygenation. This has been estimated to vary between 1.2 and 1.8 protons from pH 6.9 to 7.9 in human blood (86) and also appears to be a function of O_2 saturation (54).

Hemoglobin, which is the principal source of protons for both reactions, provides H^+ by two mechanisms. First, the intracellular contents are potent buffers, releasing ~3 mol of proton per mole of Hb monomer with a unit pH change (134). Second, the pK values of certain acidic groups on the Hb molecule change with oxygenation, releasing Bohr protons (113). The number of hydrogen ions released with binding of a molecule of O_2 can be computed from the relationship between two linked functions, as described by Wyman (145)

$$\left(\frac{\partial H^+}{\partial HbO_2}\right)_{pH} = -\left(\frac{\partial \log P_{O_2}}{\partial pH}\right)_{HbO_2} \quad (24)$$

where the term on the right side of the equation is the Bohr factor. As an approximation, one proton is released with binding of two O_2 molecules under normal circumstances, but this ratio varies significantly, depending on pH, P_{CO_2}, 2,3-DPG concentration, and even the O_2 saturation of blood (7, 54, 71, 134).

PLASMA. Dissolved CO_2 rapidly leaves plasma as blood reaches the pulmonary capillary. As discussed in CARBAMATE FORMATION IN PLASMA, p. 179, the difference between arterial and venous carbamate concentrations is infinitesimal and there is no production of CO_2 via carbamate reactions. Most CO_2 liberated from plasma is generated from plasma HCO_3^-. There is no evidence that carbonic anhydrase is present in plasma (99). Without catalysis the contribution of the dehydration reaction (Fig. 10, dashed arrows) is negligible. Recent evidence (98, 131) suggests that a relatively small concentration of carbonic anhydrase is localized to the capillary endothelium in some tissues and can catalyze the hydration-dehydration reaction to some extent (31, 39, 89). The quantities present are probably far too small (16) to provide the tremendous catalysis required for rapid conversion of HCO_3^- to free CO_2 (72, 86). The major pathway for mobilization of plasma HCO_3^- is through the action of intracellular carbonic anhydrase. As intracellular HCO_3^- decreases, plasma HCO_3^- enters the cell in exchange for Cl^- and the production of free CO_2 by the dehydration reaction occurs within the cell. Although the contribution of plasma to total blood CO_2 content is greater than that of the erythrocyte, almost all CO_2 excreted from the plasma must first enter the cell so that it can be processed to a form (molecular CO_2) that is readily excreted.

Haldane Effect

The role of the Haldane effect in CO_2 exchange was emphasized in the chapter by Roughton (129) in the 1964 edition of the *Handbook* section on the respiratory system. His estimate of the role of oxylabile carbamate in this event was too great because the influence of 2,3-DPG on carbamate formation had not been described. Although this modifies the relative importance of the mechanisms involved, it has no effect on his conclusions regarding the physiological impact of this phenomenon.

The quantities of oxylabile CO_2 exchange occurring via the carbamate and HCO_3^- reactions are functions of P_{CO_2}, pH, and the concentration of 2,3-DPG (86). The influence of pH on the Haldane effect under conditions of normocarbia and normal organic phosphate levels is shown in Figure 11. The Haldane effect is small under acidemic conditions but increases with increasing pH and reaches a maximum under normal acid-base circumstances. Below pH 7.5, oxylabile HCO_3^- is the predominant mechanism. Bohr protons released with oxygenation combine with HCO_3^- to form carbonic acid, which then dehydrates to CO_2 and water. The relative role of oxylabile carbamate in the Haldane effect increases with alkalemia for two reasons. First, at higher pH a greater portion of the α-amino groups involved in the carbamate reaction is present in the uncharged -NH_2 form, which binds CO_2 (62, 126). Second, binding of 2,3-DPG to the NH_2-terminal of the β-chains of Hb decreases with increasing pH (53), thereby lessening the inhibition of carbamate formation by the organic phosphate. As the carbamate reaction becomes more prominent, fewer Bohr protons are available for the HCO_3^- reaction. This factor is magnified because carbamate formation consumes more than one proton for each CO_2 molecule released. Consequently, with progressive increase in pH the participation of oxylabile HCO_3^- in the Haldane effect diminishes and eventually ceases.

Hill et al. (69) have calculated that the Haldane effect is responsible for 46% of normal resting CO_2 exchange. This is in contrast to the Bohr effect, which accounts for only 2% of O_2 exchange. The contribution of the Haldane effect is also influenced by ventilation-perfusion ($\dot{V}A/\dot{Q}$) abnormalities. In alveoli with low $\dot{V}A/\dot{Q}$, the respiratory exchange ratio is lower as CO_2 excretion decreases more than O_2 uptake. Hence a greater fraction of CO_2 exchange is oxylabile. On the other hand, the exchange ratio can be much greater than 1.0 in alveoli with an elevated $\dot{V}A/\dot{Q}$, and most

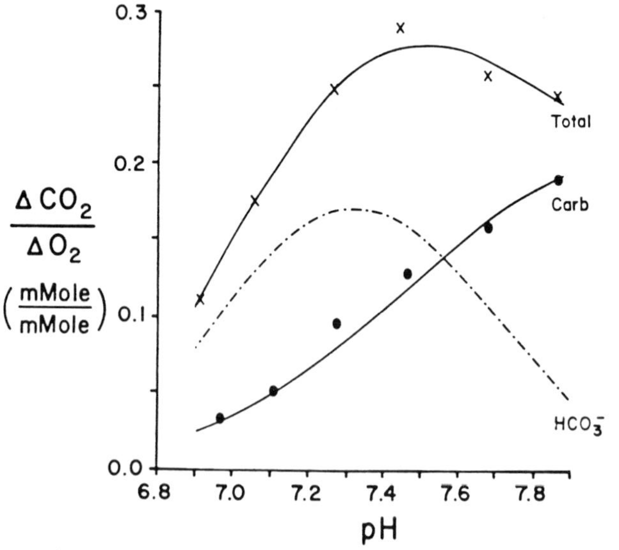

FIG. 11. Variation in Haldane effect as function of extracellular pH at P_{CO_2} of 42.5 Torr in erythrocyte suspensions. ●, Data obtained with carbonic anhydrase inhibition. ×, Data obtained without carbonic anhydrase inhibition. Contributions of oxylabile carbamate and HCO_3^- to total Haldane effect are indicated. [From Klocke (86).]

CO_2 is linked to the alteration in blood P_{CO_2} and pH rather than the oxylabile mechanism.

Grant (56) has investigated the influence of the Haldane effect on gas transport in a model that considers gas exchange both in the blood and during alveolar ventilation. He demonstrated that loss of the Haldane effect would not reduce CO_2 excretion to the same degree as its normal participation in gas exchange but would influence tissue P_{CO_2} and acid-base status. It appears that the Haldane effect does not greatly augment the quantity of CO_2 excreted but is instrumental in minimizing changes in tissue and venous P_{CO_2}; this led Christiansen, Douglas, and Haldane (27) to search for its existence.

Relative Contributions to CO_2 Exchange

Dissolved CO_2, carbamates, and HCO_3^- are responsible for 5%, 7%, and 88%, respectively, of the CO_2 content of arterial blood (Table 4). However, the relative contributions of each of these forms to CO_2 exchange in the lungs and tissues are not necessarily proportional to their concentrations. The arterial and venous CO_2 contents of blood of the resting human are fractionated in Table 4, based on available data that best approximate physiological conditions. The relative importance of each form in CO_2 excretion is provided by the venous-arterial difference and can vary significantly from its overall concentration.

As seen in Table 4, 1.02 mM of the 1.91 mM of excreted CO_2, 53% of the total, results from changes in plasma concentrations. However, most of this CO_2 content is in the form of HCO_3^-, and this ion must first enter the cell to be converted to free CO_2 before it can be excreted. In this sense the overwhelming majority of CO_2 molecules leaving blood in the lung involve intracellular reactions, a factor of prime importance when considering the kinetics of CO_2 exchange.

Changes in blood HCO_3^- account for 1.51 mM or 79% of the total CO_2 excreted. The value for dissolved CO_2 is 0.16 mM (8.4%) and for carbamate is 0.24 mM (12.6%). The latter is much less than Roughton's estimate (129) of 29.1% calculated from data obtained on blood devoid of 2,3-DPG but is quite similar to the calculations of Bauer and Schröder (12) concerning the role of carbamate in CO_2 excretion.

The fraction of CO_2 excreted via the Haldane mechanism can be calculated by assuming that the CO_2 dissociation curve does not shift its position with oxygenation. If a standard dissociation curve (2) is used, CO_2 content of arterial blood is 48.5 ml/100 ml at P_{CO_2} 40 Torr and 51.3 ml/100 ml at P_{CO_2} 46 Torr. The difference between these two, 2.8 ml/100 ml, is 65% of total CO_2 exchange. The remaining 35% of CO_2 excretion occurs via the Haldane mechanism. However, if the CO_2 dissociation curve did not shift with oxygenation, mixed venous P_{CO_2} in resting humans would have to increase to ~50 Torr to transport the same quantity of CO_2 and maintain arterial P_{CO_2} at 40 Torr. This estimate of the Haldane mechanism is slightly less than that calculated by Hill et al. (69). However, this type of computation and other estimates of the importance of different mechanisms of CO_2 exchange are quite sensitive to small changes in assumed values. For example, a change in venous plasma pH of 0.01 units would only change venous HCO_3^- concentration 2% but would affect the calculated venous-arterial difference by one-third. The precise fraction of CO_2 exchange occurring via different pathways depends on the conditions present in a given situation.

TABLE 4. *Carbon Dioxide Transport in Blood of Resting Human*

	Arterial	Venous	Venous-Arterial Difference
Plasma			
pH	7.40	7.37	−0.03
P_{CO_2}, Torr	40.0	46.0	6.0
Dissolved CO_2, mM	0.68	0.77	0.09
HCO_3^-, mM	13.48	14.41	0.93
Carbamate, mM	0.30	0.30	0.00
Total CO_2 content, mM	14.46	15.48	1.02
Erythrocytes			
pH	7.22	7.20	−0.02
P_{CO_2}, Torr	40.0	46.0	6.0
Hb, g/100 ml	15.0	15.0	0.0
Hematocrit, %	45.0	45.2	0.2
O_2 content, ml/100 ml	20.22	15.22	−5.00
Dissolved CO_2, mM	0.42	0.49	0.07
HCO_3^-, mM	5.65	6.23	0.58
Carbamate, mM	1.20	1.44	0.24
Total CO_2 content, mM	7.27	8.16	0.89

All concentrations are expressed in millimoles per liter of blood. Dissolved CO_2 in plasma was calculated from its solubility in plasma (8). The CO_2 dissolved in intracellular contents was calculated on the basis of water content (0.717) of cells (132). Plasma HCO_3^- was calculated with the dissociation constant reported by Rispens et al. (124). Erythrocyte HCO_3^- was computed with plasma (0.93) and cell water (0.717) fractions and the Donnan relationship (r) reported by Fitzsimons and Sendroy (48) (assuming a linear relationship between r and O_2 saturation). Plasma and erythrocyte carbamate concentrations were computed from published values of equilibrium constants (60, 111). Linear relationship between O_2 saturation and carbamate formation was assumed (46). Changes in cell volume with oxygenation were calculated from the work of Dill et al. (36), with a linear relationship between O_2 saturation and cell volume.

TIME-DEPENDENT FACTORS IN CO_2 EXCHANGE

Carbon dioxide exchange involves multiple interrelated physical and chemical events, which are depicted in Figure 10. Although each of these processes is relatively rapid, they are entwined in a complex manner. Forster (49) has pointed out that in this situation the combination of processes might proceed at a rate substantially slower than any single step. A great deal of data dealing with the kinetics of individual events in CO_2 exchange is available. Unfortunately it has not been technically feasible to study the kinetics of the integrated system as it occurs in vivo. As a result, insights into the interactions of the various steps in CO_2 exchange have been achieved largely through computational models (14, 69).

Diffusion of CO_2

Movement of large volumes of CO_2 from one body compartment to another depends almost exclusively on diffusion of molecular CO_2. During CO_2 excretion there are three barriers to diffusion of the gas—the viscous interior of the cell, the erythrocyte membrane, and the alveolar-capillary membrane.

Diffusive movement of CO_2 proceeds rapidly in aqueous solutions in comparison with O_2 because of its greater solubility. Inside the cell, diffusion of any gas is hampered by the closely packed Hb molecules. Gros and Moll (61) measured diffusion of CO_2 through thin layers of Hb solutions under conditions in which there was little facilitated diffusion by HCO_3^-. They found a fairly linear relationship between CO_2 diffusivity and Hb concentration. These findings agreed well with the work of previous investigators; the reduction of CO_2 diffusivity in any tissue appears to be a linear function of protein concentration. In concentrated Hb solution (33 g/100 ml) at 38°C, CO_2 diffusivity is 1.14×10^{-5} cm^2/s, ~35%–40% of its value in water (61). This reduction does not hinder CO_2 exchange. For example, if reactions of CO_2 are neglected, with a step change in P_{CO_2} at the exterior of the cell, equilibrium in the center of the erythrocyte would be achieved with a half time of 0.3 ms.

The issue of the importance of CO_2 permeability of the erythrocyte membrane is more controversial. There have been no accurate measurements of erythrocyte permeability to CO_2. Forster (50) used relative lipid solubilities and masses of the two compounds to calculate a value of 0.58 cm/s by extrapolation from measurements of erythrocyte permeability to ammonia. Gros and Moll (61) measured CO_2 diffusion in thin layers of Hb solutions and erythrocytes; they found a difference of only 0%–3% between the two. From these data they estimated that the permeability was >3.0 cm/s, although their measurements admittedly did not have the accuracy necessary to define the permeability with precision.

Silverman et al. (137) measured the rate of depletion of isotopic O_2-enriched CO_2 in erythrocyte suspensions. Based on the observation that the rate of degradation of isotopic CO_2 was not affected until over 80% of intracellular carbonic anhydrase activity was inhibited, they concluded that erythrocyte permeability to CO_2 was rate limiting rather than the kinetics of the hydration reaction. From these data they calculated an erythrocyte permeability for CO_2 of 0.0076 cm/s. In contrast, Itada and Forster (76), using basically the same technique, assumed that the effect of membrane permeability on the reaction rate was negligible and calculated the intracellular activity of carbonic anhydrase from their data. If the low estimate of CO_2 permeability of Silverman et al. (137) were correct, the erythrocyte membrane would significantly hinder CO_2 excretion. Computations of CO_2 exchange indicate that end-capillary equilibrium between alveolar gas and capillary blood is barely reached if CO_2 permeability is assumed to be infinite (14). Reducing erythrocyte CO_2 permeability to 0.0076 cm/s would lead to significant end-capillary disequilibrium. Most likely the reduced estimate of CO_2 permeability resulted from artifacts caused by unstirred layers of fluid on the exterior surface of the erythrocyte. Coin and Olson (28) demonstrated the presence of such artifacts under conditions optimal for measuring cell kinetics in a stopped-flow reaction apparatus. The isotopic CO_2 studies were conducted under circumstances much more conducive to this artifact, a possibility recently acknowledged (136).

Gutknecht et al. (65) measured permeability to CO_2 in artificial lipid bilayers. Carefully controlling for the effect of stagnant layers on the surfaces of the membrane, they obtained a CO_2 permeability of 0.35 cm/s, very similar to Forster's calculated value of 0.58 cm/s (50). Although these membranes are not identical to the erythrocyte membranes, these data provide the best experimental estimate of permeability available.

The alveolar-capillary membrane is extremely permeable to CO_2. Conditions of diffusion limitation to CO_2 exchange by the membrane have not been achieved under physiological conditions. Using an isolated perfused lung preparation, Effros et al. (40) have established diffusion disequilibrium for CO_2 in the lung. Large sinks for radiolabeled CO_2 were created in the perfusion fluid and liquid placed in the alveolar space by raising the pH of both to 8.4 and adding carbonic anhydrase. Under these circumstances the authors observed end-capillary disequilibrium for CO_2. They concluded that pulmonary blood flow would have to reach extremely high, nonphysiological values before an alveolar–end-capillary P_{CO_2} gradient would occur as a result of diffusion limitation.

Hyde et al. (75) attempted to measure the diffusing capacity for CO_2 in humans with $^{13}CO_2$. During rest and exercise they found either minimal or no $^{13}CO_2$ end-capillary gradients and could only estimate that pulmonary diffusing capacity was >200 $ml \cdot min^{-1} \cdot Torr^{-1}$. In addition, most of this resistance to gas exchange appeared to be the result of chemical reaction rates rather than diffusive movement of CO_2 through the membrane. On the basis of available data, the calculated half time for CO_2 diffusion from blood to the alveolar gas is 2.4 ms, too rapid a process to limit gas exchange (91).

Dehydration of Carbonic Acid

As gas exchange is initiated in the pulmonary capillary, there are two stimuli to conversion of HCO_3^- to carbonic acid with subsequent dehydration to CO_2. The decrease in dissolved CO_2 with exposure to alveolar gas lessens end-product inhibition of the dehydration-hydration reaction. In addition, oxygenation of Hb is associated with the intracellular release of Bohr protons, leading to an instantaneous increase in carbonic acid via reaction (2).

INTRACELLULAR DEHYDRATION. Once the equilibrium between HCO_3^- and CO_2 is disturbed, the initial rate of CO_2 production is limited by the speed of the dehydration reaction. The change in free CO_2 is directly proportional to the degree of catalysis provided by carbonic anhydrase, whether the equilibrium is altered by a step change in P_{CO_2} (80) or release of oxylabile H^+ (86). The catalysis observed under these circumstances, a factor of ~10,000–16,000, is similar to that predicted from kinetic observations obtained in dilutions of cell lysates (79). The importance of carbonic anhydrase is underscored by the observation of Holland and Forster (72) that no change in P_{CO_2} occurs in the first 40 ms after a step change in P_{CO_2} if the enzyme is inhibited.

After the first 50–100 ms of disequilibrium and rapid CO_2 production, the dehydration reaction slows due to substrate depletion (72, 86). From this point in time, the major limiting factor in release of CO_2 appears to be the replenishment of intracellular stores of HCO_3^- by transmembrane Cl^--HCO_3^- exchange.

The very large quantities of carbonic anhydrase in the erythrocyte have led to postulates of an excess of enzyme activity beyond that needed for CO_2 exchange (129, 141). In a sense this is true because overall CO_2 exchange can be maintained despite partial or even complete inhibition of the enzyme (23, 141). However, the relative importance of different mechanisms of CO_2 exchange are markedly altered under these circumstances; dissolved CO_2 and carbamate compounds account for a larger fraction of total exchange. Experimental (72, 86) and theoretical (14, 69) evidence indicates that the initial portion of CO_2 exchange under normal circumstances is limited by carbonic anhydrase activity.

PLASMA DEHYDRATION. Carbonic anhydrase is absent from plasma (99), and in the past the dehydration reaction was thought to proceed at its uncatalyzed rate in plasma. Because of the short duration of capillary transit, the uncatalyzed reaction was thought to provide a negligible contribution to overall CO_2 exchange. However, recently three different laboratories using isolated, blood-free lungs provided data that indicate that plasma HCO_3^- has access to carbonic anhydrase in the pulmonary capillary. Effros et al. (39) injected radiolabeled carbon into the pulmonary circulation either as a bolus of CO_2 or HCO_3^-. Venous recovery of the label in either case was essentially the same under control circumstances, indicating rapid conversion of HCO_3^- to CO_2. In the presence of acetazolamide, the labeled CO_2 was lost into the alveolar space but labeled HCO_3^- was recovered in a manner similar to an intravascular marker. Crandall and O'Brasky (31) studied slow downstream pH changes after buffer containing CO_2 passed through the pulmonary circulation. With excretion of CO_2, perfusate pH would be expected to change slowly after capillary transit as the uncatalyzed dehydration proceeded to reestablish equilibrium. These changes were absent under control circumstances but were noted with enzyme inhibition. Klocke (89) quantitated CO_2 excretion in isolated lungs perfused with HCO_3^- buffer and estimated expected elimination of dissolved CO_2 from simultaneous measurements of acetylene excretion. Under conditions of carbonic anhydrase inhibition (Fig. 12), observed CO_2 excretion was only slightly greater than expected, as a result of uncatalyzed dehydration of carbonic acid. In control experiments performed without enzyme inhibition, CO_2 excretion was substantially greater, indicating catalysis during pulmonary capillary transit. Analysis of alveolar and pulmonary venous P_{CO_2} indicates attainment of virtual equilibrium of the dehydration reaction in blood-free lungs perfused with buffer (90).

Lönnerholm (98) provided anatomical evidence that carbonic anhydrase is localized to the pulmonary capillary endothelium. Effros et al. (41) utilized radiolabeled acetazolamide to show that this enzyme was

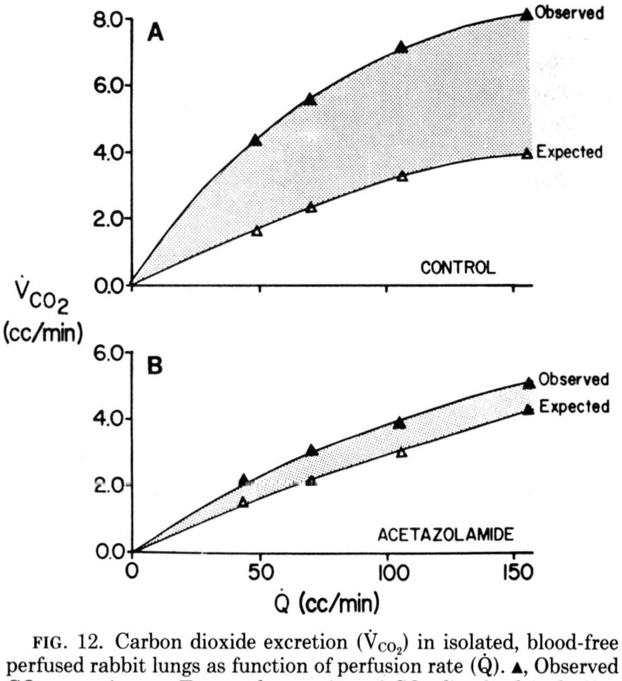

FIG. 12. Carbon dioxide excretion ($\dot{V}_{CO_2}$) in isolated, blood-free perfused rabbit lungs as function of perfusion rate ($\dot{Q}$). ▲, Observed CO_2 excretion. △, Expected excretion of CO_2 dissolved in buffer, calculated from simultaneous measurements of excretion of acetylene dissolved in buffer. *Shaded areas*, CO_2 generated in pulmonary capillary from HCO_3^- contained in perfusate. Small amount of CO_2 generated in presence of acetazolamide (*B*) is result of uncatalyzed dehydration reaction. Larger amount formed under control conditions (*A*) is due to catalysis of dehydration by capillary endothelial carbonic anhydrase. [From Klocke (89).]

accessible to plasma constituents during a single circulation. The carbonic anhydrase that is localized to the vascular endothelium is the result of active synthesis of the enzyme and does not represent adsorption of enzyme liberated into plasma by hemolysis. Ryan et al. (131) used specific antibodies to carbonic anhydrase and demonstrated its presence on the membranes of endothelial cells that had been passed through repeated generations of culture in blood-free media.

The presence of enzyme on the pulmonary capillary endothelium raises the possibility that plasma HCO_3^- can participate directly in the dehydration reaction without entering the erythrocyte in exchange for Cl^-. If true, this would radically alter conventional concepts of CO_2 exchange (129). In an elegant study Bidani et al. (16) have quantitated the amount of enzyme present on the endothelium and characterized its biochemical properties. They measured postcapillary pH changes after CO_2 elimination in isolated rat lungs perfused with HCO_3^- buffer containing varying concentrations of acetazolamide. The magnitudes of these observed pH changes were matched to those changes expected in a mathematical model of gas exchange with differing catalytic factors. The resulting initial velocities of the dehydration reaction under these circumstances were plotted as a function of substrate (HCO_3^-) concentration with the Lineweaver-Burk format (Fig. 13). Acetazolamide inhibition of pulmonary vascular carbonic anhydrase is noncompetitive, with an inhibition constant of 1.3×10^{-3} mM.

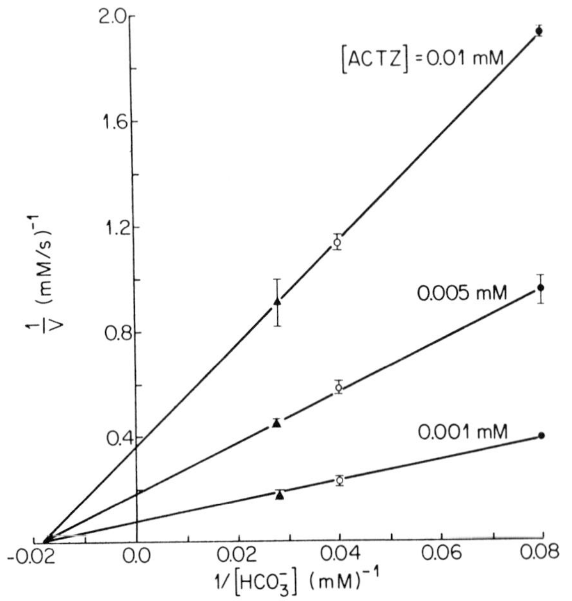

FIG. 13. Lineweaver-Burk plot of reciprocals of reaction velocity (V) and substrate (HCO_3^-) concentration in presence of different concentrations of acetazolamide (ACTZ). ●, 12 mM HCO_3^- in perfusate; ○, 25 mM HCO_3^- in perfusate; ▲, 35 mM HCO_3^- in perfusate. Data obtained in isolated perfused rat lungs in absence of blood carbonic anhydrase. Catalysis is result of activity of pulmonary vascular carbonic anhydrase. [From Bidani et al. (16).]

The maximum reaction velocity (Vmax) and K_m obtained from the data are 25 mM/s and 55 mM, respectively, suggesting that the enzyme has properties most similar to human CA I. The calculated turnover number (k_{cat}) is 25,000 at 37°C and pH 7.4–7.5. The authors calculated that endothelial enzyme activity is sufficient to catalyze the dehydration reaction by a factor of 130–150, far less than the erythrocyte catalysis of 13,000. Thus pulmonary vascular carbonic anhydrase probably has a very minor role in CO_2 exchange but is present in sufficient quantities to prevent end-capillary disequilibrium of the plasma dehydration reaction and resulting postcapillary pH changes (14).

Vascular carbonic anhydrase activity has also been demonstrated in other organs. The hindlimb musculature of the cat (42) and rabbit (106) contains sufficient enzyme to prevent most or all postcapillary disequilibrium. The rabbit liver appears to have intermediate activity (106), but the guinea pig liver has no apparent vascular enzyme (107). Studies of pulmonary vascular carbonic anhydrase indicate sufficient activity to abolish all postcapillary disequilibrium in the rabbit (39, 90), rat (31), and guinea pig (106). No significant physiological role has been attributed to vascular carbonic anhydrase.

Bicarbonate-Chloride Exchange

Participation of plasma HCO_3^- in the intracellular dehydration reaction requires rapid entry of the ion into the cell during the relatively short capillary transit time. This occurs in conjunction with simultaneous movement of Cl^- in the opposite direction to maintain electrical neutrality.

SPEED OF BICARBONATE-CHLORIDE SHIFT. Prior to 1970, estimates of the time required for 90% completion of this exchange ranged from 0.1 to >1.0 s (117). Technical difficulties in measuring kinetic events were largely responsible for the variability. More recent data indicate that the effective erythrocyte permeability at 37°C is ~10^{-4} cm/s for Cl^- and two- to fivefold greater for HCO_3^- (26, 87). Thus, after a step change in transmembrane HCO_3^- concentration, a new equilibrium is approached with a half time of ~0.1 s. Although this process seems sufficiently rapid to prevent end-capillary disequilibrium, HCO_3^--Cl^- exchange cannot be considered a single event acting independently of other elements of CO_2 elimination. The interaction of the dehydration reaction, release of Bohr protons after oxygenation, and Cl^- shift result in overall exchange that is much slower than any single event in the chain.

Crandall and Bidani (29) modeled CO_2 exchange to investigate the importance of the kinetics of HCO_3^--Cl^- exchange. Figure 14 illustrates the influence of effective membrane permeability on CO_2 excretion. Computed CO_2 excretion increases 8% as membrane permeability is increased from 10^{-4} to 10^{-3}

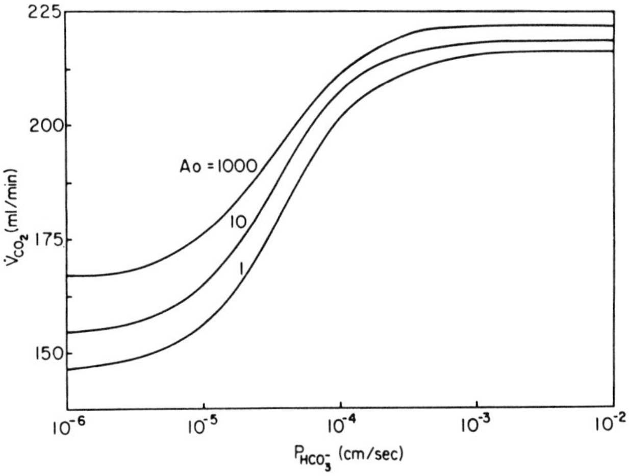

FIG. 14. Computed effect of erythrocyte HCO_3^- permeability ($P_{HCO_3^-}$) and plasma catalysis (A_0) of dehydration reaction on pulmonary CO_2 exchange in resting human. [From Crandall and Bidani (29).]

cm/s. Although this increase is minimal, a similar decrement in HCO_3^- permeability has a more substantial negative effect. Because of shorter capillary transit and increased CO_2 production, changes in permeability have greater effects during exercise. A 10-fold change in permeability is computed to produce a 14% change in CO_2 excretion. Interestingly the presence of extracellular carbonic anhydrase activity has relatively little effect on CO_2 exchange. As illustrated in Figure 14, CO_2 elimination increases with enhancement of plasma carbonic anhydrase activity, but the maximum increment in CO_2 elimination is only 7%, even with catalysis similar to that present inside the cell. Crandall and Bidani (29) demonstrated that this paradox results from compartmentalization of blood buffers. Plasma protein buffering power is only 10% that of the erythrocyte interior, and with rapid dehydration of plasma HCO_3^- there is a concomitant reduction in H^+ concentration, which reduces the speed of the dehydration reaction. Both enzyme activity and buffering of pH changes are necessary to maintain a rapid rate of CO_2 production from HCO_3^-.

Crandall et al. (30) have confirmed the importance of the HCO_3^--Cl^- shift in experiments in isolated lungs perfused with suspensions of erythrocytes. Steady-state CO_2 elimination was significantly reduced when facilitated erythrocyte HCO_3^--Cl^- exchange was blocked with 4,4′-diisothiocyano-2,2′-disulfonic stilbene (DIDS). Despite addition of extracellular carbonic anhydrase to the perfusate, steady-state CO_2 excretion was less than control, confirming the role of intracellular buffering in maintenance of the dehydration reaction.

In high doses both salicylates (32) and furosemide (17), drugs frequently used in clinical medicine, can inhibit HCO_3^--Cl^- exchange. The effect of lower therapeutic levels on CO_2 exchange is not clear. Inhibition of this important mechanism probably does not limit CO_2 exchange in the intact organism but leads to augmentation of CO_2 excretion by other pathways, such as increased elimination of dissolved CO_2 through hyperventilation (29). This type of adaptation occurs when the dehydration reaction is blocked by inhibition of carbonic anhydrase (23).

MECHANISM OF ANIONIC EXCHANGE. For many years anionic movement across the erythrocyte membrane has been viewed as a passive diffusion phenomenon down an electrochemical gradient (55). Presumably HCO_3^- movement was tied to simultaneous Cl^- exchange by considerations of electroneutrality rather than any direct transport process. Passow (108) postulated that fixed cationic charges in membrane pores restricted cation movement but facilitated anion diffusion.

Initial doubt concerning the validity of this mechanism was raised by the demonstration that the electrical resistance of the membrane of the *Amphiuma* erythrocyte was orders of magnitude greater than would be expected if anion exchange occurred by simple diffusion (96). Shortly thereafter, Gunn et al. (63) reported that self-exchange of labeled Cl^- displayed saturation kinetics. In addition, they demonstrated that Cl^- flux was pH dependent, with a peak flux at pH 7.8, behavior that was incompatible with the fixed-charge hypothesis. These findings led the authors to postulate that exchange is accomplished by a membrane carrier that reacts with the anion and has a fixed number of sites. Cabantchik and Rothstein (21, 22) developed a series of disulfonic stilbene derivatives that inhibit anion exchange when bound to the apparent membrane carrier, a protein with a molecular mass of 95,000 daltons. The carrier, known as band 3 protein because of its position on acrylamide gel electrophoresis, constitutes one-third of the total membrane protein and spans the membrane, with binding sites on both the interior and exterior of the membrane (127). Approximately 10^6 sites are present on the surface of a single cell, with each site having a turnover number of 5×10^4 ions/s (93).

The carrier system is inhibited by both HCO_3^- and halides, leading Dalmark (33) to postulate the existence of a separate "modifier" site on the carrier that interacts with the transport site and prevents translocation of an anion bound to the transport site. Gunn and Fröhlich (64) demonstrated that the carrier is asymmetric, with an apparent K_m for the exterior site that is 20-fold less than that for the interior site. Their data support a "Ping-Pong" mechanism in which the carrier transports a single anion through the membrane followed by transport of another ion in the opposite direction. They hypothesize that the carrier cannot revert to its initial configuration without transport of a second ion in the opposite direction, so there is no net transfer of electrical charge. This facilitated process contrasts with a frequently observed exchange mechanism in which two ions of like charge are simultaneously exchanged in opposite directions. Knauf (93) summarizes the current knowledge of the anion-exchange mechanism in his excellent review.

Interaction of CO_2 and O_2 Exchange

Carbon dioxide elimination in the lung depends on two events. The first is exposure to an alveolar P_{CO_2} less than mixed venous P_{CO_2}. Carbon dioxide diffuses from blood, and HCO_3^- is mobilized until capillary and alveolar P_{CO_2} values are equal. The processes of CO_2 diffusion, catalysis of carbonic acid dehydration, buffering, and transmembrane HCO_3^--Cl^- exchange appear to be sufficiently rapid to achieve end-capillary equilibrium. The second factor is oxygenation of Hb with resulting elimination of oxylabile CO_2. This introduces a complicating factor in that O_2 uptake must precede CO_2 elimination.

OXYLABILE CARBAMATE KINETICS. The binding of CO_2 to proteins is rapid. Plasma carbamate formation occurs with a half time of 0.047 s but does not contribute to oxylabile CO_2 exchange (60). Binding of CO_2 to Hb also is accomplished quickly, and the studies of Forster et al. (51) indicate that carbamate formation in Hb is complete in 0.1–0.2 s. These investigations were conducted in previously oxygenated or reduced Hb solutions. However, when CO_2 bound to Hb in intact erythrocytes is released after oxygenation, the rate appears to be substantially slower (86). This process follows an exponential time course with a half time of 0.12 s and requires 0.5–0.6 s for completion (Fig. 15). This reaction should reach completion in the pulmonary capillary, but the margin for error is small. In the experiment shown in Figure 15, oxygenation of the cell suspension was complete in 0.1 s, but oxygenation in the pulmonary capillary is thought to require 0.2–0.3 s under normal conditions (69, 143, 144). Thus mobilization of oxylabile carbamate may require close to the full time that blood remains in the pulmonary capillary under resting conditions. With the shorter capillary transit time associated with exercise, CO_2 exchange via the carbamate pathway may not quite reach completion, although any end-capillary disequilibrium should be small.

The cause of the discrepancy between the oxylabile carbamate kinetics in erythrocytes illustrated in Figure 15 (86) and previous data obtained in Hb solution (51) is not clear. Both were obtained with the same continuous-flow–P_{CO_2} electrode technique. The viscous cell interior could theoretically slow diffusion of CO_2, but this is unlikely because Kernohan and Roughton (80) reported that the initial portion of the carbamate reaction is identical in cell suspensions and solutions. Carbamate kinetics are usually measured during binding of CO_2 to Hb, and the data in Figure 15 was obtained during release of CO_2. However, the kinetics of carbamate formation or degradation are given by (51)

$$d[\text{R-NHCOOH}]/dt = k'[\text{R-NH}_2][CO_2] - k[\text{R-NHCOOH}] \quad (25)$$

Substituting Equations 19–22 and integrating (assuming $[CO_2]$ and $[H^+]$ are constant) yields

$$\frac{[\text{R-NHCOOH}] - [\text{R-NHCOOH}]_\infty}{[\text{R-NHCOOH}]_0 - [\text{R-NHCOOH}]_\infty} = e^{-bt} \quad (26)$$

where subscript 0 is initial concentration and ∞ is equilibrium concentration. The first-order rate constant, b, equals

$$b = k'\left\{\frac{[CO_2]K_z([H^+] + K_x)}{[H^+]([H^+] + K_z)} + \frac{K_x}{K_c}\right\} \quad (27)$$

Hence the approach to equilibrium should be identical despite the direction of reaction (25).

Another feasible explanation of this discrepancy is the possibility that bound CO_2 cannot be released prior to the occurrence of a slow conformational change of the Hb molecule that accompanies oxygenation. Oxylabile carbamate kinetics then would differ from carbamate kinetics not associated with concurrent oxygenation. However, the kinetics of most conformational changes appear quite rapid and this postulated behavior would be anomalous (4).

Oxylabile carbamate kinetics involve multiple ionic species and reactions. The interactions of these processes are complex, and the rate of release of CO_2 from carbamate compounds may be influenced by experimental circumstances. Hemoglobin solutions, dilute erythrocyte suspensions, and whole blood have differing buffering powers, reactant concentrations, and compartmentalization of chemical species. Discrepancies in carbamate kinetics may be the result of differing experimental conditions rather than any in-

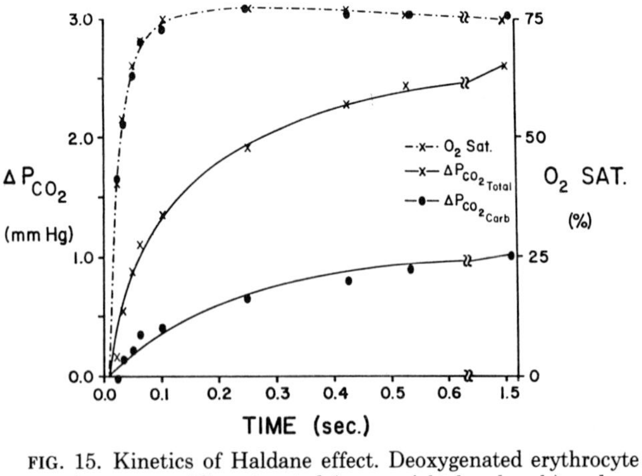

FIG. 15. Kinetics of Haldane effect. Deoxygenated erythrocyte suspension was rapidly saturated (-·-·-·, *right-hand scale*) and resulting liberation of CO_2 (—, *left-hand scale*) monitored in continuous-flow rapid-reaction apparatus. *Lower solid curve* was obtained during carbonic anhydrase inhibition and represents carbamate formation. *Upper solid curve* was obtained without enzyme inhibition and represents sum of changes due to both oxylabile HCO_3^- and carbamate. [From Klocke (86).]

trinsic change in reaction kinetics (E. Hill, unpublished observations).

Another potential cause for the difference between carbamate kinetics in solution and cell suspension is suggested by the recent demonstration that the rate of reactions in a stopped-flow apparatus may be affected by a stagnant layer of fluid on the cell surface (28). The presence of a stagnant layer would slow diffusion of CO_2 out of the cell. The concurrent rapid changes of O_2 during the experiment illustrated in Figure 15 argue against this possibility, but it is difficult to compare exchange of the two gases because the partial pressure gradients for diffusion were quite different. An additional uncertainty arises from the use in these experiments of a continuous-flow apparatus, an instrument that is less likely to develop an expanding stagnant layer. Further investigation is needed to clarify the issue.

OXYLABILE BICARBONATE KINETICS. Bohr protons are liberated rapidly (58) and are available to react with HCO_3^- almost simultaneously during oxygenation. The rate of mobilization of HCO_3^- initially depends on intracellular carbonic anhydrase activity and is later limited by the speed of transmembrane HCO_3^--Cl^- exchange (86). As illustrated in Figure 15, production of oxylabile CO_2 from HCO_3^- does not appear to be complete by the time blood leaves the capillary, especially considering the more rapid oxygenation in that experiment compared to the usual in vivo rate (143). The full Haldane effect may not be realized before blood leaves the pulmonary capillary. Abnormalities of O_2 exchange that delay or prevent completion of the oxygenation process would only exacerbate this phenomenon. In addition, reduction of capillary transit time during exercise could also impair the Haldane mechanism. Even if end-capillary equilibrium is not reached, CO_2 excretion is probably not compromised in vivo. A slight increase in alveolar ventilation would lower alveolar P_{CO_2} sufficiently to promote increased exchange, which would compensate for the lack of attainment of equilibrium of the oxylabile reaction.

Models of Gas Exchange

Events occurring in the lung are difficult to duplicate experimentally, and extrapolation of in vitro data is hazardous because gas exchange can be affected by complex interactions that are not apparent in an experimental situation. This has led numerous investigators to attempt to model gas exchange. Hlastala (70) has analyzed the effect of Haldane kinetics and concluded that oxylabile CO_2 exchange is not complete by the time blood leaves the capillary. Wagner (143) has raised issue with this conclusion on the basis of the values of kinetic parameters used in the simulation. However, all models of gas exchange that include O_2-linked CO_2 excretion indicate that even if end-capillary equlibrium is achieved, there is much less margin of safety than previously assumed (14, 15, 69, 70, 144). Certainly CO_2 exchange proceeds much more slowly than O_2 exchange, a fact appreciated only in the last decade (143). Under conditions of abnormal diffusion or ventilation-perfusion difficulties, end-capillary disequilibrium may exist for both O_2 and CO_2 (144).

Computations of gas exchange are limited by the model chosen and the data used to characterize the model. Earlier attempts to describe the kinetics of gas exchange used lumped-parameter models. For example, the events involved in intracapillary exchange were usually characterized by a single phenomenological constant θ. This approach is clearly inappropriate for models of CO_2 exchange because it does not include interactions of the different processes involved. More recent work (14, 69) has focused on individual rate-limiting steps. In addition, failure to incorporate unknown factors into a model can lead to erroneous conclusions. The prediction of slow postpulmonary capillary pH changes (52, 69) resulting from disequilibrium of the dehydration reaction in plasma occurred because the presence of pulmonary vascular carbonic anhydrase had not yet been established (31, 39, 89). Similarly this lack of slow pH changes in the lung cannot be extrapolated to all tissues because slow postcapillary pH changes can occur in tissues without vascular carbonic anhydrase (107). Appropriate conclusions depend on the choice of a proper model, a truism more easily stated than achieved.

Finally, accuracy of the data used to characterize models of gas exchange may not apply to the in vivo situation. All kinetic data have been obtained under in vitro conditions (91). In addition, successful application of a two-phase gas-liquid system has not been achieved; as a result the time course of gas tensions and chemical concentrations has poorly mimicked the events occurring in the pulmonary capillary. This is particularly important when exchange is characterized by phenomenological, rather than true chemical, constants. Extrapolation of these data to in vivo circumstances is tenuous. Recent evidence (28) strongly suggests that in vitro estimates of cellular O_2 association constants are too low because of artifacts caused by stagnant layers of unstirred fluid on cellular surfaces. Because this type of artifact depends on experimental conditions and the kinetic event that is being characterized (92), no simple correction factor can be applied to previously acquired data. Furthermore, if stagnant layers exist on cell surfaces and affect the rate of gas exchange in a reaction apparatus, then these factors must be even more important in the pulmonary capillary where the linear velocity is 3–4 orders of magnitude smaller and the Reynolds number almost zero. The effects of stagnant layers and mixing of intracellular contents (146), events that almost certainly occur in vivo, have never been incorporated into theoretical models because sufficient information concerning these factors is not available. Soni et al. (139) have provided the only available in vivo data concerning the kinetics of CO_2 exchange. They utilized body plethysmography to measure changes in pulmonary alveolar gas volume in dogs after injection of a bolus of acid. The excretion of CO_2 in the pulmonary capillary bed proceeded with a half time of 0.4 s. Further experiments from the same laboratory indicated that a bolus of HCO_3^- solution takes slightly >2 s to traverse the capillary, possibly the result of movement of the ion into pericapillary tissues (45). These fragmentary pieces of information underscore the need for kinetic measurements in the intact lung to fully understand the dynamics of CO_2 exchange.

The author appreciates the assistance of Anne Coe and Marsha Barber in the preparation of this manuscript.

This work was supported by Grant HL-15194 from the National Heart, Lung, and Blood Institute.

REFERENCES

1. ALTMAN, P. L., AND D. S. DITTMER (editors). *Respiration and Circulation.* Bethesda, MD: Fed. Am. Soc. Exp. Biol., 1971, p. 211–217.
2. ALTMAN, P. L., J. F. GIBSON, JR., AND C. C. WANG. *Handbook of Respiration.* Philadelphia, PA: Saunders, 1958, p. 64.
3. ANDERSSON, B., P. O. NYMAN, AND L. STRID. Amino acid sequence of human erythrocyte carbonic anhydrase B. *Biochem. Biophys. Res. Commun.* 48: 670–677, 1972.
4. ANTONINI, E., AND M. BRUNORI. Ligand-dependent conformational changes. In: *Hemoglobin and Myoglobin in Their Reactions with Ligands.* New York: Elsevier, 1971, p. 135–152.
5. ARNONE, A. X-ray studies of the interaction of CO_2 with human deoxyhemoglobin. *Nature Lond.* 247: 143–145, 1974.
6. ARNONE, A., P. H. ROGERS, AND P. D. BRILEY. The binding of CO_2 to human deoxyhemoglobin: an x-ray study using low-salt crystals. In: *Biophysics and Physiology of Carbon Dioxide,* edited by C. Bauer, G. Gros, and H. Bartels. New York: Springer-Verlag, 1980, p. 67–74.
7. ARTURSON, G., L. GARBY, B. WRANNE, AND B. ZAAR. Effect of 2,3-diphosphoglycerate on the oxygen affinity and on the proton- and carbamino-linked oxygen affinity of hemoglobin in human whole blood. *Acta Physiol. Scand.* 92: 332–340, 1974.
8. AUSTIN, W. H., E. LACOMBE, P. W. RAND, AND M. CHATTERJEE. Solubility of carbon dioxide in serum from 15 to 38 C. *J. Appl. Physiol.* 18: 301–304, 1963.
9. BAUER, C. Antagonistic influence of CO_2 and 2,3-diphosphoglycerate on the Bohr effect of human haemoglobin. *Life Sci. Part II Biochem. Gen. Mol. Biol.* 8: 1041–1046, 1969.
10. BAUER, C. Reduction of the carbon dioxide affinity of human haemoglobin solutions by 2,3-diphosphoglycerate. *Respir. Physiol.* 10: 10–19, 1970.
11. BAUER, C., R. BAUMANN, U. ENGELS, AND B. PACYNA. The carbon dioxide affinity of various human hemoglobins. *J. Biol. Chem.* 250: 2173–2176, 1975.
12. BAUER, C., AND E. SCHRÖDER. Carbamino compounds of haemoglobin in human adult and foetal blood. *J. Physiol. Lond.* 229: 457–471, 1972.
13. BENESCH, R., AND R. E. BENESCH. The effect of organic phosphates from the human erythrocyte on the allosteric properties of hemoglobin. *Biochem. Biophys. Res. Commun.* 26: 162–167, 1967.
14. BIDANI, A., E. D. CRANDALL, AND R. E. FORSTER. Analysis of postcapillary pH changes in blood in vivo after gas exchange. *J. Appl. Physiol.* 44: 770–781, 1978.
15. BIDANI, A., R. W. FLUMERFELT, AND E. D. CRANDALL. Analysis of pulsatile capillary blood flow and volume on gas exchange. *Respir. Physiol.* 35: 27–42, 1978.
16. BIDANI, A., S. J. MATHEW, AND E. D. CRANDALL. Pulmonary vascular carbonic anhydrase activity. *J. Appl. Physiol.* 55: 75–83, 1983.
17. BRAZY, P. C., AND R. B. GUNN. Furosemide inhibition of chloride transport in human red blood cells. *J. Gen. Physiol.* 68: 583–599, 1976.
18. BROWN, E. B., JR., AND R. L. CLANCY. In vivo and in vitro CO_2 blood buffer curves. *J. Appl. Physiol.* 20: 885–889, 1965.
19. BUNN, H. F., AND R. W. BRIEHL. The interaction of 2,3-diphosphoglycerate with various human hemoglobins. *J. Clin. Invest.* 49: 1088–1095, 1970.
20. BURSAUX, E., C. POYART, P. GUESNON, AND B. TEISSEIRE. Comparative effects of CO_2 on the affinity for O_2 of fetal and adult erythrocytes. *Pfluegers Arch.* 378: 197–203, 1979.
21. CABANTCHIK, Z. I., AND A. ROTHSTEIN. The nature of the membrane sites controlling anion permeability of human red blood cells as determined by studies with disulfonic stilbene derivatives. *J. Membr. Physiol.* 10: 311–330, 1972.
22. CABANTCHIK, Z. I., AND A. ROTHSTEIN. Membrane proteins related to anion permeability of human red blood cells. I. Localization of disulfonic stilbene binding sites in proteins involved in permeation. *J. Membr. Biol.* 15: 207–226, 1974.
23. CAIN, S. M., AND A. B. OTIS. Carbon dioxide transport in anesthetized dogs during inhibition of carbonic anhydrase. *J. Appl. Physiol.* 16: 1023–1028, 1961.
24. CARTER, M. J. Carbonic anhydrase: isoenzymes, properties, distribution, and functional significance. *Biol. Rev. Camb. Philos. Soc.* 47: 465–513, 1972.
25. CHANUTIN, A., AND R. R. CURNISH. Effect of organic and inorganic phosphates on the oxygen equilibrium of human erythrocytes. *Arch. Biochem. Biophys.* 121: 96–102, 1967.
26. CHOW, E. I.-H., E. D. CRANDALL, AND R. E. FORSTER. Kinetics of bicarbonate-chloride exchange across the human red blood cell membrane. *J. Gen. Physiol.* 68: 633–652, 1976.
27. CHRISTIANSEN, J., C. G. DOUGLAS, AND J. S. HALDANE. The absorption and dissociation of carbon dioxide by human blood. *J. Physiol. Lond.* 48: 244–277, 1914.
28. COIN, J. T., AND J. S. OLSON. The rate of oxygen uptake by human red blood cells. *J. Biol. Chem.* 254: 1178–1190, 1979.
29. CRANDALL, E. D., AND A. BIDANI. Effects of red blood cell HCO_3^-/Cl^- exchange kinetics on lung CO_2 transfer: theory. *J. Appl. Physiol.* 50: 265–271, 1981.
30. CRANDALL, E. D., S. J. MATHEW, R. S. FLEISCHER, H. I. WINTER, AND A. BIDANI. Effects of inhibition of RBC HCO_3^-/Cl^- exchange on CO_2 excretion and downstream pH disequilibrium in isolated rat lungs. *J. Clin. Invest.* 68: 853–862, 1981.
31. CRANDALL, E. D., AND J. E. O'BRASKY. Direct evidence for participation of rat lung carbonic anhydrase in CO_2 reactions. *J. Clin. Invest.* 62: 618–622, 1978.
32. CRANDALL, E. D., H. I. WINTER, J. D. SCHAEFFER, AND A. BIDANI. Effects of salicylate on HCO_3^-/Cl^- exchange across the human erythrocyte membrane. *J. Membr. Biol.* 65: 139–145, 1982.
33. DALMARK, M. Effects of halides and bicarbonate on chloride transport in human red blood cells. *J. Gen. Physiol.* 67: 223–234, 1976.
34. DENNARD, A. E., AND R. J. P. WILLIAMS. The catalysis of the reaction between carbon dioxide and water. *J. Chem. Soc. Lond. A*: 812–816, 1966.
35. DEVOE, H., AND G. B. KRISTIAKOWSKY. The enzyme kinetics of carbonic anhydrase from bovine and human erythrocytes. *J. Am. Chem. Soc.* 83: 274–280, 1961.

36. DILL, D. B., H. T. EDWARD, AND W. V. CONSOLAZIO. Blood as a physicochemical system. XI. Man at rest. *J. Biol. Chem.* 118: 635–648, 1937.
37. DONALDSON, T. L., AND J. A. QUINN. Kinetic constants determined from membrane transport measurements: carbonic anhydrase activity at high concentrations. *Proc. Natl. Acad. Sci. USA* 71: 4995–4999, 1974.
38. EDSALL, J. T. Carbon dioxide, carbonic acid, and bicarbonate ion: physical properties and kinetics of interconversion. In: *CO_2: Chemical, Biochemical, and Physiological Aspects*, edited by R. E. Forster, J. T. Edsall, A. B. Otis, and F. J. W. Roughton. Washington, DC: NASA, 1969, SP-188, p. 15–27.
39. EFFROS, R. M., R. S. Y. CHANG, AND P. SILVERMAN. Acceleration of plasma bicarbonate conversion to carbon dioxide by pulmonary carbonic anhydrase. *Science Wash. DC* 199: 427–429, 1978.
40. EFFROS, R. M., G. MASON, AND P. SILVERMAN. Role of perfusion and diffusion in $^{14}CO_2$ exchange in the rabbit lung. *J. Appl. Physiol.* 51: 1136–1144, 1981.
41. EFFROS, R. M., L. SHAPIRO, AND P. SILVERMAN. Carbonic anhydrase activity of rabbit lungs. *J. Appl. Physiol.* 49: 589–600, 1980.
42. EFFROS, R. M., AND M. L. WEISSMAN. Carbonic anhydrase activity of the cat hind leg. *J. Appl. Physiol.* 47: 1090–1098, 1979.
43. EIGEN, M., K. KUSTIN, AND G. MAASS. Die Geschwindigkeit der Hydration von SO_2 in wassriger Lösung. *Z. Phys. Chem.* 30: 130–136, 1961.
44. FAURHOLT, C. Etudes sur les aqueuses de carbamates et de carbonates. *J. Chim. Phys.* 22: 1–44, 1925.
45. FEISAL, K. A., M. A. SACKNER, AND A. B. DUBOIS. Comparison between the time available and the time required for CO_2 equilibration in the lung. *J. Clin. Invest.* 42: 24–28, 1963.
46. FERGUSON, J. K. W. Carbamino compounds of CO_2 with human haemoglobin and their role in the transport of CO_2. *J. Physiol. Lond.* 88: 40–55, 1936.
47. FERGUSON, J. K. W., AND F. J. W. ROUGHTON. The direct chemical estimation of carbamino compounds of CO_2 with haemoglobin. *J. Physiol. Lond.* 83: 68–86, 1934.
48. FITZSIMONS, E. J., AND J. SENDROY, JR. Distribution of electrolytes in human blood. *J. Biol. Chem.* 236: 1595–1601, 1961.
49. FORSTER, R. E. Rate of gas uptake by red cells. In: *Handbook of Physiology. Respiration*, edited by W. O. Fenn and H. Rahn. Washington, DC: Am. Physiol. Soc., 1964, sect. 3, vol. I, chapt. 32, p. 827–837.
50. FORSTER, R. E. The rate of CO_2 equilibrium between red cells and plasma. In: *CO_2: Chemical, Biochemical, and Physiological Aspects*, edited by R. E. Forster, J. T. Edsall, A. B. Otis, and F. J. W. Roughton. Washington, DC: NASA, 1969, SP-188, p. 275–286.
51. FORSTER, R. E., H. P. CONSTANTINE, M. R. CRAW, H. H. ROTMAN, AND R. A. KLOCKE. Reaction of CO_2 with human hemoglobin solution. *J. Biol. Chem.* 243: 3317–3326, 1968.
52. FORSTER, R. E., AND E. D. CRANDALL. Time course of exchanges between red cells and extracellular fluid during CO_2 uptake. *J. Appl. Physiol.* 38: 710–718, 1975.
53. GARBY, L., AND C.-H. DE VERDIER. Affinity of human hemoglobin A to 2,3-diphosphoglycerate. Effect of hemoglobin concentration and of pH. *Scand. J. Clin. Lab. Invest.* 27: 345–350, 1971.
54. GARBY, L., M. ROBERT, AND B. ZAAR. Proton- and carbamino-linked oxygen affinity of normal human blood. *Acta Physiol. Scand.* 84: 482–492, 1972.
55. GOLDMAN, D. E. Potential, impedence and rectification in membranes. *J. Gen. Physiol.* 27: 37–60, 1943.
56. GRANT, B. J. B. Influence of Bohr-Haldane effect on steady-state gas exchange. *J. Appl. Physiol.* 52: 1330–1337, 1982.
57. GRAY, B. A. The rate of approach to equilibrium in uncatalyzed CO_2 hydration reactions: the theoretical effect of buffering capacity. *Respir. Physiol.* 11: 223–234, 1971.
58. GRAY, R. D. The kinetics of the alkaline Bohr effect of human hemoglobin. *J. Biol. Chem.* 245: 2914–2921, 1970.
59. GROS, G., AND C. BAUER. High pK value of the N-terminal amino group of the γ-chain causes low CO_2 binding of human fetal hemoglobin. *Biochem. Biophys. Res. Commun.* 80: 56–62, 1978.
60. GROS, G., R. E. FORSTER, AND L. LIN. The carbamate reaction of glycylglycine, plasma, and tissue extracts evaluated by a pH stopped flow apparatus. *J. Biol. Chem.* 251: 4398–4407, 1976.
61. GROS, G., AND W. MOLL. The diffusion of carbon dioxide in erythrocytes and hemoglobin solutions. *Pfluegers Arch.* 324: 249–266, 1971.
62. GROS, G., H. S. ROLLEMA, AND R. E. FORSTER. The carbamate equilibrium of α- and ϵ-amino groups of human hemoglobin at 37°C. *J. Biol. Chem.* 256: 5471–5480, 1981.
63. GUNN, R. B., M. DALMARK, D. C. TOSTESON, AND J. O. WIETH. Characteristics of chloride transport in human red blood cells. *J. Gen. Physiol.* 61: 185–206, 1973.
64. GUNN, R. B., AND O. FRÖHLICH. Asymmetry in the mechanism for anion exchange in human red blood cell membranes. *J. Gen. Physiol.* 74: 351–374, 1979.
65. GUTKNECHT, J., M. A. BISSON, AND F. C. TOSTESON. Diffusion of carbon dioxide through lipid bilayer membranes: effects of carbonic anhydrase, bicarbonate, and unstirred layers. *J. Gen. Physiol.* 69: 779–794, 1977.
66. HAMBURGER, H. J. Anionenwanderungen in serum und Blut unter dem Einfluss von CO_2, Säure und Alkali. *Biochem. Z.* 86: 309–324, 1918.
67. HENDERSON, L. E., D. HENRIKSSON, AND P. O. NYMAN. Primary structure of human carbonic anhydrase C. *J. Biol. Chem.* 251: 5457–5463, 1976.
68. HENRIQUES, O. M. Die Bindungsweise des Kohlendioxyds im Blute. *Biochem. Z.* 200: 1–24, 1928.
69. HILL, E. P., G. G. POWER, AND L. D. LONGO. Mathematical simulation of pulmonary O_2 and CO_2 exchange. *Am. J. Physiol.* 224: 904–917, 1973.
70. HLASTALA, M. P. Significance of the Bohr and Haldane effects in the pulmonary capillary. *Respir. Physiol.* 17: 81–92, 1973.
71. HLASTALA, M. P., AND R. D. WOODSON. Saturation dependency of the Bohr effect: interactions among H^+, CO_2, and DPG. *J. Appl. Physiol.* 38: 1126–1131, 1975.
72. HOLLAND, R. A. B., AND R. E. FORSTER II. Effect of temperature on rate of CO_2 uptake by human red cell suspensions. *Am. J. Physiol.* 228: 1589–1596, 1975.
73. HOLMES, R. S. Mammalian carbonic anhydrase isoenzymes: evidence for a third locus. *J. Exp. Zool.* 197: 289–295, 1976.
74. HOLMES, R. S. Purification, molecular properties and ontogeny of carbonic anhydrase isoenzymes. *Eur. J. Biochem.* 78: 511–520, 1977.
75. HYDE, R. W., R. J. M. PUY, W. F. RAUB, AND R. E. FORSTER. Rate of disappearance of labeled carbon dioxide from the lungs of humans during breath holding: a method for studying the dynamics of pulmonary CO_2 exchange. *J. Clin. Invest.* 47: 1535–1552, 1968.
76. ITADA, N., AND R. E. FORSTER. Carbonic anhydrase activity in intact red blood cells measured with ^{18}O exchange. *J. Biol. Chem.* 252: 3881–3890, 1977.
77. JEFFERY, S., Y. EDWARDS, AND N. CARTER. Distribution of CAIII in fetal and adult human tissue. *Biochem. Genet.* 18: 843–849, 1980.
78. KEILIN, D., AND T. MANN. Carbonic anhydrase. Purification and nature of the enzyme. *Biochem. J.* 34: 1163–1176, 1940.
79. KERNOHAN, J. C., W. W. FORREST, AND F. J. W. ROUGHTON. The activity of concentrated solutions of carbonic anhydrase. *Biochim. Biophys. Acta* 67: 31–41, 1963.
80. KERNOHAN, J. C., AND F. J. W. ROUGHTON. Thermal studies of the rates of the reactions of carbon dioxide in concentrated haemoglobin solutions and in red blood cells. A. The reactions catalysed by carbonic anhydrase. B. The carbamino reactions of oxygenated and deoxygenated haemoglobin. *J. Physiol. Lond.* 197: 345–361, 1968.

81. KHALIFAH, R. G. The carbon dioxide hydration activity of carbonic anhydrase. Stop-flow kinetic studies on the native human isoenzymes B and C. *J. Biol. Chem.* 246: 2561–2573, 1971.
82. KHALIFAH, R. G. Carbon dioxide hydration activity of carbonic anhydrase: paradoxical consequences of the unusually rapid catalysis. *Proc. Natl. Acad. Sci. USA* 70: 1986–1989, 1973.
83. KILMARTIN, J. V., J. FOGG, M. LUZZANA, AND L. ROSSI-BERNARDI. Role of the α-amino groups of the α and β chains of human hemoglobin in oxygen-linked binding of carbon dioxide. *J. Biol. Chem.* 248: 7039–7043, 1973.
84. KILMARTIN, J. V., AND L. ROSSI-BERNARDI. The binding of carbon dioxide by horse haemoglobin. *Biochem. J.* 124: 31–45, 1971.
85. KLOCKE, R. A. Influence of oxygenation, pH, and 2,3-diphosphoglycerate on carbon dioxide exchange. *Chest* 61, Suppl.: 20S–22S, 1972.
86. KLOCKE, R. A. Mechanism and kinetics of the Haldane effect in human erythrocytes. *J. Appl. Physiol.* 35: 673–681, 1973.
87. KLOCKE, R. A. Rate of bicarbonate-chloride exchange in human red cells at 37°C. *J. Appl. Physiol.* 40: 707–714, 1976.
88. KLOCKE, R. A. Carbon dioxide transport. In: *Lung Biology in Health and Disease. Extrapulmonary Manifestations of Respiratory Disease*, edited by E. D. Robin. New York: Dekker, 1978, vol. 8, chapt. 9, p. 315–343.
89. KLOCKE, R. A. Catalysis of CO_2 reactions by lung carbonic anhydrase. *J. Appl. Physiol.* 44: 882–888, 1978.
90. KLOCKE, R. A. Equilibrium of CO_2 reactions in the pulmonary capillary. *J. Appl. Physiol.* 48: 972–976, 1980.
91. KLOCKE, R. A. Kinetics of pulmonary gas exchange. In: *Pulmonary Gas Exchange. Ventilation, Blood Flow, and Diffusion*, edited by J. B. West. New York: Academic, 1980, vol. 1, p. 174–218.
92. KLOCKE, R. A., AND F. FLASTERSTEIN. Kinetics of erythrocyte penetration by aliphatic acids. *J. Appl. Physiol.* 53: 1138–1143, 1982.
93. KNAUF, P. Erythrocyte anion exchange and the band 3 protein: transport kinetics and molecular structure. In: *Current Topics in Membranes and Transport*, edited by F. Bronner and A. Kleinzeller. New York: Academic, 1979, vol. 12, p. 249–363.
94. KNOCHE, W. Chemical reactions of CO_2 in water. In: *Biophysics and Physiology of Carbon Dioxide*, edited by C. Bauer, G. Gros, and H. Bartels. New York: Springer-Verlag, 1980, p. 3–11.
95. KOESTER, M. K., A. M. REGISTER, AND E. A. NOLTMANN. Basic muscle protein: a third genetic locus isoenzyme of carbonic anhydrase. *Biochem. Biophys. Res. Commun.* 76: 196–204, 1977.
96. LASSEN, U. V. Membrane potential and membrane resistance of red cells. In: *Oxygen Affinity of Hemoglobin and Red Cell Acid Base Status*, edited by P. Astrup and M. Rørth. New York: Academic, 1972, p. 291–306. (Alfred Benzon Symp., 4th, 1971.)
97. LILJAS, A., K. K. KANNAN, P.-C. BERGSTÉN, I. WAARA, K. FRIDBORG, B. STRANDBERG, U. CARLBOM, L. JÄRUP, S. LÖVGREN, AND M. PETEF. Crystal structure of human carbonic anhydrase C. *Nature Lond. New Biol.* 235: 131–137, 1972.
98. LÖNNERHOLM, G. Pulmonary carbonic anhydrase in the human, monkey, and rat. *J. Appl. Physiol.* 52: 352–356, 1982.
99. MAREN, T. H. Carbonic anhydrase: chemistry, physiology, and inhibition. *Physiol. Rev.* 47: 595–781, 1967.
100. MAREN, T. H., C. S. RAYBURN, AND N. E. LIDDELL. Inhibition by anions of human red cell carbonic anhydrase B: physiological and biochemical implications. *Science Wash. DC* 191: 469–472, 1976.
101. MATTHEW, J. B., J. S. MORROW, R. J. WITTEBORT, AND F. J. N. GURD. Quantitative determination of carbamino adducts of α and β chains in human adult hemoglobin in presence and absence of carbon monoxide and 2,3-diphosphoglycerate. *J. Biol. Chem.* 252: 2234–2244, 1977.
102. MCHARDY, G. J. R. The relationship between the differences in pressure and content of carbon dioxide in arterial and venous blood. *Clin. Sci. Lond.* 32: 299–309, 1967.
103. MELDRUM, N. U., AND F. J. W. ROUGHTON. Carbonic anhydrase. Its preparation and properties. *J. Physiol. Lond.* 80: 113–142, 1933.
104. MORROW, J. S., J. B. MATTHEW, R. S. WITTEBORT, AND F. R. N. GURD. Carbon 13 resonances of $^{13}CO_2$ carbamino adducts of α and β chains in human adult hemoglobin. *J. Biol. Chem.* 251: 477–484, 1976.
105. NICHOLS, G., JR. Serial changes in tissue carbon dioxide content during acute respiratory acidosis. *J. Clin. Invest.* 37: 1111–1122, 1958.
106. O'BRASKY, J. E., AND E. D. CRANDALL. Organ and species differences in tissue vascular carbonic anhydrase activity. *J. Appl. Physiol.* 49: 211–217, 1980.
107. O'BRASKY, J. E., T. MAURO, AND E. D. CRANDALL. Postcapillary pH disequilibrium after gas exchange in isolated perfused liver. *J. Appl. Physiol.* 47: 1079–1083, 1979.
108. PASSOW, H. Passive ion permeability of the erythrocyte membrane. *Prog. Biophys. Mol. Biol.* 19: 425–467, 1969.
109. PERRELLA, M., D. BRESCIANA, AND L. ROSSI-BERNARDI. The binding of CO_2 to human hemoglobin. *J. Biol. Chem.* 250: 5413–5418, 1975.
110. PERRELLA, M., G. GUGLIELMO, AND A. MOSCA. Determination of the equilibrium constants for oxygen-linked CO_2 binding to human hemoglobin. *FEBS Lett.* 78: 287–290, 1977.
111. PERRELLA, M., J. V. KILMARTIN, J. FOGG, AND L. ROSSI-BERNARDI. Identification of the high and low affinity CO_2-binding sites of human haemoglobin. *Nature Lond.* 256: 759–761, 1975.
112. PERRELLA, M., L. ROSSI-BERNARDI, AND F. J. W. ROUGHTON. The carbamate equilibrium between CO_2 and bovine haemoglobin at 25°C. In: *Oxygen Affinity of Hemoglobin and Red Cell Acid Base Status*, edited by P. Astrup and M. Rørth. New York: Academic, 1972, p. 177–207. (Alfred Benzon Symp., 4th, 1971.)
113. PERUTZ, M. F., H. MUIRHEAD, L. MAZZARELLA, R. A. CROWTHER, J. GREER, AND J. V. KILMARTIN. Identification of residues responsible for the alkaline Bohr effect in haemoglobin. *Nature Lond.* 222: 1240–1243, 1969.
114. PETERS, J. P. Studies of the carbon dioxide absorption curve of human blood. III. A further discussion of the form of the absorption curve plotted logarithmically, with a convenient type of interpolation chart. *J. Biol. Chem.* 56: 745–750, 1923.
115. PETERS, J. P., H. A. BULGER, AND A. J. EISENMAN. Studies of the carbon dioxide absorption curve of human blood. IV. The relation of the hemoglobin content of blood to the form of the carbon dioxide absorption curve. *J. Biol. Chem.* 58: 747–768, 1924.
116. PETERS, J. P., H. A. BULGER, AND A. J. EISENMAN. Studies of the carbon dioxide absorption curve of human blood. V. The construction of the CO_2 absorption curve from one observed point. *J. Biol. Chem.* 58: 769–771, 1924.
117. PIIPER, J. Rates of chloride-bicarbonate exchange between red cells and plasma. In: *CO_2: Chemical, Biochemical, and Physiological Aspects*, edited by R. E. Forster, J. T. Edsall, A. B. Otis, and F. J. W. Roughton. Washington, DC: NASA, 1969, SP-188, p. 267–273.
118. PINSENT, B. R. W., L. PEARSON, AND F. J. W. ROUGHTON. The kinetics of carbon dioxide with hydroxide ions. *Trans. Faraday Soc.* 52: 1512–1520, 1956.
119. PLEWES, J. L., A. J. OLSZOWKA, AND L. E. FARHI. Amount and rates of CO_2 storage in lung tissue. *Respir. Physiol.* 28: 359–370, 1976.
120. POCKER, Y., AND D. W. BJORKQUIST. Comparative studies of bovine carbonic anhydrase in H_2O and D_2O. Stopped-flow studies of the kinetics of interconversion of CO_2 and HCO_3^-. *Biochemistry* 16: 5698–5707, 1977.
121. POCKER, Y., AND S. SARKANEN. Carbonic anhydrase: structure, catalytic versatility, and inhibition. *Adv. Enzymol. Relat. Areas Mol. Biol.* 47: 149–274, 1978.

122. REEVES, R. B. Temperature-induced changes in blood acid-base status: Donnan r_{Cl} and red cell volume. *J. Appl. Physiol.* 40: 762–767, 1976.
123. RIDDERSTRÅLE, Y. Observations on the localization of carbonic anhydrase in muscle. *Acta Physiol. Scand.* 106: 239–240, 1979.
124. RISPENS, P., C. W. DELLEBARRE, D. ELEVELD, W. HELDER, AND W. G. ZIJLSTRA. The apparent first dissociation constant of carbonic acid in plasma between 16 and 42.5°. *Clin. Chim. Acta* 22: 627–637, 1968.
125. RODKEY, F. L., H. A. COLLISON, J. D. O'NEAL, AND J. SENDROY, JR. Carbon dioxide absorption curves of dog blood and plasma. *J. Appl. Physiol.* 30: 178–185, 1971.
126. ROSSI-BERNARDI, L., AND F. J. W. ROUGHTON. The specific influence of carbon dioxide and carbamate compounds on the buffer power and Bohr effects in human haemoglobin solutions. *J. Physiol. Lond.* 189: 1–29, 1967.
127. ROTHSTEIN, A., Z. I. CABANTCHIK, AND P. KNAUF. Mechanism of anion transport in red blood cells: role of membrane proteins. *Federation Proc.* 35: 3–10, 1976.
128. ROUGHTON, F. J. W. Recent work on carbon dioxide transport by the blood. *Physiol. Rev.* 15: 241–296, 1935.
129. ROUGHTON, F. J. W. Transport of oxygen and carbon dioxide. In: *Handbook of Physiology. Respiration*, edited by W. O. Fenn and H. Rahn. Washington, DC: Am. Physiol. Soc., 1964, sect. 3, vol. I. chapt. 31, p. 767–825.
130. ROUGHTON, F. J. W. Some recent work on the interactions of oxygen, carbon dioxide and haemoglobin. *Biochem. J.* 117: 801–812, 1970.
131. RYAN, U. S., P. L. WHITNEY, AND J. W. RYAN. Localization of carbonic anhydrase on pulmonary artery endothelial cells in culture. *J. Appl. Physiol.* 53: 914–919, 1982.
132. SAVITZ, D., V. W. SIDEL, AND A. K. SOLOMON. Osmotic properties of human red cells. *J. Gen. Physiol.* 48: 79–94, 1964.
133. SHAW, L. A., AND A. C. MESSER. The transfer of bicarbonate between the blood and tissues caused by alterations of the carbon dioxide concentration in the lungs. *Am. J. Physiol.* 100: 122–136, 1932.
134. SIGGAARD-ANDERSEN, O. Oxygen-linked hydrogen ion binding of human hemoglobin. Effects of carbon dioxide and 2,3-diphosphoglycerate. I. Studies on erythrolysate. *Scand. J. Clin. Lab. Invest.* 27: 351–360, 1971.
135. SILVERMAN, D. N., AND C. K. TU. Buffer dependence of carbonic anhydrase catalyzed oxygen-18 exchange at equilibrium. *J. Am. Chem. Soc.* 97: 2263–2269, 1975.
136. SILVERMAN, D. N., C. K. TU, AND N. ROESSLER. Diffusion-limited exchange of ^{18}O between CO_2 and water in red cell suspensions. *Respir. Physiol.* 44: 285–298, 1981.
137. SILVERMAN, D. N., C. K. TU, AND G. C. WYNNS. Depletion of ^{18}O from $C^{18}O_2$ in erythroycte suspensions. The permeability of the erythrocyte membrane to CO_2. *J. Biol. Chem.* 251: 4428–4435, 1976.
138. SIRS, J. A. Electrometric stopped flow measurements of rapid reactions in solution. Part 1. Conductivity measurements. *Trans. Faraday Soc.* 54: 201–206, 1958.
139. SONI, J., K. A. FEISAL, AND A. B. DUBOIS. The rate of intrapulmonary blood gas exchange in living animals. *J. Clin. Invest.* 42: 16–23, 1963.
140. STADIE, W. C., AND H. O'BRIEN. The catalysis of the hydration of carbon dioxide and dehydration of carbamic acid by an enzyme isolated from red blood cells. *J. Biol. Chem.* 103: 521–529, 1933.
141. SWENSON, E. R., AND T. H. MAREN. A quantitative analysis of CO_2 transport at rest and during maximal exercise. *Respir. Physiol.* 35: 129–159, 1978.
142. VISSER, B. F. Pulmonary diffusion of carbon dioxide. *Phys. Med. Biol.* 5: 155–166, 1960.
143. WAGNER, P. D. Diffusion and chemical reaction in pulmonary gas exchange. *Physiol. Rev.* 57: 257–312, 1977.
144. WAGNER, P. D., AND J. B. WEST. Effects of diffusion impairment on O_2 and CO_2 time courses in pulmonary capillaries. *J. Appl. Physiol.* 33: 62–71, 1972.
145. WYMAN, J. Linked functions and reciprocal effects in haemoglobin: a second look. *Adv. Protein Chem.* 19: 223–286, 1964.
146. ZANDER, R., AND H. SCHMID-SCHÖNBEIN. Intracellular mechanisms of oxygen transport in flowing blood. *Respir. Physiol.* 19: 279–289, 1973.
147. ZBOROWSKA-SLUIS, D. T., A. L'ABBATE, AND G. A. KLASSEN. Evidence of carbonic anhydrase activity in skeletal muscle: a role for facilitative carbon dioxide transport. *Respir. Physiol.* 21: 341–350, 1974.
148. ZBOROWSKA-SLUIS, D. T., A. L'ABBATE, R. R. MILDENBERGER, AND G. A. KLASSEN. The effect of acetazolamide on myocardial carbon dioxide space. *Respir. Physiol.* 23: 311–316, 1975.

Ventilation-perfusion relationships

LEON E. FARHI | *Department of Physiology, State University of New York at Buffalo, Buffalo, New York*

CHAPTER CONTENTS

BODY ORGANS THAT EXCHANGE GAS with the environment usually rely on many capillary beds, arranged in parallel, each of which performs part of the total task. In this respect the lung is far from unique; it is, however, different because some specific constraints are introduced by the combination of two additional factors. First, the various microcirculations do not come into contact with a common pool of inspired gas: each of the millions of alveoli receives a specific fraction of the total ventilation. Second, blood-gas exchange is not dependent on active transport mechanisms; O_2 and CO_2 move across the alveolar-capillary membrane solely on the basis of diffusion due to differences in partial pressure. As a consequence, the composition of the end products of the process (i.e., alveolar gas and end-capillary blood) is based strictly on the composition and amount of the two media (inspired gas and mixed venous blood) that exchange with each other. This chapter deals with the subtle and not-so-subtle ways in which the relationship between the flows of gas and blood affects gas exchange. First the mechanism in its simplest form, a single alveolus, is described. Then I proceed to describe the complex lung (made up of a myriad of alveoli), gas exchange in that "real" lung, how this gas exchange can be used to obtain some information on the system, and how the system is affected by a variety of conditions. Finally the role of ventilation and perfusion in tissue homeostasis is discussed.

Many authors (11, 46, 64, 65) have reviewed portions of this subject. Several pages in the 1964 edition of the *Handbook* on respiration were devoted to this topic (47). Much of the earlier material, important as it is, is either omitted here or sketched broadly where duplication is necessary to ensure continuity of the text.

GAS EXCHANGE IN A SINGLE ALVEOLUS

Oxygen and Carbon Dioxide

The effects of the relationship between ventilation and perfusion (commonly expressed as their ratio, $\dot{V}A/\dot{Q}$) on alveolar gas pressures and respiratory gas exchange of a normal resting subject breathing air can be described qualitatively. An average alveolus, which serves as reference, has a $\dot{V}A/\dot{Q}$ of approximately unity and returns end-capillary blood to the left heart with a partial pressure of O_2 (P_{O_2}) of 100 mmHg and a partial pressure of CO_2 (P_{CO_2}) of 40 mmHg. Let us now examine gas exchange in two hypothetical cases, one in which ventilation is much higher than in the standard alveolus and the other in which it is considerably reduced. In the former the excess ventilation provides a large sink for CO_2, elimination of which can increase substantially above control level, since the reference alveolus eliminates only ~10% of the CO_2 reaching it via the mixed venous blood. Thus the end-capillary blood contains less CO_2, and equilibrium P_{CO_2} is reduced. For example, if $\dot{V}A/\dot{Q} = 5$, then CO_2

output ($\dot{V}_{CO_2}$) more than doubles while alveolar P_{CO_2} (PA_{CO_2}) drops to approximately half the control value. In the same alveolus, in contrast, O_2 uptake ($\dot{V}_{O_2}$) can rise only insignificantly, since O_2 saturation is practically complete at normal ventilatory levels. The obvious consequence is that virtually all the additional O_2 introduced into the system by the excess ventilation remains in the gas phase and raises the P_{O_2}. In summary, an alveolus with a high $\dot{V}A/\dot{Q}$ can be expected to have an elevated P_{O_2}, a reduced P_{CO_2}, and an increased gas-exchange ratio (R). The same laws of supply and demand are operative when the element with a low $\dot{V}A/\dot{Q}$ is considered; here PA_{O_2} drops, P_{CO_2} rises, and R is decreased. Note that *1)* the rise in P_{CO_2} is limited since the maximum P_{CO_2} is that of mixed venous blood and *2)* as long as the reduction in P_{O_2} remains moderate, blood O_2 saturation does not decrease appreciably.

To define more exactly the gas pressures and exchange levels that correspond to the various $\dot{V}A/\dot{Q}$ values, a rigorous mathematical analysis can be used, based on the following assumptions:

1. All respiratory elements are supplied with the same inspired gas and the same mixed venous blood.
2. There is perfect equilibrium across the alveolar membrane, so that end-capillary P_{O_2} equals alveolar P_{O_2} (PA_{O_2}) and the end-capillary P_{CO_2} is the same as PA_{CO_2}.
3. Lung metabolism is only a minute fraction of whole-body metabolism. As a consequence, $\dot{V}_{O_2}$ by alveolar gas from air is considered to equal the $\dot{V}_{O_2}$ by the pulmonary capillary blood. A similar postulate is required for CO_2.

On that basis

$$\dot{V}_{CO_2} = \dot{V}A\,\frac{PA_{CO_2}}{863} = \dot{Q}(C\bar{v}_{CO_2} - Cc_{CO_2}) \qquad (1)$$

where $\dot{Q}$ is blood flow, $C\bar{v}_{CO_2}$ is the concentration of CO_2 in mixed venous blood, and Cc_{CO_2} is the concentration of CO_2 in capillary blood. From this

$$\frac{C\bar{v}_{CO_2} - Cc_{CO_2}}{PA_{CO_2}} = \frac{1}{863}\,\frac{\dot{V}A}{\dot{Q}} \qquad (2)$$

The transformation allows graphic demonstration of the role $\dot{V}A/\dot{Q}$ plays in CO_2 exchange. In Figure 1 a CO_2 dissociation curve is drawn with a point $C\bar{v}$ on the vertical axis at $C\bar{v}_{CO_2}$. If a point A on the dissociation curve represents the alveolar-arterial CO_2 level in a respiratory element, the slope of the line joining A to $C\bar{v}$ is $(C\bar{v}_{CO_2} - CA_{CO_2})/PA_{CO_2}$, or, according to Equation 2, $(1/863)(\dot{V}A/\dot{Q})$. It is also possible to assume various values of $\dot{V}A/\dot{Q}$, calculate the corresponding slope, draw the appropriate line from A, and determine the P_{CO_2} at the intersection of that line with the dissociation curve. A plot of P_{CO_2} versus $\dot{V}A/\dot{Q}$ is given in Figure 2. In this and in all subsequent figures where a dependent variable is shown against $\dot{V}A/\dot{Q}$, the latter is plotted on a logarithmic scale. As Rahn (45) indicated, this is the logical way to look at $\dot{V}A/\dot{Q}$, which can have values from zero to infinity, with a mean normal value of approximately one. A similar graphic analysis for O_2 (Fig. 3) yields the PA_{O_2}-$\dot{V}A/\dot{Q}$ relationship shown in Figure 3 and the O_2 curve of Figure 2.

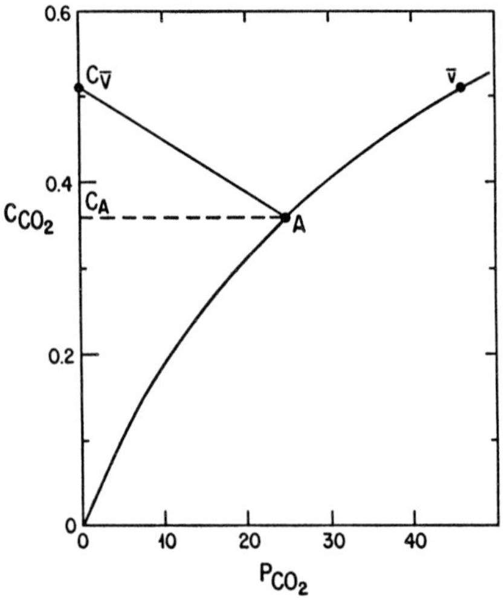

FIG. 1. Calculation of ventilation-perfusion ratio ($\dot{V}A/\dot{Q}$) from CO_2 exchange. Plot of CO_2 concentration (C_{CO_2}) versus CO_2 partial pressure (P_{CO_2}) with a standard dissociation curve. *Point $C\bar{v}$*, CO_2 concentration in mixed venous blood. Any given point on the curve, e.g., *A*, can be joined to *$C\bar{v}$*, providing a line in which the vertical distance between $\bar{v}$ and *A* is given by $C\bar{v} - CA$ (where CA is the CO_2 concentration in alveolar capillary blood), while the distance from *A* to the ordinate is by definition the alveolar partial pressure of CO_2 (PA_{CO_2}). Slope of the line is therefore $(C\bar{v}_{CO_2} - CA_{CO_2})/PA_{CO_2}$ or $1/863 \times \dot{V}A/\dot{Q}$. Note that C_{CO_2} must be in milliliters/milliliter and PA_{CO_2} in torr.

A major shortcoming of the preceding determinations is that they treat O_2 and CO_2 independently, ignoring the Bohr and Haldane effects. A more accurate approach was developed independently by Rahn (45) and by Riley and Cournand (50–52). In both cases the procedure requires a corollary of assumption 3, namely that if $\dot{V}_{O_2\,gas} = \dot{V}_{O_2\,blood}$ and $\dot{V}_{CO_2\,gas} = \dot{V}_{CO_2\,blood}$, it must follow that $R_{gas} = R_{blood}$. The modus operandi is to then *1)* assume arbitrarily a value of R, *2)* determine the P_{O_2}-P_{CO_2} combinations that can occur in a given inspired gas exchanging at that R, *3)* determine the P_{O_2}-P_{CO_2} sets that can result when the given mixed venous blood exchanges at the same R, *4)* find if there is a combination that is common to both groups of data, and *5)* repeat steps *1–4* for different values of R.

As a result of this iterative procedure, Table 1, which provides the P_{O_2} and P_{CO_2} that obtain at a number of preselected R values, was generated. From these pressures it is possible to calculate additional information for each of these combinations, including blood O_2 and CO_2 concentrations (and hence $Ca_{O_2} - Cv_{O_2}$ and $Cv_{CO_2} - Ca_{CO_2}$) and the ventilatory

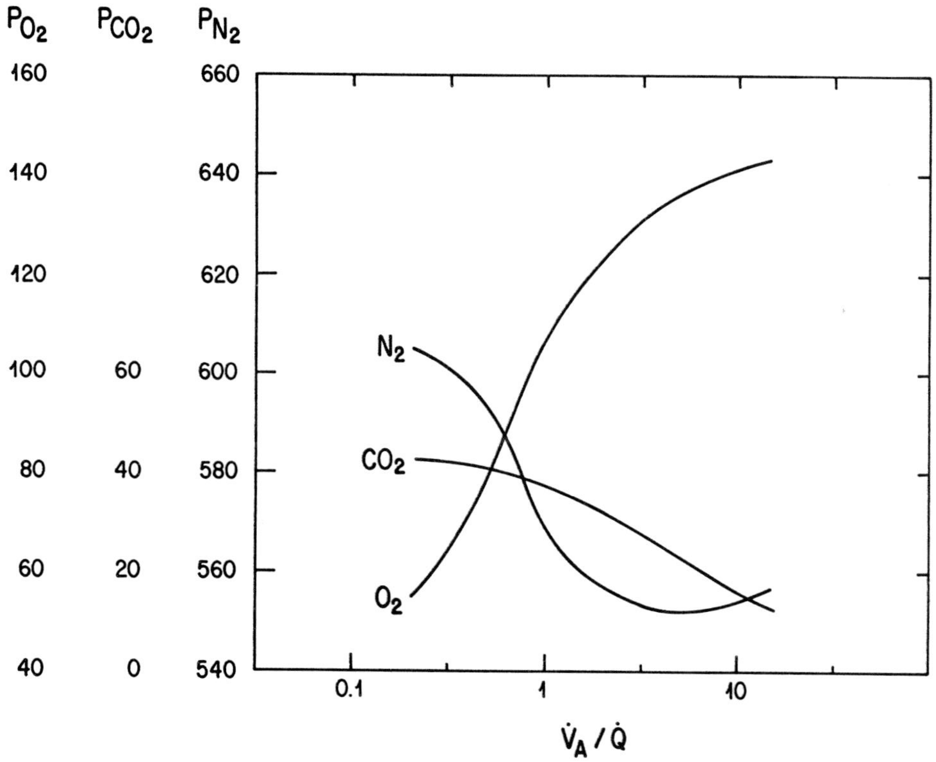

FIG. 2. Alveolar and end-capillary gas pressures as a function of $\dot{V}_A/\dot{Q}$. As $\dot{V}_A/\dot{Q}$ increases, O_2 partial pressure (P_{O_2}) and CO_2 partial pressure (P_{CO_2}) move toward inspired gas values; i.e., P_{O_2} increases and P_{CO_2} decreases. Because the rate of change of these two pressures is not identical, N_2 is concentrated at low $\dot{V}_A/\dot{Q}$ values and diluted if the gas-exchange ratio is >1.

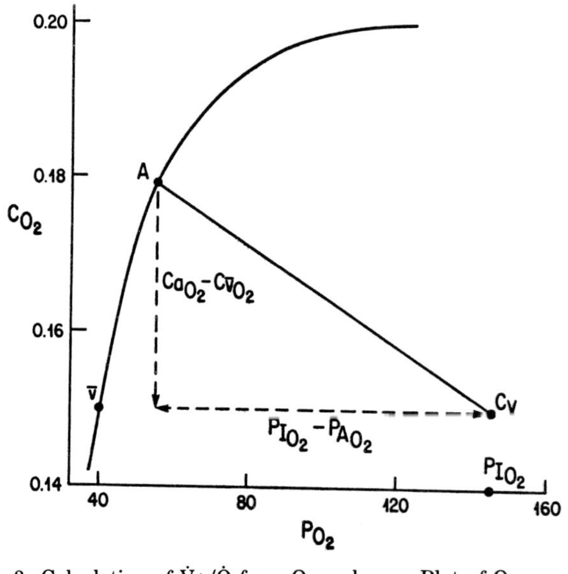

FIG. 3. Calculation of $\dot{V}_A/\dot{Q}$ from O_2 exchange. Plot of O_2 concentration (C_{O_2}) versus P_{O_2}. To determine $\dot{V}_A/\dot{Q}$, a *point Cv* is plotted at coordinates $P_{I_{O_2}}$, $C\bar{v}_{O_2}$. When this point is joined to *point A* (on the line that represents blood returning from a given alveolus) the A-C$\bar{v}$ slope is $(Ca_{O_2} - C\bar{v}_{O_2})/(P_{I_{O_2}} - P_{A_{O_2}})$ and represents therefore $1/863 \times \dot{V}_A/\dot{Q}$. $P_{I_{O_2}}$, inspired partial pressure of O_2; $C\bar{v}_{O_2}$, O_2 concentration in mixed venous blood; Ca_{O_2}, O_2 concentration in arterial blood; $P_{A_{O_2}}$, alveolar partial pressure of O_2.

equivalents for O_2 and CO_2, $\dot{V}_A/\dot{V}_{O_2}$ and $\dot{V}_A/\dot{V}_{CO_2}$, respectively. The $\dot{V}_A/\dot{Q}$ value is usually computed from Equation 2 combined with a similar relationship for O_2 to yield

$$\dot{V}_A/\dot{Q} = \frac{863R(Cc_{O_2} - C\bar{v}_{O_2})}{P_{A_{CO_2}}} \qquad (3)$$

Values of $\dot{V}_A/\dot{Q}$ range from zero to infinity, the first extreme corresponding to the mixed venous point (see EFFECT OF INERT-GAS DILUENT, p. 206). Simply stated, if blood flows through the lung without meeting any gas flow it will emerge unchanged. In an alveolus with an infinite $\dot{V}_A/\dot{Q}$, i.e., no blood flow, alveolar gas would have the same composition as inspired gas. Note that R does not increase to infinity but is limited to the ratio of $C\bar{v}_{CO_2}$ (which represents the maximum possible CO_2 loss) to the highest achievable $Ca_{O_2} - Cv_{O_2}$, i.e., the difference between blood O_2 concentrations at P_{CO_2} and $P\bar{v}_{O_2}$ (partial pressure of O_2 in mixed venous blood).

Table 1 pertains to a specific set of input conditions. Should any of these change, the information in Table 1 would be invalid and a new table would have to be generated. Besides requiring time, this may necessitate a new set of dissociation curves, if these have

TABLE 1. *Gas Pressures and Ventilation-Perfusion Ratios at Different Gas-Exchange Ratios*

R	$P_{A_{O_2}}$	$P_{A_{CO_2}}$	$P_{A_{N_2}}$	Ca_{O_2}	Ca_{CO_2}	$\dot{V}_A/\dot{Q}$
	39.5	43.0	630.5	14.6	51.6	0
0.4	55.5	42.5	650.0	17.4	50.5	0.22
0.5	75.5	41.3	596.2	18.8	49.5	0.44
0.6	87.6	40.1	585.3	19.2	48.8	0.60
0.7	96.7	39.0	577.3	19.5	48.1	0.78
0.8	103.5	38.0	571.5	19.6	47.6	0.91
0.9	108.5	37.0	567.5	19.7	47.0	1.07
1.0	113.5	35.8	563.3	19.8	46.4	1.25
1.2	119.7	33.8	559.5	19.9	45.3	1.61
1.5	126.2	30.9	555.9	19.9	43.7	2.20
2.0	133.0	26.5	553.5	20.0	40.8	3.56
3.0	140.0	19.5	553.5	20.0	35.4	7.36
4.0	143.5	13.0	556.5	20.0	29.8	14.80
	149	0	564	20.0	0	0

R, gas-exchange ratio; $P_{A_{O_2}}$, alveolar partial pressure of O_2; Ca_{O_2}, concentration of O_2 in arterial blood; $\dot{V}_A/\dot{Q}$, ventilation-perfusion ratio.

changed (as could occur if a resting subject started to exercise beyond the anaerobic threshold). It is not surprising therefore that computer programs that can develop a table of values for a very wide range of circumstances have been developed (41).

Neither the pen-and-paper nor the computer approach allows one to start with a $\dot{V}_A/\dot{Q}$ value and end up with the numbers describing gas exchange in the alveolus so defined, since $\dot{V}_A/\dot{Q}$ is one of the output values. To find the information pertaining to alveoli not described by Table 1, it is necessary to interpolate. This is customarily done by using the O_2-CO_2 diagram (48), plotting the points from the table, and drawing a smooth line to form a continuum (Fig. 4). The curve is rather flat in the low $\dot{V}_A/\dot{Q}$ range, which means that alveoli with reduced $\dot{V}_A/\dot{Q}$ values differ from each other much more in terms of P_{O_2} than in terms of P_{CO_2}. The opposite is true at the extreme right of the curve, i.e., at very high $\dot{V}_A/\dot{Q}$. Another consideration is that, because of the shape of the O_2 dissociation curve and the position of the normal alveolar point on that curve, the O_2 concentration in elements with a low $\dot{V}_A/\dot{Q}$ may drop considerably, whereas it cannot rise significantly in high $\dot{V}_A/\dot{Q}$ areas, despite the elevated P_{O_2}. This point had not escaped Haldane (22) in his early description of the alveolar-arterial O_2 difference.

Nitrogen

The drop in P_{O_2} without an appreciable rise in P_{CO_2} when $\dot{V}_A/\dot{Q}$ is reduced can occur only when there is enough atmospheric N_2. As the fraction of that gas is decreased, while the inspired P_{O_2} ($P_{I_{O_2}}$) is maintained, the $\dot{V}_A/\dot{Q}$ line becomes steeper (16). When 100% O_2 is inspired, the line is reduced to a straight line originating at the inspired point and having a slope of −1. This is actually a logical constraint: if the alveolar gas is composed of only O_2 and CO_2, then the sum of P_{O_2} and P_{CO_2} must always equal $P_B - 47$, where P_B is the barometric pressure. In other words, any change in P_{CO_2} must be matched by an equal and opposite change in P_{O_2}.

The effect of $\dot{V}_A/\dot{Q}$ on N_2 levels is shown in Figure 2. When $R > 1$ the influx of CO_2 more than counterbalances the $\dot{V}_{O_2}$, and N_2 is diluted. On the other hand, at low R values there must be a marked rise in P_{N_2}, since the total gas volume is now shrinking and N_2 must be concentrated. At one point, and at one point only, $P_{A_{CO_2}}$ exactly matches $P\bar{v}_{N_2}$ (partial pressure of N_2 in mixed venous blood).

Inert Gases

Although the main role of the gas-exchange system is to provide O_2 and eliminate CO_2, the lung can also take up or vent to the atmosphere other gases and volatile substances; it is required to perform this func-

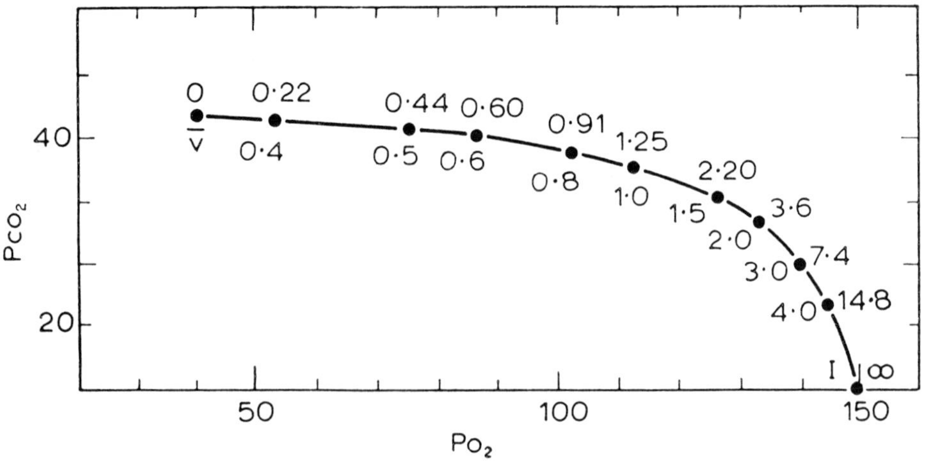

FIG. 4. Ventilation-perfusion ratio plotted on O_2-CO_2 diagram. Line is drawn for a resting subject, breathing air at sea level. Numbers *above* and to *right* of line indicate $\dot{V}_A/\dot{Q}$; other numbers show gas-exchange ratio (CO_2 output/O_2 uptake). [From Farhi (11).]

tion in a variety of circumstances, e.g., during anesthesia (induction and recovery phases) or when inert gases are infused for diagnostic purposes.

Uptake of an inert-gas x ($\dot{V}_x$) is given by

$$\dot{V}_x = \dot{V}_I(FI_x - \dot{V}_E)FE_x \quad (4)$$

where the difference between inspired uptake ($\dot{V}_I$) and expired minute ventilation ($\dot{V}_E$) is due to the combination of $\dot{V}_{O_2}$, $\dot{V}_{CO_2}$, and $\dot{V}_x$; FI_x is inspired fraction of gas x; and FE_x is expired fraction of gas x. The equation can be transformed into

$$\dot{V}_x = \frac{\dot{V}_A(FI_x - FE_x) + \dot{V}_{O_2}[FI_x(1 - R)]}{1 - FI_x} \quad (5)$$

Thus prediction of $\dot{V}_x$ in an alveolus requires knowledge of the local $\dot{V}_{O_2}$ and R. Although it is possible to perform these calculations with a digital computer (15), Equation 5 is clearly not the easiest to handle. For this reason most of the quantitative work on inert-gas exchange deals with elimination rather than uptake, a condition to which Equation 6 can be applied

$$\dot{V}_x = \frac{\dot{V}_A PA_x}{863} = \dot{Q}(C\bar{v}_x - Cc_x) \quad (6)$$

Note the similarity to Equation 1, where x is replaced by CO_2.

If x is chemically inert (i.e., does not combine with any of the blood components), its concentration must equal the amount physically dissolved, in accordance with Henry's law, with a solubility coefficient of α_x. Equation 6 can thus be restated as

$$\dot{V}_x = \frac{\dot{V}_A PA_x}{863} = \frac{\dot{Q}\alpha_x}{760}(P\bar{v}_x - PA_x) \quad (7)$$

where $P\bar{v}_x$ is the partial pressure of gas x in mixed venous blood, and, assuming equilibrium between alveolar gas and arterial blood

$$\dot{V}_x = \frac{\dot{V}_A PA_x}{863} = \frac{\dot{Q}\alpha_x}{760}(P\bar{v}_x - Pc'_x) \quad (8)$$

where Pc'_x is the pressure in end-capillary blood.

Because $863\alpha/760$ is the partition coefficient of the gas, usually expressed as λ, the equation leads to

$$PA_x/P\bar{v}_x = \lambda_x/(\lambda_x + \dot{V}_A/\dot{Q}) \quad (9)$$

Because $PA_x = Pc_x$, the left side of the equation is the equivalent of $[(\dot{Q}\alpha_x Pc_x)/760]/[(\dot{Q}\alpha_x P\bar{v}_x)/760]$, which in turn is the ratio of the amount of x in the gas leaving the element to the amount present in the incoming blood and represents the fractional retention of the gas. It is usually shown as R, but to avoid confusion with the same designation for gas-exchange ratio it appears in Figure 5 as $P'A$, as a function of $\dot{V}_A/\dot{Q}$ for a variety of gases. Figure 5 reinforces what is intuitively evident: poorly soluble gases are cleared

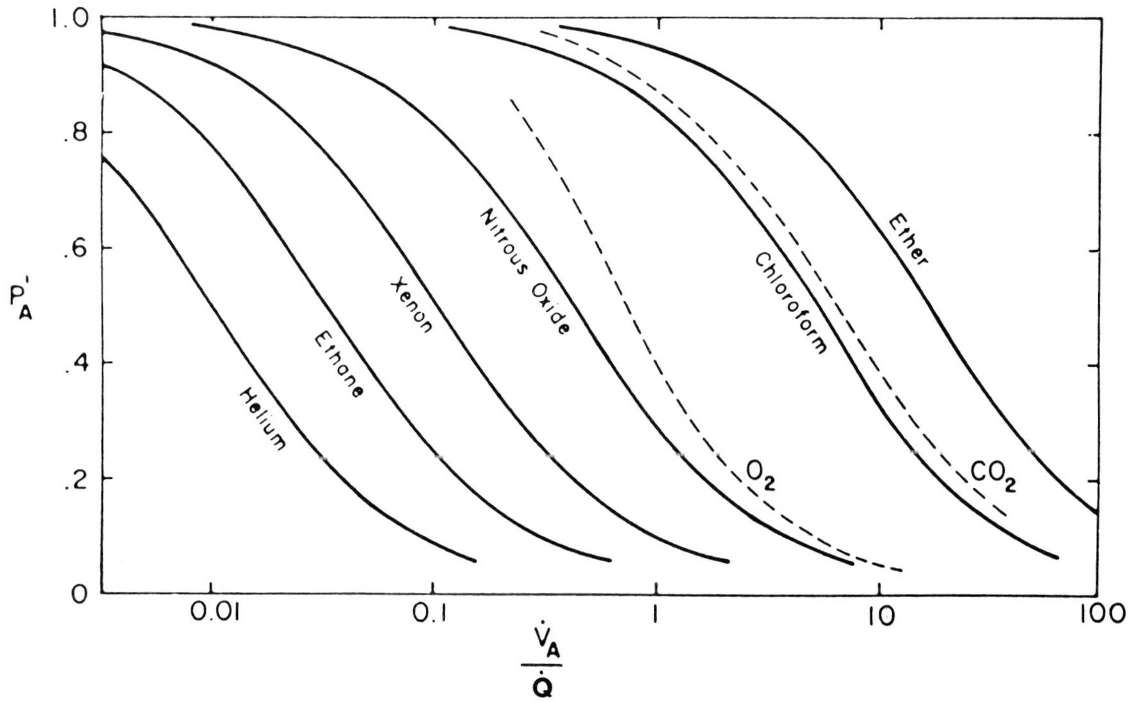

FIG. 5. Equilibrium pressures for elimination of inert gas from the lungs. Curves are normalized by showing alveolar pressure divided by pressure of the gas in the incoming mixed venous blood ($P'A$). O_2 and CO_2 are also shown to indicate that they behave appropriately if their dissociation curve is taken into account. O_2 is normalized as $(PI_{O_2} - PA_{O_2})/(PI_{O_2} - P\bar{v}_{O_2})$, where $P\bar{v}_{O_2}$ is the mixed venous partial pressure of O_2. [From Farhi (12).]

from mixed venous blood practically entirely ($P'_A \simeq 0$), even when $\dot{V}_A/\dot{Q}$ is small. The low solubility implies that the amount of gas that can evolve from the blood phase is too small to generate a back pressure that could limit seriously further diffusion. If almost all the gas is extracted from every volume of blood, elimination of inert gases of low solubility will reflect the blood flow through the lung, or, in the accepted parlance, elimination will be perfusion limited.

At the opposite end of the scale, when a very soluble gas reaches the lung, it is enough that a small fraction of the amount presented moves into the gas phase to produce an equilibrium at a level that will therefore be very close to that of mixed venous blood. An increase in blood flow is of only minor consequence: gas elimination depends on the rate at which the tracer can be removed from the alveolar gas; i.e., gas elimination is ventilation limited.

Figure 6 expands this idea by indicating how two gases—one very soluble and one poorly soluble—are eliminated as a function of both ventilation and perfusion. Besides illustrating the difference between the two excretion patterns, Figure 6 shows that the terms *perfusion limited* and *ventilation limited* should not be taken too literally: even poorly soluble gases require a modicum of ventilation to reach the atmosphere, and very soluble gases have to be delivered to the lung by the circulation.

Between the two extremes there are numerous gases whose elimination is exquisitely dependent on $\dot{V}_A/\dot{Q}$. The peak sensitivity expressed as $dP'_A/(d \log \dot{V}_A/\dot{Q})$ is maximum when $\dot{V}_A/\dot{Q} = \lambda$; this is also the condition in which 50% of the gas is eliminated. At any $\dot{V}_A/\dot{Q}$, there is a gradation of elimination of gases, as a function of λ. This makes it possible to return to Figure 5 and read the value of P'_A for two selected gases at any $\dot{V}_A/\dot{Q}$ over a wide range of $\dot{V}_A/\dot{Q}$. When $\dot{V}_A/\dot{Q}$ is extremely low (i.e., much smaller than the lesser of the two λ values), retention of both gases is practically complete. As increasingly higher $\dot{V}_A/\dot{Q}$ values are considered, P'_A will drop, but the P'_A of the less soluble gas will drop faster. Finally, at very high $\dot{V}_A/\dot{Q}$, P'_A approaches zero for both tracers. The relationship between the two elimination patterns is best demonstrated by plotting one P'_A against the other (Fig. 7). This presentation, which yields a curve similar in shape to the $\dot{V}_A/\dot{Q}$ line for every pair of gases studied, is the basis for the analysis of $\dot{V}_A/\dot{Q}$ distribution on the basis of simultaneous elimination of different inert gases (see DETERMINATION OF $\dot{V}_A/\dot{Q}$ DISTRIBUTION, p. 208).

For a more detailed analysis of the elimination of inert gases, consult references 12 and 17.

Review of Assumptions

The above approach is the basis of countless studies to which we owe our present knowledge; it is therefore appropriate to review the validity and limitations of the basic assumptions.

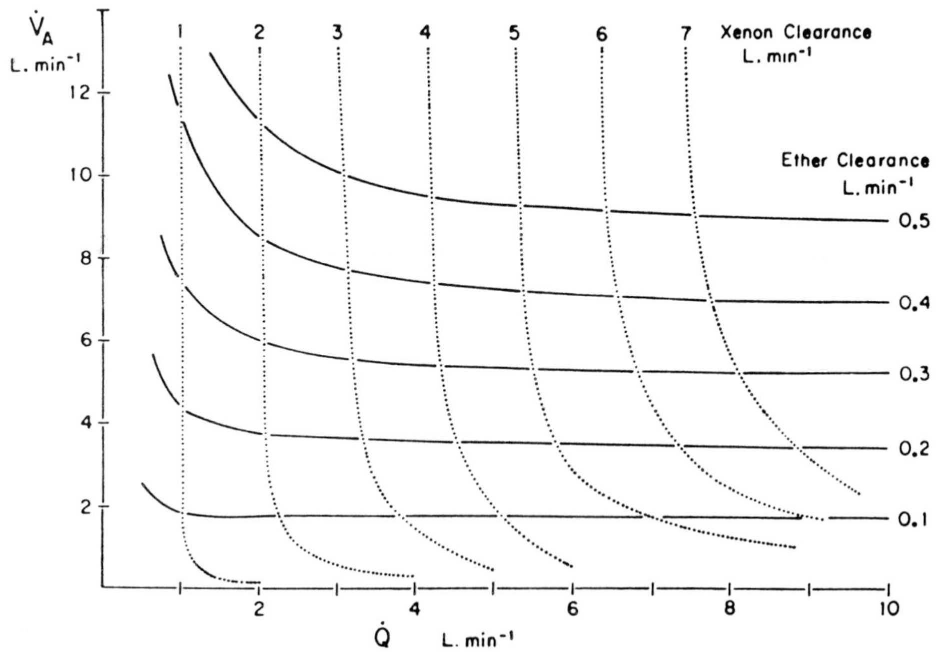

FIG. 6. Effect of solubility on inert-gas elimination. Abscissa is pulmonary blood flow ($\dot{Q}$), in liters/minute; ordinate is alveolar ventilation ($\dot{V}_A$) in liters/minute. Isoclearance lines indicate virtual blood flow cleared of the inert gas for any combination of $\dot{V}_A$ and $\dot{Q}$, the two gases combined having a λ (partition coefficient) of ~0.1 for xenon and 15 for ethyl ether. When $\dot{V}_A$ exceeds 2 liters/min, ether clearance is perfusion dependent, while elimination of xenon is a function of $\dot{V}_A$. [From Farhi (12).]

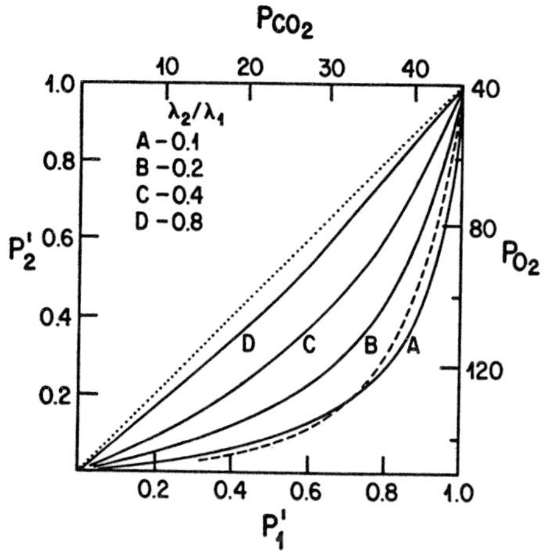

FIG. 7. $\dot{V}_A/\dot{Q}$ curves for various pairs of gases. P_1', P'_A of gas 1; P_2', P'_A of gas 2. *Solid curves A–D* correspond to λ_2/λ_1 (ratio of partition coefficients of 2 gases) values shown and use the *bottom* and *left scales*. Although only the ratio λ_2/λ_1 (and not one of the specific partition coefficients) determines the shape of the curves, the $\dot{V}_A/\dot{Q}$ value for any point on a curve is a function of the absolute λ. *Dashed curve*, $\dot{V}_A/\dot{Q}$ curve for O_2 and CO_2, with appropriate pressures shown *above* and *right*. *Dotted line*, identity line. [From Farhi and Yokoyama (17).]

UNIFORMITY OF INSPIRED GAS COMPOSITION. The classic view of alveolar ventilation postulates that a certain fraction of the volume inspired by the alveoli during each breath is in reality alveolar gas that is stored in the dead space at the end of the preceding expiration. Similarly, part of the expired volume is simply inspirate that failed to reach the gas-exchanging elements at the end of the preceding breath. One can therefore act as if that fraction of the expiration had never left the alveoli and describe a virtual alveolar ventilation, i.e., a flux representing only the inspiration of fresh gas from the environment and only that part of the expiratory volume that is vented to the outside.

If the idea is accepted that the $\dot{V}_A/\dot{Q}$ of the various alveoli may be different, and therefore that alveolar gas composition is not identical throughout the lung, the simple concept of alveolar ventilation is more difficult to apply. Insofar as the gas filling the dead space at the end of expiration originates from millions of alveoli, the gas taken in by any of these at the beginning of inspiration is not exactly the same composition as its own alveolar gas. For example, assume that 10% of the alveoli are not perfused. Because they cannot eliminate any CO_2, their $P_{A_{CO_2}}$ must be zero, according to the standard analysis. If, however, these elements receive one-third of their inspired volume from the dead space (90% of which originates from normally perfused alveoli, in which $P_{A_{CO_2}} = 40$, giving a $P_{CO_2} = 36$ in the end-expiratory dead-space gas), the unperfused alveoli have a $P_{CO_2} = 12$. The problem is further complicated: *1*) the composition of each segment of the dead space may be different from that of another segment, to which a different set of alveoli will have contributed; and *2*) one cannot assume that all alveoli reinspire from the dead space the same fraction of their total intake.

The effect of this variability in the nature of the gas actually inspired by each alveolus has been discussed in detail by Ross and Farhi (53), who concluded that the range of alveolar gas composition is not limited to the $\dot{V}_A/\dot{Q}$ line but covers a substantial area of the O_2-CO_2 diagram (Fig. 8). The net effect of reinspiration of mixed alveolar gas from the dead space is to reduce the difference in alveolar gas composition throughout the lung, since each alveolus is influenced by the mean gas exchange, or at least the mean end-expiratory gas exchange.

West (63), who extended this analysis, described gas exchange as it would occur in alveoli that were ventilated entirely through collateral ventilation from other elements. As West noted, this is the extreme case in the preceding analysis, equivalent to having the ventilation of one alveolus supplied entirely by dead-space gas coming from another alveolus.

UNIFORMITY OF PULMONARY ARTERIAL BLOOD COMPOSITION. There is little doubt that pulmonary arterial blood is well mixed and hence that the blood perfusing the different alveoli enters all gas-exchange areas at the same gas pressures. There may, however, be a difference in composition, in that various degrees of erythrocyte skimming may lead to different hematocrit and hemoglobin concentrations in separate areas (28). Such an occurrence would give rise to a situation where various $\dot{V}_A/\dot{Q}$ lines within the same lung should be considered, each one based on a different set of dissociation curves. These differences in hematocrit affect not only O_2 and CO_2 but also inert gases, since gas solubility in plasma and erythrocytes might be different, but appear to be of only minor consequence with the tracers usually studied (69).

EQUILIBRIUM ACROSS THE ALVEOLAR MEMBRANE. In their original papers, Riley and Cournand (51, 52) considered the possibility that diffusion limitations might prevent O_2 equilibrium across the alveolar membrane and discussed how this would be reflected in the $\dot{V}_A/\dot{Q}$ line. The topic was taken up again by King and Briscoe (27) in a very elegant article. It is, however,

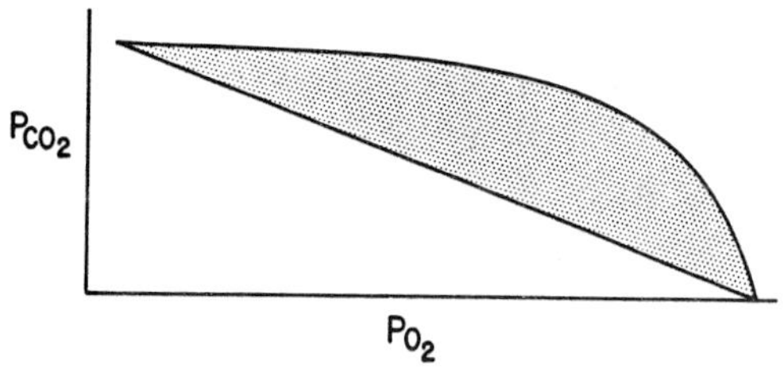

FIG. 8. *Shaded area*, $\dot{V}/\dot{Q}$ area drawn assuming that alveoli rebreathe some gas from dead space. As opposed to the standard $\dot{V}_A/\dot{Q}$ line, all points in *shaded area* can occur. Overall gas-exchange ratio (R) is a combination of dead-space R and alveolar R. [From Ross and Farhi (53).]

generally accepted that diffusing capacity (D) must be reduced to extremely low levels to have significant effects. In 1961 Piiper and his co-workers (42–44) discussed the $D/\dot{Q}$ concept and pointed out clearly that the diffusing capacity of each alveolus must be closely matched to its perfusion to optimize gas exchange.

More recently, evidence from several laboratories has indicated that gas composition within the respiratory elements may not be uniform. Bulk flow ventilation delivers inspired gas up to a finite distance from the alveolar wall. From that point on a diffusion gradient is responsible for movement of the gases. The effect of this gas diffusion limitation is difficult to establish in theory, since much depends on assumed local (i.e., in the acinus) distribution of blood flow. If the bulk of the perfusion goes to the distal part (i.e., the part farthest away from the terminal bronchus), O_2 would have to travel a measurable distance before it reaches the vascular section of the alveoli. If the opposite is true, i.e., if the central part of the secondary lobule is better perfused [as Wagner et al. (59a) demonstrated in the rat], diffusion in the gas phase may be less important.

EFFECT OF INERT-GAS DILUENT. To obtain the $\dot{V}A/\dot{Q}$ line, one needs to draw the gas R lines (45, 51) or incorporate the equation for such lines in the computer program (41). Either procedure calls for a formula for calculating $\dot{V}_{O_2}$, a step in which it is normally assumed that no N_2 (or whatever inert-gas diluent is present) is exchanged. The P_{N_2} of an air-breathing subject varies from alveolus to alveolus, depending on the local R, so that there is in fact inert-gas exchange, given by

$$\dot{V}_x = \dot{Q}\alpha_x(PA_x - P\bar{v}_x) \quad (10)$$

where x is the inert-gas species and $\dot{V}_x$ may be positive or negative, depending on whether PA_x exceeds $P\bar{v}_x$. Thus the assumption that $\dot{V}_x = 0$ is mathematically tenable only if $\lambda_x = 0$ (a condition that exists for no known gas) or if $PA_x = P\bar{v}_x$ (an equality that is found only in alveoli exchanging at one value of R). Canfield and Rahn (10) discussed the fact that there is continuous N_2 uptake from alveoli where P_{N_2} is high and an equal output of N_2 from alveoli where P_{N_2} is low. The low solubility of N_2 makes it possible to neglect the N_2 exchange, as is done traditionally in calculating $\dot{V}_{O_2}$; when other gases replace N_2, the error may be considerable. How the solubility of the inert gas affects the $\dot{V}A/\dot{Q}$ line in either the unsteady state (when the inert gas is either taken up or eliminated) or the steady state (when the net exchange is zero) is discussed next.

Unsteady state. The anesthesiologists have long been aware of the arterial hypoxemia that can occur during recovery from N_2O anesthesia, a phenomenon for which Fink (18) coined the term *diffusion hypoxia* to indicate that it was due to the diffusion of N_2O in the alveoli, leading to dilution of O_2 and hypoxia. The exact relationship between N_2O and O_2 exchange was described by Farhi and Olszowka in 1967 (15). In essence, if a soluble inert gas is present in the inspirate and not found, or found at a lower pressure in the mixed venous blood, it will be absorbed and will thereby concentrate both O_2 and CO_2. As a matter of fact, under certain conditions PA_{O_2} may exceed PI_{O_2}, despite $\dot{V}_{O_2}$ (Fig. 9). When alveoli contain a mixture of several gases, the one with the lowest solubility acts as the slow gas: some of it is taken up by (or eliminated from) mixed venous blood as the latter reaches equilibrium with alveolar gas. The exchange is limited by the low solubility, which allows the alveoli to maintain an inert-gas pressure that is substantially different from the pressure of that gas in mixed venous blood or in other alveoli. Such a gas becomes the swing species, its fractional concentration exceeding that in the inspirate if there is net uptake of the other gases or falling below inspired concentration if it is diluted by net output of the remaining gases. Under normal circumstances, N_2 is the slow gas. If, however, it is replaced by a much more soluble gas, O_2 can become the slow gas, as shown in Figure 9. During elimination of inert gas, PA_{O_2} may in theory fall below $P\bar{v}_{O_2}$ (Fig. 10).

Steady state. In the steady state the range of alveolar–to–mixed venous pressure differences is much smaller than during the unsteady state, because $P\bar{v}$ must fall in the midrange of the individual values. Nevertheless, if the inert-gas diluent is sufficiently soluble, there is a measurable net uptake from alveoli with low $\dot{V}A/\dot{Q}$ (thereby concentrating O_2 in these elements) and elimination into those with high $\dot{V}A/\dot{Q}$, thereby diluting O_2. The consequence is a reduced range of P_{O_2}.

The effect of the nature of the inert gas on alveoli with a $\dot{V}A/\dot{Q} = 0$ is now considered. These alveoli can be divided into three groups: *1*) collapsed alveoli with no blood-gas interface, *2*) open but unventilated alveoli, and *3*) closed gas-filled elements. Clearly the

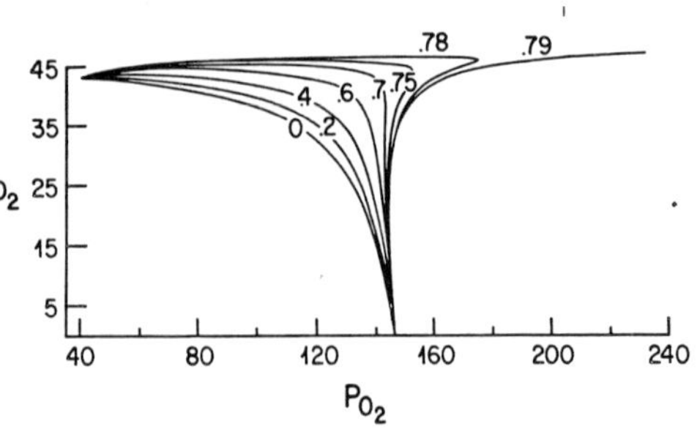

FIG. 9. $\dot{V}A/\dot{Q}$ curves for a subject breathing 21% O_2 and various N_2O fractions. Fraction of inspired N_2O (FI_{N_2O}) is shown on each curve; remainder of inspired gas is N_2. Mixed venous gas assumed to be free of N_2O. When FI_{N_2O} exceeds 0.7, PA_{O_2} will be higher than PI_{O_2} because of shrinkage in gas volume. [From Farhi and Olszowka (15).]

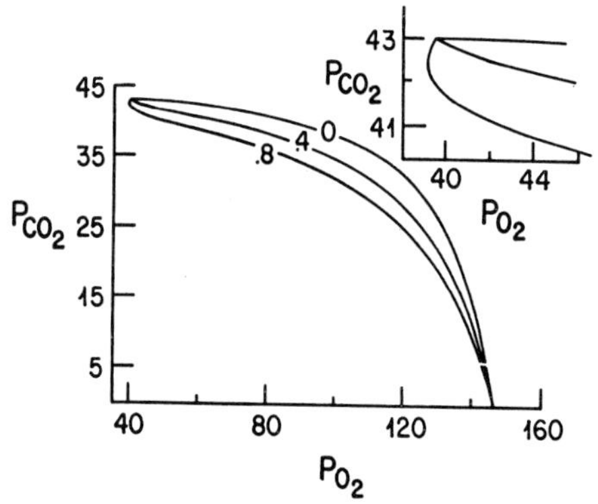

FIG. 10. $\dot{V}A/\dot{Q}$ curves during elimination of N_2O on the O_2-CO_2 diagram. *Curves*, $\dot{V}A/\dot{Q}$ curves of a subject who has previously breathed a mixture containing some N_2O and is then suddenly switched to air breathing. Fraction of N_2O in initial mixture is 0 (control, standard $\dot{V}A/\dot{Q}$ curve), 0.4, or 0.8. Curve area that lies near the $\dot{V}A/\dot{Q}$ = 0 area is expanded in the *inset* and shows that it is theoretically possible to have a PA_{O_2} lower than $P\bar{v}_{O_2}$. [From Farhi and Olszowka (15).]

first type returns mixed venous blood to the left heart, acting as a physiological right-to-left shunt.

In the second group, CO_2 rapidly achieves the level at which it no longer exchanges with blood. Oxygen and the inert gas are taken up continuously and replaced by outside air entering the alveoli. The rate of gas exchange is limited by blood flow through the alveolar walls and by the solubility of the inert gas. The $\dot{V}A/\dot{Q} = 0$ point is located in the blood R = 0 line originating from the mixed venous blood point. If the solubility of the inert gas is small, as is the case for N_2, these two points are extremely close to each other and can be assumed to be the same for all intents and purposes. If, however, the solubility is high, P_{O_2} of the unventilated areas may exceed substantially that of venous blood. As an example, when breathing 21% O_2 in N_2O, the difference is as high as 4 Torr (41).

Finally, in closed alveoli, O_2 and CO_2 exchange until they reach pressures that are close to those in the mixed venous blood. Because the sum of these two pressures is much lower than PI_{O_2}, while total pressure must be atmospheric, the partial pressure of the inert-gas diluent must rise, causing uptake of that gas and further resorption of O_2 and CO_2. Blood therefore exchanges at a negative R, and the $\dot{V}A/\dot{Q} = 0$ point is above and to the right of the mixed venous point, on a blood R line having the slope of $-PA_{CO_2}/PA_{O_2}$. The distance between the two points is a function of the solubility of the inert gas.

Conclusions

Although the mathematical approach to analysis of gas pressures and exchange in different alveoli as a function of $\dot{V}A/\dot{Q}$ retains enormous importance and has led to giant strides in our understanding of respiratory physiology, such an analysis requires that many assumptions be made. Some of these are either mathematically correct or introduce only a minor error (e.g., the omission of N_2 exchange from the calculation); others, such as the assumption that all alveoli are ventilated only with fresh outside air, yield errors that are often substantial. In view of these limitations, one cannot be too cautious when interpreting quantitative conclusions based on the classic concepts.

GAS EXCHANGE IN THE WHOLE LUNG

The preceding development, dealing with gas exchange in a single alveolus, applies to the whole lung only if all its elements have the same $\dot{V}A/\dot{Q}$, an identical inspired gas composition (including rebreathing from the dead space), an equal circulating hematocrit, and similar geometry, thus replicating the gas-diffusing pathway. Such an ideal lung does not exist. There is a considerable range of $\dot{V}A/\dot{Q}$ values in the lung of the resting individual and experimental animal. This statement is based on different types of evidence.

Direct Measurement of Lobar Differences in Gas Exchange

Martin and his co-workers (33, 34) modified the Carlens tracheal divider to obtain samples of gas from various lobes in humans. They demonstrated differences in ventilation, perfusion, and $\dot{V}A/\dot{Q}$ and showed that these were affected by posture. Rahn et al. (49) reached similar conclusions in their studies of anesthetized dogs, in which they sampled gas returning from different lobar bronchi and assessed distribution of inspired gas by measuring deposition of radioactive particles.

Regional Differences in Gas Exchange in the Vertical Lung

The advent of accurate techniques for measuring small concentrations of radioactive gases allowed Ball et al. (4) and West and Dollery (66) to determine ventilation and perfusion at different lung levels along the apex-to-base axis. With the principles that are universally accepted today, the radioactivity at different heights is assessed by external counting. A γ-emitting gas is delivered to the lung either by addition to the inspirate or by intravenous injection. The first route allows determination of the distribution of ventilation; the second yields data on the distribution of blood flow.

In the erect subject the bases of the lungs are better ventilated than the apices. Milic-Emili et al. (37) demonstrated that this is due to the weight of the lung, which compresses the lowermost alveoli and—by decreasing their volume—allows them to operate on the steep part of their pressure-volume curve. The apical alveoli are relatively distended and therefore have a lower compliance. The vertical distribution of blood flow, which is also due to gravity, was described by Anthonisen and Milic-Emili (2) in a companion paper; West et al. (67) explained this on the basis of a complex relationship linking pulmonary arterial, pulmonary venous, and alveolar pressures. The analysis led to the functional division of the lung into three zones. The topmost zone, zone I, is characterized by the fact that alveolar pressure exceeds the local arterial pressure (i.e., the pressure at the root of the pulmonary artery minus the difference in height between the point considered and the origin of the pulmonary artery); therefore zone I is not perfused. The middle zone, zone II, is one in which a Starling resistor system, caused by the fact that alveolar pressure is intermediate between local arterial and venous pressures, throttles blood flow. Finally, in zone III, where the alveolar pressure is the lowest of the triad, flow is continuous and unimpeded. The gradient of distribution of perfusion is much steeper than that of ventilation and, as a consequence, $\dot{V}A/\dot{Q}$ decreases from apex to base (62).

These regional differences are not due to intrinsic local properties of lung tissue but are caused entirely by gravity. Kaneko et al. (26) studied subjects in a variety of postures and demonstrated that the distribution gradients are always set along the axis on which gravity acts, regardless of body position.

Gas Exchange

The assumption of gas pressure equilibrium between gas and end-capillary blood implies that in a homogeneous lung these pressures should be identical in the mixed alveolar gas as collected at the mouth and in the pulmonary venous blood, if appropriate corrections are made for anatomical right-to-left shunts. This would not be the case in a nonhomogeneous lung, as explained in 1922 by Haldane (22), who reasoned that each alveolus contributes to the mixed alveolar gas as a function of its ventilation, whereas it contributes to the mixed blood as a function of its perfusion. As a consequence the gas is more influenced by alveoli with a high $\dot{V}A$, whereas the blood reflects more closely the better perfused elements, and gas-to-blood pressure differences occur. These alveolar-arterial differences have formed the classic basis for our understanding of the effects of lung inhomogeneity.

These various demonstrations of $\dot{V}A/\dot{Q}$ inhomogeneity do not duplicate each other but provide independent evidence. Even more important, the results are complementary. For example, using a very ingenious technique, Lenfant (32) demonstrated the existence of alveoli with a $\dot{V}A/\dot{Q}$ far lower than that detected with radioactive tracers, clearly showing that in addition to regional differences there are important intraregional variances.

DETERMINATION OF $\dot{V}A/\dot{Q}$ DISTRIBUTION

Interpretation of data obtained by external counting of γ-emitting tracers is straightforward and requires no elaboration. This is not true for techniques based on the analysis of gas exchange, where one starts with solid figures (the alveolar and arterial gas pressures) and proceeds to construct a mathematical model of the lung that would yield the same gas and blood compositions. Before some of these manipulations are described, two points need to be emphasized.

1. The model that is obtained explains only the data at hand. Use of another set of values, obtained at the same time on the same subject but dealing with other gases, might yield an entirely different analogue. Even when the same set of numbers is considered, an infinity of models can be derived, since the number of alveoli is several orders of magnitude higher than the number of data points, leading to an underdetermined system. In general the analogue proposed is the simplest combination of $\dot{V}A/\dot{Q}$ values that explains the actual findings.

2. All models are based—implicitly or explicitly—on the mathematical relationship described earlier or on their graphic representation, the $\dot{V}A/\dot{Q}$ line. Because of the assumptions and simplifications discussed earlier, all the models must be viewed as conceptual rather than true descriptions of the lung.

Three-Compartment Model

The first serious attempt to quantitate the degree of $\dot{V}A/\dot{Q}$ inhomogeneity was made by Riley and Cournand and co-workers (51, 52). Although the assumptions and procedures may appear crude by today's standards, these papers, which still stand as superb examples of an incisive analytical approach, have probably had more effect than any other paper. The concept of equivalent shunt and alveolar dead space, which they proposed, is still widely used. One of the cornerstones of the approach is that the PA_{O_2} level does not affect the $\dot{V}A/\dot{Q}$ distribution, the true shunt, or the diffusing capacity of the lung. The PA_{O_2} does, however, alter the effects of these three independent variables. For example, the same anatomic shunt produces a much higher alveolar-arterial difference when PA_{O_2} is elevated, because of the shape of the O_2 dissociation curve.

The approach requires the observer to study the subject or preparation at a PA_{O_2} approaching normal values as well as at a PA_{O_2} of ~40 Torr. In each of these two conditions, Pa_{CO_2} serves to calculate dead space (in combination with mixed expired P_{CO_2} and minute volume, using the Bohr equation) as well as PA_{O_2}, using the alveolar gas equation and assuming equality between PA_{CO_2} and Pa_{CO_2}. In a second step, one determines graphically the combination of shunt and diffusing capacity that would yield the same $PA_{O_2} - Pa_{O_2}$ values as those obtained experimentally at the two oxygenation levels. The model that emerges from the calculations consists of *1*) an ideal compartment, having the same $\dot{V}A/\dot{Q}$ throughout; *2*) a dead-space compartment that includes anatomic dead space and an alveolar dead space resulting from ventilation of a virtual unperfused compartment; and *3*) a shunt compartment that lumps together true anatomic right-to-left anastomosis, blood flow through atelectatic areas, and the blood flow through another virtual compartment, perfused but unventilated. In other words, all alveoli with a $\dot{V}A/\dot{Q}$ higher than the mean value for the whole lung are assumed to contribute all their blood flow and an appropriate part of their ventilation to the ideal compartment and some excess ventilation to the alveolar dead space. In a similar fashion, overperfused areas ($\dot{V}A/\dot{Q}$ lower than the mean) contribute to the ideal lung and to the shunt.

Two-Compartment Model

A different approach was taken by Briscoe and Cournand (6), who initially divided the lung into two functional compartments on the basis of the ventilation per unit volume, as assessed by N_2 washout. The blood flow to the slow and fast areas was then calculated. Although this method has obvious limitations (two alveoli with the same $\dot{V}A/\dot{Q}$ are placed in different compartments if one alveolus has high $\dot{V}A$ and $\dot{Q}$ values per unit volume and the other has low values), it deserves special mention because it separates the effects of uneven distribution from those of true shunt and anatomic dead space.

Nitrogen Difference

The next major step was taken when Canfield and Rahn (10) described the effects of $\dot{V}A/\dot{Q}$ on N_2 exchange, as shown in Figure 2. The basic mechanism that leads to alveolar-arterial differences applies to N_2. An arterial-alveolar N_2 difference must occur in the nonhomogeneous lung, because the various elements contribute to mixed gas and blood leaving the lung to a different extent. Note that PA_{N_2} falls appreciably in low $\dot{V}A/\dot{Q}$ areas but does not rise much in high $\dot{V}A/\dot{Q}$ elements.

Canfield and Rahn (10) pointed out two major advantages of the N_2 approach, both based on the fact that the body neither consumes nor produces N_2. As a consequence, venous blood N_2 concentration must equal arterial N_2 concentration, making $Pa_{N_2} - PA_{N_2}$ insensitive to shunt. In addition, during the steady state, P_{N_2} must be the same throughout the body and determination of this variable in any body fluid yields Pa_{N_2}. Indeed some of the pioneering work that validated the concept and demonstrated a sizable increase in $Pa_{N_2} - PA_{N_2}$ in patients with pulmonary emphysema was conducted with urine (29, 30).

Triple Gradient

Once the principle of the N_2 difference was described and technical means to obtain good analytical blood N_2 data were reported (14), it became possible to combine this measurement with determination of O_2 and CO_2 differences. In principle this allows determination of maldistribution and true shunt separately.

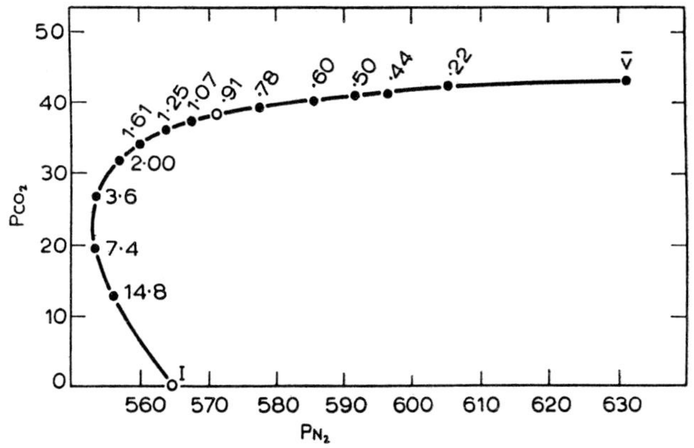

FIG. 11. $\dot{V}A/\dot{Q}$ curve on P_{CO_2}-P_{N_2} diagram. Inspired curve was presented by Canfield and Rahn (10). Curve shown here gives $\dot{V}A/\dot{Q}$ values for a resting subject breathing air at sea level. $\bar{v}$, Mixed venous. [From Farhi (11).]

Nitrogen–Carbon Dioxide Relationship

The data from Figure 2 pertaining to CO_2 and N_2 have provided another way to assess $\dot{V}A/\dot{Q}$ distribution. A $\dot{V}A/\dot{Q}$ line can be drawn that relates the P_{CO_2} and P_{N_2} that obtain at various $\dot{V}A/\dot{Q}$ values (Fig. 11), as proposed by Canfield and Rahn (10). If this curve is set aside, the P_{CO_2}-P_{N_2} diagram can be used to illustrate a simple property of gas mixing (Fig. 12). If one is given two primary gas mixtures in which P_{CO_2} and P_{N_2} are known, these two gases can be plotted as points L and M. Any secondary mixture of L and M, in any proportion, can also be plotted as a point X, which must fall on the straight line joining L to M. The relative distance to L and M is dictated by the ratio in which M and L contribute to the secondary mix. Obviously, if two such secondary mixes are generated, both points, X and Y, will fall on LM. If only X and Y are known, it is impossible to back-calculate the composition of L and M, but they must lie on the extrapolation of XY.

Figure 13 shows how this principle was first used to analyze $\dot{V}A/\dot{Q}$ distribution on the basis of CO_2-N_2 relationships (11). The $\dot{V}A/\dot{Q}$ line for the subject being tested was plotted on the diagram, as were the alveolar and arterial points. Joining these two points and extending the line to the intersections with the $\dot{V}A/\dot{Q}$ line led to the identification of two points, L and M, both of which have the following characteristics: *1*) they describe possible P_{CO_2}-P_{N_2} combinations that can exist in the lung, and *2*) mixing of the gas and blood leaving the alveoli can generate both the mixed alveolar gas and the arterial points.

The lung can now be described in terms of two compartments. In addition to the standard assumptions on which the $\dot{V}A/\dot{Q}$ line is based, the CO_2 dissociation curve is considered to be linear between L and M, a reasonable simplification over a short portion of the curve, i.e., for $\dot{V}A/\dot{Q}$ values from 0 to 10 in a resting subject with a mixed venous P_{CO_2} ($P\bar{v}_{CO_2}$) of ~50 Torr.

When this analysis is applied to the normal lung, it yields a model in which one compartment receives

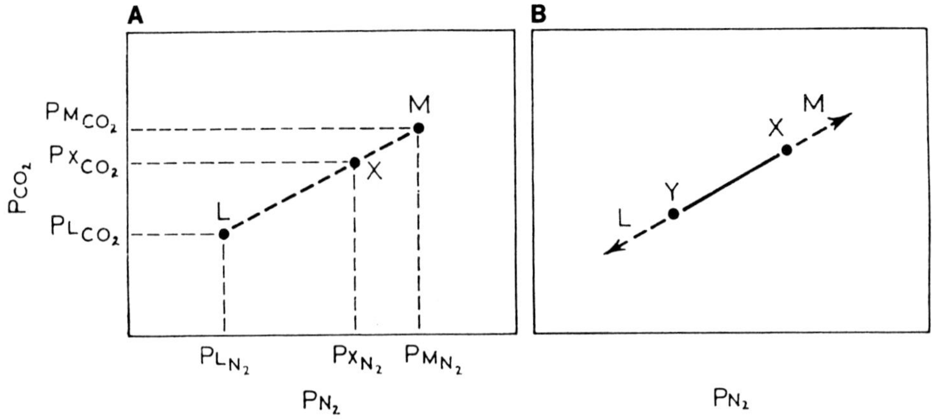

FIG. 12. Principle used to determine $\dot{V}A/\dot{Q}$ distribution on the P_{CO_2}-P_{N_2} diagram. *A*: if two gases, L and M, are mixed in any proportion, yielding gas X, *points L, M,* and *X* must be on a straight line. *B*: if two secondary mixtures, X and Y, are plotted, the primary components must lie on the extrapolation of *XY*. PM_{CO_2}, partial pressure of CO_2 in gas M; PX_{CO_2}, partial pressure of CO_2 in gas X; PL_{CO_2}, partial pressure of CO_2 in gas L. [From Farhi (11).]

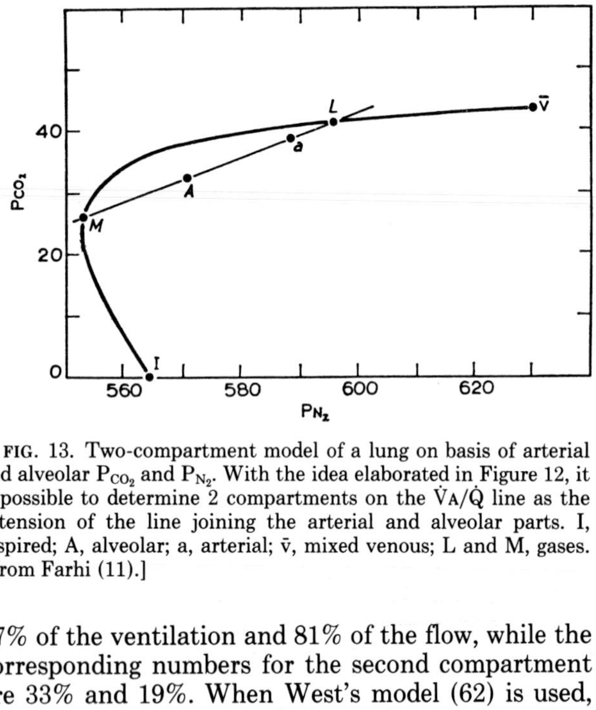

FIG. 13. Two-compartment model of a lung on basis of arterial and alveolar P_{CO_2} and P_{N_2}. With the idea elaborated in Figure 12, it is possible to determine 2 compartments on the $\dot{V}A/\dot{Q}$ line as the extension of the line joining the arterial and alveolar parts. I, inspired; A, alveolar; a, arterial; v̄, mixed venous; L and M, gases. [From Farhi (11).]

67% of the ventilation and 81% of the flow, while the corresponding numbers for the second compartment are 33% and 19%. When West's model (62) is used, the first compartment includes the bottom four slices and the second compartment includes the top four.

Inert-Gas Elimination

Much of the recent progress in the determination of $\dot{V}A/\dot{Q}$ distribution is based on study of the elimination of inert gases of different solubilities. In their fundamental paper, Farhi and Yokoyama (17) applied the approach shown in Figure 13 to the $\dot{V}A/\dot{Q}$ line for two inert gases, as shown in Figure 7. In practice, they studied the elimination of three inert gases (68), from which they could obtain three sets of $\dot{V}A/\dot{Q}$ lines, each one of which divided the lungs into two compartments. Because each set of gases is particularly sensitive to the $\dot{V}A/\dot{Q}$ range that is the geometric mean between the λ of the two gases, it is possible to select gas pairs that emphasize different $\dot{V}A/\dot{Q}$ ranges.

The use of inert gases was expanded in a major way by Wagner et al. (61), who refined the approach in several respects. *1*) They used six inert gases, the solubility of which increases at nearly equal increments (on a logarithmic scale). *2*) Determinations were made during steady state. [Yokoyama and Farhi (68) preloaded the animals and studied them during washout.] *3*) A much improved gas chromatographic technique was used for analysis (60). *4*) The results were expressed in terms of dead space, a shunt, and 48 compartments.

The initial mathematical approach was inadequate (25, 40) and has been replaced. For an excellent review, see Hlastala (23).

Although the modified approach of Wagner et al. remains the most commonly used technique for analyzing multiple inert-gas elimination, several alternatives have been proposed (24, 38).

Gas Solubility, Dead Space, and Shunt

One of the most useful models that analyze the effects of nonuniformity of $\dot{V}A/\dot{Q}$ is the original three-compartment representation of Riley and Cournand (51, 52), whose approach led to the concepts of physiological dead space and physiological shunt. In view of the differential pattern of gas elimination as a function of gas solubility, it is important to examine the relationships of solubility, high $\dot{V}A/\dot{Q}$, and dead space on one hand and that of solubility, low $\dot{V}A/\dot{Q}$, and shunt on the other.

If one assumes a normal value for $\dot{V}A/\dot{Q}$, all alveoli with a higher $\dot{V}A/\dot{Q}$ have in effect an excess ventilation that can be defined quantitatively on the basis of the calculated ideal ventilation, $\dot{V}'A$, which would have been required to yield the same $\dot{V}A/\dot{Q}$ as in the normal elements. The relative excess ventilation can then be said to be the difference between $\dot{V}_A$ and $\dot{V}'_A$, divided by $\dot{V}_A$. For example, if the reference $\dot{V}_A/\dot{Q}$ is 0.9, an alveolus with a $\dot{V}_A/\dot{Q}$ of 3.6 would have an excess ventilation of (3.6 − 0.9)/3.6 or 75%, which simply says that 75% of the $\dot{V}_A$ is above what is needed to maintain the mean $\dot{V}_A/\dot{Q}$. In a second step, to consider the effects of this hyperventilation, one starts by determining the equilibrium partial pressure of a gas being cleared by the lung in both the control alveolus and the hyperventilated one. From these two numbers the fraction of the ventilation that would be reported as dead-space ventilation is deduced. For example, if retention of a gas is 80% in the control alveolus and 60% in the hyperventilated one, 25% of the latter's ventilation would be attributed to dead-space ventilation. These computations are repeated for several high $\dot{V}_A/\dot{Q}$ values and for multiple gases. The compound results are plotted in Figure 14, where excess ventilation appears as the abscissa and calculated dead space as the ordinate. As expected, solubility is paramount. A poorly soluble gas is eliminated practically entirely at normal $\dot{V}_A/\dot{Q}$; any additional ventilation increases clearance only minimally and is therefore largely wasted, appearing as dead space. This is not true for very soluble gases, for which additional gas flow is quite successful in extracting more tracer gas, resulting in a lower dead space at the same level of hyperventilation.

Similar reasoning can be applied to hyperperfused alveoli (low $\dot{V}_A/\dot{Q}$) and shunt. The results of this set of calculations appear in Figure 15, which shows that poorly soluble gases do not contribute extensively to shunt, since additional blood flow can easily be cleared of tracer. On the other hand, very soluble gases, when introduced in high-perfusion areas, are retained and lead to a sizable shuntlike effect.

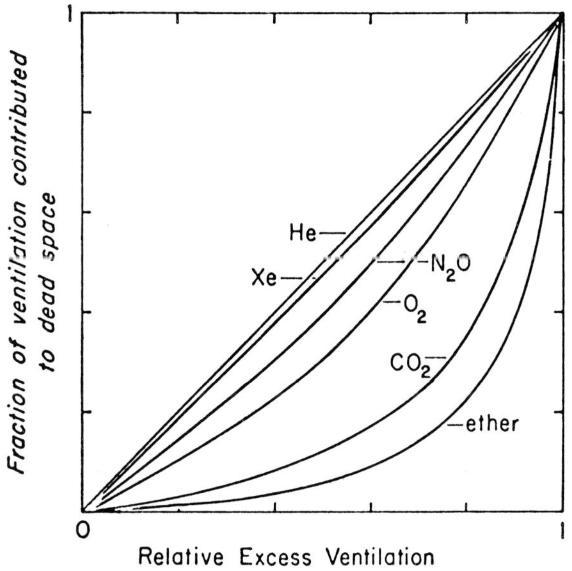

FIG. 14. Relation between excess ventilation and dead-space ventilation. [From Farhi and Yokoyama (17).]

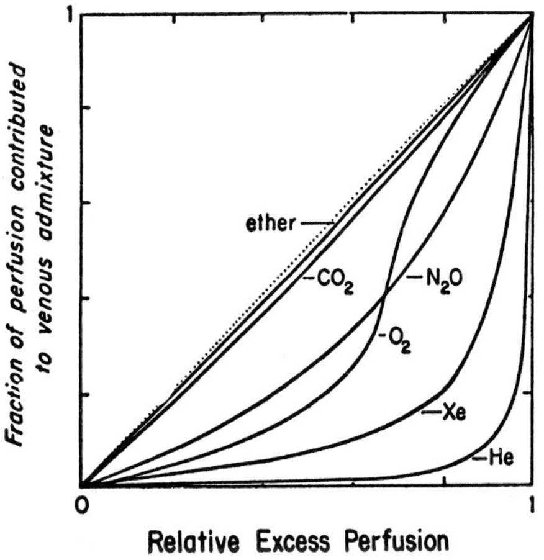

FIG. 15. Relation between excess perfusion and shunt. [From Farhi and Yokoyama (17).]

ALVEOLAR-ARTERIAL DIFFERENCES

It is now established that, even in the normal subject, there are arterial-alveolar differences for CO_2 and N_2 and an alveolar-arterial O_2 difference. The magnitude of these three differences is now compared and whether the information they provide is redundant or complementary is determined.

Haldane (22) had already predicted that, even in the presence of inhomogeneity, Pa_{CO_2} would be close to the ideal value, because retention of CO_2 in low $\dot{V}_A/\dot{Q}$ alveoli can be balanced by increased elimination from areas with high $\dot{V}_A/\dot{Q}$. The arterial-alveolar CO_2 difference is due mainly to the fact that alveoli with high $\dot{V}_A/\dot{Q}$ contribute proportionately more than others to the expirate and thereby lower $P_{A_{CO_2}}$. Thus the CO_2 difference manifests itself by a drop in $P_{A_{CO_2}}$ and reflects high $\dot{V}_A/\dot{Q}$ values.

Nitrogen pressure in high $\dot{V}_A/\dot{Q}$ alveoli remains close to the ideal value (see Fig. 2) because in that $\dot{V}_A/\dot{Q}$ range the increase in P_{O_2} is accompanied by a decrease in P_{CO_2}, leaving P_{N_2} close to $P_{I_{N_2}}$. Blood returning from alveoli with a low $\dot{V}_A/\dot{Q}$ has an elevated P_{N_2} and predominates in the mixed pulmonary venous blood. Nitrogen is therefore the opposite of CO_2: arterial-alveolar differences are due mainly to a shift in blood level away from ideal and are the reflection of low $\dot{V}_A/\dot{Q}$ alveoli.

The O_2 relationships are somewhat more complex. Whereas the CO_2 dissociation curve is practically rectilinear in the physiological range and the N_2 dissociation curve is absolutely linear, the O_2 dissociation curve is not. The alveolar-arterial O_2 difference is therefore affected by the P_{O_2} of the alveoli. For any distribution pattern, the alveolar-arterial O_2 difference is maximal when the mean $\dot{V}_A/\dot{Q}$ is at the "knee" of the curve. Under these conditions, low $\dot{V}_A/\dot{Q}$ alveoli

		(A − a)D_{O_2} on air	(A − a)D_{O_2} on 100% O_2	(A − a)D_{O_2} on low O_2	(a − A)D_{CO_2}	(a − A)D_{N_2}
Venous admixture		++	++++	+	◌	O
Diffusion limitation		+	◌	++	◌	O
Uneven $\dot{V}_A/\dot{Q}$	High $\dot{V}_A/\dot{Q}$	++	+	+	++++	+
	Low $\dot{V}_A/\dot{Q}$	++	+	+	+	++++

FIG. 16. Contribution of various factors to arterial-alveolar differences in P_{CO_2} and P_{N_2} [(a − A)D] and alveolar-arterial differences in P_{O_2} [(A − a)D]. Contributions are shown as going from O (no effect of factor on the right on the difference shown above the symbol) to ++++. ◌, Effect is too small to be measured accurately. ▨, Differences that are specific to a certain factor. [From Farhi (11).]

fall on the steep part of the curve and their saturation is reduced, while alveoli with an elevated $\dot{V}_A/\dot{Q}$ cannot make up for the O_2 deficiency, as their P_{O_2} puts them on the flat part of the dissociation curve. The O_2 difference is due to both an increase in mean $P_{A_{O_2}}$ above the ideal value and a decrease in Pa_{O_2}.

Other factors, namely diffusion limitations and true shunt, can also create alveolar-arterial differences. Figure 16 shows the relationship among all the factors involved.

FACTORS AFFECTING $\dot{V}_A/\dot{Q}$ DISTRIBUTION

Practically every change in ventilation and/or in perfusion affects distribution of $\dot{V}_A/\dot{Q}$ to some extent. The following list is not intended to be comprehensive nor is the coverage within each area meant to be all-inclusive; instead this section is a guide to some of the possible alterations in distribution pattern.

Posture

As mentioned earlier, Kaneko et al. (26) demonstrated that the vertical gradient of $\dot{V}_A/\dot{Q}$ distribution is due solely to the direction of the gravity gradient. Because the anteroposterior diameter of the human chest wall is somewhat shorter than the apex-to-diaphragm distance, a decrease in the alveolar-arterial O_2 difference in the supine subject is expected. In fact, the accumulated evidence (see ref. 1) shows that recumbency leads to a drop in O_2 saturation that cannot be attributed only to hypoventilation. The accepted explanation is that some of the dorsal alveoli collapse, increasing the shunt. Abernethy et al. (1) showed a slight but significant rise in urinary-alveolar P_{N_2} difference after one hour of recumbency, indicating that some of the alveolar-arterial O_2 difference must be due to areas of low $\dot{V}_A/\dot{Q}$. The logical explanation is that some of the alveoli close to the dorsal gutter are so compressed by the weight of the lung that they either are grossly underventilated or collapse altogether. In experimental animals, anesthetized dogs, either in the supine or lateral position, develop atelectasis (19) and have to be subjected to periodic reinflation of the lungs. There is evidence that it is indeed the alveoli with a very high $\dot{V}_A/\dot{Q}$ that are unstable (58).

Gravity

Clearly, another way to affect the vertical distribution of $\dot{V}_A/\dot{Q}$ is to alter the gravitational acceleration. A temporary reduction in $+G_z$ (foot-to-head acceleration) was achieved by Michels and West (36), using parabolic flight profiles. Although the exposure was far too short to allow development of a steady state, it was sufficiently long to permit the investigators to predict that distribution of both ventilation and blood flow should become uniform at zero gravity.

There is much more information on what happens when gravity is increased, most of which is summarized in a recent review article (13). Much of our knowledge is due to the work of Barr (5) and in particular to the excellent studies of Bryan et al. (8, 9), who demonstrated a sharper gradient in distribution of both perfusion and ventilation at high G_z. There is an increase in both dead space and alveolar-arterial O_2 differences (5, 39, 59). The effects of maldistribution are potentiated by a drop in total pulmonary blood flow and a consequent decrease in $P\bar{v}_{O_2}$.

Exercise

The increased pulmonary blood flow that occurs during muscular exercise is directed in a large measure to the lung apices, which are normally hypoperfused. As a consequence, distribution of $\dot{V}_A/\dot{Q}$ becomes more uniform, as can be demonstrated with radioactive gas tracers (7). In fact the arterial-alveolar N_2 difference drops to practically zero (3).

Altitude

The decrease in $P_{I_{O_2}}$ encountered in altitude raises pulmonary arterial pressure and should be expected to decrease $\dot{V}_A/\dot{Q}$ inhomogeneity. Although Sylvester et al. (56) reported this, it has not been confirmed by all investigators. In an early study of the effects of altitude on alveolar-arterial O_2 differences, Kreuzer et al. (31) found that there may actually be a wider distribution of $\dot{V}_A/\dot{Q}$ ratios and questioned whether this harmful effect was not due to other adaptive mechanisms with higher priority. Later, Haab et al. (21) also reported an apparent increase in inhomogeneity in subjects acutely exposed to altitude, studied by the arterial-alveolar N_2 method.

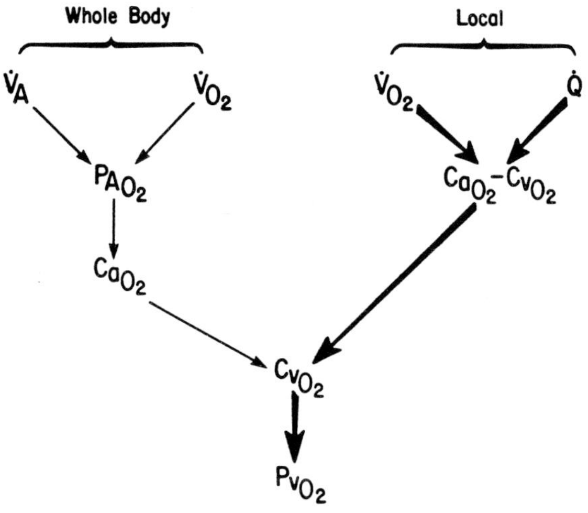

FIG. 17. Control of local P_{O_2}, assumed to be closely related to P_{O_2} of the venous blood that has equilibrated with the tissue or organ. Because arterial O_2 concentration (Ca_{O_2}) is not very responsive to changes in PA_{O_2} in the normal P_{O_2} range, the main factor affecting Cv_{O_2} (and hence Pv_{O_2}) is the local regulation of blood flow to match O_2 needs. $\dot{V}_{O_2}$, O_2 consumption.

Liquid Breathing

When an animal is made to breathe liquids, a new λ is established for all gases and the pattern of exchange is altered. If the new respiratory medium has different O_2 and CO_2 solubilities, as is usually the case, the standard $\dot{V}A/\dot{Q}$ can be modified drastically (35). In particular, when the ratio of CO_2 solubility in the inspirate to that of the O_2 solubility exceeds the ratio of the slopes of the blood dissociation curves, the $\dot{V}A/\dot{Q}$ line acquires an upward concavity. It is also possible to have the same gas-exchange ratio in alveoli with different $\dot{V}A/\dot{Q}$ values.

Compensatory Mechanisms

Hypoxic vasoconstriction provides an excellent feedback loop, the effect of which is to reduce blood flow to hypoventilated areas, moving $\dot{V}A/\dot{Q}$ toward normal values. Grant et al. (20) measured the effectiveness of this response and found it to be optimal in the physiological range. Insofar as the effects of hypoxia on pulmonary vascular resistance are described in detail in the first volume of this *Handbook* section on the respiratory system (19a), they are not detailed here.

Unilateral pulmonary artery occlusion causes bronchoconstriction and a shift of ventilation away from the unperfused lung (54). This appears to be due to the decrease in CO_2 on the unperfused side.

VENTILATION, PERFUSION, AND TISSUE HOMEOSTASIS

If the function of the lung is simply to ensure that the blood supplied to the organism through the arterial tree is of adequate composition in terms of O_2 and CO_2, the role of the total gas-exchange system is to allow each cell of the body to maintain adequate local P_{O_2} and P_{CO_2}. These premises are not only different in various tissues and in distinct locations of the same organ but also vary with time at one site. Actual measurement of local P_{O_2} is therefore not only technically arduous, it is also devoid of significance as a global indicator. For lack of a better definition, Pv_{O_2} and Pv_{CO_2} are accepted as reflections of P_{O_2} and P_{CO_2} in the organ perfused by that blood. In a classic paper, Tenney (57) has indeed shown that under well-defined conditions the P_{O_2} of blood leaving a capillary mirrors that of the tissue supplied by that vessel. The question addressed here is not what the proper pressure of O_2 and CO_2 is in tissues but rather how ventilation and blood flow affect local P_{O_2} and P_{CO_2}, using end-capillary blood as an indicator. This topic was first treated by Suskind and Rahn (55).

The cascade of O_2 from the inspired gas to end-capillary (or venous) blood includes two major drops, the first from PI_{O_2} to PA_{O_2} and the second from Pa_{O_2} to Pv_{O_2}, and one minor drop from PA_{O_2} to Pa_{O_2}. The first of these is linked to the relationship between $\dot{V}_{O_2}$ and $\dot{V}A$, according to

$$PI_{O_2} - PA_{O_2} = 863\dot{V}_{O_2}/\dot{V}A \qquad (11)$$

a simplified statement that neglects the small correction required by the effect of the gas-exchange ratio.

The drop in P_{O_2} across the peripheral capillary reflects $Ca_{O_2} - Cv_{O_2}$, which is dictated by the ratio of local blood flow to local $\dot{V}_{O_2}$. If one neglects the $PA_{O_2} - Pa_{O_2}$, which is small in comparison to the others, all the factors involved can be grouped as in Figure 17, which shows how Pv_{O_2} is determined by Cv_{O_2}, which is in turn dictated by Ca_{O_2} and $Ca_{O_2} - Cv_{O_2}$. The first of these depends on the interplay

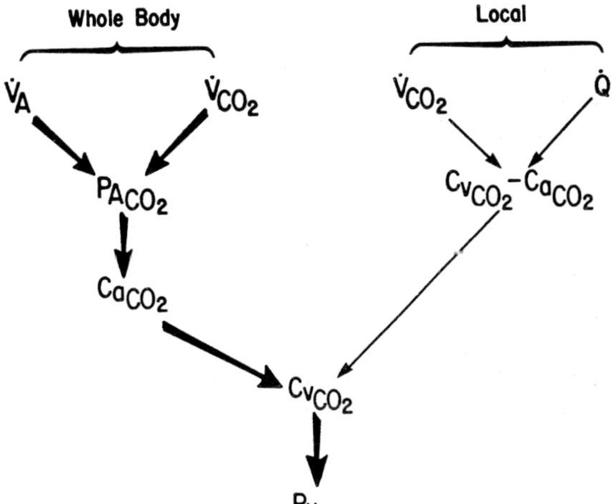

FIG. 18. Control of local P_{CO_2}. Venous-arterial CO_2 difference ($Cv_{CO_2} - Ca_{CO_2}$) normally represents only ~10% of Ca_{CO_2}; Ca_{CO_2} is therefore the dominant factor in setting tissue P_{CO_2}. $\dot{V}_{CO_2}$, CO_2 output.

between total body $\dot{V}_{O_2}$ and $\dot{V}_A$, as indicated in Equation 11, but because $P_{A_{O_2}}$ falls on the flat part of the O_2 dissociation curve—in a normal subject breathing air at sea level—Ca_{O_2} is relatively constant despite variations in Pv_{O_2} and hence is not very dependent on the body's ventilatory response to the O_2 demand. The main factor governing Pv_{O_2} remains therefore Ca_{O_2} − Cv_{O_2}, i.e., the local blood flow per unit $\dot{V}_{O_2}$.

Figure 18 shows a similar scheme for CO_2 exchange. It also incorporates a ventilatory side, based on the equation

$$P_{A_{CO_2}} = 863\dot{V}_{CO_2}/\dot{V}_A \quad (12)$$

and the Fick equation for CO_2

$$Cv_{CO_2} - Ca_{CO_2} = \dot{V}_{CO_2}/\dot{Q} \quad (13)$$

In this case, however, $Cv_{CO_2} - Ca_{CO_2}$ is small in comparison to the Ca_{CO_2}. As a consequence, even sizable changes in local blood flow per unit $\dot{V}_{CO_2}$ have little effect on Cv_{CO_2} and hence Pv_{CO_2}, which is dictated mainly by the ventilation per unit $\dot{V}_{CO_2}$.

It is therefore appropriate to conclude that although both CO_2 and O_2 are transported by the same media—gas flow and blood flow—their tissue levels can be regulated independently of each other by appropriate readjustments of ventilation and local perfusion; CO_2 responds to ventilation and O_2 responds to local perfusion.

REFERENCES

1. ABERNETHY, J. D., J. J. MAURIZI, AND L. E. FARHI. Diurnal variations in urinary-alveolar N_2 difference and effects of recumbency. *J. Appl. Physiol.* 23: 875–879, 1967.
2. ANTHONISEN, N. R., AND J. MILIC-EMILI. Distribution of pulmonary perfusion in erect man. *J. Appl. Physiol.* 21: 760–766, 1966.
3. BACHOFEN, H., H. J. HOBI, AND M. SCHERRER. Alveolar-arterial N_2 gradients at rest and during exercise in healthy men of different ages. *J. Appl. Physiol.* 34: 137–142, 1973.
4. BALL, W. C., P. B. STEWART, L. G. S. MENSHAM, AND D. V. BATES. Regional pulmonary function studied with xenon^{133}. *J. Clin. Invest.* 41: 519–531, 1962.
5. BARR, P. O. Pulmonary gas exchange in man, as affected by prolonged gravitational stress. *Acta Physiol. Scand.* 28, Suppl. 207: 1–46, 1963.
6. BRISCOE, W. A., AND A. COURNAND. The degree of variation of blood perfusion and of ventilation within the emphysematous lung and some related considerations. In: *Pulmonary Structure and Function*, edited by A. V. S. de Reuck and H. O'Connor. Boston, MA: Little, Brown, 1962, p. 304–326. (Ciba Found. Symp.)
7. BRYAN, A. C., L. G. BENTIVOGLIO, F. BEEREL, H. MACLEISH, A. ZIDULKA, AND D. V. BATES. Factors affecting regional distribution of ventilation and perfusion in the lung. *J. Appl. Physiol.* 19: 395–402, 1964.
8. BRYAN, A. C., W. D. MACNAMARA, J. SIMPSON, AND H. N. WAGNER. Effect of acceleration on the distribution of pulmonary blood flow. *J. Appl. Physiol.* 20: 1129–1132, 1965.
9. BRYAN, A. C., J. MILIC-EMILI, AND D. PENGELLY. Effect of gravity on the distribution of pulmonary ventilation. *J. Appl. Physiol.* 21: 778–784, 1966.
10. CANFIELD, R. E., AND H. RAHN. Arterial-alveolar N_2 gas pressure differences due to ventilation-perfusion variations. *J. Appl. Physiol.* 10: 165–172, 1957.
11. FARHI, L. E. Ventilation-perfusion relationship and its role in alveolar gas exchange. In: *Advances in Respiratory Physiology*, edited by C. G. Caro. London: Arnold, 1966, p. 148–197.
12. FARHI, L. E. Elimination of inert gas by the lung. *Respir. Physiol.* 3: 1–11, 1967.
13. FARHI, L. E. Physiological shunts: effects of posture and gravity. In: *Cardiovascular Shunts*, edited by K. Johansen and W. Burggren. Copenhagen: Munskgaard, 1985, p. 322–333. (Alfred Benzon Symp., 21st, 1984.)
14. FARHI, L. E., A. W. T. EDWARDS, AND T. HOMMA. Determination of dissolved N_2 in blood by gas chromatography and (a-A)N_2 difference. *J. Appl. Physiol.* 18: 97–106, 1963.
15. FARHI, L. E., AND A. J. OLSZOWKA. Analysis of alveolar gas exchange in the presence of soluble inert gases. *Respir. Physiol.* 5: 53–67, 1968.
16. FARHI, L. E., AND H. RAHN. A theoretical analysis of the alveolar-arterial O_2 difference with special reference to the distribution effect. *J. Appl. Physiol.* 7: 699–703, 1955.
17. FARHI, L. E., AND T. YOKOYAMA. Effects of ventilation-perfusion inequality on elimination of inert gases. *Respir. Physiol.* 3: 12–20, 1967.
18. FINK, B. R. Diffusion anoxia. *Anesthesiology* 16: 511–519, 1955.
19. FINLEY, T. N., C. LENFANT, P. HAAB, J. PIIPER, AND H. RAHN. Venous admixture in the pulmonary circulation of anesthetized dogs. *J. Appl. Physiol.* 15: 418–424, 1960.

19a. FISHMAN, A. P., AND A. B. FISHER (editors). *Handbook of Physiology. The Respiratory System. Circulation and Nonrespiratory Functions.* Bethesda, MD: Am. Physiol. Soc., 1985, sect. 3, vol. I.

20. GRANT, B. J. B., E. E. DAVIES, H. A. JONES, AND J. M. B. HUGHES. Local regulation of pulmonary blood flow and ventilation-perfusion ratios in the coatimundi. *J. Appl. Physiol.* 40: 216–228, 1976.
21. HAAB, P., D. R. HELD, H. ERNST, AND L. E. FARHI. Ventilation-perfusion relationships during high-altitude adaptation. *J. Appl. Physiol.* 26: 77–81, 1969.
22. HALDANE, J. S. *Respiration.* New Haven, CT: Yale Univ. Press, 1922.
23. HLASTALA, M. P. Multiple inert gas elimination technique. *J. Appl. Physiol.* 56: 1–7, 1984.
24. HLASTALA, M. P., AND H. T. ROBERTSON. Inert gas elimination characteristics of the normal and abnormal lung. *J. Appl. Physiol.* 44: 258–266, 1978.
25. JALIWALA, S. A., R. E. MATES, AND F. J. KLOCKE. An efficient optimization technique for recovering ventilation-perfusion distributions from inert gas data. Effects of random experimental error. *J. Clin. Invest.* 55: 188–192, 1975.
26. KANEKO, K., J. MILIC-EMILI, M. B. DOLOVICH, A. DAWSON, AND D. V. BATES. Regional distribution of ventilation and perfusion as a function of body position. *J. Appl. Physiol.* 21: 767–777, 1966.
27. KING, T. K. C., AND W. A. BRISCOE. Bohr integral isopleths in the study of blood gas exchange in the lung. *J. Appl. Physiol.* 22: 659–674, 1967.
28. KING, T. K. C., AND D. MAZAL. Alveolar-capillary CO_2 and O_2 gradients due to uneven hematocrits. *J. Appl. Physiol.* 40: 673–678, 1976.
29. KLOCKE, F. J., AND H. RAHN. A method for determining inert gas ("N_2") solubility in urine. *J. Clin. Invest.* 40: 279–285, 1961.
30. KLOCKE, F. J., AND H. RAHN. The arterial-alveolar inert gas ("N_2") difference in normal and emphysematous subjects, as indicated by the analysis of urine. *J. Clin. Invest.* 40: 286–294, 1961.
31. KREUZER, F., S. M. TENNEY, J. C. MITHOEFER, AND J. REMMERS. Alveolar-arterial oxygen gradient in Andean natives at high altitude. *J. Appl. Physiol.* 19: 13–16, 1964.

32. LENFANT, C. Measurement of factors impairing gas exchange in man with hyperbaric pressure. *J. Appl. Physiol.* 19: 189–194, 1964.
33. MARTIN, C. J., F. CLINE, AND H. MARSHALL. Lobar alveolar gas concentrations: effect of body position. *J. Clin. Invest.* 32: 617–621, 1953.
34. MARTIN, C. J., AND A. C. YOUNG. Ventilation-perfusion variations within the lung. *J. Appl. Physiol.* 11: 371–376, 1957.
35. MATALON, S. V., AND L. E. FARHI. Ventilation-perfusion lines and gas exchange in liquid breathing: theory. *J. Appl. Physiol.* 49: 262–269, 1980.
36. MICHELS, D. B., AND J. B. WEST. Distribution of pulmonary ventilation and perfusion during short periods of weightlessness. *J. Appl. Physiol.* 45: 987–998, 1978.
37. MILIC-EMILI, J., J. A. M. HENDERSON, M. B. DOLOVICH, D. TROP, AND K. KANEKO. Regional distribution of inspired gas in the lung. *J. Appl. Physiol.* 21: 749–759, 1966.
38. NEUFELD, G. R., J. J. WILLIAMS, P. L. KLINEBERG, AND B. E. MARSHALL. Inert gas a-A differences: a direct reflection of $\dot{V}/\dot{Q}$ distribution. *J. Appl. Physiol.* 44: 277–283, 1978.
39. NUNNELEY, S. A. Gas exchange in man during combined $+G_z$ acceleration and exercise. *J. Appl. Physiol.* 40: 491–495, 1976.
40. OLSZOWKA, A. J. Can $\dot{V}_A/\dot{Q}$ distribution in the lung be recovered from inert gas retention data? *Respir. Physiol.* 25: 191–198, 1975.
41. OLSZOWKA, A. J., AND L. E. FARHI. A digital computer program for constructing ventilation-perfusion lines. *J. Appl. Physiol.* 26: 141–146, 1969.
42. PIIPER, J. Unequal distribution of pulmonary diffusing capacity and the alveolar-arterial PO_2 differences: theory. *J. Appl. Physiol.* 16: 493–498, 1961.
43. PIIPER, J. Variations of ventilation and diffusing capacity to perfusion determining the alveolar-arterial O_2 difference: theory. *J. Appl. Physiol.* 16: 507–510, 1961.
44. PIIPER, J., P. HAAB, AND H. RAHN. Unequal distribution of pulmonary diffusing capacity in the anesthetized dog. *J. Appl. Physiol.* 16: 499–506, 1961.
45. RAHN, H. A concept of mean alveolar air and the ventilation-blood flow relationships during gas exchange. *Am. J. Physiol.* 158: 21–30, 1949.
46. RAHN, H., AND L. E. FARHI. Ventilation-perfusion relationship. In: *Pulmonary Structure and Function*, edited by A. V. S. de Reuck and H. O'Connor. Boston, MA: Little, Brown, 1962, p. 137–153. (Ciba Found. Symp.)
47. RAHN, H., AND L. E. FARHI. Ventilation, perfusion and gas exchange—the $\dot{V}_A/\dot{Q}$ concept. In: *Handbook of Physiology. Respiration,* edited by W. O. Fenn and H. Rahn. Washington, DC: Am. Physiol. Soc., 1964, sect. 3, vol. 1, chapt. 30, p. 735–766.
48. RAHN, H., AND W. O. FENN. *A Graphical Analysis of the Respiratory Gas Exchange.* Washington, DC: Am. Physiol. Soc., 1955.
49. RAHN, H., P. SADOUL, L. E. FARHI, AND J. SHAPIRO. Distribution of ventilation and perfusion in the lobes of the dog's lung in the supine and erect position. *J. Appl. Physiol.* 8: 417–426, 1956.
50. RILEY, R. L., AND A. COURNAND. "Ideal" alveolar air and the analysis of ventilation-perfusion relationships in the lungs. *J. Appl. Physiol.* 1: 825–847, 1949.
51. RILEY, R. L., AND A. COURNAND. Analysis of factors affecting partial pressures of oxygen and carbon dioxide in gas and blood of lungs: theory. *J. Appl. Physiol.* 4: 77–101, 1951.
52. RILEY, R. L., A. COURNAND, AND K. W. DONALD. Analysis of factors affecting partial pressures of oxygen and carbon dioxide in gas and blood of lungs: methods. *J. Appl. Physiol.* 4: 102–120, 1951.
53. ROSS, B. B., AND L. E. FARHI. Dead-space ventilation as a determinant in the ventilation-perfusion concept. *J. Appl. Physiol.* 15: 363–371, 1960.
54. SEVERINGHAUS, J. W., E. W. SWENSON, T. N. FINLEY, M. T. LATEGOLA, AND J. WILLIAMS. Unilateral hypoventilation produced in dogs by occluding one pulmonary artery. *J. Appl. Physiol.* 16: 53–60, 1961.
55. SUSKIND, M., AND H. RAHN. Relationship between cardiac output and ventilation and gas transport, with particular reference to anesthesia. *J. Appl. Physiol.* 7: 59–65, 1954.
56. SYLVESTER, J. T., A. CYMERMAN, G. GURTNER, O. HOTTENSTEIN, M. COTE, AND D. WOLFE. Components of alveolar-arterial O_2 gradient during rest and exercise at sea level and high altitude. *J. Appl. Physiol.* 50: 1129–1139, 1981.
57. TENNEY, S. M. A theoretical analysis of the relationship between venous blood and mean tissue oxygen pressures. *Respir. Physiol.* 20: 283–296, 1974.
58. VELASQUEZ, T., AND L. E. FARHI. Effect of negative-pressure breathing on lung mechanics and venous admixture. *J. Appl. Physiol.* 19: 665–671, 1964.
59. VON NIEDING, G., H. KREKELER, K. KOPPENHAGEN, AND S. RUFF. Effect of acceleration on distribution of lung perfusion and respiratory gas exchange. *Pfluegers Arch.* 342: 159–176, 1973.
59a. WAGNER, P., J. MCRAE, AND J. REED. Stratified distribution of blood flow in secondary lobule of the rat lung. *J. Appl. Physiol.* 22: 1115–1123, 1967.
60. WAGNER, P. D., P. F. NAUMANN, AND R. B. LARAVUSO. Simultaneous measurement of eight foreign gases in blood by gas chromatography. *J. Appl. Physiol.* 36: 600–605, 1974.
61. WAGNER, P. D., H. A. SALTZMAN, AND J. B. WEST. Measurement of continuous distributions of ventilation-perfusion ratios: theory. *J. Appl. Physiol.* 36: 588–599, 1974.
62. WEST, J. B. Regional differences in gas exchange in the lung of erect man. *J. Appl. Physiol.* 17: 893–898, 1962.
63. WEST, J. B. Gas exchange when one lung region inspires from another. *J. Appl. Physiol.* 30: 479–487, 1971.
64. WEST, J. B. *Ventilation, Blood Flow and Gas Exchange* (3rd ed.). Oxford, UK: Blackwell, 1977.
65. WEST, J. B. Ventilation-perfusion relationships. *Am. Rev. Respir. Dis.* 116: 919–943, 1977.
66. WEST, J. B., AND C. T. DOLLERY. Distribution of blood flow and ventilation-perfusion ratio in the lung, measured with radioactive CO_2. *J. Appl. Physiol.* 15: 405–410, 1960.
67. WEST, J. B., C. T. DOLLERY, AND A. NAIMARK. Distribution of blood flow in isolated lung; relation to vascular and alveolar pressures. *J. Appl. Physiol.* 19: 713–724, 1964.
68. YOKOYAMA, T., AND L. E. FARHI. Study of ventilation-perfusion ratio distribution in the anesthetized dog by multiple inert gas washout. *Respir. Physiol.* 3: 166–176, 1967.
69. YOUNG, I. H., AND P. D. WAGNER. Effect of intrapulmonary hematocrit maldistribution on O_2, CO_2, and inert gas exchange. *J. Appl. Physiol.* 46: 240–248, 1979.

Diffusing-capacity heterogeneity

MICHAEL P. HLASTALA | *Departments of Medicine and of Physiology and Biophysics, University of Washington, Seattle, Washington*

CHAPTER CONTENTS

MEASUREMENTS OF THE PULMONARY diffusing capacity of O_2 and of CO have had a major influence in physiological studies and in the practice of clinical medicine. However, these measurements often have been difficult to interpret because of the many physiological components that interact to comprise the final measured value. The classic approach has been to analyze separately the membrane diffusing capacity (Dm) and the red blood cell components (70) by use of a homogeneous lung model and to interpret physiological and clinical findings within this restricted framework. The results and interpretations are affected by heterogeneity in alveolar ventilation ($\dot{V}_A$), alveolar volume (V_A), alveolar perfusion ($\dot{Q}$), and pulmonary diffusing capacity (D_L). The relative importance of each of these heterogeneities and of their interactions varies according to individual characteristics and the particular method chosen to measure D_L. In general, measured D_L usually underestimates true D_L (actual D_L of the lung); however, there are examples of heterogeneities that can result in an overestimate of true D_L. Recently some new approaches have been developed to permit reexamination of the familiar concept of diffusing capacity in an attempt to understand better the physiological information contained in these measurements. This chapter first addresses the interrelationships among blood flow, ventilation, gas solubility, and diffusing capacity in a homogeneous lung, then considers data demonstrating the importance of heterogeneities on measured D_L, and finally considers the influence of gas-phase diffusion limitation.

Several terms have been used to express deviation from uniform behavior in the lung, including *heterogeneity*, *inhomogeneity*, *nonhomogeneity*, *nonuniformity*, and *maldistribution*. Because these terms are generally considered synonymous, the term *heterogeneity* is used throughout this chapter. The modifier L (referring to the whole lung) is dropped; D means D_L unless specifically noted.

GAS EQUILIBRATION ACROSS ALVEOLAR-CAPILLARY MEMBRANE

Movement of gas between the alveolar gas phase and pulmonary capillary blood is thought to be a passive process governed by the simple laws of diffusion. Equilibration of gas in pulmonary capillary blood flowing past the alveolus and separated by a diffusion barrier is described by the homogeneous lung model shown in Figure 1. Over any increment of distance along the capillary, the flux of gas into the blood is defined by Fick's law of diffusion

$$d\dot{M} = dD_x(P_A - Pb) \quad (1)$$

where $d\dot{M}$ is the uptake of gas by blood in the infinitesimal capillary element dx, dD_x is the diffusing capacity of the element of diffusion barrier, and P_A and Pb are the partial pressures of the gas in the alveolus and in capillary blood. The flux of gas across the barrier increment creates an infinitesimal change in blood gas content (C) in the element

$$d\dot{M} = \dot{Q} \cdot dC = \dot{Q}\beta b \cdot dPb \quad (2)$$

where βb is the capacitance coefficient (effective solubility) of the gas in blood. Many investigators have used such basic principles to describe the equilibration

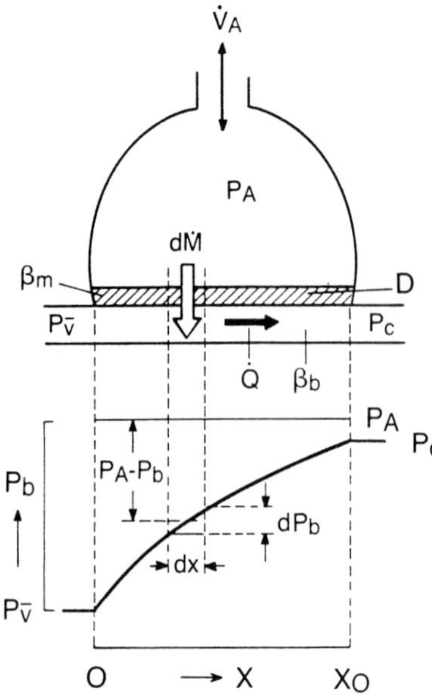

FIG. 1. Factors affecting equilibration of gas in pulmonary capillary of homogeneous lung. βb, Capacitance coefficient of blood; βm, capacitance coefficient of membrane; D, diffusing capacity; dṀ, differential transport rate of gas; dPb, differential partial pressure of gas in blood; dx, infinitesimal capillary element; PA, alveolar partial pressure; Pb, partial pressure of gas in blood; Pc, partial pressure of gas in capillary; Pv̄, partial pressure of mixed venous blood; Q̇, perfusion; V̇A, alveolar ventilation; O, X, and X_0, points along pulmonary capillary. [Adapted from Piiper and Scheid (65).]

kinetics across the alveolar-capillary membrane. Piiper and Scheid (64) have presented a useful summary approach. The equilibration between end-capillary blood and alveolar gas can be determined by combining Equations 1 and 2 (assuming D is distributed uniformly with respect to blood volume along the capillary) and integrating along the length of the capillary

$$(P_A - P_{c'})/(P_A - P_{\bar{v}}) = e^{-D/\dot{Q}\beta b} \quad (3)$$

where Pc′ is end-capillary partial pressure of gas, and Pv̄ is mixed venous partial pressure of gas.

The relative equilibration is directly dependent on the ratio D/Q̇βb, the balance between diffusing capacity and perfusion (Fig. 2). Piiper and Scheid (65) described a total mass-transfer conductance that can be divided into two components: a perfusion conductance (Gperf) and a diffusion conductance (Gdiff)

$$D/\dot{Q}\beta b = \text{Gdiff}/\text{Gperf} \quad (4)$$

Relative equilibration across the alveolar-capillary membrane depends on the Gdiff/Gperf ratio. The conductance ratio varies for different gases according to the physical properties of the gas in the diffusion membrane and in the blood. Diffusing capacity depends on the diffusion coefficient (*D*), the solubility of the gas in the membrane (βm), the area of the membrane (*A*), and its thickness (*h*)

$$D = D\beta m A/h \quad (5)$$

When the D/Q̇βb for two gases (1 and 2) are compared, factors describing anatomical relationships and blood flow cancel out

$$\frac{D_2/\dot{Q}\beta_2 b}{D_1/\dot{Q}\beta_1 b} = \frac{D_2(\beta m/\beta b)_2}{D_1(\beta m/\beta b)_1} \quad (6)$$

Relative equilibration of gas in the pulmonary capillary is strongly dependent on the βm/βb ratio. For example, gases that bind with hemoglobin (e.g., O_2 and CO) have a very small βm/βb compared with inert gases (e.g., N_2 and He), which have a βm/βb near unity. During conditions of hypoxia, the βm/βb of CO may be as low as 2.5×10^{-5} (65). Some inert gases (e.g., SF_6) are highly lipid soluble and have a βm/βb greater than unity. Less important is the diffusion coefficient for gases in tissue, which is approximately inversely proportional to the molecular weight of the gas [cf. Kawashiro et al. (36)]. Diffusion coefficients for very heavy gases, e.g., SF_6, and very light gases, e.g., H_2, may differ by a factor of 8. When both the diffusion coefficient and the βm/βb factors are considered together, it is evident that a gas such as CO has a small D/Q̇βb (a small Gdiff/Gperf ratio) and is usually diffusion limited in its exchange properties in the lung except when its partial pressure is increased over ~20 mmHg. Inert gases have a large D/Q̇βb (a large Gdiff/Gperf ratio) and are perfusion limited in the lung. Oxygen and CO_2 fall in between and may demonstrate both perfusion limitation and diffusion limitation.

REGIONAL DIFFUSING-CAPACITY HETEROGENEITY

The characteristics of a single alveolar region that is sufficiently small to result in uniformity have been

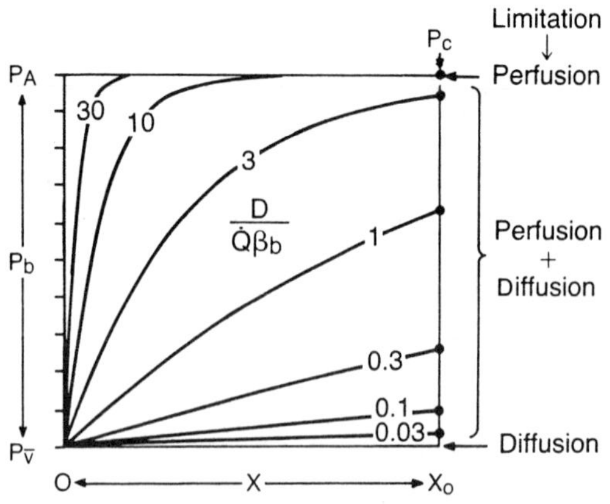

FIG. 2. Equilibration profiles for blood transiting pulmonary capillary for various values of diffusive conductance–to–perfusive conductance ratio. (D/Q̇βb). Partial pressure of gas is plotted as function of relative distance along pulmonary capillary. High values of D/Q̇β show perfusion limitation; low values show diffusion limitation. PA, alveolar partial pressure; Pb, partial pressure of gas in blood; Pc, partial pressure of gas in capillary; Pv̄, partial pressure of mixed venous blood; O, X, and X_0, points along pulmonary capillary. [Adapted from Piiper and Scheid (64).]

examined. However, lung perfusion has been shown to be dependent on gravity (95) as well as other intraregional stress factors. The higher perfusion pressure in the bottom of the lung results in greater recruitment of capillaries and therefore a larger capillary volume and capillary surface area for diffusion. In addition, large regional differences in lung volume and in alveolar ventilation are known to occur. Hamer (25) demonstrated, using the breath-hold technique, that overall D_{CO}, Dm, and capillary volume vary as a function of lung volume. Although these variations may result from several potential methodological limitations, they nevertheless suggest that there may be regional differences due to regional lung-volume differences. Morphologically it has been shown that there are local variations in membrane thickness (alveolar epithelium, basement membrane, and capillary endothelium) and in the diffusion distances within blood (90). This may result in significant local variations in diffusing capacity.

The significance of differences in distribution of alveolar ventilation to alveolar volume ($\dot{V}A/VA$) and in distribution of alveolar ventilation to perfusion ($\dot{V}A/\dot{Q}$) is described in the chapters by Anthonisen and Fleetham and by Farhi in this *Handbook.* Quantitation of the distribution of $\dot{V}A/\dot{Q}$ adequately describes the exchange of gases that are perfusion limited (large $D/\dot{Q}\beta b$ ratio). Inert gases fall into this category, but for gases that are either partially or completely diffusion limited (small $D/\dot{Q}\beta b$), such as CO or O_2 (in hypoxia), the heterogeneous distribution of diffusing capacity is also an important determinant of overall gas exchange.

Theoretical Considerations

In reviewing the Bohr integration approach to the analysis of pulmonary capillary O_2 equilibration, Visser and Maas (84) emphasized the importance of the balance between diffusing capacity and perfusion and suggested that $D/\dot{Q}$ heterogeneity in the lung must affect the partial pressure of O_2 in arterial blood (Pa_{O_2}). As a result, several model studies of the influence of $D/\dot{V}A$ or $D/\dot{Q}$ heterogeneity have been performed with the steady-state, single-breath, and rebreathing methods used to analyze the established measurement techniques for their sensitivity to heterogeneities.

STEADY-STATE METHOD. The influence of regional heterogeneity on calculation of values for both D_{O_2} and D_{CO} was assessed by Chinet et al. (9). The lung was divided into 15 parallel compartments with different $\dot{V}A/\dot{Q}$ ratios and with either $D/\dot{V}A$ or $D/\dot{Q}$ differing as well. An apparent diffusing capacity ("D"), as would be measured experimentally, was calculated and compared with the true diffusing capacity (D) for both O_2 and CO, resulting in the observation that the "D"/D ratio is smaller than unity for most cases. This indicates that the effect of regional heterogeneities on determination of diffusing capacity by the steady-state method results in an underestimation of true diffusing capacity (Fig. 3). This underestimation becomes progressively worse as the degree of heterogeneity (described as σ) is increased. The calculation of diffusing capacity by the ideal-alveolar-gas approach [estimating the partial pressure of alveolar CO (PA_{CO}) from the CO_2-determined physiological dead space] results in apparent diffusing-capacity values that deviate less from the true diffusing capacity than does the calculation of diffusing capacity by means of the average alveolar partial pressure. An important exception is that, under certain conditions, D_{CO} may be overestimated when the ideal-alveolar-gas approach is used. This is so apparently because of the higher blood-gas partition coefficient (λ) for CO than for CO_2 that results in a different venous admixture (due to $\dot{V}A/\dot{Q}$ heterogeneity) for CO than for CO_2 and an underestimation of PA_{CO_2}. The value of λ for O_2 is closer to that for CO_2, and the resulting venous admixtures of O_2 and CO_2 are closer than those of CO and CO_2. [For discussion of λ dependence of physiological dead space and venous admixture, see Hlastala and Robertson (30)].

SINGLE-BREATH METHOD. There are at least two types of heterogeneity that affect the single-breath D_{CO} method. Piiper and Sikand (66) have analyzed the influences of both D/VA and $\dot{V}A/VA$ heterogeneity. The importance of D/VA heterogeneity is depicted in Figure 4, which shows a lung with two compartments with different D/VA. The semilogarithmic plot of the alveolar CO fraction versus the length of breath-hold time is the sum of two exponentials with rate constants corresponding to the D/VA of the two compartments. When calculating diffusing capacity on the basis of a homogeneous lung model, the values of apparent diffusing capacity are obtained from the slope of the chord that extends from the initial point to any point on the overall lung curve, resulting in lower apparent diffusing-capacity values for longer breath-hold times. At the limit of zero breath-hold time, apparent diffusing capacity approaches true diffusing capacity; however, practical limitations prevent breath-hold times of less than ~5 s. Supporting data were obtained by Sikand and Piiper (77) in dogs. The first evidence of this type of curvilinear semilogarithmic decrease in PA_{CO_2} was demonstrated in 1954 by Forster et al. (20), who concluded that "a four-or-five-fold variation in D/VA throughout the lung is not unreasonable" and "is the most likely single cause of curvature of the plot of log F_{A_E} against time" (F_{A_E}, fractional concentration of expired alveolar gas). Similar data were obtained several years later in the same laboratory (78). Piiper and Sikand (66) also showed a similar decrease in apparent diffusing capacity given a theoretical heterogeneous distribution of $\dot{V}A/VA$ to regions of identical D/VA. The error, which could be corrected if VA were measured by an independent technique such as inert-gas washout, was attributed

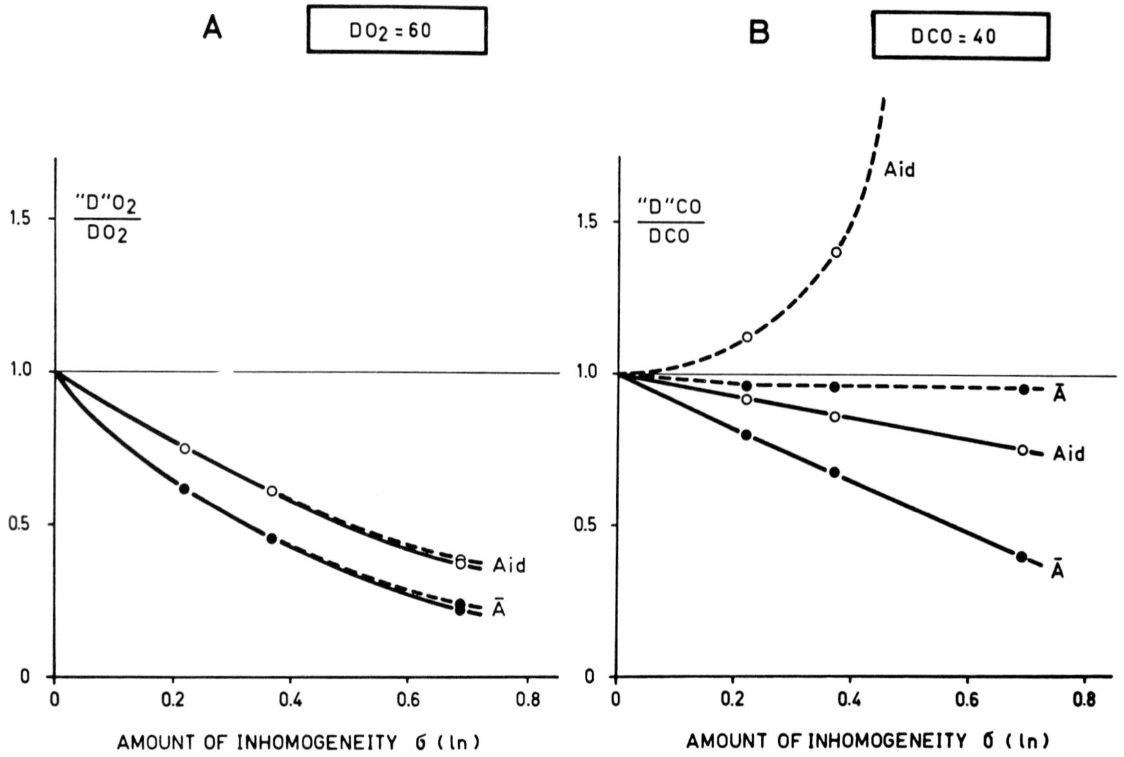

FIG. 3. Apparent diffusing capacity ("D") normalized by true diffusing capacity (D) for O_2 (*A*) and CO (*B*) plotted against relative heterogeneity (σ). ●, "D" calculated from average alveolar partial pressures ($\bar{A}$); ○, "D" calculated from ideal alveolar partial pressures (Aid); ——, D distributed in proportion to $\dot{Q}$; – – – –, D distributed according to $\dot{V}_A$. [Adapted from Chinet et al. (9).]

to inaccuracies in estimating V_A from the dilution of an indicator gas. The curved semilogarithmic plot of $P_{A_{CO_2}}$ versus breath-hold time might also be caused by back pressure of CO in blood.

REBREATHING METHOD. Rebreathing methods tend to equilibrate gas concentrations throughout the lung and minimize the effects of any regional heterogeneities in $\dot{V}_A$, $\dot{Q}$, D, or V_A that might be present. However, because of limitations in mixing during rebreathing, there is still a separation between the mixed rebreathing bag and the individual regions of the lung where the heterogeneities exist [as demonstrated by Scheid et al. (72)]. In all the cases of regional heterogeneity examined, the calculated apparent diffusing capacity underestimated true diffusing capacity. The authors concluded that the rebreathing and steady-state methods are similar in their degree of underestimating D_{O_2}.

The degree to which a diffusing-capacity measurement is diminished by heterogeneity depends on *1*) the type and magnitude of heterogeneity, *2*) the test method used, and *3*) the test gas used (O_2 or CO). Because gas transfer is independent of lung volume, V_A heterogeneity does not affect steady-state D_{O_2} or D_{CO}. Inasmuch as CO transfer is virtually exclusively diffusion limited, perfusion heterogeneity with respect to diffusing capacity has a minimal effect on D_{CO} in either the steady-state or non-steady-state methods. However, non-steady-state O_2 methods are influenced by all types of heterogeneity, and steady-state O_2 methods are sensitive primarily to perfusion heterogeneity.

Experimental Evidence for Diffusing-Capacity Heterogeneity

Distribution of $D/\dot{Q}$ was analyzed by Piiper (58), who showed that heterogeneity of $D/\dot{Q}$ increases the resulting alveolar-arterial O_2 difference ($P_{A_{O_2}} - Pa_{O_2}$). Moreover the functional relationship of $P_{A_{O_2}} - Pa_{O_2}$ versus $P_{A_{O_2}}$ varied with different $D/\dot{Q}$ distributions. At any $P_{A_{O_2}}$, $P_{A_{O_2}} - Pa_{O_2}$ increased with increasing $D/\dot{Q}$ heterogeneity. Supporting data were obtained in dogs (62). The $P_{A_{O_2}} - Pa_{O_2}$ increased from 6.0 Torr to 41.6 Torr, and the venous admixture decreased from 20.7% to 1.7% as $P_{A_{O_2}}$ increased from 45 Torr to 255 Torr. The authors were unable to explain the data with any fixed combination of $\dot{V}_A/\dot{Q}$ and pure shunt distribution; they concluded that the data could only be explained by invoking the presence of a heterogeneity in $D/\dot{Q}$. It was suggested that $D/\dot{Q}$ heterogeneity might be manifested both regionally and temporally (because of pulsatile pulmonary perfusion). This analysis was performed with the assumption that $\dot{V}_A/\dot{Q}$ distribution remains constant at different $P_{A_{O_2}}$, but it is now known that $\dot{Q}$ and $\dot{V}_A$ distributions are both

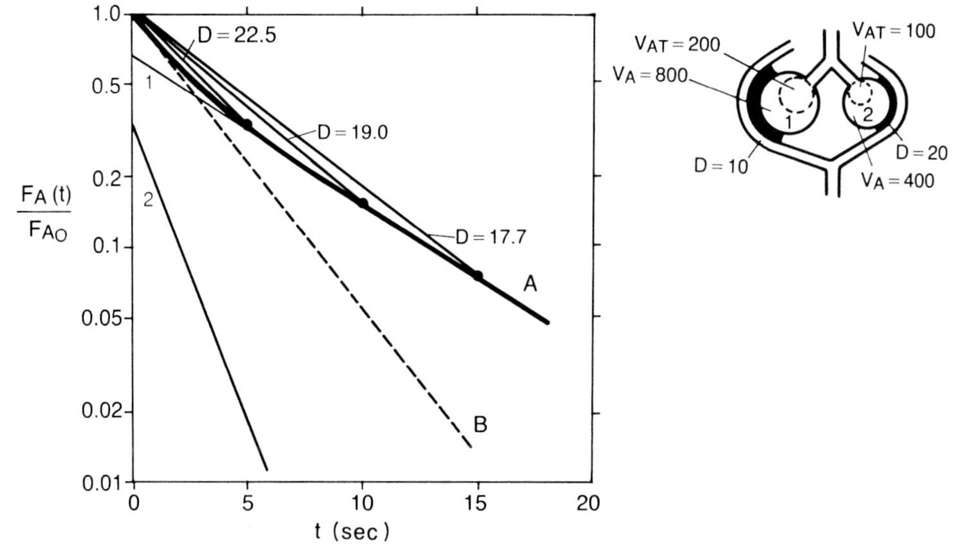

FIG. 4. *Curve A*, alveolar partial pressure vs. time (*t*) during a single-breath diffusing-capacity measurement (D) as function of breath-hold time with unequal distribution of diffusing capacity–to–alveolar volume ratio (D/V_A). *Lines 1* and *2*, CO profile for compartments 1 and 2. *Curve B*, homogeneous lung with same overall D. Measured D is determined from slope of chord between alveolar fraction at a specific time [$F_A(t)$] and original point F_{A_0}. V_{AT}, tidal alveolar ventilation. [From Piiper and Sikand (66).]

affected by the $P_{A_{O_2}}$, which invalidates the boundary conditions of the model used.

Lewis et al. (43) attempted to demonstrate an effect of $\dot{V}_A$ heterogeneity on diffusing capacity by utilizing the inherent differences between the steady-state and rebreathing methods. A methacholine-histamine aerosol of sufficient concentration to alter ventilation distribution was administered to normal subjects. Steady-state D_{CO} fell, whereas rebreathing D_{CO} remained unchanged. On the assumption that rebreathing methods tend to minimize apparent results of $\dot{V}_A$ distribution, it was reasoned that the decreased steady-state D_{CO} must have been due to a more heterogeneous $\dot{V}_A$ distribution.

Burrows et al. (6, 7) designed a method for determination of diffusing-capacity heterogeneity by analysis of the equilibration kinetics of He and CO during washout. The major disadvantages of this approach were that the mathematical solutions were nonunique and that a time-consuming graphic iterative method was required. Mittman (53) obtained additional data points by analyzing both the washin and washout curves for CO and for He. The mathematical approach also provided more flexibility, allowing for a range of derived diffusing-capacity values rather than specific, nonunique values. Results were always consistent with the presence of D/$\dot{V}_A$ heterogeneity. The washin-washout method was updated by Lewis et al. (44), who added three important improvements. *1*) Both mixed expired and end-tidal CO data were used for each breath. *2*) An improved mathematical transformation technique was used. *3*) In an attempt to better define behavior of the poorly ventilated spaces, equilibrated resident inert gas was used rather than an inspired, washed-in inert gas. The results again showed that diffusing capacity was always heterogeneously distributed. A major assumption of this technique, which is likely to limit precision, is that the two compartments determined for $\dot{V}_A$ distribution adequately describe diffusing-capacity distribution. This is unlikely to be true because different processes govern $\dot{V}_A$ and D distribution. However, this assumption will not invalidate the qualitative observation of diffusing-capacity heterogeneity. Another disadvantage of a washout approach is the requirement for steady-state behavior. Variability must occur in vivo with pulsatile blood flow and periodic ventilation, each of which is controlled independently.

An alternative method for measuring pulmonary diffusing capacity has been proposed by Newth et al. (56). This single-exhalation technique utilizes exhaled P_{CO} measured at the mouth as a function of time. The rationale is that, given a constant expired flow rate, the $P_{A_{O_2}}$-time function is the same as the mouth P_{CO}-time function. When this approach was used with normal subjects, the D_{CO} was calculated to be independent of lung volume, a finding that contrasts sharply with the volume dependence of D_{CO} determined by the single-breath method (25). The findings were unaffected by inhalation time, prior breath-holding time, or lung volume. However, D_{CO} did become slightly volume dependent in subjects in the prone position and with high rates of exhalation (situations that might be expected to alter $\dot{V}_A/V_A$ distribution). Indeed, slow exhalation may result in an overestimate of D_{CO} (18). Ventilation distribution is certainly disrupted in chronic obstructive lung disease, in which Newth et al. (56) found a marked reduction in D_{CO} as lung volume declined. However, during exhalation, gas is contributed from different lung regions to a variable extent (83) and the relative importance of each region changes as a function of several variables, including lung volume. Thus it is remarkable that the single-exhalation method shows a general volume independence. Perhaps sequential-ventilation heterogeneity superimposes on $D/\dot{V}_A$ or $D/\dot{Q}$ heterogeneity to yield apparent diffusing-capacity homogeneity. Cotton et al. (12) showed an apparent heterogeneity in $D/\dot{V}_A$ at very high and very low lung volumes due to exaggerated $\dot{V}_A/V_A$ heterogeneity in such extreme volumes. A recent theoretical study by Cotton and Graham (11) has shown that the single-exhalation method can be affected severely by diffusing-capacity heterogeneity. Theoretically, an advantage of the washout method (44) is that such effects of sequencing and $\dot{V}_A$ distribution may be discernible.

Part of the explanation for differences in D_{CO} values determined with such diverse techniques may be the difference in volume history of the lung. Cassidy et al. (8) used a modified breath-hold technique and concluded that the higher D_{CO} seen when a specific lung volume is reached by exhalation could be explained by a larger alveolar surface area (due to unfolding of pleats) than is achieved by inhalation to the same lung volume. Using morphological techniques, Weibel et al. (94) showed a folding of the alveolar surface that, at any given lung volume, depended on whether lung volume was increasing or decreasing. They demonstrated unfolding of pleats in the alveolar-capillary membrane during lung inflation that resulted in increased alveolar surface. Refolding of the membrane during exhalation did not occur until lower lung volumes were reached or until some time had elapsed. However, the physiological measurements of Cassidy et al. (8) may be affected by a very different distribution of inspired CO under the two conditions. It is possible that full inspiration provides a more uniform distribution of inspired CO or, in other words, a more homogeneous $D/\dot{V}_A$ and a more uniform distribution of $P_{A_{CO}}$. This possibility was discounted by Rose et al. (69) on the assumption that the rebreathing technique minimizes the effect of heterogeneities. As noted earlier, this may not be an appropriate assumption (72).

Differential Effect of Diffusing-Capacity Heterogeneity on O_2 and CO Transfer

Heterogeneity of $D/\dot{Q}$ has different effects on O_2 and on CO by virtue of the different $D/\dot{Q}\beta b$ ratios. The analysis of Piiper and Scheid (64) in Figure 2 shows that the relative equilibration is a nonlinear function of $D/\dot{Q}\beta b$. However, for a diffusion-limited gas such as CO, relative end-capillary disequilibrium is nearly linearly related to $D/\dot{Q}\beta b$. In the presence of $D/\dot{Q}\beta b$ heterogeneity, the CO content of mean end-capillary blood will closely reflect the mean $D/\dot{Q}\beta b$. For typical $D/\dot{Q}\beta b$ ratios encountered in vivo, O_2 is usually completely equilibrated. An increase in $D/\dot{Q}\beta b$ will result in no change in end-capillary O_2 content, but a reduced $D/\dot{Q}\beta b$ may be sufficient to reduce end-capillary O_2 content. Relative end-capillary disequilibrium for O_2 is nonlinearly related to $D/\dot{Q}\beta b$. Therefore the mean end-capillary blood may have a lower O_2 content than would correspond to the mean $D/\dot{Q}\beta b$, and the result would be an apparent reduction in diffusing capacity caused by $D/\dot{Q}\beta b$ heterogeneity. Using the breath-hold technique, Hyde et al. (34) capitalized on this idea by measuring D_{CO} and D_{O_2} simultaneously. To measure O_2 uptake in an analogous manner with CO uptake, a stable O_2 isotope ($^{34}O_2$) was used. Because $D/\dot{Q}$ heterogeneity affects D_{O_2} but not D_{CO}, estimated *true* D_{O_2} was calculated from measured D_{CO}. The discrepancy between true D_{O_2} and measured D_{O_2} was used to indicate the relative importance of $D/\dot{Q}$ heterogeneity. The average measured D_{O_2} was 58% of the average true D_{O_2}, indicating a considerable degree of uneven $D/\dot{Q}$ distribution in normal subjects. The major drawback of this approach, however, is the number of potential errors in measuring both D_{O_2} and D_{CO}. In a similar study in dogs, Savoy et al. (71) concluded that the discrepancy between D_{O_2} and D_{CO} was primarily due to heterogeneities in both $D/\dot{V}_A$ and $D/\dot{Q}$. These authors also pointed out that considerable uncertainty is added by the lack of detailed data on the interaction of O_2 and CO with hemoglobin.

The relative nonlinearity of gas equilibrium as a function of $D/\dot{Q}$ was further utilized by Hyde et al. (33), using two different inspired CO concentrations: 0.2% and 4.0%. The end-capillary CO content is nearly linearly related to $D/\dot{Q}$ in the normal range for a fractional inspired CO ($F_{I_{CO}}$) of 0.2%. Therefore measured D_{CO} is not affected by $D/\dot{Q}$ heterogeneity with $F_{I_{CO}} = 0.2\%$. However, when inspired CO is increased to 4%, end-capillary CO content becomes nonlinearly related to $D/\dot{Q}$ because enough CO is taken up in the pulmonary capillary to reach the nonlinear portion of the carboxyhemoglobin dissociation curve. Therefore end-capillary CO content will be nonlinearly related to $D/\dot{Q}\beta b$ and measured D_{CO} will be affected by $D/\dot{Q}$ heterogeneity with $F_{I_{CO}} = 4.0\%$. In supine normal subjects, analysis of the data suggested that 19% of the perfusion was distributed to a region with 50% of the diffusing capacity. In seated normal subjects, 25% of the perfusion was distributed to a region with 50% of the diffusing capacity. Because the relative heterogeneity changed very little with the change in position, the authors concluded that the cause of the uneven $D/\dot{Q}$ was not related to gravitational forces but had to be a manifestation of intraregional (local) heterogeneity in perfusion (and therefore $D/\dot{Q}$) distribution.

The differential effect of diffusing-capacity heterogeneity on D_{CO} and D_{O_2} was used by both Cross et al. (13) and Gong et al. (23) to explain the changes in D_{O_2} and D_{CO} occurring with exercise. These authors used a modified single-exhalation method to measure simultaneously $\dot{Q}$, D_{CO}, and D_{O_2}. When subjects changed from rest to moderate exercise, the cardiac output nearly doubled from 6.9 to 12.9 liters·min^{-1}, D_{O_2} increased from 24 to 43 ml·min^{-1}·$mmHg^{-1}$, but the D_{CO} only increased slightly (from 45 to 49 ml·min^{-1}·$mmHg^{-1}$). It was concluded that the rise in D_{O_2} during exercise was due to a more homogeneous $D/\dot{Q}$ distribution within the individual gas-exchange units.

Exercise

Measured values for diffusing capacity increase with exercise. The question of whether diffusing capacity rises steadily with severity of exercise or ultimately reaches a plateau has important implications with regard to the mechanism of the increase, but insufficient data have been obtained to answer this question. The rise in diffusing capacity during exercise is thought to be caused by an increase in diffusion area due to *1)* an increase in the diameter of capillary vessels caused by increased transmural pressure and *2)* recruitment of capillaries not perfused during rest. However, two other mechanisms leading to an increase in apparent diffusing capacity (with constant true D) may also play a role: *1)* functional heterogeneity of diffusing capacity may be decreased at exercise, resulting in a greater underestimation of true diffusing capacity at rest, and *2)* the effects of heterogeneity on the measurement of steady-state D_{O_2} are reduced at higher O_2 uptake despite a constant degree of heterogeneity.

Heterogeneity of $D/\dot{V}_A$ and $D/\dot{Q}$ was analyzed by Johnson and Miller (35, 52), who measured D_{CO} at different lung volumes and at varying levels of exercise using the previously described method of Lilienthal et al. (45). They analyzed the distribution of $D/\dot{Q}$ in terms of variation in $D/\dot{Q}\beta b$. It was concluded that normal subjects exhibit a marked heterogeneity of $D/\dot{Q}$ at rest and that this heterogeneity improves with exercise. As described earlier, this conclusion was supported by Cross et al. (13). Johnson and Miller also concluded that ventilation may be unevenly distributed with respect to capillary surface area but that this needs to improve to explain the sharp increase in measured D_{O_2} from rest to exercise. Gurtner and Fowler (24) obtained similar data showing an increase in D_{CO} with exercise and concluded that this increase was due to an improvement in D/V_A distribution resulting from recruitment of capillaries.

In a theoretical study of the increase in apparent diffusion capacity of O_2 with exercise, Piiper (60) showed that $D/\dot{Q}$ heterogeneity results in an apparent diffusing capacity that is much lower than the true diffusing capacity. The relative difference between apparent diffusing capacity and true diffusing capacity decreases as O_2 uptake increases. It was concluded that a rise in D_{O_2} occurring with increases in O_2 uptake may reflect the presence of $D/\dot{Q}$ heterogeneity rather than an actual rise in diffusing capacity. This theoretical construct was supported by experimental findings from the same laboratory (41, 63). Later, using a rebreathing technique, Meyer et al. (50) found an increase in D_{CO} in parallel with an increase in D_{O_2} with exercise. It was concluded that functional diffusing-capacity heterogeneity may play a smaller role than other factors, such as hemoglobin reaction-rate limitation, in limiting O_2 and CO exchange. However, use of the rebreathing technique limited sensitivity to diffusing-capacity heterogeneity.

Pulmonary Capillary Transit Time

There is evidence for heterogeneous perfusion distribution and heterogeneous pulmonary capillary transit-time distribution within individual gas-exchange units that are small enough for effective gas-phase diffusional equilibrium. Wagner et al. (89) have observed a heterogeneity of perfusion within the individual rat lung lobule with greater perfusion in the proximal region than in the peripheral region. Because perfusion is equal to capillary volume divided by transit time, a heterogeneous distribution of $D/\dot{Q}$ implies a heterogeneous distribution of transit time if diffusing capacity is related to capillary volume. Heterogeneity in pulmonary transit time has been found by Wagner et al. (92) and Knopp and Bassingthwaighte (40) using different preparations. This implies, but does not prove, the presence of $D/\dot{Q}$ heterogeneity. The capillary network around the alveolus has been examined and found to be diffuse and heterogeneous (87, 93). Although the overall distribution of lung capillary filling may be governed largely by vertical, gravitational factors (95), the capillaries are still sensitive to local factors. Within a given horizontal plane, there is a significant heterogeneity in capillary length (93). Even within a single alveolus, the distance traveled by a red cell in transiting the alveolus may vary considerably. Transit times varying between 0.79 s and 1.78 s have been measured in a single lung (within a 9-cm distance) (32). A different study estimated pulmonary capillary transit times ranging between 0.35 s and 1.7 s (79). This anatomical evidence suggests that a considerable heterogeneity in $D/\dot{Q}$ should be expected on the basis of a heterogeneity in red cell transit time.

Another source of $D/\dot{Q}$ heterogeneity is the time-dependent pulsation in pulmonary perfusion. Using a sensitive, water-filled plethysmograph, Menkes et al. (49) showed distinct pulsations in the uptake of CO from the alveolar gas that were due to changes in pulmonary capillary blood volume during the cardiac cycle. Although the gas-exchange significance of these pulsations would be lessened by the fact that the average pulmonary capillary transit time is about the same as the cardiac period (3, 27), there may still be a time-dependent heterogeneity in $D/\dot{Q}$ due to pulsatile perfusion that may vary from region to region.

Vertical Distribution of Diffusing Capacity

One potential explanation for diffusing-capacity heterogeneity is the vertical distribution of perfusion caused by gravity. The first attempt to quantitate this vertical distribution in diffusing capacity was made in 1960 by Dollery et al. (15), who used ^{15}O-labeled CO. Regional anatomic distribution of CO uptake was determined with external counters. In normal subjects at rest, a vertical gradient in D/V_A was found with the highest values in the base of the lung, whereas during exercise the vertical distribution of D/V_A became more uniform. It was concluded that the improvement in D/V_A heterogeneity was a direct result of an improvement in vertical perfusion distribution. Increased perfusion to the upper zones resulted in capillary recruitment and hence increased upper-zone diffusing capacity. West et al. (96) also reported that clearance rates of inhaled radioactive CO were faster from the lung base than from the apex but were dependent on both regional blood flow and $D/\dot{V}_A$, leading to uncertainty in the interpretation of radioactive CO data.

Supporting evidence for a vertical distribution of diffusing capacity has also been obtained by bolus techniques. Because the distribution of inspired gas is dependent on lung volume and inspiratory flow rate, injection of a CO and acetylene bolus at the mouth at different times during inspiration changes the distribution of the CO and acetylene. Michaelson et al. (51) constructed a lung model to determine the D/V_A and $\dot{Q}/V_A$ distribution that came closest to predicting their actual data. Because of a limitation in the number of gases, the authors were restricted to the assumption of linear vertical gradients. They found a steep gradient in $\dot{Q}/V_A$, increasing from apex to base, and a similar (but less steep) gradient in D/V_A. Therefore a vertical gradient in $D/\dot{Q}$ was found. The authors concluded that the relative degree of vertical unevenness of D/V_A compared with $\dot{Q}/V_A$ could account only in part for previous observations attributed to heterogeneity of $D/\dot{V}_A$ and $D/\dot{Q}$. Therefore a more generalized unevenness of $D/\dot{V}_A$ and $D/\dot{Q}$ must exist throughout the lung, independent of gravity. This may be due to a variation in pulmonary capillary transit time, or it may be due to a gradient of perfusion from the center to the periphery of the secondary lobule at a specific vertical level (68, 89).

Using the single-exhalation technique, Denison et al. (14) inserted a fiberoptic bronchoscope into lobar bronchi to measure regional $\dot{V}_A/V_A$, D_{CO}/V_A, and $\dot{Q}/V_A$ within each lobe of normal human subjects. Care was taken to minimize perturbation of the measurements due to the presence of the bronchoscope by staying within large airways and by keeping the mass spectrometer sampling rate small compared with the regional exhaled flow rate. Vertical gradients for $\dot{V}_A/V_A$, $\dot{Q}/V_A$, and D/V_A were found in the lateral decubitus (both left and right) and the sitting positions. The magnitude of the vertical difference was greatest for $\dot{Q}/V_A$ and smallest for $\dot{V}_A/V_A$ (Fig. 5). Because the vertical gradients for D/V_A and $\dot{Q}/V_A$ were different, there must also have been a vertical gradient in $D/\dot{Q}$ (highest in the lower lobes), although this ratio was not calculated. These data show a specific anatomical distribution of diffusing capacity, which is related to gravitational factors. This observation in normal lungs sharply contrasts with the apparent homogeneity of diffusing capacity observed with the single-exhalation technique (56).

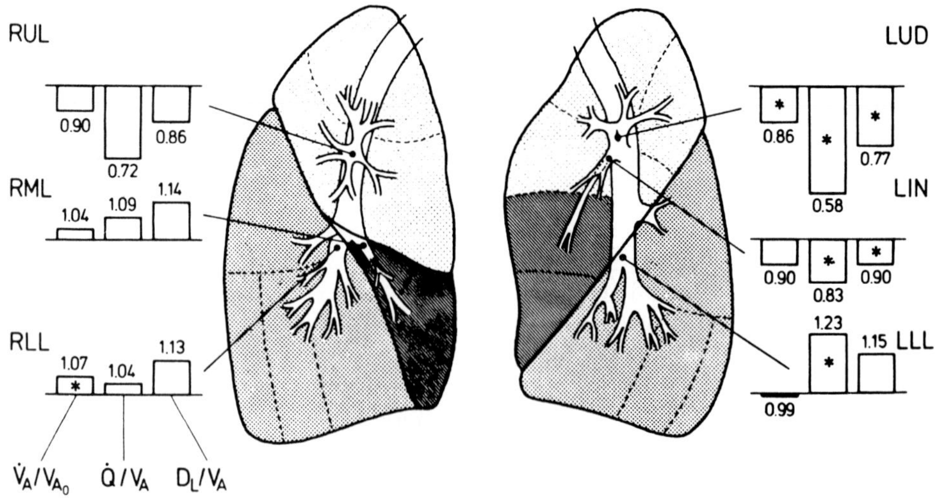

FIG. 5. Average results for relative alveolar ventilation-to-alveolar volume ratio ($\dot{V}_A/V_{A_0}$), perfusion-to-alveolar volume ratio ($\dot{Q}/V_A$), and pulmonary diffusing capacity-to-alveolar volume ratio (D_L/V_A) obtained from lobar bronchi in seated humans. Values are expressed relative to value obtained for whole lung. RUL, right upper lobe; RML, right middle lobe; RLL, right lower lobe; LUD, left upper bronchial division; LIN, lingula; LLL, left lower lobe; *, significant difference at 5% level of confidence compared to value for whole lung. [From Denison et al. (14).]

Carrier-Gas Density

An important observation was made by Kvale, Davis, and Schroter (42). When the steady-state method was used in normal human subjects, the D_{CO} increased with increasing carrier-gas density at any ventilation. This is in direct contrast to an earlier study by Nairn et al. (54), who found no density dependence of the single-breath D_{CO}, and to the initial working hypothesis of the authors in establishing the experimental protocol. They expected that the D_{CO} would be highest in the He (low-density) environment because of faster gas-phase diffusion. It was concluded that the results could best be explained by Taylor diffusion, although the importance of this phenomenon has been substantially discounted (74). Altered gas density might affect ventilation distribution (98), but this possibility now seems unlikely also (10). An alternative explanation can be proposed for the findings of Kvale et al. (42) based on the calculations of Paiva and Engel (57), who showed that inspired gas (such as CO) may be distributed differently from overall alveolar ventilation by virtue of the interaction between convection and diffusion in the airways. This mechanism suggests that with SF_6 (high-density gas), inspired CO may be distributed more homogeneously with respect to diffusing capacity, which would result in a more homogeneous, effective $D/\dot{V}_A$ and thus a higher measured apparent D_{CO}. This possibility is supported by the calculations of Chinet et al. (9), who showed that, for CO, $D/\dot{V}_A$ heterogeneity has a greater effect on apparent D_{CO} than on $D/\dot{Q}$ heterogeneity.

Magnussen (48) measured the single-breath D_{CO} with background gases of He or SF_6 separately. In patients with asthma both the He D_{CO} and SF_6 D_{CO} decreased with breath-hold time, which is consistent with the presence of D/V_A and/or $\dot{V}_A/V_A$ heterogeneity. In patients with emphysema, He D_{CO} decreased and SF_6 D_{CO} increased with increasing breath-hold time. It was concluded that these very different findings could be explained by a dominance of parallel heterogeneity in asthma but a dominance of series heterogeneity in emphysema. The mechanisms involved in this approach need clarification.

Comparison of Physiological and Morphological Measurements of Diffusing Capacity

Diffusing-capacity heterogeneity has the basic property of altering measured apparent diffusing capacity compared with true diffusing capacity. A resulting dilemma is that it becomes difficult to correlate measurements of diffusing capacity made by different methods. A morphometric estimation of human lung diffusing capacity has been presented by Gehr et al. (21). The maximum possible D_{O_2} of 263 $ml \cdot min^{-1} \cdot Torr^{-1}$ and a minimum D_{O_2} of 125 $ml \cdot min^{-1} \cdot Torr^{-1}$ were estimated. These values are higher than the range of normal resting D_{O_2} of 20–30 $ml \cdot min^{-1} \cdot Torr^{-1}$. However, the estimated D_{O_2} corresponds to the totally inflated and unfolded lung. Correction for the available area in vivo for gas exchange yields estimated D_{O_2} values of between 61 and 190 $ml \cdot min^{-1} \cdot Torr^{-1}$, which are closer to physiological measurements of D_{O_2} in exercise.

Part of the difference between morphometric and physiological measurements of diffusing capacity can be explained by diffusing-capacity heterogeneity. Geiser et al. (22) used a log-normal distribution pattern for both $\dot{V}_A/\dot{Q}$ and diffusing capacity and showed that correction for diffusing-capacity heterogeneity results in an estimated diffusing capacity of about twice the value obtained by the classic steady-state method. This relative value depends on the specific type of diffusing-capacity heterogeneity assumed by Geiser et al., who point out that the resulting estimate would be increased to a value much nearer (within 50%) the morphometric measurements (93).

An approach to the measurement of Dm by physiological means was developed by Burns and Shepard (5), who perfused isolated lungs with blood containing sodium dithionite, which rapidly binds with O_2 so that the blood P_{O_2} is always near zero. Therefore the complexities of hemoglobin-O_2 interaction are eliminated. The rebreathing technique decreases but does not eliminate the influence of $D/\dot{V}_A$ heterogeneity (72). Membrane D_{O_2} (Dm_{O_2}) was found to be in the range of 6–43 $ml \cdot min^{-1} \cdot Torr^{-1}$ for the left lower lobe of the dog. This value corresponds more closely to the dog D_{O_2} that was morphologically estimated by Siegwart et al. (76), suggesting that lower physiological measurements may be due to the presence of $D/\dot{V}_A$ and $D/\dot{Q}$ heterogeneity.

INTERACTION OF VENTILATION-PERFUSION HETEROGENEITY WITH DIFFUSING-CAPACITY HETEROGENEITY

A major step in the understanding of diffusing-capacity heterogeneity came with the realization that both $\dot{V}_A/\dot{Q}$ distribution and diffusing-capacity distribution interact to determine the exchange of O_2 and CO (as well as other gases). Piiper (59) first showed that $\dot{V}_A/\dot{Q}$ distribution and $D/\dot{Q}$ distribution interact to influence arterial oxygenation. The effects are not independent and are not additive. Piiper suggested that the same two factors would influence CO_2 exchange as well as O_2 exchange and that it might be possible to separate the two mechanisms.

A significant effort at integrating $\dot{V}_A/\dot{Q}$ heterogeneity with diffusing-capacity heterogeneity was made by Briscoe and colleagues. King and Briscoe (37, 38) described a graphic method using Bohr integral isopleths and $\dot{V}_A/\dot{Q}$ isopleths superimposed on the O_2 dissociation curve. The lung was divided into two finite $\dot{V}_A/\dot{Q}$ compartments (a fast space and a slow space) based on N_2 washout. When 100% O_2 is breathed, the Pa_{O_2} tension is used to determine shunt.

Dead-space volume, $\dot{V}_A$, $\dot{Q}$, and D are determined in the fast and slow spaces from arterial blood gases measured at three different inspired O_2 fractions (21%, 24%, and 30%). A sequence of papers was published describing the distributions obtained in various respiratory diseases (2, 4, 26, 39). Unfortunately several assumptions incorporated in this approach produce significant errors. The O_2 dissociation curve was taken to be a linear function with no Bohr effect; this can have a major influence on derived capillary O_2 profiles (28). Because pulmonary capillary O_2 equilibration is virtually complete except for very low $D/\dot{Q}$, the calculated diffusing capacity is extremely sensitive to experimental error in Pa_{O_2}. Moreover changes in inspired P_{O_2} almost certainly result in changes in $\dot{V}_A$ and $\dot{Q}$ distribution, thus negating the steady-state assumption.

A separate attempt to interrelate the influence of several types of heterogeneity was published by Thews and Vogel (81, 85). After a steady state was reached breathing a gas containing 0% CO_2, 12% O_2, and 30% He, the breathing mixture was changed to 4.8% CO_2, 16% O_2, and 0% He. Helium washout was used to obtain the distribution of $\dot{V}_A/V_A$ into four separate compartments. By combining He washout with CO_2 washin, the $\dot{V}_A/\dot{Q}$ was obtained for each compartment. Because O_2 washin deviated from CO_2 washin only by diffusion limitation, the diffusing capacity for each compartment was obtained from the difference in time constants between the washin of O_2 and of CO_2. This method has been applied to analyze data in three cases (75, 80, 86). Although in principle the method offers a useful approach, it suffers from several limitations. One is the assumption of steady-state behavior, which is unlikely with the administration of 5% CO_2 (particularly during hypoxia). Another is the assumption of linear O_2 and CO_2 dissociation curves when the inspired O_2 fraction was increased from 12% to 16%. Furthermore the analysis assumes constancy of mixed venous P_{O_2} and P_{CO_2} for ~1 min after the change, but recirculation occurs after 15 s. Perhaps the most significant drawback is the sensitivity of the derived values to small errors in measurement.

SOLUBILITY DEPENDENCE OF GAS EXCHANGE

Inert gases exhibit a distinct advantage for analysis of $\dot{V}_A/\dot{Q}$ heterogeneity because their $\beta m/\beta b$ approaches unity and minimizes diffusion limitation in the alveolar-capillary membrane. When an inert gas in physical solution in the venous blood is delivered to the lung, the relative elimination of gas is dependent on the λ of the gas, $\dot{V}_A$, and $\dot{Q}$ (16). For any gas, as λ increases, the retention of the gas increases; as the $\dot{V}_A/\dot{Q}$ ratio increases, the relative retention decreases, as the $\dot{V}_A/\dot{Q}$ ratio approaches λ the relative sensitivity of the gas retention to $\dot{V}_A/\dot{Q}$ increases.

The relationship between retention and solubility was extended by Farhi and Yokoyama (17, 99), who used two gases to analyze the lung as a two-compartment system. Theoretically the most sensitive approach to analyzing the $\dot{V}_A/\dot{Q}$ distribution of the lung would be to examine the elimination characteristics of an infinite number of gases with λ spread across the entire scale from zero to infinity. However, availability of gases and practical limitations in analysis prevent such an approach. A realistic compromise approach has been developed by Wagner et al. (90), who used six inert gases that are spread across the solubility scale in order to be sensitive to the range of physiological $\dot{V}_A/\dot{Q}$ units that exist in the lung, both in health and in disease. This multiple–inert-gas–elimination technique involves the infusion of SF_6, ethane, cyclopropane, halothane, diethyl ether, and acetone and the subsequent analysis of the concentrations of these gases in mixed venous blood, arterial blood, and mixed expired gas. Using knowledge of the relative retention and excretion of these six gases, one can determine the general pattern of the $\dot{V}_A/\dot{Q}$ distribution in the lung. An alternative approach is to consider the lung in terms of a transformer of the partial pressure of mixed venous inert gas into specific excretion and retention values. If one knows the excretion and retention of each of the six gases, then it is possible to predict the behavior of any other gas of known finite λ (30, 55, 97).

The multiple–inert-gas analysis is based on three important assumptions: *1*) gas exchange is in a steady-state mode, *2*) alveolar gas is in diffusion equilibrium with end-capillary blood, and *3*) different lung compartments interact independently in a parallel fashion. These assumptions are not completely valid but are used for simplicity of analysis. Steady-state behavior is often assumed despite the inherent periodicity of respiration. Parallel and independent behavior of lung units is not an unusual assumption in a physiological analysis in which "as-if" behavior is considered. However, diffusion equilibrium of alveolar gas and end-capillary blood may not be a uniformly valid assumption. The following sections present a basic format for analyzing the interactive influences of $\dot{V}_A/\dot{Q}$ heterogeneity and diffusing-capacity heterogeneity.

MOLECULAR-WEIGHT DEPENDENCE OF GAS EXCHANGE

The classic assumption of diffusion equilibrium between alveolar gas and end-capillary blood has been questioned on several occasions. There are two potential regions of diffusion disequilibrium: the gas phase and the alveolar-capillary membrane. There has been little doubt that, except for extremely low Dm, inert gases always equilibrate across the alveolar-capillary membrane (19, 88). However, diffusion equilibrium in the gas phase is more controversial. Early on, Rauwerda (67) initiated the controversy with his excellent thesis evaluating the soluble–inert-gas–rebreathing technique for measuring cardiac output. In this comprehensive thesis he considered the influence of gas-phase heterogeneity within the lung and concluded that inspired gas quickly mixes and equilibrates with alveolar gas within the period of one breath. Since these early calculations, several investigators have confirmed theoretically the basic finding of gas-phase diffusion equilibrium [for review, see Scheid and Piiper (74)]. However, experimental evidence has now been obtained indicating that gases of different molecular weights equilibrate at different rates in the gas phase. Such experiments involve examination of the expired plateau of two gases of different molecular weights after a single inspiration or during washout of gases previously equilibrated within the lung. These studies were summarized by Scheid and Piiper (74), who concluded that the diffusion-dependent disequilibrium can be explained by stratified inhomogeneity (gas-phase diffusion disequilibrium within the alveolar region).

An alternative explanation for gas-phase diffusion-dependent disequilibrium has been presented by Paiva and Engel (57) and by Luijendijk et al. (47). By modeling the interaction between convection and diffusion in the airways, they were able to simulate the molecular-weight–dependent disequilibrium without invoking the presence of stratified inhomogeneity. This theoretical construct may provide a potential explanation for the discrepancy between the theoretical diffusion calculations and the experimental findings. These two mechanisms are not mutually exclusive; it may be that diffusion-dependent heterogeneity exists both in the airways and at the alveolar level.

Diffusion-dependent heterogeneity means that the gas phase exhibits characteristics that would retard the exchange of gas in the lung to a degree that is dependent on the molecular weight of that gas. Graham's law states that the average velocity (and ability to diffuse) is proportional to the inverse of the square root of the molecular weight. Inert-gas elimination would then be dependent on molecular weight as well as λ. The theory describing the interactive influence of these two parameters has been elaborated on by Scheid et al. (73), who concluded that gas-phase diffusion limitation is more important for gases with high λ and the decrement in gas exchange is more apparent in the excretion of the gas. The authors also described the relative importance of gas-phase diffusion limitation on recovery of data from a multiple–inert-gas–elimination technique (31). Discrepancies were seen in recovered distributions after moderate degrees of diffusion limitation.

Evidence supporting the existence of a measurable gas-phase diffusion limitation has been observed in only one study that involves elimination of the usual six trace inert gases. Truog et al. (82) showed a significant retardation of elimination of the high-molecular-weight gases in rats; these data were used to calculate an effective gas-phase diffusing capacity (31). Evidence of molecular-weight dependence has not been observed in the studies of Wagner and West (91), but the multiple–inert-gas–elimination technique is relatively insensitive to detection of gas-phase diffusion limitation because the gases are spread out on the solubility scale. Any molecular-weight dependence of excretion and retention can usually be modeled as $\dot{V}A/\dot{Q}$ heterogeneity in the presence of experimental error because, in normal lungs, molecular-weight dependence is relatively small compared with the effects of $\dot{V}A/\dot{Q}$ heterogeneity.

A far more sensitive approach to evaluating gas-phase diffusion limitation is to examine the elimination characteristics of gases with similar λ but widely varied molecular weights. Gases of similar solubility should have identical retention and excretion regardless of $\dot{V}A/\dot{Q}$ heterogeneity if gas-phase diffusion limitation is negligible. When acetylene and Freon 22 (2 gases with virtually identical solubility) have been used in dogs, a molecular-weight dependence of gas elimination has been shown (29), substantiating the earlier preliminary findings of Adaro and Farhi (1). The equivalent gas-phase diffusing capacity ($D'/\beta g\dot{V}A$) calculated at 5.05 accounted for ~2.5 Torr of the $PA_{O_2} - Pa_{O_2}$ in that study. Gas-phase diffusion resistance was greater with the administration of positive end-expiratory pressure, presumably because of the higher lung volumes and greater diffusion distances between mean alveolar gas and the alveolar-capillary membrane.

COMBINED SOLUBILITY AND MOLECULAR-WEIGHT DEPENDENCE

In addition to the well-described distribution of $\dot{V}A/\dot{Q}$ in the lung, one must also consider a distribution of gas-phase diffusing capacity as well as a distribution of alveolar-capillary Dm. Consider a series three-compartment model with steady-state gas exchange (Fig. 6). The proximal alveolar compartment (A) is constantly and continuously ventilated. The unventilated distal alveolar compartment (A′) exchanges gas with compartment A by diffusion through an alveolar gas-diffusion barrier (with diffusive conductance D′) and exchanges gas with the blood by diffusion through an alveolar-capillary membrane diffusion barrier (with diffusive conductance D). The alveolus is perfused with constant blood flow ($\dot{Q}$). A test gas is infused into venous blood so that mixed venous partial pressure ($P\bar{v}$) is constant, and the gas is eliminated through the lung.

Gas transport between compartment A and the environment (I) is described by the relationship

$$\dot{M} = \beta g\dot{V}A(PA - PI) \qquad (7)$$

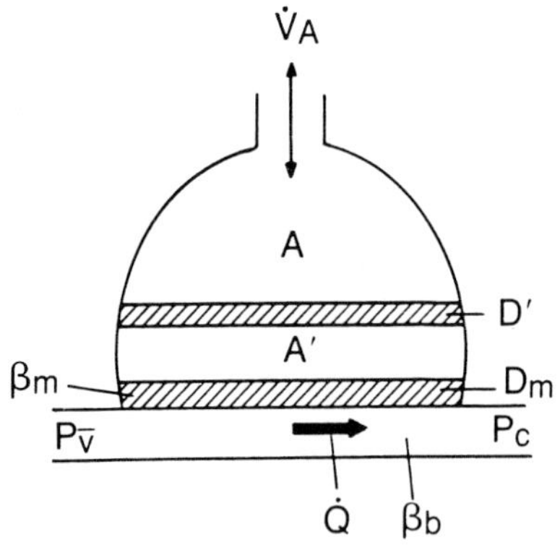

FIG. 6. Diffusion limitation model of homogeneous lung with alveolar ventilation (V̇A) and perfusion (Q̇). Alveolar compartment A exchanges gas by convection to outside and by diffusion with compartment A′ through gas-phase diffusive conductance (D′). Compartment A′ also exchanges gas with blood by diffusion through alveolar-capillary membrane diffusion conductance (Dm). βb, Effective solubility of blood; βm, solubility of gas in membrane; Pc, partial pressure of gas in the capillary; Pv̄, partial pressure of mixed venous blood.

where Ṁ is the transport rate of gas; βg is the capacitance coefficient of the gas in the gas phase [for all ideal gases, equal to 1.16 ml (STPD)·liter^{-1} (BTPS)·Torr^{-1} at 37°C; see ref. 62]; PA is the partial pressure of alveolar gas in compartment A; and PI is the partial pressure of inspired gas.

Diffusional exchange between the alveolar gas compartments A and A′ occurs according to Fick's law of diffusion

$$\dot{M} = D'(P_{A'} - P_A) \tag{8}$$

The diffusive conductance is proportional to the diffusion constant of the gas in the gaseous medium, is specific for the gas species, and depends on the composition of the gaseous medium and on the total gas pressure.

Gas transport by blood depends on blood flow and the solubility of gas in the blood

$$\dot{M} = \dot{Q}\beta b(P\bar{v} - Pc') \tag{9}$$

Equilibration between the blood and compartment A′ is a diffusive process through the alveolar-capillary membrane diffusive conductance and is governed by Fick's law of diffusion

$$\dot{M} = Dm(P_A - Pb) \tag{10}$$

Integration of Equation 10 across the length of the pulmonary capillary, as performed for Equation 2 earlier, yields

$$(P\bar{v} - Pc')/(P\bar{v} - P_{A'}) = 1 - e^{-Dm/\dot{Q}\beta b} \tag{11}$$

Substitution of Equation 11 into Equation 9 yields

$$\dot{M} = \dot{Q}\beta b(P\bar{v} - P_{A'})(1 - e^{-Dm/\dot{Q}\beta b}) \tag{12}$$

Equations 7, 8, and 12 describe gas transport through three serial interfaces of the lung. In the steady state, all three transport rates must be equal. Combining Equations 7, 8, and 12 and using the identity $\lambda = \beta g/\beta b$, the unknowns Ṁ and PA′ can be eliminated to yield equations describing the excretion (E = PA/Pv̄) and retention (R = Pa/Pv̄) of inert gas

$$R = \frac{\lambda FG + (\dot{V}_A/\dot{Q})(1 - G)}{\lambda FG + (\dot{V}_A/\dot{Q})} \tag{13}$$

$$E = \frac{\lambda G}{\lambda FG + (\dot{V}_A/\dot{Q})} \tag{14}$$

where $F = 1 + \beta g\dot{V}_A/D'$ and $G = 1 - e^{-Dm/\dot{Q}\beta b}$.

At the limit of no diffusion limitation (both D′ and Dm $\rightarrow \infty$), F and G become unity and

$$R = E = \frac{\lambda}{\lambda + (\dot{V}_A/\dot{Q})} \tag{15}$$

which is the equation derived by Farhi (16) for steady-state inert-gas elimination in the homogeneous lung with complete diffusional equilibrium.

At the limit of no alveolar-capillary membrane diffusion limitation (Dm $\rightarrow \infty$), G becomes unity and

$$R = \frac{\lambda F}{\lambda F + (\dot{V}_A/\dot{Q})} \tag{16}$$

$$E = \frac{\lambda}{\lambda F + (\dot{V}_A/\dot{Q})} \tag{17}$$

which were described by Scheid et al. (73) for elimination of inert gas in the presence of stratified inhomogeneity. The behavior of inert gases eliminated by the lung in the presence of V̇A/Q̇ heterogeneity and gas-phase diffusion limitations has been analyzed in detail (31,73).

At the limit of no gas-phase diffusion limitation (D′ $\rightarrow \infty$), F becomes unity and

$$R = \frac{\lambda G + (\dot{V}_A/\dot{Q})(1 - G)}{\lambda G + (\dot{V}_A/\dot{Q})} \tag{18}$$

$$E = \frac{\lambda G}{\lambda G + (\dot{V}_A/\dot{Q})} \tag{19}$$

The retention and excretion described in Equations 18 and 19 illustrate the expected elimination properties of an alveolar-capillary membrane diffusion-limited gas (e.g., O_2 or CO) that is being eliminated from a single alveolus. Appropriate transformations must be made for uptake of inspired gases.

For inert gases, which are not membrane diffusion limited (βm/βb ratio near unity), G is unity. To exert an equivalent diffusion limitation for an inert gas, Dm must be considerably lower than D′. Figure 7 shows the relative values of Dm and D′ for equivalent diffusion limitation. The relationship is dependent on λ, but for any gas a lower Dm is required to exert the same degree of diffusion limitation as a given D′. For a gas with λ = 1.0, a D′ of 10^8 will exert the same influence as a Dm of 10^4. In the gas phase the D′ for different gases is related to the molecular weight; thus D′ for O_2 is similar to D′ for N_2. In the alveolar-

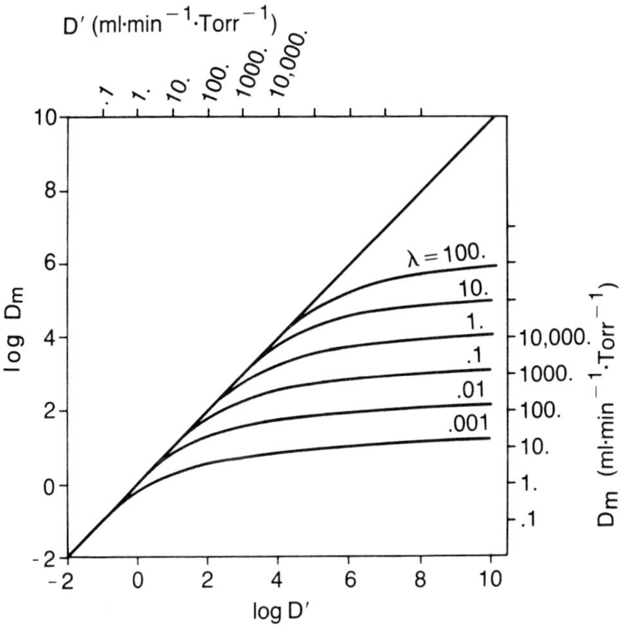

FIG. 7. Equivalent values of membrane diffusing capacity (Dm) and gas-phase diffusive conductance (D′) for equal diffusion limitation plotted on log scale. *Lines*, hypothetical gases with given blood-gas partition coefficient (λ). *Diagonal line*, line of identity.

capillary membrane, the Dm for different gases is primarily related according to $\beta m/\beta b$ (see Eq. 6), so that the Dm for O_2 is considerably less than the Dm for N_2. Therefore the relative influence of diffusion limitation on different gases is dependent on whether that limitation is in the gas phase or the membrane.

The concepts contained within Equations 18 and 19 have been used by Lodato (46) to quantitate D_{O_2} in excised dog lobes. The approach combines $\dot{V}A/\dot{Q}$ distribution and alveolar-capillary membrane diffusion limitation in normal lungs. Lodato used an isolated, perfused dog lung lobe with zero inspired O_2. The elimination characteristics of O_2 were compared with those of inert gases of similar λ. Because inert gases are not subject to membrane diffusion limitation due to the high $\beta m/\beta b$ and high $D/\dot{Q}\beta b$ (see Fig. 2), any difference between the retention and excretion of O_2 and the inert gas reflects diffusion limitation (as described by the difference between Eq. 18 and Eq. 15). A D_{O_2} determined for the lobe was 2.7 $ml \cdot min^{-1} \cdot Torr^{-1}$, which corresponds to a lung D_{O_2} of 13.6 $ml \cdot min^{-1} \cdot Torr^{-1}$. For intact dogs, this value is within the range of 10–32 $ml \cdot min^{-1} \cdot Torr^{-1}$ taken from the literature. The approach used in this study was quite sophisticated, yet it was necessarily limited to an apparent D_{O_2} without consideration of diffusing-capacity heterogeneity.

FUTURE DIRECTIONS

Our understanding of diffusing-capacity heterogeneity is quite rudimentary. Based on the known anatomy and physiology of the lung, it is reasonable to assume that pulmonary diffusing capacity is distributed heterogeneously. Indeed, many experimental results can be explained by such a hypothesis. At present the state of the art is such that diffusing-capacity heterogeneity has been suggested, but its existence has not been proved. The first order of business is to demonstrate that significant diffusing-capacity heterogeneity exists.

Some data suggest that diffusion limitation within the gas phase of the lung contributes significantly to overall lung diffusing capacity. The importance of gas-phase diffusion limitation must be quantitated by different experimental approaches. Quantitative separation of gas-phase and alveolar-capillary membrane diffusion limitation is important because the behavior of each with different types of gases is quantitatively different. Different types of respiratory disease may have different individual effects on these two components.

Better understanding of the distribution of diffusing capacity cannot be achieved without the development of a new method for separating and quantifying the importance of Dm and gas-phase D′ distribution. A promising approach will be to utilize gases with different λ and different diffusion properties, although there are at present relatively few gases available that have the requisite characteristics and that are physiologically usable.

Assuming that a precise and sensitive method of analysis can be developed, it then will be possible to examine the various factors that affect the distribution of diffusing capacity. The important advantage will be in separating changes in apparent diffusing capacity due to variations in diffusing-capacity heterogeneity from changes in true diffusing capacity. Once these interactions are firmly established, they may provide a much better understanding of and confidence in pulmonary diffusing capacity as a physiological marker and a clinical tool.

REFERENCES

1. ADARO, F., AND L. E. FARHI. Effects of intralobular gas diffusion on alveolar gas exchange (Abstract). *Federation Proc.* 30: 437, 1971.
2. ARNDT, H., T. K. C. KING, AND W. A. BRISCOE. Diffusing capacities and ventilation perfusion ratios in patients with the clinical syndrome of alveolar capillary block. *J. Clin. Invest.* 49: 408–422, 1970.
3. BIDANI, A., R. W. FLUMERFELT, AND E. D. CRANDALL. Analysis of the effects of pulsatile capillary blood flow and volume on gas exchange. *Respir. Physiol.* 35: 27–42, 1978.
4. BRISCOE, W. A., AND T. K. C. KING. The diffusing capacity of the lung in obstructive disease studied with the aid of Bohr integral isopleths. *Am. Rev. Respir. Dis.* 95: 891–893, 1967.
5. BURNS, B., AND R. H. SHEPARD. DL_{O_2} in excised lungs perfused

phometric estimation of pulmonary diffusion capacity. IV. Effect of varying positive pressure inflation of air spaces. *Respir. Physiol.* 18: 285–308, 1973.
95. West, J. B. Regional differences in gas exchange in the lung of erect man. *J. Appl. Physiol.* 17: 893–898, 1962.
96. West, J. B., R. A. B. Holland, C. T. Dollery, and C. M. E. Matthews. Interpretation of radioactive gas clearance rates in the lung. *J. Appl. Physiol.* 17: 14–20, 1962.
97. West, J. B., P. D. Wagner, and C. M. W. Derks. Gas exchange in distributions of $\dot{V}A/\dot{Q}$ ratios: partial pressure-solubility diagram. *J. Appl. Physiol.* 37: 533–540, 1974.
98. Wood, L. D. H., A. C. Bryan, S. K. Bau, T. R. Weng, and H. Levison. Effect of increased gas density on pulmonary gas exchange in man. *J. Appl. Physiol.* 41: 206–210, 1976.
99. Yokoyama, T., and L. E. Farhi. Study of ventilation-perfusion ratio distribution in the anesthetized dog by multiple inert gas washout. *Respir. Physiol.* 3: 166–176, 1967.

CHAPTER 13

Measurement of cardiac output by alveolar gas exchange

MARVIN A. SACKNER | *Department of Medicine, Mount Sinai Medical Center, Miami Beach, Florida*

CHAPTER CONTENTS

THE RATE OF UPTAKE or excretion of physiological gases (e.g., O_2 and CO_2) or chemically inert, soluble gases (e.g., acetylene, nitrous oxide, Freon), determined from analysis of alveolar gas exchange without sampling the blood, can be used to calculate pulmonary capillary blood flow ($\dot{Q}c$). In normal subjects, $\dot{Q}c$ constitutes the output of the right heart minus right-to-left shunts due to anatomic and/or physiological communications as a result of blood flow through underventilated or nonventilated alveoli. Invasive measurements of cardiac output ($\dot{Q}T$) requiring blood sampling based on the Fick O_2 or indicator-dilution principles include the blood flow due to venous admixture. However, venous admixture normally represents <6% of the $\dot{Q}T$ at rest and <3% during exercise (50), a value within the experimental range of error of all currently available noninvasive and invasive methods. Therefore in this chapter, $\dot{Q}T$ and $\dot{Q}c$ are used interchangeably except when circumstances indicate a large difference between the two.

In Butler's (12) chapter in the 1965 edition of the *Handbook* section on respiration, the historical progress toward development of ideal alveolocapillary gas-exchange methods was reviewed. In the two decades since publication of this chapter, many technological refinements have taken place, although few new principles have been described. This chapter is a review of the advances that have taken place since 1965. References prior to that time are cited only as necessary for understanding the methodology reported since then.

MEASUREMENT OF PULMONARY CAPILLARY BLOOD FLOW WITH PHYSIOLOGICAL GASES

Both CO_2 and O_2 have been used as the markers for measuring $\dot{Q}c$. Under steady-state conditions, according to the Fick principle

$$\dot{Q}c = \dot{V}_x/(Ca_x - C\bar{v}_x)$$

where Ca_x is the arterial blood concentration of O_2 or CO_2, $C\bar{v}_x$ is the mixed venous blood concentration of O_2 or CO_2, and $\dot{V}_x$ is the uptake of the gas from the lung. The $\dot{V}_x$ is easily determined by monitoring the inspired and expired volumes of the gas over a finite period or on a breath-by-breath basis with the use of *1)* manometric methods, *2)* gas chromatography, or *3)* the more popular, rapid responding analyzers of physical gas, which include polarographic, infrared, and mass spectrometer devices. Although Ca_x can be determined directly from the arterial blood, it is more convenient to measure the partial pressure from alveolar gas and convert it to the equivalent arterial gas content with the use of the dissociation curve for O_2 or CO_2. The main problem with using O_2 and CO_2 as markers for $\dot{Q}c$ is the determination of their mixed venous concentration. Of the two, CO_2 poses less of a problem than O_2; several methods have been proposed to estimate $C\bar{v}_{CO_2}$, but only one method has been reported for indirect estimation of $C\bar{v}_{O_2}$.

Measurement With O_2

For estimation of $C\bar{v}_{O_2}$, the subject rebreathes from a bag with a volume equivalent to functional residual capacity containing 8%–9% CO_2 in N_2. This produces alveolar partial pressures of O_2 and CO_2 ($P_{A_{O_2}}$ and $P_{A_{CO_2}}$) that become stable 4–8 s from onset of rebreathing, with a plateau maintained up to an additional 6 s (Fig. 1). Values for the partial pressure of O_2 (P_{O_2}) at rest range from 35 to 52 mmHg and are believed to reflect mixed venous P_{O_2} ($P\bar{v}_{O_2}$) (14). To convert $P\bar{v}_{O_2}$ to $C\bar{v}_{O_2}$, the hemoglobin concentration and venous plasma pH must be taken into account. The rebreathing method exposes the subject to severe, potentially hazardous hypoxia. The method also requires a trial and error approach to the value of the O_2 concentration (C_{O_2}) in the bag, since the plateau of O_2 equilibration must be reached before recirculation takes place, an important factor in exercise studies. Furthermore, shifts in the oxyhemoglobin dissociation curve during exercise studies must be considered because of pH and temperature changes, and these can only be obtained by invasive means. Finally, the method has not been reported in conditions involving inequalities of the ventilation/perfusion ratio ($\dot{V}A/\dot{Q}$) that might prevent attainment of an equilibration plateau prior to recirculation. Measurement of Ca_{O_2} must be obtained by arterial puncture. For these reasons the measurement of $P\bar{v}_{O_2}$ by rebreathing during induced hypoxia has little to recommend it in view of the variety of indirect methods for assessment of $\dot{Q}c$.

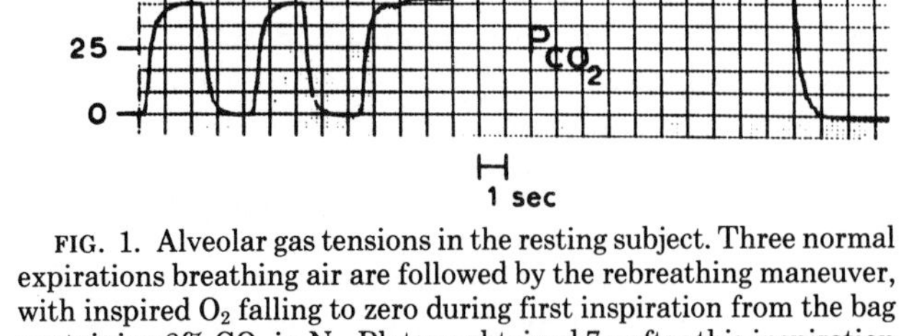

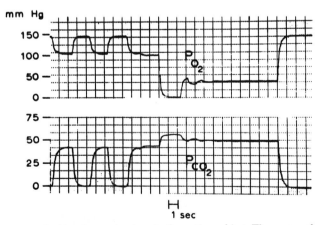

FIG. 1. Alveolar gas tensions in the resting subject. Three normal expirations breathing air are followed by the rebreathing maneuver, with inspired O_2 falling to zero during first inspiration from the bag containing 8% CO_2 in N_2. Plateau obtained 7 s after this inspiration is maintained for 6 s. In practice, sensitivity of O_2 channel is increased during measurement of equilibrium value. P_{O_2}, partial pressure of O_2; P_{CO_2}, partial pressure of CO_2. [From Cerretelli et al. (14).]

Measurement With CO_2

Employment of CO_2 as a marker for measurement of $\dot{Q}c$ has several attractive features: *1)* CO_2 is simple to deal with because it is virtually absent from the inspired air, *2)* CO_2 is so soluble that end-capillary partial pressure of CO_2 (P_{CO_2}) is almost equivalent to $P_{A_{CO_2}}$, *3)* the slope of the CO_2 dissociation curve is so steep that nonuniformity of $P_{A_{CO_2}}$ in the lung causes an alveolar-arterial difference in partial pressure of CO_2 ($P_{A_{CO_2}} - Pa_{CO_2}$) of <1 mmHg, *4)* $P\bar{v}_{CO_2} - Pa_{CO_2}$ is so small that the effect of right-to-left shunts is minimal, *5)* the slope of the CO_2 dissociation curve is linear over the physiological range, and *6)* although standard or individual dissociation curves may vary considerably in position when plotted on linear coordinates, this has little effect on the relationship between pressure difference and content difference, provided appropriate correction for hemoglobin concentration and O_2 saturation are applied (12, 63). Therefore P_{CO_2} can be easily converted to the CO_2 concentration (C_{CO_2}), as long as the pH and oxyhemoglobin concentrations are known or unchanged during the determination of $\dot{Q}c$.

Carbon dioxide has major disadvantages as a tracer for measurement of $\dot{Q}c$. *1)* The difference between Pa_{CO_2} and $P\bar{v}_{CO_2}$ for a C_{CO_2} difference of 4 ml/100 ml is only 4–5 mmHg; a measurement error as small as 1 mmHg P_{CO_2} would affect the calculation of resting $\dot{Q}c$ by 20%–25%. *2)* The $P\bar{v}_{CO_2} - Pa_{CO_2}$ can be increased from 6 to 8 mmHg if the mixed venous blood is fully saturated with O_2 (a situation common to several methods used to estimate $P\bar{v}_{CO_2}$) and the oxygenated dissociation curve must be employed. *3)* Lung tissue contains carbonic anhydrase, which buffers alveolar CO_2 fluctuations. This causes the equivalent lung volume for CO_2 to be considerably larger than alveolar volume; e.g., ~2.0 ml CO_2 [standard temperature and pressure, dry (STPD)] go into lung tissues for a Pa_{CO_2} rise of 1 mmHg, whereas only 0.45 ml enters the pulmonary capillary blood. *4)* Although $Pa_{CO_2} - P_{A_{CO_2}}$ under normal resting conditions is small and accurate values are unavailable, if not taken into account a $Pa_{CO_2} - P_{A_{CO_2}}$ of only 0.5 mmHg would lead to a nearly 10% error in calculation of $\dot{Q}c$. *5)* Changes of body position, exercise, and pulmonary disease may affect $Pa_{CO_2} - P_{A_{CO_2}}$ substantially. *6)* The temperature of pulmonary arterial blood may fluctuate to a minor extent during the respiratory cycle, but the consequent changes in mixed venous composition at rest are so small that negligible error is introduced. *7)* The $P\bar{v}_{CO_2} - Pa_{CO_2}$ and CO_2 output ($\dot{V}_{CO_2}$) are very sensitive to changes in ventilation but very insensitive to changes in systemic blood flow, and inaccurate determinations of $\dot{Q}c$ occur when there are slight deviations from the steady state (12, 19, 25, 62, 77).

All methods that use CO_2 for estimation of $\dot{Q}c$ have as their basis the indirect determination of $P\bar{v}_{CO_2}$. These methods include analyses during three respiratory maneuvers: *1*) breath holding, *2*) rebreathing, and *3*) single expirate.

BREATH-HOLDING METHODS. Breath holding requires a high degree of subject cooperation and is probably suitable only for trained normal subjects. During breath holding, $P_{A_{CO_2}}$ rises rapidly as the reduced hemoglobin is oxygenated until it reaches and then exceeds the initial $P\bar{v}_{CO_2}$ when it tapers off. This rise of $P_{A_{CO_2}}$ toward $P\bar{v}_{CO_2}$ is described by the following equation (12)

$$P_{A_{CO_2}} = P\bar{v}_{CO_2} - \lambda CO_2(P\bar{v}_{CO_2} - P_{A_{CO_2}})e^{-Kt}$$

where

$$K = \frac{\lambda_{CO_2} \cdot \dot{Q}c(P_B - 47)}{ELV(CO_2)}$$

where t is time, λ_{CO_2} is the slope of the blood CO_2 dissociation curve, P_B is the barometric pressure, and $ELV(CO_2)$ is the equivalent lung volume for CO_2, i.e., the alveolar volume plus the CO_2 dissociation slope of lung tissue times $P_{A_{CO_2}}$.

The $P\bar{v}_{CO_2}$ can be estimated after inspiring air or O_2 and breath holding at different intervals. As long as $P_{A_{O_2}}$ remains high, O_2 uptake ($\dot{V}_{O_2}$) is unchanged, and the gas-exchange ratio (R) is a direct function of $\dot{V}_{CO_2}$ during that period. The $P_{A_{CO_2}}$ is plotted against R and the line extrapolated to the point where R = 0. This gives the $P_{A_{CO_2}}$ value at which CO_2 exchange would stop, i.e., the equilibrium P_{CO_2}. This latter represents oxygenated $P\bar{v}_{CO_2}$, but true $P\bar{v}_{CO_2}$ can be calculated from it. Alternatively, different $P_{A_{CO_2}}$ levels can be obtained by varying inspired CO_2 and breath-holding times and plotting the data in the same way (25). A variation of the breath-holding method has been described for patients on mechanical ventilators in which the respirator can be preset to give predetermined inspiratory and pause-time fractions (32).

The breath-holding methods assume that both $\dot{Q}c$ and $\dot{V}_{CO_2}$ remain constant over the time necessary to construct the slope for calculation of $P\bar{v}_{O_2}$, an assumption that seems unlikely. During heavy exercise the breath-holding maneuvers cannot be readily accomplished even by trained subjects. Because of problems with both analysis and performance, there is little interest in utilizing breath holding methods for determination of $\dot{Q}c$.

REBREATHING METHODS. In contrast to breath-holding maneuvers, rebreathing over a short interval from a bag containing a CO_2 mixture is usually easily accomplished by both trained and untrained subjects. Rebreathing is a more natural maneuver during both resting and exercising conditions and promotes more even mixing between lung regions having $\dot{V}A/\dot{Q}$ inequalities. Rebreathing from a bag containing air is almost equivalent to the breath-holding technique for estimating the plateau $P\bar{v}_{O_2}$. The CO_2 equilibrium cannot be reached prior to recirculation, and an extrapolation method must be employed (25). The bag gas is diluted by the residual volume of the subject at the start of each new rebreathing cycle, and the final steady $P_{A_{CO_2}}$ reached depends as much on the duration of each rebreathing cycle as the $P\bar{v}_{CO_2}$ (12). For estimating $P\bar{v}_{CO_2}$, this technique is not acceptable.

Methods that appear to be useful to estimate $P\bar{v}_{CO_2}$ include rebreathing a mixture of CO_2 at a concentration expected near $C\bar{v}_{CO_2}$, nominally 5% at rest and 10%–15% during exercise. The gas in the bag must be at a concentration such that the $P_{A_{CO_2}}$ reached after the first inspiration is within 2 mmHg of $P\bar{v}_{CO_2}$. A spurious plateau of CO_2 may occur if the dead-space gas of the lung is breathed to and fro, but this is usually recognized. If the initial concentration of CO_2 in the gas is too high, an apparent plateau may be reached late when O_2 absorption by the lung concentrates $P_{A_{CO_2}}$ and the $P\bar{v}_{O_2}$ has risen due to recirculation (12).

Plateau or equilibrium value. In this method the subject rebreathes from a bag containing 2–4 liters of a mixture of CO_2 in O_2. At the end of a normal expiration the subject is connected to the bag and rebreathes deeply and regularly at ~30 breaths/min. End-tidal CO_2 is recorded continuously at the mouth with an infrared analyzer or mass spectrometer. A perfect plateau, indicating cessation of CO_2 exchange between mixed venous blood and alveolar gas, is indicated by <0.5-mmHg change in P_{CO_2} during a complete rebreathing cycle begun with inspiration from the bag (Fig. 2). A correct plateau value of oxygenated $P\bar{v}_{CO_2}$ appears within 6 s from the start of rebreathing and is broken by recirculation at 10 s. The equilibrium value of oxygenated $P\bar{v}_{CO_2}$ can be estimated to within ±0.8 mmHg (49, 55).

Extrapolation value. If the bag does have a sufficiently greater P_{CO_2} than the end-tidal value, the recording of $P_{A_{CO_2}}$ is marked by phase reversal below the sustained equilibrium value. After this phase reversal, P_{CO_2} rises toward the equilibrium value (Fig. 2). It is impractical to predict this value from equations involving tidal volume, lung volume, initial $P_{A_{CO_2}}$, and the small changes of $P_{A_{CO_2}}$ with each breath. Jones et al. (49) derived an empirical equation based on inspired CO_2 and end-tidal CO_2 for its calculation.

Both from actual data and analysis of a mathematical model, the extrapolation method estimates oxygenated $P\bar{v}_{CO_2}$ to within ±2 mmHg during exercise (55, 57). The major reason for the greater variability of the extrapolation compared to the equilibrium method is technological. It is difficult to analyze four or five breaths within the time interval of 10 s of rebreathing, and the construction of the graph for these points is somewhat arbitrary. The adequacy of fit in some published graphs is more apparent than real because the scales reflect CO_2 percentages and must be multiplied approximately sevenfold for conversion into tensions. There is also a potential error in deciding on the

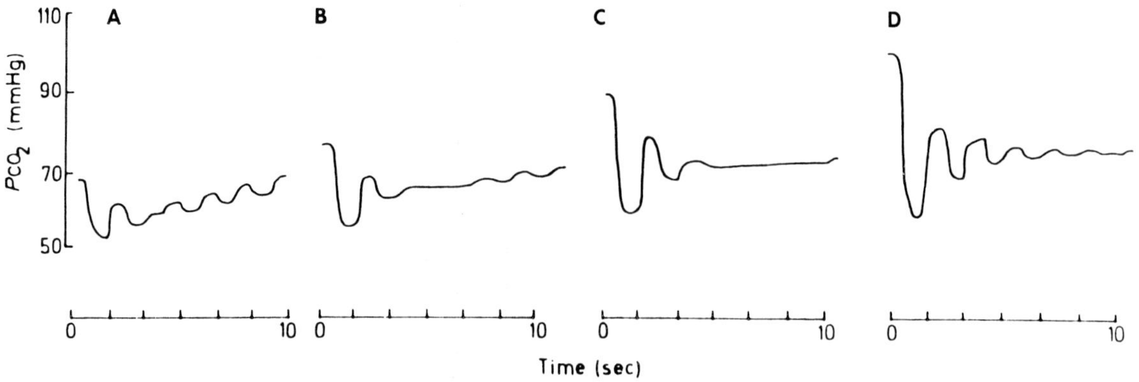

FIG. 2. Records of partial pressure of CO_2 (P_{CO_2}) during rebreathing. Four different patterns are shown, obtained with successively increasing initial bag CO_2 concentrations in a normal subject exercising at a work load of (600 kp·m)/min (CO_2 output 1.5 liters/min). *Pattern C*, a sustained equilibrium; *patterns A* and *B*, unsustained, phase reversal, which occurs at a lower P_{CO_2}; *pattern D*, delayed equilibrium at a higher P_{CO_2}. Despite wide variation in initial bag P_{CO_2}, P_{CO_2} after 10-s rebreathing is similar and 6 mmHg separates the 10-s end-tidal value of the two extremes (*A* and *D*). [From Jones et al. (49). Reprinted by permission from *Clinical Science*, © 1967, The Biochemical Society, London.]

proper end-tidal CO_2 value because the mixed expired CO_2 tracing as measured with the rapid responding CO_2 analyzers (37, 50) has an upward slope with superimposed cardiogenic oscillations.

Interpolation value. If the CO_2 equilibrium value is not sustained or if the equilibration is delayed to beyond 10 s, then the mean of two values of end-tidal CO_2 at 10 s between the two rebreathings can be used, if not >2% CO_2 separates the initial bag concentrations. If these conditions are met, this value should fall within ±1 mmHg of equilibrium P_{CO_2} (49).

Appraisal of different rebreathing methods. In young adults and patients with cardiopulmonary disease who can sustain steady-state exercise, oxygenated $P\bar{v}_{O_2}$ can be estimated in 90% of trials. In 60%–70% of trials, the more desirable plateau pattern is obtained from one or two rebreathing trials, whereas in the remainder the extrapolation or interpolation approach must be employed. In practice, underestimation rather than overestimation of oxygenated $P\bar{v}_{O_2}$ is the major problem; thus the aim is to obtain one rebreathing estimate that is too high (equilibration delayed until after 10 s), even if an early rebreathing had given a satisfactory estimate (49). In most middle-aged adults, $P\bar{v}_{CO_2}$ determined with rebreathing methods is accurate and reproducible only during exercise and in the absence of pulmonary disease (18). In patients with moderate-to-severe obstructive airway disease, the rebreathing technique for measuring $\dot{Q}_T$ is accurate only if Pa_{CO_2} is measured directly rather than estimated from end-tidal P_{CO_2} (PET_{CO_2}) (62).

Downstream correction for oxygenated mixed venous CO_2 tension. Jones et al. (49) compared the P_{CO_2} of the blood in the pulmonary artery during equilibrium rebreathing and found that it was higher than the P_{CO_2} that would be found in blood during prolonged equilibration such as used for determination of the CO_2 dissociation curve by in vitro tonometry. The PET_{CO_2} during rebreathing was compared with blood in the pulmonary capillaries by sampling blood after it had passed to the brachial artery. This demonstrated a fall in P_{CO_2} after blood left the lungs, implying that the equilibrium P_{CO_2} could not be related directly to mixed venous CO_2 content ($C\bar{v}_{CO_2}$) with the use of in vitro blood CO_2 dissociation curves. This effect was not influenced by the initial CO_2 concentration in the rebreathing bag nor by the duration of rebreathing but was related to duration of exercise level. An empirical regression equation was derived: $P_{CO_2} = 1.4 + 2.6\ \dot{V}_{CO_2}$ (liters·min^{-1}·mmHg^{-1}). The latter is subtracted from oxygenated $P\bar{v}_{CO_2}$ measured at equilibrium and together with Pa_{CO_2} converted to $C\bar{v}_{CO_2} - Ca_{CO_2}$. Some authors have not applied this correction, and their values of resting $\dot{Q}c$ are generally too low because $C\bar{v}_{CO_2} - Ca_{CO_2}$ may be overestimated by 2 mmHg. At high levels of exercise the correction becomes less important, i.e., a ±4 mmHg error at a $\dot{V}_{CO_2}$ of 2.5 liters/min would cause an error of only ±10% in $\dot{Q}c$ (49).

Arterial partial pressure of CO_2. This value can be determined with arterial puncture, but such a procedure detracts from the noninvasive advantages of the method. In resting normal subjects, the difference between PET_{CO_2} and Pa_{CO_2} is virtually zero and the PET_{CO_2} can be used as the Pa_{CO_2}. With exercise the slope of expired P_{CO_2} increases because of the increased excretion of CO_2 into a falling lung volume (Fig. 3). Any estimate of Pa_{CO_2} from PET_{CO_2} depends on the level of work and on the pattern of breathing. Jones et al. (50) developed an empirical regression equation for this correction: $PET_{CO_2} - Pa_{CO_2} = 0.004\ \dot{V}_{CO_2} - 0.13$ breaths/min + 0.75 mmHg. This equation allows estimation of Pa_{CO_2} from PET_{CO_2} in normal subjects during exercise but is imprecise and cannot be used if distribution of ventilation is uneven. Alternatively, Pa_{CO_2} during exercise in normal subjects can

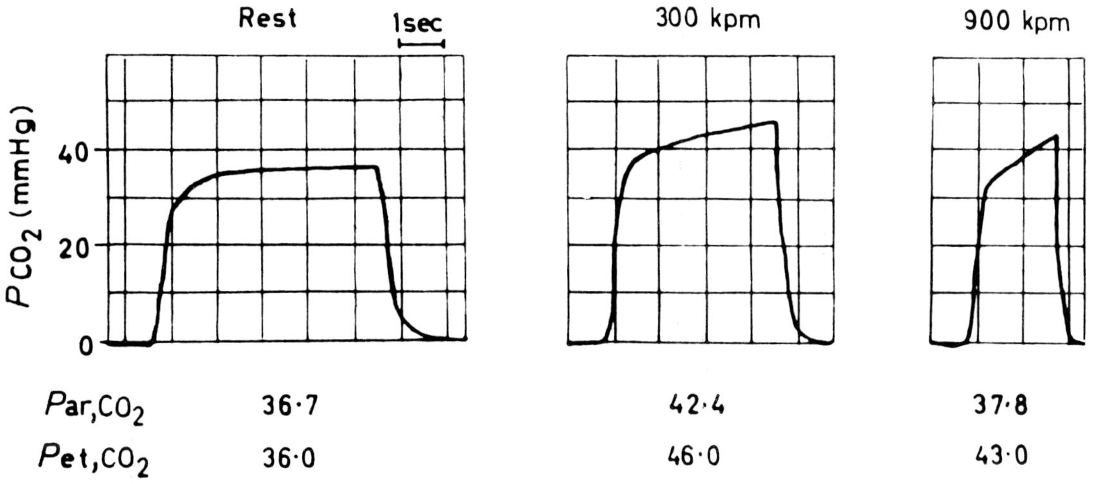

FIG. 3. Mass spectrometer record of expired CO_2 showing increase in slope of alveolar P_{CO_2} with increasing exercise. Par_{CO_2}, arterial P_{CO_2}. Pet_{CO_2}, end-tidal P_{CO_2}. [From Jones et al. (50).]

be calculated with an assumed dead space and the Bohr equation (18).

Blood CO_2 dissociation curve. A standard CO_2 dissociation curve is used for the conversion of $P\bar{v}_{CO_2} - Pa_{CO_2}$ into CO_2 content. During moderate-to-intense exercise, coexisting metabolic acidosis affects the CO_2 dissociation curve. Values for such changes can be assumed, and equations have been developed suitable for incorporation into a digital computer program for manipulation of the CO_2 dissociation curve at varying levels of hemoglobin and base excess. Neglect of this correction (37) can introduce errors up to 5%–10% into $\dot{Q}c$ determination.

Cardiac output estimation. The $\dot{V}_{CO_2}$ is usually determined by collection of mixed expired air over a minute or two before or after estimation of $C\bar{v}_{CO_2} - Ca_{CO_2}$ and application of the Fick principle for calculation of $\dot{Q}c$

$$\dot{Q}c = \dot{V}_{CO_2}/(C\bar{v}_{CO_2} - Ca_{CO_2})$$

Values of $\dot{Q}c$ reported in the literature tend to be too low unless the "downstream" correction determined by equilibration for oxygenated $P\bar{v}_{CO_2}$ is applied. The $\dot{Q}T$ calculated in this way agrees closely both at rest and during exercise with more direct methods, but the extrapolation method usually gives spuriously high results (38, 43, 49).

SINGLE-BREATH EXPIRATE METHOD. *Theory.* During a slow exhalation, Pa_{CO_2} and PA_{CO_2} begin to rise. If it is assumed that during this process $C\bar{v}_{CO_2}$ and Ca_{O_2} remain unchanged, then Ca_{CO_2} will approach and become equal to $C\bar{v}_{CO_2}$ such that CO_2 exchange ceases and R = 0. At this point the difference between the arterial and mixed venous blood is the O_2 content, and therefore Pa_{CO_2} will be higher than $P\bar{v}_{CO_2}$ by virtue of the Haldane effect. During the equilibration period, $\dot{V}_{CO_2}$ from the blood diminishes while $\dot{V}_{O_2}$ remains constant. Thus, while Pa_{CO_2} rises, R falls. Since at the beginning of the slow expiration, Pa_{CO_2} is lower and the equilibrium point higher than $P\bar{v}_{CO_2}$, there is a time when $P\bar{v}_{CO_2} = Pa_{CO_2}$. This occurs when R = 0.32, since for every unit volume of O_2 taken up by hemoglobin of venous blood, 0.32 vol of CO_2 is displaced without change in P_{CO_2} [Fig. 4; (56)].

During a slow exhalation (10 s), PA_{O_2} and PA_{CO_2} (as measured by discrete gas samples or continuously by mass spectrometry) are plotted against each other and the instantaneous R (Rinst) values are calculated. The P_{CO_2} values are then plotted against Rinst. The Pa_{CO_2} is determined by the R of a previously collected breath or by analysis of the same breath used to plot the PA_{O_2} versus PA_{CO_2} relationship or by integrating the expired CO_2 over volume with a suitable measuring device (spirometer or pneumotachograph) (56). For R values the corresponding Pa_{CO_2} can be located from the plot of PA_{O_2} versus PA_{CO_2}. With this method the P_{CO_2} of the arterial blood (from mixed expired R), true mixed venous blood (R = 0.32), and oxygenated mixed venous blood (R = 0) is established. The arteriovenous

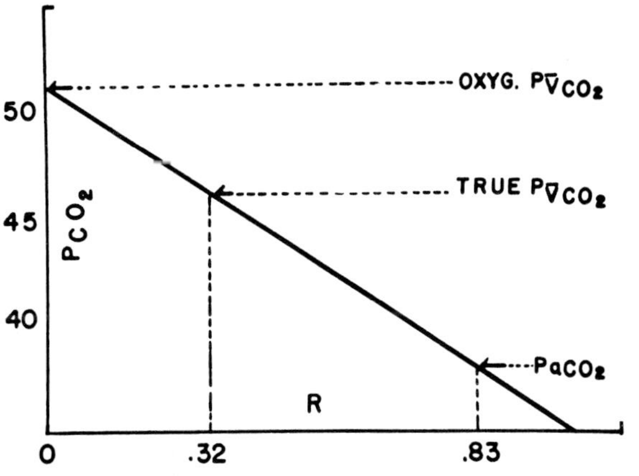

FIG. 4. Linear relationship between P_{CO_2} of arterial blood (Pa_{CO_2}) and the instantaneous exchange ratio R when the breath is held for one circulation time. Oxyg. $P\bar{v}_{CO_2}$, oxygenated mixed venous P_{CO_2}. [From Kim et al. (56).]

content difference can be obtained by multiplying the difference in oxygenated $P\bar{v}_{CO_2}$ and Pa_{CO_2} by the slope of the CO_2 dissociation curve (assumed to be 0.47 ml·100 ml^{-1}·mmHg^{-1}). If R = 0.32 is used as the location of the Haldane effect, true $P\bar{v}_{CO_2}$ can be calculated and the equation for $\dot{Q}c$ can be delineated (56)

$$\dot{Q}c = \frac{\dot{V}_{CO_2} - 0.32\dot{V}_{O_2}}{S_{CO_2}(P\bar{v}_{CO_2} - Pa_{O_2})}$$

or

$$\dot{Q}c = \frac{\dot{V}_{O_2}(R - 0.32)}{S_{CO_2}(P\bar{v}_{CO_2} - Pa_{CO_2})}$$

where $\dot{V}_{CO_2}$ is the CO_2 output, $\dot{V}_{O_2}$ is the O_2 consumption, R is the gas-exchange ratio minus 0.32 (the Haldane effect), and S_{CO_2} is the slope of the CO_2 dissociation curve for blood (assumed to be 0.47 ml·100 ml^{-1}·mmHg^{-1}).

Problems with single-expirate method assumptions. The relationship between PA_{CO_2} and Rinst is critically dependent on the shape of the PA_{CO_2} versus PA_{O_2} curve. Hlastala et al. (44), with a representative curve (Fig. 5) comprising 405 data points, showed that utilizing all the data points gave a calculated $\dot{Q}c$ of 9.5 liters/min. Deletion of the first 25 data points resulted in a calculated $\dot{Q}c$ of 8.4 liters/min, whereas deletion of the last 50 data points resulted in a value of 7.4 liters/min. Although it is visually difficult to detect a difference between the fitted curves, the difference in $\dot{Q}c$ is ~25%. Thus the decision as to when dead-space air is fully eliminated and alveolar gas is being expired is crucial. Hlastala et al. (44) used tidal volume for their measurements, whereas Kim et al. (56) used a larger volume, but this difference is not responsible for the assertions of Hlastala et al. Grønlund (41) demonstrated that the rigorous attempt at curve fitting by the latter to evaluate the single-expirate method is a source of major systemic and random errors. The random errors depend heavily on such experimental circumstances as the duration of the expiration and the analytic precision of the measured PA_{O_2} and PA_{CO_2}. The problem is that the relation between PA_{CO_2} and PA_{O_2} is not a polynomial function, although Hlastala et al. (44) attempted to fit the curve with a third-order polynomial. The curve can be fitted with a complicated differential equation, but no analytical solution exists. Finally, Grønlund (41) found that the single-expirate method is quite sensitive to imperceptibly visible differences in the curve shape because the algorithm used to calculate $\dot{Q}c$ uses curve slope rather than absolute values of PA_{CO_2} versus PA_{O_2}.

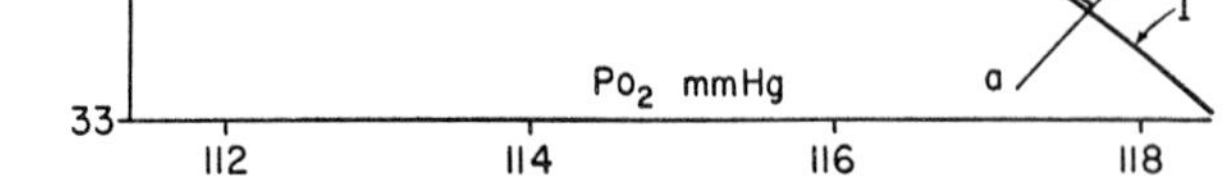

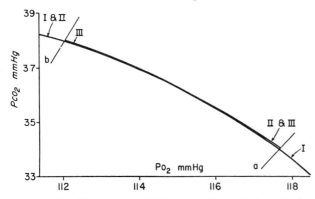

FIG. 5. Partial pressure of CO_2 versus P_{O_2} typical expiration against an airway resistor. *Curve I*, 3rd-order polynomial fit to all 405 data points. *Curve II*, polynomial fit after deletion of 25 data points to *right* of *line a*. *Curve III*, polynomial fit after deletion of 50 data points to *left* of *line b* in addition to those to *right* of *line a*. [From Hlastala et al. (44).]

Chen et al. (15) selected a value of $\dot{R}$ = 0.38 to represent the point of true $P\bar{v}_{CO_2}$ in contrast to R = 0.32 utilized by Kim et al. (56). The Chen group achieved a good fit for the PA_{CO_2} versus Rinst plot by excluding points corresponding to $PA_{CO_2} < 30$ mmHg and by eliminating points that lay farther than 0.7 mmHg from the quadratic regression of PA_{CO_2} on PA_{O_2} and then recalculating the regression equation. The latter was used to determine the regression of PA_{CO_2} on Rinst, which was slightly curved and was well fitted by a quadratic regression equation. These investigators attributed the nonlinearity to such factors as *1)* contamination of alveolar gas during expiration by dead-space gas or uneven emptying of alveoli and *2)* storage of some expired CO_2 in lung tissue, giving a lower than expected value of PA_{CO_2} measured at the mouth. The authors could simulate the increase of curvature of Rinst versus PA_{CO_2} plots in normal subjects by adding dead space to the mouthpiece or continuously adding air to the breathing tube. Mean values of $\dot{Q}T$ at rest in patients with cardiac disease obtained with the modified single-expirate method and direct Fick measurements with cardiac catheterization showed excellent agreement.

One assumption of the single-expirate method is that there is a linear relation between R and PA_{CO_2}, but pulsatility of $\dot{Q}c$ suggests that there may be oscillations in O_2 and CO_2 transfer between the blood and alveolar air. This induces slight irregularities in alveolar gas pressures as a function of time. Another factor potentially affecting the slope of the PA_{O_2} versus PA_{CO_2} curve is the cardiogenic oscillations in the expired-gas plateaus. However, smoothing out these variations with a computer has no significant effect on the computation of $\dot{Q}c$. Although the Haldane effect may vary with blood pH and 2,3-diphosphoglycerate level, these changes do not influence the calculation of $\dot{Q}c$, since it is the slope of the R versus PA_{CO_2} curve and the absolute values of R that are important (44).

Another assumption of the single-expirate technique is that the lung tissue does not buffer significant amounts of CO_2 during the test and therefore can be ignored. This assumption is invalid because significant amounts of carbonic anhydrase are present in lung tissue. If the values reported by Sackner et al. (77) are used, i.e., 438 ml for lung tissue volume and 0.38 ml CO_2·100 ml^{-1} tissue·mmHg^{-1} for tissue CO_2 dissociation curve, it can be calculated that 1.66 ml CO_2/mmHg are taken up by lung tissue. For a 2.5-liter alveolar volume, 3.28 ml CO_2 are required to raise the $P_{A_{CO_2}}$ alone by 1 mmHg. To raise P_{CO_2} in the lung by 1 mmHg, 1.66 + 3.23 = 3.94 ml CO_2 are required. Thus the lung would retain 34% (1.66/4.94) of the CO_2. In a lung computer model using such values, fluctuations in alveolar gas R of 0.4–2.3 correspond to fluctuations in blood R of 0.7–1.2 (44). Since completion of the reaction of CO_2 with lung tissue is only a few seconds because the lung tissue contains carbonic anhydrase (28, 45), neglect of the CO_2 solubility in lung tissue introduces a significant error into the calculation of $C\bar{v}_{CO_2} - Ca_{CO_2}$.

A crucial assumption of the single-expirate method is that the continuous change in composition of expired alveolar gas is not due to sequential emptying of alveoli but reflects points at which gas exhaled later in the expiration represents gas that has had a longer lung residence time. This assumption has been confirmed in normal resting subjects but does not hold under conditions involving uneven distribution of ventilation and perfusion (25). Although a potential advantage of the single-expirate method is that it provides a noninvasive means of estimating Pa_{CO_2} in addition to $P\bar{v}_{CO_2}$, it is unlikely to apply to patients with pulmonary disease because of the errors produced by sequential emptying of alveoli with different $\dot{V}A/\dot{Q}$.

Appraisal of cardiac output measured with single-expirate method. Hlastala et al. (44) measured $\dot{Q}c$ in normal subjects and concluded that the method was not suitable during tidal breathing because of the range of values calculated, i.e., from −47 to 173 liters/min. Buderer et al. (11) instituted restraints into the data processing of the $P_{A_{O_2}}$ versus $P_{A_{CO_2}}$ relationship and obtained much less variability with the method during exercise. Compared to direct Fick measurements of $\dot{Q}c$, the values found with the single-expirate method were consistently lower; part of this discrepancy was attributed to the subjects performing a modified Valsalva maneuver during exhalation. Inman et al. (46) found significantly lower values of Pa_{CO_2} for the single-expirate method in normal exercising subjects than $P_{ET_{CO_2}}$ measured during rebreathing and concluded that the single-expirate method should not be used in exercise testing. In contrast, Gilbert and Auchincloss (33) found good agreement between the single-expirate method and dye-dilution $\dot{Q}T$ during exercise. However, they noted several disadvantages to the single-expirate method: requirements for a high degree of cooperation; difficulty in performing the long, slow expiratory maneuver; tedious calculations; complex respiratory circuit design; and unsuitability in patients with uneven $\dot{V}A/\dot{Q}$.

In anesthetized dogs, direct comparison of systemic and pulmonary arterial blood analysis with the single-expirate method at twice the tidal volume revealed no systematic error in Pa_{CO_2} estimates of 32–48 mmHg or $P\bar{v}_{CO_2}$ estimates of 23–59 mmHg. The random errors of arterial and venous estimates were ±1.5 and ±1.2 mmHg (±2 SD), respectively (65). Furthermore there was no systematic error in the comparison of the single-expirate method to the dye-solution method, even when $\dot{Q}c$ was increased by joining the circulation of two dogs (66).

ONE-STEP REBREATHING METHOD. *Principles.* Recognizing the problems associated with the single-expirate and standard rebreathing methods for estimation of $\dot{Q}c$, Farhi et al. (26) reported a sophisticated analysis of a rebreathing maneuver designed to overcome the limitations of the standard techniques. They recognized that the volume of CO_2 added to the alveolar gas measures CO_2 movement out of the pulmonary capillary blood only if $P_{A_{CO_2}}$ is constant. If $P_{A_{CO_2}}$ varies, lung tissue gas stores readjust and the amount of CO_2 gained is given by the algebraic difference between the CO_2 eliminated from blood and the CO_2 gained by the gas phase. These changes can be large enough to produce significant errors in methods based on CO_2 exchange during breath holding, prolonged expiration, or rebreathing.

To circumvent the problem of changing lung tissue CO_2 stores, Farhi et al. (26) proposed a one-step rebreathing method. Tidal volume and frequency are chosen to increase alveolar ventilation and cause an initial drop in $P_{A_{CO_2}}$ (Fig. 6). During the subsequent rise of $P_{A_{CO_2}}$ with each breath, during which $P_{A_{CO_2}}$ returns to the value of $P_{ET_{CO_2}}$ immediately prior to the first inspiration from the rebreathing bag, this moment represents equivalence of P_{CO_2} lung tissue to the base-line value, signifying that net CO_2 change of the lung stores is zero. Best results were obtained when the subsequent rise of $P_{A_{CO_2}}$ is restored to its initial level within 10 s. Hence the volume of CO_2 gained by the combination of alveolar gas and bag gas equals the cumulative loss of CO_2 from the pulmonary circulation during this time interval. A graphic analysis of the time course of alveolar CO_2 with each breath

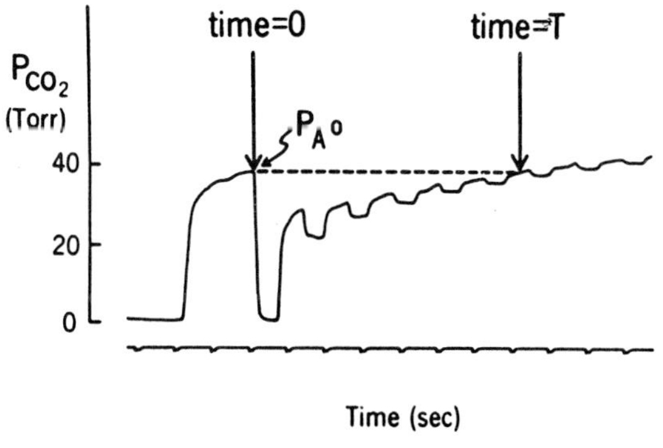

FIG. 6. Partial pressure of CO_2 at the mouth versus time. P_{A_0}, end-expiratory CO_2 pressure of the last control breath. T, time required for alveolar P_{CO_2} to return to P_{A_0} after the initial fall. [From Farhi et al. (26).]

during the rebreathing procedure allowed calculation of the equilibrium $C\bar{v}_{CO_2}$ and the $\dot{V}_{O_2}$. The calculation of the capillary arterial CO_2 content ($C\bar{c}_{CO_2}$) is based on the implicit assumption that $PA_{CO_2} - Pa_{CO_2}$ is negligible during rebreathing. The $C\bar{c}_{CO_2}$ is calculated from PA_{CO_2} during rebreathing and from the CO_2 dissociation curve. Farhi et al. (26) have rigorously derived equations for the determination of $\dot{Q}c$ with this one-step rebreathing method.

Other rebreathing methods based on the Fick principle require two steps: in nearly every case, *1)* $\dot{V}_{CO_2}$ is measured in the steady state and *2)* $\dot{V}_{CO_2}$ and Pa_{CO_2} are changed to permit estimation of $P\bar{v}_{CO_2}$ (Pa_{CO_2} is usually obtained during the first part of the test). This sequential approach requires considerable time and prevents repeated determinations of $\dot{Q}c$ in rapid succession. The one-step rebreathing technique requires only 20–25 s; ventilation, $\dot{V}_{CO_2}$, and PA_{CO_2} are restored rapidly after the maneuver, normally within 30–45 s. In contrast to two-step rebreathing methods, the one-step technique does not require multiple runs and does not rely on the equilibrium assumption. Finally, in nearly all CO_2 techniques, Ca_{CO_2} obtained from PET_{CO_2} during free breathing is taken to be identical to Pa_{CO_2}, with the assumption that $Pa_{CO_2} - PA_{CO_2} = 0$. However, an error of only 1 mmHg in Pa_{CO_2} in the resting subjects leads to a 10% error in $\dot{Q}c$.

Appraisal of one-step rebreathing method. During rest and exercise on a treadmill, the values with the one-step CO_2 rebreathing method are 2% higher than those with an acetylene (C_2H_2) rebreathing method obtained simultaneously (26). The method has not been reported in patients with uneven $\dot{V}A/\dot{Q}$ in whom the sloping tracing of expired PA_{CO_2} may introduce large errors and preclude use of this technique. Finally, the graphic analysis of breath-by-breath variations of CO_2 during the rebreathing maneuver used to obtain the pre-rebreathing value of PA_{CO_2} is tedious and not readily reducible to digital computer data processing. The validity of the method has not been reported on by other groups.

MEASUREMENT OF PULMONARY CAPILLARY BLOOD FLOW WITH CHEMICALLY INERT SOLUBLE GASES

Many techniques for measurement of $\dot{Q}c$ are based on the Bornstein modification of the Fick principle. These depend on measuring the uptake of a chemically inert, soluble gas as a function of its alveolar concentration and lung volume. The rationale of these methods rests on the premise that the mixed venous content of the tracer gas is zero. The most widely used methods involve breath-holding and rebreathing procedures and are based on *1)* analyzing the exponential fall of the soluble gas measured by a rapid responding analyzer, *2)* considering the lung volume at which the soluble gas is taken up by the blood through measurement of dilution with an inert, poorly soluble gas, and *3)* correcting for the volume of soluble gas that equilibrates with lung tissue (12, 13, 80). Other methods involving steady-state open-circuit approaches and solutions of $\dot{Q}c$ based on agreement with computer lung model simulations (16, 61, 85) are not popular. Ideally the change in amount and concentration of the inspired soluble gas should be measured prior to the recirculation of the venous blood that might contain the gas. This time is ~13 s at rest and 8 s at heavy exercise (74, 93). Finally, neither the respiratory maneuvers nor the soluble gas utilized should alter $\dot{Q}c$.

As Butler (12) noted, the ideal gas for measurement of $\dot{Q}c$ should be soluble in blood, relatively insoluble in lung tissue, easily analyzed, and completely removed in the body so that the problem of recirculation would not arise. Its solubility should not be influenced by the concentration of hemoglobin. No such gas has been found. The following gases together with their Bunsen solubility coefficients (ml gas/ml blood/760 mmHg at 37°C) fulfill many of the characteristics: *1)* C_2H_2 (0.75), *2)* nitrous oxide (N_2O; 0.47), and *3)* Freon 22 (0.74). At the low concentrations employed in testing, none of these gases appears to affect $\dot{Q}T$ (5, 75, 80). All can be measured with rapid responding devices such as infrared analyzers or mass spectrometers. Gases with higher solubilities, e.g., dimethyl ether, acetone, and ethyl iodide, dissolve in the mucosa of the airways during inspiration and evaporate from the airway wall during expiration, thereby introducing an uncertain error into the measured concentration of their alveolar gas fraction (12, 13, 61). This error appears to be relatively small for dimethyl ether (81). The high lipid solubility of such gases also creates problems because their solution into blood varies with the hematocrit value. Helium and nitrogen are too insoluble in the blood to obtain an accurate measurement of alveolar gas fraction prior to recirculation (9, 12, 13, 64).

Rebreathing, Multiple-Breath-Hold, and Single-Breath Constant Expiratory Methods

The first practical method for measuring $\dot{Q}c$ by analysis of inert-gas uptake was reported by Grollman and associates (40) over half a century ago. It involved rebreathing of C_2H_2 from a bag of ~2.8 liters and analyzing C_2H_2 and O_2 concentrations from two samples obtained ~10 and 20 s after initiation of the rebreathing procedure. The difference between the two samples corrected for solubility of C_2H_2 in blood was assumed to be proportional to the venoarterial difference for O_2. The $\dot{Q}T$ was calculated by dividing this difference into the $\dot{V}_{O_2}$ measured by an open-circuit method prior to rebreathing. No corrections were made for solubility of C_2H_2 in lung tissue. The method generally showed good correlations with the direct Fick method and indicator-dilution methods both at rest and during exercise, but its values were systematically lower, a difference unrelated to venous admixture (1, 93). Cander and Forster (13) pointed out that Grollman's failure to account for solution of C_2H_2 in lung tissue might introduce a 10% underestimation of $\dot{Q}c$. Added to this factor was contamination of the late sample by recirculation, which might cause a 30% underestimation of $\dot{Q}c$. Yuba (94), using gas chromatography for analysis, found agreement between group mean values for the Grollman method and direct Fick method in patients with mitral valve disease and emphysema. However, inspection of their raw data reveals a wide scatter of the Grollman data relative to the Fick data in individuals.

MULTIPLE-BREATH-HOLDING METHOD. Recognizing the problems associated with the Grollman method, Cander and Forster (13) measured the alveolar disappearance of several soluble gases by varying the breath-holding time up to 20 s and analyzing alveolar samples. The alveolar gas fraction of the soluble gas was corrected for dilution by lung volume during breath holding by analyzing the concentration of helium, an insoluble tracer gas. The corrected alveolar gas concentration fraction of its initial alveolar value was plotted against time of breath holding and fitted with a single exponential slope. Acetylene and N_2O were found to be satisfactory test gases and showed a rapid (<1.5 s) initial fall in alveolar concentration, resulting from solution of the gas into pulmonary tissue and capillary blood volume (Vti,c) and a subsequent more gradual decrease related to uptake by $\dot{Q}c$. The capillary blood volume is included in the measurement because the blood in the capillaries but not in the larger vessels equilibrates with soluble gases over the time interval of breath (78, 80).

The equation for solving $\dot{Q}c$ by this method as well as the rebreathing method is

$$\dot{Q}c = \frac{V_A \times 760}{\alpha_{C_2H_2}[F_{A_{C_2H_2}}\text{ intercept}/F_{A(C_2H_2)_0}](P_B - P_{H_2O})} \times \frac{\ln[F_{A_{C_2H_2}}/F_{A(C_2H_2)_0}]}{t}$$

where $\dot{Q}c$ is pulmonary capillary blood flow determined with C_2H_2, V_A is alveolar volume determined by helium dilution, $\alpha_{C_2H_2}$ is the Bunsen solubility coefficient for C_2H_2, $F_{A_{C_2H_2}}$ is the alveolar fraction of C_2H_2 corrected for helium dilution, $F_{A(C_2H_2)_0}$ is the initial fraction, $F_{A_{C_2H_2}}$ intercept is the intercept value corrected for timing from the intercept of $C^{18}O$ disappearance curve, $P_B - P_{H_2O}$ is barometric pressure minus water vapor pressure, and t is time. For calculation of $\dot{Q}c$ with N_2O, values appropriate for this gas would be substituted into the equation. The average values of $\dot{Q}c$ with C_2H_2 and N_2O in five subjects were 3.34 liters·min^{-1}·M^{-2} and 3.28 liters·min^{-1}·M^{-2}, respectively, values similar to those reported by the Fick or indicator-dilution methods. The coefficient of variation for $\dot{Q}c$ was 14% and for pulmonary Vti,c was 22% (13). The multiple-breath-holding technique using C_2H_2 or N_2O has also been used to measure $\dot{Q}c$ in normal subjects during moderate exercise (48).

Inspection of the raw data points depicted in figures published by Cross et al. (22) and Johnson et al. (48) reveals marked uncertainty of the regression slope unless at least four data points are obtained. Values for pulmonary Vti,c in animals on whom postmortem examinations have been performed indicate that the multiple-breath-holding method may underestimate true lung weight in normal dogs by 33% and overestimate it in pulmonary edema by 30% (35, 36). However, this discrepancy would produce an almost imperceptible error in the calculation of $\dot{Q}c$ (81). The multiple-breath-holding procedure is useful for accurately determining the CO disappearance curve from the alveoli, which in turn is used to calculate diffusing capacity (Fig. 7). Since the disappearance curve should intercept at unity, this offers a means to accurately time the start of the disappearance curve of soluble gases to estimate pulmonary tissue volume (34).

Appraisal of multiple-breath-holding method. The advantage of this method is that no assumptions need be made regarding the timing of the start and termination of the breath-holding maneuver, which could be a problem if only one breath-holding time were used. Because in each maneuver the length of breath-holding time (e.g., from the start of breath-hold maneuver at the beginning of expiration or at the point where half the volume has been inspired to the point where the alveolar sample has been collected) can be kept constant, valid slopes and intercepts of the alveolar gas disappearance curve can be obtained. Errors in disregarding the equilibration of the gas with lung tissue and carrying out breath holding beyond recirculation can also be avoided. However, the method has several disadvantages. *1)* The multiple breath holds (4–7) required to construct a gas disappearance curve take a minimum of 20–35 min to accomplish, and duplicate trials at given steady-state conditions would double this time. *2)* It is assumed that a steady state is present during collection for each data point, but this is highly unlikely, particularly during prolonged exercise. *3)* The subject must be highly motivated. *4)* True alveolar samples may be difficult to obtain in patients with $\dot{V}A/\dot{Q}$ inequalities. *5)* Untrained subjects often perform a Valsalva maneuver during breath holding, which might modify $\dot{Q}c$. *6)* Breath holding is difficult for subjects to perform during exercise. *7)* Patients with lung disease may not be able to breath hold even at rest.

REBREATHING METHOD. *Procedure.* Rebreathing from a bag containing C_2H_2, N_2O, dimethyl ether, or Freon 22 with continuous gas sampling or discrete

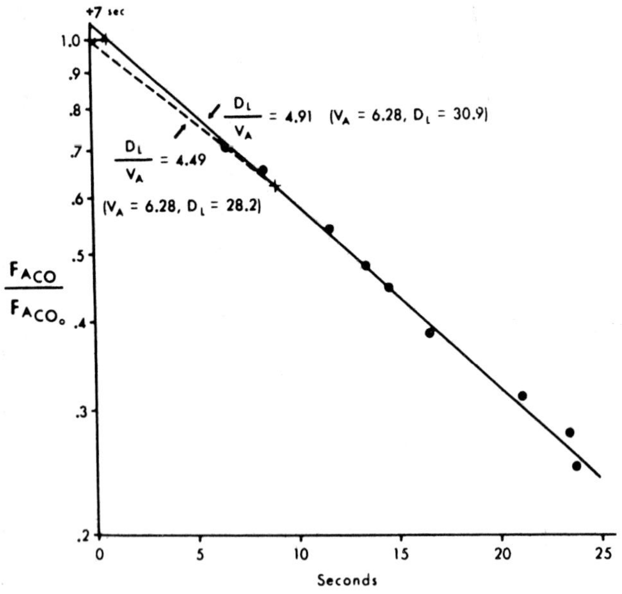

FIG. 7. Carbon monoxide disappearance curve in a normal subject obtained with multiple-breath-holding times. •, Individual data points; +, another data point that might be used to calculate a single-breath diffusing capacity (DL), in which breath-holding varies between 8 and 12 s; ----, slope used for calculation of the latter, because it was assumed that the zero intercept was unity. Because the value at unity was actually +0.7 s, the standard calculation in this example underestimated diffusing capacity by 9%. VA, alveolar volume; $F_{A_{CO}}$, alveolar fraction of CO; $F_{A_{CO_0}}$, intercept value of $F_{A_{CO}}$. [From Sackner et al. (80).]

sampling over selected parts of the breath on a breath-by-breath basis has several advantages over the multiple-breath-holding technique. Estimation of $\dot{Q}c$ and pulmonary Vti,c by rebreathing provides *1)* either a continuous recording, a four- to seven-point alveolar disappearance curve, or a mean integral of the expired soluble gas concentrations, *2)* a recording of the initial and final volumes or continuous recording of volume of the lung-bag system by the dilution of an inert, poorly soluble gas, *3)* collection of the data necessary to calculate $\dot{Q}c$ in 15 s or less, *4)* duplicate values of $\dot{Q}c$ and pulmonary Vti,c from two runs in as short a time as 3–5 min, *5)* minimization of $\dot{V}A/\dot{Q}$ inequalities, *6)* a more natural respiratory maneuver during exercise than breath holding, *7)* simultaneous estimation of $\dot{V}_{O_2}$ as an independent assessment of the steady state, and *8)* application to both healthy and sick infants and adults (3, 9, 16, 20, 69, 80, 87, 88, 94–96). In practice the rebreathing bag is filled with a test gas mixture containing trace amounts of either C_2H_2, N_2O, dimethyl ether, or Freon 22; poorly soluble gases such as He or Ar; and O_2 and N_2. Addition of CO allows calculation of diffusing capacity and a means to estimate timing of the onset of the rebreathing maneuver. The gas mixture is rebreathed, the gases are analyzed with a mass spectrometer, and alveolar disappearance curves for the soluble gases are corrected for dilution and plotted as an exponential function over time. The volume of the rebreathing bag can range from just above the subject's tidal volume to 3.5 liters; this value has not been standardized among investigators. Nominal gas concentrations used in the rebreathing bag range from 0.4% to 1% for C_2H_2, from 5% to 10% for N_2O, and from 3% to 14% for Freon 22. A variation of the rebreathing maneuver to achieve earlier mixing has been reported by Nishida and associates (67, 68). The first breath from the bag is inspired to total lung capacity, and then six-to-seven breaths of one liter are rebreathed and sampled for gas analyses. This modification does not appear to offer any advantage over standard procedures and requires greater cooperation.

The mechanical setup for the rebreathing procedure is simple: a collapsible bag (preferably fabricated from an impermeable material such as Teflon) is connected to a three-way valve that permits the subject to be turned into the system at a desired point in the breathing cycle. For gas analysis a sampling port is located at the mouthpiece and the tubing from this port is connected to a rapid responding gas analyzer. The mass spectrometer is the ideal instrument since its response time is rapid enough to measure changing gas concentrations at rates up to 60 breaths/min or greater and multiple gases can be analyzed. The device removes gas from the bag-lung system at a rate of 15 ml/min; this volume is so small that it can be disregarded in adult testing but not in babies or small animals. Specific infrared analyzers for C_2H_2, N_2O, and Freon 22 have slower response times, and their continuous recording introduces distortions in the slope of the gas disappearance curves at rapid respiratory rates. The equation for solving $\dot{Q}c$ is the same as for the multiple-breath-holding method (see MULTIPLE-BREATH-HOLDING METHOD, p. 241).

The characteristics of soluble gases used in rebreathing estimation of $\dot{Q}c$ include the following. Acetylene has a disagreeable taste, but this tends to disappear with repeated trials. Its solubility coefficient in blood has been determined by many investigators and lies within a narrow range (64). A potential disadvantage is its explosive hazard, but this occurs at concentrations of 2%; lesser concentrations are employed in testing (9). Nitrous oxide has a slightly sweet taste and is nonexplosive but supports combustion and has a well-defined solubility coefficient. Its analysis by mass spectrometry presents a problem when diffusing capacity for CO needs to be determined simultaneously. The mass of CO is near that of N_2O, which prevents the simultaneous estimation of these gases in the usual pulmonary laboratory analyzers. Freon 22 has the advantage of being nonexplosive, but its solubility coefficient has not been well defined. A comparison of $\dot{Q}c$ measured with C_2H_2 or the Fick principle to that measured with Freon 22 reveals that Freon 22 values are systematically lower (9, 42). Bonde-Peterson et al. (9) note that this difference might relate to differences between in vivo and in vitro Bunsen solubility coefficients caused by gas stratification. As Freon molecules are heavier (86.5 g/mol) than C_2H_2 molecules (26.0 g/mol), Freon 22 may concentrate more in the central parts of the acinus. Because end-expiratory gas comes from the peripheral parts of the unit, $\dot{Q}c$ will be underestimated and a spuriously high solubility coefficient will be produced. To reconcile the $\dot{Q}c$ data determined with Freon 22 to standard techniques, the effective Bunsen solubility coefficient should be 0.67 rather than 0.74 as determined in vitro.

Pulmonary tissue volume. The rebreathing method for $\dot{Q}c$ depends in part on the accurate determination of pulmonary Vti,c. Measurement of the latter is based on certain assumptions regarding the time at which the soluble gas dissolves in lung tissue. There is fairly good evidence that once gas has arrived at the level of lung tissue and the capillary blood, its solution is almost instantaneous; the problem is deciding on the exact point of arrival. At the onset of the rebreathing procedure the tracer gas does not reach the tissues as a square wave. The following approaches to timing have been utilized: *1*) the beginning of inspiration, *2*) 0.5 or 0.7 s after the beginning of inspiration, *3*) when half of the inspired volume passes through the combined dead space of the apparatus and an assumed value for the subject's anatomic dead space (body weight in kg × 2.2), and *4*) when the intercept value of the CO disappearance slope equals unity. The last method assumes that at time 0, transfer of CO to the pulmonary capillary blood by the combination of diffusion and chemical reaction is instantaneous, thereby signaling the start of equilibration of the soluble gas with lung tissue (Fig. 8). The stable isotope $C^{18}O$ is used as the tracer because the molecular weights of

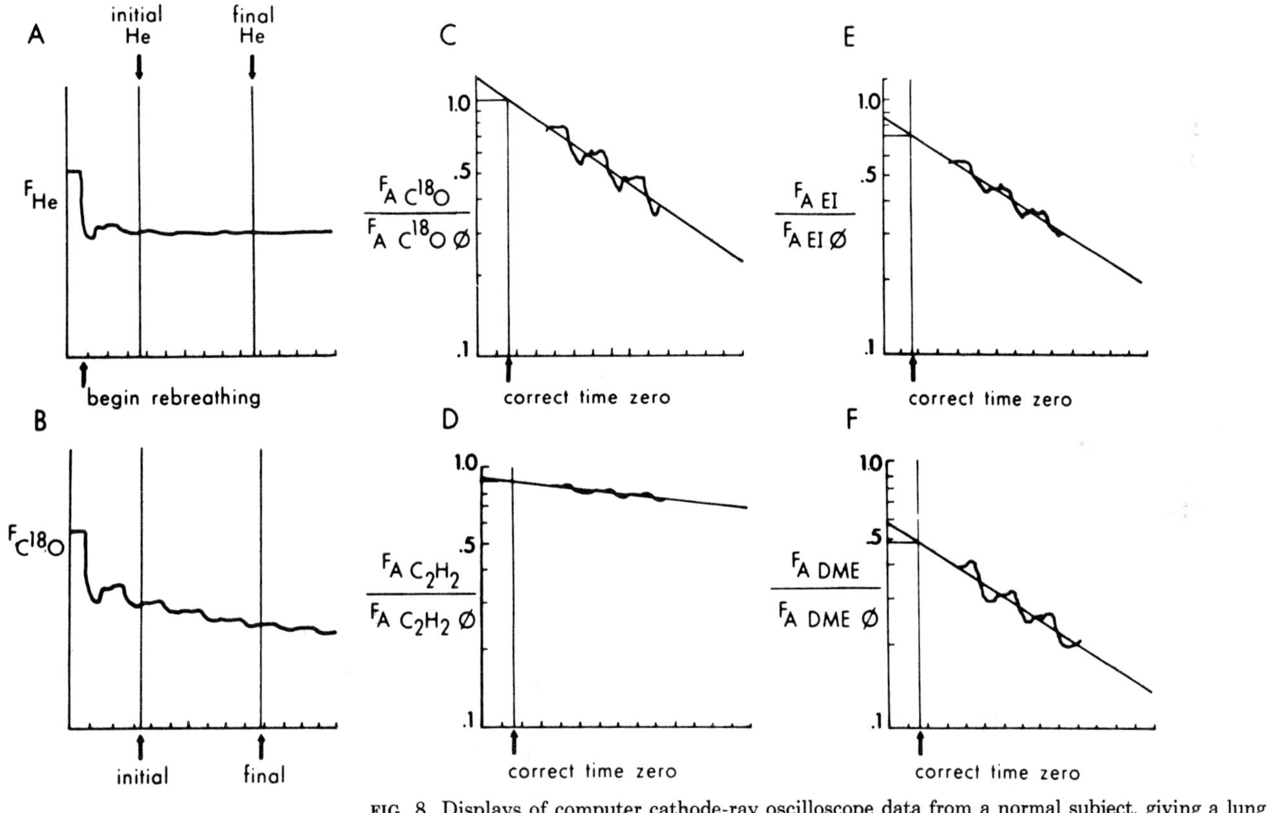

FIG. 8. Displays of computer cathode-ray oscilloscope data from a normal subject, giving a lung volume of 3.16 liters, $\dot{V}_{O_2}$ of 324 ml/min, CO diffusing capacity of 36.7 ml CO·min^{-1}·Torr^{-1}, C_2H_2 $\dot{Q}c$ of 6.37 liters/min, C_2H_2 pulmonary tissue plus capillary blood volume (Vti,c) of 564 ml, and dimethyl ether pulmonary Vti,c of 467 ml. *A*: helium tracing during rebreathing. Oscillations are minimal by third breath. *B*: $C^{18}O$ tracing during rebreathing; *vertical lines*, which delineate least-squares best fit of data, are under program control and modification by operator. Lines are midway between inspiratory and expiratory $C^{18}O$ excursion over an interval of 3 breaths. Incorrect placement of cursors at trough of first and peak of last of these 3 breaths changed least-squares-fit equation to effect an increase in C_2H_2 pulmonary Vti,c of 6%, a decrease in dimethyl ether pulmonary Vti,c of 4%, a fall in C_2H_2 $\dot{Q}c$ of 11%, and a fall in diffusing capacity of 12%. *C*: $C^{18}O$ disappearance curve with least-squares-fit line; real time 0 does not intercept at unity. *D*: C_2H_2 disappearance curve with least-squares-fit line; time 0 is 1.58 s after beginning of rebreathing corrected from $C^{18}O$ intercept of 1.0. Pulmonary Vti,c corrected for time by $C^{18}O$ is 564 ml compared with 404 ml with a real time 0. *E*: ethyl iodide (EI) disappearance curve with its least-squares-fit line. *F*: dimethyl ether (DME) disappearance curve with its least-squares-fit line. Time 0 is 1.58 s after beginning of rebreathing. Pulmonary Vti,c corrected for time by $C^{18}O$ is 457 ml compared with 318 ml with real time 0. [From Sackner et al. (81).]

CO and N_2 are nearly identical at 28 and cannot be distinguished by mass spectrometer analysis (80).

In addition to the problem of deciding on time 0, the least-squares regression equation through all or selected portions of the alveolar disappearance slope of the soluble gas modifies the intercept value and the calculated pulmonary Vti,c. Thus the slope has been computed from *1)* end-tidal values, *2)* last 40 s of expiration data, *3)* last 0.3 s of expiration, *4)* a volume-weighted average of end-inspiratory and end-expiratory concentrations, and *5)* all the points sampled continuously (at 7–20 points/s) (31, 80, 87). Friedman et al. (30) utilized these algorithms to compare the values of pulmonary Vti,c to postmortem lung water measured in control animals and those with oleic acid–induced pulmonary edema. The best correlation among the various methods (96% ± 14% pulmonary Vti,c of lung water) was obtained with the use of all the data points and the $C^{18}O$ intercept determination for fixing time 0.

Both sampling of expiratory data and using the first breath with an assumed dead space overestimates pulmonary Vti,c. The correction of the disappearance slope of $C^{18}O$ to obtain time 0 appears to be more important than utilizing all the samples during rebreathing, since good agreement of pulmonary Vti,c and lung weight during moderate pulmonary edema has been obtained with the use of end-tidal gas concentrations only (29).

The $C^{18}O$ intercept correction for time 0 has also been used for the multiple-breath-holding technique (35), but the values for pulmonary Vti,c so obtained were ~35% higher than with the standard breath-holding method (13) and the rebreathing method (81). This might relate to slight changes in the hemodynamic state during collection of the data, causing slight alterations of the slope of alveolar disappearance of the soluble gas. This would greatly affect the intercept value and have almost no effect on the slope of the disappearance curve and hence the calculated $\dot{Q}c$, because the calculation of pulmonary Vti,c is quite sensitive to slight variations in the intercept value. For example, a coefficient of variation of −5% produces an overestimation of C_2H_2 by 62%. Despite the large variation of pulmonary Vti,c in individuals, the mean values reported by different investigators using different assumptions are similar, i.e., 560 ml with a range from 412 to 692 ml (81). As shown in Figure 9, errors in estimating pulmonary Vti,c by C_2H_2 have minimal impact on calculation of $\dot{Q}c$.

Overland et al. (70) proposed that two soluble gases be used with the multiple-breath-holding or rebreathing procedures. Theoretically this enables calculation of a unique solution of pulmonary Vti,c without resorting to imprecise estimation of the intercept value of one gas by assuming that both gases would give the same pulmonary Vti,c value. However, because of the uncertainty of the tissue and blood solubilities among various combinations of gases (e.g., C_2H_2, dimethyl

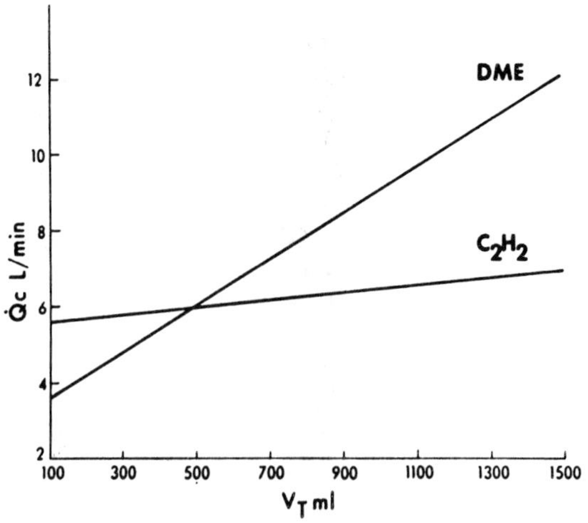

FIG. 9. Theoretical change in pulmonary Vti,c (V_T) on calculation of $\dot{Q}c$. Initial value of $\dot{Q}c$ was taken as 6 liters/min and pulmonary Vti,c as 500 ml. $\dot{Q}c$ data were calculated by keeping the slope of disappearance curves of C_2H_2 and dimethyl ether (DME) constant while varying the value of pulmonary Vti,c. Diagram shows that C_2H_2 $\dot{Q}c$ values are relatively insensitive to changes in pulmonary Vti,c compared with dimethyl ether $\dot{Q}c$. [From Sackner et al. (81).]

ether, and ethyl iodide), this method actually gives less precise and less accurate values than the intercept of alveolar disappearance of C_2H_2 using $C^{18}O$ to estimate time 0 (81). In one study in normal subjects, both C_2H_2 and dimethyl ether were equally acceptable gases for measuring pulmonary Vti,c during rebreathing with $C^{18}O$ as a marker (81). In another study, in both normal subjects and patients with pulmonary edema, C_2H_2 was more suitable than dimethyl ether (71).

Accuracy of rebreathing method. Although much attention has been directed toward accurate estimation of pulmonary Vti,c as a means for early detection of pulmonary edema, inclusion of its value into the equation for $\dot{Q}c$ contributes minimally to the final value of $\dot{Q}c$. If the normal value of 600 ml for pulmonary Vti,c is disregarded, a 7%–12% underestimation of $\dot{Q}c$ at rest for both C_2H_2 and N_2O and <1%–2% at heavy work loads is produced (47, 81, 95). If pulmonary Vti,c in infants is disregarded, $\dot{Q}c$ as measured by Freon 22 might be underestimated by 14% (17). Alternatively, constant values of pulmonary Vti,c can be assumed with little alteration of $\dot{Q}c$ as calculated from the slope of the alveolar disappearance curve of the soluble gas (90). Simultaneous comparisons between the rebreathing method and the indicator-dilution method agree in normal humans and anesthetized animals (80, 88). In isolated perfused lung preparations, $\dot{Q}c$ is consistently greater than pump flow because C_2H_2 disappearance from the lungs is increased by diffusion across the pleura into room air. However, pulmonary Vti,c is still measured with the same degree of reproducibility as in intact animals (21, 29).

Errors of rebreathing method. Petrini et al. (72)

analyzed the errors in $\dot{Q}c$ and pulmonary Vti,c in lung models due to dead space, volume rebreathed, rebreathing frequency, uneven distribution among pulmonary Vti,c and $\dot{Q}c$, ventilation, and alveolar volume. Increases in dead space cause underestimation of $\dot{Q}c$ and overestimation of pulmonary Vti,c, but these errors are minimized by rapid rebreathing with high volumes. However, rebreathing of large tidal volume may produce hemodynamic alterations and a new source of error. Calculations from the lung model indicate that the uneven distribution due to gravitational forces in normal subjects causes <1% error in $\dot{Q}c$. A mathematical lung model of obstructive lung disease constructed from data in the literature indicates that $\dot{Q}c$ might be underestimated by −1% to −18%. Errors in $\dot{Q}c$ in restrictive lung diseases are smaller but are associated with greater errors in computation of pulmonary Vti,c. In vivo data suggest that even fewer errors in $\dot{Q}c$ might occur with the rebreathing method in airway obstruction than predicted by Petrini et al. (72). Thus histamine-induced bronchospasm in sheep, amounting to a sixfold increase of airway resistance, does not affect the simultaneous equality of $\dot{Q}c$ and $\dot{Q}_T$ by rebreathing and thermodilution, respectively, despite marked unevenness of distribution of ventilation (73).

The mean coefficient of variation for multiple determinations of $\dot{Q}c$ with C_2H_2 is 8% with continuous sampling and $C^{18}O$ for time 0 (81) and 12% with a computer analysis least-squares fit of selected points with time 0 defined as the time at which half the tidal volume had passed the combined dead space of the subject and apparatus (69). Corresponding values of $\dot{Q}c$ with dimethyl ether are 12% and 12%, respectively.

Appraisal of rebreathing method. The major problems with the rebreathing method relate to its lack of standardization between normals and patients with cardiopulmonary disease. Thus rebreathing bag volumes ranging from a few hundred milliliters above resting tidal volume to 4 liters have been employed at respiratory frequencies from 12 to 50 breaths/min. Different bag volumes and respiratory rates are selected to maintain a large rebreathing volume for minimization of dead-space volume error and a rapid enough respiratory rate to obtain sufficient data points prior to recirculation. However, both of these variables affect $\dot{Q}c$ estimations. In one study an increase of rebreathing rate from 16 to 38 breaths/min increased $\dot{Q}c$ 34% at a volume of 2 liters and 18% at 4 liters. Doubling of rebreathing volume at 16 breaths/min increased $\dot{Q}c$ 36%, but at 38 breaths/min there was no significant change (58). The rise of $\dot{Q}c$ with increase in rebreathing volumes at the lower respiratory rate is real and not an artifact, since $\dot{V}_{O_2}$ also increases. Larger rebreathing volumes markedly reduce the variability of pulmonary Vti,c measurements (58). Resting values of $\dot{Q}c$ with the rebreathing method are generally higher than with the Fick or indicator-dilution methods because voluntary hyperventilation increases heart rate and $\dot{Q}c$ (23, 51, 72, 80). The latter can be corrected by multiplying $\dot{Q}c$ by the ratio of the $\dot{V}_{O_2}$ during steady-state conditions prior to rebreathing to the $\dot{V}_{O_2}$ during rebreathing (51).

Because an increased respiratory frequency occurs during exercise and this variable must be controlled, an excessive frequency at rest must be employed to keep this variable constant. In one study in which it was desired to compare resting values of $\dot{Q}c$ to exercise values of $\dot{Q}c$, spurious values of pulmonary Vti,c were obtained at rates of 24 breaths/min during exercise due to insufficient collection of data points prior to recirculation at 10 s; therefore a rate of 50 breaths/min was used both at rest and exercise. This caused a rise of resting $\dot{Q}c$ and a falsely greater slope of $\dot{Q}c$ versus $\dot{V}_{O_2}$ (30). In retrospect this effect might have been minimized by maintaining a slower respiratory rate and assuming a value for pulmonary Vti,c. Finally, the rebreathing method requires subject cooperation. The bag must be emptied with each inspiration and respiratory frequency kept constant with the aid of a metronome or a breath-sound simulator (80). However, this is generally not a problem since even patients with moderate-to-severe airway obstruction usually achieve this maneuver with minimal training.

When all the variables of the rebreathing procedure are controlled, the method is ideally suited for studying serial changes in $\dot{Q}c$ over time. With computer data processing, the results of a study are almost immediately available to the investigator. The procedure is far easier for the subject to accomplish and presents less difficulty with data processing than any other method for measuring $\dot{Q}c$ by analysis of alveolar gas exchange. In normal subjects an excellent approximation of $\dot{Q}c$ can be achieved from measuring the slope of the disappearance curve of the soluble gas and assuming a value for pulmonary Vti,c, thereby markedly simplifying the data processing. The method has been utilized to assess serial changes of $\dot{Q}c$ over minutes to hours in the following situations: water immersion (8), intravenous saline loading (27, 60), exercise at ambient and stressful environmental conditions (31, 58), after administration of aerosolized bronchodilators (79), during anesthesia (83), and with cigarette smoking (86).

SINGLE-BREATH CONSTANT EXPIRATORY METHOD. *Procedure.* After exhalation to near residual volume, the subject inspires a test gas mixture consisting of He, O_2, N_2, and trace quantities of C_2H_2 and ^{18}C-labeled CO to near total lung capacity, breath holds two seconds, and then exhales at a constant rate that varies from 200 to 500 ml/s. Theory predicts that $\dot{Q}c$ during a constant expiratory flow can be calculated from the following equation (24)

$$\dot{Q}c = \frac{\dot{V}_E}{\alpha b} \frac{\ln F_A/F_{A_0}}{\ln[(V_A + \alpha tiVti)/(V_{A_0} + \alpha tiVti)]}$$

where $\dot{V}_E$ is expiratory flow rate; αb is the Bunsen coefficient for blood; αti is the Bunsen solubility coefficient for pulmonary tissue; F_A is the alveolar fraction of C_2H_2; $F_{A_0} = F_I \cdot F_{I_{He}}^{-1} \cdot F_{A_{He}}^{-1}$ (where F_I is inspired fraction of C_2H_2, $F_{I_{He}}$ is inspired fraction of He, and $F_{A_{He}}$ is alveolar fraction of He); V_A is alveolar volume; V_{A_0} is V_A at full inspiration and calculated from the formula $V_{A_0} = (V_I - V_{DS})/(F_{I_{He}}/F_{A_{He}})$, where V_I is the inspired volume and V_{DS} is the dead-space volume; and Vti is pulmonary parenchymal tissue volume. Since F_A and V_A can be constantly measured during expiratory flow and the other indices are constant, the slope and intercept for C_2H_2 during expiration may be calculated on the basis of linear regression. Pulmonary parenchymal tissue volume can be measured directly, but because it has only a small effect on the calculation of $\dot{Q}c$ it can be estimated (3.5 g/cm height).

Appraisal of single-breath constant expiratory method. This new method has been reported by a single group of investigators (24) and agrees with thermodilution $\dot{Q}_T$ determinations at rest in cardiac patients. In patients with severe chronic obstructive lung disease (<60% of forced vital capacity expired in 1 s), $\dot{Q}c$ cannot be reproducibly measured. Furthermore, constant expiratory flow during strenuous exercise is difficult to achieve.

Body Plethysmographic Methods

PROCEDURE. In this method the subject is enclosed in an airtight chamber, the body plethysmograph. The soluble gas N_2O, at an inspired concentration of 60%–80%, is inhaled, and its instantaneous beat-by-beat uptake by blood flowing through the pulmonary capillaries is sensed by a sensitive pressure transducer because the chamber pressure becomes negative with respect to atmospheric pressure. Nitrous oxide is the only gas that can be used with this method, since it is nontoxic in the high concentration necessary to sense the small changes in plethysmographic pressure (equivalent to a volume change of ±1 ml). The mean alveolar fraction of N_2O at the time of the study is obtained by a rapid-responding gas analyzer. Pulmonary capillary blood flow is calculated by the Bornstein modification of the Fick principle (59, 75, 91). This assumes that there is no significant recirculation and that the partial pressure of N_2O (P_{N_2O}) in the blood leaving any pulmonary capillary is the same as that in the corresponding alveolus at any instant in time. The formula used is

$$\dot{Q}c = \frac{\dot{V}_{N_2O} \times K \times HR}{\alpha_{N_2O} \times F_{A_{N_2O}}}$$

where $\dot{Q}c$ is the pulmonary capillary blood flow per minute, $\dot{V}_{N_2O}$ is the volume of N_2O absorbed per heartbeat, HR is the heart rate per minute, α_{N_2O} is the Bunsen solubility coefficient of N_2O in blood at 37°C and 1 atm pressure and equals 0.47 ml/ml blood, and $F_{A_{N_2O}}$ is the fraction of N_2O in alveolar gas expressed as the fraction of 1 atm (760 mmHg). The constant K includes the following three corrections. A volume of N_2 approximately equal to 3% of $\dot{V}_{N_2O}$ will diffuse from the blood into the alveoli. This is the result of the P_{N_2} gradient of 250–350 mmHg created by taking the breath of the N_2O-O_2 gas mixture. This volume is predictable from the ratio of solubility coefficients of the two gases and must be added to the measured volume of N_2O absorbed. Because the gas inspired is at room temperature (22°C ± 1°C), the volume must be increased by ~5% to correct it to 37°C. Nitrous oxide leaves the pulmonary parenchyma and enters the alveoli or blood as the alveolar N_2O concentration decreases. Based on a pulmonary Vti,c of 600 ml and a fall of 0.5% in $F_{A_{N_2O}}$ per second when the $\dot{V}_{N_2O}$ is 15 ml/s, this correction is ~8% of $\dot{V}_{N_2O}$. This factor will not change with changes of blood flow since concentration changes parallel volume changes, the proportion remaining constant. This volume also must be added to the volume change. The total of these factors, K, amounts to ~1.16.

CONSIDERATION OF PLETHYSMOGRAPHIC PRESSURE. In addition to the estimation of mean $\dot{Q}c$, the plethysmographic method provides a recording of individual $\dot{Q}c$ pulses. Configuration of these waveforms has potential usefulness regarding the pulmonary hemodynamic status (90). Although this feature is attractive and the principles of the method are simple, major problems with instrumentation and data processing have severely curtailed its application. Sensing of changes in plethysmographic pressure (calculated as a volume with Boyle's law) requires extremely sensitive transducers that respond to the minor environmental pressure changes. Because the subject functions as a heat sink, temperature and relative humidity are altered within the chamber, producing drifts of the DC component of the plethysmographic pressure signal. Therefore the subject must remain within the chamber several minutes until equilibration is achieved. Differential pressure gradients within the chamber are caused by strenuous body movements, and large pressure oscillations occur that cannot be electronically filtered since they lie in the same frequency band as the signal. Subtle alterations of barometric pressure and vibrations from remote machinery within the building can produce low- and high-frequency artifacts.

During breath holding or slow expiration, oscillations of the pressure in the body plethysmograph (calculated as volume) occur as a result of the heartbeat. These oscillations when the lungs are inflated with air are also present with N_2O and must be subtracted on a beat-by-beat basis from the N_2O recording to exclude this mechanical artifact and derive the instantaneous $\dot{V}_{N_2O}$ by the pulmonary capillaries. The subtracting process can be done by hand, but for the method to be practical an interactive computer analysis program is necessary (75).

IMPROVEMENT OF PLETHYSMOGRAPHIC VOLUME AND FLOW SENSING. Several systems have been devised to obtain more stable recordings of the rate of gas uptake. The system devised by Bosman et al. (10) consists of a pneumatic servomechanism that injects or removes air from the body plethysmograph to maintain a constant pressure. The rate of air transfer by the device is recorded continuously. The base line for zero gas uptake is a straight horizontal line, and slow drift due to temperature, humidity, or respiratory quotient effects is seen as a slight displacement of the base line. This approach gives a graphic beat-by-beat display of the $\dot{V}_{N_2O}$, which in turn is proportional to stroke output (Fig. 10). With this method the subject can exhale slowly so that a simultaneous record of the rate of $\dot{V}_{N_2O}$ and alveolar N_2O concentration can be obtained.

The pneumatic servomechanism was later modified and simplified to enable utilization of commercially available components in its fabrication. It initially incorporated a sensitive optical pressure-sensing unit with an operational amplifier. A modified commercially available electropneumatic servomechanism was substituted for the purely pneumatic system (53). Recently a commercially available variable-reluctance differential transducer was substituted for the hand-fabricated optical pressure-sensing unit (75). The electropneumatic servomechanism gives a flat frequency response up to 6–10 Hz, which is more than ample for valid recordings of the $\dot{Q}c$ pulse.

To directly record the derivative of pressure without using a servomechanism, Karatzas et al. (52) designed a pneumatic differentiating circuit. It consisted of a glass capillary tube acting as a pneumatic resistance in the line to one side of a differential pressure transducer connected to the body plethysmograph; the other side was connected directly to the plethysmograph. The size of the capillary tube was chosen to give a frequency response flat to 10 Hz. In this system, plethysmographic pressure was allowed to vary.

Another approach to measurement of the instantaneous rate of $\dot{V}_{N_2O}$ is to utilize a body plethysmograph with a pneumotachograph or fine mesh screen in its wall (54, 89, 90). The differential pressure across the resistance of the screen is calibrated to the rate of airflow in or out of the chamber, permitting plethysmographic pressure to remain approximately atmospheric (Fig. 11). Flow into the box is measured as the primary signal. This produces less noise on the recording than the estimation of flow obtained by calculating or electronically differentiating the volume signal, as originally described by Lee and DuBois (59). However, the frequency response is flat to only 3.5 Hz in contrast to the higher values of 6–10 Hz reported for the electropneumatic servomechanism and pneumatic differentiating methods (52, 53, 75). Furthermore the signal in the flow box is quite sensitive to slight changes in pressure gradients in the room caused by heating and cooling. Frequency response is an indirect function of chamber volume, and the method is only advocated for the small constant-pressure body plethysmographs, i.e., ~350 liter capacity. Since 85%–90% of the harmonic content of the instantaneous $\dot{Q}c$ pulse can be represented by the first five harmonics [Fig. 12; (75)], the flow body plethysmograph might not faithfully depict the wave configuration in the presence of tachycardia. For example, at a pulse rate of 120/min, the plethysmographic pressure or flow transducer should have a flat frequency response to 10 Hz to accurately display the waveform. However, either transducer would still provide accurate estimates of mean $\dot{Q}c$.

RESPIRATORY MANEUVER. Measurement of $\dot{Q}c$ can be obtained with the breath held and glottis open (59) and during slow exhalation and inhalation (10, 75, 76, 89). To ensure stable expiratory or inspiratory flow rates and prevent artifacts from variation in airway resistance, it is best to sense flow with a pneumotachograph and provide the subject with this information through a visual or auditory metering device. Flow rates are generally held between 2 and 3 liters/min (75). The $\dot{Q}c$ has also been measured during normal breathing, but the subject must rebreathe gas from a

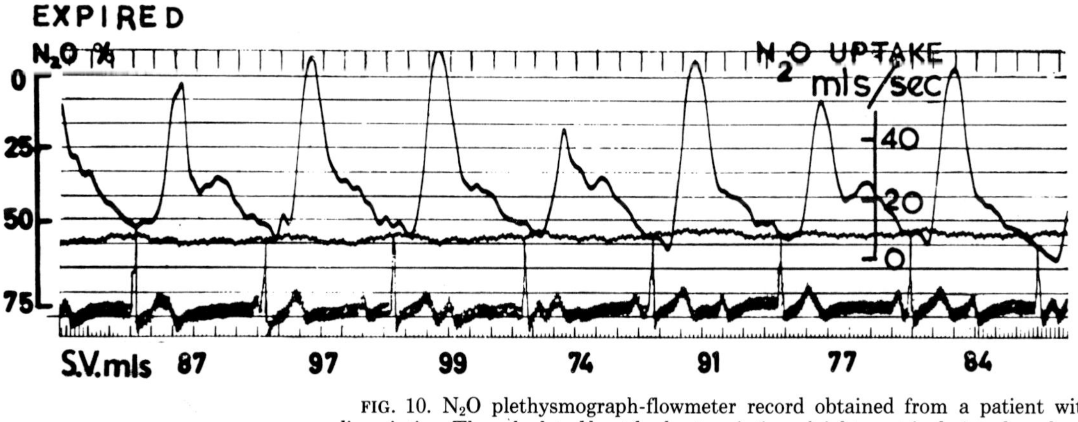

FIG. 10. N_2O plethysmograph-flowmeter record obtained from a patient with atrioventricular dissociation. The calculated beat-by-beat variation of right ventricular stroke volume (S.V., milliliters) is shown below each cardiac cycle. [From Bosman et al. (10). Reprinted by permission from *Clinical Science*, © 1964, The Biochemical Society, London.]

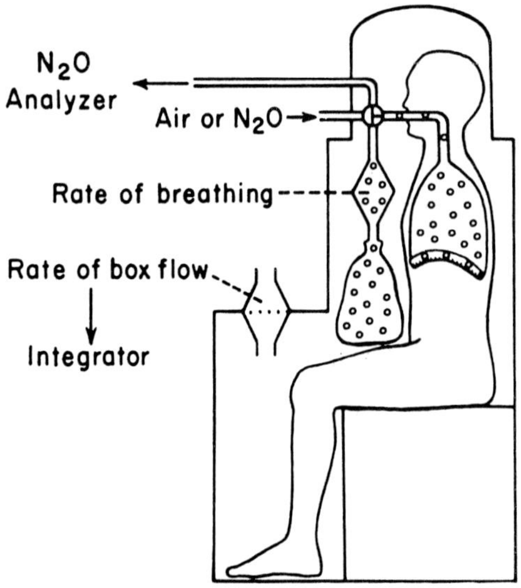

FIG. 11. Flow body plethysmograph. Airflow into box to replace N_2O (○) absorbed is measured by the flowmeter (rate of box flow). Rate of inhalation from or exhalation into bag containing N_2O is measured by the other flowmeter (rate of breathing). Concentration of N_2O at lips is measured by an infrared analyzer. [From Vermeire and Butler (89), by permission of the American Heart Association, Inc.]

bag within the body plethysmograph, which is heated to 37°C by heating coils and saturated with water vapor to minimize pressure fluctuations due to heating and cooling of gas. Wasserman and Naimark (92) believed that $\dot{Q}c$ could not be determined with a closed glottis because the cardiogenic oscillations were accentuated too greatly during air inflation. Since calculated $\dot{Q}c$ is the same whether the glottis is opened or closed in apneic dogs, the problems associated with glottal closure in humans may relate to different degrees of straining between the air and N_2O maneuvers (75).

DATA PROCESSING. During breath holding or slow expiration, oscillations of flow in the body plethysmograph and at the mouth occur as a result of the heartbeat. These mechanical oscillations during breath holding on air are also present during breath holding with N_2O and must be subtracted from the oscillatory signals after inspiration of N_2O to derive the instantaneous uptake of this gas by the pulmonary capillaries. Sackner et al. (75) adopted the following approach to data processing. Since each N_2O pulse is synchronous with the heartbeat but the heart rate is not usually exactly regular, air pulses must be subtracted from N_2O pulses on a beat-by-beat basis. It is assumed that the onset of these pulses bears a constant time relationship to the QRS complex of the electrocardiogram. Therefore the subtraction process is begun from the R wave of the electrocardiogram and terminated with the R wave accompanying the next N_2O pulse. If the air pulse is longer than the N_2O pulse, the subtraction terminates at the end of the N_2O pulse and the remaining data of the air pulse are discarded. If the air pulse is shorter than the N_2O pulse, an average level from the end of the air pulse is subtracted from the N_2O pulse. This produces a degree of uncertainty for the flow at the end of a heartbeat, which is not important since at this time $\dot{V}_{N_2O}$ is near the minimum. Unless there is an irregular cardiac rhythm, it is easier to average several pulses on air and to subtract this average pulse from the average of several N_2O pulses, being careful to select the pulses from the same time periods of the run. The average instantaneous rate of $\dot{V}_{N_2O}$ is then converted to $\dot{Q}c$ by dividing each data point by the mean FA_{N_2O} times α_{N_2O}. The average FA_{N_2O} is obtained by taking the mean FA_{N_2O} of the initial or beginning exhalate with the final concentration at termination of the maneuver or from the continuous recording of FA_{N_2O} as the subject slowly exhales and adjusting the values of FA_{N_2O} for each pulse to account for the time delay of gas analysis. The integral of the instantaneous blood flow with each pulse is stroke volume, which when multiplied by heart rate equals $\dot{Q}c$.

REPRODUCIBILITY AND ACCURACY. Sackner et al. (75) measured $\dot{Q}c$ at intervals over a 25- to 35-min period in normal adults in the sitting and supine positions. For the supine position the average deviation from the mean of two determinations of $\dot{Q}c$ was 3% and for the sitting position 9%. In anesthetized dogs there is excellent agreement between $\dot{Q}c$ plus right-to-left shunt and $\dot{Q}T$ measured by indicator dilution (16, 75). Compared to the rebreathing estimates of resting $\dot{Q}c$, values determined with body plethysmographic measurements are generally lower and more comparable to indicator-dilution and direct Fick methods. This difference is related to the respiratory maneuvers in this method, which are analogous to quiet breathing, in contrast to the rapid rebreathing of large volumes in the rebreathing techniques for estimating $\dot{Q}c$.

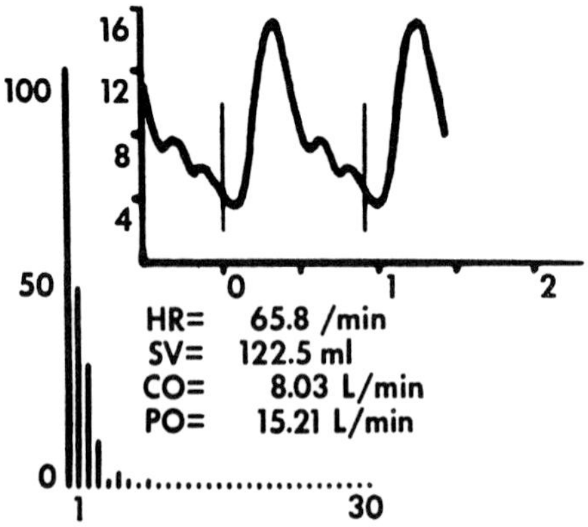

FIG. 12. Computer display (*upper right*) of average pulmonary capillary blood flow pulse from 6 supine normal subjects together with the Fourier analysis. *Two vertical bars*, R-R interval; *y*-axis, blood flow in liters per minute; *x*-axis, time in seconds. HR, heart rate; SV, stroke volume; CO, mean pulmonary capillary blood flow; PO, peak pulmonary capillary blood flow. *Bar graph* (*left*), Fourier analysis: *y*-axis, percent of total harmonic content; *x*-axis, harmonics from 1 to 30. [From Sackner et al. (75).]

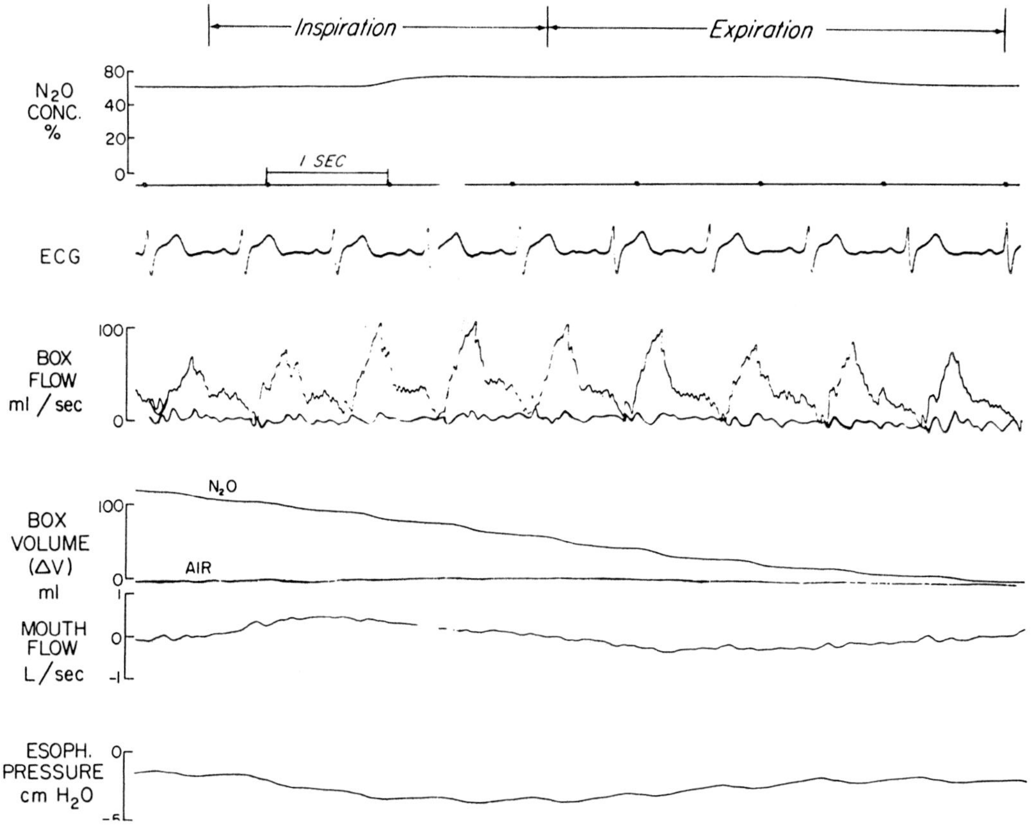

FIG. 13. Effect of respiration on pulmonary capillary blood flow. Plethysmographic tracing during one respiratory cycle. Control (air) box flow and volume recordings are traced on the N_2O record. Difference between 2 box flow tracings represents instantaneous capillary blood flow. [From Astrom et al. (2).]

APPLICATIONS. During inspiration, expiration, and changes in body posture, $\dot{Q}c$ has been measured with the body plethysmographic techniques. The $\dot{Q}c$ generally rises during tidal inspiration and falls with expiration (Fig. 13). With deep inspiration and expiration, there is no clear relationship between intrapleural pressure and $\dot{Q}c$ (2, 89). Passive tilting to the upright position produces marked falls in $\dot{Q}c$, which can be blunted by inflation of an antigravity suit [Fig. 14; (7, 84)]. Several investigators (75, 76, 90) have analyzed the configuration of the pulmonary capillary waveform to indirectly assess the mechanical properties of the pulmonary blood vessels, but discussion of the interpretation of waveform changes is not included in this chapter. Serial measurements of $\dot{Q}c$ have also been made during administration of pharmacologic agents affecting $\dot{Q}$T (76, 89). Measurements of $\dot{Q}c$ have been obtained immediately after isometric or limited isotonic exercise but not during active isotonic exercise (84).

APPRAISAL. The advantages of measuring $\dot{Q}c$ with the N_2O body plethysmographic method include *1*) the ability to estimate $\dot{Q}c$ under basal conditions, *2*) high reproducibility and repeatability at short intervals, *3*) assessment of postural changes that are not masked by increases of $\dot{Q}c$ induced by rebreathing, *4*) estimations within selected portions of the tidal volume, *5*) analysis of stroke volume on a beat-by-beat basis, and *6*) display of the $\dot{Q}c$ waveform. The disadvantages include *1*) the subject must be confined to an airtight chamber, *2*) the breathing maneuvers require training, *3*) two identical breathing maneuvers must be performed in sequence, one on air and one on N_2O, *4*) $\dot{Q}c$ cannot be determined during moderate-to-heavy isotonic exercise, *5*) sensations produced by N_2O inhalation may be unpleasant, and *6*) complex data processing and sophisticated instrumentation are required.

Substitution of Thorax for Body Plethysmograph

GLOTTIS OPEN, THORACIC VOLUME CONSTANT. *Principles.* In the conventional body plethysmographic method a sensitive gauge measures the decrease in gas pressure in an airtight chamber as N_2O molecules leave the alveolar gas and dissolve in the pulmonary capillary blood. In the spirometric or pneumotachographic methods the rigid body plethysmograph is replaced with the subject's own thorax. As molecules of N_2O leave the alveoli and dissolve in the pulmonary

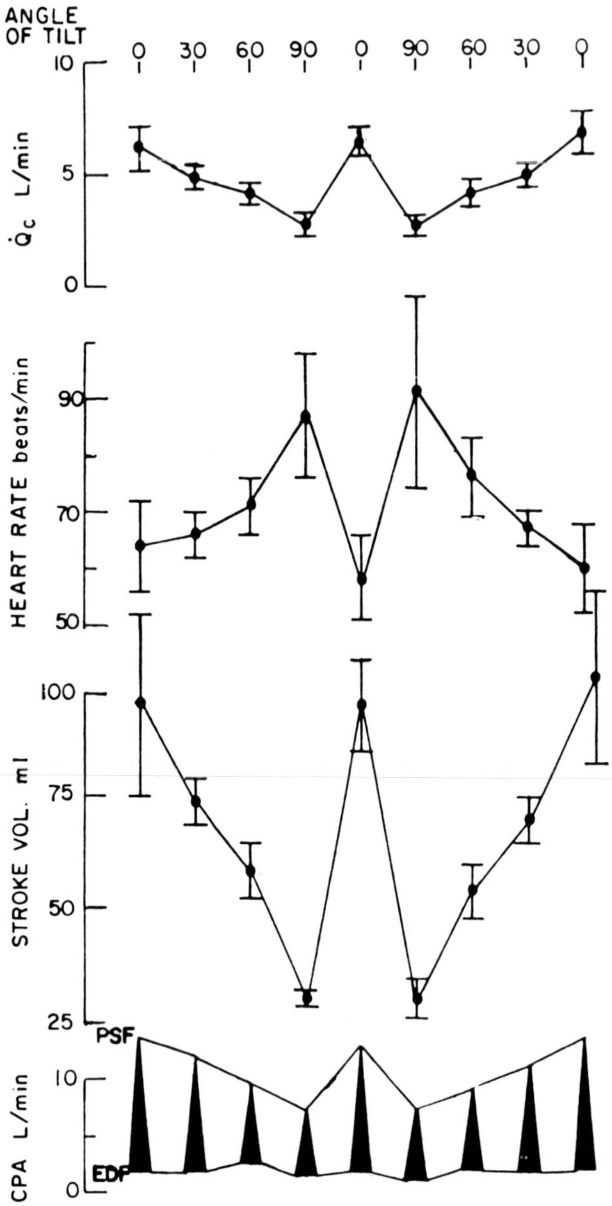

FIG. 14. Effects of tilting from supine (0°) to vertical position (90°) on pulmonary capillary blood flow ($\dot{Q}c$), heart rate, stroke volume, peak systolic flow (PSF), end-diastolic flow (EDF), and capillary pulse amplitude (CPA). Values are means in 4 normal subjects. *Vertical bars*, standard deviations. [From Segel et al. (84).]

capillary blood, alveolar gas pressure decreases and draws gas into the the alveoli from the airway, which can be recorded with the spirometer or pneumotachograph. The actual change in alveolar gas pressure is insignificant because of the low impedance of this system. The change in spirometric volume or pneumotachographic airflow reflects the exchange of gas molecules between alveoli and blood as the thoracic volume remains constant. An important requirement of the method is that the subject hold the breath at constant thoracic volume so that the change in volume or airflow reflects gas uptake only.

Figure 15 shows the spirometric, thoracic volume pneumographic, and electrocardiographic recordings during a control period of breath holding. Both the thoracic volume pneumographic and spirometric tracings show oscillations synchronous with the heartbeat, but the thoracic volume remains almost constant from beat to beat at comparable points in the heart cycle. With N_2O the thoracic volume remains constant but the spirometric tracing shows a rapid decrease in volume, with superimposed oscillations synchronous with the heartbeat. Overall the Krogh spirometer during air breath holding moves upward and then slowly downward as a function of R, whereas with N_2O it moves downward as N_2O is taken up in the pulmonary capillaries (90). It is important that the spirometer be the Krogh type, since inertia of conventional water displacement or rolling seal models prevents response to the small volume changes produced by cardiogenic oscillations and $\dot{V}_{N_2O}$. On the other hand, any small pneumotachograph can be used if it is desired to monitor airflow rather than volume change during breath holding.

This method is difficult to utilize in conscious subjects who require much training to relax their respiratory muscles while maintaining the glottis opened but does not pose a problem in the anesthetized, paralyzed state (16, 39, 75). The flow into the airway after a breath of either air or N_2O, as measured with pneumotachography, has a much greater pulsatility than is seen during conventional body plethysmography. The difference between the air and N_2O recordings may be difficult to discern (Fig. 16). However, subtraction of the flow tracing during breath holding on air from that after N_2O produces a pulsatile waveform of $\dot{Q}c$. Because of the low signal-to-noise ratio in the recordings (i.e., small signal due to $\dot{V}_{N_2O}$ and large signal due to cardiogenic oscillations) the final waveform is often distorted, although the stroke volume agrees with the indicator-dilution method (39, 77).

Appraisal. This method has three advantages: *1)* the instrumentation is simpler than the body plethysmograph, *2)* the subject is not confined to a small enclosed space, and *3)* $\dot{Q}c$ can be measured in anesthetized, paralyzed patients in the operating room and in selected patients on mechanical ventilators. It has four disadvantages: *1)* much training of the conscious subject is required, i.e., the glottis must be kept open and the rib cage–abdominal musculature relaxed so that a constant thoracic volume is maintained, *2)* the method can only be used during breath holding, *3)* it cannot be utilized during exercise, and *4)* there is a tendency for distortion of the $\dot{Q}c$ waveform, particularly when $\dot{Q}c$ is reduced.

GLOTTIS CLOSED, THORACIC VOLUME VARIABLE. *Principles.* In these methods, the $\dot{V}_{N_2O}$ is reflected by a shrinking of thoracic volume, which is sensed by an external device placed over the rib cage–abdominal system. As in conventional methods, a recording is

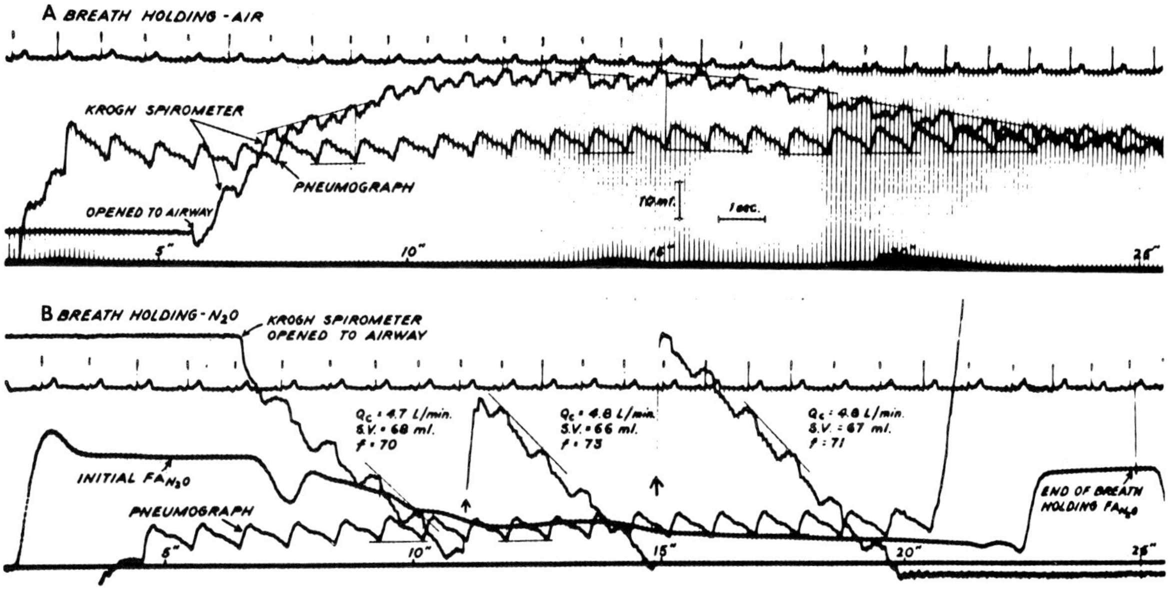

FIG. 15. Typical record of a well-trained subject during breath holding after a breath of air (*A*) and N_2O (*B*). *Horizontal lines* drawn on the pneumograph tracing indicate that breath holding was precise. Lines perpendicular to *x*-axis are drawn to the spirometer tracing through corresponding points of successive heartbeats. Slope drawn through points where perpendiculars intercept the spirometer tracing is a measure of the net rate of gas exchange. Spirometer tracing was replaced in position when it reached the lower edge of the record. $\dot{Q}c$, capillary blood flow; SV, stroke volume; f, frequency; FA_{N_2O}, alveolar fraction of N_2O. [From Wasserman and Comroe (91).]

first made during breath holding with air and then with N_2O. The volume changes on air are subtracted from N_2O and $\dot{Q}c$ is calculated with the Bornstein equation.

Capacitance plethysmography. This method has been utilized only in anesthetized dogs. A sensitive, temperature-stable meter is connected to a wire mesh screen (30 × 15 cm) shielded at the top and sides (4). The screen is positioned ~25 cm above the dog's torso, and the meter is also connected directly to the dog via a skin electrode. The test animal serves as a variable surface-area component (variable capacitor electrode) and the wire screen as a constant-reference component (fixed capacitor electrode) in a two-plate capacitor system. The principles of capacitance plethysmography are similar to those for a parallel-plate capacitor system where the dielectric properties of living tissue are used as part of the capacitor. Capacitance varies inversely with the distance between the plates and directly with changes in surface area and physical characteristics of the dielectric material. Respiratory movements alter the capacitance of the system by varying the area, separation, and distribution of the dielectric material. The distance from the torso to the fixed electrode is adjusted by trial and error to produce a nearly linear calibration and a large signal-to-noise ratio. To calibrate the device, air volumes ranging from 5 to 100 ml are introduced into the endotracheal tube of the anesthetized dog (4).

The testing procedure consists of passively hyperventilating the dog for 10 s with ambient air and then allowing passive exhalation to the functional residual capacity level. The endotracheal tube is clamped for 15 s and changes of thoracic volume are recorded. Hyperventilation and passive expiration are repeated and a 500-ml bolus of a mixture of 80% N_2O and 20% O_2 is then introduced through the endotracheal tube, 300 ml are withdrawn, and a 20-ml pre-breath-holding sample of alveolar gas is collected for FA_{N_2O} analysis. The dog is allowed to passively return to functional residual capacity and the endotracheal tube is clamped for 15 s while thoracic volume changes are recorded. Gas is then withdrawn for analysis of FA_{N_2O} and $\dot{Q}c$ is

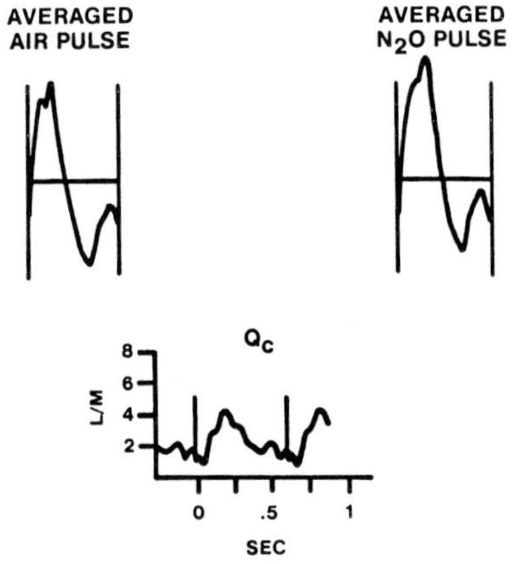

FIG. 16. Computer displays of pneumotachographic tracings at airway in an anesthetized, paralyzed patient. *Upper left*, air pulse; *upper right*, N_2O pulse. *Bottom*: pulmonary capillary blood flow ($\dot{Q}c$) obtained by subtracting air pulse from N_2O pulse and converting to $\dot{Q}c$ through the standard N_2O equation; *y*-axis, $\dot{Q}c$ in liters/minute; and *x*-axis, time in seconds. *Vertical bars*, R-R interval of electrocardiogram. [From Greenberg et al. (39).]

calculated by the Bornstein equation. There is good agreement between this method and the indicator-dilution method for estimation of $\dot{Q}_T$ (4).

Appraisal. This method has not been reported in conscious humans in whom slight shifts of body position might alter the volume calibration of the device.

Respiratory inductive plethysmography. This device consists of two coils of Teflon-insulated wire sewn onto elastic cloth bands encircling the rib cage and the abdomen. The leads from the wires are connected to an oscillator module. Changes in cross-sectional area of the rib cage and abdominal compartments change the self-inductance of electrical oscillations from the coils, which is demodulated. These signals can be calibrated to volume change with spirometry. To increase the sensitivity for detection of $\dot{V}_{N_2O}$ during breath holding, a further gain adjustment is made by equating the volume of air inspired from a spirometer exactly equivalent to the volume added to the respiratory inductive plethysmograph during the air breath-holding maneuver. This gain is kept constant during the N_2O run. The subject first inspires air to total lung capacity, exhales to functional residual capacity, and a valve is turned to produce closure of the airway; the subject relaxes against the closed airway with the glottis open so that mouth pressure can be recorded to ensure that the patient is not straining. The mean slope of the thoracic volume is measured over the first 4–8 s of breath holding. This maneuver is repeated with inspiration of a mixture of 80% N_2O and 20% O_2. The breath-holding slope of air is subtracted from N_2O and the result divided by the product of the $F_{A_{N_2O}}$ and solubility coefficient of N_2O in blood to yield $\dot{Q}c$. For measurement of the pulsatility of $\dot{Q}c$, the signals are passed through analog or digital differentiators (82).

Simultaneous measurements of $\dot{Q}c$ with body plethysmography and respiratory inductive plethysmography fall within 20% of a line of identity. For analysis of waveform, respiratory inductive plethysmography accentuates pulse amplitude probably because of underdampening of the signal by the chest wall; i.e., the rib cage–abdominal system coupled to the respiratory inductive plethysmograph functions as a semirigid body plethysmograph.

In addition to measurement of $\dot{Q}c$, analysis of $\dot{V}_{N_2O}$ at end inspiration can be used to calculate pulmonary Vti,c. The respiratory inductive plethysmographic volume after N_2O inhalation is smaller than the volume of gas recorded with spirometry. By utilizing $F_{A_{N_2O}}$ and α_{N_2O} and correcting for $\dot{V}_{N_2O}$ by $\dot{Q}c$, pulmonary Vti,c can be calculated. Although values similar to those reported with the rebreathing procedure are obtained, the variability of this method is much greater than with the rebreathing technique (82).

Appraisal. The advantages and disadvantages of this method are similar to those of the spirometric-pneumotachographic methods carried out with the glottis open and thoracic volume kept constant during breath holding. With both these methods there is a distinct advantage over the standard body plethysmographic method. The latter requires the subject to be confined to a chamber for several minutes to achieve temperature and humidity stability. Even then, variability in the slope of the recording with air due to temperature and humidity alterations can be marked. The subtraction of the air from the N_2O slope can cause an error in the estimation of $\dot{V}_{N_2O}$. Respiratory inductive plethysmography eliminates this problem since the changes in the air control slope during breath holding are solely related to changes in the gas-exchange ratio and not to the external environment. The method requires training to achieve relaxation against a closed airway and cannot be used in the anxious, tachypneic patient. Furthermore the breath-holding procedure does not allow the method to be utilized during exercise. Finally, the shape of the $\dot{Q}c$ pulse is distorted.

Vital Capacity N_2O Spirometric Method

PRINCIPLE. When a subject performs a vital capacity maneuver with air as the test gas, the volume expired essentially equals the volume inspired and the spirographic tracing returns to the original base line; when N_2O is substituted for air in the spirometer, the volume expired is less than the volume inspired and the spirographic tracing does not return to its original base line. This difference can be attributed to *1)* absorption of N_2O by blood perfusing the pulmonary capillaries and *2)* absorption of N_2O by the lung tissues. Rigatto et al. (74) reported that the lung tissues did not absorb "a significant amount of N_2O during a single breath of this gas." Therefore they believed that the difference between the volume of N_2O inspired and the volume expired during the vital capacity maneuver measured the volume of N_2O taken up by pulmonary blood flow. Although others have convincingly demonstrated that lung tissue takes up N_2O (13, 21, 77), their neglect of this correction to $\dot{Q}c$ would introduce an error amounting to <10%.

PROCEDURE. The volume of N_2O absorbed during the test is obtained by *1)* measuring the difference between initial and final base lines when the vital capacity maneuver was performed with N_2O as the test gas, *2)* subtracting from that value the difference between initial and final base lines observed when the vital capacity had been performed with air as the test gas, and *3)* multiplying the difference between *1)* and *2)* by the correction factor for nitrogen eliminated during the test on inspiring N_2O. The duration of the vital capacity maneuver is measured from the spirographic tracing. To the measured time, 0.75 s is added to correct for the N_2O absorbed by the blood remaining in the pulmonary capillary bed at the test termination. This correction factor corresponds to the mean time that blood is believed to spend in the pulmonary capillary bed.

From the volume of N_2O absorbed during the test and the duration of the test, the volume of N_2O absorbed per minute ($\dot{V}_{N_2O}$) is calculated. This is divided by the Bunsen solubility coefficient of N_2O times the calculated value of FA_{N_2O} during inspiration. The latter is measured from an equation that involves the inspired concentration of N_2O, the volume of N_2O inspired, and the residual volume. The values of $\dot{Q}c$ determined in this way correlate well with the direct Fick method and are reproducible.

APPRAISAL. The method has the advantages of *1)* simplicity of instrumentation and *2)* fairly simple data processing. Its disadvantages include *1)* excellent cooperation is required for accurate performance of the vital capacity maneuver, *2)* N_2O equilibration with tissue volume is neglected, *3)* it cannot be used in patients with lung disease who have uneven distribution of $\dot{V}A/\dot{Q}$, and *4)* it cannot be used during exercise.

SUMMARY

The ideal method for estimation of mean $\dot{Q}c$ from analysis of alveolar gas exchange has not been discovered. From the standpoint of ease of performance and reproducibility under diverse conditions and in health and disease, the rebreathing of the chemically inert soluble gas C_2H_2, with appropriate corrections for dilution by the lung volume and absorption by lung tissue, appears to offer the best approach. Standardization and publication of $\dot{Q}c$ values in normal humans utilizing this procedure remain a priority.

This study was supported partly by Grant HL-10622 from the National Heart, Lung, and Blood Institute.

REFERENCES

1. ASMUSSEN, E., AND M. NIELSEN. The cardiac output in rest and work determined simultaneously by the acetylene and the dye injection methods. *Acta Physiol. Scand.* 27: 217–230, 1953.
2. ASTROM, H. R., K.-H. LIN, AND M. B. MCILROY. Pulmonary capillary blood flow during normal spontaneous breathing in man. *J. Appl. Physiol.* 35: 823–829, 1973.
3. AYOTTE, B., J. SEYMOUR, AND M. B. MCILROY. A new method for measurement of cardiac output with nitrous oxide. *J. Appl. Physiol.* 28: 863–866, 1970.
4. BARROW, R. E., AND M. D. SHULT. Atraumatic measuring of pulmonary capillary blood flow in dogs. *J. Appl. Physiol.* 42: 980–984, 1977.
5. BAYLEY, T., J. A. CLEMENTS, AND A. J. OSBAHR. Pulmonary and circulatory effects of fibrinopeptides. *Circ. Res.* 21: 469–485, 1967.
6. BECKLAKE, M. R., C. J. VARVIS, L. D. PENGELLY, S. KENNING, M. MCGREGOR, AND D. V. BATES. Measurement of pulmonary blood flow during exercise using nitrous oxide. *J. Appl. Physiol.* 17: 579–586, 1962.
7. BEGIN, R., R. DOUGHERTY, E. D. MICHAELSON, AND M. A. SACKNER. Effect of sequential anti-G suit inflation on pulmonary capillary blood flow in man. *Aviat. Space Environ. Med.* 47: 937–941, 1976.
8. BEGIN, R., M. EPSTEIN, M. A. SACKNER, R. LEVINSON, R. DOUGHERTY, AND D. DUNCAN. Effects of water immersion to the neck on pulmonary circulation and tissue volume in man. *J. Appl. Physiol.* 40: 293–299, 1976.
9. BONDE-PETERSEN, F., P. NORSK, AND Y. SUZUKI. A comparison between Freon and acetylene rebreathing for measuring cardiac output. *Aviat. Space Environ. Med.* 51: 1214–1221, 1980.
10. BOSMAN, A. R., A. J. HONOUR, G. DE J. LEE, R. MARSHALL, AND F. D. STOTT. A method for measuring instantaneous pulmonary capillary blood flow and right ventricular stroke volume in man. *Clin. Sci.* 26: 247–260, 1964.
11. BUDERER, M. C., J. A. RUMMEL, C. F. SAWIN, AND D. G. MAULDIN. Use of the single-breath method of estimating cardiac output during exercise-stress testing. *Aerospace Med.* 44: 756–760, 1973.
12. BUTLER, J. Measurement of cardiac output using soluble gases. In: *Handbook of Physiology. Respiration*, edited by W. O. Fenn and H. Rahn. Washington, DC: Am. Physiol. Soc., 1965, sect. 3, vol. II, chapt. 62, p. 1489–1503.
13. CANDER, L., AND R. E. FORSTER. Determination of pulmonary parenchymal tissue volume and pulmonary capillary blood flow in man. *J. Appl. Physiol.* 14: 541–551, 1959.
14. CERRETELLI, P., J. C. CRUZ, L. E. FARHI, AND H. RAHN. Determination of mixed venous O_2 and CO_2 tensions and cardiac output by a rebreathing method. *Respir. Physiol.* 1: 258–264, 1966.
15. CHEN, H., N. P. SILVERTON, AND R. HAINSWORTH. Evaluation of a method for estimating cardiac output from a single breath in humans. *J. Appl. Physiol.* 53: 1034–1038, 1982.
16. CHENEY, F. W., S. TAKAHASHI, AND J. BUTLER. Comparison of two methods of measuring pulmonary capillary blood flow in dogs. *J. Appl. Physiol.* 27: 127–131, 1969.
17. CHU, J., J. A. CLEMENTS, E. K. COTTON, M. H. KLAUS, A. Y. SWEET, W. H. TOOLEY, B. L. BRADLEY, AND L. C. BRANDORFF. Neonatal pulmonary ischemia. I. Clinical and physiological studies. *Pediatrics* 40, Suppl.: 709–728, 1967.
18. CLAUSEN, J. P., O. A. LARSEN, AND J. TRAP-JENSEN. Cardiac output in middle-aged patients determined with CO_2 rebreathing method. *J. Appl. Physiol.* 28: 337–342, 1970.
19. CLODE, M., T. J. H. CLARK, AND E. J. M. CAMPBELL. The immediate CO_2 storage capacity of the body during exercise. *Clin. Sci.* 32: 161–165, 1967.
20. COTTON, E. K., J. J. COGSWELL, B. CHIR, G. J. A. CROPP, AND R. LOSEY. Measurements of effective pulmonary blood flow in the normal newborn human infant. *Pediatrics* 47: 520–528, 1971.
21. CRAPO, R. O., J. D. CRAPO, A. H. MORRIS, S. L. BERLIN, AND W. C. DEVRIES. Pulmonary tissue volume in isolated perfused dog lungs. *J. Appl. Physiol.* 48: 799–801, 1980.
22. CROSS, C. E., H. GONG, JR., C. J. KURPERSHOEK, J. R. GILLESPIE, AND R. W. HYDE. Alterations in distribution of blood flow to the lung's diffusion surfaces during exercise. *J. Clin. Invest.* 52: 414–421, 1973.
23. DONEVAN, R. E., N. M. ANDERSON, P. SEKELJ, O. PAPP, AND M. MCGREGOR. Influence of voluntary hyperventilation on cardiac output. *J. Appl. Physiol.* 17: 487–491, 1962.
24. ELKAYAM, U., A. F. WILSON, J. MORRISON, P. MELTZER, J. DAVIS, P. KLOSTERMAN, J. LOUVIER, AND W. L. HENRY. Noninvasive measurement of cardiac output by a single breath constant expiratory technique. *Thorax* 39: 107–113, 1984.
25. FARHI, L. E., AND P. HAAB. Mixed venous blood gas tensions and cardiac output by "bloodless" methods; recent developments and appraisal. *Respir. Physiol.* 2: 225–233, 1967.
26. FARHI, L. E., M. S. NESARAJAH, A. J. OLSZOWKA, L. A. METILDI, AND A. K. ELLIS. Cardiac output determination by simple one-step rebreathing technique. *Respir. Physiol.* 28: 141–159, 1976.

27. FARNEY, R. J., A. H. MORRIS, R. M. GARDNER, AND J. D. ARMSTRONG, JR. Rebreathing pulmonary capillary and tissue volume in normals after saline infusion. *J. Appl. Physiol.* 43: 246–253, 1977.
28. FEISAL, K. A., M. A. SACKNER, AND A. B. DUBOIS. Comparison between the time available and the time required for CO_2 equilibration in the lung. *J. Clin. Invest.* 42: 24–28, 1963.
29. FELTON, C. R., AND W. G. JOHANSON, JR. Lung tissue volume during development of edema in isolated canine lungs. *J. Appl. Physiol.* 48: 1038–1044, 1980.
30. FRIEDMAN, M., S. H. KAUFMAN, AND S. A. WILKINS, JR. Analysis of rebreathing measurements of pulmonary tissue volume in pulmonary edema. *J. Appl. Physiol.* 48: 66–71, 1980.
31. FRIEDMAN, M., K. L. KOVITZ, S. D. MILLER, M. MARKS, AND M. A. SACKNER. Hemodynamics in teenagers and asthmatic children during exercise. *J. Appl. Physiol.* 46: 293–297, 1979.
32. GEDEON, A., L. FORSLUND, G. G. HEDENSTIERNA, AND E. ROMANO. A new method for noninvasive bedside determination of pulmonary blood flow. *Med. Biol. Eng. Comput.* 18: 411–418, 1980.
33. GILBERT, R., AND J. H. AUCHINCLOSS, JR. Comparison of single-breath and indicator-dilution measurement of cardiac output. *J. Appl. Physiol.* 29: 119–122, 1970.
34. GLAUSER, F. L., AND A. F. WILSON. Pulmonary parenchymal tissue volume in normal subjects. The effect of age and sex. *Chest* 72: 207–212, 1977.
35. GLAUSER, F. L., A. F. WILSON, L. CAROTHERS, J. HIGI, D. WHITE, AND J. DAVIS. Pulmonary parenchymal tissue volume measurements in graded degrees of pulmonary edema in dogs. *Circ. Res.* 36: 229–235, 1975.
36. GLAUSER, F. L., A. F. WILSON, M. HOSHIKO, M. WATANABE, AND J. DAVIS. Pulmonary parenchymal tissue (Vt) changes in pulmonary edema. *J. Appl. Physiol.* 36: 648–652, 1974.
37. GODFREY, S. Manipulation of the indirect Fick principle by a digital computer program for calculation of exercise physiology results. *Respiration* 27: 513–532, 1970.
38. GODFREY, S., AND E. WOLF. An evaluation of rebreathing methods for measuring mixed venous P_{CO_2} during exercise. *Clin. Sci. Mol. Med.* 42: 345–353, 1972.
39. GREENBERG, J. J., F. J. HILDNER, S. MILLER, F. N. FIRESTONE, AND M. A. SACKNER. Preoperative and postoperative cardiac output determinations using an instantaneous pulmonary capillary blood flow method. *Ann. Thorac. Surg.* 12: 639–648, 1971.
40. GROLLMAN, A. The determination of the cardiac output of man by the use of acetylene. *J. Biol. Chem.* 88: 432–445, 1929.
41. GRØNLUND, J. Errors due to data reduction in single-breath method for measurement of pulmonary blood flow. *J. Appl. Physiol.* 52: 104–108, 1982.
42. HENEGHAN, C. P. H., AND M. A. BRANTHWAITE. Non-invasive measurement of cardiac output during anaesthesia. An evaluation of the soluble gas uptake method. *Br. J. Anaesth.* 53: 351–355, 1981.
43. HERWAARDEM, A. VAN, R. A. BINKHORST, J. F. M. FENNIS, AND A. VAN'T LAAR. Reliability of the cardiac output measurement. The indirect Fick-principle for CO_2 during exercise. *Pfluegers Arch.* 385: 21–23, 1980.
44. HLASTALA, M. P., B. WRANNE, AND C. J. LENFANT. Single-breath method of measuring cardiac output—a reevaluation. *J. Appl. Physiol.* 33: 846–848, 1972.
45. HYDE, R. W., R. J. M. PUY, W. F. RAUB, AND R. E. FORSTER. Rate of disappearance of labeled carbon dioxide from the lungs of humans during breath holding: a method for studying the dynamics of pulmonary CO_2 exchange. *J. Clin. Invest.* 47: 1535–1552, 1968.
46. INMAN, M. D., R. L. HUGHSON, AND N. L. JONES. Comparison of cardiac output during exercise by single-breath and CO_2-rebreathing methods. *J. Appl. Physiol.* 58: 1372–1377, 1985.
47. JERNERUS, R., G. LUNDIN, AND L. G. C. F. PUGH. Solubility of acetylene in lung tissue as an error in cardiac output determination with the acetylene method. *Acta Physiol. Scand.* 59: 1–6, 1963.
48. JOHNSON, R. L., JR., W. S. SPICER, J. M. BISHOP, AND R. E. FORSTER. Pulmonary capillary blood volume, flow and diffusing capacity during exercise. *J. Appl. Physiol.* 15: 893–902, 1960.
49. JONES, N. L., E. J. M. CAMPBELL, G. J. R. MCHARDY, B. E. HIGGS, AND M. CLODE. The estimation of carbon dioxide pressure of mixed venous blood during exercise. *Clin. Sci.* 32: 311–327, 1967.
50. JONES, N. L., G. J. R. MCHARDY, A. NAIMARK, AND E. J. M. CAMPBELL. Physiological dead space and alveolar-arterial gas pressure differences during exercise. *Clin. Sci.* 34: 19–29, 1966.
51. KANSTRUP, I. L., AND I. HALLBÄCK. Cardiac output measured by acetylene rebreathing technique at rest and during exercise. Comparison of results obtained by various calculation procedures. *Pfluegers Arch.* 390: 179–185, 1981.
52. KARATZAS, N. B., J. A. CLEMENTS, AND M. B. MCILROY. A pressure plethysmograph with a pneumatic differentiator for pulmonary capillary flow measurements. *J. Appl. Physiol.* 26: 385–388, 1969.
53. KARATZAS, N. B., G. DE J. LEE, AND F. D. STOTT. A new electropneumatic flowmeter for the body plethysmograph. *J. Appl. Physiol.* 23: 276–278, 1967.
54. KAWAKAMI, Y., A. SHIDA, AND M. MURAO. The effects of posture on capillary blood flow pulse and gas exchange in the lungs of man. *Jpn. Circ. J.* 44: 327–333, 1980.
55. KIBBY, P. M. A mathematical model for CO_2 exchange during the initial stages of rebreathing. *Respir. Physiol.* 3: 243–255, 1967.
56. KIM, T. S., H. RAHN, AND L. E. FARHI. Estimation of true venous and arterial P_{CO_2} by gas analysis of a single breath. *J. Appl. Physiol.* 21: 1338–1344, 1966.
57. KLAUSEN, K. Comparison of CO_2 rebreathing and acetylene methods for cardiac output. *J. Appl. Physiol.* 20: 763–766, 1965.
58. KÜNG, M., L. TACHMES, S. J. BIRCH, R. J. FERNANDEZ, W. M. ABRAHAM, AND M. A. SACKNER. Hemodynamics at rest and during exercise in comfortable, hot and cold environments. Measurement with a rebreathing technique. *Bull. Eur. Physiopathol. Respir.* 16: 429–441, 1980.
59. LEE, G. DE J., AND A. B. DUBOIS. Pulmonary capillary blood flow in man. *J. Clin. Invest.* 36: 1380–1390, 1955.
60. LEVINSON, R., M. EPSTEIN, M. A. SACKNER, AND R. BEGIN. Comparison of the effects of water immersion and saline infusion on central haemodynamics in man. *Clin. Sci. Mol. Med.* 52: 343–350, 1977.
61. LUIJENDIJK, S. C. M., A. ZWART, A. M. VAN DER KOOIJ, AND W. R. DE VRIES. Evaluation of alveolar amplitude response technique for determination of lung perfusion in exercise. *J. Appl. Physiol.* 50: 1071–1078, 1981.
62. MAHLER, D. A., R. A. MATTHAY, P. E. SNYDER, R. K. NEFF, AND J. LOKE. Determination of cardiac output at rest and during exercise by carbon dioxide rebreathing method in obstructive airway disease. *Am. Rev. Respir. Dis.* 131: 73–78, 1985.
63. MCHARDY, G. J. R. The relationship between the differences in pressure and content of carbon dioxide in arterial and venous blood. *Clin. Sci.* 32: 299–309, 1967.
64. MEYER, M., AND P. SCHEID. Solubility of acetylene in human blood determined by mass spectrometry. *J. Appl. Physiol.* 48: 1035–1037, 1980.
65. MOHAMMED, M. M. J., AND R. HAINSWORTH. Evaluation using dogs of a method for estimating mixed venous and arterial P_{CO_2} from a single breath. *J. Appl. Physiol.* 50: 196–199, 1981.
66. MOHAMMED, M. M. J., L. M. WOOD, AND R. HAINSWORTH. Evaluation using dogs of a method for estimating cardiac output from a single breath. *J. Appl. Physiol.* 50: 200–202, 1981.
67. NISHIDA, O. Determination of pulmonary parenchymal tissue volume and pulmonary blood volume by the partial rebreathing technique. *Saishin Igaku* 26: 1184–1190, 1971.
68. NISHIDA, O., M. TAKANO, T. YOSHIMI, N. SEWAKE, AND Y. NISHIMOTO. Determination of pulmonary diffusing capacity, membrane diffusing capacity, and pulmonary capillary blood volume by partial rebreathing technique. *Hiroshima J. Med. Sci.* 22: 17–28, 1973.

69. OVERLAND, E. S., R. N. GUPTA, G. J. HUCHON, AND J. F. MURRAY. Measurement of pulmonary tissue volume and blood flow in persons with normal and edematous lungs. *J. Appl. Physiol.* 51: 1375–1383, 1981.
70. OVERLAND, E. S., G. M. OZANNE, AND J. W. SEVERINGHAUS. A single-breath method for determining lung weight and pulmonary blood flow from the differential uptake of two soluble gases (Abstract). *Physiologist* 18: 341, 1975.
71. PETERSON, B. T., M. F. PETRINI, R. W. HYDE, AND B. F. SCHREINER. Pulmonary tissue volume in dogs during pulmonary edema. *J. Appl. Physiol.* 44: 782–794, 1978.
72. PETRINI, M. F., B. T. PETERSON, AND R. W. HYDE. Lung tissue volume and blood flow by rebreathing: theory. *J. Appl. Physiol.* 44: 795–802, 1978.
73. REINHART, M. E., J. R. HUGHES, M. KÜNG, W. M. ABRAHAM, T. AHMED, P. EYRE, AND A. WANNER. Determination of pulmonary blood flow by the rebreathing technique in airflow obstruction. *Am. Rev. Respir. Dis.* 120: 533–540, 1979.
74. RIGATTO, M., G. M. TURINO, AND A. P. FISHMAN. Determination of the pulmonary capillary blood flow in man. *Circulation* 9: 945–962, 1961.
75. SACKNER, M. A., R. DOUGHERTY, N. ATKINS, D. CULVER, D. POOLE, F. D. STOTT, AND A. WANNER. Techniques of pulmonary capillary blood flow determination. *Bull. Physio-Pathol. Respir.* 9: 1189–1202, 1973.
76. SACKNER, M. A., R. DOUGHERTY, H. WATSON, AND A. WANNER. Hemodynamic effects of epinephrine and terbutaline in normal man. *Chest* 68: 616–624, 1975.
77. SACKNER, M. A., K. A. FEISAL, AND A. B. DUBOIS. Determination of tissue volume and carbon dioxide dissociation slope of the lungs in man. *J. Appl. Physiol.* 19: 374–380, 1964.
78. SACKNER, M. A., K. A. FEISAL, AND D. N. KARSCH. Size of gas exchange vessels in the lung. *J. Clin. Invest.* 43: 1847–1855, 1964.
79. SACKNER, M. A., M. FRIEDMAN, G. SILVA, AND R. FERNANDEZ. The pulmonary hemodynamic effects of aerosols of isoproterenol and ipratropium in normal subjects and patients with reversible airway obstruction. *Am. Rev. Respir. Dis.* 116: 1013–1022, 1977.
80. SACKNER, M. A., D. GREENELTCH, M. S. HEIMAN, S. EPSTEIN, AND N. ATKINS. Diffusing capacity, membrane diffusing capacity, capillary blood volume, pulmonary tissue volume, and cardiac output measured by a rebreathing technique. *Am. Rev. Respir. Dis.* 111: 157–165, 1975.
81. SACKNER, M. A., G. MARKWELL, N. ATKINS, S. J. BIRCH, AND R. J. FERNANDEZ. Rebreathing techniques for pulmonary capillary blood flow and tissue volume. *J. Appl. Physiol.* 49: 910–915, 1980.
82. SACKNER, M. A., A. RAO, M. J. BROUDY, H. JONES, H. WATSON, AND M. A. COHN. Measurement of pulmonary tissue volume and capillary blood flow by a single breath respiratory inductive plethysmograph method. *Prog. Respir. Res.* 16: 271–274, 1981.
83. SALT, J. C., J. W. W. GOTHARD, AND M. A. BRANTHWAITE. Pulmonary blood flow and tissue volume. *Anesthesia* 35: 1054–1059, 1980.
84. SEGEL, N., R. DOUGHERTY, AND M. A. SACKNER. Effects of tilting on pulmonary capillary blood flow in normal man. *J. Appl. Physiol.* 35: 244–249, 1973.
85. STOUT, R. L., H. U. WESSEL, AND M. H. PAUL. Pulmonary blood flow determined by continuous analysis of pulmonary N_2O exchange. *J. Appl. Physiol.* 38: 913–918, 1975.
86. TACHMES, L., R. J. FERNANDEZ, AND M. A. SACKNER. Hemodynamic effects of smoking cigarettes of high and low nicotine content. *Chest* 74: 243–246, 1978.
87. TEICHMANN, J., F. ADARO, A. VEICSTEINAS, P. CERRETELLI, AND J. PIIPER. Determination of pulmonary blood flow by rebreathing of soluble inert gases. *Respiration* 31: 296–309, 1974.
88. TRIEBWASSER, J. H., R. L. JOHNSON, JR., R. P. BURPO, J. C. CAMPBELL, W. C. REARDON, AND C. G. BLOMQVIST. Noninvasive determination of cardiac output by a modified acetylene rebreathing procedure utilizing mass spectrometer measurements. *Aviat. Space Environ. Med.* 48: 203–209, 1977.
89. VERMEIRE, P., AND J. BUTLER. Effect of respiration on pulmonary capillary blood flow in man. *Circ. Res.* 22: 299–308, 1968.
90. WASSERMAN, K., J. BUTLER, AND A. VAN KESSEL. Factors affecting the pulmonary capillary blood flow pulse in man. *J. Appl. Physiol.* 21: 890–900, 1966.
91. WASSERMAN, K., AND J. H. COMROE, JR. A method for estimating instantaneous pulmonary capillary blood flow in man. *J. Clin. Invest.* 41: 401–410, 1962.
92. WASSERMAN, K., AND A. NAIMARK. Effect of a closed glottis on pressure oscillations in the body plethysmograph. *J. Appl. Physiol.* 17: 574–575, 1962.
93. WERKO, L., S. BERSEUS, AND H. LAGERLOF. A comparison of the direct Fick and the Grollman methods for determination of the cardiac output in man. *J. Clin. Invest.* 28: 516–520, 1949.
94. YUBA, K. A study on the pulmonary functions and the pulmonary circulation in cardio-pulmonary diseases. II. Pulmonary capillary blood flow and pulmonary capillary mean transit time in cardio-pulmonary diseases. *Jpn. Circ. J.* 35: 1399–1409, 1971.
95. ZEIDIFARD, E., AND C. T. DAVIES. An assessment of a N_2O rebreathing method for the estimation of cardiac output during severe exercise. *Ergonomics* 21: 567–572, 1978.
96. ZEIDIFARD, E., S. GODFREY, AND E. E. DAVIES. Estimation of cardiac output by an N_2O rebreathing method in adults and children. *J. Appl. Physiol.* 41: 433–438, 1976.

Peripheral inert-gas exchange

PETER D. WAGNER | *Department of Medicine, Section of Physiology, University of California at San Diego, La Jolla, California*

CHAPTER CONTENTS

AT FIRST GLANCE it might seem that the subject of inert-gas exchange in peripheral body tissues is of limited interest and relevant only to a few specialized areas of research. However, the literature abounds with concepts, situations, therapeutic measures, phenomena, and experimental techniques that are critically dependent on how inert gases are taken up or cleared from one or more tissue elements. This vast field is brought together in Table 1. The table lists categories in which inert gases are used simply as tools (tissue blood flow and volume estimates) and in which the behavior of inert gases is studied to learn about fundamental factors involved in peripheral gas exchange and anesthesia. Accordingly, knowledge of peripheral inert-gas exchange is important to scientists interested in tissue physiology, to physiologists concerned with several aspects of diving and altitude function and safety, to clinicians interested in assessing organ blood flow and function, and to anesthesiologists concerned with mechanisms of, rates of induction of, and recovery from anesthesia.

Not all of these diverse areas can be discussed in a single chapter. Thus this chapter deals with the fundamental concepts of tissue inert-gas exchange first under the simplest assumptions and subsequently by incorporating more realistic features. In this way the reader should develop an understanding of how the kinetic aspects of tissue inert-gas exchange are determined. This should have the natural consequence of allowing the reader to critically evaluate popular methods that use tissue inert-gas exchange as a tool for studying organ function. The chapter proceeds by presenting basic principles and integrating them with references to the wealth of supporting original research.

BASIC PRINCIPLES OF PERIPHERAL TISSUE EXCHANGE

This section develops a simple mathematical model of peripheral tissue inert-gas exchange in accordance with the assumptions listed below. The model is by no means original and in fact is no more than the application of simple pharmacokinetic principles of mass balance to perfusion-limited (rather than diffusion-limited) systems. This model or its variants have been published previously by many workers. The most well-known contributions to the field, listed chronologically, are

Zuntz (95)	1897
Von Schrotter (90)	1906
Haggard (30)	1924
Teorell (86)	1937
Smith and Morales (83)	1944
Jones (37)	1950
Kety (41)	1951
Mapleson (56)	1963
Eger (24)	1963
Landahl (46)	1963
Crane et al. (20)	1968
Cowles et al. (17)	1968
Ashman et al. (3)	1970
Waud and Waud (91)	1970
Zwart et al. (96)	1972

TABLE 1. *Areas of Application of Peripheral Tissue Inert-Gas Exchange*

Study of Fundamental Factors in Peripheral Gas Exchange
Basic principles of uptake or elimination by convection
Multicompartment considerations (functional heterogeneity within/between tissues)
Roles of diffusion and of perfusion in gas exchange
Perfusional and diffusional tissue "shunts"
Hyperbaric and Hypobaric Considerations
Decompression consequences
Narcosis
Central nervous system effects
Effect on body cavities
Counterdiffusion
Anesthetic Considerations
Quantitative factors in anesthetic uptake and elimination
Molecular mechanisms of anesthesia
Applications of Tissue Inert-Gas Exchange
Estimation of tissue compartment volumes
Estimation of organ perfusion
Skeletal muscular
Gastrointestinal tract
Myocardial
Cerebral
Renal
Placento-uterine
Fat
Skin and subcutaneous
Prostatic
Pancreatic
Joint
Hepatic
Splenic
Bone
Bladder
Testicular
Oral mucosa
Maxillary sinus
Radioactive Gas Tissue Dosimetry
Krypton
Xenon

The simplest construct for studying peripheral tissue exchange is shown in Figure 1. A single capillary perfuses a single tissue element. The following assumptions are made: *1*) at any point in time, the tissue element is spatially (both radially and axially) homogeneous with respect to the inert-gas partial pressure in tissue (Pti); *2*) at any point in time, inert-gas partial pressure in capillary blood (Pc) is homogeneous along the capillary and equals the effluent partial pressure in the venous blood (Pv) draining the tissue, i.e., Pc = Pv; *3*) Pti and Pc, although separately defined, are in diffusive equilibrium at any point in time, i.e., Pti = Pc; *4*) a single tissue-blood partition coefficient (λti) exists for all components of the tissue elements; *5*) there is no shunting of blood around the tissue element directly from arterial to venous sites; *6*) the inflow arterial and outflow venous vessels are sufficiently thick walled and distant enough from each other that there is no diffusion of inert gases directly between arterial and venous vessels, i.e., no "diffusional shunt"; *7*) there is no diffusion of gas between the tissue under consideration and any neighboring tissue; *8*) a single homogeneous capillary-tissue element is sufficient to account for peripheral gas exchange—there are no parallel (or serial) tissue elements of different functional characteristics simultaneously present; *9*) global variables important to inert-gas exchange are constant in time [specifically these are capillary blood flow ($\dot{Q}$), λti, and tissue volume (Vti)]; and *10*) capillary blood volume is negligibly small compared with Vti. These assumptions essentially ignore geometry, rates of diffusion, inhomogeneity of tissue blood flow and blood volume, and potential direct movement of gases between inflow arterial and outflow venous channels.

If we accept for now these simplifying assumptions, mass-balance principles can be applied to the washin (or washout) of an inert gas to determine the rate of rise (or fall) of Pti. Consider that before washin arterial partial pressure (Pa), Pti, and Pv (Fig. 1) are zero. Then, at time $t = 0$, suppose Pa is increased to a constant value >0. The question posed is, What will be the rate of rise of inert-gas Pti (which will, by assumption *3*, identically equal the rate of rise of Pc)? The question can be answered with mass-balance equations.

1. The rate of delivery of gas to the tissue element from arterial blood ($\dot{V}$in) is

$$\dot{V}\text{in} = \text{Pv} \times \beta \times \dot{Q} \tag{1}$$

2. The rate of removal of gas by means of effluent venous blood ($\dot{V}$out) is

$$\dot{V}\text{out} = \text{Pc} \times \beta \times \dot{Q} \tag{2}$$

3. The rate of buildup of gas into the tissue element ($\dot{V}$b) is

$$\dot{V}\text{b} = \frac{d\text{Pti}}{dt} \times \alpha \times \text{Vti} \tag{3}$$

where α and β are the tissue and blood solubilities of the gas, respectively, such that $\lambda\text{ti} = \alpha/\beta$ (or tissue-blood partition coefficient). As long as the units for Pa, Pv, and Pti are all the same, it does not matter what units are chosen. The same is true for the units of time and for the volume elements ($\dot{Q}$ and Vti) in Equations 1–3. Thus, if $\dot{Q}$ is given in liters/minute, Vti should be in liters and time (t in Eq. 3) should be in minutes. Similarly the units of α and β should be the same.

To conserve mass at all points in time, delivery (Eq. 1) must equal the sum of removal (Eq. 2) and storage (Eq. 3). Thus

$$\text{Pa} \times \beta \times \dot{Q} = (\text{Pv} \times \beta \times \dot{Q}) + \left(\frac{d\text{Pti}}{dt} \times \alpha \times \text{Vti}\right) \tag{4}$$

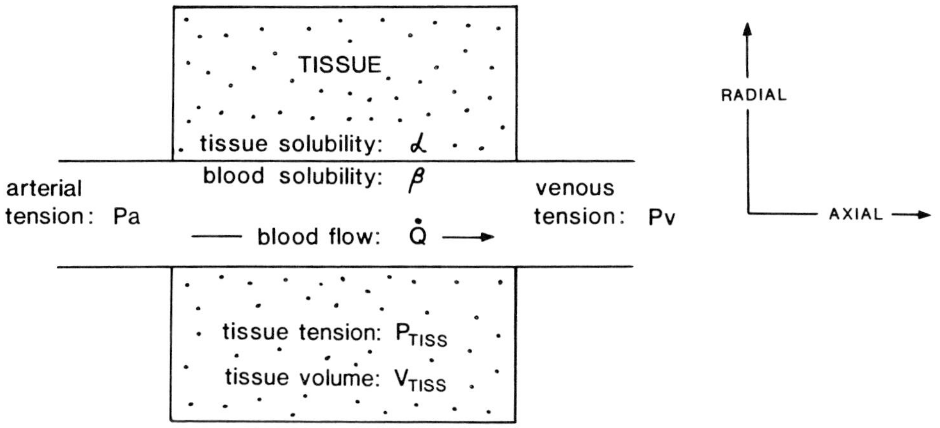

FIG. 1. Important variables in peripheral tissue gas exchange. In this simplest model, tissue tension (Pti) of a gas is uniform both in radial and in axial directions at any point in time. Tissue is characterized by its volume (Vti), blood flow ($\dot{Q}$), and solubility (α) for the gas. For blood solubility β, ability of blood to transport gas is $\beta\dot{Q}$. Storage capability of tissue for gas is αVti. Washin or washout of gas in such tissue is exponential, and exponent is $\dot{Q}/(\lambda\text{ti}\text{Vti})$, where λti is ratio of α to β and is known as tissue-blood partition coefficient of gas. Pa, inflowing arterial tension of gas; Pv, outflowing venous tension of gas.

We can simplify this equation considerably by replacing Pv by Pti (assumption *3*) and α/β by λti and then rearranging terms

$$\frac{d\text{Pti}}{dt} \times \lambda\text{ti} \times \text{Vti} = (\text{Pa} - \text{Pti})\dot{Q} \quad (5)$$

Because Pa is by assumption constant in time, (dPa/dt) = 0, so that adding $-(d\text{Pa}/dt) \times \lambda\text{ti} \times \text{Vti}$ to the left side of Equation 5 still allows equality. Hence

$$\frac{d(\text{Pti} - \text{Pa})}{dt} \times \lambda\text{ti} \times \text{Vti} = (\text{Pa} - \text{Pti})\dot{Q} \quad (6)$$

If we further simplify Equation 6 by setting $Y = \text{Pa} - \text{Pti}$, we have

$$\frac{dY}{dt} = -\frac{Y\dot{Q}}{\lambda\text{ti}\text{Vti}} \quad (7)$$

In Equation 7, which is a simple linear first-order differential equation of Y as a function of t, the variables $\dot{Q}$, λti, and Vti are constant. Of fundamental importance is the realization that $\beta\dot{Q}$ is by definition the conductance capability of the system [i.e., $\beta\dot{Q}$ represents transporting capacity (per mmHg inert-gas partial pressure) of blood for inert gas], whereas αVti is the capacitance of the tissue [i.e., αVti represents storage capacity of tissue (per mmHg inert-gas partial pressure) for inert gas]. Because $\beta\dot{Q}/(\alpha\text{Vti}) = \dot{Q}/(\lambda\text{ti}\text{Vti})$, the coefficient of Y on the right side of Equation 7 is the ratio of the conductance to the capacitance of the tissue system depicted in Figure 1. This ratio may be modified in more complex treatments of the subject, but the kinetics of inert-gas exchange between a compartment (tissue, lung) and its environment (ignoring diffusion limitation) is always governed by an exponential equation (see Eq. 9) whose exponent(s) represents some form of the conductance-capacitance ratio(s).

This is easy to understand intuitively as well: for a highly perfused tissue of small volume and a low ratio of tissue to blood solubility (low λti), one would expect rapid equilibration of blood and tissue. The converse would apply to a poorly perfused tissue of large volume and high λti. Thus, during anesthetic uptake of a fat-soluble gas such as halothane, one would expect the heart tissue to equilibrate with arterial blood levels far more rapidly than would fat tissue.

However, Equation 7 shows that what is important are not the absolute values of tissue blood flow, volume, or partition coefficient but the compound ratio $\dot{Q}/(\lambda\text{ti}\text{Vti})$. To return to Equation 7, this differential expression can be easily integrated to give a useful relationship

$$\int \frac{dY}{dt}\,dt = -\int \frac{Y\dot{Q}}{\lambda\text{ti}\text{Vti}}\,dt$$

or

$$\int \frac{dY}{Y} = -\int \frac{\dot{Q}}{\lambda\text{ti}\text{Vti}}\,dt$$

which after integration yields

$$\ln(Y) = -\frac{\dot{Q}t}{\lambda\text{ti}\text{Vti}} + k \quad (8)$$

where k is the constant of integration; k is determined from the boundary conditions, which in this example specify that at $t = 0$ (start of washin) the value of Pti is zero. Consequently, at $t = 0$, $Y = \text{Pa}$, and thus $k = \ln(\text{Pa})$. Substituting Pa − Pti for Y gives from Equation 8

$$\ln(\text{Pa} - \text{Pti}) = \ln(\text{Pa}) - \frac{\dot{Q}t}{\lambda\text{tiVti}}$$

that when exponentiated yields

$$\frac{\text{Pa} - \text{Pti}}{\text{Pa}} = \exp\left(-\frac{\dot{Q}t}{\lambda\text{tiVti}}\right)$$

or after rearrangement

$$\begin{aligned}\text{Pti} &= \text{Pa}\left[1 - \exp\left(-\frac{\dot{Q}t}{\lambda\text{tiVti}}\right)\right] \\ &= \text{Pc} = \text{Pv}\end{aligned} \tag{9}$$

Notice that Equation 9 predicts correctly that, when $t = 0$ at the very start of the washin, Pti = 0 and that, when $t = \infty$, Pa = Pc = Pti. That is, when $t = \infty$, there will be equilibration of partial pressure between tissue and inflowing arterial blood or in other words the tissue will have been saturated with the inert gas.

The interested reader could derive the corresponding result for the washout of a gas from an equilibrated tissue element under the same assumptions by following the identical sequence of steps beginning with the mass-balance statement of Equations 1–3, redefined for the case of a washout. If at time $t > 0$ the inflowing arterial blood is totally devoid of inert gas, the mass-balance statement would simply equate Equations 2 and 3 (because Pa = 0). Similar treatment thereafter will lead to

$$\text{Pti} = \text{Pti}_0 \times \exp\left(-\frac{\dot{Q}t}{\lambda\text{tiVti}}\right) \tag{10}$$

where Pti_0 is the tissue inert-gas partial pressure immediately before the start of the washout.

A number of important conclusions should be made from inspection of Equations 9 and 10. *1)* Washin and washout of homogeneous tissues in which diffusive equilibration is instantaneous and in which geometrical factors are negligible are both monoexponential functions. *2)* The exponent of the washout (or its half time, $t_{1/2} = 0.693\lambda\text{tiVti}/\dot{Q}$) depends only on the ratio $\dot{Q}/(\lambda\text{tiVti})$. This is the ratio of tissue perfusion (conductance) to the product of λti and Vti (capacitance). *3)* The half time is independent of the boundary conditions. In other words, Pti_0 for the washout and Pa for the washin do not affect the rate at which equilibration between inflowing blood and tissue partial pressures come together. Doubling Pa (Eq. 9) will not enhance the fractional degree of equilibration ratio at any time *t*. *4)* Boundary conditions will linearly affect the quantity of gas moved in either direction between tissue and blood. In other words, if Pa is doubled, Pti (Eq. 9) will be twice as high at the same

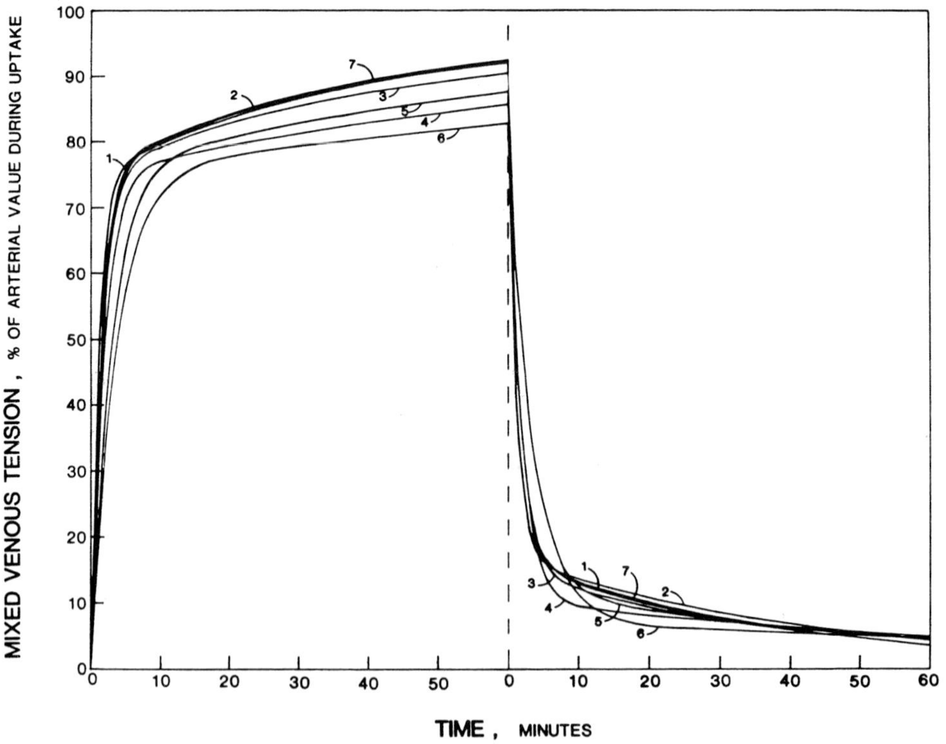

FIG. 2. Calculated concentration-time profiles for uptake (*left graph*) and elimination (*right graph*) of 7 gases in mixed venous blood. During 60 min of uptake, arterial concentration is constant and mixed venous values are given as percentage of that level. Gases are *1)* N_2, *2)* N_2O, *3)* cyclopropane, *4)* fluroxene, *5)* enflurane, *6)* halothane, and *7)* diethyl ether. Note how similar both uptake and elimination curves are for all gases, despite differences in their partition coefficients (Table 2) when arterial levels are held constant.

time t. *5*) The washin and washout boundary conditions chosen in the above derivations are the simplest [increase from 0 to Pa (washin) or decrease from Pti_0 to 0 (washout)]. By choosing nonzero initial or final steady-state boundary conditions and following through the logic of Equations 1 et seq., it can be seen that

$$(Pti - Pin) = (Pa - Pin)\left[1 - \exp\left(-\frac{\dot{Q}t}{\lambda ti Vti}\right)\right] \quad (11)$$

and

$$(Pti - Pti_\infty) = (Pti_0 - Pti_\infty) \times \exp\left(-\frac{\dot{Q}t}{\lambda ti Vti}\right) \quad (12)$$

where for the washin (Eq. 11) Pin is some initial nonzero arterial gas tension. For the washout (Eq. 12) Pti_∞ is some nonzero steady-state value reached at $t = \infty$. Conclusions *1–4* above still hold for Equations 11 and 12, except that all statements in conclusions *3* and *4* should be rephrased in terms of the difference between Pa and Pin [not just Pa (Eq. 11)] and the difference between Pti_0 and Pti_∞ [not just Pti_0 (Eq. 12)].

Figure 2 shows for both the washin and the washout processes of seven common gases how rapidly equilibration occurs for the body as a whole by using values from the literature as summarized in Table 2. Of course, Figure 2 is based for each gas on the assumptions listed earlier, and thus the curves are only approximations to reality. In particular, Figure 2 shows Pti changes subsequent to a step change in inflowing Pa.

To this point, the emphasis has been on kinetic aspects of peripheral tissue inert-gas exchange: how rapidly a gas will equilibrate between blood and tissue. Rate of equilibration was seen to depend on the conductance-capacitance ratio $\dot{Q}/(\lambda ti Vti)$. Also of interest is the quantity of a gas that a given tissue will store at equilibrium. This will be the product of the equilibrium values of Pti and λtiVti. To compare the storage

TABLE 2. *Static and Dynamic Characteristics of Several Gases in the Four Tissue Groups*

Variable	Gas	Vessel-Rich Group	Muscle	Fat	Vessel-Poor Group
$\dot{Q}$, liters/min		4.5	1.1	0.32	0.08
Vti,L, liters		6.0	36.0	15.2	13.0
λti	N_2	1.1	~1.0	5.2	1.0
	N_2O	0.8	1.15	2.3	1.0
	Cyclopropane	1.16	1.16	12.9	1.2
	Fluroxene	1.37	2.3	23.0	2.0
	Enflurane	2.1	1.7	36.2	2.0
	Halothane	2.6	3.5	60.0	3.0
	Ether	1.01	1.0	3.7	1.0
$\dot{Q}/(\lambda ti Vti)$, min^{-1}	N_2	0.68	0.031	0.0041	0.0062
	N_2O	0.94	0.027	0.0093	0.0062
	Cyclopropane	0.65	0.026	0.0017	0.0051
	Fluroxene	0.55	0.013	0.0009	0.0031
	Enflurane	0.36	0.018	0.0006	0.0031
	Halothane	0.29	0.009	0.0006	0.0021
	Ether	0.74	0.031	0.0058	0.0062
$t_{1/2}$, min	N_2	1.02	22.7	169	113
	N_2O	0.74	26.1	75	113
	Cyclopropane	1.07	26.3	419	135
	Fluroxene	1.27	52.2	747	225
	Enflurane	1.94	38.6	1,176	225
	Halothane	2.40	79.4	1,949	338
	Ether	0.93	22.7	120	113
λtiVti	N_2	6.6	36.0	78.0	13.0
	N_2O	4.8	41.4	34.5	13.0
	Cyclopropane	7.0	41.8	193.5	15.6
	Fluroxene	8.2	82.8	345.0	26.0
	Enflurane	12.6	61.2	543.0	26.0
	Halothane	15.6	126.0	900.0	39.0
	Ether	6.1	36.0	55.5	13.0
λtiVti, % of total	N_2	5	27	58	10
	N_2O	5	44	37	14
	Cyclopropane	3	16	75	6
	Fluroxene	2	18	74	6
	Enflurane	2	10	84	4
	Halothane	1	12	83	4
	Ether	6	32	50	12
	Means	3.4	22.7	65.9	8.0
Vti, % of total		9	51	21	19

$\dot{Q}$, blood flow; Vti,L, lung tissue volume; λti, tissue-blood partition coefficient; Vti, tissue volume; $t_{1/2}$, half time. [Values adapted from Eger (24).]

capacity of various tissues that are all equilibrated with the same circulating blood, thus all with the same Pti, one may simply compare αVti for the various tissues. In fact, because $\lambda ti = \alpha/\beta$, one gets the same result by comparing λtiVti for the various tissues. Table 2 focuses on the four typical tissue groups (24) and presents average values for their blood flow and Vti normalized to a 70-kg man with a 6-liter cardiac output. In addition, λti values for several gases of interest are given, and at the bottom the static and dynamic characteristics of each tissue for each gas are given. The dynamic and static properties are characterized by the conductance-capacitance ratio (representing rate of equilibration) and by capacitance (representing amount of gas stored in tissue), respectively. For ease of assimilation, equilibration half times are also presented, and the capacitance values are normalized (to add to 100).

The numbers in this table are striking. They are based on simple mass-balance concepts and are of fundamental importance, both in understanding the physiology of inert-gas exchange and in the clinical application of anesthesia and hyperbaric medicine. Although there are some major differences among gases, the overall message is clear: the half time for equilibration of gases in vessel-rich tissues such as heart, kidney, and liver is of the order of only 1–2 min. Put another way, because four half times permit 94% equilibration, it requires only 4–8 min to essentially equilibrate a vessel-rich tissue with most inert gases. The skeletal muscles equilibrate an order of magnitude more slowly, with half times in the range of 20–80 min. This is accounted for by the much larger tissue mass and lower resting blood flow per unit tissue mass than in the vessel-rich group. Perhaps the most striking data are for fatty tissues, where the shortest half time is 1¼ h and the longest is >1¼ days (halothane). Thus it would take ~5 full days to almost fully saturate (94%) the fat stores of an average person (assuming constant arterial halothane level in blood supply of fat). It would require the same time to eliminate halothane from these stores (assuming no halothane in entering arterial blood). These figures have enormous practical implications for the anesthesiologist.

Table 2 further points out the distribution of an inert gas among the four typical tissue compartments once equilibrium has been reached. Thus, although the actual volume of the three nonfat compartments is essentially 80% of the total body volume, only ~35% of the stored gas (averaged for 7 gases in Table 2) is held in that volume. The remaining 65% is stored in fat, comprising only 20% of the body volume.

An instructive exercise is to calculate for the gases in Table 2 the uptake and elimination time courses for each of the four tissue compartments of Table 2, as shown in Figure 3. Durations of uptake and elimination are each 60 min, and the important questions

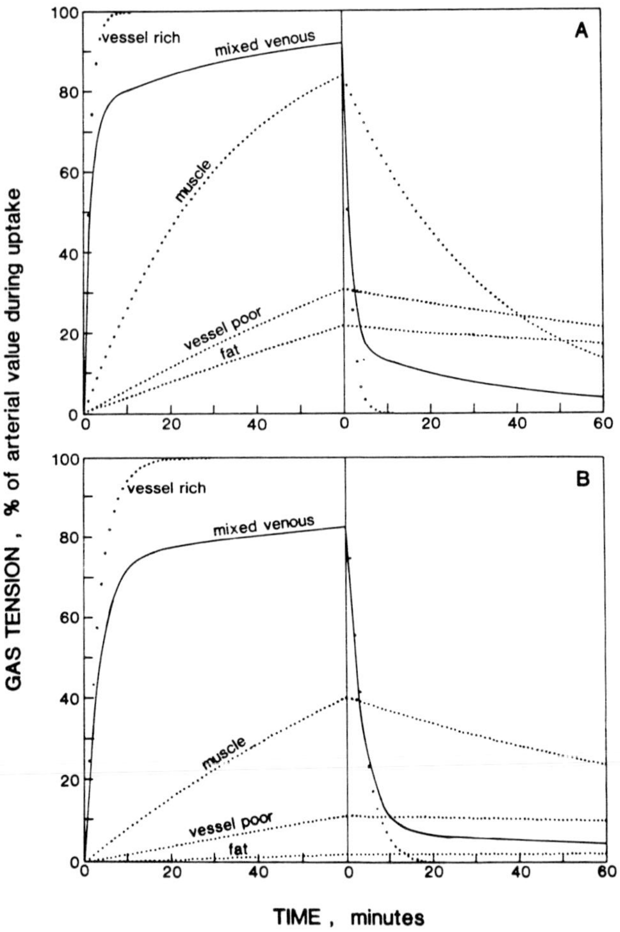

FIG. 3. Gas tension–time profiles for uptake (*left graphs*) and elimination (*right graphs*) of N_2 (*A*) and N_2O (*B*) in mixed venous blood under conditions identical to those of Fig. 2 (*solid lines*). *Dotted lines* for each gas indicate gas tensions in each of 4 standard tissues as labeled. Vessel-rich tissues equilibrate with inflowing arterial blood in ~10 min (N_2), whereas muscle, vessel-poor, and fat tissues fail to reach arterial levels within 1 h of uptake (or elimination). Rate of equilibration is determined by conductance-capacitance ratio of gas in each tissue.

concern the tissue and mixed venous levels reached as a function of time. Although somewhat removed from reality, this calculation was done by imposing a constant arterial level of each gas during the uptake period and arterial blood devoid of the gas during the subsequent washout. What is not accounted for (even allowing the earlier assumptions) is venous return of inert gases from the tissue to the lung, uptake or elimination by the lung, and subsequent return to the arterial circulation. To model uptake, Equation 9 was used for each of the four tissues to compute Pti (for each gas at each time point, using the data of Table 2). The returning mixed venous blood is the perfusion-weighted average of those four values of Pti. Similarly, Equation 10 was used for the elimination phase. Figure 3 shows the results of these calculations for an insoluble gas (N_2) and a soluble gas (N_2O) and indicates clearly how differently the four basic tissue types equilibrate, with vessel-rich areas rapidly reaching arterial levels during both washin and washout. In contrast, the equilibration of the fatty and vessel-poor tissues is much slower, and there is apparent "asymmetry" between uptake and elimination. That is, although 60 min of washin elevates Pti in vessel-poor areas to ~30% of Pa (Fig. 3), the same time period of elimination does not return the Pti of the vessel-poor group to zero (cf. vessel-rich group). The straightforward explanation of this phenomenon is that during uptake the multiplier (Pa) of Equation 9 is 100 arbitrary units, whereas on the same scale the starting Pti for elimination (Pti_0 of Eq. 10) is only ~30 units, as noted above. Consequently, the rate of fall of the Pti of the vessel-poor group during washout will be only 30% of the rate of rise during uptake. If one looks at this in terms of percentage rather than absolute changes, uptake and elimination do become symmetrical. During uptake, Pti rises by ~30% of the initial difference (of 100 units) between Pa and Pti; during elimination, Pti falls by the same 30% of the initial difference (of 30 units) between Pti and Pa. It is important to understand the subtleties of considering absolute and percentage changes in gas tensions to avoid any confusion.

Figure 3 is based on the four-compartment model of Eger (24). One of its major virtues is its simplicity. More extensive measurements and estimates of organ and tissue blood flow, volumes, and λti values have been published. Compilations can be found in Kety (41), Larson (47), and Cowles et al. (18). Ashman et al. (3), Smith et al. (82), and Davis and Mapleson (23) have tabulated comprehensive lists of tissue volumes, flows, and partition coefficients, and many original measurements have been reported (2, 9, 43, 48, 49, 54, 60, 62, 69, 92).

Inclusion of Pulmonary Gas Exchange in Tissue Inert-Gas Uptake and Elimination

The analysis so far has been limited not only by the listed assumptions but by the very unrealistic imposition of constant inert-gas Pa after step changes therein. It becomes important to consider pulmonary gas exchange simultaneously with tissue gas exchange because this moves the entire discussion a large step closer to reality (41). The usual circumstance in which tissue inert-gas exchange (uptake or elimination) is considered is one in which the inspired partial pressure (PI) of the gas is altered as a step change. When this is done, pulmonary gas exchange is altered over time to reflect the sudden change in PI. This in turn leads to a more gradual change in effluent pulmonary venous partial pressure (Ppv) (and hence systemic Pa) than heretofore considered. Furthermore, by adding pulmonary gas exchange to the system, we allow for venous return of inert gases from the tissues to the lungs (recirculation), which has a further modulating effect on both arterial and tissue gas levels.

Figure 4 is a simple diagram illustrating the interconnected nature of the lungs and tissues, showing how each "feeds" and thus affects the other. In this more realistic system, it is important to understand how to determine Pa, peripheral Pti, and mixed venous inert-gas partial pressure ($P\bar{v}$) responses to a step change in PI.

The same general assumptions about tissue exchange listed earlier (p. 258) are imposed here, and it is also assumed that the lungs are functionally perfect; i.e., they can be regarded as a one-compartment gas exchange unit in which alveolar (PA) and end-capillary (Pc′) (and hence arterial) partial pressures are identical at any point in time. Constancy of ventilation and blood flow is also assumed; no attempt to account for the tidal nature of ventilation or the beat-by-beat nature of blood flow is made.

ALGEBRAIC ANALYSIS. A relatively simple analysis can be carried out if it is limited to the consideration of a single tissue compartment interacting with the lungs.

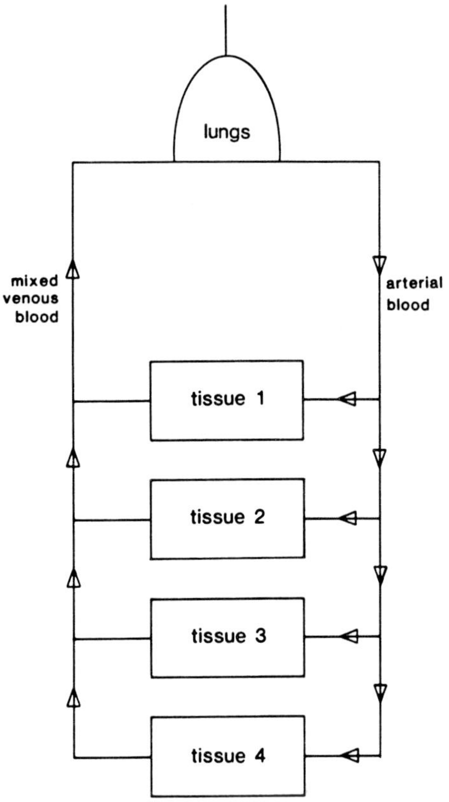

FIG. 4. Organizational arrangement of lungs, circulation, and several tissues, demonstrating their interdependence. For determining gas tensions in lungs, blood, and tissues, *1*) the key pulmonary variables are inspired gas tension, alveolar gas tension and volume, pulmonary tissue volume, alveolar ventilation, cardiac output, and blood-gas partition coefficient and *2*) the key tissue variables are tissue gas tension, tissue volume and blood flow, and tissue-blood partition coefficient.

To include several tissue compartments is still feasible, but this considerably complicates the mathematics and is not attempted here.

To derive the equations that give Pa and Pti (here, equal to $P\bar{v}$ because there is only 1 tissue in the system), one again begins with the principles of mass balance. However, by adding the lungs the system is expanded to one with two unknowns (Pa and Pti or $P\bar{v}$). Two mass-balance equations, one for the lungs and one for the tissues, must therefore be written. The result is two equations in two unknowns that can be analytically solved for both unknowns in a relatively straightforward manner.

For the lungs, the mass-balance expression equates the sum of rates of delivery and removal of gas with the rate of accumulation of the gas in the pulmonary gas stores

$$(V_L + \lambda Vti_{,L}) \frac{dP_A}{dt} = (\dot{V}_A P_I + \lambda \dot{Q}_T P\bar{v}) - (\dot{V}_A P_A + \lambda \dot{Q}_T Pa) \quad (13)$$

where V_L is lung gas volume, $Vti_{,L}$ is lung tissue volume, and λ is lung tissue-gas partition coefficient [which will for simplicity be taken to be equal to blood-gas partition coefficient, although this may not be quite true for some gases (9, 48, 49, 93)]; P_A and Pa are assumed to be equal; alveolar ventilation ($\dot{V}_A$) and total blood flow ($\dot{Q}_T$) are expressed in liters/minute, whereas V_L and $Vti_{,L}$ are in liters, giving gas partial pressures as a function of t in minutes. Equation 13 preserves mass balance: the left side represents change in lung gas stores per unit time, assuming gas and tissue volume are constant. Addition of gas to the lungs by ventilation ($\dot{V}_A P_I$) and by mixed venous blood ($\lambda \dot{Q}_T P\bar{v}$) is counteracted by its removal by ventilation ($\dot{V}_A P_A$) and blood flow ($\lambda \dot{Q}_T Pa$), and the difference must represent the rate of change of lung gas stores.

When P_A is set equal to Pa, as indicated above, and the terms are rearranged, the new equation is

$$\frac{dPa}{dt} = AP_I + BP\bar{v} - (A + B)Pa \quad (14)$$

where

$$A = \frac{\dot{V}_A}{V_L + \lambda Vti_{,L}}$$

and

$$B = \frac{\lambda \dot{Q}_T}{V_L + \lambda Vti_{,L}}$$

Recall that the goal of this analysis is to derive two expressions, one each for $P\bar{v}$ and Pa, as explicit functions of t and the constants P_I, A, B, and C (below).

For the single peripheral tissue, a mass-balance expression similar to Equation 5 is used. Thus

$$\lambda ti Vti \frac{dP\bar{v}}{dt} = (Pa - P\bar{v})\dot{Q}_T \quad (15)$$

Equation 15 is identical to Equation 5; $P\bar{v}$ has been used instead of Pti, but because they are assumed to be equal this does not alter the equation. Rewriting Equation 15 gives

$$\frac{dP\bar{v}}{dt} = CPa - CP\bar{v} \quad (16)$$

where

$$C = \frac{\dot{Q}_T}{\lambda ti Vti}$$

Equations 14 and 16 are two simultaneous linear first-order differential equations in the two unknowns $P\bar{v}$ and Pa as functions of t. To solve these equations, use a combination of the traditional method of elimination of one variable used in solving simple simultaneous linear equations and the techniques of solution of differential equations.

From Equation 14, $P\bar{v}$ is expressed in terms of Pa, dPa/dt, P_I, A, and B, and this is substituted into Equation 16, differentiating Equation 14 with respect to t to express $dP\bar{v}/dt$ in terms of dPa/dt, d^2Pa/dt^2, P_I, A, and B. This gives

$$\frac{d^2Pa}{dt^2} + (A + B + C)\frac{dPa}{dt} + ACPa - ACP_I = 0 \quad (17)$$

This more complicated linear second-order differential equation does not contain $P\bar{v}$ and so can be directly solved for Pa as a function of t by conventional techniques. The result is given in Equation 18 for inert gas Pa as a function of t for uptake ($P_I > 0$)

$$Pa = P_I[1 - W_1 \exp(+\gamma_1 t) + W_2 \exp(+\gamma_2 t)] \quad (18)$$

where

$$\gamma_1 = \frac{-(A + B + C) + \sqrt{(C - A)^2 + 2(C + A)B + B^2}}{2}$$

$$\gamma_2 = \frac{-(A + B + C) - \sqrt{(C - A)^2 + 2(C + A)B + B^2}}{2}$$

$$W_1 = (A + \gamma_2)/(\gamma_2 - \gamma_1)$$

$$W_2 = (A + \gamma_1)/(\gamma_2 - \gamma_1)$$

By substituting Equation 18 into Equation 14, the corresponding term for $P\bar{v}$ during uptake is derived

$$P\bar{v} = P_I\left[1 - W_1 \frac{(A + B + \gamma_1)}{B} \exp(+\gamma_1 t) + W_2 \frac{(A + B + \gamma_2)}{B} \exp(+\gamma_2 t)\right] \quad (19)$$

Recall that in Equations 18 and 19

$$A = \frac{\dot{V}A}{VL + \lambda Vti,L}$$

$$B = \frac{\lambda \dot{Q}T}{VL + \lambda Vti,L}$$

$$C = \frac{\dot{Q}T}{\lambda ti Vti}$$

Before discussing the implications of Equations 18 and 19, the corresponding expressions for elimination of gas from the lung and peripheral tissue system should be presented. One cannot simply substitute $P_I = 0$ (for elimination) into Equations 18 and 19; as can be seen, this would give $Pa = P\bar{v} = 0$ at all times. One must return to Equations 14 and 16, set $P_I = 0$ in Equation 14, and rework the subsequent solution process above. Thus for elimination Equations 14 and 16 become, respectively

$$\frac{dPa}{dt} = BP\bar{v} - (A + B)Pa \qquad (20)$$

and

$$\frac{dP\bar{v}}{dt} = CPa - CP\bar{v} \qquad (21)$$

Substituting $P\bar{v}$ from Equation 20 into Equation 21 as before yields

$$\frac{d^2Pa}{dt^2} + (A + B + C)\frac{dPa}{dt} + ACPa = 0 \qquad (22)$$

Solution of this differential equation gives

$$Pa = \left[\frac{Pa_0(A + B + \gamma_2) - BP\bar{v}_0}{\gamma_2 - \gamma_1}\right]\exp(\gamma_1 t) - \left[\frac{Pa_0(A + B + \gamma_1) - BP\bar{v}_0}{\gamma_2 - \gamma_1}\right]\exp(\gamma_2 t) \qquad (23)$$

and

$$P\bar{v} = \left\{\frac{[Pa_0(A + B + \gamma_2) - BP\bar{v}_0](A + B + \gamma_1)}{B(\gamma_2 - \gamma_1)}\right\}\exp(\gamma_1 t) - \left\{\frac{[PA_0(A + B + \gamma_1) - BP\bar{v}_0](A + B + \gamma_2)}{B(\gamma_2 - \gamma_1)}\right\}\exp(\gamma_2 t) \qquad (24)$$

P_I is assumed to be 0, and Pa_0 and $P\bar{v}_0$ are the arterial and tissue (or mixed venous) inert-gas partial pressures at the start of washout when $t = 0$.

Equations 18 and 19 (uptake) and 23 and 24 (elimination) give analytical expressions for inert-gas Pa and $P\bar{v}$ as functions of t for the simple system of a single perfect lung in series with a single peripheral tissue. Although the mathematics may seem formidable, the four equations are each just the sum of two exponential terms, and all of the constants involved are determined by the lung and tissue ratios of conductance to capacitance (constants A, B, and C) together with boundary-condition gas partial pressures (P_I, Pa_0, and $P\bar{v}_0$).

Some comments should be made about these equations. *1*) The exponents γ_1 and γ_2 can never be equal because the square-root terms always sum to a positive number. This is because A, B, and C are themselves made up of real (positive) biological variables. *2*) It is easily shown that the value of $A + B + C$ must always exceed the value of $[(C - A)^2 + 2(C + A)B + B^2]^{1/2}$. Consequently both γ_1 and γ_2 must always be negative, no matter what numerical values are chosen for A, B, and C (as long as these are, of course, positive). *3*) It is not difficult to show for uptake that $Pa = P\bar{v} = 0$ at $t = 0$ and that $Pa = P\bar{v} = P_I$ at true equilibration ($t = \infty$). Similarly, at $t = 0$ for elimination, Equations 23 and 24 reduce to $Pa = Pa_0$ and $P\bar{v} = P\bar{v}_0$, whereas at $t = \infty$, $Pa = P\bar{v} = 0$. Thus the equations satisfy the imposed boundary conditions. *4*) For uptake and elimination, both Pa and $P\bar{v}$ are linearly related to the boundary values (P_I for uptake and Pa_0 and $P\bar{v}_0$ for elimination). *5*) The exponents γ_1 and γ_2 are the same for Pa and $P\bar{v}$ during both uptake and elimination. In other words, the system behaves in a manner determined by γ_1 and γ_2, which in turn are made up of the conductance-capacitance ratios A and B for the lung and C for the tissues. The boundary conditions (P_I, Pa_0, $P\bar{v}_0$) determine uptake or elimination by contributing to the constants multiplying the exponential components of Equations 18, 19, 23, and 24.

NUMERICAL APPROACH. *Consideration of multiple body tissue compartments.* The analytical expressions given in Equations 18, 19, 23, and 24 are very useful *1*) in understanding the principles of tissue exchange with blood and *2*) for directing calculations of Pa and $P\bar{v}$ at any point in time.

However, being limited to a single peripheral tissue, they cannot predict total-body inert-gas exchange because the heterogeneity of tissue conductance-capacitance ratios is so important (see Table 2). To now incorporate, for example, the four characteristic tissue compartments requires writing the following set of mass-balance equations. Although in principle no more complicated than the single tissue case, the analysis is in practice very difficult. The equations are

$$\frac{dPa}{dt} = AP_I + BP\bar{v} - (A + B)Pa \qquad (25)$$

$$\frac{dPv_1}{dt} = C_1(Pa - Pv_1) \tag{26}$$

$$\frac{dPv_2}{dt} = C_2(Pa - Pv_2) \tag{27}$$

$$\frac{dPv_3}{dt} = C_3(Pa - Pv_3) \tag{28}$$

$$\frac{dPv_4}{dt} = C_4(Pa - Pv_4) \tag{29}$$

$$P\bar{v} = (\dot{Q}_1Pv_1 + \dot{Q}_2Pv_2 + \dot{Q}_3Pv_3 + \dot{Q}_4Pv_4)/\dot{Q}_T \tag{30}$$

Equation 25 is exactly as before and represents pulmonary gas exchange (still in context of a one-compartment lung). Equations 26–29 are (as for Eq. 16) descriptions of tissue exchange in one of the four tissues whose conductance-capacitance ratios are respectively C_1–C_4; Pv_1–Pv_4 are the effluent (tissue) partial pressures from the four tissues. Equation 30 states that $P\bar{v}$ is the flow-weighted average of the four tissue partial pressures ($\dot{Q}_1$–$\dot{Q}_4$ are flows in each compartment). Thus Equations 25–30 form a set of five simultaneous linear first-order differential equations and one simultaneous linear equation for a total of six equations in six unknowns. In principle, by the same general approach given for the single-tissue case, it would be possible to obtain an analytical solution for the six variables (Pa, $P\bar{v}$, Pv_1, Pv_2, Pv_3, and Pv_4) as functions of t. They would all be multiexponential sums, such as in Equations 18, 19, 23, and 24, but would contain a greater number of terms with very complicated coefficients.

This point is stressed because the problem can be circumvented by numerical analytical approaches. In other words, Equations 25–30 can be solved by computer-performed numerical (rather than analytical) methods. This general approach is a powerful tool applicable to many kinds of difficult multivariate biological modeling problems. It is also simple, both in principle and execution (provided one has access to a digital computer for doing the calculations). The solution proceeds as follows.

Equations 25–29 are rewritten as what can be called finite difference equations

$$\Delta Pa = [AP_I + BP\bar{v} - (A + B)Pa]\Delta t \tag{31}$$

$$\Delta Pv_1 = C_1(Pa - Pv_1)\Delta t \tag{32}$$

$$\Delta Pv_2 = C_2(Pa - Pv_2)\Delta t \tag{33}$$

$$\Delta Pv_3 = C_3(Pa - Pv_3)\Delta t \tag{34}$$

$$\Delta Pv_4 = C_4(Pa - Pv_4)\Delta t \tag{35}$$

whereas Equation 30 remains as before. Next, the starting conditions must be defined; i.e., initial values must be set down for all constants (A, B, C_1–C_4) and for P_I, Pa, Pv_1–Pv_4, and $P\bar{v}$. For uptake a value of $P_I > 0$ is selected, and generally $Pa = Pv_1 = Pv_2 = Pv_3 = Pv_4 = P\bar{v} = 0$. Then, for some very small time increment Δt (perhaps of the order of 1 s), Equations 30–35 are evaluated by computer because all terms on the right side are known at $t = 0$. This gives new values for the six partial pressures at $t = \Delta t$. The entire process is then repeated, but this time the just-calculated values of Pa, Pv_1–Pv_4, and $P\bar{v}$ are used in the right sides of Equations 30–35, and new values for these six partial pressures are computed (for $t = 2\Delta t$). By repeating this cyclical maneuver n times until the total time t ($=n\Delta t$) reaches some desired value, the partial pressure–time profiles of the inert gas in arterial and mixed venous blood as well as the four tissue compartments are obtained. The potential difficulty with this method is that if Δt is not small enough, the calculation will be in error. Specifically, Δt must be small enough that the true gradient of the partial pressure–time curve over Δt is essentially constant. Two general approaches are used to deal with this issue. The simplest is to repeat the entire sequence of partial pressure–time profile determinations with a smaller value of Δt. If the resulting profiles are not significantly different in the two cases, the larger value of Δt is sufficiently small to ensure an accurate result. Alternatively (or in addition), a more sophisticated procedure such as the Runge-Kutta forward integration technique (64, 73) can be used to perform the calculations more accurately using less computer time.

The great advantage of such numerical approaches is that systems of almost any complexity can be dealt with fairly easily. Thus to add several more tissues or to incorporate pulmonary inhomogeneity into the system simply means adding the appropriate mass-balance equations and treating them exactly as Equations 30–35 above. Furthermore, it is easy to change boundary conditions (starting values of gas partial pressure) as often as desired. The disadvantage is that only numerical results and not theoretical principles can be deduced directly from the computed values.

Figure 5 shows sample profiles of arterial and mixed venous tissue partial pressures computed with the aid of Equations 30–35 in a homogeneous lung–four-tissue system, based on the tissues in Table 2. The mixed venous curves should be compared with those of Figure 2, which is an identical simulation except that Pa values in Figure 2 were constant at 100 (uptake) or 0 (elimination) arbitrary units.

Circulation time delays between peripheral tissues and lung. In all the preceding analyses, it was implicitly assumed that circulation time from the lungs to tissue and back to the lungs was zero. For most purposes, these times (being on the order of a few seconds) are not at all important for considerations of tissue uptake or elimination over times of minutes to days. However, these delays can be taken into account by using appropriate values (in Eqs. 30–35) for gas partial pressure. For example, for uptake, where Pa =

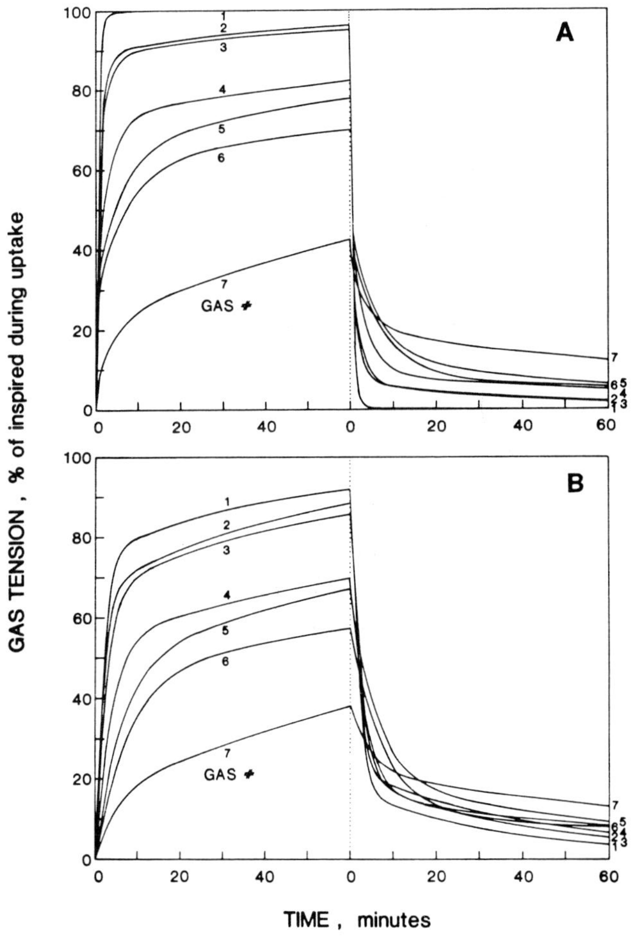

FIG. 5. Gas tension–time profiles for uptake (*left graphs*) and elimination (*right graphs*) of 7 gases of Fig. 2 computed during 60 min of uptake at constant inspired tension and during 60 min of elimination (0 inspired tension). Tissue variables are as in Fig. 2; however, this figure allows for pulmonary gas exchange and recirculation from tissues to lungs according to model of Fig. 4. Time-course calculations are shown for both arterial (*A*) and mixed venous (*B*) gas tensions. Rate of equilibration is inversely related to blood-gas partition coefficient, with large differences among gases. In all cases, true equilibrium would be reached when tensions were 100% (uptake) or 0% (elimination) of inspired.

$Pv_1 = Pv_2 = Pv_3 = Pv_4 = P\bar{v} = 0$ initially, Equation 31 is evaluated with Pv_1–Pv_4 and $P\bar{v}$ all kept at zero, not just for the first time interval Δt but for as many cycles as it takes for the total time to equal the desired sum of lung-to-tissue and tissue-to-lung circulation times. Thereafter a similar delay is maintained in the numerical evaluation of Equation 31. Similar tactics are used when evaluating the other equations in the system. Mapleson (57) evaluated the consequences of failing to allow for circulation time. He concluded that significant errors were confined to the first 2 min or so of uptake or elimination when circulation time was ignored.

Allowances for fluctuating ventilation and cardiac output. The numerical analytical approach of Equations 30–35 is also well suited to studying the effects of time-varying ventilation and/or cardiac output. Thus, if the quantitative nature of the ventilation-time or perfusion-time relationship is known, appropriate values can be used in Equations 30–35 in the computations of gas partial pressures. It should be apparent that to additionally include tidal ventilation and beat-to-beat perfusion variation in the analytical scheme of Equations 25–30 would make an already very complicated problem intractable and certainly impractical.

SUMMARY OF MATHEMATICAL ANALYSIS. To this point, the entire chapter has focused on the mathematical behavior of inert gases exchanging convectively between blood and tissues. Formulations of increasing complexity have been presented and two general approaches—analytical and numerical—have been discussed at some length. All of these analyses have operated within the constraints of the many assumptions listed at the beginning of the chapter. The purposes of such a lengthy treatment are several: *1*) most importantly, to illustrate the principles involved in convective peripheral tissue inert-gas exchange; *2*) to illustrate the factors that govern rates of uptake and elimination and the determination of whole-body (arterial and mixed venous) levels of gases as a function of uptake and elimination time; *3*) to provide tools for the interested reader to further pose and answer questions about tissue inert-gas exchange; *4*) to present general mathematical tools that go beyond inert-gas exchange in tissues and that can be applied to a large number of biological systems that can be modeled as a set of interconnecting functional compartments; and *5*) to provide the theoretical insight necessary for a critical evaluation of techniques (described in APPLICATION OF INERT GASES TO MEASUREMENT OF ORGAN PERFUSION, p. 273) that use tissue inert-gas exchange as tools in the functional evaluation of tissue mass or blood flow.

Comparison of Multicompartment Models With Actual Data

Given the models developed above and the framework of assumptions on which they were built, it is appropriate to ask how well such models predict uptake and elimination of inert gases by the body. Before examining published data, obtained mostly by anesthesiologists, it is worth pointing out that predictability of actual washin or washout curves depends not only on whether the listed assumptions are reasonable but also on numerical values for conductance-capacitance terms. Clearly, even if the assumptions hold, curves predicted from incorrect values for ventilation, cardiac output, tissue-compartment volumes, blood flow, and partition coefficient will not match measured curves. Unfortunately measurement of all of these variables is not generally made on the particular subject whose washin or washout is being measured, and in fact most of the variables must be taken as average values from the literature. This is especially true of tissue volumes, flows, and tissue-blood partition coefficients. These caveats notwithstanding, uptake and/or elimination curves presented in the literature are compared with those predicted from the numerical analytical approach with four tissue compartments (Table 2). The necessary average data of Table 2 were used in the predictions, and Figures 6–8 show the comparisons. In general it is easier to compare uptake data because a critical variable in comparing elimination curves is the prior duration of uptake, which is not always indicated. The comparisons shown are for three commonly used gases, N_2O (Fig. 6), cyclopropane (Fig. 7), and halothane (Fig. 8), encompassing the midrange of blood-gas partition coefficients.

Given the inability to precisely match most of the variables, the expired or arterial comparisons are surprisingly good when "average 70-kg man" variable values are used. It is not unreasonable to conclude that for washin or washout of inert gases from the entire body over time frames of minutes to hours the analyses given earlier approximate real data and probably allow for the major components in inert-gas exchange between the tissues, blood, lungs, and external environment. Such a conclusion is especially useful to anesthesiologists wishing to model tissue uptake-elimination ratios of anesthetic gases. Eger (24) arrived at similar conclusions using data from Sechzer and coworkers (75, 76), Onchi and Asao (65), and Severinghaus (81).

Further comparisons can be made using the data of Beneken Kolmer et al. (7) for halothane uptake and elimination in the dog. For their illustrated case (dog 12), concentrations of halothane in arterial and mixed venous blood are compared in Table 3. Considering the coarseness of parameter choices for the predictions, the agreement is remarkably good for both arterial and venous blood. Cowles et al. (19) tabulate uptake half times for three of the gases in Table 2 (cyclopropane, halothane, and ether). Their data also pertain to the anesthetized dog, and the comparison with values predicted from Equations 30–35 is given in Table 4. To a first approximation, there is general agreement, especially if the three gases are compared with each other. Although the halothane values seem quite different, the time course of uptake is quite slow, such that the percentage of equilibration of halothane is not far off 50% at the measured half times, as indicated in the table.

However, considerable caution should be used before concluding that the simple convective kinetic approach in homogeneous tissue completely accounts for real data. For example, simply studying washin or

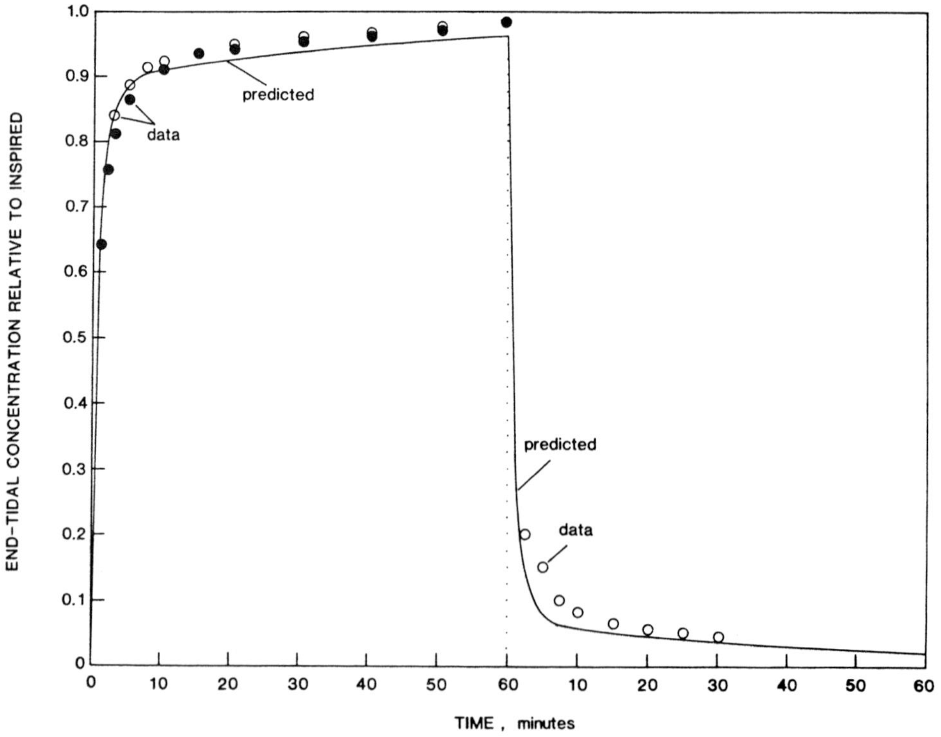

FIG. 6. Comparison of measured and predicted end-tidal N_2O concentrations during uptake (*left*) and elimination (*right*). Predictions come from model of Fig. 4 and Eqs. 30–35 in text. Excellent agreement is noted during both phases, indicating that 4 basic tissue compartments and simple convective mass-balance principles are sufficient to explain actual data. [Measured data from Rackow et al. (70) and Salanitre et al. (72).]

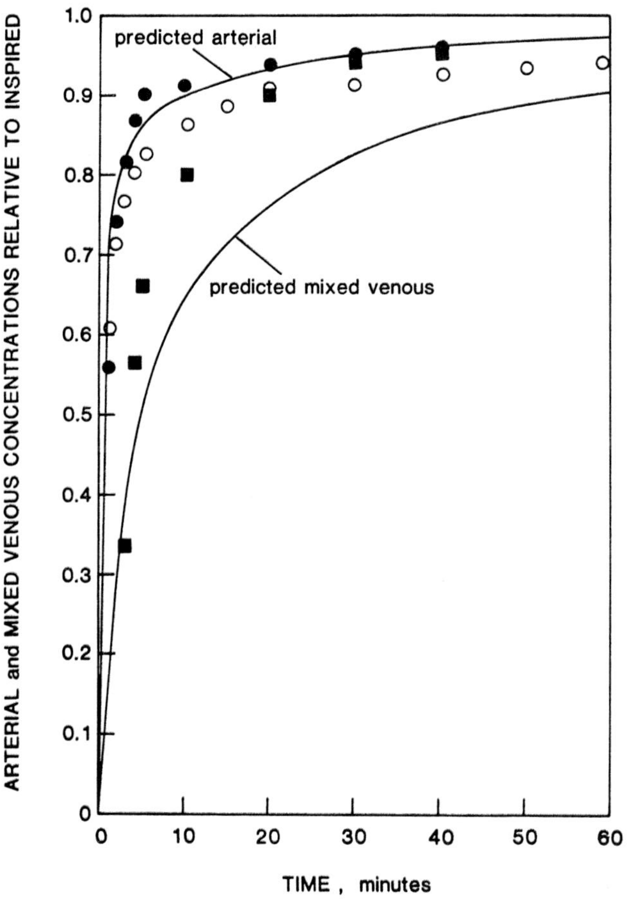

FIG. 7. Comparison of real arterial and mixed venous cyclopropane concentrations with those predicted from numerical analysis described in text (prediction based on considering 4 tissue compartments and homogeneous lung). From 2 studies (70, 75), it is evident that arterial data (●, ○) are quite well followed by simple model. However, there is unexplained difference between actual and predicted mixed venous levels (■). Tables 3 and 4 give additional comparisons with better agreement between measured and predicted mixed venous levels.

washout of single gases in arterial or mixed venous blood over minutes to hours provides insufficient data to critically evaluate some of the originally listed assumptions, particularly those related to whether intratissue, intertissue, or tissue-blood diffusion of gases is rate limiting to peripheral inert-gas exchange.

CONSIDERATION OF TISSUE-BLOOD DIFFUSION OF INERT GASES

Although the preceding sections deal only with convective kinetic processes, explicitly assuming diffusional equilibrium in the tissues (i.e., gas partial pressure throughout any one tissue is uniform at any instant and equal to that in effluent venous blood from the tissue), there have been many theoretical and experimental studies that have questioned these assumptions. Clearly the physical process by which tissue-blood inert-gas exchange occurs has to be diffusion along a concentration gradient, and so the question is quite relevant. Kety's review (41) summarizes the theoretical approach to tissue diffusion. He shows how Fick's law in its simplest form leads to an exponential result

$$\text{Pti} = \text{Pc}(1 - e^{-kt}) \qquad (36)$$

where Pc and Pti are instantaneous capillary and tissue partial pressures, respectively, at any time t. Here, on the continuing assumption of a homogeneous Pti but a finite "barrier" to diffusion between capillary blood and tissue, Pti exponentially equilibrates with Pc over time t, depending on the value of the exponent k.

The important observation from Equation 36 is its exponential nature. We have already seen how convective kinetic exchange follows exponential patterns, and moreover in the whole body they must be multiexponential due to the heterogeneity of tissue conductance-capacitance ratios. Consequently it is not possible to determine whether tissue diffusion rates have a measurable effect on tissue gas exchange simply by the appearance of the tissue washin or washout curves—exponentiality will be observed whether or not diffusion rates are important. If one were confident that a given tissue were functionally homogeneous and moreover if one could accurately determine the conductance-capacitance ratio for the tissue, one could argue that tissue exchange should follow a predictable monoexponential form. Departure from the predicted rate or multiexponentiality might therefore suggest diffusion limitation. However, in practice, one

TABLE 3. *Arterial and Mixed Venous Halothane Levels During Elimination. Comparison of Data With Predictions of Equations 30–35*

Time, min	Arterial Data	Level Prediction	Mixed Venous Data	Level Prediction
0	100	100	100	100
10	37	30	50	49
20	28	21	34	34
30	21	18	27	29
40	15	16	21	26
50	13	15	18	25
60	11	14	15	23

[Data from Beneken Kolmer et al. (7).]

TABLE 4. *Half Times of Uptake in Dog. Comparison of Data with Predictions of Equations 30–35*

	Cyclopropane	Halothane	Ether
Arterial			
Measured	2.1	27.1*	92.5
Predicted	1	7	93
Mixed venous			
Measured	7.5	58.4†	>100
Predicted	4	27	115

Values are in minutes. * At 27.1 min, equations predict 65% rather than 50% of equilibration. † At 58.4 min, equations predict 57% rather than 50% of equilibration. [Data from Cowles et al. (19).]

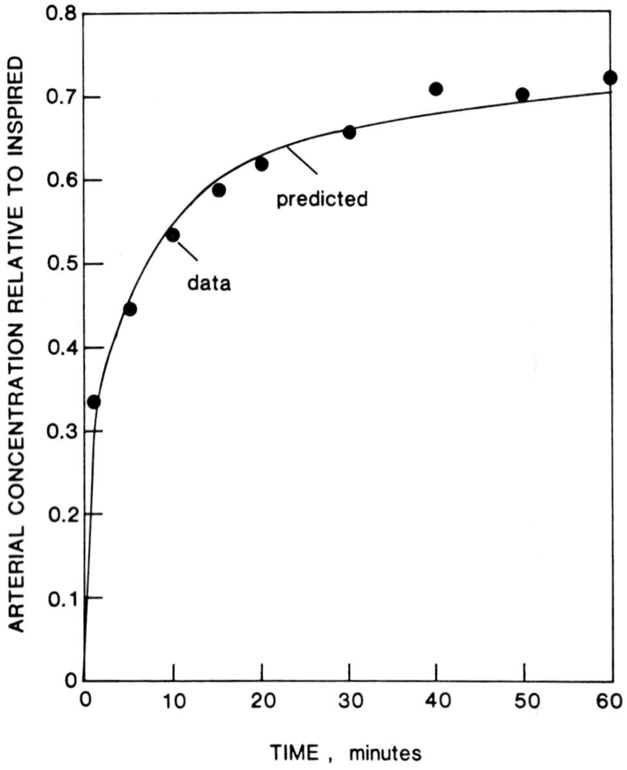

FIG. 8. Comparison of measured and predicted arterial halothane concentrations during uptake. Again, Eqs. 30–35 were used for predictions. Figure emphasizes that standard variable values from Table 2 and 4-compartment model satisfactorily account for observed arterial values. [Data from Sechzer et al. (77).]

cannot be sure of either of the above requirements, and on purely logical grounds it is highly unlikely that any tissue is spatially uniform in terms of its conductance-capacitance ratio: different regions will probably exhibit different flows per unit tissue mass.

To study the potential overall effect of diffusion limitation in a tissue, the most useful approach is to compare the washin or washout of two or more gases with similar partition coefficients but very different molecular weights. Only diffusive and not convective processes are presumed to be sensitive to molecular weight. Thus a gas of higher molecular weight will exhibit slower exchange kinetics than one of lower molecular weight [with the same partition coefficient(s)] if diffusion limitation is important.

The bulk of theoretical evidence supports the notion that diffusive processes in the tissues are mostly very rapid and not rate limiting. Thus Kety (41) has closely examined diffusion distances in many tissues and, on the basis of Copperman's calculations (16) for rates of diffusion radially away from a capillary, has concluded that equilibrium between blood and tissue should be essentially complete within 1 s. In the context of whole-body washin or washout over minutes to hours, even an order-of-magnitude error in this conclusion would be of little significance. Forster (27) has examined the rate of tissue-blood diffusion equilibration theoretically using available geometric data and commonly accepted values for tissue inert-gas diffusion coefficients of $\sim 10^{-5}$ cm^2/s and reached similar conclusions in well-vascularized tissues. However, in resting skeletal muscle, assuming a conductance-capacitance ratio of 0.02, Forster calculated the half time for diffusive equilibration to be ~55 s, which is not neglectable. However, Forster reached the same conclusions as above, i.e., that even if equilibration is incomplete its detection is not possible by inspection of the tissue washin or washout curve alone.

Although Goresky et al. (29) apparently agree that tissue inert-gas diffusion is unlikely to be rate limiting based on their modeling, Hills (33) strongly disagrees. Hills believes that tissue diffusion coefficients have been grossly overestimated; i.e., rather than being 10^{-5} cm^2/s, they are 10^{-8} cm^2/s or less. He bases his argument on the fact that the figure of 10^{-5} reflects diffusion in water, whereas real tissues include cellular material that may greatly impede diffusion of gas molecules. Direct measurement of diffusion of inert gases in rat abdominal muscle by Kawashiro et al. (38), however, yields values ~50% that in water. Moreover, as discussed in APPLICATION OF INERT GASES TO MEASUREMENT OF ORGAN PERFUSION, p. 273, inert-gas washout from local tissues does reflect and depend on local blood flow rate, and under many conditions perfusion determined in this way relates well to direct measurement of blood flow by other methods.

Most but not all theoretical evidence then suggests that diffusion equilibration is not a factor significantly limiting tissue gas exchange. This is just as well because, as so aptly stated by Kety (41) in discussing the modeling of tissue diffusion outward from capillary cylinders:

> Such a model might be satisfactory if all the capillaries were disposed in parallel and oriented so that all the arterial ends were on one side. Where the arrangement is more or less random with the arterial end of one cylinder adjacent to the venous end of another, there would be gradients not only within but also between the cylinders, introducing almost hopeless complexity into an attempt at mathematical treatment.

We are little further ahead in dealing with such a difficult issue today, and it has really become the province of the experimentalist to determine the importance of diffusion limitation at the tissues. For the mathematically inclined reader, there are several expositions of the mathematical treatment of tissue inert-gas diffusion. The Krogh cylinder–like model of Copperman (16) is an early but complicated treatment of radial diffusion from capillaries to tissues. The much simpler lumped-parameter approach of Forster (27) is also followed by Piiper et al. (68). Hills (33) considered diffusion into heterogeneous tissues, and his work was later extended by Hennessy (31, 32). Scheid et al. (74) presented an overview of approaches that includes both perfusion-limited and diffusion-limited exchange in heterogeneous tissues.

Experimental data generally (but not entirely) support the conclusion that tissue diffusion equilibration is not rate limiting. Jones (37) found no systematic difference between N_2 and ^{133}Xe body washout rate constants. Clearance of inert gases and other tracers such as ^{24}Na from local tissues is sensitive to local blood flow, suggesting that diffusion limitation is at least not dominant in inert-gas exchange (39). Measurement of local blood flow (see APPLICATION OF INERT GASES TO MEASUREMENT OF ORGAN PERFUSION, p. 273) by inert-gas clearance correlates well with measured values over a wide range (79). Ohta et al. (61) found whole-body Ar and N_2 clearance to be identical despite their different molecular weights. These workers also found cerebral washout of Ar and methane to be identical (63).

Inert-gas absorption from the bowel lumen into mucosal blood vessels has been studied for mixtures of insoluble gases (H_2, He, CH_4, SF_6, and ^{133}Xe) by measuring pulmonary elimination after injection of the gas mixture into the lumen of the small bowel, colon, and stomach (53), one at a time. For the small bowel, the data were compatible with perfusion-limited absorption; however, to some extent for the colon and to a major extent for the stomach, pulmonary elimination followed diffusion coefficients for the several gases.

Thus, for considerations of exchange between solid tissues and their perfusing blood, evidence indicates that diffusion limitation is not important; in special circumstances, such as gas uptake from the stomach or transcutaneous exchange (21) (taking place over relatively long distances between supplying blood and surface of skin), diffusion limitation may become important.

Diffusional Shunts

The preceding comments are concerned with a form of diffusion between tissue and nutrient capillary that would favor equilibration of a low-molecular-weight gas over one of higher molecular weight but similar solubility. Another way in which diffusion could affect tissue equilibration is through so-called "diffusional shunts," a form of countercurrent diffusional exchange between tissue vessels in a way so as to short-circuit tissue exchange. This is shown in Figure 9. If such short-circuiting occurred, it would delay tissue-blood equilibration for the gas in question. Because it would be more evident for a low-molecular-weight gas

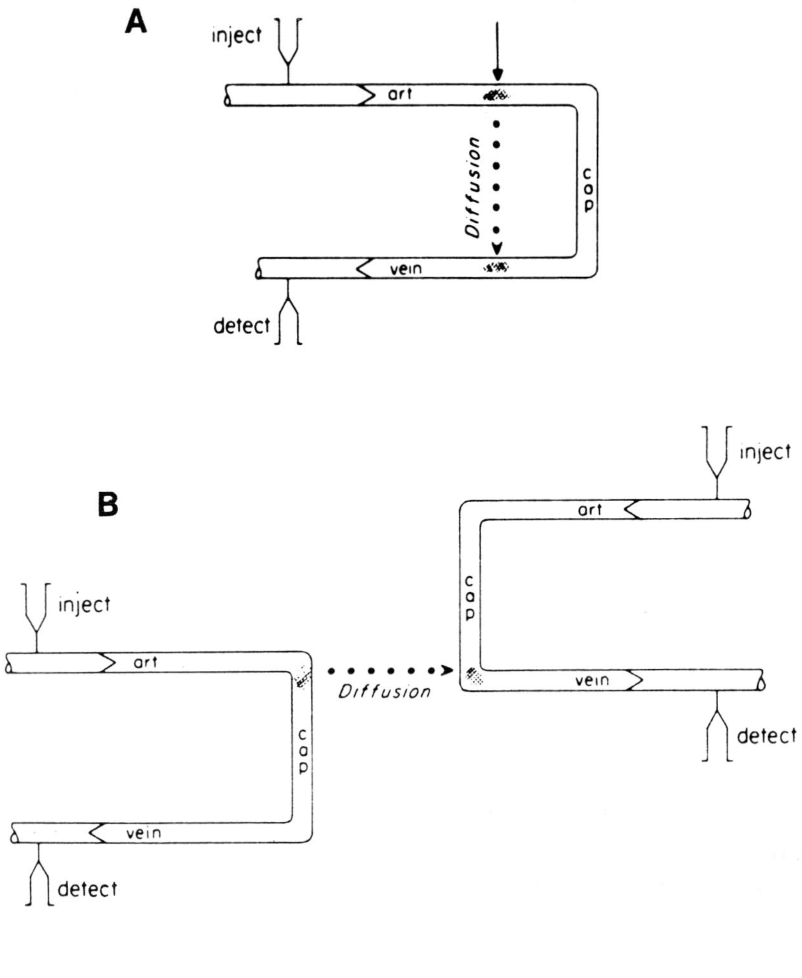

FIG. 9. Two possible models to explain "diffusional shunts" in tissue. *A*: there is direct diffusion between inflowing arteriole and outflowing venule. *B*: arterioles and venules within tissue may be arranged spatially so that they are conducive to significant diffusion between arterioles and venules. [From Roth and Feigl (71).]

(because of its higher diffusion coefficient), the result would be to delay equilibration of low- compared with high-molecular-weight gases. Note that this effect is precisely the opposite of the effect that diffusion limitation within the tissue at the capillary level would have, where a low-molecular-weight gas would equilibrate faster.

Sejrsen and Tonnesen (80) found that when a bolus of a mixture of labeled red cells, labeled plasma, and ^{133}Xe was injected into the cat gastrocnemius muscle arterial supply, ^{133}Xe appeared up to 1 s earlier than the intravascular markers. This was interpreted as evidence of a diffusional shunt for ^{133}Xe between vessels supplying and draining the muscle. Under the conditions of their experiment, Sejrsen and Tonnesen calculated that the diffusional shunt was equivalent to a real shunt of ~10%.

Other workers report evidence of diffusional shunts for inert gases in various tissues, generally by the observation of earlier venous appearance times of gaseous versus cellular tracers injected together into the artery of an organ. Thus this was seen by Roth and Feigl (71) at low flows in dog myocardium, by Aukland et al. (4) in skeletal muscle, and by Brodersen et al. (8) and Stosseck (85) in the brain. Bassingthwaighte and Yipintsoi (6) found similar evidence in cardiac muscle. Whether this evidence is taken to represent diffusional exchange between possibly randomly arranged microscopic vessels within the organ or countercurrent exchange between larger arterioles and vessels lying in close proximity, the data are difficult to explain on any other basis. Sejrsen and Tonnesen (79) interpreted multiexponential washout of indicators from local tissue sites as further evidence for diffusional shunting, but as pointed out by Sparks and Mohrman (84), local flow heterogeneity could equally well explain the data.

It therefore appears that if the early appearance of gaseous markers in effluent tissue venous blood is not due to other unexplained phenomena, there is general agreement that there may be a small but significant countercurrent exchange or diffusional shunt in many body tissues. Such a phenomenon would cause tissue perfusion measured by monitoring local gas washout to be underestimated (see APPLICATION OF INERT GASES TO MEASUREMENT OF ORGAN PERFUSION, p. 273), as pointed out by Piiper et al. (68). This is because some of the gas, as it washed out in venous blood, would diffuse into the tissue's arterial blood and then reappear in the venous effluent, causing an overall delay in washout.

Intertissue Diffusion

A third and entirely different manner in which tissue diffusion of inert gases could play a significant role in body uptake or elimination is by means of diffusion between adjacent but structurally separate tissues with different conductance-capacitance ratios. The most likely situations for such intertissue diffusion are between well-perfused organs and neighboring fat. Suggested candidates are *1*) gut and omental fat, *2*) kidneys and perirenal fat, *3*) skin and subcutaneous fat, *4*) heart and pericardial fat, and *5*) grey and white matter in the brain.

Perl et al. (66) suggested the possibility of such a phenomenon in 1960, pointed out how it would increase the overall rate of uptake or elimination of a fat-soluble gas, and provided evidence for it by comparing N_2O and cyclopropane uptake (67). Eger (26) questions the interpretation of the data because of a questionable assumption about cyclopropane solubility made by these authors. However, subsequent work has generally shown that intertissue diffusion is measurable. Allott et al. (1) directly measured halothane levels in perirenal fat and found them much higher (20- to 35-fold) in the fat close to the kidney as compared with the most distant fat; this strongly supports the existence of intertissue diffusion. The alternative interpretation that juxtarenal fat is enormously well perfused is not supported by observations. The data of Eger (25) further support the concept, as do the data of Cohen et al. (13) for diffusion between grey and white matter in the brain. Sejrsen (78) found evidence of intertissue diffusion for ^{133}Xe in the skin.

Just how important intertissue diffusion is quantitatively is difficult to evaluate. That it is measurable indicates a significant role that should not be neglected; however, it is probably of importance only to fat-soluble gases being taken up or eliminated over long periods of time (hours to days rather than minutes).

Evaluation of Assumptions

At the beginning of this chapter the ground rules for analysis of inert-gas uptake and elimination are laid out as a series of 10 assumptions. These assumptions required: *1*) tissue functional homogeneity geometrically and temporally, *2*) diffusional equilibrium without diffusional shunt or intertissue diffusion, and *3*) time invariant values of the important variables (pulmonary and tissue conductance-capacitance ratios).

How good these assumptions are depends to a large extent on what questions are being asked and what tissues and gases are being studied. By and large, the simple four-tissue kinetic (convective) models described in BASIC PRINCIPLES OF PERIPHERAL TISSUE EXCHANGE, p. 257, do a good job of predicting for most gases the overall uptake and elimination. This is probably because *1*) the lungs can be well defined mathematically and play a large role in gas uptake and elimination; *2*) the major tissue flows, volumes, and partition coefficients are fairly well known and also play a major role in gas exchange; and *3*) incomplete diffusion equilibration within or between tissues and diffusional shunt are either nonexistent (in some tissues) or of fairly small overall effects compared with the effect of the variables in *1* and *2* above.

Unless one is interested in rapid changes (over a time frame of seconds), the assumptions of time-invariant ventilation and blood flow are quite reasonable. However, research aimed at intraorgan heterogeneity of conductance and/or capacitance values or at diffusion-related phenomena cannot afford to uncritically accept such assumptions. Such a conclusion is also true for those concerned with estimating tissue blood flow by inert-gas uptake or clearance. In any one case, clearance curves may be affected by all three varieties of diffusion limitation (see CONSIDERATION OF TISSUE-BLOOD DIFFUSION OF INERT GASES, p. 269). As a result the clearance will reflect these effects as well as blood flow. Interpretation of clearance data may well then require some caution.

In the next section, we examine the application of inert gases to the measurement of tissue or organ blood flows and look at the assumptions in considerably more detail.

APPLICATION OF INERT GASES TO MEASUREMENT OF ORGAN PERFUSION

Seymour Kety (39–42) is responsible for laying down much of the theory pertinent to tissue blood flow measurement and for devising the techniques for making them. A readable summary of the several approaches is presented by Lassen and Larsen (51) and is briefly reiterated here.

Presentation of the principles of each method is important because the necessary assumptions can be identified, and this aids subsequent interpretation of data and the establishment of limits on the value of the techniques in actual practice. Each of the methods described is based on the same guiding principle that underlies all of the preceding material in this chapter: the conservation of mass.

Technique 1: Average Organ Blood Flow by Measurement of Prolonged Inert-Gas Uptake

In 1948 Kety and Schmidt (42) applied the Fick principle (integrated over time) to measure cerebral blood flow. A gas of medium to low solubility in blood is breathed at constant P_I for ~15 min, and the concentration-time profiles in arterial and draining cerebral venous blood are measured in intermittent samples. If the gas has a relatively low brain-blood partition coefficient, cerebral Pti equilibrium will essentially be reached within this time. Over the 15 min, the difference between the total amount of gas delivered by arterial blood and that removed in the effluent venous blood must equal the amount delivered to and stored in cerebral tissue. If at 15 min equilibrium is assumed between tissue and effluent venous blood, the following mass-balance equation expresses the above principle

$$\text{Pti}\ \alpha\text{Vti} = \int_{t=0}^{t=15} (\text{Pa},t\ \beta\dot{\text{Q}})dt - \int_{t=0}^{t=15} (\text{Pv},t\ \beta\dot{\text{Q}})dt \quad (37)$$

The left side of this equation expresses the total gas content of the tissue at 15 min; Pti is assumed to be equal to Pv at 15 min. The right side contains two integral terms, one for arterial and one for venous blood. They represent cumulative delivery and removal, respectively, of gas from the tissue, and their difference therefore equals total gas stored in the tissue over the 15 min. Because the tissue-blood partition coefficient (λti) is the ratio of tissue to blood solubilities, Equation 37 can be rearranged to give

$$\frac{\dot{\text{Q}}}{\text{Vti}} = \text{Pv}\ \lambda\text{ti} \Big/ \int_{t=0}^{t=15} (\text{Pa},t - \text{Pv},t)dt \quad (38)$$

Note that in this equation gas partial pressure terms appear in both the numerator and the denominator so that units are unimportant. Also, λti is a dimensionless constant. If *t* is in minutes and Vti is in milliliters, the term $\dot{\text{Q}}$/Vti is cerebral blood flow in units of milliliters per minute per milliliter of tissue.

Figure 10 illustrates the principle and its simplicity applied to another organ, the kidney. The height of the partial pressure–time curves at equilibrium (5 min in this case) is divided by the area between the two curves and the result is multiplied by λti to give blood flow per milliliter tissue.

The method is elegantly simple in concept. It is of major importance that it is model independent; i.e., no mathematical model of uptake is required for its execution because it simply uses cerebral inflow and outflow concentration data and processes them numerically. The method is noninvasive of the tissue, although sufficiently frequent samples of arterial and cerebral venous blood must be obtained to faithfully construct the partial pressure–time profiles. It is not necessary to calibrate the gas partial pressure–measuring device (as long as it is linear through zero) because gas partial pressure units are unimportant, as shown above.

There are, however, critical assumptions required. *1*) Cerebral blood flow is assumed constant over the washin period; in other words, the result is an average over the 5–15 min of data collection. *2*) Partial pressure equilibration between tissue and effluent venous blood is necessary. *3*) The tissue under study must account wholly for the effluent venous blood: to the extent that blood from other organs and/or tissues contaminates the sample, the result will partly reflect perfusion per unit volume of those tissues also. *4*) For purposes of interpretation, the tissue should be ho-

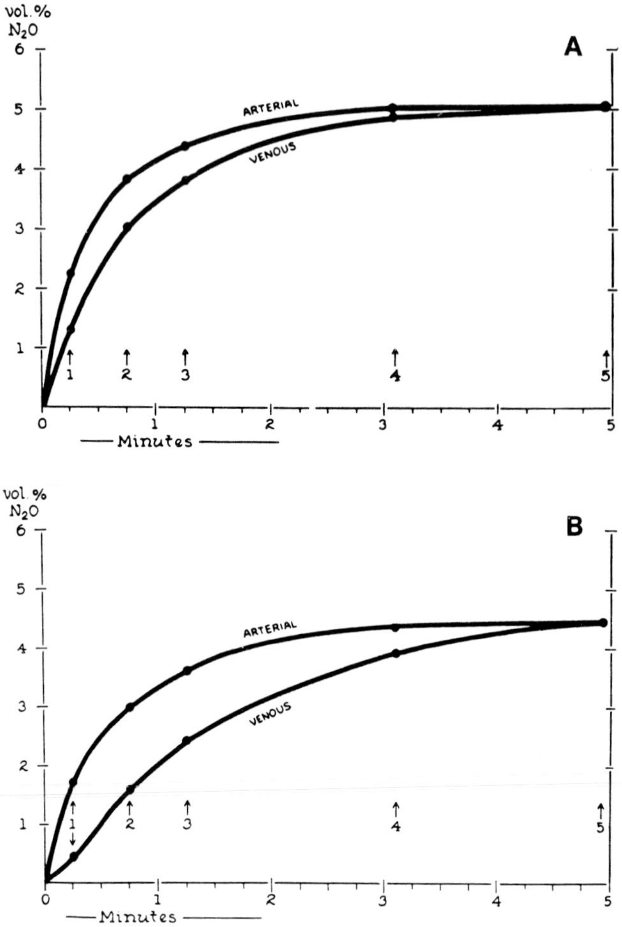

FIG. 10. Nitrous oxide uptake method of Kety and Schmidt (42) applied to kidneys for measuring organ blood flow. The N_2O levels are recorded over several minutes in both arterial and venous blood of organ until they are equal. Blood flow per unit tissue volume is then given by product of tissue-blood partition coefficient and equilibrium concentration of N_2O divided by area between arterial and venous curves. *A*: normal renal flow, 290 ml·100 g^{-1}·min^{-1}. *B*: slow renal flow, 122 ml·100 g^{-1}·min^{-1}. [From Conn et al. (15).]

mogeneous with respect to λti and blood flow per unit volume. If this is not the case, the result is an "as-if" equivalent perfusion of a homogeneous organ with a uniform value of λti and uniform blood flow. Moreover, any nonuniformity raises the potential problem of whether the venous sampling site is representative of the tissue. *5*) Equation 37 must be appropriate: there must be no unaccounted sources of delivery or removal of the tracer gas. Thus intertissue diffusion must be negligible, as must collateral perfusion to adjacent tissues or other forms of gas loss such as lymphatic drainage and loss via specific routes (e.g., in urine for the kidneys).

Although Kety and Schmidt (42) originally applied their technique to the brain, it has been used for other organs. Thus, as illustrated in Figure 10, Conn et al. (15) applied it to patients with anuria to study renal blood flow. Despite lymphatic drainage, urinary losses, and possible diffusional loss of tracer into perirenal fat (1), the method is especially well suited to the kidney. As a relatively fat-free organ with a λti value of ~1 for tracers such as N_2O, the conductance-capacitance ratio is ~(1,200 ml/min perfusion)/300 g mass or ~4/min. Thus tissue-blood equilibration is theoretically ~98% complete in 1 min ($1 - e^{-4} = 0.98$). Figure 10 shows that rapid equilibration in the kidney does occur: 98% equilibrium has in fact occurred within 3 min for the normal case, as judged by the shape and confluence of the renal arterial and venous curves for the tracer (in this case, N_2O).

It is interesting to estimate the potential error of loss of gas in urine. If one assumes at all times that urine gas partial pressure equals Pa (worst case), takes normal values for renal and urinary flow of 1,200 ml/min and 1 ml/min, respectively, and assumes equal solubility in urine and blood, the rate of loss via urine is only 1/1200 of the rate of delivery. More importantly, however, the rate of uptake by the kidney at any point in time is the product of instantaneous blood flow and the arterial (Ca) and venous (Cv) gas concentration difference, whereas urine loss is the product of instantaneous urine flow and Ca. Thus the ratio (*R*) of urine loss to renal tissue uptake at any instant is

$$R = \frac{\text{urine flow} \times \text{Ca}}{\text{blood flow} \times (\text{Ca} - \text{Cv})} \tag{39}$$

From Figure 10, at $t = 15$ s in the upper panel, Ca is ~2.2 ml/100 ml and Cv is ~1.3 ml/100 ml, so $R = 0.00075$. Thus <1/10 of 1% of the gas being stored in the kidney is being released into urine at 15 s, a negligible rate. At 3 min, data from the same figure show Ca = 5.0 ml/100 ml and Cv = 4.8 ml/100 ml, so $R = 0.02$. Here, urine losses equal 2% of renal accumulation, and the error is still small. Finally, when the tissues are fully saturated, *R* should approach unity if the only loss of tracer is in urine. This would lead to an arteriovenous steady-state difference (Eq. 39) of ~5/1200 or 0.004 ml/100 ml. This difference cannot be measured. Consequently, because of the very low urine flow rate, urinary losses are insignificant for the purpose of blood flow. Equation 38 raises another issue, i.e., the consequence of experimental error. As the equation states, and as shown in Figure 10, the key variable is the area between the two concentration-time profiles, which is determined by subtracting the areas under each curve from one another. The larger the time required to reach equilibrium and the more soluble the tracer gas is in blood, the larger will be the areas under each curve and the smaller will be the relative difference between the two areas. Measurement errors will be magnified therefore if the tracer is unduly soluble or if the time required for equilibration is too long, and this will result in potentially large errors in flow estimation.

As a result, the method generally employs gases such as N_2O, Ar, Ne, H_2, ^{85}Kr, or ^{133}Xe. The method is naturally inappropriate for measuring flows to organs or tissues with small conductance-capacitance ratios because equilibration times will be too long to permit sufficient accuracy in the area determination. The organs for which the approach works best are the brain, kidney, and myocardium.

Finally, compared with indicator-dilution flow measurements, it should be recognized that the gas uptake approach *1*) measures average perfusion, *2*) because of its nature is not rapidly repeatable, and *3*) cannot be used to measure short-term variations or transients in flow.

Technique 2: Blood Flow by Arterial Bolus Injection and Subsequent Tissue Washout Analysis

If a bolus of a relatively insoluble tracer (^{133}Xe or ^{85}Kr) is injected into the artery of an organ and radioactivity over that organ is subsequently measured, the rate of washout of the tracer from the organ is related to the rate of blood flow through the organ. If the tissue is homogeneous with respect to conductance-capacitance ratios and if the tracer is freely diffusible (not diffusion limited in its exchange between blood and tissue), a monoexponential washout of tracer from the tissue should be obtained. The equation for this is the same as Equation 10, from which it is apparent that

$$\frac{\text{perfusion}}{\text{volume}} = \lambda\text{ti}\,\frac{0.693}{t_{1/2}} \tag{40}$$

where $t_{1/2}$ is the half time in minutes of the exponential washout and perfusion/volume is in milliliters per minute per milliliter tissue.

In sharp contrast to the integral method described in the previous section, the bolus approach is a transient technique that can be repeated at fairly frequent intervals. It does require intra-arterial injection of the dissolved tracer, but subsequent measurement by external counters renders the sampling of tissue effluent venous blood unnecessary. By using a relatively insoluble tracer that is essentially totally eliminated by the lungs, recirculation to the tissues (which would render the washout nonmonoexponential) does not occur.

Also in contrast to the integral approach, a mathematical model of tissue exchange must be assumed, in particular, one in which tissue-blood exchange is not diffusion limited. If diffusion limitation occurred, the washout would at least partly reflect the rate of diffusive equilibration rather than perfusion. The method is potentially well suited to studying regional differences in blood flow, limited by the spatial resolution of the radioactivity counters for the tracer being used. The integral method can only give whole-organ blood flow (per milliliter tissue) unless venous sampling can be accomplished from different areas within the organ, which is not generally possible.

A major issue associated with the bolus injection method is that often the observed washout is multiexponential. Lassen and Larsen (51) suggest that this can be put to advantage because each component of the multiexponential curve can be separately analyzed by means of Equation 40 after some sort of stripping or curve-peeling procedure to separate the observed curve into its monoexponential components. When this is done, functional "compartments" with estimatable flows can be determined; however, note that association of any such virtual compartments with a physiologically distinct tissue compartment is a dangerous procedure. Before accepting such a conclusion, some sort of verification must be attempted, and this is often not possible.

In an attempt to apply the principles of the approach in a totally noninvasive manner, Mallett and Veall (55) had subjects rebreathe the tracer before recording the tissue washout, avoiding the potentially serious risks of carotid arterial puncture, especially in patients with atherosclerotic arterial disease. The difficulties introduced by their approach are *1*) the extracranial radioactive interferences caused by the nonselective method of introducing the tracer and *2*) significant recirculation of the tracer back to the tissues. However, on the basis of equations allowing for recirculation (e.g., Eqs. 25–30), this effect can be approximately corrected for. Moreover, on the assumption that the extracranial component is associated with a long time constant, this complication is amenable to mathematical correction also.

Technique 3: Blood Flow by Arterial Bolus Injection and Measurement of Height-Area Ratio of Concentration-Time Curve

A similar method of gas introduction by arterial bolus injection can be used to measure tissue blood flow by an analysis different from that for technique 2. Meier and Zierler (59, 94) showed that for an indicator-dilution curve recorded after rapid intra-arterial injection, the following relationship holds

$$\dot{Q} = \lambda\text{ti}\,\frac{\text{height}}{\text{area}} \tag{41}$$

where height and area are for the indicator-dilution curve recorded. The equation rests on many of the usual assumptions and is well discussed by Tonnesen and Sejrsen (88).

Thus this approach varies from technique 2 in that the entire curve is analyzed, not just the downslope reflecting washout after delivery. Importantly, technique 3 does not depend on assumptions of diffusive equilibrium or homogeneous perfusion within the tissue, but clearly a single average value is obtained for the region under measurement. Just as with techniques 1 and 2 and the corresponding variables involved, it is not necessary to determine the height or area of the curve in absolute units because height and area appear as a ratio. Thus counts per minute of radioactivity will suffice.

Unlike the washout analysis of technique 2, this method cannot be made noninvasive by inhaling the gas because Equation 41 strongly depends on the rapid appearance of a bolus of tracer at the measurement site. As with the preceding techniques, the method has been used mostly in the brain, kidney, and heart; it has also been used in skeletal muscle (88).

Technique 4: Local Injection of Tracer and Measurement of Blood Flow by Monitoring Subsequent Removal

In this approach, first used by Kety (40) in 1949 and later by Lassen et al. (52), a dissolved radioactive tracer is injected directly into the tissue under study, and its local concentration is subsequently measured over time during its washout. The measurement is made either by external counting of radioactivity or via a probe inserted into the injection site.

The principle is identical to that of technique 2, and the assumptions about diffusive equilibrium and the uniformity of conductance-capacitance ratios within the tissue are just as important as for technique 2. Two factors make this approach different from technique 2: *1*) the time course of the washout is usually considerably slower than when the tracer is given intra-arterially and *2*) most importantly there is the question of whether local tissue damage resulting from the injection itself changes the flow pattern. Lassen and Larsen (51) note that there is a transient hyperemic response to injection per se that lasts several minutes and may well interfere with the interpretation of results.

This method has been used for measurements of flow in skeletal muscle, heart, uterus, brain, subcutaneous fatty tissue, and many other organs (see Table 1). It has been applied frequently to the clinical problem of assessing peripheral blood flow in ischemic vascular disease, where large differences between normal and abnormal state can be demonstrated, as shown in Figure 11 for muscle flow after a period of ischemic exercise.

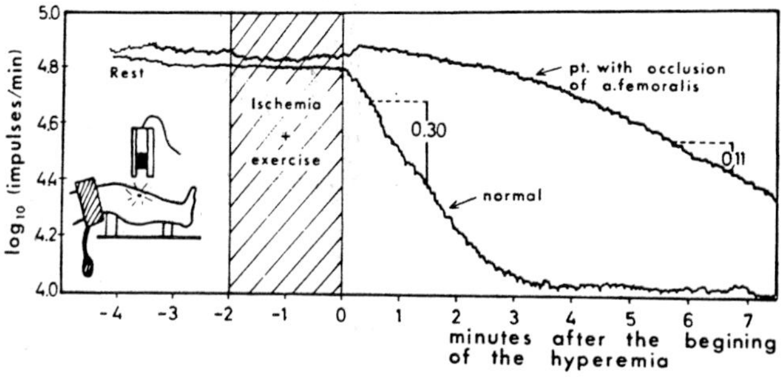

FIG. 11. The ^{133}Xe washout technique for measuring calf muscle blood flow. Small volume (0.1 ml) of ^{133}Xe dissolved in saline is injected directly into muscle, and its subsequent washout is monitored externally by scintillation detector after 2-min period of ischemic exercise. In normal case washout is rapid, and difference between normal curve and data from patient with occlusive arterial disease is striking. The ^{133}Xe counts on ordinate are on log scale, and blood flow is calculated from log slope of washout curve. [From Lassen and Larsen (51).]

Evaluation of Methods for Measuring Tissue Perfusion With Inert Gases

The preceding sections present the principles and assumptions of the four approaches that use inert gases as tracers in evaluating tissue perfusion. This section is a review of published experiences in which major advantages and limitations of the approaches as they occur in practice are summarized. This section therefore reviews not only the qualitative limit placed on the methods by the necessary assumptions but also the magnitude of such effects and thus their actual importance.

As with most techniques in physiology, one can find numerous papers that claim validity and at the same time many that point out flaws. Both kinds must themselves be critically examined, both for logical errors and for placing appropriate emphasis on flaws in proportion to their actual significance. In general, conclusions about any of the methods are determined by *1*) the technical sensitivity and accuracy needed to answer the particular physiological questions posed; *2*) the type of organ under study, which may or may not be suitable for any one of the four basic methods; *3*) the physiological state of the organ under study; *4*) the available equipment for making the measurements; *5*) the experience of the investigative team; and *6*) the agreement (or lack thereof) with concurrently implemented independent flow measurements. It is therefore clear that critical evaluation of inert-gas methods for tissue flow measurement is a difficult and noisy task in itself. Those caveats notwithstanding, the following general comments seem to reflect opinions and data in the literature.

TECHNIQUE 1. This method, the integral approach of Kety first developed for N_2O and cerebral blood flow, seems generally reliable for organs with high conductance-capacitance ratios such as the brain, heart, and kidney (15, 42). It is clearly inappropriate for tissues that equilibrate slowly such as fat. The method is relatively invasive (arterial and venous serial sampling), measures an average flow over 5–15 min, and requires equilibrium assumptions by the end of the 5- to 15-min washin. The method cannot be applied very frequently to a given tissue.

TECHNIQUES 2 AND 3. These methods, somewhat similar in that they use inert-gas washout profiles to calculate flow after arterial injection of the tracer, meet with varying success, depending on the several factors mentioned in discussing the two approaches. The approach with Zierler's theory (94) (technique 3, so-called stochastic approach) has mostly been found adequate with ^{133}Xe as the tracer in isolated muscle experiments when compared with microsphere or direct outflow measurements (58, 88). Tonnesen and Sejrsen (88) had less success with the exponential washout analysis (technique 2), even in the simplest setting of the isolated skeletal muscle, and in fact they express considerable skepticism with the exponential washout approach. Similarly, Hulten et al. (36) found good agreement between direct venous outflow measurement and that obtained by technique 3 using arterial injection of ^{85}Kr to measure flow in the isolated small bowel.

For intact animal studies, the results have been generally disappointing. Hirzel and Krayenbuehl (34) found good agreement between electromagnetic flow-probe measurements and ^{133}Xe washout-determined perfusion for canine heart only below 100 ml/min. However, when flow-probe values exceeded 100 ml/min, the ^{133}Xe technique badly underestimated perfusion by up to 60% (i.e., indicating flow of 200 ml/min when by flow probe the perfusion was at 500 ml/min). Marcus et al. (58) found that cerebral blood flow was badly underestimated by ^{133}Xe clearance (compared with that obtained with microspheres), except at very low flow rates of 10 $ml \cdot min^{-1} \cdot 100\ ml^{-1}$. This was despite elaborate surgical procedures designed to optimize the comparison (external carotid artery ligation, removal of soft tissues of head, lead shielding, and ^{133}Xe injection into internal carotid artery).

Using a modification of technique 2 (where instead of tracer bolus, steady-state infusion was used to first saturate tissues under study), Klocke et al. (45) studied heart blood flow with H_2 as the tracer gas. The washout was recorded after cessation of the infusion, and in normal dogs and humans the washouts were essentially monoexponential and permitted reasonable flow estimates to be obtained (although no independent method of flow measurement was used). However, in patients with coronary artery disease and in dogs with experimental arterial occlusion, multiexponential curves were obtained. The authors had great difficulty in attaching significance to the components of these curves, other than to make the general conclusion that they were probably the result of heterogeneous flow distribution. Their final comment was that "flows calculated from inert gas data can be heavily dependent upon the details of the technique which is employed when flow is heterogeneous."

These comments by Klocke et al. (45) cannot be emphasized strongly enough: the "compartmentalization" of multiexponent washout (or washin) curves must be performed with extreme caution. Although there is little risk in descriptive curve fitting with sums of exponentials to match actual data, there is enormous risk in subsequently attempting to attach structural significance to the parameters of any virtual compartment so derived. Because of the complexity and multifactorial nature of tissue gas exchange evident throughout this review (several types of potential diffusion-limited exchange, structurally and functionally determined heterogeneity of conductance-capacitance ratio, etc.), compartmental analysis of multiexponential washout curves should probably not be attempted unless the investigator has a great deal of experience and knowledge of the pitfalls.

TECHNIQUE 4. This method, calculating flow from the exponential washout of a tracer that has been injected directly into the tissue, has been the most frequently used of the four methods and has come closest to regular clinical application. The literature abounds with reports of the use of ^{133}Xe clearance from the lower limbs of humans (and animals) as a method of assessing blood flow in peripheral vascular disease. Figure 11 clearly demonstrates very different clearance rates of injected ^{133}Xe in normal subjects and patients with arterial occlusive disease. Other papers agree that such differences are large (22, 50), and positive conclusions have been drawn about the validity of the approach (35). However, when well-controlled comparisons are made between the ^{133}Xe clearance method and other established techniques, such as direct volumetric recording or venous occlusion plethysmography, two major problems emerge with the ^{133}Xe technique: *1*) usually the values obtained with ^{133}Xe are ~50% of directly or plethysmographically measured flows (10, 44, 58, 89) or they frankly fail to correlate under some conditions of importance such as during reactive hyperemia (Fig. 12) and *2*) even when there is general agreement the variability of the ^{133}Xe measurement is quite large (Fig. 12). For example, Tonnesen (87) reported a 63% coefficient of variation, and Kjellmer et al. (44) found a 53% coefficient of variation (for differences between flow measured directly and by ^{133}Xe at the same time). Such large inherent uncertainties considerably reduce the confidence of individual measurements in a given subject or experimental preparation and strongly suggest that meticulous technical execution is imperative when making measurements.

Although the clearance from an injected depot leads to disappointing results in most cases, as described above, some authors have had success in certain situations. Tonnesen (87) found quite good agreement for normal human calf muscle flow after exercise comparing venous occlusion plethysmography with ^{133}Xe clearance. In other tissues, there are favorable reports, albeit with technical modifications resulting from particular anatomic peculiarities of the tissues under study. Thus Fraser et al. (28) found that clearance of ^{133}Xe from the nonpregnant sheep uterine lumen yielded excellent results compared with microsphere measurements of endometrial blood flow [although they assumed a ^{133}Xe partition coefficient of 1.0 compared with the generally used value of 0.7 (14)]. Chi-

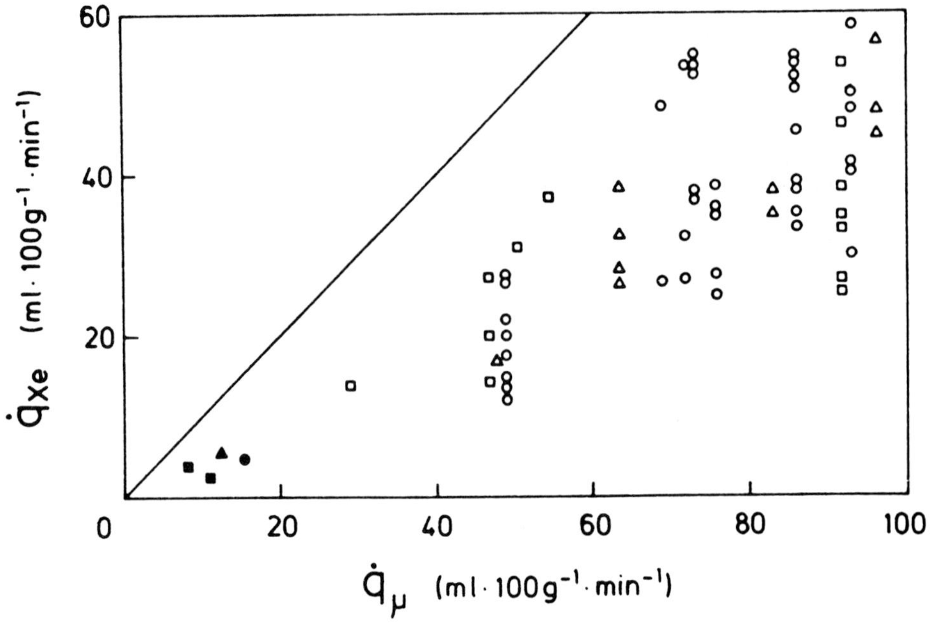

FIG. 12. Comparison of muscle blood flow (q̇) measured by ^{133}Xe washout (see Fig. 11) and that measured by radioactive microspheres injected into muscle's arterial supply. Latter measurements correlate well with direct volumetric measurements of venous outflow. Figure shows *1*) correlation between 2 methods; *2*) much scatter, indicating that individual measurements may be considerably in error; and *3*) underestimation of blood flow by about a factor of 2 when ^{133}Xe method is used. *Open symbols*, muscle stimulated; *closed symbols*, muscle resting; *circles*, gastrocnemius; *squares*, vastus lateralis; *triangles*, triceps. [From Cerretelli et al. (10).]

moskey (11) found good agreement between skin blood flow measured by ^{133}Xe and by plethysmography, as did Aust et al. (5) for maxillary sinus blood flow in humans. The data of Aust et al. (5) further indicate the large amount of variability in the data; although the mean values were 0.88 $ml \cdot ml^{-1} \cdot min^{-1}$ for plethysmography and 0.93 $ml \cdot ml^{-1} \cdot min^{-1}$ for ^{133}Xe clearance, the standard deviation of the differences between the two measurements, case by case, was 0.22 $ml \cdot ml^{-1} \cdot min^{-1}$, or 25% of the plethysmographic value.

One of the particular problems of the tissue injection approach is the potential of local trauma due to injection and the unknown consequences this may have for subsequent ^{133}Xe washout. Although Christensen (12) found clearance to be independent of injected volume over the range of 0.05–0.2 ml, most workers agree that a hyperemic initial period must be allowed to pass before washout measurement can be made. Why it appears (fairly universally) that the ^{133}Xe approach underestimates flow by perhaps two times (Fig. 12) is not clear, but there are several potential factors. *1*) Researchers may be using a value too low for the ^{133}Xe tissue-blood partition coefficient. In 1961 Conn (14) suggested a value of 0.7, which most workers have adopted. The data of Andersen and Ladefoged (2) agree. Cerretelli et al. (10) recently suggested that if capillary hematocrit was low due to the Fahraeus-Lindqvist effect the tissue-blood partition coefficient might actually be 20% higher and explain part of the discrepancy. *2*) The possibility that local flow reduction occurs because of injected tracer fluid compressing capillaries is not supported by the data of Christensen (12) in which ^{133}Xe clearance did not depend on the fluid volume injected. *3*) The possibility of clearance that is partially limited by diffusion would be consistent with the fairly common finding that the ^{133}Xe method best correlates with other methods at low flows (Fig. 12) and progressively underestimates perfusion at higher flows. This would be supported by the theoretical argument of Hills (33) that the diffusion coefficients relevant for gases in tissues are related to movement through a dense cellular matrix and not water. If this is the case, the operative coefficient would not be in the range of 10^{-5} cm^2/s but would be as low as $\sim 10^{-8}$ cm^2/s. The interesting possibility of partial diffusion limitation is still open. *4*) Heterogeneity of flow may cause disparity between direct measurements, which reflect whole-organ flow, and those of the ^{133}Xe technique, which measure local flows over a few cubic millimeters.

SUMMARY

Tissue inert-gas exchange is an important issue to a variety of clinicians and physiologists for many diverse reasons (see Table 1). The literature contains many fairly simple as well as more complex theoretical treatments of multicompartment kinetic (convective) models that predict whole-body inert-gas uptake and elimination fairly well over time frames of minutes to hours (see BASIC PRINCIPLES OF PERIPHERAL TISSUE

EXCHANGE, p. 257). Such a model is developed and presented in detail in this chapter, incorporating several levels of complexity. Evaluating the predictions of these models by both algebraic (analytical) and numerical means is demonstrated. Three potential effects of diffusion-limited tissue gas exchange are presented with evidence for and against their practical existence and importance.

Perhaps the major (isobaric) utilization of inert-gas exchange at the tissues pertains to methods for measuring tissue perfusion, a variable of interest both to the physiologist and the clinician. Four classic methods are presented, together with the assumptions implicit in their applicability, and a review of their appropriateness to various tissues is given. The general conclusion from these methods is that they are naturally susceptible to considerable variability and often correlate poorly with direct measurements of flow, except under the most favorable conditions in isolated organs. Part of the problem with such methods is that the basic relative roles of perfusion limitation and diffusion limitation in various settings of interest remain quite unclear; to the extent that diffusion-limited exchange exists, the methods are fundamentally in error. It would be a major advance to determine in all the situations and tissues and for the gases of interest the degree to which tissue exchange is limited, even partially, by diffusive processes.

REFERENCES

1. ALLOTT, P. R., A. STEWARD, AND W. W. MAPLESON. Pharmacokinetics of halothane in the dog. *Br. J. Anaesth.* 48: 279–295, 1976.
2. ANDERSEN, A. M., AND J. LADEFOGED. Partition coefficient of 133-xenon between various tissues and blood in vivo. *Scand. J. Clin. Lab. Invest.* 19: 72–78, 1967.
3. ASHMAN, M. N., W. B. BLESSER, AND R. B. EPSTEIN. A nonlinear model for the uptake and distribution of halothane in man. *Anesthesiology* 33: 419–429, 1970.
4. AUKLAND, K., S. AKRE, AND S. LERAAND. Arteriovenous countercurrent exchange of hydrogen gas in skeletal muscle. *Scand. J. Clin. Lab. Invest. Suppl.* 99: 72–75, 1967.
5. AUST, R., L. BACKLUND, B. DRETTNER, B. FALCK, AND B. JUNG. Comparative measurements of the mucosal blood flow in the human maxillary sinus by plethysmography and by xenon. *Acta Oto-Laryngol.* 85: 111–115, 1978.
6. BASSINGTHWAIGHTE, J. B., AND T. YIPINTSOI. The emergence function: effects of flow and capillary-tissue exchange in the heart. In: *Capillary Permeability*, edited by C. Crone and N. A. Lassen. Copenhagen: Munksgaard, 1970, p. 580–585. (Alfred Benzon Symp. 2.)
7. BENEKEN KOLMER, H. H., A. G. BURM, C. A. CRAMERS, J. M. RAMAKERS, AND H. L. VADER. The uptake and elimination of halothane in dogs: a two- or multicompartment system? II: Evaluation of wash-in and wash-out curves. *Br. J. Anaesth.* 47: 1169–1175, 1975.
8. BRODERSEN, P., P. SEJRSEN, AND N. A. LASSEN. Diffusion bypass of xenon in brain circulation. *Circ. Res.* 32: 363–369, 1973.
9. CANDER, L. Solubility of inert gases in human lung tissue. *J. Appl. Physiol.* 14: 538–540, 1959.
10. CERRETELLI, P., C. MARCONI, D. PENDERGAST, M. MEYER, N. HEISLER, AND J. PIIPER. Blood flow in exercising muscles by xenon clearance and by microsphere trapping. *J. Appl. Physiol.* 56: 24–30, 1984.
11. CHIMOSKEY, J. E. Skin blood flow by ^{133}Xe disappearance validated by venous occlusion plethysmography. *J. Appl. Physiol.* 32: 432–435, 1972.
12. CHRISTENSEN, N. J. The significance of work load and injected volumes in $xenon^{133}$ measurement of muscular blood flow. *Acta Med. Scand.* 183: 445–447, 1968.
13. COHEN, E. N., K. L. CHOW, AND L. MATHERS. Autoradiographic distribution of volatile anesthetics within the brain. *Anesthesiology* 37: 324–331, 1972.
14. CONN, H. L., JR. Equilibrium distribution of radioxenon in tissue: xenon-hemoglobin association curve. *J. Appl. Physiol.* 16: 1065–1070, 1961.
15. CONN, H. L., JR., W. ANDERSON, AND S. ARENA. Gas diffusion technique for measurement of renal blood flow with special reference to the intact, anuric subject. *J. Appl. Physiol.* 5: 683–689, 1953.
16. COPPERMAN, R. The theory of inert gas exchange at the lung and tissues. [Cited in Kety (41), p. 9.]
17. COWLES, A. L., H. H. BORGSTEDT, AND A. J. GILLIES. An electric analog for the uptake, distribution and excretion of inhalation anesthetics. *Data Acquis. Process. Biol. Med.* 5: 75–92, 1968.
18. COWLES, A. L., H. H. BORGSTEDT, AND A. J. GILLIES. Tissue weights and rates of blood flow in man for the prediction of anesthetic uptake and distribution. *Anesthesiology* 35: 523–526, 1971.
19. COWLES, A. L., H. H. BORGSTEDT, AND A. J. GILLIES. The uptake and distribution of four inhalation anesthetics in dogs. *Anesthesiology* 36: 558–570, 1972.
20. CRANE, R., M. YATES, AND S. N. STEEN. An improved electronic simulator for the study of the distribution of anaesthetic agents. *Br. J. Anaesth.* 40: 936–942, 1968.
21. CULLEN, B. F., AND E. I. EGER II. Diffusion of nitrous oxide, cyclopropane, and halothane through human skin and amniotic membrane. *Anesthesiology* 36: 168–173, 1972.
22. DAVIES, W. T. Blood flow measurement in patients with intermittent claudication. *Angiology* 31: 164–175, 1982.
23. DAVIS, N. R., AND W. W. MAPLESON. Structure and quantification of a physiological model of the distribution of injected agents and inhaled anaesthetics. *Br. J. Anaesth.* 53: 399–405, 1981.
24. EGER, E. I., II. A mathematical model of uptake and distribution. In: *Uptake and Distribution of Anesthetic Agents*, edited by E. M. Papper and R. J. Kitz. New York: McGraw-Hill, 1963, chapt. 7, p. 72–87.
25. EGER, E. I., II. Intertissue diffusion of anesthetics (Letter to the editor). *Anesthesiology* 38: 201, 1973.
26. EGER, E. I., II. Diffusion may limit or may increase anesthetic uptake. In: *Anesthetic Uptake and Action*, edited by E. I. Eger II. Baltimore, MD: Williams & Wilkins, 1974, chapt. 15, p. 249–257.
27. FORSTER, R. E., II. Diffusion factors in gases and liquids. In: *Uptake and Distribution of Anesthetic Agents*, edited by E. M. Papper and R. J. Kitz. New York: McGraw-Hill, 1963, chapt. 2, p. 20–29.
28. FRASER, I. S., B. W. BROWN, P. E. MATTNER, AND B. F. HUTTON. Measurements of endometrial blood flow in anaesthetized ewes by $xenon^{133}$ clearance and microsphere techniques. *Q. J. Exp. Physiol. Cogn. Med. Sci.* 67: 531–535, 1982.
29. GORESKY, C. A., W. H. ZIEGLER, AND G. G. BACH. Capillary exchange modeling. Barrier-limited and flow-limited distribution. *Circ. Res.* 27: 739–764, 1970.
30. HAGGARD, A. W. The absorption, distribution and elimination of ethyl ether. II. Analysis of the mechanism of absorption and elimination of such a gas or vapor as ethyl ether. *J. Biol. Chem.* 59: 753–770, 1924.
31. HENNESSY, T. R. Inert gas diffusion in heterogeneous tissue I:

without perfusion. *Bull. Math. Biophys.* 33: 235–248, 1971.

32. HENNESSY, T. R. Inert gas diffusion in heterogeneous tissue II: with perfusion. *Bull. Math. Biophys.* 33: 249–257, 1971.
33. HILLS, B. A. Diffusion versus blood perfusion in limiting the rate of uptake of inert non-polar gases by skeletal rabbit muscle. *Clin. Sci. Lond.* 33: 67–87, 1967.
34. HIRZEL, H. O., AND H. P. KRAYENBUEHL. Validity of the ^{133}xenon method for measuring coronary blood flow. *Pfluegers Arch.* 349: 159–169, 1974.
35. HOFFMANN, D. C. An assessment of the xenon-133 method of measuring muscle blood flow. *Aust. NZ J. Surg.* 38: 66–70, 1968.
36. HULTEN, L., M. JODAL, J. LINDHAGEN, AND O. LUNDGREN. Colonic blood flow in cat and man as analyzed by an inert gas washout technique. *Gastroenterology* 70: 36–44, 1976.
37. JONES, H. B. Respiratory system: nitrogen elimination. In: *New Medical Physics*, edited by O. Glasser. Chicago, IL: Year Book, 1950, vol. 2, p. 855–871.
38. KAWASHIRO, T., A. C. CARLES, S. F. PERRY, AND J. PIIPER. Diffusivity of various inert gases in rat skeletal muscle. *Pfluegers Arch.* 359: 219–230, 1975.
39. KETY, S. S. Measurement of regional circulation by the local clearance of radioactive sodium. *Am. Heart J.* 38: 321–328, 1949.
40. KETY, S. S. Quantitative determination of cerebral blood flow in man. In: *Methods in Medical Research*, edited by V. R. Potter. Chicago, IL: Year Book, 1949, vol. 1, p. 204–217.
41. KETY, S. S. The theory and applications of the exchange of inert gas at the lungs and tissues. *Pharmacol. Rev.* 3: 1–41, 1951.
42. KETY, S. S., AND C. F. SCHMIDT. The nitrous oxide method for the quantitative determination of cerebral blood flow in man: theory, procedure and normal values. *J. Clin. Invest.* 27: 476–484, 1948.
43. KIRK, W. P., P. W. PARISH, AND D. A. MORKEN. In vivo solubility of ^{85}Kr in guinea pig tissues. *Health Phys.* 28: 249–261, 1975.
44. KJELLMER, I., I. LINDBJERG, I. PREROVSKY, AND H. TONNESEN. The relation between blood flow in an isolated muscle measured with the Xe^{133} clearance and a direct recording technique. *Acta Physiol. Scand.* 69: 69–78, 1967.
45. KLOCKE, F. J., R. C. KOBERSTEIN, D. E. PITTMAN, I. L. BUNNELL, D. G. GREENE, AND D. R. ROSING. Effects of heterogeneous myocardial perfusion on coronary venous H_2 desaturation curves and calculations of coronary flow. *J. Clin. Invest.* 47: 2711–2724, 1968.
46. LANDAHL, H. D. On mathematical models of distribution: In: *Uptake and Distribution of Anesthetic Agents*, edited by E. M. Papper and R. J. Kitz. New York: McGraw-Hill, 1963, chapt. 16, p. 191–214.
47. LARSON, C. P., JR. Solubility and partition coefficients. In: *Uptake and Distribution of Anesthetic Agents*, edited by E. M. Papper and R. J. Kitz. New York: McGraw-Hill, 1963, chapt. 1, p. 5–19.
48. LARSON, C. P., JR., E. I. EGER II, AND J. W. SEVERINGHAUS. Solubility of halothane in blood and tissue homogenates. *Anesthesiology* 23: 349–355, 1962.
49. LARSON, C. P., JR., E. I. EGER II, AND J. W. SEVERINGHAUS. Ostwald solubility coefficient for anesthetic gases in various fluids and tissues. *Anesthesiology* 23: 686–689, 1962.
50. LASSEN, N. A. Muscle blood flow in normal man and in patients with intermittent claudication evaluated by simultaneous Xe^{133} and Na^{24} clearances. *J. Clin. Invest.* 43: 1805–1812, 1964.
51. LASSEN, N. A., AND O. A. LARSEN. Measurement of blood flow with freely diffusible indicators as inert gases, antipyrine, labelled water and rubidium. *Acta Endocrinol. Suppl.* 158: 95–111, 1972.
52. LASSEN, N. A., J. LINDBJERG, AND O. MUNCK. Measurement of blood-flow through skeletal muscle by intramuscular injection of xenon^{133}. *Lancet* 1: 686–689, 1964.
53. LEVITT, M. D., AND D. G. LEVITT. Use of inert gases to study the interaction of blood flow and diffusion during passive absorption from the gastrointestinal tract of the rat. *J. Clin. Invest.* 52: 1852–1862, 1973.
54. LOWE, H. J., AND K. HAGLER. Determination of volatile organic anesthetics in blood, gases, tissues, and lipids: partition coefficients. In: *Gas Chromatography in Biology and Medicine*, edited by R. Porter. London: Churchill, 1969, p. 86–112. (Ciba Symp.)
55. MALLETT, B. L., AND N. VEALL. Investigation of cerebral bloodflow in hypertension, using radioactive xenon inhalation and extracranial recording. *Lancet* 1: 1081–1082, 1963.
56. MAPLESON, W. W. An electric analogue for uptake and exchange of inert gases and other agents. *J. Appl. Physiol.* 18: 197–204, 1963.
57. MAPLESON, W. W. Circulation-time models of the uptake of inhaled anaesthetics and data for quantifying them. *Br. J. Anaesth.* 45: 319–333, 1973.
58. MARCUS, M. L., C. J. BISCHOF, AND D. D. HEISTAD. Comparison of microsphere and xenon-133 clearance method in measuring skeletal muscle and cerebral blood flow. *Circ. Res.* 48: 748–761, 1981.
59. MEIER, P., AND K. I. ZIERLER. On the theory of the indicator-dilution method for measurement of blood flow and volume. *J. Appl. Physiol.* 6: 731–744, 1954.
60. MEYER, M., U. TEBBE, AND J. PIIPER. Solubility of inert gases in dog blood and skeletal muscle. *Pfluegers Arch.* 384: 131–134, 1980.
61. OHTA, Y., A. AR, AND L. E. FARHI. Solubility and partition coefficients for gases in rabbit brain and blood. *J. Appl. Physiol.* 46: 1169–1170, 1979.
62. OHTA, Y., AND L. E. FARHI. Cerebral gas exchange: perfusion and diffusion limitations. *J. Appl. Physiol.* 46: 1164–1168, 1979.
63. OHTA, Y., S. H. SONG, A. C. GROOM, AND L. E. FARHI. Is inert gas washout from the tissues limited by diffusion? *J. Appl. Physiol.* 45: 903–907, 1978.
64. OLSZOWKA, A. J., AND P. D. WAGNER. Numerical analysis in gas exchange. In: *Pulmonary Gas Exchange*, edited by J. B. West. New York: Academic, 1980, vol. 1, chapt. 8, p. 263–306.
65. ONCHI, Y., AND Y. ASAO. Absorption, distribution and elimination of di-ethyl ether in man. *Br. J. Anaesth.* 33: 544–548, 1961.
66. PERL, W., G. T. LESSER, AND J. M. STEELE. The kinetics of distribution of the fat-soluble inert gas cyclopropane in the body. *Biophys. J.* 1: 111–135, 1960.
67. PERL, W., H. RACKON, E. SALANITRE, G. L. WOLF, AND R. M. EPSTEIN. Intertissue diffusion effect for inert fat-soluble gases. *J. Appl. Physiol.* 20: 621–627, 1965.
68. PIIPER, J., M. MEYER, AND P. SCHEID. Dual role of diffusion in tissue gas exchange: blood-tissue equilibration and diffusion shunt. *Respir. Physiol.* 56: 131–144, 1984.
69. POWER, G. G. Solubility of O_2 and CO in blood and pulmonary and placental tissue. *J. Appl. Physiol.* 24: 468–474, 1968.
70. RACKOW, H., E. SALANITRE, R. M. EPSTEIN, G. L. WOLF, AND W. PERL. Simultaneous uptake of N_2O and cyclopropane in man as a test of compartment model. *J. Appl. Physiol.* 20: 611–620, 1965.
71. ROTH, A. C., AND E. O. FEIGL. Diffusional shunting in the canine myocardium. *Circ. Res.* 48: 470–480, 1981.
72. SALANITRE, E., H. RACKOW, L. T. GREENE, D. KLONYMUS, AND R. M. EPSTEIN. Uptake and excretion of subanesthetic concentrations of nitrous oxide in man. *Anesthesiology* 23: 814–822, 1962.
73. SCHEID, F. *Schaum's Outline of Theory and Problems of Numerical Analysis.* New York: McGraw-Hill, 1968. (Schaum's Outline Ser.)
74. SCHEID, P., M. MEYER, AND J. PIIPER. Elements for modeling inert gas washout from heterogeneous tissues. In: *Proc. ISOTT Meetings, Ruston, Louisiana, 1983*, p. 1–8.
75. SECHZER, P. H., R. D. DRIPPS, AND H. L. PRICE. Uptake of cyclopropane by the human body. *J. Appl. Physiol.* 14: 887–890, 1959.
76. SECHZER, P. H., H. W. LINDE, AND R. D. DRIPPS. Uptake of halothane by the human body (Abstract). *Anesthesiology* 23: 161, 1962.

77. SECHZER, P. H., H. W. LINDE, R. D. DRIPPS, AND H. L. PRICE. Uptake of halothane by the human body. *Anesthesiology* 24: 779–783, 1963.
78. SEJRSEN, P. Blood flow in cutaneous tissue in man studied by washout of radioactive xenon. *Circ. Res.* 25: 215–229, 1969.
79. SEJRSEN, P., AND K. H. TONNESEN. Inert gas diffusion method for measurement of blood flow using saturation techniques. *Circ. Res.* 22: 679–693, 1968.
80. SEJRSEN, P., AND K. H. TONNESEN. Shunting by diffusion of inert gas in skeletal muscle. *Acta Physiol. Scand.* 86: 82–91, 1972.
81. SEVERINGHAUS, J. W. The rate of uptake of nitrous oxide in man. *J. Clin. Invest.* 33: 1183–1189, 1954.
82. SMITH, N. T., A. ZWART, AND J. E. W. BENEKEN. Interaction between the circulatory effects and the uptake and distribution of halothane: use of a multiple model. *Anesthesiology* 37: 47–58, 1972.
83. SMITH, R. E., AND M. F. MORALES. On the theory of blood-tissue exchanges. I. Fundamental equations. *Bull. Math. Biophys.* 6: 125–131, 1944.
84. SPARKS, H. V., AND D. E. MOHRMAN. Heterogeneity of flow as an explanation of the multiexponential washout of inert gas from skeletal muscle. *Microvasc. Res.* 13: 181–184, 1977.
85. STOSSECK, K. Hydrogen exchange through the pial vessel wall and its meaning for the determination of the local cerebral blood flow. *Pfluegers Arch.* 320: 111–119, 1970.
86. TEORELL, T. Kinetics of distribution of substances administered to the body. *Arch. Int. Pharmacodyn. Ther.* 57: 205–224, 1944.
87. TONNESEN, K. H. Simultaneous measurement of the calf blood flow by strain-gauge plethysmography and the calf muscle blood flow measured by ^{133}xenon clearance. *Scand. J. Clin. Lab. Invest.* 21: 65–76, 1968.
88. TONNESEN, K. H., AND P. SEJRSEN. Inert gas diffusion method for measurement of blood flow. *Circ. Res.* 20: 552–564, 1967.
89. TONNESEN, K. H., AND P. SEJRSEN. Washout of ^{133}xenon after intramuscular injection and direct measurement of blood flow in skeletal muscle. *Scand. J. Clin. Lab. Invest.* 25: 71–81, 1970.
90. VON SCHROTTER, H. Der Sauerstoff in der Prophylaxe und Therapie der Luftdruckerkrankungen in M. Michaelis. In: *Handbuch der Sauerstofftherapie*, edited by V. A. Hirschwald. Berlin. 1906, p. 155.
91. WAUD, B. E., AND D. R. WAUD. Calculate kinetics of distribution of nitrous oxide and methoxyflurane during intermittent administration in obstetrics. *Anesthesiology* 32: 306–316, 1970.
92. YEH, S.-Y., AND R. E. PETERSON. Solubility of krypton and xenon in blood, protein solutions, and tissue homogenates. *J. Appl. Physiol.* 20: 1041–1047, 1965.
93. YOUNG, I. H., AND P. D. WAGNER. Solubility of inert gases in homogenates of canine lung tissue. *J. Appl. Physiol.* 46: 1207–1210, 1979.
94. ZIERLER, K. L. Equations for measuring blood flow by external monitoring of radioisotopes. *Circ. Res.* 16: 309–321, 1965.
95. ZUNTZ, N. Zur Pathogenese und Therapie der durch rasche Luftdruckanderungen Erzeugten. *Fortschr. Med.* 15: 632–639, 1897.
96. ZWART, A., N. T. SMITH, AND J. E. W. BENEKEN. Multiple model approach to uptake and distribution of halothane: the use of an analog computer. *Comput. Biomed. Res.* 5: 228–238, 1972.

CHAPTER 15

Gas exchange in body cavities

STEPHEN H. LORING | Department of Physiology, Harvard School of Public Health,
JAMES P. BUTLER | Boston, Massachusetts

CHAPTER CONTENTS

THE PROBLEM OF GAS EXCHANGE in body cavities has stimulated some of the best thought and most elegant experiments in the field of respiration. Artificially produced gas cavities in the body provide an opportunity to examine gas diffusion in tissue and gas transport by the blood in systems that are simpler and thus easier to analyze than the lungs (22, 38). As experimental models, these cavities have achieved an importance in physiology far exceeding the importance of gas exchange in naturally occurring cavities. Gas exchange in body cavities does have direct physiological significance, and the absorption of gas from cavities and the elaboration of gas into them contribute to disease. For example, absorption of gas from alveoli distal to closed airways in the lungs leads to atelectasis, and elaboration of gas into various body cavities like the middle ear, bowel, and cerebral ventricles can be a hazard of anesthetic gas administration (6, 18, 20, 27, 29).

Artificially produced gas cavities have been used to measure the gaseous environment and properties of surrounding tissues. Under certain conditions the CO_2 and O_2 in tissue have been shown to equilibrate rapidly and nearly completely with those gases in tissue gas cavities (38). Thus gas cavities have provided a convenient way to measure the average pressures of the respiratory gases in tissue (33, 39, 40). Sørensen (30) has used gas tensions in subcutaneous gas pockets to estimate the average arterial partial pressure of CO_2 (Pa_{CO_2}) in uninstrumented unrestrained animals. Uptake of CO from gas cavities by the blood in surrounding tissues has been used to estimate the blood flow in bladder and intestinal mucosa (2, 8) and to demonstrate the increased vascularity in tissues of animals acclimatized to high altitude (34).

This chapter has two primary intents: *1*) to provide a theoretical perspective from which to approach problems of gas movements in and around body cavities and *2*) to describe briefly some of the more recent studies in this area. The following presentation is largely complementary to the excellent chapter by Piiper (22) in the 1965 edition of the *Handbook* section on respiration, which we recommend for a different perspective on the underlying physiology of gas cavities and for a discussion of earlier work.

TYPES OF GAS CAVITIES

Piiper (22) has divided gas cavities in the body into four functional types. We do not consider open ventilated gas cavities like the lungs in this chapter. There remain three main types of gas cavities: *1*) open nonventilated cavities, *2*) closed rigid cavities, and *3*) closed collapsible cavities. For these cavities the flux of gases into or out of the cavity is determined by gas transport in the blood perfusing tissues adjacent to the cavities (perfusion limitation), or by diffusion of gases through these tissues (diffusion limitation), or by both. The three cavities differ mainly in the consequences of net gas transfer into or out of the cavity and not in the principles or mechanisms of gas exchange.

Open Nonventilated Cavities

Open nonventilated cavities remain at or near am-

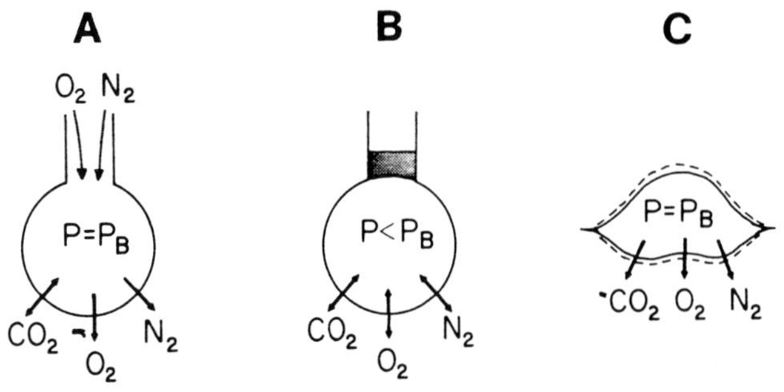

FIG. 1. Three types of gas cavities in the body. *A*: open nonventilated cavity. *B*: closed rigid cavity. *C*: closed collapsible cavity. *Arrows*, net gas flux (*single-headed*) or equilibrium (*double-headed*) in state of constant composition. P, total pressure of gas; P_B, barometric pressure. [Adapted from Piiper (22).]

bient pressure, and gas flows into or out of the cavity (Fig. 1*A*). When there is net gas absorption, the gas entering the cavity is usually different from the resident gas, and the steady-state concentrations and flux rates reflect this continuous bulk movement. Examples of open nonventilated cavities include the paranasal sinuses (18, 27) and perhaps the unventilated lung. When the cavity opening becomes blocked, pressure within the cavity changes and the cavity usually behaves like a closed rigid cavity.

Closed Rigid Cavities

Closed rigid cavities have a fixed volume, and net gas flux results in a change in gas pressure (Fig. 1*B*). As in the closed collapsible cavities, a transient state is usually succeeded by steady-state absorption of gas. Gas pressure in the cavity may become low enough to cause transudation of liquid that replaces the departing gas and may eventually fill the cavity. Rigid cavities that are completely closed are uncommon in nature, occurring as a transient phenomenon when an open nonventilated cavity like a paranasal sinus becomes closed. The middle ear is a closed rigid cavity that, though closed for most of the time, is intermittently opened to allow air to enter and therefore functions normally as an open nonventilated cavity. Pathological obstruction of the eustachian tube prevents the periodic return of middle ear pressure to atmospheric, and fluid transudation eventually obliterates the air space. Artificial closed rigid cavities can be made airtight and relatively impermeable to water, and Lategola (16) has measured the pressure within such cavities as an index of the total gas pressure within the tissues.

Closed Collapsible Cavities

Closed collapsible cavities remain at or near ambient pressure, while gas fluxes cause a change in cavity volume (Fig. 1*C*). Usually gas concentrations reach steady-state concentrations early in the cavity's life, after which net gas absorption causes pocket volume to decrease until all the gas is gone. Closed collapsible gas pockets occur naturally (e.g., intestinal gas) in the course of diagnostic procedures like laparoscopy, and with disease. The N_2 in intestinal gas comes in part from swallowed air and in part from blood. Bacterial degradation of intestinal contents releases other gases (CO_2, H_2, CH_4) that dilute intestinal N_2 enough to favor the diffusion of blood-borne N_2 into the intestinal lumen (17, 26). In the lungs, gas absorption in alveoli beyond occluded airways results in atelectasis. Other pathological closed gas cavities include pneumothorax and tissue emphysema. Bubbles formed in blood and tissues by lung disruption, decompression, or isobaric supersaturation (10) are a special type of collapsible gas cavity and are of great practical importance to diving medicine. An unusual example of a closed collapsible cavity is the fish swim bladder (25). Swim bladders have a relatively constant volume but are unlike most collapsible pockets in that gases (O_2 and CO_2) are secreted into the lumen by the gas gland. In these respects the fish swim bladder is similar to open nonventilated cavities in which gas convection into the cavity proceeds simultaneously and continuously with gas absorption by the cavity walls. Closed collapsible gas cavities like subcutaneous gas pockets (24) have been extensively used as preparations in physiological studies.

THEORY

It may be useful at this point to summarize the theoretical basis of most of the current approaches to gas transport in pockets (14, 24). In this section we emphasize the essential physics underlying such transport rather than the sometimes complex mathematical forms that arise. We first consider a closed pocket that contains some inert gas. This gas diffuses into the surrounding tissue and is convected away by capillary blood flow. The interplay between the diffusive process leading from the gas phase source and the removal process of convection in the blood constitutes the fundamental problem of gas transport in pockets.

In a quasi steady state (where all relevant gradients have been temporally established), Fick's first law of diffusion states that the partial pressure gradient driving the transport is proportional to the actual flux of the molecular species. (There is an immediate analogy to Ohm's law, wherein a potential gradient drives an electron current.) More precisely, the rate at which inert gas is transported ($-d^2\dot{V}$) from the gas phase to a differentially small capillary section is given by

$$-d^2\dot{V} = \delta_{ti}\alpha_{ti}d^2S(Pg - Pc)/h \qquad (1)$$

where δ_{ti} is the diffusion coefficient of the molecular species in the tissue, α_{ti} is the solubility coefficient in the tissue, and d^2S is the differential area serving the capillary (normal to the diffusive gas flux). The ratio of the partial pressure differences between pocket and

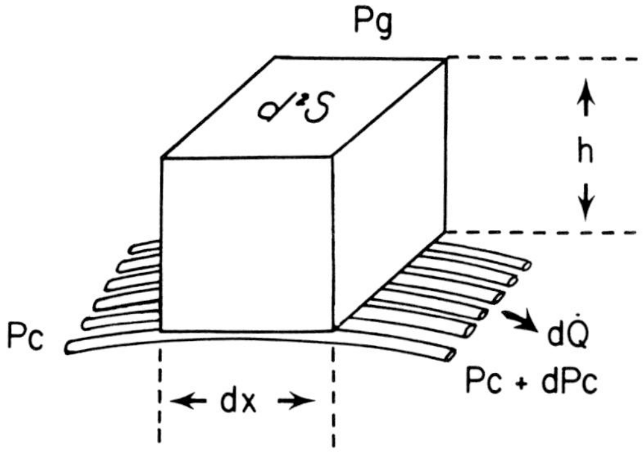

FIG. 2. Differential surface of gas cavity wall with its blood supply. *h*, Tissue thickness; Pc, blood partial pressure; Pg, pocket partial pressure; d^2S, differential area serving capillary; $d\dot{Q}$, differential blood flow; dx, differential length.

blood (Pg − Pc) to the tissue thickness *h* is the gradient term that drives the flux. (Fig. 2 shows the geometric model considered here.)

The net rate of convective transport out of that section of capillary, according to the Fick principle, is simply the difference in the rate entering and the rate leaving

$$-d^2\dot{V} = \alpha_c dPc\ d\dot{Q} \qquad (2)$$

where α_c is the solubility coefficient in the capillary blood, dPc is the differential partial pressure difference from entering to leaving, and $d\dot{Q}$ is the differential blood flow through that segment. At this point we explicitly assume that any flux contribution to or from the capillary in the direction away from the pocket is negligible. Under these circumstances the conservation of mass implies that the two fluxes above must be equal

$$\alpha_c dPc\ d\dot{Q} = \delta_{ti}\alpha_{ti} d^2S(Pg - Pc)/h \qquad (3)$$

Typically one proceeds by integrating this relation across the capillary bed, first at right angles to the blood flow and then along the capillaries themselves. This yields a global relation between the external parameters (partial pressures in the gas phase, the entering blood, and the exiting blood) and the net rate of transport.

Note, however, that there are a number of assumptions implicit in Equations 1–3. We list some of these, argue for their plausibility, and remark on the circumstances under which some of them might be violated.

Homogeneity of Geometric Parameters

The first integral indicated above is essentially a sum over all the capillaries at a fixed point along the axis of blood flow. At each equivalent point in all capillaries, one assumes that the axial differential pressure difference (or the gradient along the capillary), the absolute partial pressure, and the barrier thickness are the same. The differential volume flux from the cavity is then given by

$$-d\dot{V} = \alpha_c dPc\ \dot{Q} \qquad (4)$$

$$= \delta_{ti}\alpha_{ti} dx\ w\ (Pg - Pc)/h \qquad (5)$$

where w is width perpendicular to blood flow and x is distance along the capillaries. If the axial differential pressure, the pressure, and the thickness are not constant, then this relation must be replaced by an equivalent one, wherein one interprets the blood flow and the gradients as effectively laterally weighted quantities. This in itself is not a problem; however, subsequent integrations and their interpretations become more problematic. In particular the detailed mathematical structure of the final results becomes compromised. The essential features of those results, however, are expected to hold nevertheless.

Equations 4 and 5 form the starting point for the attention of most investigators. These equations are still differential; one would like global relations between gas, arterial, and venous partial pressures; blood flow; and net gas transport. Consider integrating along the capillary. Equation 4 yields a relation between the overall flux and the partial pressure differences in the entering and exiting blood; Equation 5 yields a further relation to the partial pressure in the gas pocket. Note that the ratio $\delta_{ti}/\dot{Q}$ will appear quite naturally, modified by some geometric considerations from integrations over x. This is the source of the diffusion-perfusion ($D/\dot{Q}$) ratio, where

$$D = \delta_{ti}A/h \qquad (6)$$

and *A* is the area available for diffusion. We return to these points in MODELS OF GAS FLUX FROM CAVITIES—PERFUSION VERSUS DIFFUSION LIMITATION, p. 290.

Steady-State and Spatially Uniform Gas Phase

It is commonly assumed that the species in the gas phase (actually within the pocket) is at a uniform partial pressure. If the pocket is filled with a single species, then thermodynamic equilibrium assures us that the partial pressure (here the absolute dry pressure) is indeed spatially uniform. If, further, the pocket is sufficiently compliant, then the gas pressure is the constant ambient pressure. For gas mixtures, however, the partial pressures cannot be strictly uniform because gas is being diffusively transported from the pocket volume to the pocket surface, where tissue diffusion takes over. In this circumstance we may ask how quickly steady-state conditions are reached. The time scale for diffusive events to stabilize in any phase is given by $l^2/4\delta$, where *l* is the total length of capillary contact region in appropriate length scale, and δ is the diffusivity of the species within the medium. For gases in the gas phase, δ is ~0.2 cm^2/s, and a typical gas pocket linear dimension might be 1 cm. The time scale for equilibrium conditions to be established within the pocket is thus ~5 s. This is very short in comparison with the time scale of all experimental investigations, and we may thus consider the steady-state assumption to be valid.

However, steady state does not imply uniformity of partial pressure (unless only a single species is present). In particular the gradient for a tracer gas can be approximated by using Fick's law. Nitrous oxide is the most quickly eliminated of all the gases listed in Table 1. Tucker and Tenney (37) measured a flux of 20 ml in 3 h in a pocket at 1 atm N_2O. Because this gas is essentially diffusion limited, that flux will scale approximately with its absolute pressure. If we assume a pocket surface area of 10 cm^2 and a maximal distance in the gas phase of 2 cm, we find an upper bound on the nonuniformity of partial pressure in the gas phase of around two parts per thousand. Thus even in this worst case the pocket may be assumed to be *1*) in steady state after a few seconds and *2*) uniform in partial pressure.

Steady-State and Spatially Linear Tissue Phase

An exactly analogous assumption is made for the species diffusing within the tissue. Here the relevant dimension is the barrier thickness, bounded above by ~1 mm (42). The diffusion coefficients are $\sim 10^{-5}$ cm^2/s. The time scale for the diffusive process to reach steady state is therefore ~4 min, which again is much shorter than the time scales of interest. The assumption of steady state is therefore on firm ground.

Is the partial pressure linear with distance from the pocket to the capillary? If one neglects transport in the axial direction, then the flux is essentially one-dimensional (from pocket to capillary). After a steady state has been reached, the flux is spatially constant; Fick's law then implies that a constant gradient (i.e., linear pressure profile) has been established. One can then simplify by replacing the more general gradient term with the simple ratio of the pressure differences between the pocket and the capillary to the barrier thickness. (See VERY SMALL COLLAPSIBLE CAVITIES: BUBBLES, p. 293, for comments on radially disposed flux in a spherical geometry.) This whole approach fails however, if the species is not inert but is biologically active. Specifically, if sources or sinks are present within the tissue, then the flux is no longer given by just a gradient term. Thus, even in steady state, this gradient is not spatially uniform. [Van Liew (38) discusses O_2 transport in this context.]

TABLE 1. *Solubility and Diffusion Coefficients of Inert Gases in Tissue*

Gas	α_{ti}, $ml \cdot ml^{-1} \cdot mmHg^{-1}$	δ_{ti}, cm^2/s
N_2	1.7×10^{-5}	0.68×10^{-5}
H_2	2.0	1.2
He	1.2	1.4
Ar	3.8	0.57
N_2O	63.0	0.55
SF_6	0.51	0.30

Data from Tucker and Tenney (37) and Piiper et al. (24).

Convective Blood Transport

The axial transport of gas at the capillary level, given by Equation 2, is explicitly assumed to be solely convective. Yet this is not strictly true because the inert gas can diffuse in blood as well. That is, the flux density is proportional to $Pu - \delta_{ti}\,\mathrm{grad}(P)$, where u is the linear velocity of the convecting fluid. The first term corresponds to convection (see Eq. 2); the second is just the Fick term. If the gradients scale like $1/l$, where l is the capillary length, then the ratio of the two terms describes which is the more important. This dimensionless number, often called the Péclet number (Pe) [by its heat transfer analogue (28)], is given by

$$Pe = ul/\delta_{ti} \tag{7}$$

When Pe is large (small) compared to unity, convection (diffusion) is the dominant transport mechanism. For capillary transport, l, u, and δ_{ti} are ~0.1 cm, 0.1 cm/s, and 10^{-5} cm^2/s, respectively, and therefore Pe is expected to be $\sim 10^3$. Thus convection dominates and the use of the mass flow term alone in Equation 2 is justified.

Unidirectional Tissue Transport

This assumption is slightly more problematical. Indeed our fundamental formula, Equation 1 (Fick's first law), assumes that the net transport to the capillary arises solely from the gradient established from the pocket to the capillary. We have neglected any transport in the tissue that is axially disposed. How valid is this? Here an argument on time scales does not help us. Rather, this assumption may be argued simply on the basis that net transport is an extensive phenomenon with respect to the area over which it takes place. Now the area seen by the capillary bed in the direction of the pocket is rather large in comparison with the axially projected tissue area in the direction of capillary blood flow. Thus the ratio of the areas determines the extent to which this assumption of unidimensionality for diffusion (the lateral dimension from the capillary) is valid. (For a discussion of axial diffusion and its implications, see refs. 21 and 35.)

Perfusion Versus Diffusion Domination (Limitation)

We now examine the essential implications of Equations 4 and 5. The immediate integration with respect to the axial distance x along the capillary yields

$$\int_{Pa}^{Pv} 1/(Pg - Pc)dPc = \int_0^l (\alpha_{ti}/\alpha_c)(\delta w/h)dx = (\alpha_{ti}/\alpha_c)(D/\dot{Q}) \tag{8}$$

Here is an immediate analogy to the Bohr integral. In that case, the lack of an analytic relation between the content and the partial pressure requires a sophisticated analysis to make progress. However, it is fundamentally the same as the equations for inert gases.

Here Henry's law saves us. That is, because the content is linearly related to the partial pressure by the solubility, one obtains the analytically integrable expression above. In particular

$$\dot{V} = -\dot{Q}\Gamma(Pg - Pa) \quad (9)$$

where $\Gamma = \alpha_c[1 - \exp(-\lambda)]$, $\lambda = \alpha_{ti}D/\alpha_c\dot{Q}$, and Pa is the partial pressure in arterial blood. This notation is from Tucker and Tenney (37), who refer to λ as the diffusion:circulation coefficient. What is the physics here? Rather than engaging in a complex mathematical exercise (which has been done by others) we focus on two limiting cases: diffusion limitation and convection (or perfusion) limitation. In the first case, one has that Pa ≅ Pv (partial pressure in venous blood); convection is so high that either capillary residence time is sufficiently short or capillary residence volume is sufficiently high that the partial pressure does not change significantly. Then it is clear that $\dot{V}$ is approximately given by

$$\dot{V} \cong -\alpha_{ti}D(Pg - Pv) \quad (10)$$

where λ approaches zero and Γ approaches $\alpha_{ti}D/\dot{Q}$. This is then consistent with Equation 1, integrated over the pocket surface, with capillary pressure approximated by venous pressure.

By contrast, if the residence time in the capillary is sufficiently large, or if the capillary volume is sufficiently small, then the blood equilibrates with the pocket gas (Pv ≅ Pg) and the characteristics of its diffusive behavior become unimportant. The net transport is given essentially by

$$\dot{V} = -\alpha_c\dot{Q}(Pg - Pa) \quad (11)$$

Here λ approaches infinity and Γ approaches α_c. Again this is consistent with Equation 2, with the integral of dPc approximated by Pg − Pa.

It is interesting to inquire why the ratio $D/\dot{Q}$ appears as an important parameter. If one simply looks at the ratio of the two limiting cases of transport that are possible, immediately $D/\dot{Q}$ governs which of the two is dominant. The molecular species is diffusing laterally away from the pocket and is being convected axially away by the capillary blood flow; the magnitude of $D/\dot{Q}$ governs this interaction.

These principles apply to specific aspects of gas exchange in body cavities. When gas cavities are created, total gas volume (or pressure) and gas concentrations and gradients all change at varying rates and may or may not approach limiting values. We attempt to explain what actually occurs by separately addressing different aspects of the experimental results rather than by following many aspects as they change simultaneously.

MEASUREMENTS OF GAS FLUX IN CAVITIES

Gas flux is usually determined by measuring the volume of gas in a collapsible cavity. After transients of gas composition have subsided, gas leaves the cavity at a constant rate; the pocket volume does not seem to influence absorption rate much until almost all of the gas is gone (22). Analysis is relatively simple when volume is measured at intervals during this steady-state phase of gas absorption. Individual gas fluxes in the transient phases of gas absorption are determined by simultaneous measurements of gas concentration and volume. Occasionally tracers have been used to estimate changes in gas volume (2). Gas fluxes have also been studied in closed rigid gas cavities, where both the rate of pressure change (18, 27, 36) and the maximal pressure achieved (5, 19) have been measured, although the latter is strongly influenced by the characteristics of leaks into the cavity. Net gas flux into an open nonventilated cavity can be measured directly (18, 27) or indirectly (7). Because most studies of gas fluxes have utilized closed collapsible cavities, we use collapsible cavities to illustrate the principles involved. Conclusions concerning gas fluxes drawn from studies of closed collapsible gas cavities usually apply with minor modifications to the other types of cavities.

COMPOSITION OF GAS IN CAVITIES

The composition of gas in the body cavities depends on many variables, but certain generalizations can be made that apply to air and several other inert gases. Gas composition of a pocket initially filled with air is summarized below. [For a more detailed description, see Piiper (22).]

When a gas mixture is introduced into a cavity, fluxes of gas into and out of the cavity occur at different rates for different gases until a steady-state concentration is reached or approached or until all the gas is absorbed. If the gas is initially air, there is a transient unsteady state in which water vapor and CO_2 diffuse into the pocket until their partial pressures in the gas become nearly equal to those in surrounding tissues. The solubility of H_2O and CO_2 in tissue and blood is so high that diffusion of these species is fast and equilibration is rapid (22). When N_2 or another relatively insoluble inert gas is predominant in the cavity, O_2 behaves like CO_2 and H_2O, and partial pressure of O_2 (P_{O_2}) in the cavity approaches that in the tissue. Tissue O_2 tension is usually nearly equal to that in mixed venous blood (22, 31). Thereafter the concentrations of N_2, O_2, CO_2, and water vapor remain constant in a "state of constant composition" (22). The initial transients were studied by Van Liew and described by Piiper [Fig. 3; (22)].

The partial pressure of N_2 (P_{N_2}) in the cavity is substantially greater than in the blood, and there is a gradient for N_2 to diffuse from the cavity into the blood and subsequently into the alveoli. This partial pressure difference arises from the shapes and slopes of the O_2 and CO_2 content curves of blood and from the relative rates of CO_2 production and O_2 consump-

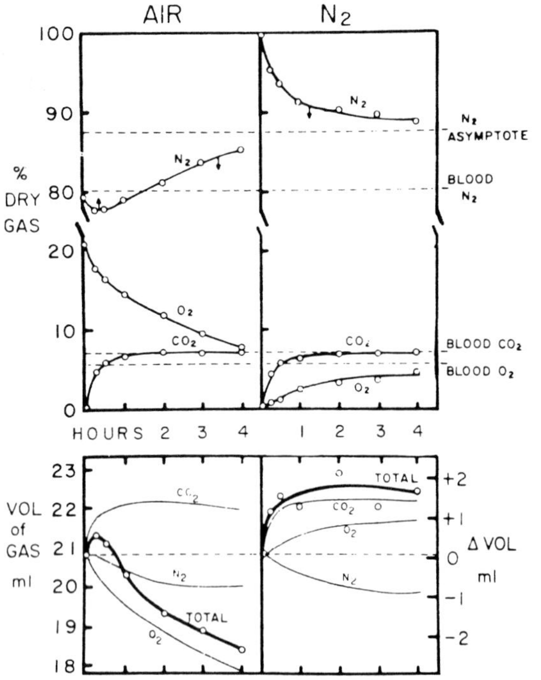

FIG. 3. Changes in composition (*top*) and volume (*bottom*) of subcutaneous gas pockets for first 4 h after injection with air (*left*) and N_2 (*right*). *Top: broken lines* mark the steady-state composition approached, which for CO_2 and O_2 is practically identical with corresponding venous blood values; for N_2 it is higher. *Bottom: heavy lines*, total gas volume; *light lines*, change of dry gas volumes of CO_2, O_2, and N_2. [From Piiper (22).]

tion by the tissues (Fig. 4). Between the alveoli and the tissues of air-breathing animals, the P_{O_2} falls from ~101 Torr to 41 Torr, a drop of 60 Torr. The comparable rise for the partial pressure of CO_2 (P_{CO_2}) is from 40 Torr to ~46 Torr, a rise of 6 Torr. The total pressure of the respiratory gases in tissues is therefore 54 Torr below that in the alveoli. If one assumes that P_{O_2} and P_{CO_2} of the pocket equals that in the tissues and that the gas in both pockets and alveoli is essentially at atmospheric pressure, then the P_{N_2} in the cavity must be 54 Torr higher than that in the alveoli and arterial blood. This partial pressure gradient drives N_2 from the cavity into blood. As N_2 leaves the pocket, the concentrations and partial pressures of the other species tend to rise, establishing gradients that assure that the gas will eventually be completely absorbed.

Figure 4 shows typical values for partial pressures of gases in air, alveoli, arterial blood, mixed venous blood, and a collapsible pocket during steady-state gas absorption in an air-breathing animal. In this example N_2 limits the rate of gas absorption as it diffuses from the pocket and is transported from the tissues by the blood. The preceding analysis applies equally to situations where other relatively insoluble inert gases are introduced into cavities as long as there is only one inert gas present. (Multiple-inert-gas fluxes are analyzed in MULTIPLE INERT GASES, p. 291.) The analysis of respiratory gas flux is more complicated because CO_2 is evolved by tissues and O_2 is consumed by them. Another complication arises because the O_2 content of blood is not a linear function of its partial pressure. When the cavity contains either no inert gas or a highly soluble one that can be rapidly absorbed, the fluxes of CO_2 and O_2 become rate limiting and contribute to pressure gradients. These special cases are addressed in EXCHANGE OF O_2 AND CO_2 (see next page).

TOTAL GAS PRESSURE IN TISSUE

The sum of the partial pressures of all gases in tissue is a convenient measure of the tendency of a gas pocket to be absorbed. Regardless of the gases breathed or injected into a cavity, the state of constant composition will be characterized by partial pressure differences that favor gas absorption. (Isobaric supersaturation is an exception that is discussed in SUPERSATURATION AND BUBBLE GROWTH, p. 293.) As just discussed, P_{O_2} and P_{CO_2} in tissue can be thought of as contributing to a total tissue gas pressure that is subatmospheric by ~54 Torr (22). Lategola (16) measured total gas pressure in subcutaneously implanted rigid capsules permeable to N_2, O_2, and CO_2 but relatively impermeable to H_2O. He found pressures at equilibrium to be 40–50 Torr below atmospheric pressure, in agreement with theory. For animals breathing pure O_2, total gas pressure in tissues would be ~610 Torr below atmospheric pressure (22).

NONSTEADY STATE

Before the steady state of constant composition is reached, gas concentrations within the cavity must achieve their steady-state values. During this period

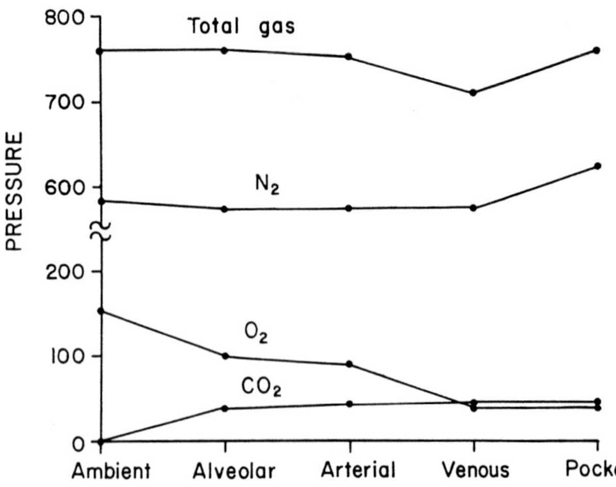

FIG. 4. Pressures of gases in air, alveoli, arterial blood, mixed venous blood, and subcutaneous gas pocket of an air-breathing animal. Total gas pressure gradient from pocket to blood is due principally to N_2 gradient. Water vapor pressure is assumed to be 20 Torr in air and 47 Torr in the body. [Data from Piiper (22) and Tenney and Ou (34).]

of adjustment, gas pocket volume may increase or may decrease at rates different from steady-state absorption rates. For example, when N_2 is injected subcutaneously the initial rapid influx of water vapor, CO_2, and O_2 into the pocket far exceeds the efflux of N_2, and the pocket volume increases (22). When pockets in air-breathing animals are initially filled with relatively insoluble non-N_2 inert gases, N_2 influx causes a prolonged period of volumetric expansion that complicates analysis of gas absorption (32, 37). As discussed earlier in THEORY, p. 284, the flux rate of inert gases out of gas cavities depends on two potentially rate-limiting processes: *1*) diffusion through tissues and *2*) removal by blood. The relative importance of perfusion and diffusion in determining the rate of gas flux is discussed in MODELS OF GAS FLUX FROM CAVITIES—PERFUSION VERSUS DIFFUSION LIMITATION (see next page).

EXCHANGE OF O_2 AND CO_2

In considering inert gases one assumes that gas solubilities are constant and that gases are neither produced nor consumed. For respiratory gases one must examine additional factors, including the metabolic consumption of O_2 and production of CO_2 and hemoglobin saturation kinetics.

Of the two respiratory gases, CO_2 is the first to equilibrate in tissues and gas spaces because of its very high solubility in tissues and blood. The ability of blood to carry CO_2 is greater than its ability to carry O_2, and CO_2 is ~23 times more permeant in tissues. (By permeant we mean the $\alpha_{ti}\delta_{ti}$ product is large.) Thus, in the presence of O_2 or some relatively insoluble inert gas like N_2, the P_{CO_2} values in pocket, blood, and tissues are essentially in equilibrium in the steady state (38).

The excised cat bladder is an excellent preparation for studying the interplay between the metabolic and diffusional fluxes of the respiratory gases. Van Liew (45) used this preparation to study the diffusion of CO_2. He estimated the Krogh permeation coefficient of CO_2 in the bladder wall by a method that allows computation of the metabolic production of CO_2 by the tissue. Van Liew points out that the permeation coefficient (in $cm^2 \cdot min^{-2} \cdot atm^{-1}$) is well suited to describe diffusion through inhomogeneous tissues whose solubility coefficients and Fick diffusion coefficients might not accurately reflect the diffusion rates of gas through them. The permeation coefficient for CO_2 was 23–43 times those of O_2, N_2, and CO measured in the same preparation (1, 47).

The metabolic production of CO_2 by the bladder tissue acts as an additional source of CO_2 and must be considered when the CO_2 gradients from the lumen to the gas outside the bladder are small. However, CO_2 diffuses so readily that CO_2 flux from the lumen is usually much greater than metabolic production of CO_2, rendering metabolic production unimportant in determining CO_2 flux.

In the same preparation, Van Liew and Chen (47) later found this is not the case for O_2 diffusion and metabolism. Because O_2 diffuses less readily than CO_2, O_2 utilization by the tissues is significant when compared to O_2 flux rates from the bladder lumen. Figure 5 shows experimental data plotted to determine the Krogh diffusion constant and metabolic O_2 consumption. The authors replot their data in idealized form and discuss in detail the O_2 economy of the excised bladder (47).

The flux rates of O_2 in subcutaneous gas pockets in vivo are further complicated by the nonlinearity of the oxyhemoglobin saturation curve. Van Liew and coworkers (49) have examined O_2 flux from gas pockets whose P_{O_2} extends up to ~3,000 Torr. They divide the pocket P_{O_2} into three ranges. Between 40 Torr and ~350 Torr, O_2 diffusing from the pocket is insufficient to meet the metabolic requirements of adjacent tissue, and O_2 is supplied by the perfusing blood. An increase in pocket P_{O_2} causes a large increase in O_2 flux into the tissue. The increased O_2 flux reduces desaturation of capillary blood with a relatively small increase in tissue P_{O_2} (because the hemoglobin saturation curve is relatively steep in this range). The net O_2 diffusing into a volume of tissue can be equated with the decrease in O_2 delivered by the perfusing blood.

With a pocket P_{O_2} of 350–800 Torr, O_2 flux from the pocket is sufficient to meet metabolic demands, and the hemoglobin in blood perfusing the tissue remains saturated. An increase in pocket P_{O_2} causes O_2 to diffuse further into the tissue, while O_2 uptake in each tiny volume of tissue close to the pocket remains fixed by the metabolic rate. In this range or

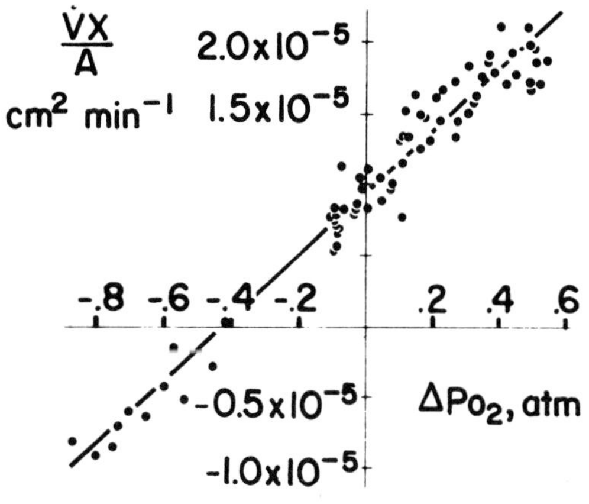

FIG. 5. Exit rate of O_2 from bladders suspended in air (*right*) or pure O_2 (*left*) vs. P_{O_2} difference, inside minus outside. Exit rate is normalized by thickness/area (x/A) to decrease variability due to bladder dimensions and to allow estimation of Krogh diffusion constant. At *y*-intercept, all O_2 leaving the pocket is consumed in inner half of bladder tissue. At the *x*-intercept, O_2 diffusing from external gas is sufficient to meet metabolic requirements of tissue, and there is no P_{O_2} gradient or O_2 flux at the inner surface of bladder wall. [From Van Liew and Chen (47).]

pocket P_{O_2}, where only small amounts of O_2 are exchanged with blood (those carried in physical solution in the blood), O_2 flux is equal to pocket pressure by the curvilinear function $K\sqrt{(Pg - Pti)}$, where Pg is P_{O_2} in the pocket, Pti is P_{O_2} in the tissue beyond the influence of the pocket, and K is a constant. If perfusion stops entirely (38, 42) or is increased fourfold (44), the O_2 flux stays nearly constant because metabolic consumption of O_2 by the tissue close to the pocket is constant.

When pocket P_{O_2} is >800 Torr, the flux of O_2 from the pocket is more than sufficient to meet metabolic needs of the surrounding tissue, and blood perfusing the tissue carries away significant amounts of dissolved O_2. As pocket P_{O_2} increases to >800 Torr, the relationship between pocket P_{O_2} and O_2 flux is increasingly linear, like that of inert gases. The characteristics of O_2 absorption from pockets provide strong support for models of gas exchange in which perfusion is distributed uniformly in the tissue, as described in the next section.

Nonlinearity in the carboxyhemoglobin dissociation curve affects CO flux from gas cavities in a way analogous to that for O_2. Coburn et al. (2) studied the uptake of CO from dog bladders in vivo and found that when the partial pressure of CO (P_{CO}) in the pocket was <450 Torr, uptake was limited by diffusion. At higher partial pressures, hemoglobin became saturated and uptake was limited by perfusion of mucosal vessels.

The ability of blood to contain O_2 or CO_2 depends on the presence of other gases, and this dependence affects flux rates from cavities. Van Liew and Chen (47) measured O_2 efflux from gas pockets when O_2 was diluted in either N_2 or CO. At moderately high pocket P_{O_2}, CO reduced O_2 efflux; when pocket P_{O_2} fell below ~250 Torr, the CO diffusing into the blood displaced sufficient O_2 from hemoglobin to cause a net flux of O_2 into the pocket. Coburn et al. (2) noted the same phenomenon in studies on dog bladders. A similar effect (the Haldane effect) is seen when O_2 displaces CO_2 from capillary blood (49), causing pocket P_{CO_2} to be greater for higher pocket P_{O_2} values. The interaction of O_2, CO, and CO_2 in their combination with hemoglobin and solution in blood has been used to study blood flow distribution in tissues, as discussed next.

MODELS OF GAS FLUX FROM CAVITIES—PERFUSION VERSUS DIFFUSION LIMITATION

Gas leaves cavities by diffusing through surrounding tissues and by dissolving in blood, which carries it away. For most inert gases under most conditions, these processes are all that need to be considered. Metabolic consumption and production of respiratory gases were considered in the preceding section. Cutaneous gas exchange, except in the special circumstances of isobaric supersaturation or hyperbaria, is usually negligible. Extremely permeant gases may diffuse far into tissues surrounding a gas cavity (2). However, most models of gas exchange in subcutaneous gas pockets have considered the gas, the perfusing blood, and the tissue as a closed system. In purely diffusion-determined or purely perfusion-determined exchange, flux rates are described by the Fick equation (Eq. 10) for diffusion or the Fick principle (Eq. 11) for perfusion.

The question of perfusion versus diffusion limitation of gas flux, nicely presented by Piiper (22), has continued to spark interest. The original analysis presented by Piiper et al. (24) for the inert gases N_2, He, H_2, and Ar showed the importance of both diffusion and perfusion in determining flux rate. In this analysis a uniform diffusion barrier was interposed between the gas and blood flowing through a capillary (Fig. 6*A*). Absorption rates of various gases were compared according to a form of Equation 9, and the ratio of diffusion limitation to perfusion limitation $[(A/h)(D/\dot{Q})]$ was computed for each gas. Experimental data fit the model fairly well for the relatively insoluble inert gases they studied.

Van Liew (42) has proposed an alternate model for gas exchange in subcutaneous gas pockets. Based on

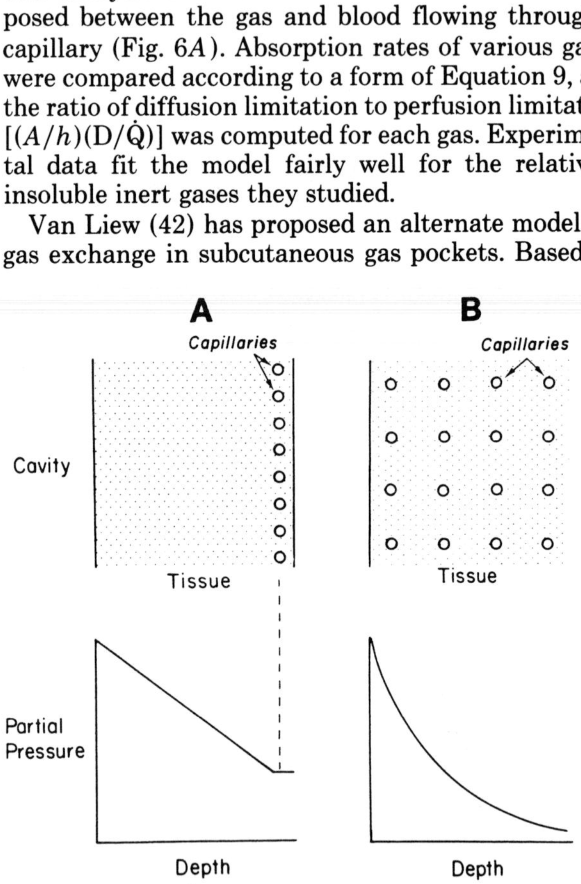

FIG. 6. Two basic models for analysis of gas exchange in body cavities. Diagrams of cavity wall with capillaries cut in cross section are shown with plots of partial pressure of gas diffusing from cavity into blood. *A*: model with uniform diffusion barrier separating the cavity from a vascular bed. Gas in pericapillary tissue is in equilibrium with that in blood. Gradients are uniform, and flux is a linear function of partial pressure in the pocket. *B*: basic model with perfused capillaries uniformly distributed in a homogeneous diffusion barrier. Gradients are not uniform, and flux is not a linear function of partial pressure in the pocket. (Model includes an additional diffusion barrier, not shown here, which accounts for incomplete equilibration of partial pressure in blood and pericapillary tissue.) [*A* adapted from Piiper et al. (23); *B* adapted from Van Liew (42).]

data obtained from studies of O_2 absorption from subcutaneous pockets, he proposed that the tissue surrounding a pocket comprises a uniform diffusion barrier in which the capillaries and perfusion are uniformly distributed (Fig. 6*B*). A model incorporating distributed perfusion could explain why O_2 flux continued to increase as P_{O_2} was increased above levels necessary to saturate hemoglobin in the capillaries (49). This model could also explain the interaction of O_2 and CO in gas pockets (43) and the effects of a fourfold increase in perfusion on flux of N_2 and O_2 (44). For H_2 and He, Van Liew estimated the effluent blood to be nearly in equilibrium with the local tissue partial pressure, whereas there was an end-capillary–to–tissue gradient for N_2 and Ar. He also computed the partial pressure of end-capillary blood relative to local tissue partial pressures and included this estimate in the factor *K*.

Piiper (23) later examined models of gas exchange from pockets and tested the models with data from the original study of Piiper et al. (24). He concluded that a model of uniformly distributed perfusion with complete blood-tissue equilibration (Fig. 6*B*) was less able to predict inert-gas transport than the earlier, simpler model (Fig. 6*A*). (The distributed-perfusion model would have been equally able to fit the data if it had been afforded the same number of variables as competing theories.) Piiper also examined two hybrid models that included distributed perfusion and a discrete diffusion barrier, both of which are consistent with Van Liew's finding that blood-tissue equilibration was sometimes incomplete. Piiper concluded that although the more complex models were able to explain the inert-gas data as effectively as the simplest model, they were needlessly complex and had no special advantage in explaining the limited set of experimental data of Piiper et al. (24).

Although the models discussed by Piiper can explain data from subcutaneous gas pockets, other types of gas cavities behave differently. Coburn et al. (2) found that CO uptake from the urinary bladder of dogs is limited by diffusion at low P_{CO} and limited by perfusion at higher P_{CO}, but they discovered no evidence for increased fluxes at the highest P_{CO}, as had been found for O_2 in subcutaneous pockets (49). They concluded that the exchange of CO occurred in a superficial mucosal vascular bed that was physiologically separate from deeper vessels and tissues. They obtained different results when highly soluble (and thus permeant) gases like N_2O or C_2H_2 were placed in the lumen. Flux rates of these gases were not limited by the perfusion of the superficial mucosal vascular bed, and the gases diffused rapidly into deeper tissues even after all perfusion was stopped. A model of this preparation would include a superficial diffusion barrier and mucosal vascular bed similar to Figure 6*A* with a deeper diffusion barrier and perfused tissue reservoir as seen only by more soluble gases.

As more data have been gathered in a greater variety of experimental conditions, more complicated models have been created to explain all the findings. Our understanding has evolved with these models. Flux of certain inert gases out of subcutaneous gas pockets seems to be adequately predicted by a simple model of a diffusion barrier in series with a convective sink (23), whereas data on oxygen flux and fluxes of O_2 and CO from pockets require a more complex model in which perfusion is distributed and in which gas diffuses a variable distance into tissues and variably saturates blood (49). Other experimental preparations are adequately explained only with other, often more complicated models.

MULTIPLE INERT GASES

When there is more than one inert gas in the gas cavity and surrounding tissues, total gas flux equals the sum of fluxes of individual gases. Analysis is complicated because the concentration of one gas in the cavity may importantly depend on the fluxes of other gases. Tenney et al. (32) offered an early illustration of this phenomenon in their study of gas transfers in SF_6 and N_2 pneumoperitoneums in air-breathing animals. After the rapid equilibration of water vapor, O_2, and CO_2, the influx of N_2 exceeds the efflux of SF_6, which is relatively insoluble and slow to diffuse; gas volume therefore doubles before beginning to decrease. In air-breathing animals the efflux of N_2 is slowed because of the high partial pressure of N_2 in arterial blood (Pa_{N_2}), so the less soluble SF_6 is absorbed faster than N_2. In the final steady-state condition the pocket is filled with N_2, CO_2, and O_2 only. When a highly soluble gas like N_2O is initially present in the cavity, the rapid absorption of this gas causes the concentration of other gases within the cavity to rise, as in the lungs during breath holding ["second gas effect" (13)]. For a number of inert gases Tucker and Tenney (37) worked out in theory and demonstrated experimentally similar examples of multiple gas transfers in the transient non–steady state.

To qualitatively illustrate some of these points, consider an infinitely compliant pocket initially filled with 50% N_2 and 50% SF_6 in an O_2-breathing animal. Figure 7 shows the time course of the pocket volume and the partial pressures of the relevant gases. (Fig. 7 is not quantitative; we use it only to illustrate the principles of multiple-gas elimination.) There are essentially three phases where different phenomena dominate. In phase I, which may last hours, there is an influx of the respiratory gases H_2O, CO_2, and O_2 in order of decreasing speed. These gases are much faster than N_2 or SF_6, and therefore the pocket volume increases. As it does so, the partial pressures of N_2 and SF_6 correspondingly decrease. This continues until the respiratory gases equilibrate at approximately venous partial pressures. In phase II, which may last days, there is competition between the efflux of N_2 and SF_6. Because N_2 is faster, its partial pressure

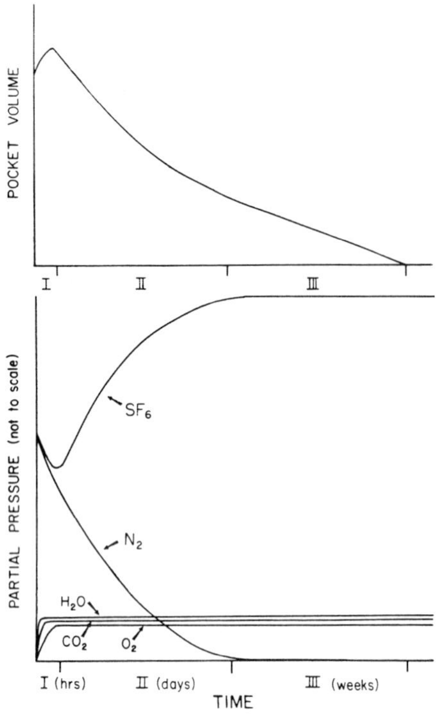

FIG. 7. Qualitative behavior of pocket volume and partial pressures of H_2O, CO_2, O_2, N_2, and SF_6 as a function of time in an O_2-breathing animal. Pocket is initially composed of 50% N_2 and 50% SF_6. Scales are arbitrary.

drops, while that of SF_6 rises because of the volume drop. We enter phase III after this interaction has stopped because of total N_2 elimination. Now all the gases remain at essentially a fixed partial pressure, and the volume of the pocket falls linearly in time, its rate being governed by the slowest gas. For SF_6 this final phase may last weeks. In phase III the partial pressures are constant so the partial volumes of each gas remain at a fixed proportion of the total volume.

Although Tucker and Tenney (37) successfully calculated the behavior of two inert gases in the pocket, their results are severely complicated by the nonlinear interactions between the two gases. That is, volumetric changes due to absorption of either gas profoundly influence the behavior (via the partial pressure) of the other. Here we develop the theory underlying a situation with multiple tracer gases. Specifically we assume that the pocket is filled with N_2 and also any number of inert gases in trace amounts. (The pocket will of course contain O_2, CO_2, and water vapor, but their partial pressures can be taken as constant and then need not be considered here.) The pocket volume's temporal dependence is governed by N_2 only, and it therefore contributes simply one additional term in the equations describing the driving of the inert tracer gases.

We adopt the notation of Tucker and Tenney (37). The equation describing the absorption of gas X (a tracer, any inert gas except N_2) is given by

$$d(Pg_X V)/P_I dt = \dot{V}_X = -\Gamma_X \dot{Q} Pg_X \qquad (12)$$

where V is the volume of gas and P_I is the total inert-gas pressure in the pocket, approximately given by Pg_N because the other gases are present in trace amounts only. Expanding the derivative gives

$$\dot{P}g_X = -(Pg_I \Gamma_X \dot{Q}/V + \dot{V}/V) Pg_X \qquad (13)$$

In solving for Pg_X one sees immediately that $\dot{P}g_X$ is dependent not just on Pg_X but on V and $\dot{V}$. That is, the first term on the right side of Equation 13 is essentially the first-order kinetic exchange term (with a time-dependent coefficient); it is trying to drive Pg_X down as gas X is lost. The second term (recall that $\dot{V} < 0$) is opposite in sign; it is trying to drive Pg_X up as volume is lost. Now the volume, because gas X is present in trace amounts only, is completely dominated by the dependence of V on N_2. Thus V depends on t only and not on Pg_X. This is what vastly simplifies Tucker's work; indeed it allows for multiple tracer gases to be used simultaneously.

Because V and N_2 are essentially unaffected by the presence of X, the simple theory applies for the volumetric dependence on time. That is, by Equation 9

$$\dot{V} = -\Gamma_{N_2} \dot{Q} Pg_I \omega \qquad (14)$$

or

$$V(t) = V_0 - \Gamma_{N_2} \dot{Q} Pg_I \omega t \qquad (15)$$

where ω is the driving pressure coefficient, given by $\omega = (Pg_I - Pa_{N_2})/Pg_I$. Note that $\omega = 0.077$ for air-breathing animals, and $\omega = 1.0$ for O_2-breathing animals. This linear dependence of pocket volume on time may then be substituted into Equation 13. Elementary calculus shows that

$$Pg_X/Pg_{X_0} = (V/V_0)^{(\theta/\omega - 1)} \qquad (16)$$

where θ is the exchange coefficient, $\theta = \Gamma_X/\Gamma_{N_2}$, and the zero subscript refers to time zero. This is the final result for the behavior of any inert gas present in the pocket in trace amounts.

One immediately sees from this that the partial pressure of the tracer and the pocket volume are related by a power law that depends uniquely on the characteristics of the gas and the pocket. If the exchange coefficient is large compared with the driving pressure coefficient, then the tracer gas X is absorbed from the pocket much faster than N_2. This would occur if the solubility of the tracer were large. Conversely, if the exchange coefficient is small compared with the driving pressure coefficient, then Pg_X actually rises as the pocket volume decreases. This would be the case for a relatively insoluble gas such as SF_6 in an animal breathing O_2, where $\omega = 1$ (no arterial back pressure). (Fig. 8 is an example of partial pressure rise.) Of course that is expected in a circumstance where the change of pocket volume dominates the behavior of Pg_X rather than its own absorption characteristics. [This relation holds only so long as gas X

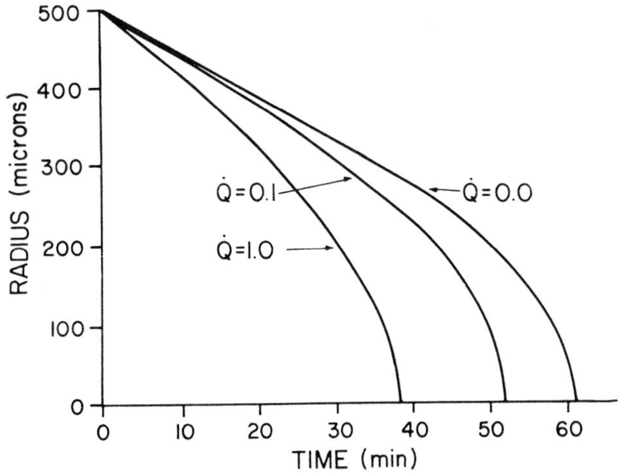

FIG. 8. Theoretical predictions of shrinkage of an N_2 bubble at various rates of perfusion of tissue (ml/min) for an animal breathing O_2. $\dot{Q}$, blood flow rate. [From Hlastala and Van Liew (12).]

remains in tracer amounts; when Pg_X rises too far, the full theory of Tucker and Tenney (37) must be invoked.]

VERY SMALL COLLAPSIBLE CAVITIES: BUBBLES

Bubbles of trapped gas in tissues and blood, e.g., those of decompression sickness and venous air embolism, provide medically relevant examples of closed collapsible gas cavities. An early analysis of gas flux from bubbles by Van Liew (41) sets the external boundary condition of the bubble to be homogeneous and constant, and gas flux is limited by diffusion. Geometric factors cancel conveniently, and bubble diameter is predicted to decrease linearly with time.

The assumption of pure diffusion limitation is no longer valid if gas flux from bubbles affects the partial pressure of gas in surrounding capillaries. Surface tension increases the pressure within bubbles and can increase absorption rates of the smallest bubbles (41). Furthermore in very small bubbles the gas diffusing through shells of tissue follows radiating and therefore divergent paths, thus increasing the rate of gas flux. These complicating influences were included in a later theoretical model of gas bubble resorption by Van Liew and Hlastala (48). Bubble diameter decreases fastest when diameters are smallest, just before the bubble disappears. These authors subsequently made quantitative predictions of bubble resorption using the distributed-diffusion model and data from experiments on various inert gases (12). Figure 8 shows the radius of an N_2 bubble as a function of time for various rates of perfusion (12).

Bubble disappearance rates and flux rates of gas out of pockets depend on ambient pressure. Compression substantially changes the fractional composition of gas in pockets or bubbles because water vapor pressure is invariant with total pressure, and P_{O_2} and P_{CO_2} change proportionately less than ambient pressure, whereas inert-gas pressure changes more (41, 46, 50). Compression therefore increases the pocket-to-blood pressure difference for the rate-limiting gas, thereby tending to accelerate absorption. On the other hand, the decrease in surface area of a bubble as it is compressed reduces absorption rates.

SUPERSATURATION AND BUBBLE GROWTH

Bubbles can form de novo tissues under conditions of isobaric supersaturation. This intriguing phenomenon, described by Graves and others (3, 9, 10, 15), results from diffusion of two or more inert gases in opposite directions and has inspired a number of explanations. Regional supersaturation and bubble growth can occur transiently as a result of changing breathing gas mixtures or in the steady state as a result of breathing one gas mixture while exposing the skin to another. Cowley et al. (4) directly measured the elevated gas pressure in tissues during steady-state isobaric supersaturation.

Graves et al. (9) described one possible mechanism of supersaturation termed *counterdiffusion supersaturation*. When two gases diffuse in opposite directions through composite tissues whose layers are differently permeable to the gases, the sum of the partial pressures and hence the total gas pressure may be greater or less than the ambient pressure. In the example illustrated by Graves et al. (9), the total gas pressure in the tissue is maximal at the interface between tissue layers. In the model of inert-gas counterperfusion and diffusion supersaturation proposed by Hills (11) there is a single homogeneous tissue diffusion barrier adjacent to a zone of limited convective capacity. When the more diffusible gas is adjacent to the diffusion barrier, or the more soluble gas is transported by convection, supersaturation can occur. Tepper et al. (35) presented a more detailed model that considered local tissue gas tensions in tissue cylinders surrounding capillaries. Diffusion of gas in tissue in a direction paraxial with the capillaries could increase local supersaturation when breathing mixtures are changed. Supersaturation is of great importance in diving medicine.

SUMMARY

Gas cavities in the body are sufficiently diverse in their anatomy and physiology that no simple description can apply to all cavities under all conditions. It is clear, however, that gas fluxes can be analyzed by model systems incorporating diffusion and convection. These models vary from a simple uniform diffusion resistance separating a uniform gas from a vascular sink to complex models incorporating distributed perfusion, axial diffusion in tissue surrounding capillaries, and hemoglobin saturation kinetics. The simplest model (see Fig. 6*A*) is adequate to describe fluxes of air or other relatively insoluble inert gases from subcutaneous gas pockets. For the study of O_2 or CO uptake, a more elaborate model is required that incorporates perfusion distributed in tissue with incomplete equilibration of gas between tissue and capillary blood (see Fig. 6*B*). The urinary bladder is modeled by two distinct diffusion barriers: *1*) a proximal limited mucosal vascular bed and *2*) a distal tissue reservoir. Finally, in isobaric supersaturation more complicated models have been invoked with tissue inhomogeneous in its diffusion resistance (counterdiffusion), homogeneous tissue with limited perfusion (counterperfusion), and gas diffusion paraxial with capillaries. The analysis of multiple-gas flux is complex even with the simplest of models unless tracer techniques are used. Knowledge of the physiology of gas exchange in body cavities is useful in other areas of medicine and physiology, and gas cavities will probably continue to provide useful preparations for the study of gas movements within the body.

REFERENCES

1. Chen, P.-Y., and H. D. Van Liew. Krogh constants for diffusion of nitrogen and carbon monoxide in bladder tissue. *Respir. Physiol.* 24: 43–49, 1975.
2. Coburn, R. F., M. Swerdlow, K. J. Luomanmäki, R. E. Forster, and K. Powell. Uptake of carbon monoxide from the urinary bladder of the dog. *Am. J. Physiol.* 215: 1010–1023, 1968.
3. Collins, J. M. Isobaric inert gas supersaturation: observations, theory, and predictions. *J. Appl. Physiol.* 44: 914–917, 1978.
4. Cowley, J. R. M., C. Allegra, and C. J. Lambertsen. Subcutaneous tissue gas space pressure during superficial isobaric counterdiffusion. *J. Appl. Physiol.* 47: 224–227, 1979.
5. Dueker, C. W., C. J. Lambertsen, J. J. Rosowski, and J. C. Saunders. Middle ear gas exchange in isobaric counterdiffusion. *J. Appl. Physiol.* 47: 1239–1244, 1979.
6. Eger, E. I., II, and L. J. Saidman. Hazards of nitrous oxide anesthesia in bowel obstruction and pneumothorax. *Anesthesiology* 26: 61–66, 1965.
7. Elner, A. Indirect determination of gas absorption from the middle ear. *Acta Oto-Laryngol.* 74: 191–196, 1972.
8. Forster, R. E. Measurement of gastrointestinal blood flow by means of gas absorption. *Gastroenterology* 52: 381–386, 1967.
9. Graves, D. J., J. Idicula, C. J. Lambertsen, and J. A. Quinn. Bubble formation resulting from counterdiffusion supersaturation: a possible explanation for isobaric inert gas urticaria and vertigo. *Phys. Med. Biol.* 18: 256–264, 1973.
10. Graves, D. J., J. Idicula, C. J. Lambertsen, and J. A. Quinn. Bubble formation in physical and biological systems: a manifestation of counterdiffusion in composite media. *Science Wash. DC* 179: 582–584, 1973.
11. Hills, B. A. Supersaturation by counterperfusion and diffusion of gases. *J. Appl. Physiol.* 42: 758–760, 1977.
12. Hlastala, M. P., and H. D. Van Liew. Absorption of in vivo inert gas bubbles. *Respir. Physiol.* 24: 147–158, 1975.
13. Johnson, T. S., G. D. Swanson, I. E. Sodal, J. T. Reeves, and R. W. Virtue. A closed lung system study of inert gas absorption. *J. Appl. Physiol.* 47: 240–244, 1979.
14. Kety, S. The theory and applications of the exchange of inert gas at the lungs and tissues. *Pharmacol. Rev.* 3: 1–41, 1951.
15. Lambertsen, C. J., and J. Idicula. A new gas lesion syndrome in man, induced by "isobaric gas counterdiffusion." *J. Appl. Physiol.* 39: 434–443, 1975.
16. Lategola, M. T. Measurement of total pressure of dissolved gas in mammalian tissue in vivo. *J. Appl. Physiol.* 19: 322–324, 1964.
17. Levitt, M. D. Volume and composition of human intestinal gas determined by means of an intestinal washout technic. *N. Engl. J. Med.* 284: 1394–1398, 1971.
18. Loring, S. H., and S. M. Tenney. Gas absorption from frontal sinuses. *Arch. Otolaryngol.* 97: 470–474, 1973.
19. Matz, G. J., C. G. Rattenborg, and D. A. Holaday. Effects of nitrous oxide on middle ear pressure. *Anesthesiology* 28: 948–950, 1967.
20. Munson, E. S., and H. C. Merrick. Effects of nitrous oxide on venous air embolism. *Anesthesiology* 27: 783–787, 1966.
21. Perl, W., and F. P. Chinard. A convection-diffusion model of indicator transport through an organ. *Circ. Res.* 22: 273–298, 1968.
22. Piiper, J. Physiological equilibria of gas cavities in the body. In: *Handbook of Physiology. Respiration*, edited by W. O. Fenn and H. Rahn. Washington, DC: Am. Physiol. Soc., 1965, sect. 3, vol. II, chapt. 48, p. 1205–1218.
23. Piiper, J. Various models for analysis of the absorption of inert gases from gas cavities in the body. *Respir. Physiol.* 9: 74–85, 1970.
24. Piiper, J., R. E. Canfield, and H. Rahn. Absorption of various inert gases from subcutaneous gas pockets in rats. *J. Appl. Physiol.* 17: 268–274, 1962.
25. Piiper, J., H. T. Humphrey, and H. Rahn. Gas composition of pressurized, perfused gas pockets and the fish swim bladder. *J. Appl. Physiol.* 17: 275–282, 1962.
26. Pogrund, R. S., and F. R. Steggerda. Influence of gaseous transfer between the colon and blood stream on percentage gas compositions of intestinal flatus in man. *Am. J. Physiol.* 153: 475–482, 1948.
27. Rasmussen, P. E. Middle ear and maxillary sinus during nitrous oxide anesthesia. *Acta Oto-Laryngol.* 63: 7–16, 1967.
28. Rohsenow, W. M., and H. Y. Choi. *Heat, Mass, and Momentum Transfer.* Englewood Cliffs, NJ: Prentice-Hall, 1961.
29. Saidman, L. J., and E. I. Eger II. Change in cerebrospinal fluid pressure during pneumoencephalography under nitrous oxide anesthesia. *Anesthesiology* 26: 67–72, 1965.
30. Sørensen, S. C. Arterial P_{CO_2} in awake cats calculated from gas tensions in subcutaneous pockets. *Respir. Physiol.* 3: 261–265, 1967.
31. Tenney, S. M. A theoretical analysis of the relationship between venous blood and mean tissue oxygen pressures. *Respir. Physiol.* 20: 283–296, 1974.
32. Tenney, S. M., F. G. Carpenter, and H. Rahn. Gas transfers in a sulfur hexafluoride pneumoperitoneum. *J. Appl. Physiol.* 6: 201–208, 1953.
33. Tenney, S. M., and D. H. Morrison. Tissue gas tensions in small wild mammals. *Respir. Physiol.* 3: 160–165, 1967.
34. Tenney, S. M., and L. C. Ou. Physiological evidence for increased tissue capillarity in rats acclimatized to high altitude. *Respir. Physiol.* 8: 137–150, 1970.
35. Tepper, R. S., E. N. Lightfoot, A. Baz, and E. H. Lanphier. Inert gas transport in the microcirculation: risk of isobaric supersaturation. *J. Appl. Physiol.* 46: 1157–1163, 1979.
36. Thomsen, K. A., K. Terkildsen, and I. Arnfred. Middle ear pressure variations during anesthesia. *Arch. Otolaryngol.* 82: 609–611, 1965.
37. Tucker, R. W., and S. M. Tenney. Inert gas exchange in subcutaneous gas pockets of air-breathing animals: theory and measurement. *Respir. Physiol.* 1: 151–171, 1966.
38. Van Liew, H. D. Oxygen and carbon dioxide permeability of

subcutaneous pockets. *Am. J. Physiol.* 202: 53–58, 1962.
39. VAN LIEW, H. D. Tissue gas tensions by microtonometry; results in liver and fat. *J. Appl. Physiol.* 17: 359–363, 1962.
40. VAN LIEW, H. D. Tissue pO_2 and pCO_2 estimation with rat subcutaneous gas pockets. *J. Appl. Physiol.* 17: 851–855, 1962.
41. VAN LIEW, H. D. Factors in the resolution of tissue gas bubbles. In: *Underwater Physiology*, edited by C. J. Lambertsen. New York: Academic, 1966, p. 191–204.
42. VAN LIEW, H. D. Coupling of diffusion and perfusion in gas exit from subcutaneous pocket in rats. *Am. J. Physiol.* 214: 1176–1185, 1968.
43. VAN LIEW, H. D. Interaction of CO and O_2 with hemoglobin in perfused tissue adjacent to gas pockets. *Respir. Physiol.* 5: 202–210, 1968.
44. VAN LIEW, H. D. Effect of a change of perfusion on exit of nitrogen and oxygen from gas pockets. *Respir. Physiol.* 12: 163–168, 1971.
45. VAN LIEW, H. D. Diffusion constant for CO_2 through urinary bladders of cats. *Respir. Physiol.* 13: 372–377, 1971.
46. VAN LIEW, H. D., B. BISHOP, P. D. WALDER, AND H. RAHN. Effects of compression on composition and absorption of tissue gas pockets. *J. Appl. Physiol.* 20: 927–933, 1965.
47. VAN LIEW, H. D., AND P.-Y. CHEN. Interaction of O_2 diffusion and O_2 metabolism in cat urinary bladder tissue. *Am. J. Physiol.* 229: 444–448, 1975.
48. VAN LIEW, H. D., AND M. P. HLASTALA. Influence of bubble size and blood perfusion on absorption of gas bubbles in tissues. *Respir. Physiol.* 7: 111–121, 1969.
49. VAN LIEW, H. D., W. H. SCHOENFISCH, AND M. M. GOLDBERG. Diffusion of oxygen from gas pockets to capillaries. *Microvasc. Res.* 1: 257–265, 1969.
50. VAN LIEW, H. D., W. H. SCHOENFISCH, AND A. J. OLSZOWKA. Exchanges of N_2 between a gas pocket and tissue in a hyperbaric environment. *Respir. Physiol.* 6: 23–28, 1968.

CHAPTER 16

Gas exchange in exercise

PAOLO CERRETELLI
PIETRO E. DI PRAMPERO | *Department of Physiology, School of Medicine, University of Geneva, Geneva, Switzerland*

CHAPTER CONTENTS

EXERCISE IS THE MOST POTENT STRESS to the body oxidative machinery, i.e., to the muscle system and the functions concerned with external and alveolar gas exchange, gas transport, and tissue respiration. In fact the ventilatory pump may need to increase its mechanical power >50-fold to provide maximum external gas exchange, the circulatory pump may have to raise its resting metabolic rate up to 8-fold to assure maximum output, and most muscles have to sustain oxidation rates >100-fold the resting level. Thus exercise is the most suitable variable for studying the limits of the mechanisms underlying lung and tissue gas exchange, transport, utilization, and removal and other performance characteristics of the organism as a whole.

Until the 1970s the respiratory and cardiovascular responses to exercise were correlated typically with work load and/or steady-state O_2 consumption. Recently, with the improvement and speed of most analytical techniques, analysis of the unsteady state of exercise (the rest-to-work transient and the recovery phase) has been emphasized. This dynamic approach has been very rewarding and is a primary source of information for exercise physiologists. In fact the study of the transients allows sorting out, on the basis of their different time courses, the components of the multifactorial regulation mechanism operating at exercise, thus providing insight into the processes coupling muscle contraction to gas exchange.

This chapter summarizes the work done over the past 20 years on the many direct and indirect aspects of gas exchange, with a focus on exercise. Priority is given to the functions involved in gas exchange characterized by energetic constraints, such as the energetics of the respiratory and cardiac pumps as well as muscle energetics, with emphasis on metabolic transients. Reviews (oriented exclusively toward exercise) of traditional subjects, such as arterial gas tensions, alveolar-arterial gas gradients, pulmonary diffusing capacity, and maximum O_2 transport and utilization, are included. This statistical appraisal may be useful not only for the knowledge it provides of the state of the art but also for a critical and constructive approach to some problems that are still debatable. Recent work on the regulation of the cardiovascular function at exercise is also presented.

STEADY STATE

External Gas Exchange

PULMONARY VENTILATION, WORK OF BREATHING, AND ENERGY COST. Heavy exercise imposes a potent stress on the ventilatory pump. In fact, pulmonary expired minute ventilation ($\dot{V}_E$) may attain values of >150 liters/min, ~25 times those at rest and 60%–70% of the subject's maximum voluntary ventilation (MVV) (352, 364). Such ventilatory rates are brought about by a 3-fold increase of the resting frequency and by increasing ~6 times the tidal volume (VT) up to ~60% of the subject's vital capacity (VC).

Volume changes of the respiratory apparatus imply work performed on the respiratory system (Wrs), mainly expanding or compressing the gas in the lungs and displacing it in and out of the airways. The driving forces exerted by the respiratory muscles are opposed mainly by static forces (elastic, gravitational, and surface) and flow-resistive forces (viscous and turbulent resistance of the gas and viscous resistance of the tissues); the inertial forces are negligible except at very high levels of $\dot{V}$E. The diaphragm carries out the major part of Wrs, both at rest (70% of the total) and during exercise hyperpnea (60%). At low ventilatory rates, in addition to the diaphragm, only the external intercostals and in some subjects the scaleni are active. When $\dot{V}$E > 50 liters/min, the sternomastoids and the extensor of the vertebral column also come into action toward the end of inspiration. The muscles of the abdominal wall and the internal intercostals contract only at the end of expiration. At high $\dot{V}$E levels all respiratory muscles become active. In the latter case the dynamic component represents most of Wrs, with the exception of *1*) the work done to overcome the flow resistance of the chest wall, *2*) part of the work done by the inspiratory muscles to overcome the elastic resistance of the lung, and *3*) the negative work done by the inspiratory muscles during the first part of the expiration (4). The Wrs may be determined from the area of pressure-volume loops (351). The mechanical work per unit time, i.e., the power ($\dot{W}$rs), increases from a resting value of ~0.02 W to a maximum ($\dot{W}$rs,max) of 12 W; the latter value is found in trained subjects breathing >180 liters/min (352).

During quiet breathing, ~50% of the total dynamic resistance is opposed by nose passages; the remaining 50% is equally shared between lung (tissue and airways) and chest (rib cage and abdomen) resistance (4). During exercise, when $\dot{V}$E > 40 liters/min, there is a switch from nasal to oronasal breathing, which is determined not only by increased nasal resistance but also by psychological factors (425).

The $\dot{W}$rs,max is only slightly affected by added inspiratory and expiratory resistances (95, 132) and appears even to decrease in subjects breathing air at 3 and 6 ATA, in the latter case apparently because of depletion of energy stores in the inspiratory muscles (229). In both cases the expiratory peak transpulmonary pressure never exceeds 30% of the values observed during MVV and forced vital capacity (FVC) maneuvers (229, 364). The $\dot{W}$rs,max recorded during a 15-s maximum breathing capacity (MBC) maneuver is threefold greater than that measured during maximum aerobic exercise; the difference is attributed to a more powerful performance of the inspiratory muscles and greater dissipation of energy due to dynamic compression of intrathoracic airways (229).

The energy cost of breathing has been either measured or estimated from Wrs, assuming an efficiency value η. The principle employed for the direct measurement is that introduced in 1918 by Liljestrand (318), whereby total body O_2 consumption ($\dot{V}_{O_2}$) is measured at different levels of $\dot{V}$E either imposed voluntarily, or obtained by increasing the dead space of the subject, or by adding CO_2 to inspired air. Resting $\dot{V}_{O_2}$ of the respiratory pump ($\dot{V}resp_{O_2}$) obtained by back extrapolation varies widely, from 0.25 to ~1 ml O_2/liter ventilation (4). The $\dot{V}resp_{O_2}$ increases progressively with increasing $\dot{V}$E. The ratio $\Delta\dot{V}resp_{O_2}$/$\Delta\dot{V}$E varies among authors: 1–2.5 ml/liter for $\dot{V}$E ranging from 40 to 60 liters/min, 1.2–5 ml/liter for $\dot{V}$E ranging from 60 to 80 liters/min, and 4–5.5 ml/liter for $\dot{V}$E ranging from 90 to 130 liters/min (40, 345; see ref. 4 for a review).

The $\dot{W}$rs,max may become a limiting factor in severe exercise. This is true when a given increase in $\dot{V}$E does not lead to an increase but rather to a decrease of O_2 availability to working muscles, because respiratory muscles take up all or more than the additional O_2 provided by hyperpnea, i.e., when $\Delta\dot{V}resp_{O_2}/\Delta\dot{V}E = \Delta\dot{V}tot_{O_2}/\Delta\dot{V}E$ ($\dot{V}tot_{O_2}$, total O_2 consumption) (369). In sedentary subjects characterized by a $\dot{V}$E of ~90 liters/min at a work load of 0.8 maximum $\dot{V}_{O_2}$ ($\dot{V}max_{O_2}$), this "useful" ceiling seems to occur at a $\dot{V}$E of 120 liters/min (442), i.e., above the $\dot{V}$E level spontaneously selected during maximum aerobic exercise. Similarly, respective ceilings of 130 and 170 liters/min were identified for two subjects whose cost of breathing was estimated from measured $\dot{W}$rs,max and an assumed efficiency value of 25% for the respiratory muscles (336). Thus, in healthy individuals working in normal environments, maximum sustained activity of the limb muscles does not appear to be limited for practical purposes by the energy requirement of the respiratory pump. In fact, maximum aerobic performance is attained at ventilation levels corresponding to ~50%–60% of the individual MVV, a rate at which ventilation can be sustained indefinitely (178, 469) and that is usually below the critical ceiling for the individual. The $\dot{V}$E attained during maximum sustained activity can approach the ceiling only when the ventilatory pump is overloaded relative to $\dot{V}_{O_2}$ (e.g., in hypoxia) (Fig. 1). At this point, respiratory muscles must compete for O_2 with other muscles and both respiratory and/or locomotion (limb) work must be reduced. This is observed at very high altitude where not only $\dot{V}max_{O_2}$ but also maximum exercise ventilation tends to drop (390). In most subjects maximum exercise ventilation may be even higher in hypoxia [up to barometric pressure (PB) = 0.5 atm] than in normoxia (81); this indicates that in normoxia the fraction of the absolute $\dot{V}max_{O_2}$ available for useful work is slightly greater than in hypoxia (423).

Alveolar Gas Exchange

ARTERIAL O_2 AND CO_2 TENSIONS AND ALVEOLAR-ARTERIAL O_2 AND CO_2 GRADIENTS. An extensive review

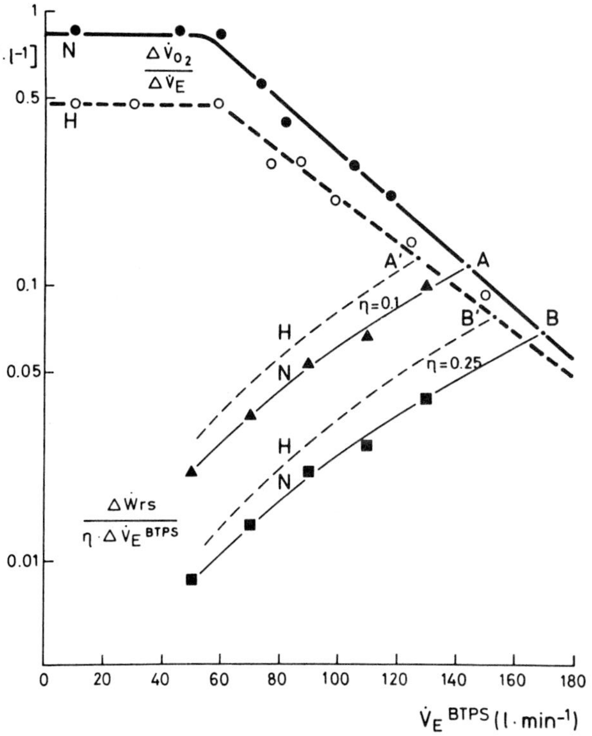

FIG. 1. Increase of overall O_2 uptake per unit increase of expired minute ventilation ($\Delta\dot{V}_{O_2}/\Delta\dot{V}_E$, kJ/liter) in normoxia (N, ●, —) and in chronic hypoxia (H, ○, – – –; 5,800 m). [Data from Pugh et al. (390).] O_2 cost of ventilation ($\Delta\dot{W}rs/\eta\Delta\dot{V}_E$) in normoxia (N, —, ■, ▲) and in chronic hypoxia (H, - - -), as calculated on the basis of efficiency values (η) of 0.25 (*lower curves*) and 0.1 (*upper curves*). [Data from Cruz (114), Margaria et al. (336), and Thoden et al. (470).] Pulmonary ventilation expressed at body temperature, ambient pressure, saturated with water vapor ($\dot{V}_E^{BTPS}$) in liters per minute. "Critical level" for exercise ventilation is ~15 liters/min lower in hypoxia (*A'* and *B'*) than in normoxia (*A* and *B*). This indicates that in hypoxia the fraction of absolute $\dot{V}max_{O_2}$ utilized by respiratory muscles is necessarily greater than in normoxia.

of the literature (Table 1) indicates that arterial O_2 partial pressure (Pa_{O_2}) in 175 resting moderately active young subjects studied by 17 different authors (see refs. in Table 1) averaged 91.5 ± 4.9 (SD) mmHg. Submaximum and maximum aerobic exercise did not affect significantly Pa_{O_2} (Fig. 2). The observed constancy of Pa_{O_2} over a wide metabolic range seems to rule out the possibility that at sea level in normal nonathletic individuals the alveolar-capillary membrane limits O_2 transfer. By contrast, it has been recently shown (133a) that in endurance athletes characterized by very high (72 ml·kg^{-1}·min^{-1}) maximum aerobic power ($\dot{V}max_{O_2}$) levels, Pa_{O_2} during maximum short-term exercise may drop as low as 75 ± 2.3 mmHg. This finding, according to the authors, may be the consequence of diffusion limitation secondary to very short red cell transit times in the lungs. Resting arterial CO_2 partial pressure (Pa_{CO_2}) measured by 14 authors in 147 subjects (Table 1) averaged 38.2 ± 1.8 mmHg. After a modest but significant increase observed at ~35% of $\dot{V}max_{O_2}$ (Fig. 2), Pa_{CO_2} decreased sharply with further increases of work load. Near $\dot{V}max_{O_2}$, Pa_{CO_2} averaged 33.3 ± 3.5 mmHg (data from many subjects, 12 authors, Table 1). Thus nonathletic subjects hyperventilated even during submaximum exercise. This seems to be the case also for endurance athletes whose Pa_{CO_2} level at maximum exercise may range between 30 and 35 mmHg (133a).

The alveolar-arterial difference in partial pressure of O_2 ($PA_{O_2} - Pa_{O_2}$), which at rest in young male subjects averaged 11.0 ± 3.1 mmHg (15 authors, 143 subjects, Table 1), is unchanged when work load is increased up to ~40% of $\dot{V}max_{O_2}$ (Fig. 2). A further increase of work intensity produced larger $PA_{O_2} - Pa_{O_2}$ values up to an average maximum of 24.8 ± 7.2 mmHg (5 authors, 30 subjects, Table 1). In 16 endurance athletes, mean $PA_{O_2} - Pa_{O_2}$ at $\dot{V}max_{O_2}$ was found to be 33 mmHg (133a).

As is well known, the observed widening of $PA_{O_2} - Pa_{O_2}$ at exercise could be attributed to incomplete O_2 equilibration from alveoli to end capillary. However, Staub (453) indicates that this occurrence for normal sedentary subjects is highly improbable. The increased $PA_{O_2} - Pa_{O_2}$ at exercise may also be caused by *1)* ill-matching of ventilation ($\dot{V}A$) and blood flow ($\dot{Q}$) in the lung, *2)* true shunts, and *3)* uneven distribution of the lung diffusing capacity (DL) and uneven distribution of the DL/$\dot{Q}$ ratio in the lungs or certain lung areas (268).

The distribution of the ventilation-perfusion ($\dot{V}A/\dot{Q}$) ratio becomes more homogeneous during exercise, as a result of an increased $\dot{Q}$ relative to $\dot{V}A$ in the upper lobes of the lungs (72, 268, 492), while the distribution of $\dot{V}A$ to lung volume tends to become more homogeneous along the lung vertical axis. These changes should reduce rather than increase $PA_{O_2} - Pa_{O_2}$. The improved evenness of $\dot{V}A$ and $\dot{Q}$ during exercise is documented by experiments with radioactive gases (493) and is supported by two observations. *1)* Cardiogenic oscillations [i.e., the opposite-phase ripples of the PA_{CO_2} (alveolar partial pressure of CO_2) and PA_{O_2} tracings synchronous to heart rate (HR) and attributed to cyclic changes of expirate composition because of a variable contribution of gas from the dependent part of the lung at each heartbeat] practically disappear. *2)* The alveolar-arterial pressure difference for nitrogen ($PA_{N_2} - Pa_{N_2}$), an indicator of the lung $\dot{V}A/\dot{Q}$ inhomogeneity (76, 164, 165, 391), becomes negligible (31). Recently Gledhill et al. (191) have shown a significant reduction of the observed $PA_{O_2} - Pa_{O_2}$ both at rest and at exercise when replacing the N_2 fraction of the inspired air with dense sulfur hexafluoride (SF_6). These results, which argue against a diffusion limitation of the O_2 transport across the membrane (which, because of the reduction of the diffusivity of O_2 in SF_6, should widen $PA_{O_2} - Pa_{O_2}$), are explained with an SF_6-induced decrease of a preexisting inhomogeneity of $\dot{V}A/\dot{Q}$ distribution that can only exist within regions (intraregional) rather than

TABLE 1. *Partial Pressure of O_2 and CO_2 in Arterial Blood and Corresponding Alveolar-Arterial Differences at Rest and Exercise*

Year	Age Range, yr	Observations	Rest					Exercise						Ref.
			n	Pa_{O_2}, mmHg	$PA_{O_2} - Pa_{O_2}$, mmHg	Pa_{CO_2}, mmHg	$Pa_{CO_2} - PA_{CO_2}$, mmHg	n	$\dot{V}_{O_2}$, liters/min, or % max	Pa_{O_2}, mmHg	$PA_{O_2} - Pa_{O_2}$, mmHg	Pa_{CO_2}, mmHg	$Pa_{CO_2} - PA_{CO_2}$, mmHg	
1946	28–36		6	94.2	8.9			6	1.66	88.9	16.6			317, 404
1950	22–37	8 M, 2 F	10	98.0	9	36.0	2.1	10	1.00	88.0	7	40.9	−2.0	463
1954	23–60		19	85.1	9.7	38.8		34	1.07	82.5	19.6	42.0		168
1955	20–33	10 M, 4 F	14	89.1	6.9	39.8		14	1.58	91.6	10.1	38.1		39
1958	17–19	Athletic	14	101.9		35.0		14	0.8 max	84.9		34.0		247
									max	78.8		30.1		
1959	17–39			97 ($n = 7$)	12 ($n = 6$)	36.0 ($n = 12$)			1.90 ($n = 12$)	90.0 ($n = 6$)	11 ($n = 5$)	38.0 ($n = 12$)		323
1956, 1960	Young			87.6	17	36.9	0.2		1.49	88.7	17.1	40.1		19, 20
									1.82	84.7	20	39.1		
									2.89	83.8	26.2	37.3		
									3.30	87.6	24.1	36.7		
									3.49	87.9	35	29.1		
1962	21–27		5	92.6	8.4	39.5	0.8							57
1963	21–26		7	87.0		37.9		7	1.59	92.7		41.0		340
1964	20–24		8	93.0		37.1		8	0.3 max	98.3		39.6		37
									0.5 max	97.9				
1965	20–26		7	87.0	14.7	37.9		7	0.4 max	92.1	11	41.0		230
			8	92.8	13.2	36.6		8	0.75 max	98.0	10	38.3		
1966	21–37		17		12.7		0.7	17	2.00		19		−6.0	270
1967	22–25							5	1.46	91	8.7	39.4	−3.3	214
		Airway obstruction							1.45	87	5.1	40.8	−5.8	
1969	20–28		5	97	7.4	40	2.8	5	0.61	97	7	39.0	1.4	497
									0.99	97	4.3	39.0	−0.9	
									1.64	98	3.8	39.0	−3.8	
									2.42	97	6.3	38.0	−3.0	
									3.30	97	10.8	35.0	−2.8	
1969	38–55	U	15	87	15	39		13	0.3 max	92	14	36		217
		T		87	14	39		13	0.3 max	91	15	35		
		U						9	0.6 max	97	18	29		
		T						9	0.6 max	86	27	33		
		U						8	0.8 max	94	23	26		
		T						8	0.8 max	85	26	34		
		U						13	max	93	26	33		
		T						13	max	89	28	33		
1971	28		10	92	7	42		10	0.85	94	7	42		134
									1.3	95	10	42		
									1.8	94	14	41		
									2.3	95	17	39		
									2.7	95	22	36		
									3.0	95	24	33		
1973	24	$PA_{N_2} - Pa_{N_2}$	10	85.5	9.5	38.5		10	1.4	87	9	39.8		31
	44		8	81.0	18	35.7		8	1.35	83	14	38.7		
	68		7	74.5	23	36.3		7	1.07	79	19.5	32.2		
1978	23–33		5	86.9	10.9			5	1.8	87.5	15.5			191
		80% SF_6		91.0	4.2				1.9	88.4	10.1			
1978			3	93		38		3	max	84		34		464
		Acetazolamide		107		38			max	88	35			
1979	24–34	f = 15/min						5	1.02	97		35.7	−1.8	271
		f = 30/min							0.91	98.4		37.7	−0.3	
		f = 45/min							1.07	97.2		37.1	0.4	
		f = 15/min							1.63	90.4		41.6	−4.5	
		f = 30/min							1.65	93.8		38.3	−1.7	
		f = 45/min							1.67	96.2		37.4	−1.3	
1984	20–45	Endurance-trained subjects	16	91	8	38.9		16	max	75.0	33.0	32.5		133a

n, Number of subjects; Pa_{O_2}, partial pressure of O_2 in arterial blood; $PA_{O_2} - Pa_{O_2}$, alveolar-arterial difference in partial pressure of O_2; Pa_{CO_2}, arterial partial pressure of CO_2; $Pa_{CO_2} - PA_{CO_2}$, arterial-alveolar difference in partial pressure of CO_2; $\dot{V}_{O_2}$, O_2 consumption; M, male; F, female; U, untrained; T, trained; $PA_{N_2} - Pa_{N_2}$, alveolar-arterial difference in partial pressure of N_2; SF_6, sulfur hexafluoride; f, respiratory frequency.

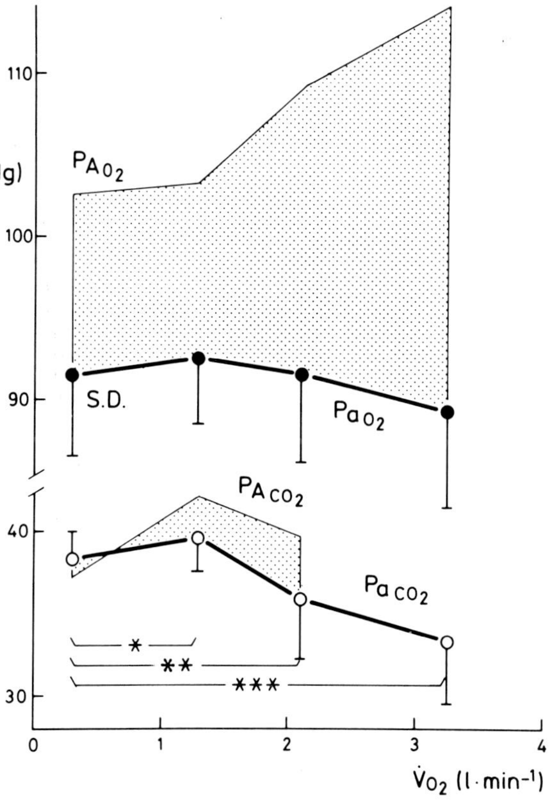

FIG. 2. Mean arterial O_2 partial pressure (Pa_{O_2}, ●) and Pa_{CO_2} (○) values (±SD) as a function of O_2 consumption ($\dot{V}_{O_2}$). *Thin lines*, calculated alveolar values. *Shaded areas*, alveolar-arterial difference in partial pressure of O_2 ($P_{A_{O_2}} - Pa_{O_2}$) and CO_2 ($Pa_{CO_2} - P_{A_{CO_2}}$.) *, $P < 0.05$. **, $P < 0.01$. ***, $P < 0.001$. [Data from Table 1 (ref. 133a not included).]

between regions (interregional); the latter is reduced at exercise.

True shunt (venous admixture) could be responsible partly for the observed exercise-induced increase of $P_{A_{O_2}} - Pa_{O_2}$. The percent of venous admixture, after a reduction at moderate work loads, tends to increase (497) with increasing $\dot{V}_{O_2}$. Concurrently, mixed venous blood O_2 partial pressure ($P\bar{v}_{O_2}$) undergoes most of its reduction as a function of increased metabolism below 40% $\dot{V}max_{O_2}$. These two changes could qualitatively (if not quantitatively) describe the shape of the curve appearing in Figure 2. In addition to the factors outlined above, it is possible that part of the observed increase of $P_{A_{O_2}} - Pa_{O_2}$ with exercise is due to a more uneven regional distribution of diffusing capacity in the lung (377) and/or a more uneven distribution of diffusing capacity to blood flow (497).

Training does not seem to affect $P_{A_{O_2}} - Pa_{O_2}$ at rest or at exercise (217). The same is true for airway obstruction (214). Aging, however, appears to widen both resting and exercise $P_{A_{O_2}} - Pa_{O_2}$. Because $P_{A_{N_2}} - Pa_{N_2}$ was the same in elderly subjects as in young individuals (31), the suggestion was made that with aging the number of lung units with low $\dot{V}_A/\dot{Q}$ ratio is not increased. Because this conclusion contrasts with previous results obtained by scanning the distribution of radioactive gases in the lung (236), the larger $P_{A_{O_2}} - Pa_{O_2}$ was attributed to the combined effect of $\dot{V}_A/\dot{Q}$ and $D_L/\dot{Q}$ inequalities, a situation compatible with a narrow $P_{A_{N_2}} - Pa_{N_2}$ (31).

The differences in CO_2 partial pressure (P_{CO_2}) between pulmonary capillary blood and alveolar gas ($Pa_{CO_2} - P_{A_{CO_2}}$) due to the high diffusivity of CO_2 across the alveolar membrane should be essentially zero. However, there are physicochemical and physiological reasons why in real lungs positive $Pa_{CO_2} - P_{A_{CO_2}}$ could arise (e.g., the presence of unperfused alveoli) (435). Recent experimental evidence also suggests that paradoxical negative P_{CO_2} gradients may exist between blood and alveolar gas (175, 205). Table 2 is a review of the literature limited to the studies in which $Pa_{CO_2} - P_{A_{CO_2}}$ was measured at rest and at exercise on the same individuals; average results are plotted in Figure 2 as a function of $\dot{V}_{O_2}$. The average $Pa_{CO_2} - P_{A_{CO_2}}$ measured on >40 subjects at rest by five authors is not significantly different from zero. Also, at work loads corresponding to average $\dot{V}_{O_2}$ values of ~1.5 and 2.5 liters/min, mean $Pa_{CO_2} - P_{A_{CO_2}}$ values were only slightly negative. Scheid and Piiper (435) attribute negative $P_{A_{CO_2}} - Pa_{CO_2}$ values to measurement artifacts or inadequate techniques.

LUNG DIFFUSING CAPACITY. Meyer (348) and Piiper and Scheid (383) recently extensively analyzed and critically reviewed the literature on DL at rest and at exercise. Mean resting and exercise DL values for CO ($D_{L_{CO}}$), as assessed by steady-state, single-breath, and rebreathing methods, appear in Table 3. Despite the large differences among $D_{L_{CO}}$ values obtained at rest by the various methods, there is no doubt that $D_{L_{CO}}$ increases with an increase in the rate of gas exchange. The same conclusion can be drawn from the measurements of DL for O_2 ($D_{L_{O_2}}$), irrespective of the technique used (Table 4). However, the entity of the DL rise depends on the work load and partly on the method employed for the determination. The highest DL levels and the largest scatter among measurements occur for steady-state $D_{L_{O_2}}$ estimates (cf. refs. 208, 405, 440, 478). The increase of DL observed during exercise is due to broadening of the effective gas-blood

TABLE 2. *Alveolar-Arterial Difference in P_{O_2} and P_{CO_2} as Function of O_2 Consumption at Rest and Exercise*

$\dot{V}_{O_2}$, liters/min	$P_{A_{O_2}} - Pa_{O_2}$, mmHg	$Pa_{CO_2} - P_{A_{CO_2}}$, mmHg
0.3	11 ± 3.1	1.1 ± 1.1
1.1–1.3	11.3 ± 4.8	−2.7 ± 2.4
2.3–2.6	17.4 ± 6.7	−3.9 ± 1.8
3–4	24.9 ± 7.2	

$\dot{V}_{O_2}$, O_2 consumption; $P_{A_{O_2}} - Pa_{O_2}$, alveolar-arterial difference in partial pressure of O_2; $Pa_{CO_2} - P_{A_{CO_2}}$, arterial-alveolar difference in partial pressure of CO_2. Data from Table 1.

TABLE 3. *Pulmonary Diffusing Capacity of CO at Rest and at Exercise*

Method	D_{LCO}, $ml \cdot min^{-1} \cdot mmHg^{-1}$	*n*	Age Range, yr	Years of Coverage	Ref.
Rest					
Steady-state	22.0 ± 5.2 (20.5)	457	16–69	1954 →	11, 12, 43, 56, 125, 156, 176, 204, 296, 297, 314, 315, 398, 421, 441, 460
Single-breath	31.0 ± 8.2 (31.1)	819	15–79	1956 →	12, 14, 64, 74, 116, 117, 126, 173, 176, 183, 186, 212, 259, 310, 315, 316, 337, 338, 344, 360, 361, 388, 411, 412, 447, 485
Rebreathing	24.1 ± 7.6 (25.8)	101	15–60	1954 →	166, 300, 449, 596
Exercise					
Steady-state	44 ± 14 (38.5)	558	15–66	1954 →	13, 14, 35, 41, 42, 55, 115, 149, 169, 180, 199, 207, 213, 237, 243, 244, 246, 265, 266, 322, 337, 359, 387, 392, 402, 415, 440, 461
Single-breath	46.2 ± 6.16 (42.2)	122	18–52	1957 →	2, 33, 48, 75, 119, 177, 199, 269, 301, 326, 353, 363, 403, 416, 481
Rebreathing	44.0 ± 15 (41.7)	25	24–60	1969 →	309, 420

Population mean (±SD) and subjects' average (number in parentheses) D_{LCO} values at rest and at exercise, measured by steady-state, single-breath, and rebreathing methods. *n*, Number of subjects.

TABLE 4. *Pulmonary Diffusing Capacity of O_2 at Rest and at Exercise*

Method	D_{LO_2}, $ml \cdot min^{-1} \cdot mmHg^{-1}$	*n*	Age Range, yr	First Year Studied	Ref.
Rest					
Steady-state	28.8 ± 5.4 (30.3)	87	19–66	1909	38, 60, 297, 436
Single-breath	28.6 ± 4.3 (29.3)	28	20–46	1966	196, 258
Rebreathing	27.7 ± 12 (26.4)	22	27–43	1970	98, 350
Exercise					
Steady-state	67.2 ± 8.2 (65.6)	85	19–66	1915	54, 61, 106, 208, 298, 317, 405, 440, 446, 478
Single-breath	42.3 (41.5)	14	22–42	1970	113, 184, 197
Rebreathing	49.7 ± 28 (45.6)	13	27–43	1970	87, 195, 380, 482

Population mean (±SD) and subjects' average (number in parentheses) D_{LO_2} values at rest and at exercise, measured by steady-state, single-breath, and rebreathing methods. *n*, Number of subjects.

contact surface caused by the dilation of pulmonary vessels down to the capillaries, a consequence of increased transmural pressure and recruitment of previously nonperfused vascular districts. So far it has been impossible to quantitate the individual role of the above factors. Two additional mechanisms lead to an apparent increase of DL: *1)* the more homogeneous vertical distribution of blood perfusion in the lungs during exercise (493), whereby, due to the decrease of the lung functional inhomogeneity, DL is less underestimated than at rest and *2)* the reduced negative effect on the estimate of D_{LO_2} of a given degree of lung inhomogeneity when $\dot{V}_{O_2}$ is high, such as during exercise (378). It is not known whether DL rises steadily with increasing metabolism and/or whether a plateau level is attained, which is a problem of considerable interest for characterizing the maximum capacity of the lungs for diffusive gas exchange across the gas-blood barrier. A statistical analysis of the data of the literature does not settle the question, as can be seen in Figure 3, in which mean D_{LCO} and D_{LO_2} values obtained by several authors using different methods are plotted against $\dot{V}_{O_2}$. The DL appears to increase with increasing work load, but the scatter of the data does not establish or rule out the existence of a plateau. Note, however, that several authors have demonstrated a leveling off of DL with increasing $\dot{V}_{O_2}$ (41, 54, 106, 169, 180, 243, 245, 246, 326, 405). Recently Meyer et al. (349) determined rebreathing D_{LCO} and D_{LO_2} from alveolar–mixed venous equilibration kinetics of $C^{18}O$ and $^{18}O_2$. Their results show in all cases relatively high DL resting values (47 ± 11 and 54 ± 10 $ml \cdot min^{-1} \cdot mmHg^{-1}$) and only a modest rise of DL with increasing work load, at least in the range covered by Figure 3. The observation (see Fig. 2) that $P_{AO_2} - Pa_{O_2}$ is increased only twofold when $\dot{V}_{O_2}$ is increased to the maximum levels (12–15-fold) implies also that DL should keep increasing with increasing metabolism even in the upper $\dot{V}_{O_2}$ range. By contrast, the drop of Pa_{O_2} found in highly trained athletes at very heavy work loads (133a, 144, 247) would be compatible with a leveling off of DL. The problem could possibly be settled by simultaneous measurements of Pa_{O_2}, DL, and $\dot{Q}$ during maximum exercise in athletes characterized by very high maximum aerobic power.

The results in Figure 3 may suggest that the D_{LO_2}/D_{LCO} average ratio is above unity at all work loads except rest. A more accurate analysis of the literature, whereby only the ratios of simultaneously measured D_{LO_2} and D_{LCO} are considered (113, 184, 195–197, 258, 297, 441, 478), sets the above average values at 0.77 ± 0.25 (SD) for rest and 1.08 ± 0.33 for exercise, thus considerably below the ratio of the Krogh's diffusion constants K_{O_2}/K_{CO}, which is 1.23.

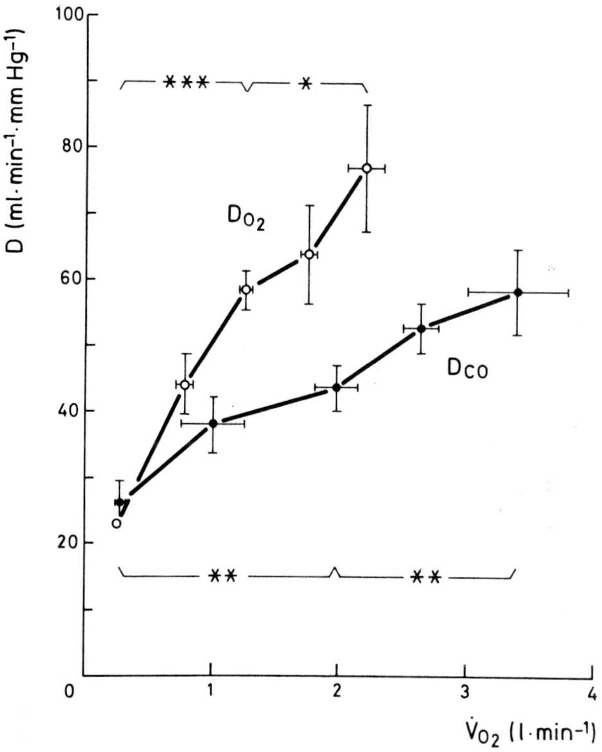

FIG. 3. Mean (±SD) diffusing capacity for O_2 (D_{O_2}; 44 subj.) and D_{CO} (318 subj.) as a function of $\dot{V}_{O_2}$ by various methods. *, $P < 0.05$. **, $P < 0.01$. ***, $P < 0.001$. (Data from refs. 13, 35, 48, 55, 75, 119, 149, 169, 199, 265, 269, 326, 337, 359, 363, 387, 392, 402, 415, 461, 478, 511.)

Meyer et al. (349) recently measured DL for isotopic O_2 and CO and found a value for the above ratio of ~1.2 both for rest and exercise. Such a value is compatible with the assumption that diffusion between the gas phase and Hb is the major resistive component to O_2 transfer in the lung.

Pulmonary diffusing capacity for CO_2 (DL_{CO_2}) was assessed in humans by the single-breath technique with the stable isotope $^{13}CO_2$ (260). Resting values were not significantly different from infinity (223–∞). Recent measurements (382) carried out by rebreathing yielded DL_{CO_2} values of 179 ± 13 ml·min^{-1}·mmHg^{-1} (SD) at rest and of 306 ± 6 ml·min^{-1}·mmHg^{-1} at moderate exercise (75 W). From these measurements the authors predict a practically imperceptible diffusion limitation for pulmonary CO_2 exchange at rest but a considerable $Pa_{CO_2} - PA_{CO_2}$ (~7 mmHg) at maximum exercise because of equilibration deficit.

Blood O_2-Carrying Capacity

Blood O_2 transport during or after acute and/or chronic exercise may undergo appreciable changes as a consequence of physiological circulatory and physicochemical adjustments, such as *1)* a change and/or redistribution of blood volume and flow, respectively, *2)* an alteration of the red blood cell (RBC) geometry, *3)* a change of [Hb] and of hematocrit (Hct), and *4)* a shift of the oxyhemoglobin dissociation curve (ODC).

CHANGE AND/OR REDISTRIBUTION OF BLOOD VOLUME AND FLOW. Short intensive muscular exercise causes fluid to leak out of the vascular compartment and plasma volume may drop 15% (45); when exercise is carried out in normal environmental conditions, mean corpuscular volume is only slightly affected, despite observed remarkable increases in plasma osmolarity and acidification (44, 46). By contrast, in prolonged heavy exercise [e.g., a 45-km walk (389) or 85-km race in cross-country skiing (28)], plasma volume and mean corpuscular volume do not vary substantially. Regular exercise training [e.g., running 3 miles in 30 min 3 times/wk for 16 wk (367) or pedaling 2 h/day for 8 consecutive days at a load corresponding to 65% of individual $\dot{V}max_{O_2}$ (107)] increased blood volume 338 ml and 457 ml, respectively, mainly because of an expansion of plasma volume, because mean corpuscular volume was essentially constant. Training-induced hypervolemia was associated with an increase of renin and vasopressin activity, which facilitates Na^+ and H_2O retention, and with a progressive increase in plasma albumin content (107). Because the main determinant of maximum whole-body aerobic power is maximum cardiac output ($\dot{Q}_T$,max) (see FACTORS LIMITING MAXIMUM O_2 CONSUMPTION, p. 309), whose level may be influenced to a various extent by blood volume and viscosity, measurements of $\dot{V}max_{O_2}$ carried out 2–10 min after intensive performances or after a training program are likely to vary significantly. These changes, however, because of the many concomitant biochemical modifications induced by exercise, cannot be attributed exclusively to hemodynamics. Conversely, the reduction of performance capacity observed after exhausting efforts cannot be ascribed to cardiovascular factors (28).

Rowell (418) recently and extensively reviewed the problem of redistribution of blood flow during exercise. Unlike dogs (480), humans respond to exercise up to $\dot{V}max_{O_2}$ with a drastic reduction of splanchnic blood flow [from 1.6 to 0.4 liters/min (418)] and renal blood flow [60% reduction from resting control (202)]. Blood is directed preferentially to working muscles, which may therefore increase their $\dot{V}_{O_2}$ without a corresponding increase of $\dot{Q}_T$ and with a considerable saving of energy by the circulatory pump (see next section). A further contribution to the reduction of the cost of O_2 transport to the contracting muscles can also be expected from the blood shift from the skin and from resting muscles (~1 liter/min), the latter assessed by plethysmographic and ^{133}Xe-clearance measurements.

RED BLOOD CELL GEOMETRY. Evidence that in vitro RBCs change their volume according to the chemical potential of the surrounding fluid, although not as much as expected from simple theory (434), and the observation that important changes of osmolarity and of plasma [H^+] occur as a consequence of work and/or heat stress have led to the conclusion that there are conditions in which the RBC geometry must be altered even in vivo (109). A change of RBC size, affecting its rheology, may impair gas exchange in working muscles.

HEMOGLOBIN CONCENTRATION AND HEMATOCRIT. Prolonged heavy exercise appears to increase RBC fragility. This change has been attributed to increases in circulatory rate, temperature, plasma acidity, and possibly cell compression. Despite this, trained athletes are characterized by larger RBC mass and total Hb per kilogram body weight (281), even though RBC concentration, Hct, and [Hb] are lower than in sedentary subjects (71). For instance, in a group of 11 world-class professional bicycle riders checked repeatedly (i.e., off-season and during their competitive season after 9 mo of heavy physical activity), RBC concentration was 4.6 ± 0.2 and 4.7 ± 0.2 × $10^6/\mu l$, respectively, whereas Hct was 45.0 and 45.1 and [Hb] was 14.5 and 15.1 (482a). These relatively low values are likely due to training-induced expansion of blood volume. Whether hemodilution is a positive feature for increasing $\dot{Q}_{T,max}$ and thus maximum Hb flow, still needs investigation. The athletes indicated above had very high $\dot{V}max_{O_2}$ values, particularly at top condition. Acute (158, 506) and maintained (506) isovolemic or hypovolemic (−800 ml) anemia does not affect significantly the maximum levels of $\dot{V}_E$, $\dot{Q}_T$, and HR, whereas the $\dot{Q}_T/\dot{V}_{O_2}$ and $\dot{V}_E/\dot{V}_{O_2}$ ratios are increased and $P\bar{v}_{O_2}$ for a given $\dot{V}_{O_2}$ is below control levels. With both acute and established anemia, $\dot{V}max_{O_2}$ is reduced proportionally to the drop of [Hb] (158, 506). Inhalation of low [CO] (225 ppm), on the other hand, induces, together with anoxemia (HbCO = 18%–20%), a leftward shift of the ODC and a higher $\dot{Q}_T/\dot{V}_{O_2}$ ratio than in control conditions (483).

The effect of blood infusion (normovolemic or slightly hypervolemic) on maximum aerobic power ($\dot{V}max_{O_2}$), as appears from a review of the literature, is still rather controversial. In fact, results showing that a 2 g/100 ml increase of [Hb] raises $\dot{V}max_{O_2}$ (Table 5) have been obtained with an average initial Hb level ($[Hb]_{in}$) of 13.5 ± 1 g/100 ml, i.e., well below the physiological range. Furthermore the function $\Delta\dot{V}max_{O_2}/\Delta[Hb]$ vs. $[Hb]_{in}$ appears to be a decreasing exponential, approaching the abscissa at 18 g/100 ml. Even at an $[Hb]_{in}$ level of ~16 g/100 ml, $\Delta\dot{V}max_{O_2}$ for an increase of 1 g/100 ml in $[Hb]_{in}$ is marginal (~2%), i.e., within the limits of the measurement error by conventional techniques. Besides, there are authors who challenge the above results. Williams et al. (504, 505) do not find significant effects from whole-blood (500 ml), RBC (275 ml), or plasma (225 ml) infusion on endurance capacity as well as on resting, submaximum, and maximum HR. Measurements carried out on 13 members of a Himalayan team before and 4 wk after leaving high altitude, when [Hb] was still 11.6% higher than control, show an insignificant increase of $\dot{V}max_{O_2}$ (79). From a general functional standpoint even a modest increase (5%) of $\dot{V}max_{O_2}$ as a consequence of blood infusion should improve drastically the endurance performances and cause a solution of continuity in the curve of athletic records. This break in the curves cannot be observed. Training at medium altitude aimed at improving maximum aerobic performances based on increased [Hb] has also resulted in equivocal conclusions.

TABLE 5. *Increase of Maximum Aerobic Power After Autologous Blood Infusion in Humans*

n	$[Hb]_{in}$, g/100 ml	Δ[Hb], g/100 ml	$\Delta\dot{V}max_{O_2}$, %	$\Delta\dot{V}max_{O_2}/\Delta$[Hb], %	Ref.
Male					
3	13.2	1.7	8	4.7	153
4	12.2	2.9	21	7.2	153
5	13.1	1.3	8	6.2	158
11	15.1	1.2	4	3.3	73
4	14.6	2.0	7	3.5	451a
5	13.8	3.8	13	3.4	406b
Female					
9	12.7	2.0	10	5.0	406a
Mean	13.5 ± 1	2.0 ± 1	10.1 ± 5.5	4.7 ± 1.5	
			9.1*		
13	14.6	1.7†	5	2.9	79

n, Number of subjects; $[Hb]_{in}$, initial concentration of Hb in blood; Δ[Hb], increase of [Hb] after infusion; $\Delta\dot{V}max_{O_2}$, increase of maximum aerobic power; $\Delta\dot{V}max_{O_2}/\Delta$[Hb], gain in $\dot{V}max_{O_2}$ per 1 g increase in [Hb]. * Weighted mean. † Δ[Hb] obtained by altitude exposure.

In the dog, extremely high Hct levels (60%) associated with increased blood volume, as found in man at high altitude, have important bearings on hemodynamics such as relative and absolute drops of $\dot{Q}_T$ and HR. This condition, however, is not associated with a reduction of O_2 delivery nor does it interfere with peripheral O_2 extraction during exercise. In fact, in normoxia, for any given $\dot{V}_{O_2}$ level the observed decrease of $\dot{Q}_T$ appears to be fully compensated for by a greater $Pa_{O_2} - P\bar{v}_{O_2}$, and $\dot{V}max_{O_2}$ is practically unaffected (436a).

SHIFT OF OXYHEMOGLOBIN DISSOCIATION CURVE. It is well known that Hb in the RBC functions in conjunction with intracellular polyphosphates, particularly with 2,3-diphosphoglycerate (2,3-DPG). The main function of this compound appears to be the maintenance of Hb affinity for O_2 within the physiologically useful range for the various conditions that may be encountered by the body. This, for instance, appears true for altitude natives as well as for lowlanders acclimatized to altitude (135, 432). These subjects, despite a decreased Pa_{CO_2}, appear to keep their Hb-O_2 affinity, as determined from the O_2 half-saturation pressure of Hb (P_{50}), rather constant by an average 20% increase of their 2,3-DPG/Hb ratio (432). A situation that with respect to blood oxygenation shares some analogies with chronic hypoxia is that

TABLE 6. *Effects of Exercise and Endurance Training on P_{50} and 2,3-DPG Concentrations*

	Subject Condition	Concentration		Ref.
		P_{50}	2,3-DPG	
Exercise				
Anaerobic	U	↑		452
	U + T		↑	167
	U + T	=	=	439
	T	↑	↑	466
	U + T	=	=	66
	U	↑	↑	283
Aerobic	U + T		↑	150
	U + T		↑	167
	T	=	=	466
	U	=	=	472
Endurance training		=	↑	439
		↑	↑	466
		=	=	394
		↑	=	188
		↑	↑	66
		=	↑	482a

P_{50}, O_2 half-saturation pressure of Hb; 2,3-DPG, 2,3-diphosphoglycerate; U, untrained; T, trained; ↑, increases; =, unchanged.

induced by heavy maintained aerobic exercise. An example of this is an athlete (such as a professional road bicycle rider) accustomed to work up to 10 h a day over several months and characterized by a prolonged very low $P\bar{v}_{O_2}$ (~20–25 mmHg) and mixed venous blood O_2 content ($C\bar{v}_{O_2}$ ~ 10 ml/100 ml). Because venous blood is ~75%–80% of the whole-blood volume, the average Hb insaturation level in this subject is quite comparable to that of high-altitude residents, and certain blood adaptations appear to be similar [e.g., 20% increase of the 2,3-DPG/Hb ratio, constant P_{50} (97)]. Because many variables (e.g., changes of temperature, [H^+], and P_{CO_2}) interfere with Hb-O_2 affinity, the values reported in the literature for P_{50} and [2,3-DPG] in athletes and in exercising untrained and trained subjects are very controversial [(66, 150, 167, 188, 283, 302, 394, 439, 452, 466, 472); Table 6]. Variables that should be carefully accounted for are exercise load (aerobic vs. anaerobic, for the obvious implications concerning blood acidification), exercise duration, and training. An interesting observation on the possibly homeostatic role of 2,3-DPG was made by Woodson et al. (506), who found in maintained isovolemic anemia (7–9 days) an 18% rise of 2,3-DPG and a 2-mmHg increase in P_{50}, which probably afforded some compensation for decreased O_2 transport. The 2,3-DPG/Hb ratio was not significantly affected, however, after autologous blood reinfusion (73).

Energy Cost of Blood Pumping

The heart is essentially an aerobic organ characterized by an extremely high density of mitochondria (~35% of the muscle total volume) and oxidative enzymes and by a maximum oxidative potential, exceeding three- to fourfold that of skeletal muscle. Even during very heavy exercise, healthy myocardium relies very little on anaerobic glycolysis, which occurs only in the presence of anoxia or ischemia, such as after coronary artery occlusion (105) or with cardiac arrest during open-heart surgery. In the latter condition the myocardium may build a large lactic O_2 debt, as shown by direct lactate (La) estimates carried out in human bioptic samples where [La] as high as 30 μmol/g of wet tissue was found (7).

The homogeneous arterial blood supply and the relatively easy access to a major efferent vein allow assessment of substrate utilization and gas exchange in the left ventricle. Measurements in normal individuals have shown that plasma free fatty acids are the preferred substrate for the myocardium, accounting for ~50%–60% of the total metabolism both at rest and at moderate exercise (274, 306, 366). Other substrates are triglycerides, which contribute 15% of the total energy supply at rest and 10% at exercise; glucose, which provides 15% of the overall fuel at rest and 25% at exercise; and La, which contributes 10%–15% of the total substrates at rest (307) and even more [up to 60%, according to Keul et al. (279)] during heavy exercise. Steady-state myocardial $\dot{V}_{O_2}$ ($M\dot{V}_{O_2}$) has been determined in humans from catheterization of the coronary sinus (53) and from the measurement of coronary blood flow by inert-gas washout (287). In normal resting subjects, $M\dot{V}_{O_2}$ averages 8–10 ml O_2/100 g of left ventricle and per minute (68) or a total of 18–20 ml O_2 for the whole left ventricle (~200 g), to which must be added the $\dot{V}_{O_2}$ of the right ventricular and atrial mass (~140 g), estimated at ~4 ml O_2/min. Thus, at rest, myocardial metabolism accounts for ~5%–8% of the energy expenditure of the whole body.

Braunwald (67) identified six physiological determinants of myocardial energy expenditure and their relative O_2 requirement:

1. Basal metabolism, i.e., resting $\dot{V}_{O_2}$ measured in the nonbeating heart. This component is estimated in the range 1.5–2 ml·100 g^{-1}·min^{-1}, or ~20% of the total $\dot{V}_{O_2}$ of the active beating heart. This energy is used by the cell membrane to maintain the ionic environment and for other cell processes not directly related to contraction.

2. Activation metabolism. This includes at least two components: electrical activation, i.e., the energy expenditure associated with propagation of the action potential in the myocardium, estimated at ~0.5%–1% of total $M\dot{V}_{O_2}$ (286), and the release and reuptake of Ca^{2+} by the sarcoplasmic reticulum, which accounts for 10%–15% of total energy expenditure.

3. Development and maintenance of systolic pressure. This fraction can be estimated by the tension-time index (TTI), i.e., the product of left ventricular mean systolic pressure (P) and the duration of systole referred to one minute. According to Sarnoff et al. (433), in any given functional state of the beating heart, TTI is the principal determinant of $M\dot{V}_{O_2}$,

accounting for ~30% of total energy expenditure (189). The relationship between TTI and $M\dot{V}_{O_2}$ is constant, whether TTI is augmented by increased HR, increased mean systolic pressure, or longer duration of the systole. Levine and Wagman (313) note, however, that TTI measured as above overlooks the geometry of the heart. In fact, based on the law of Laplace [$T = P(R/2)$], the tension (T) depends also on the mean radius (R) of the heart chamber, which is assumed to be spheric.

4. Myocardial fiber shortening and external work, i.e., the stroke work [stroke volume (q_{st}) times mean aortic pressure] plus a kinetic energy term. In the normal heart the estimated work component due to shortening could comprise as much as 17% of the total $M\dot{V}_{O_2}$ (67).

5. Inotropic state of contractility. Assessed as peak dP/dt, this also appears to be a major determinant of $M\dot{V}_{O_2}$, as shown by the fall of $M\dot{V}_{O_2}$ induced by pharmacological agents acutely depressing left ventricular contractility (200).

6. Heart rate, to which $M\dot{V}_{O_2}$ appears to be linearly related (280, 307). The observed high correlation between $M\dot{V}_{O_2}$ and TTI is also a consequence of the above relation.

Other obvious determinants of $M\dot{V}_{O_2}$ are the myocardial mass and possibly the role of a hypothetical active relaxation of the ventricle.

As is well known, the increase of $\dot{Q}_T$ during heavy exercise in the erect position results from an increase of both HR (×2.5) and q_{st} (×2). Concurrently, $M\dot{V}_{O_2}$ may increase up to fivefold. The greater part of the increased O_2 supply to the heart is provided by higher coronary blood flow. In fact, the arteriovenous O_2 difference can increase only slightly because myocardial O_2 extraction at rest averages 70% ± 6% [(347); see also Fig. 4*C*]. The $M\dot{V}_{O_2}$ values for 100 g of left ventricular mass are plotted as a function of total energy consumption of the body ($\dot{V}_{O_2}$), of $\dot{Q}_T$, and of left ventricular blood flow ($\dot{Q}_{LV}$) in Fig. 4*A*, *B*, and *C*, respectively. There appears to be a good correlation (r = 0.88, 0.95, and 0.99, respectively) between these variables. Average maximum $M\dot{V}_{O_2}$ ($M\dot{V}max_{O_2}$) may be estimated for humans on the basis of an assumed left ventricular weight of 200 g and on the assumption that the energy cost of the remainder of the heart is ~25% that of the left ventricle. It may attain 100–120 ml/min, i.e., 4% of total aerobic metabolism at an overall $\dot{V}_{O_2}$ level of ~3 liters/min. The $M\dot{V}max_{O_2}$ per unit weight of the heart appears to range between 300 and 400 ml $O_2 \cdot kg^{-1} \cdot min^{-1}$, i.e., 3- to 4-fold higher than that for skeletal muscle.

The efficiency of the cardiac pump is conventionally estimated as

$$\eta = \frac{W}{W + H} = \frac{\dot{W}}{M\dot{V}_{O_2}} \qquad (1)$$

where W is the useful work carried out, $\dot{W}$ is the power output, and H is the heat produced (the kinetic factor of cardiac work, estimated at ~5% of the total, is usually neglected). On the basis of measured "net" $M\dot{V}_{O_2}$ (i.e., active minus nonbeating heart) for the left ventricle, η was estimated at ~18% at rest and ~21% at heavy exercise. These values appear to be higher for athletes, reaching 25% at rest and 33% at heavy work (189).

If the cost of the cardiac pump is assumed to be 120 ml O_2/min and if the relatively fast recovery kinetics of $\dot{Q}_T$ after a maximum effort are considered, the error introduced by cardiac activity in the estimate of the body total O_2 debt and/or of the kinetics of the overall $\dot{V}_{O_2}$ off-response (see next section) appears to be negligible [~30 ml O_2 and ~2% of the observed half time ($t_{1/2}$), respectively].

Cardiovascular Adjustments

Exercise appears to be the most powerful stress for the cardiovascular system. No pharmacological agent administered at rest can induce the elevation of $\dot{Q}_T$

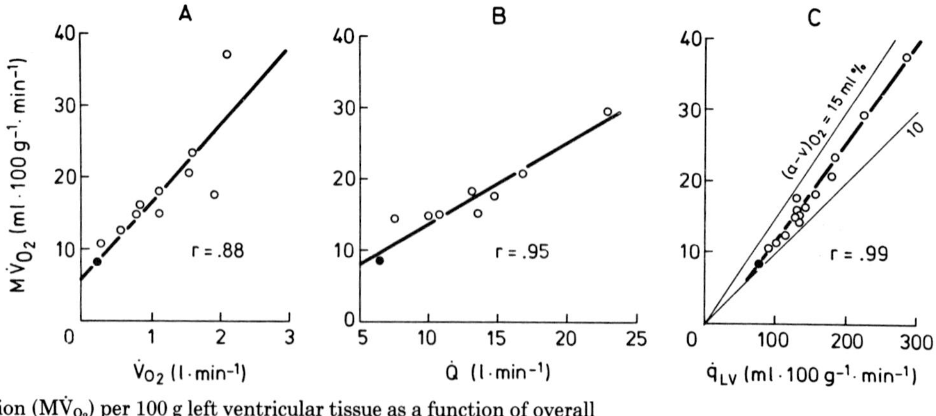

FIG. 4. Myocardial O_2 consumption ($M\dot{V}_{O_2}$) per 100 g left ventricular tissue as a function of overall O_2 consumption ($\dot{V}_{O_2}$), cardiac output ($\dot{Q}$), and left ventricular blood flow ($\dot{Q}_{LV}$) at rest (●) and exercise (○). $(a - v)_{O_2}$, Arteriovenous O_2 difference in milliliters of O_2 per 100 ml of blood. (Data from refs. 52, 241, 280, 346, 347, 397.)

observed during moderate isotonic or dynamic exercise. The changes occurring in peripheral circulation during dynamic exercise, particularly the vasodilation taking place in the vessels supplying working muscles, are directed toward increasing the capacity of the vascular bed to return blood to the right atrium (volume load) without augmenting ventricular afterload (206). Also redistribution of blood flow from nonworking vasoconstricted districts [e.g., the splanchnic region (65, 418), the kidney (202), and the skin and resting skeletal muscles (58, 418, 512, 513)] to active muscles represents in humans an important adaptive mechanism that improves O_2 transport while limiting the increase in $\dot{Q}_T$ and systemic arterial pressure. Venous return is prompted not only by increased activity of the heart but also by the rhythmic contractions of limb muscles and by alternate tensing of the abdominal and thoracic walls. The pumping action provided by leg muscles during stationary running could account for ~30% of the total energy required to circulate blood (454). The $\dot{Q}_T$ response to isotonic exercise involves the integrated effects on the myocardium of tachycardia, sympathetic stimulation, and the operation of the Frank-Starling mechanism (68, 450).

REGULATION OF CARDIAC OUTPUT. Steady-state $\dot{Q}_T$ adjustments to predominantly isotonic work appear to be proportional to the $\dot{V}_{O_2}$ of the contracting muscle mass. As is well known, the increased transport and peripheral unloading of O_2 is assured not only by increased $\dot{Q}_T$ but also by greater tissue extraction. The latter is also prompted by an increase in nutritional flow (opening of a large capillary bed) and possibly by reduced Hb affinity for O_2 at the capillary–muscle cell interface. Whether the increase of $\dot{Q}_T$ observed during aerobic isotonic work is coincidental to or driven by the increase in metabolism is unclear. It is possible that $\dot{Q}_T$ (like HR and arterial pressure) during single twitches or sustained isometric contractions is set by a neurogenic mechanism ("cortical irradiation") or, as Asmussen et al. (21) hypothesize, by a reflex originating in the contracting muscles or by both. Whereas a reflex mechanism cannot be excluded, the biochemical changes eliciting the response, the nature of the sensor, its mode of action with reference to the muscle mass involved and to the distribution of the hypothesized changes, and the possible link between metabolic events and the cardiovascular center still need investigation (see below). Note, however, that in predominantly dynamic activities the $\dot{Q}_T/\dot{V}_{O_2}$ relationship is relatively constant and independent of many relevant variables, such as age, body size, sex, exercise mode, training level, and athletic condition (Fig. 5).

Whereas the $\dot{Q}_T/\dot{V}_{O_2}$ relationship (Fig. 5) appears to be the same for all individuals in most experimental conditions (some important exceptions are considered below), the determinants of $\dot{Q}_T$ (i.e., HR and q_{st}) for any given submaximum $\dot{V}_{O_2}$ level are subject to large individual fluctuations (51, 148, 159, 290, 400, 419) that in most cases tend to be compensatory with respect to $\dot{Q}_T$. In Figure 6, HR (*A*), q_{st} (*B*), and $\dot{Q}_T$

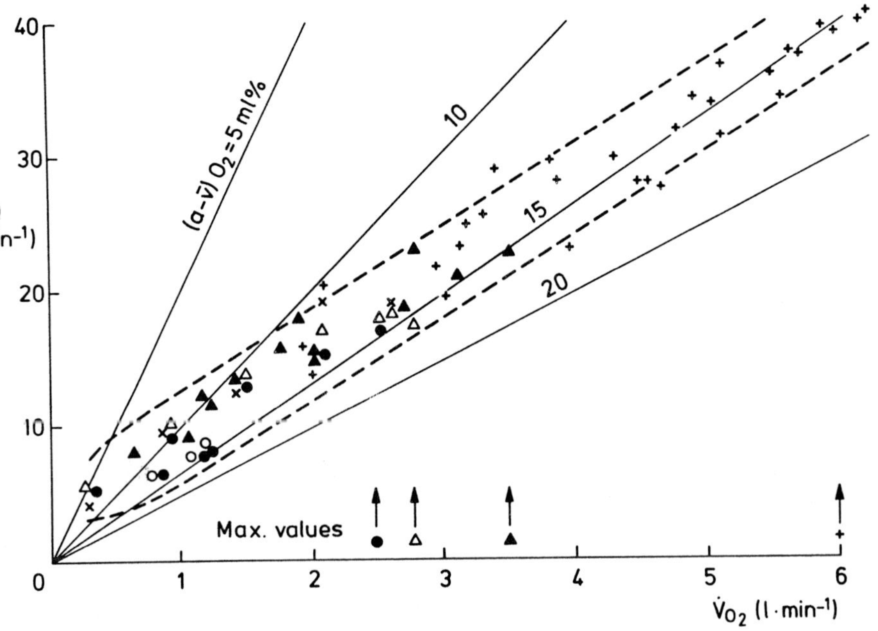

FIG. 5. Cardiac output ($\dot{Q}$) as a function of O_2 uptake ($\dot{V}_{O_2}$) for different groups of subjects: ●, boys (11–14 yr); ○, girls (11–14 yr); ▲, adult males; △, adult females; +, male athletes; ×, female athletes. Group $\dot{V}max_{O_2}$ values shown by ↑. Isopleths showing arterial–mixed-venous O_2 difference in milliliters of O_2 per 100 ml of blood, $(a\text{-}\bar{v})_{O_2}$, are also drawn. (Data from refs. 26, 36, 86, 155, 161, 201, 217, 227, 430.)

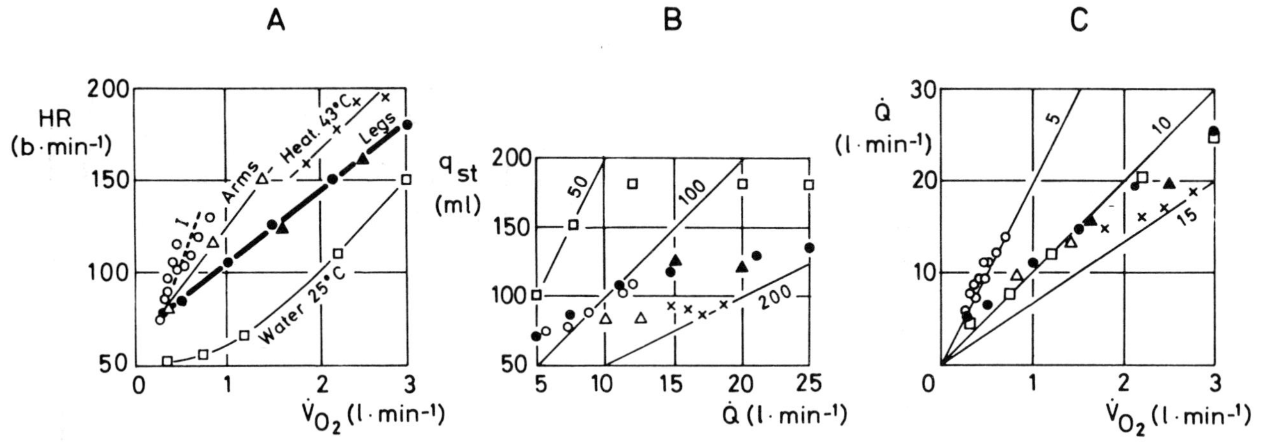

FIG. 6. *A*: heart rate (HR) as a function of $\dot{V}_{O_2}$. *B*: relationship between stroke volume (q_{st}) and cardiac output ($\dot{Q}$). Isopleth HR lines: 50, 100, 200/min. *C*: cardiac output as a function of $\dot{V}_{O_2}$. Isopleths show arterial–mixed-venous O_2 difference: 5, 10, 15 ml/100 ml. ●, Walking and running (P. Cerretelli, unpublished observations); □, during aquatic activity (400); ×, in hot environments (419); △, during arm exercise (51); ▲, during arm and leg exercise (51); ○, during isometric (I) exercise (148; P. Cerretelli, unpublished observations).

(*C*) are plotted as a function of $\dot{V}_{O_2}$ for different groups of normal subjects carrying out dynamic exercises (e.g., walking, running, pedaling, lifting light weights by the legs during immersion in 25°C water up to the neck, pedaling in a hot environment, arm cranking, and superimposing arm-to-leg exercise). Even if allowance is made for possibly large interindividual variability, at any given $\dot{V}_{O_2}$ level, HR is higher in arm cranking than in walking, pedaling, or simultaneously arm cranking and leg pedaling (Fig. 6*A*). The HR is also higher when a given load is carried out at 43.3°C than at 25.6°C (419). However, HR appears to drop when the exercise is carried out in an aquatic environment at a temperature well below body thermal neutrality for water. Homologous q_{st} changes appear to compensate for the observed HR variations (Fig. 6*B*), so that the $\dot{Q}_T/\dot{V}_{O_2}$ relationship (Fig. 6*C*) is practically identical for all conditions. Also, in swimming and during normoxic exercise in hyperbaric conditions, the relationships between $\dot{Q}_T$ and $\dot{V}_{O_2}$ are the same as the control relationships. The only known situations in which $\dot{Q}_T/\dot{V}_{O_2}$ is shifted upward are a reduction of the inspired O_2 partial pressure ($P_{I_{O_2}}$) (457) and moderate CO poisoning (483). In both cases the "error signal" affecting the $\dot{Q}_T/\dot{V}_{O_2}$ relationship could be the reduced O_2 arterial blood content, which would influence the hypothetical sensor controlling $\dot{Q}_T$. The recent observation (80) that in chronic hypoxia the $\dot{Q}_T$ response for a given $\dot{V}_{O_2}$ level tends to resume the normoxic pattern with increasing Hct despite persisting lower partial pressure of O_2 (P_{O_2}) seems to indicate the possible involvement of a metabolic detector sensitive to O_2 content or flow. With regard to heat adaptation, the contention that in hot climates a sizable fraction of $\dot{Q}_T$ may be shifted from working muscles to the skin for thermoregulation, with a consequent upper shift of the $\dot{Q}_T/\dot{V}_{O_2}$ relationship, now appears too simplistic. As a matter of fact, $\dot{Q}_T/\dot{V}_{O_2}$, in the range of submaximum work loads, remained essentially constant even when ambient air temperature was raised over 40°C (419), while the determinants of $\dot{Q}_T$ (HR and q_{st}) compensate for one another. By contrast, when skin temperature was increased by circulating hot water around it so that local blood flow was greatly enhanced and thus an error signal introduced, the $\dot{Q}_T/\dot{V}_{O_2}$ ratio increased disproportionately and measured peak $\dot{V}_{O_2}$ was lower than the subject's $\dot{V}max_{O_2}$ (417). The variable influence of a spontaneous and/or induced heat stress on the partition of regional blood flow explains the rather controversial conclusions of different investigators on the effect of heat on cardiovascular performance.

For any given value of $\dot{V}_{O_2}$, HR and $\dot{Q}_T$ are much higher in the course of sustained isometric contractions than during energetically equivalent isotonic loads (Fig. 6). This is true also for arterial pressure, which is also influenced by body posture (23) and/or muscle mass involved (182). As Lind and co-workers (319–321) note, the persisting high-pressure response to isometric exercise is probably aimed at overcoming the flow resistance opposed by the contracting muscles (pressure load). Cardiovascular reactions to sustained isometric exercise are independent of the contracting muscle mass and about proportional to the percentage of the maximum voluntary tension that the muscle mass can elicit. Most investigators (179, 343) have confirmed this observation. Recently it was shown that the cardiovascular responses to static contractions are dependent on muscle mass, provided the tension developed by the muscle is sufficiently low (355), and that the blood pressure response is almost unique to fast-twitch motor units (376). The large increase of $\dot{Q}_T$ with respect to $\dot{V}_{O_2}$ observed during isometric contractions (Fig. 6) may be just a determinant of the pressor response or, if the theory of metabolic control proves satisfactory, the response to one or more of the many disproportionate (with respect to $\dot{V}_{O_2}$) physicochemical changes occurring in muscle during static contractions (e.g., increase of extracellular K^+ and drop of high-energy phosphates) (see *Cardiovascular Transients*, p. 321).

The excessive increase of $\dot{Q}_T$ for a given level of $\dot{V}_{O_2}$ during isometric exercise introduces a practical concept in the physiological evaluation of the subject's performance, i.e., that of a myocardial load as opposed to an overall metabolic load. This notion may be relevant not only for exercise physiologists but particularly for cardiologists (356). From the increase of HR (and thus of $\dot{Q}_T$ because q_{st} is practically unchanged) (Fig. 6) and from systolic pressure it is possible to estimate $M\dot{V}_{O_2}$ for the subject involved in isometric activities (see *Energy Cost of Blood Pumping*, p. 305). For example, it may be calculated that a sustained isometric exercise, such as developing a net tension of 100 kg (20% of the maximum) by both plantar flexors [$\Delta\dot{V}_{O_2}$ = 300 ml/min (96)] by increasing HR up to ~130 beats per minute and systolic pressure to ~160 mmHg, imposes a metabolic stress on the heart equivalent to pedaling at 100 W on a bicycle ergometer or walking at 6 km/h on a +5% grade ($\dot{V}_{O_2} \cong$ 1.5 liters/min).

REGULATION OF MUSCLE BLOOD FLOW. Steady-state skeletal muscle blood flow and myocardial blood flow increase during exercise through the influence of several chemical and metabolic mediators, such as extracellular K^+ (the rise of which is associated with repetitive depolarization of the cell), changes in tissue osmolarity linked to metabolism, low P_{O_2}, increased P_{CO_2}, changes of adenosine, and neurogenic factors [e.g., the activity of intrinsic arteriolar neurons recently described by Honig and Frierson (249)]. The relative participation of these mediators of exercise hyperemia appears to depend on the pattern of exercise and on its duration (see refs. 267, 365, and 451 for reviews; see also *Cardiovascular Transients*, p. 321).

In human muscles composed of a mixture of fiber types, resting blood flow measured by venous occlusion plethysmography and by ^{133}Xe clearance (305) averages 3–5 $ml \cdot min^{-1} \cdot 100\ g^{-1}$ of tissue. In dogs standing on a treadmill the resting value was threefold higher both in respiratory and in leg muscles (170; P. Cerretelli, unpublished observations), but it is back in the range of human values after light narcosis. Because of the large vasodilatory reserve, muscle blood flow may increase to a maximum of 40–70 $ml \cdot min^{-1} \cdot 100\ g^{-1}$ of tissue in the limb muscles of trained individuals (104; P. Cerretelli, unpublished observations) and up to 100 ml in the dog diaphragm (170). All the above values may be underestimates of actual maximum flows if, as appears from recent comparative measurements with radionuclide-labeled microspheres, the ^{133}Xe-clearance method underestimates blood flow by ~50% (88) at all metabolic levels. Both in running dogs and in humans, top muscle blood flow determined from ^{133}Xe clearance in various active muscles is attained at fractions of the subject's or the animal's peak $\dot{V}_{O_2}$ for the exercise performed (running, leg pedaling, or arm cranking) well below unity (62, 104, 203, 386; P. Cerretelli, unpublished observations), a finding that is not confirmed for the miniature swine, where muscle $\dot{Q}$ increases up to $\dot{V}max_{O_2}$ (14a). Another recent finding that may have important implications in tissue gas exchange is a considerable regional inhomogeneity of muscle blood flow revealed by microsphere embolization at rest and exercise both in the isolated perfused dog gastrocnemius (382a) and in the intact animal (373a).

Oxygen Utilization and its Limiting Factors

MAXIMUM O_2 CONSUMPTION. Many studies have been devoted to the assessment of various characteristics of $\dot{V}max_{O_2}$, such as *1)* variability within the same population or among different ethnic groups (3, 9, 83, 120, 123, 138, 172, 192, 226, 293, 305, 311, 399, 401, 409, 458, 508); *2)* effects of sex and age (22, 24, 25, 218, 308, 407, 408, 444, 445); *3)* training, detraining, and athletic condition (10, 92, 109a, 124, 143, 151, 171, 174, 218, 219, 223, 276, 408, 428, 429, 431, 436b, 436c, 459, 482a); *4)* determinants: heredity versus environment (284, 285, 294, 487); and *5)* environmental effects and limiting factors (79, 82, 122, 153, 220, 221, 239, 240, 273, 332, 333, 362, 418, 506, 507). These studies are summarized in Table 7. The review by Lacour and Flandrois (303) is a more detailed discussion of these and related problems.

FACTORS LIMITING MAXIMUM O_2 CONSUMPTION. It is well known that $\dot{V}max_{O_2}$ increases with increasing $P_{I_{O_2}}$ (34, 162, 232, 273, 332, 333, 362, 465, 490, 509) and after the transfusion of RBCs (73, 79, 153, 157, 158, 406a, 406b, 451a), a finding that has not always been confirmed (504, 505) (see also *Blood O_2-Carrying Capacity*, p. 303). In addition, $\dot{V}max_{O_2}$ decreases in hypoxia (both acute and chronic), being reduced to ~0.65 the sea-level value at an altitude of 5,000 m above sea level (see refs. 82 and 303 for reviews), after CO inhalation (156, 157, 385, 395, 483), and after acute anemia (506).

It is generally inferred from these data that, at sea

TABLE 7. *Overview of Most Relevant Characteristics of $\dot{V}max_{O_2}$*

Average $\dot{V}max_{O_2}$ (20 yr), $ml \cdot kg^{-1} \cdot min^{-1}$	40–50
Average $\dot{V}max_{O_2}$ (20 yr), $\mu mol \cdot kg^{-1} \cdot s^{-1}$	30–37
$\dot{V}max_{O_2}$ per kg (male)/$\dot{V}max_{O_2}$ per kg (female)	1.15–1.20
$\dot{V}max_{O_2}$ (60 yr)/$\dot{V}max_{O_2}$ (20 yr)	0.70
$\dot{V}max_{O_2}$ (after training)/$\dot{V}max_{O_2}$ (before training)	1.10–1.20
$\dot{V}max_{O_2}$ (top athletes)/$\dot{V}max_{O_2}$ (nonathletes)	1.50–1.70
Fraction of $\dot{V}max_{O_2}$ variability explained by heredity	0.70

$\dot{V}max_{O_2}$, maximum O_2 consumption. Limiting factors: cardiac output, mitochondrial oxidizing capacity, tissue O_2 diffusion, and capillary density (see also Table 9). No ethnic differences.

level, $\dot{V}max_{O_2}$ is mostly limited by the O_2-transport system ($\dot{Q}$T times blood O_2 capacity). However, several other factors (e.g., peripheral circulation, O_2 diffusion at the muscle level, mitochondrial capacity) have also been considered among the possible factors that limit $\dot{V}max_{O_2}$, particularly during exercise with small muscle groups (122, 273, 427).

The factors limiting $\dot{V}max_{O_2}$ are described in detail next. Before discussing this controversial problem, we briefly outline the model according to which the data of the literature are interpreted.

The O_2 path from the external environment to the mitochondria can be viewed as a cascade of resistances in series, with each individual resistance (Ri) overcome by a specific O_2 pressure gradient (ΔPi). If this is true, and assuming that the system behaves linearly, the O_2 flow through each section equals the overall flow through the system, and the total resistance (Rtot) is the sum of the n resistances in series

$$\dot{V}_{O_2} = \frac{\sum_{i=1}^{n} \Delta Pi}{\sum_{i=1}^{n} Ri} = \frac{\Delta Ptot}{Rtot} \qquad (2)$$

where ΔPtot is the total O_2 pressure gradient from the environment to the mitochondria.

Equation 2 can be utilized to calculate the fraction of Rtot that can be attributed to each Ri, provided that the corresponding fraction of the O_2 pressure gradient can be estimated, together with ΔPtot and Rtot. As shown by Shephard (443), this can be done and the various terms appearing in Equation 2 or similar equations (e.g., the O_2-conductance equations) can be estimated according to data available in the literature; this procedure requires, however, several assumptions and complex calculations. A somewhat different approach is therefore developed here; i.e., the observed changes of $\dot{V}max_{O_2}$ resulting from (or accompanied by) measured changes of other physiological parameters that can be likened to Ri are entered into Equation 2. It is then possible to calculate the Ri/Rtot ratio. For a more detailed discussion of this approach, the reader is referred to di Prampero (137b).

Calculations of each ΔPi can be avoided by solving Equation 2 for conditions under which ΔPtot is constant. In this case, the changes in O_2 flow through the system, which follow a given change of resistance (ΔRtot), can be expressed in relative terms from Equation 2

$$\frac{\dot{V}_{O_2} + \Delta\dot{V}_{O_2}}{\dot{V}_{O_2}} = \frac{\Delta Ptot}{\Delta Rtot + Rtot} \cdot \frac{Rtot}{\Delta Ptot} = \frac{1}{1 + \left(\frac{\Delta R_1}{Rtot} + \frac{\Delta R_2}{Rtot} + \dots + \frac{\Delta R_n}{Rtot}\right)} \qquad (3)$$

where Rtot $= R_1 + R_2 + \dots + R_n$. For practical purposes when exercising at $\dot{V}max_{O_2}$, Equation 3 can be rearranged into the simpler form

$$\frac{\dot{V}max_{O_2} + \Delta\dot{V}max_{O_2}}{\dot{V}max_{O_2}} = \frac{1}{1 + \left(\frac{\Delta RQ}{Rtot} + \frac{\Delta Rm}{Rtot} + \frac{\Delta Rc}{Rtot}\right)} \qquad (4)$$

which can be written in the equivalent form

$$\frac{\dot{V}max_{O_2} + \Delta\dot{V}max_{O_2}}{\dot{V}max_{O_2}} = \frac{1}{1 + \left(\frac{RQ}{Rtot}\cdot\frac{\Delta RQ}{RQ} + \frac{Rm}{Rtot}\cdot\frac{\Delta Rm}{Rm} + \frac{Rc}{Rtot}\cdot\frac{\Delta Rc}{Rc}\right)} \qquad (4a)$$

where the following three individual resistances have been identified: *1*) RQ, inversely proportional to $\dot{Q}$T,max and to the average slope of the ODC; *2*) Rc, inversely proportional to peripheral diffusion and perfusion, which in turn depend on the O_2 diffusion coefficient from the capillary to the cells, on the surface and volume of the capillary bed, and on the average distance between capillary and cell; and *3*) Rm, inversely proportional to mitochondrial O_2 utilization capacity; Rm depends on the molecular conductance for O_2, the surface of the inner mitochondrial membrane, and on the total volume of mitochondria. The reader is referred to Taylor and Weibel (468) for a detailed discussion of the physiological and morphological parameters on which RQ, Rc, and Rm depend and to Shephard (443) for an analytical formulation of the corresponding pressure gradients.

By setting RQ/Rtot = FQ, Rm/Rtot = Fm, Rc/Rtot = Fc and rearranging

$$FQ\cdot\frac{\Delta RQ}{RQ} + Fm\cdot\frac{\Delta Rm}{Rm} + Fc\cdot\frac{\Delta Rc}{Rc} = \frac{1}{(\dot{V}max_{O_2}/\Delta\dot{V}max_{O_2} + 1)} - 1 \qquad (5)$$

Thus in Equation 5 the three terms FQ, Fc, and Fm indicate the fractional limitations of $\dot{V}max_{O_2}$ due to O_2 transport, peripheral perfusion and diffusion, and mitochondrial capacity, respectively; ΔRQ/RQ, ΔRc/Rc, and ΔRm/Rm are the relative changes of the appropriate resistances. The resistances will be assumed to be inversely proportional: *1*) RQ, to $\dot{Q}$T,max

$$RQ = \frac{kQ}{\dot{Q}T,max} \qquad (6)$$

2) Rc, to capillary cross-sectional area

$$Rc = \frac{kc}{\text{capillary cross section}} \qquad (7)$$

3) Rm, to mitochondrial succinate dehydrogenase (SDH) activity

$$\text{Rm} = \frac{k\text{m}}{\text{SDH}} \quad (8)$$

If only the relative changes of resistance are considered, as in Equation 5, the three constants kQ, kc, and km cancel out. However, they have to be introduced for dimensional uniformity and they can be assigned, conventionally, the value of 1.0.

It should have become apparent by now that pulmonary ventilation and lung diffusion have not been considered among the possible limiting factors, an assumption that seems well justified, at least for sea-level conditions (see PULMONARY VENTILATION, WORK OF BREATHING, AND ENERGY COST, p. 297, and LUNG DIFFUSING CAPACITY, p. 301).

We now solve Equation 5 for experimental conditions in which $\dot{V}\text{max}_{O_2}$ changes have been elicited with training, in which conditions it can be assumed that ΔPtot is substantially unchanged.

The percentage increases with training of *1)* $\dot{V}\text{max}_{O_2}$, *2)* $\dot{Q}$T,max (ΔRQ/RQ), *3)* mitochondrial enzyme activity (ΔRm/Rm), and *4)* capillary cross section per unit muscle surface (ΔRc/Rc) are reported in Table 8 from several studies. It can be calculated from this table that for two-leg (cycling) endurance training in humans, the subjects' mean increase in $\dot{V}\text{max}_{O_2}$ is 16.6%; the corresponding increase in enzymatic activity is 31.2% (24 subjects) (10, 220, 221). Thus $\Delta\dot{V}\text{max}_{O_2}/\dot{V}\text{max}_{O_2}$ = 0.166 and ΔRm/Rm = −0.312. If the increase in $\dot{V}\text{max}_{O_2}$ were only due to increased mitochondrial activity, ΔRQ/RQ = ΔRc/Rc would equal zero and substituting the above two experimental values into Equation 5, Fm could be calculated as 0.46. The latter value, however, is an obvious overestimate, because $\dot{Q}$T,max and capillary density are both increased with training [Table 8; (102, 255, 261)]. These two parameters were not measured in the above studies. Other data in Table 8 indicate, however, that $\dot{Q}$T and capillary density in two-leg endurance training increase on the average by 11.3% (12 subjects) (152, 429; see also ref. 104) and by 20% (5 subjects) (10), respectively. Thus ΔRQ/RQ = −0.113 and ΔRc/Rc = −0.20. Inserting also the above values into Equation 5

TABLE 8. *Percent Change of Level and/or Activity With Training in Humans*

Conditions	n	$\dot{V}\text{max}_{O_2}$	SDH	Cap	$\dot{Q}$T,max	Ref.
Endurance training	13	+19	+32			221
	6	+11.8	+22			220
	5	+16	+40	+20		10
	3	+35			+21	429
	9	+16			+8	152
One-leg endurance training						
Trained leg	10	+21.5	+33			431
	6	+11	+27			219
Untrained leg	10	+6	0			431
	6	+3.6	0			219
Interval training	6	+3.5	+27.5			220
One-leg sprint training						
Trained leg	10	+13	+19			431
Untrained leg	10	+3	0			431
Detraining	8	−3	−20			221

n, Number of subjects; $\dot{V}\text{max}_{O_2}$, maximum O_2 consumption; SDH, succinate dehydrogenase activity; Cap, muscle capillary density; $\dot{Q}$T,max, maximum cardiac output.

TABLE 9. *Limitation of $\dot{V}\text{max}_{O_2}$ During Maximum Exercise*

α	Two Legs FQ	Two Legs Fm	Two Legs Fc	One Leg FQ	One Leg Fm	One Leg Fc
0.1	0.85	0.14	0.01	0.56	0.40	0.04
0.5	0.82	0.12	0.06	0.53	0.31	0.16
1.0	0.80	0.10	0.10	0.50	0.25	0.25
2.0	0.76	0.08	0.16	0.47	0.18	0.35
10.0	0.70	0.03	0.27	0.43	0.05	0.52

$\dot{V}\text{max}_{O_2}$ limitation, in relative units (FQ + Fm + Fc = 1), during 1- and 2-leg exercise. Limitation due to cardiac output (FQ), mitochondrial oxidizing capacity and tissue O_2 diffusion (Fm), and capillary density (Fc). Two peripheral factors Fm and Fc are related by factor α, with Fc = αFm, and thus are assumed to be interdependent.

$$-0.113\text{FQ} - 0.312\text{Fm} - 0.20\text{Fc} = \frac{1}{0.166 + 1} - 1 \quad (9)$$

If the assumptions are made that no other factors except those taken into account intervene in limiting $\dot{V}\text{max}_{O_2}$, then

$$\text{FQ} + \text{Fm} + \text{Fc} = 1 \quad (10)$$

and that the two peripheral factors are interdependent

$$\text{Fc} = \alpha\text{Fm} \quad (11)$$

then FQ, Fm, and Fc can be calculated with the aid of Equation 9 for any given value of α (Table 9). It appears that, for a 100-fold variation of α (from 0.1 to 10), FQ changes only from 0.85 to 0.70. If, based on the data in Table 8 (10, 220, 221), the further assumption is now made that α = Fc/Fm = (ΔFc/Fc)/(ΔFm/Fm) = 0.20/0.312 = 0.64, then FQ = 0.81, Fm = 0.12, and Fc = 0.07. These values are consistent also with the upper limit of Fm that can be calculated from the data on interval training and detraining with the aid of Equation 5 [see Table 8; (220, 221)] and with the data of Gollnick et al. (193) who observed an average 13% increase of $\dot{V}\text{max}_{O_2}$ after 5 mo of endurance training in 6 humans while mitochondrial SDH activity increased on the average by 95%.

Note that the above calculated limitation of $\dot{V}\text{max}_{O_2}$ due to mitochondria (Fm = 0.12) was obtained from the changes of SDH concentration rather than from the increase of the overall mitochondrial capacity in vitro. The latter, both in humans (240) and in rats (371), increases by 50%–100%, i.e., to a larger extent than the former (~30%). On the basis of these data, therefore, the importance of mitochondria as a limiting factor would be smaller, and that of $\dot{Q}_T$ larger, than reported in Table 9.

All the available evidence suggests therefore that, during maximum whole-body exercise, $\dot{V}max_{O_2}$ is essentially limited by $\dot{Q}_T$, a conclusion that, although based on different grounds, is shared by many authors (e.g., ref. 443). This is true despite the fact that a 12% reduction in $\dot{Q}_{T,max}$ has no effect on $\dot{V}max_{O_2}$ (154) and a 22% $\dot{Q}_{T,max}$ reduction reduces $\dot{V}max_{O_2}$ by only 6% (160). These data were obtained by β-adrenergic blockade, a procedure that is unlikely to reduce blood flow to the working muscles. Ivy et al. (262), however, assign a major role to muscle respiratory capacity in determining maximum aerobic power. These authors base their conclusion on the results of a statistical analysis of 20 physically active subjects, which showed that 72% of the variance in $\dot{V}max_{O_2}$ could be explained by the combined effects of muscle respiratory capacity and percentage of slow-twitch fibers. However, because $\dot{Q}_T$ was not measured, this analysis does not exclude it as the possible limiting factor.

During one-leg exercise the $\dot{V}max_{O_2}$ limitation due to the periphery seems more important. Under these conditions, in fact, training increases $\dot{V}max_{O_2}$ by 15.8% and mitochondrial activity by 26.2% (26 subjects) (219, 429). Thus, on this basis alone, Fm (as from Eq. 5) is 0.52. However, also under these conditions the increase in $\dot{V}max_{O_2}$ is partly due to $\dot{Q}_{T,max}$ and muscle capillarization changes. The latter can be assumed to be identical with those observed in two-leg training: thus $\Delta Rc/Rc = -0.20$ (10). On the other hand, the increase in $\dot{Q}_{T,max}$ can be assumed to be identical with the increase in $\dot{V}max_{O_2}$ observed when exercising the nontrained leg (+4.3%), in which no enzymatic adaptation was observed (see Table 8): thus $\Delta RQ/RQ = -0.043$. Substituting these values into Equation 5, and on the basis of the same assumptions as above (see Eqs. 10 and 11), it can be calculated that, for a 100-fold change of α (from 0.1 to 10) FQ varies only from 0.56 to 0.43; the corresponding values of Fm and Fc are listed in Table 9. If, once again, $\alpha = (\Delta Fc/Fc)/(\Delta Fm/Fm) = 0.20/0.262 = 0.76$, than $FQ = 0.51$, $Fm = 0.28$, and $Fc = 0.21$. Thus for exercises involving small muscle groups the periphery becomes more important as a limiting factor.

In conclusion, even if the results of the above analysis should be taken with care because of the many assumptions and approximations involved in the calculations and discussed in detail elsewhere (137b), they do support the view that whole-body $\dot{V}max_{O_2}$ is mostly (70%–80%) limited by $\dot{Q}_T$, while for exercises with small muscle groups the role of $\dot{Q}_T$ becomes progressively less important, attaining ~50% during one-leg maximum exercise.

Comparative Aspects of Gas Exchange

A question that has often interested exercise physiologists is how and to what extent the working capability of humans compares with that of domestic and wild mammals. The most extensive studies of gas exchange at exercise have been carried out mainly on humans; the performance of other mammals, perhaps with the exception of the horse (514), only recently interested investigators. A thorough comparative analysis of the physiological characteristics relevant to exercise in the various species would include a qualitative and quantitative evaluation of the energy sources available, a study of the cardiorespiratory functional potential, and an examination of the specific mechanical, energetic, and thermodynamic aspects of muscle contraction. This chapter is limited to summarizing the results of the most recent studies of some comparative aspects of maximum aerobic performance. Other relevant aspects are covered by a recent series of papers (488) featuring, for a wide range of running mammals, the anatomic and functional design of the respiratory system from the lung to the mitochondria.

The measurement of gas exchange at exercise and more specifically the assessment of its maximum rate in animals has always been difficult. The difficulties derive from the wide range of body sizes (6 orders of magnitude), which per se imposes the use of different ergometric or metabolic techniques (e.g., treadmill running, swimming, or cold exposure) and varying gas analytical procedures for sampling ventilations that may range from a few milliliters to >1,000 liters per minute.

During the 1970s, $\dot{V}max_{O_2}$ data for several species have appeared in the literature; a summary is presented in Figure 7 as a function of body weight. It appears that in the body-weight range 10^2–10^5 g, $\dot{V}max_{O_2}$ per unit body weight does not differ substantially: in fact, hamsters, rats, and guinea pigs have the same $\dot{V}max_{O_2}$ as the horse, although their body weight ratio varies 2–4 orders of magnitude.

In the *upper panel* of Figure 7 the ratio between measured $\dot{V}max_{O_2}$ and resting $\dot{V}_{O_2}$ has been calculated or estimated. The contention that $\dot{V}max_{O_2}$ is a constant multiple of resting $\dot{V}_{O_2}$ regardless of the mass of the animal body does not always work as well as was the case with Taylor and Weibel's (468) data. The *upper panel* of Figure 7 also shows that the data concerning $\dot{V}max_{O_2}$ cannot be treated simply as an allometric function of the body mass of the type $y = a \cdot x^b$ (for a critical viewpoint on allometric scaling, see ref. 448).

For a correct interpretation of the data in Figure 7, however, three important points should be considered. *1*) In carrying out their measurements, all authors must have fulfilled the criteria for obtaining actual $\dot{V}max_{O_2}$ and true resting values, which might not al-

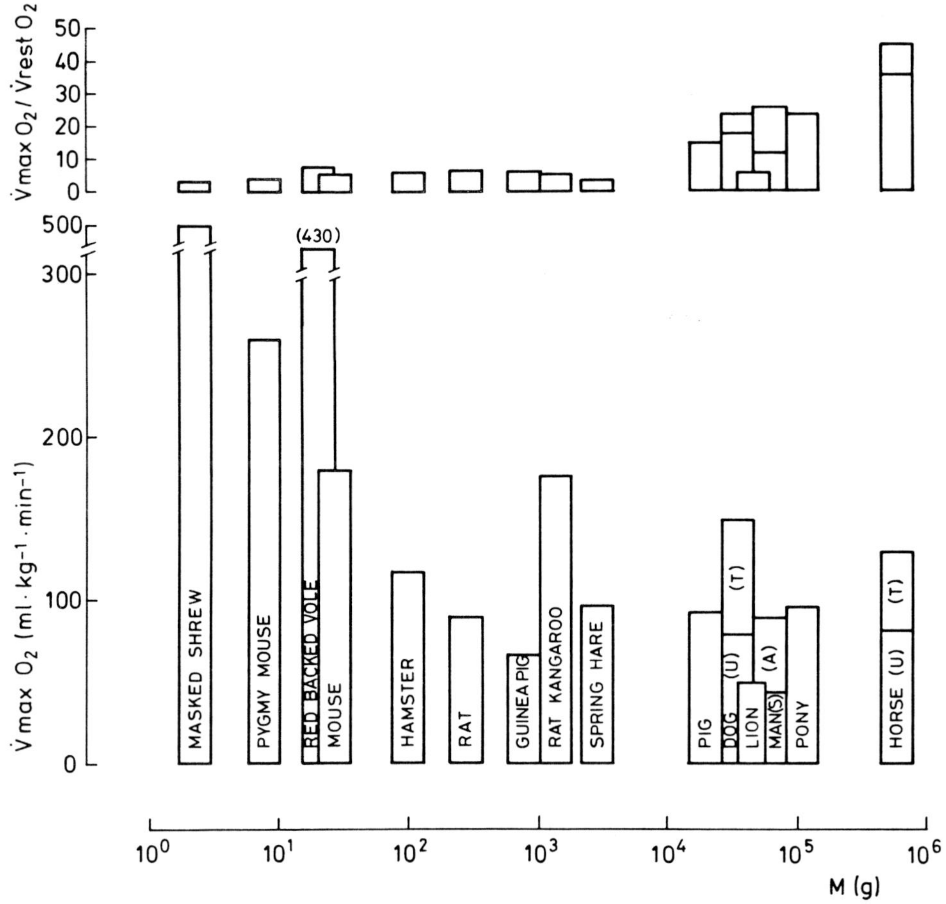

FIG. 7. Maximum O_2 consumption [$\dot{V}max_{O_2}$ ($ml \cdot kg^{-1} \cdot min^{-1}$), *lower panel*] and ratio of $\dot{V}max_{O_2}$ to resting O_2 consumption ($\dot{V}rest_{O_2}$, *upper panel*) as a function of body mass [M (g, log scale)] for various mammals. U, untrained; T, trained; S, sedentary; A, athlete. [Data for small rodents (312, 358, 370, 413, 414, 438); data for average-size mammals (springhares, pigs, baby lions: 100, 437, 438, 467); data for the dog (32, 90, 101, 145, 253, 325, 357, 368, 379, 410, 437, 438, 484, 510); data for trained horses (G. Cortili, unpublished observations); data for untrained horses (471); data for humans (303).]

ways be the case. *2*) All animals must have been appropriately trained to run on the treadmill. *3*) The results from habitual runners should not have been averaged with those from more-sedentary batches or species, because $\dot{V}max_{O_2}$ may change by a factor of 2 as a function of specific-exercise training and inborn athletic characteristics, therefore altering significantly the results.

The factors potentially limiting $\dot{V}max_{O_2}$ are *1*) respiratory (maximum exercise ventilation, DL, tissue diffusion, blood gas transport); *2*) cardiovascular ($\dot{Q}$T,max and maximum muscle blood flow); *3*) metabolic (muscle enzyme concentration, mitochondrial volume, different fiber typing); and *4*) thermal. All the above factors may actually be limiting in circumstances that are species specific. As common examples, consider *1*) pulmonary ventilation, which in the dog and in other panting animals may take a considerable fraction of the overall $\dot{V}_{O_2}$, thus limiting the maximum performance of the limb muscles and *2*) the "effective" shape of the ODC that in some species may considerably affect O_2 unloading. However, for the species (dog and horse) in which arteriovenous O_2 difference [17 ml O_2/100 ml at $\dot{V}max_{O_2}$ for the dog (90) and 13.6 ml O_2/100 ml at 0.8 $\dot{V}max_{O_2}$ for the horse (471)] and Hct (48% for the dog and 47% for the horse) have been measured, the coefficient of utilization of O_2 appears to be the same as for humans.

This suggests that, as is true for humans (see FACTORS LIMITING MAXIMUM O_2 CONSUMPTION, p. 309), in large mammals the primary factor limiting $\dot{V}max_{O_2}$ is $\dot{Q}$T.

UNSTEADY STATE

The transfer of gas between organism and environment results from the interplay of three major factors:

1) tissue metabolism, *2*) gas transport and delivery (uptake) to (from) the lungs, and *3*) gas exchange to the outside.

The primary event at the onset (offset) of muscular exercise is a sudden change in the rate of ATP splitting. The energy sources for ATP resynthesis [phosphocreatine (PC) breakdown, anaerobic glycolysis with net La production, and oxidative phosphorylation] are subsequently called on, according to their intrinsic dynamic characteristics, thus minimizing [ATP] changes. These primary events modulate gas exchange at the tissue level, which is therefore directly dictated by the energetic requirements of the working muscles. On the contrary, the gas-exchange transients at the lung level and between the lung and the atmosphere reflect the events taking place in the tissues in a distorted manner because of the intervening circulatory delays and because of the buffering effects of the gas stores (tissues, blood, and lung). In fact, the net amount of gas x leaving (or entering) a given system during a period of time t (Vx_t) is given by

$$Vx_t = Vx{,}in_t - Vx{,}out_t + \Delta Vx{,}st_t \qquad (12)$$

where in is gas inflow, out is gas outflow, and $\Delta Vx{,}st_t$ is the change, during the time t, of the gas stored in the system.

At steady state and for t sufficiently long, $\Delta Vx{,}st_t$ can be neglected. However, for short periods of time and particularly during the unsteady state, this simplification cannot be applied, as $\Delta Vx{,}st_t$ may be a significant fraction of the total amount of the transferred gas (46a, 189a). In addition, $\Delta Vx{,}st_t$ is often difficult to assess and, even when a satisfactory estimate of its amount can be made, its time course can only be approximated. Thus, although the dynamic behavior of gas exchange to the ambient can be described in terms of mathematical functions with a high level of accuracy (see refs. 324 and 500), it is often quite arduous to infer from such analyses the dynamic behavior of other body compartments (e.g., the muscle). With these limitations in mind, in this section we briefly review the dynamic behavior in the unsteady states of *1*) pulmonary gas exchange, *2*) gas transport to the lung, and *3*) gas exchange at the tissue level, aiming at a coherent picture rather than a comprehensive survey of the field. Throughout this section the symbols for $\dot{V}_{O_2}$, energy expenditure, and the like refer to net quantities, i.e., above preexercise resting values.

Pulmonary Gas-Exchange Transients

In this section an analysis is made of the time courses of ventilation, CO_2 elimination, and $\dot{V}_{O_2}$ at the onset and offset of exercise. The work intensities below the subject's $\dot{V}max_{O_2}$ (aerobic) are separated from those requiring energy expenditure greater than $\dot{V}max_{O_2}$.

AEROBIC EXERCISE. *Moderate.* The exercise intensities included in this category are those in which blood [La] does not increase above preexercise level, i.e., according to a widely used terminology, below anaerobic threshold (see ref. 495). Although the upper limit for moderate aerobic exercise is ~1.0–1.2 liters/min in active nonathletic subjects, it is substantially higher in fit subjects and also depends on the exercise mode (e.g., arms vs. legs, mass of muscles involved, body position).

Ventilation. Many authors (15, 18, 69, 118, 127, 324, 340, 486, 496a) have extensively investigated and reviewed the ventilatory responses at the onset and offset of cycloergometric and treadmill exercise. Most of the studies show an initial rapid increase, occurring substantially without delay, followed by a more gradual rise to the steady state, which is attained 3–4 min after the onset of exercise. At the offset of exercise the opposite situation is found: a sudden decrease, followed by a more gradual return to resting level. The magnitude of the initial rapid rise (or decrease) is ~50% of the overall ventilatory response for moderate work levels (<100 W) (18, 127, 324). According to Beaver and Wasserman (47), however, the initial rapid rise in $\dot{V}_E$ varies widely among subjects and is totally absent in some cases. If the initial rapid change is disregarded, as a first approximation, the ventilatory response at the onset and offset of a square-wave exercise can be described by monoexponential functions with $t_{1/2}$ = 35–45 s; faster responses are generally found in recovery (see ref. 324). Diamond et al. (136) report somewhat slower $\dot{V}_E$ responses at the onset of square-wave moderate exercise ($t_{1/2}$ = 35–63 s).

During sinusoidal or ramp increases of work load, a single exponential curve describes appropriately the response of $\dot{V}_E$, which in this case lacks the rapid initial component (78, 112, 136, 500, 501). In addition, the $\dot{V}_E$ responses observed by Casaburi et al. (78) during sinusoidal work changes were slower ($t_{1/2}$ = 35–83 s) than those observed by Diamond et al. (136) at the onset of square-wave exercise ($t_{1/2}$ = 35–63 s).

Wigertz (502) also investigated the ventilatory response at the onset of step, ramp, and sinusoidal exercise loads in a range from loadless pedaling to 210 W. In all cases the $\dot{V}_E$ response could be appropriately described by a monoexponential function with $t_{1/2}$ = 47 s, without time delays. In addition, an initial abrupt component could be demonstrated only if motionless resting served as base-line control. This observation is consistent with the data of Bennett et al. (49), who showed that the abrupt component of the $\dot{V}_E$ response is detectable only if the form of the exercise forcing function comprises high-frequency harmonics.

At the onset of moderate aerobic exercise the changes of tidal volume (V_T) follow rather closely those of $\dot{V}_E$ (128, 129, 324); the initial rapid component of $\dot{V}_E$ is almost entirely accounted for by a drop in functional residual capacity (FRC) (324). On the contrary, the secondary slow change in VT is substantially due to an increase in maximum inspiratory level, so that at steady state the increase in VT can be accounted for almost equally by inspiratory and expiratory reserve volume changes (16, 324).

Carbon dioxide output and O_2 uptake. The time courses of CO_2 output ($\dot{V}_{CO_2}$) and of $\dot{V}_{O_2}$ during the non–steady state of moderate exercise have been studied during square-wave, sinusoidal, or ramp-work changes (78, 85, 136, 139, 209, 211, 222, 224, 225, 255a, 291, 324, 494, 496a, 500; see refs. 137 and 495 for reviews). Despite some specific differences, the majority of the above studies show that, as a first approximation, both $\dot{V}_{CO_2}$ and $\dot{V}_{O_2}$ kinetics can be described by monoexponential functions, with $t_{1/2}$ = 35–50 s for $\dot{V}_{CO_2}$ and 20–30 s for $\dot{V}_{O_2}$, if the kinetics of the on- and off-responses during square-wave work-load changes are substantially equal.

As Linnarsson (324) pointed out, the analysis of the $\dot{V}_{O_2}$ and $\dot{V}_{CO_2}$ kinetics can be substantially refined by including time delays and/or second-order exponentials. With this approach for square-wave exercise, it has been possible to demonstrate the existence of an initial rapid component of the $\dot{V}_{O_2}$ and $\dot{V}_{CO_2}$ on-responses, accounting for ~30% of the overall steady-state change (324, 496a, 500). This rapid component, defined by Whipp et al. (500) as "cardiodynamic," is presumably related to the rapid changes in pulmonary blood flow. Its existence had been postulated by Krogh and Lindhard (299) and shown by Gilbert et al. (190).

Heavy aerobic exercise. The exercise intensities in this category comprise those in which muscle [La] and blood [La] increase during the initial exercise period (3–10 min) to a constant level higher than resting, eventually declining as the exercise proceeds (see ref. 257 for a review). Essentially then, for large-muscle groups, heavy aerobic exercise implies $\dot{V}max_{O_2} > \dot{V}_{O_2} > 1.2$ liters/min. A constant (higher-than-resting) La level is the result of La production accompanied by simultaneous removal (e.g., refs. 181, 228, 254, 257, 354). However, *1)* the removal of La from the body during exercise is mainly due to La oxidation in active tissues, essentially the heart and skeletal muscles (149a). Furthermore *2)* the amount of energy released in the body by complete glycogen oxidation is the same, regardless of the precise pathway (glycogen → pyruvate → CO_2 or glycogen → pyruvate → lactate → pyruvate → CO_2). As a consequence, an elevated constant blood La level, irrespective of its absolute value, although having profound influences on $\dot{V}$E, the size of CO_2 stores, and acid-base balance (257), does not indicate a steady whole-body anaerobiosis; it indicates only that a certain amount of energy has been set free from anaerobic sources at an earlier time. We therefore avoid the term *anaerobic threshold* because it may be taken to indicate the presence of an anaerobic contribution throughout the exercise rather than only during its initial phase (for a review see ref. 137).

Ventilation. The ventilatory adjustments to heavy aerobic exercise are similar to those described for moderate work. However, the relative amount of the initial rapid changes of $\dot{V}$E and VT were smaller during heavy than during moderate aerobic exercise (15%–20% vs. 50% of the overall response) (18, 130, 324, 502). In addition, a slow continuous increase in $\dot{V}$E is often observed during heavy but not during moderate aerobic exercise (324, 339, 486, 500), a finding that was confirmed also for ramp exercise (500). If the initial rapid component is disregarded, the $\dot{V}$E on- and off-responses at the onset and offset of heavy aerobic exercise can be described in terms of monoexponential functions, with $t_{1/2}$ = 45 s ($\dot{V}$E on-response) and 55 s ($\dot{V}$E off-response), independent of the absolute work load (69, 94, 502). In contrast, Linnarsson (324) reported that although the $t_{1/2}$ of the $\dot{V}$E on-response is independent of the work load, that of the off-response increases significantly at higher work loads.

Carbon dioxide output and O_2 uptake. The time courses of $\dot{V}_{CO_2}$ and $\dot{V}_{O_2}$ during the unsteady state of heavy aerobic exercise have been mostly studied during square-wave work-load changes. If the effects of La production (see *Control and Kinetics of Gas Exchange in Muscle*, p. 323) are neglected, for exercises involving large-muscle groups, the on-responses can be described by monoexponential functions, with $t_{1/2}$ = 30–40 s for $\dot{V}_{O_2}$ and somewhat longer for $\dot{V}_{CO_2}$ (85, 121, 139, 209, 232, 255a, 324, 334, 498, 500; see refs. 137 and 495 for reviews). A more detailed analysis of the $\dot{V}_{O_2}$ and $\dot{V}_{CO_2}$ on-responses (324) shows that *1)* an initial rapid "cardiodynamic" component can be identified, similar to that for moderate exercise, for both $\dot{V}_{O_2}$ and $\dot{V}_{CO_2}$ and *2)* a second-order slow component becomes apparent for $\dot{V}_{O_2}$ as the work load is increased toward its maximum level. However, because the $t_{1/2}$ of these slow components is very long (>20 min) (324), they can be well identified with linear drifts (210, 498, 500). During ramp-work changes, a cardiodynamic phase cannot be identified, and the $\dot{V}_{O_2}$ on-responses are well described by monoexponential functions with $t_{1/2}$ values of the same order of magnitude as previously described, whereas the $\dot{V}_{CO_2}$ on-responses seem to be more appropriately described by a second-order exponential function (500).

During the recovery after heavy aerobic exercise, $\dot{V}_{O_2}$ remains above preexercise levels for rather long periods of time (334). This increase in metabolism is directly related to the duration and intensity of exercise (289) and is longer in older and untrained subjects (8). It may be due to the increase of muscle temperature after exercise (70) and/or to the slow decline of intracellular muscle [H^+] after heavy exercise (137a). In all cases, however, during the first minutes of recovery the analysis of the $\dot{V}_{O_2}$ off-response allows identification of a fast component with a $t_{1/2}$ = 25–30 s (50, 133, 222, 224, 225, 324, 334).

Also the $\dot{V}_{CO_2}$ off-responses after heavy aerobic exercise are characterized by double exponentials, with $t_{1/2} \sim 40$ s for the fast component and $t_{1/2} > 8$ min for the slow component (324).

A detailed analysis of the effects of La production during the initial exercise period on the $\dot{V}_{O_2}$ on-response at the onset of square-wave exercise loads has been made by Cerretelli and co-workers (89, 93, 373). These authors introduced the term *early lactate* (eLa) to define the amount of La accumulated in blood before the attainment of the steady-state $\dot{V}_{O_2}$ ($\dot{V}s_{O_2}$) over and above that measured for the same exercise duration at a later stage, i.e., when $\dot{V}s_{O_2}$ is achieved. They have shown that in arm and leg cycloergometric exercise up to 1.5 and 3.0 liters/min, in supine and sitting position, in trained and untrained subjects, respectively, the $\dot{V}_{O_2}$ on-response is slower the larger the amount of eLa. In particular, during arm cranking at 125 W, 75 W, and 50 W, the relationship between $t_{1/2}$ (s) and eLa (mM) may be described by (89)

$$\begin{aligned} t_{1/2} &= 18.0 + 6.7 \text{ eLa} \quad (r = 0.91; n = 16; 125 \text{ W}) \\ t_{1/2} &= 21.5 + 9.1 \text{ eLa} \quad (r = 0.98; n = 6; \ 75 \text{ W}) \\ t_{1/2} &= 29.2 + 6.1 \text{ eLa} \quad (r = 0.88; n = 19; \ 50 \text{ W}) \end{aligned} \tag{13}$$

where n is the number of subjects.

On the contrary, the $\dot{V}_{O_2}$ off-response is unaffected by eLa; its $t_{1/2} = 23$–30 s for all investigated conditions. In addition, training reduces both $t_{1/2}$ and eLa (89). Finally, the O_2 deficit is significantly larger than the O_2 debt only at the work loads at which eLa > 0 (93).

Thus an increase in La production during the initial exercise period is invariably associated with a slowing of the $\dot{V}_{O_2}$ on-response.

SUPRAMAXIMUM EXERCISE. *Ventilation.* To our knowledge, only a few studies of the time course of pulmonary ventilation have been made in this work-load range. In a study of square-wave cycloergometric exercise (400 W, 2 min), Whipp et al. (500) showed that after an initial sudden jump, accounting for ~20% of the overall response, $\dot{V}E$ increased throughout the exercise period, as an approximately linear function of time, whereas in the recovery after exercise the time course of $\dot{V}E$ was closely monoexponential with $t_{1/2} \sim 60$ s. Di Prampero et al. (142) observed that after short bouts of very strenuous exercise leading to exhaustion in 15–50 s (treadmill running at 18 km/h on a +10%, +15%, and +20% grade), $\dot{V}E$ remains approximately at the level attained at the very end of exercise up to 40 s in the recovery. The subsequent decline could be approximated by an exponential with $t_{1/2} = 90$–120 s.

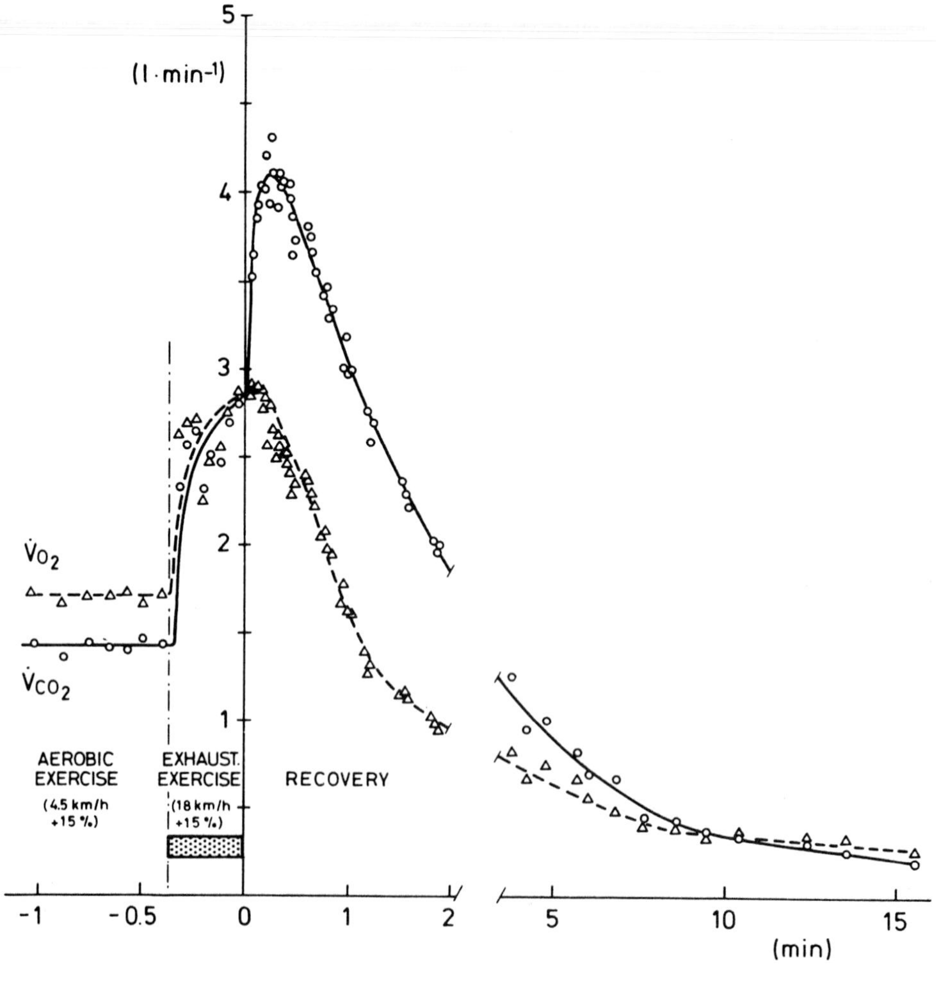

FIG. 8. Breath-by-breath O_2 uptake ($\dot{V}_{O_2}$, △) and CO_2 output ($\dot{V}_{CO_2}$, ○) as a function of time during very strenuous exercise (treadmill running at 18 km/h, on a +15% incline, exhaustion time = 22 s) and in recovery period. Exhausting exercise was preceded by ~10-min walk at 4.5 km/h on a +15% incline. (Note 3 different time scales.)

Oxygen uptake and CO_2 output. In the lower range of this exercise domain, the $\dot{V}_{O_2}$ on-responses are characterized by long $t_{1/2}$ (50–60 s) (110) and/or by double exponential functions (500). The $\dot{V}_{O_2}$ off-response can be described as the sum of a fast component ($t_{1/2}$ = 25–30 s) and a slow component ($t_{1/2}$ = 10–15 min), essentially associated with La removal (142, 278, 288, 334, 406).

For higher work intensities (>2.5 × $\dot{V}max_{O_2}$), $\dot{V}_{O_2}$ increases with the "usual" time course ($t_{1/2}$ = 25 s) tending asymptotically to the actual energy requirement of the exercise [(110, 335, 499); see Fig. 11]. Obviously this rise in $\dot{V}_{O_2}$ is interrupted abruptly when the subject's $\dot{V}max_{O_2}$ is reached. Thus $\dot{V}max_{O_2}$ is attained in a time that is shorter the heavier the exercise (27, 85, 110). After short bursts of very heavy exercise (treadmill running, 18 km/h; +10%, +15%, +20% incline) leading to exhaustion in 15–50 s, $\dot{V}_{O_2}$ remains at the maximum level for 10–35 s, depending on the exercise duration (see Figs. 8 and 11). Indeed, during recovery $\dot{V}_{O_2}$ may even increase if the subject's $\dot{V}max_{O_2}$ is not attained by the end of the exercise (142). After this initial period of recovery, $\dot{V}_{O_2}$ decreases with the same kinetics as indicated above, with the fast component $t_{1/2}$ ~ 25 s.

For work intensities well above $\dot{V}max_{O_2}$, $\dot{V}_{CO_2}$ (which during the exercise period is approximately equal to $\dot{V}_{O_2}$) increases in the first 20–40 s of recovery to a peak value that is 0.8–1.5 liters/min greater than the corresponding $\dot{V}_{O_2}$ [gas-exchange ratio (R) = 1.3–1.6], depending on the intensity and duration of the preceding exhaustive exercise. After this peak, $\dot{V}_{CO_2}$ decreases exponentially with $t_{1/2}$ ~ 100 s (Fig. 8). Because in these conditions the muscles utilize essentially carbohydrates, the difference between CO_2 volume (V_{CO_2}) and O_2 volume (V_{O_2}) (excess V_{CO_2}) is a measure of the amount of CO_2 eliminated to compensate for the acid-base balance. Indeed the excess V_{CO_2} increases with the amount of La accumulated in the body fluids at the end of the exercise; the relationship between excess V_{CO_2} and blood [La] is approximately equal in all subjects (Fig. 9). On the contrary, the relationship between excess V_{CO_2} and PA_{CO_2} during the initial (~10-min) recovery period is different in different individuals (Fig. 10), which may be due to different individual respiratory sensitivity to CO_2 and H^+.

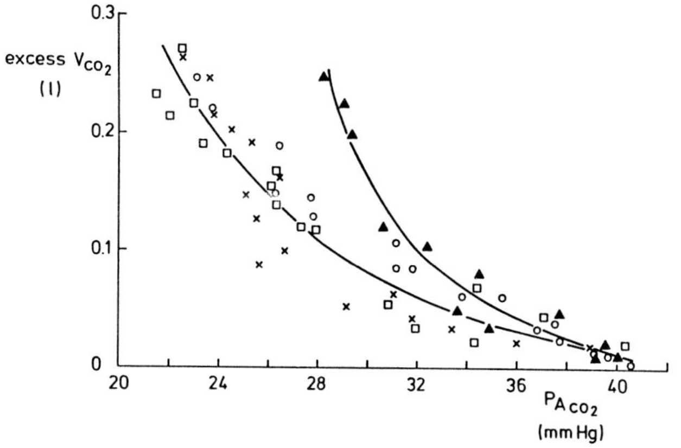

FIG. 10. Excess V_{CO_2} as a function of corresponding PA_{CO_2} in 4 subjects (□, ×, ○, ▲). Excess V_{CO_2} is here the amount of CO_2 eliminated in excess of O_2 uptake, up to the moment at which PA_{CO_2} was as indicated. Thus, as recovery proceeds, the subjects' respiratory conditions move toward the *left*, along the *curve*; points to the *extreme left* correspond to ~10 min in all subjects. Three subjects are characterized by the same function; 4th subject (▲) follows a markedly different pattern. For a given excess V_{CO_2}, drop in $[HCO_3^-]$ can be considered equal in all subjects (see Fig. 9). Therefore, this last subject (▲), having a higher PA_{CO_2} for a given excess V_{CO_2}, is presumably characterized by a lesser sensitivity to CO_2.

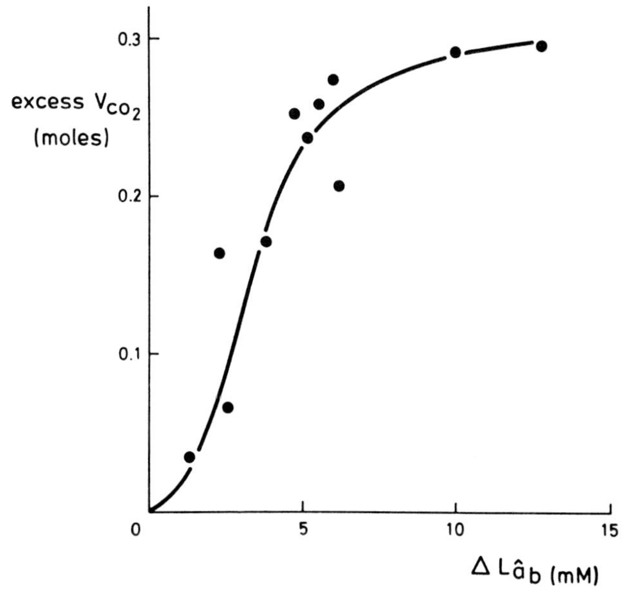

FIG. 9. Output of CO_2 in excess of O_2 uptake (excess V_{CO_2}) as a function of peak blood lactate concentration above resting ($\Delta L_{\hat{a}b}$) in recovery after very strenuous exercise (treadmill running at 18 km/h; +10%, +15%, and +20% incline; exhaustion time 14–50 s) in 4 subjects. Excess V_{CO_2} was calculated as $\int_0^{t_1} \dot{V}_{CO_2} \cdot dt - \int_0^{t_1} \dot{V}_{O_2} \cdot dt$, where t_1 is the time at which $\dot{V}_{CO_2} = \dot{V}_{O_2}$, usually ~10 min (see Fig. 8).

OXYGEN DEBT-DEFICIT. The preceding discussion shows that the $\dot{V}_{O_2}$ responses lag behind the mechanical events of the contraction, both at the onset and offset of exercise. Thus $\dot{V}_{O_2}$ through the mouth is insufficient at the onset and in excess at the offset, as compared with the muscles' requirements, and consequently an O_2 debt-deficit is incurred during the first minutes of exercise and paid in the immediate recovery period.

This section is a discussion of the O_2 debt-deficit concept. It is shown that only the fraction of the O_2 deficit that is causally related to the splitting or resynthesis of high-energy phosphates (mainly PC) is metabolism dependent and bears a fixed relation to the $\dot{V}s_{O_2}$. The remaining fractions (O_2-stores changes and eLa production) depend, on the contrary, on the interplay of several factors, such as circulatory adaptations, body posture, and size and fiber composition of the exercising muscles. The following treatment is based on the simpler case of a monoexponential $\dot{V}_{O_2}$ response, a condition that is not always met. We think, however, that this approximation, although simplifying the analysis, does not affect its significance.

In the case of square-wave aerobic exercise, the O_2 requirement can be assumed to be constant from $t = 0$ and equal to the $\dot{V}s_{O_2}$ above resting. Assuming monoexponential $\dot{V}_{O_2}$ responses, at the onset of exercise

$$\dot{V}s_{O_2} - \dot{V}t_{O_2} = \dot{V}s_{O_2} \cdot e^{-kt} \quad (14)$$

while at the offset of exercise

$$\dot{V}t_{O_2} = \dot{V}s_{O_2} \cdot e^{-kt} \quad (15)$$

where $\dot{V}t_{O_2}$ is $\dot{V}_{O_2}$ at time t, $k = 1/\tau$ is the velocity constant of the process, and $\ln 2/k = \ln 2\tau = t_{1/2}$.

The O_2 debt-deficit incurred at the onset or paid at the offset of exercise is given by the time integral of Equations 14 and 15

$$O_2 \text{ debt-deficit} = \int_0^t \dot{V}s_{O_2} \cdot e^{-kt} \cdot dt = \dot{V}s_{O_2} \cdot k^{-1} \quad (16)$$

The term *O_2 deficit* is generally confined to the onset and *O_2 debt* to the offset of exercise. Thus if the on- and off-responses have the same velocity constant (k), as is often but not always true (see AEROBIC EXERCISE, p. 314), O_2 deficit and debt are equal.

The O_2 debt-deficit can also be studied during ramp or sinusoidal exercise, when its physiological significance is obviously unchanged. Indeed, during ramp exercise followed by square-wave transition to rest, the O_2 deficit and debt [as calculated from the data in Fig. 10 of Whipp and Mahler (495) and in Fig. 5 of Whipp et al. (500)] appear to be equal.

If it is assumed that the energy requirement of the working muscles is proportional to $\dot{V}s_{O_2}$, it follows that the O_2 deficit is a measure of the energy drawn from sources other than those due to O_2 absorption through the upper airways, i.e., net PC breakdown, La production, and O_2-stores depletion. In fact *1)* muscle PC concentration at steady state is lowered in direct proportion to $\dot{V}s_{O_2}$ both in human and isolated muscles (256, 275, 277, 292, 381); *2)* a certain amount of La (eLa) is produced before the attainment of $\dot{V}s_{O_2}$ in many forms of aerobic exercise (see AEROBIC EXERCISE, p. 314, and ref. 257); and *3)* at the onset of exercise, O_2 is drawn from body stores, i.e., O_2 content of the lung, physically dissolved O_2, and O_2 bound to Mb and Hb. Thus the O_2 deficit is the sum of at least three terms

$$O_2 \text{ deficit} = V\text{PC}_{O_2} + VeLa_{O_2} + \Delta Vst_{O_2} \quad (17)$$

where $V\text{PC}_{O_2}$ is the O_2 equivalent of PC breakdown (alactic O_2 deficit-debt), $VeLa_{O_2}$ is the amount of La produced before the attainment of $\dot{V}s_{O_2}$ expressed in O_2 equivalents (89, 93, 373), and ΔVst_{O_2} is the amount of O_2 drawn from body stores. In turn, assuming that arterial O_2 content and physically dissolved O_2 do not change substantially in the rest-to-work transition

$$\Delta Vst_{O_2} = \text{FRC,r} \cdot F_{A'},r_{O_2} + \text{Vbv,r} \cdot C\bar{v},r_{O_2} + \text{MbO}_2\text{,r} - (\text{FRC,s} \cdot F_{A'},s_{O_2} + \text{Vbv,s} \cdot C\bar{v},s_{O_2} + \text{MbO}_2\text{,s}) \quad (18)$$

where FRC is the functional residual capacity of the lung, $F_{A'O_2}$ is the end-tidal alveolar O_2 fraction, Vbv is the venous blood volume, $C\bar{v}_{O_2}$ is the mixed venous blood O_2 content, MbO_2 is the O_2 bound to Mb, r is rest, and s is steady state.

At the offset of exercise, PC is resynthesized and ΔVst_{O_2} rebuilt at the expense of the extra O_2 consumed above resting without, however, any significant La production. The O_2 debt is therefore the sum of only two of the three terms of Equation 17

$$O_2 \text{ debt} = V\text{PC}_{O_2} + \Delta Vst_{O_2} \quad (19)$$

Because the time course of PC breakdown at the muscle level (i.e., the time course of $V\text{PC}_{O_2}$) is presumably dictated by the intrinsic characteristics of the muscle (see *Control and Kinetics of Gas Exchange in Muscle*, p. 323), any change of O_2 debt-deficit due to changes in ΔVst_{O_2} and/or $VeLa_{O_2}$ (Eq. 17) for a given $\dot{V}s_{O_2}$ is likely to affect k (Eq. 16), i.e., the time course of the $\dot{V}_{O_2}$ on- and off-responses at the mouth (139, 140, 331).

Oxygen debt-deficit, O_2 stores, and early lactate production. In a study on pulmonary gas exchange at the onset and offset of cycloergometric exercises (80–240 W), Linnarsson (324) showed that the $t_{1/2}$ values of the $\dot{V}_{O_2}$ on- and off-responses at the pulmonary capillary level, after correction for the lung O_2-store changes, were 3–7 s faster than at the mouth; the larger discrepancies were observed for the lower work loads. Di Prampero et al. (139) observed that the $t_{1/2}$ of the $\dot{V}_{O_2}$ on-response became faster (17–20 s) when a given step exercise ($\dot{V}s_{O_2} = 36$ ml·kg^{-1}·min^{-1}) was preceded by a base line of mild exercise ($\dot{V}s_{O_2} = 18$ ml·kg^{-1}·min^{-1}) rather than starting from rest, in which case $t_{1/2} \sim 30$ s. These results (see also ref. 121) were attributed to a substantial decrease of body O_2 stores, due to a reduction of $C\bar{v}_{O_2}$ induced by the priming exercise. Thus the term ΔVst_{O_2} in the transition from light to heavy work is proportionally smaller, leading to a faster $\dot{V}_{O_2}$ on-response (Eqs. 16 and 17). The results of di Prampero et al. (139) and of Davies et al. (121) were not confirmed by Diamond et al. (136) during square-wave work changes or by Casaburi et al. (78), who observed during sinusoidal work that the $\dot{V}_{O_2}$ on-response was essentially the same as in the transition from rest to exercise ($t_{1/2} \sim 30$ s). However, in the above experiments the priming exercise in one case and the trough of the wave in the other were presumably too mild (25 W, i.e., 300 ml/min) to yield a substantial reduction of body O_2 stores.

More recently, Hughson and Morrissey (255a) observed that during cycloergometric exercise the $\dot{V}_{O_2}$

TABLE 10. *Oxygen-Stores Contribution to O_2 Deficit at Onset of Exercise*

Work Load	$\dot{V}s_{O_2}$, liters/min	$t_{1/2}$ $\dot{V}_{O_2}$ on, s	O_2 deficit, liters	$C\bar{v}_{O_2}$, liters/liter	FRC, liters	$F_{A'O_2}$	ΔVst_{O_2}, liters	O_2 deficit − ΔVst_{O_2}, liters	$t_{1/2}$ $\dot{V}_{O_2}$ on *, s
Rest	0			0.150	3.25	0.151			
80 W	0.90	26.8	0.58	0.110	2.90	0.146	0.21	0.37	17.0
160 W	1.80	28.1	1.22	0.085	2.75	0.141	0.34	0.87	20.2
240 W	2.70	31.6	2.05	0.070	2.40	0.141	0.45	1.60	24.7

$\dot{V}s_{O_2}$, steady-state O_2 consumption above resting; $t_{1/2}$ $\dot{V}_{O_2}$ on, $t_{1/2}$ of $\dot{V}_{O_2}$ on-response; $C\bar{v}_{O_2}$, mixed venous blood O_2 content; FRC, functional residual capacity of the lung; $F_{A'O_2}$, end-tidal O_2 fraction; ΔVst_{O_2}, amount of O_2 drawn from O_2-stores changes in transition from rest to steady-state exercise (calculated according to Eq. 18 for an assumed venous blood volume of 3.7 liters); $t_{1/2}$ $\dot{V}_{O_2}$ on *, $t_{1/2}$ of $\dot{V}_{O_2}$ on-response at muscle level, assumed to be monoexponential (calculated according to Eq. 16: $t_{1/2}$ $\dot{V}_{O_2}$ on * = [(O_2 def − ΔVst_{O_2})/$\dot{V}s_{O_2}$] ln 2). [Data from Linnarsson (324), except for $C\bar{v}_{O_2}$ data, which are estimated from current literature.]

on-kinetics becomes slower in the transition from prior exercise ($t_{1/2}$ = 42–55 s) than from rest ($t_{1/2}$ = 21–27 s). The conflicting results of Hughson and Morrissey and of di Prampero et al. (139) are essentially due to the different exercise modes: step (139) versus cycloergometer (255a). Indeed, a series of experiments (P. Cerretelli and P. E. di Prampero, unpublished observations) have shown that, when starting from rest, the $\dot{V}_{O_2}$ kinetics is essentially the same for cycling and stepping exercises ($t_{1/2}$ = 21–25 s). However, when starting from work loads of increasing intensity, a divergent trend becomes apparent. In cycling, the $\dot{V}_{O_2}$ kinetics becomes monotonically slower, attaining a $t_{1/2}$ of ~60 s when starting from a work load of ~50% $\dot{V}max_{O_2}$. In stepping, for moderate work intensities, the $\dot{V}_{O_2}$ kinetics becomes faster, attaining a minimum $t_{1/2}$ of ~15.0 s when starting from ~20% $\dot{V}max_{O_2}$. For higher work intensities the $\dot{V}_{O_2}$ kinetics again becomes slower, attaining the $t_{1/2}$ of ~25 s for work loads of ~50% $\dot{V}max_{O_2}$.

These data can be explained on the basis of the different contributions of the two terms ΔVst_{O_2} and $VeLa_{O_2}$ to the O_2 deficit (see Eq. 17). In stepping, the decrease of ΔVst_{O_2} relative to the amplitude of the change of steady-state $\dot{V}_{O_2}$ ($\Delta\dot{V}s_{O_2}$) is not, or is only partially, compensated for by the increase of $VeLa_{O_2}$ for low priming exercises (<30% $\dot{V}max_{O_2}$); hence the O_2 deficit is smaller (relative to $\Delta\dot{V}s_{O_2}$) and the $\dot{V}_{O_2}$ kinetics faster than observed when starting from rest. For heavier priming exercise (~50% $\dot{V}max_{O_2}$) the increase of $VeLa_{O_2}$ is just enough to compensate for the decrease of ΔVst_{O_2}; hence the O_2 deficit (relative to $\Delta\dot{V}s_{O_2}$) and the $\dot{V}_{O_2}$ kinetics equal the values observed when starting from rest. In cycling, on the contrary, $VeLa_{O_2}$ increases substantially even for a low priming $\dot{V}_{O_2}$ (~10% $\dot{V}max_{O_2}$). Thus throughout all the starting intensity range, the decrease of the O_2 deficit (relative to $\Delta\dot{V}s_{O_2}$), due to the decreased contribution of the O_2-stores depletion, is more than compensated for by the increase of the eLa contribution; hence the $t_{1/2}$ of the $\dot{V}_{O_2}$ on-response increases.

The above data and analysis show that ΔVst_{O_2} can be a substantial fraction of the O_2 deficit and that consequently it does affect the $\dot{V}_{O_2}$ kinetics as measured at the mouth. This can also be shown as follows: Assume that *1)* the amount of venous blood for an average 70-kg human is 3.7 liters, i.e., 0.72 of the overall blood volume, both at rest and exercise; *2)* $C\bar{v},r_{O_2}$ = 0.150 liter O_2/liter; *3)* FRC,r = 3.25 liters; and *4)* $F_{A'},r_{O_2}$ = 0.15. Three increasing cycloergometric exercises requiring 0.9, 1.8, and 2.7 liters/min $\dot{V}s_{O_2}$ above resting are now considered. The corresponding values of $C\bar{v},s_{O_2}$; FRC,s; $F_{A'},s_{O_2}$; average $t_{1/2}$ of the $\dot{V}_{O_2}$ on-responses; and the O_2 deficits are listed in Table 10. The amount of O_2 drawn from the O_2 stores of the body in the transition from rest to exercise (ΔVst_{O_2}) can now be calculated with Equation 18 on the assumption that MbO_2,r = MbO_2,s. A fraction of the O_2 deficit ranging from 0.22 to 0.37 can be accounted for by ΔVst_{O_2}. As a consequence, and if a monoexponential function is assumed, the $t_{1/2}$ of the $\dot{V}_{O_2}$ on-response at the muscle level must be 7–10 s shorter than observed at the mouth (Table 10). Note also that the corrections applied in Table 10 are minimum estimates, as the Mb contribution to the O_2 deficit (Eq. 18) has been neglected. According to Honig and Gayeski (251), on transition from rest to steady-state exercise requiring 90% $\dot{V}max_{O_2}$ in the gracilis muscle of the dog, Mb desaturation releases ~5.8 ml O_2/kg muscle. On this basis, and assuming 20 kg of active muscles in humans at 90% $\dot{V}max_{O_2}$, Mb desaturation would release ~120 ml O_2. The corresponding $t_{1/2}$ at the muscle level for a work load of 240 W would then be ~2 s shorter than that reported in Table 10.

It can be concluded that *1)* the change of O_2 stores does indeed affect the $\dot{V}_{O_2}$ on-response significantly and *2)* as the events described during the on-response are reversed during the off-response, O_2 stores changes affect the O_2 debt to the same extent as the O_2 deficit (Fig. 11).

Net alactic O_2 debt-deficit. The O_2 deficit, O_2 debt, and $t_{1/2}$ of the $\dot{V}_{O_2}$ on- and off-responses are summarized in Table 11; all data here were gathered under different experimental conditions but have a common characteristic; i.e., eLa = 0. The average $t_{1/2}$ of the on- and off-responses after correction for O_2-stores changes is 15.5 ± 3.1 (SD) s. This represents the time course of $\dot{V}_{O_2}$ at the muscle level on the assumption that it is exponential. This value should be taken carefully, because it depends on the calculated changes of body

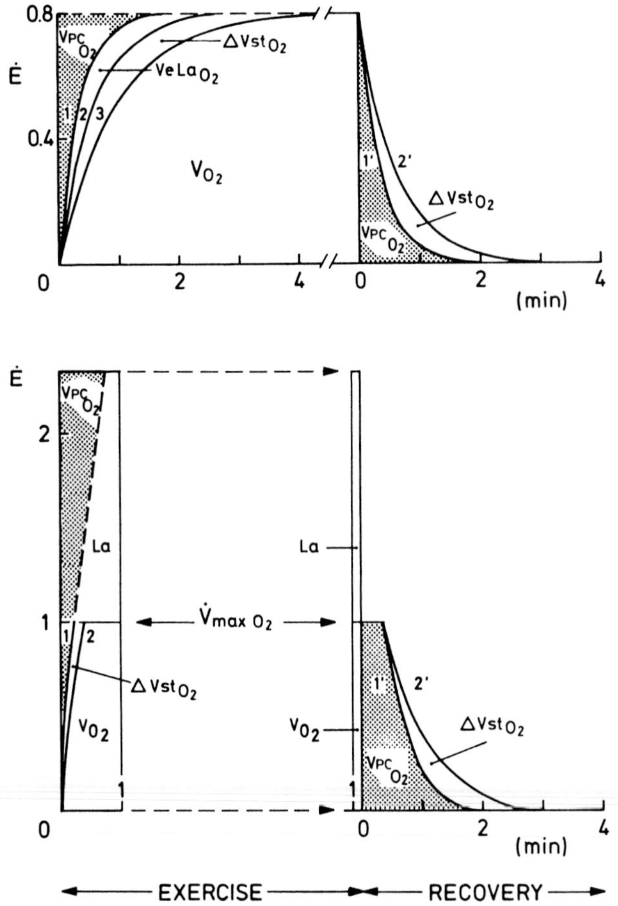

FIG. 11. Time course of energetic processes at onset of exercise in humans. Ordinate in arbitrary units: 1 = $\dot{V}max_{O_2}$. *Top*: energy requirement of exercise ($\dot{E}$) is 0.8 $\dot{V}max_{O_2}$. *Curve 1*, time course of energy yield at muscle level, resulting from sum of $\dot{V}_{O_2}$ through the mouth (*curve 3*, $t_{½}$ = 40 s), early lactate production, and O_2-stores depletion. Amount of energy contributed by latter 2 factors is indicated by areas labeled $VeLa_{O_2}$ and ΔVst_{O_2}, respectively. Area labeled V_{O_2}, amount of O_2 taken in through the mouth during exercise. (For mild aerobic exercise eLa = 0, so that *curve 3* overlaps *curve 2*.) Difference between energy requirement of exercise (constant from time 0) and *curve 1* must be supplied by net PC breakdown. Alactic O_2 debt (VPC_{O_2}), amount of phosphocreatine (PC) split in O_2 equivalents. *Curve 1*, time course of VPC_{O_2} contraction; *curve 1'*, time course of VPC_{O_2} payment; $t_{½}$ of *curves 1* and *1'* = 15 s. No La production occurs in recovery; thus *curves 2'* and *3'* coincide ($t_{½}$ of *curves 2* and *2'* = 25 s). *Bottom*: energy requirement of exercise is 2.33 $\dot{V}max_{O_2}$; duration of exercise to exhaustion is 1.15 min. *Curve 1*, time course of energy yield at muscle level, resulting from sum of $\dot{V}_{O_2}$ through the mouth (*curve 2*) and O_2-stores depletion. Lactate production (-----) begins when $\dot{V}_{O_2}$ at muscle level has reached its maximum value (*areas La*, amount of energy supplied by lactic sources). (Time course of La production, as well as time at which glycolysis begins, is hypothetical.) After exercise, VPC_{O_2} is paid by the oxidative processes that remain at maximum level for ~25 s; $t_{½}$ of *curves 1* and *1'* = 15 s (asymptote of *curve 1* = energy requirement); $t_{½}$ of *curve 2* = 30 s (asymptote = energy requirement); $t_{½}$ of *curve 2'* = 25 s. [Adapted from di Prampero (137).]

O_2 stores (Table 11). The above $t_{½}$ (for eLa and ΔVst_{O_2} = 0) is of the same order of magnitude as the values observed in isolated dog muscle in situ (381, 384), a condition characterized by negligible eLa and O_2-stores changes.

In the case of eLa and ΔVst_{O_2} = 0, because the rates of ATP splitting and resynthesis are equal (no substantial [ATP] changes occur in the transition from rest to steady state) and constant from work onset, it can reasonably be assumed that the average $t_{½}$ of the $\dot{V}_{O_2}$ on-response at the muscle level also equals that of net PC splitting. The latter is, in fact, the only energy source available to make up for the difference between ATP breakdown and its oxidative resynthesis. If this is true, the time integral of the $\dot{V}_{O_2}$ on-response at the muscle level (net alactic debt, VPC_{O_2})

$$VPC_{O_2} = \dot{V}s_{O_2}/k_{al} \qquad (20)$$

is a measure of the amount of PC broken down at the onset of exercise and expressed in O_2 equivalent units and k_{al} = ln 2/15.5 = 0.045 s^{-1} is the corresponding velocity constant. In the recovery after exercise the events are symmetrically reversed, possibly with a somewhat slower time course (Fig. 11).

Consistently with this line of reasoning, Piiper and co-workers (381, 384) have shown that VPC_{O_2} is quantitatively related to the amount of PC split (resynthesized) at the onset (offset) of exercise, with $\Delta PC/VPC_{O_2}$ = 6.5 and 5.4 (mol/mol), respectively. Experiments with the needle biopsy technique have shown that also in humans, PC is rapidly resynthesized during the first 2 min of recovery (215, 216, 256, 275, 292), concomitant with the payment of the fast component of the O_2 debt.

The estimate of VPC_{O_2} is more complicated for exercises implying eLa > 0. Nevertheless, we attempt to show that also under these conditions the experimental data are consistent with k_{al} = 0.045 s^{-1}, as calculated from Table 11. From Equations 20 and 22 the O_2 deficit is given by $\dot{V}s_{O_2}/k$ and VPC_{O_2} is given by $\dot{V}s_{O_2}/k_{al}$. Substituting in Equation 17 and rearranging

$$VeLa_{O_2} = -\Delta Vst_{O_2} + (k^{-1} - k_{al}^{-1})\dot{V}s_{O_2} \qquad (21)$$

Cerretelli et al. (93) observed that, in four moderately active subjects exercising on the bicycle ergometer, the relationship between eLa (mM) and $\dot{V}s_{O_2}$ (ml/s), resting included, could be described by

$$\begin{aligned} eLa &= -1.1 + 0.17\ \dot{V}s_{O_2} \qquad r = 0.74 \\ eLa &= -2.8 + 0.17\ \dot{V}s_{O_2} \qquad r = 0.94 \qquad (22) \\ eLa &= -2.4 + 0.14\ \dot{V}s_{O_2} \qquad r = 0.94 \end{aligned}$$

for arms (supine and sitting), legs supine, and legs sitting, respectively. If it is assumed that, in the workload range for eLa > 0, ΔVst_{O_2} is constant and that an increase of peak blood [La] of 1 mM is equivalent to a V_{O_2} of ~3 ml/kg of body weight (see ref. 137), it follows from Equations 21 and 22 that $k^{-1} - k_{al}^{-1}$ = 0.17 × 3 × 84.5 = 43 s for arms, 43 s for legs supine, and 35 s for legs sitting (avg wt of subjects = 84.5 kg).

TABLE 11. *Oxygen-Stores Contribution to O_2 Debt-Deficit and to $\dot{V}_{O_2}$ Kinetics at Onset and Offset of Exercise*

Exercise Conditions	$\dot{V}s_{O_2}$, liters/min	$t_{1/2}$ $\dot{V}_{O_2}$, s		O_2 Deficit, liters	O_2 Debt, liters	ΔVst_{O_2}, liters	$t_{1/2}$ $\dot{V}_{O_2}$*, s		n
		On	Off				On	Off	
Supine, untrained, arm, 50 W	0.61	29.0	28.0	0.418	0.404	0.160	17.9	16.9	19
Supine, trained, arm, 75 W	0.90	21.5	24.5	0.465	0.530	0.210	11.8	14.8	6
Supine and sitting, trained, arm, 125 W	1.50	18.0	23.2	0.649	0.837	0.280	10.2	15.4	16
Supine, untrained, leg, 100 W	1.20	29.5	29.0	0.851	0.837	0.260	20.5	20.0	21
							x̄ = 15.1	x̄ = 16.8	
Supine and sitting, untrained, arm, 15 W	0.15	13.0		0.045			13.0		4
Supine, untrained, leg, 30 W	0.37	24.5		0.217		0.100	13.2		4
Sitting, untrained, leg, 50 W	0.61	27.7		0.409		0.160	16.9		4
							x̄ = 14.4		4

$\dot{V}s_{O_2}$, steady-state O_2 consumption above resting; $t_{1/2}$ $\dot{V}_{O_2}$, $t_{1/2}$ of $\dot{V}_{O_2}$ on- and off-responses; ΔVst_{O_2}, O_2-stores changes in rest-to-exercise transition; $t_{1/2}$ $\dot{V}_{O_2}$*, $t_{1/2}$ of $\dot{V}_{O_2}$ on- and off-responses at muscle level; *n*, number of subjects; x̄, average value [total average (±SD) = 15.5 ± 3.1]. First 4 lines: $t_{1/2}$ $\dot{V}_{O_2}$ on-response values obtained by extrapolating to eLa = 0 the regression of $t_{1/2}$ $\dot{V}_{O_2}$ on-response vs. eLa; $t_{1/2}$ $\dot{V}_{O_2}$ off-response values measured. Last 3 lines: $t_{1/2}$, experimental conditions in which O_2 deficit = O_2 debt (thus $t_{1/2}$ $\dot{V}_{O_2}$ on = $t_{1/2}$ $\dot{V}_{O_2}$ off) and eLa = 0. ΔVst_{O_2} data obtained by interpolation from Table 10. Time course of $\dot{V}_{O_2}$* (assumed to be exponential), when eLa = 0, was calculated (see Eq. 16): $t_{1/2}$ $\dot{V}_{O_2}$* = [(O_2 deficit or O_2 debt − ΔVst_{O_2})/$\dot{V}s_{O_2}$] × ln 2.

Thus, if k_{al}^{-1} as calculated from Table 11 is 22 s, the above three figures allow calculation of the corresponding values for k^{-1} of 65, 65, and 57 s, respectively. The $t_{1/2}$ values of $\dot{V}_{O_2}$ on-responses at the mouth (ln 2/*k*) amount then to 45, 45, and 39 s, respectively, not far from the experimental values (54, 52, and 40 s) for arms, legs supine, and legs sitting, respectively.

This analysis cannot be pushed too far: in fact, *1)* the O_2 equivalent of La accumulation in blood is subject to a certain variability (see ref. 137) and *2)* ΔVst_{O_2} is not constant but increases with $\dot{V}s_{O_2}$, although at a progressively lower rate. However, the agreement between theory and experiment is satisfactory, thus supporting the view that Equation 20 (with $k_{al} = 0.045\ s^{-1}$) can describe VPC_{O_2} also when eLa > 0.

As previously indicated, since no significant La production occurs in the recovery phase, the fast component of the $\dot{V}_{O_2}$ off-response as well as the O_2 debt is independent of eLa (89, 93).

On the basis of the above analysis it can be concluded that the VPC_{O_2}, which is a measure of the amount of energy derived from PC splitting at the work onset or required for PC resynthesis at the work offset, bears a fixed relationship to $\dot{V}s_{O_2}$; the proportionality constant ($k_{al} = VPC_{O_2}/\dot{V}s_{O_2}$) amounts in all cases to ~0.045 s^{-1}. Consequently the various conditions that affect the O_2 deficit (or debt) and thus the time course of the $\dot{V}_{O_2}$ on- and off-responses at the mouth can act essentially via their effects on O_2-stores depletion and/or on eLa. It is not surprising therefore to find that at moderate work intensities (<100 W) or after training, the $\dot{V}_{O_2}$ on-response at the mouth is faster ($t_{1/2}$ ~ 20 s) than at higher work loads or in untrained subjects (89, 190, 209, 211, 231, 291). In addition, at higher work loads, longer $t_{1/2}$ values and/or double exponentials are often observed (110, 133, 324, 498). This presumably can be associated with eLa production [see Fig. 6 in Whipp and Wasserman (498)]. Indeed, Hagberg et al. (209) observed that after training (a condition known to reduce blood La accumulation), the $\dot{V}_{O_2}$ on-response became monoexponential at the same absolute work load at which before training a double exponential could clearly be detected. Finally, during cycloergometric exercise the $\dot{V}_{O_2}$ on-response is slower (and the O_2 deficit, for a given $\dot{V}_{O_2}$, larger) in the supine than in the sitting position (93). The effects of training and posture can largely be attributed to changes of eLa (89, 93), which are presumably a consequence of the improved muscle capillary supply after training (10) or of variations of muscle perfusion with changes of posture.

The hypothesis of the constancy of VPC_{O_2} relative to $\dot{V}s_{O_2}$ under all experimental conditions leads also to the prediction that at work loads for which eLa > 0, the time course of the $\dot{V}_{CO_2}$ on-response slows to a lesser extent than that of the $\dot{V}_{O_2}$ on-response, because the La production leads to a nonmetabolic CO_2 elimination. This was experimentally observed by Linnarsson (324).

The time course of the various components of the O_2-debt contraction and payment in aerobic and supramaximum exercise is schematically indicated in Figure 11.

Cardiovascular Transients

The mechanisms controlling the transport of the respiratory gases during exercise rather than from steady-state responses can better be assessed from the analysis of phasic cardiovascular adaptations, such as those occurring at the onset and offset of trains of muscle twitches or those elicited by various dynamic forcing functions. The increase of cardiac activity during transition from rest to work appears, both in humans and in the dog, to be faster than that of $\dot{V}_{O_2}$ determined at the mouth, independent of the type of muscle contraction (isotonic or isometric). Thus the stress on the cardiovascular system for a given work impulse or rectangular mechanical load [if the kinetics of the systemic pressure response are considered (5, 198, 242, 320)] may be the same or even greater than at steady state. During recovery, as a result of the previous metabolic changes occurring in the muscle, the dissociation between HR and arterial pressure on one side and $\dot{V}_{O_2}$ transients on the other is less evident, particularly if during the contraction and/or in the recovery phase muscle perfusion is arrested (5). We next examine in detail the HR response and its determinants as well as the adjustments of $\dot{Q}_T$ and muscle blood flow to sudden changes of metabolism.

HEART RATE RESPONSE. Short isometric contractions as well as light rectangular isotonic loads elicit in humans a cardiac acceleration, which for the latter case is characterized by $t_{1/2}$ = 5–10 s and in some cases by a double exponential pattern (502). This HR increase is the result of the suppression of cardiac vagal tone and not the consequence of increased sympathetic stimulation. This is proved by experiments in which HR transients were recorded after parasympathetic as well as β- and α-adrenergic blockade. After parasympathetic blockade (160, 163, 179, 238), no cardiac acceleration was observed at the onset of contraction; the resting HR, however, was substantially higher (by 35–40 beat/min) than in the controls. After adrenergic blockade (163, 179) the HR response was identical with that of the control, with the curve displaced at a lower level.

In humans the total lag time between the start of a voluntary (arm and leg) or electrically induced (arm) contraction and the first detectable change of the R-R interval in the electrocardiogram appears to be ~560 ms (63, 238, 372, 375, 501, 502), to which 45 ms must be added to include the time between cortical command and the onset of the muscle electrical activity (372). Incidentally, the lag time of the ventilatory response seems to be much shorter (~60 ms) (372). An analysis of the various components of the delay of the HR response allows allocation of ~400 ms to the efferent pathway (vagal conduction, lag time between vagal stimulation and next atrial depolarization, P-R interval) so that ~200 ms are left for the response of a hypothetical receptor, including the time for afferent transmission and cerebral conduction. The finding that the delays in the cardiac response after spontaneous and electrically induced contractions are identical (238), despite the different lengths of the pathway, is strong [although not exclusive (179, 198)] evidence that a peripheral receptor acting as a sensor of a muscle-heart reflex is involved in the response.

NATURE OF PERIPHERAL SENSOR. Two essential questions need to be answered to support the reflex hypothesis. *1*) Is there an afferent pathway for this reflex? *2*) Which is the receptor and what is the appropriate stimulus? With regard to question *1*, the analysis of the pressure response that usually parallels HR changes is very pertinent. It appears in fact that impulses conducted by small myelinated type III sensory fibers originating in free nerve endings of skeletal muscles could be responsible for both the HR and the pressure response (108, 111, 179, 198). These are abolished after preferential anesthetic block of small type III and IV afferent fibers from exercising muscles of cat limbs, despite the fact that type I, II, and large type III fibers from muscle spindles and Golgi tendon organs keep conducting proprioceptive impulses (342). Since the input from type IV unmyelinated fibers can be excluded because of their long condition time (>0.5 s), which is incompatible with the calculated 200 ms available for the stimuli to reach the reflex center, small type III fibers appear to be the most likely afferent pathway. The following observations are further indirect evidence that small type III fibers are the candidate pathway for the reflex: *a*) the constancy of the HR and pressure response when stimulating a muscle whose type I, II, and large type III afferent fibers are inactivated by anodal block in the dorsal roots and *b*) the lack of potentiation of the cardiovascular response by mechanical stimulation (vibration) of the primary afferent (type I fibers) of muscle spindles (341). In regard to question *2* (i.e., the nature of the peripheral sensor), until 1975 most authors were divided between the hypothesis of a mechanoreceptor and that of a chemoreceptor-like structure. Although it was clear that known mechanoreceptors from muscle spindles and Golgi tendon organs are not involved in the pressure and HR responses (374), the prevailing hypothesis was that free nerve endings of small type III fibers could act as mechanoreceptors or, alternatively, that the Pacinian corpuscles located within the muscle, when stimulated by the contraction, could act as mechanical sensors (238). The hypothesis that the cardiovascular response could be elicited by chemical changes and sensed by chemoreceptors was considered rather unlikely (455) because the available time (~200 ms) is supposedly too short for the detection of a chemical change in the medium and for the transmission of the signal along the afferent pathway. Recently, however, the old hypothesis (5, 21, 393) that muscle metabolic receptors may control cardiovascular and respiratory functions at exercise has acquired new vigor because several investigators established, both in animals and humans, reproducible relationships between changes of ventilation, HR, peripheral blood flow, and muscle metabolic changes at the onset of work as well as during sustained contractions. Muscle chemical changes include the increase of various electrolytes and of $[H^+]$ in the extracellular medium, high osmolarity, and relative hypoxia and hypercapnia (185, 234, 456, 476, 477). All these factors correlate to various degrees with circulatory and respiratory reactions. A decisive step in these investigations was the observation that intra-arterial infusion of KCl, raising $[K^+]$ in the muscle venous effluent to the levels observed during muscular contraction, may induce cardiovascular and respiratory reflexes (1, 503), enhancing the activity of afferent proprioceptive and nonproprioceptive fibers (235). After this finding a series of experiments was carried out to correlate exercise-induced increments of muscle $[K^+]$ (185, 282) with local as well as systemic circulatory and metabolic reactions. The results of these experiments in isolated muscles both during work transients and sustained contractions (233, 234, 473, 474) show a satisfactory correlation between the increase of $[K^+]$ in the extracellular space as a consequence of the stimulation and local circulatory adjustments. In addition, the found increase in $[K^+]$ in the extracellular space (8–10 mM) appears sufficient to depolarize the free nerve endings held responsible for the onset of the reflex (234). A good correlation is also found between $[K^+]$ and $\dot{V}s_{O_2}$, although a discrepancy is observed at the work onset and offset (233). This observation and the finding that at the onset of rectangular work loads the rate of $\dot{V}_{O_2}$ increase of isolated perfused dog muscles is slower than the adjustment of muscle blood flow (381) seem to indicate that during the on-transient, oxidative metabolism is regulated differently than blood flow. Oxidative metabolism is probably controlled by an interaction of several factors, among which the level of free creatine is important (see *Control and Kinetics of Gas Exchange in Muscle*, this page). Continuous analyses of these compounds in intact muscle preparations (e.g., by nuclear magnetic resonance spectrometers coupled with simultaneous measurements of blood flow and $\dot{V}_{O_2}$) may shed light on this important aspect of metabolic regulation.

CARDIAC OUTPUT AND MUSCLE BLOOD-FLOW TRANSIENTS. Innumerable studies have dealt with the cardiovascular changes occurring during steady-state dynamic and static exercise in humans (see *Cardiovascular Adjustments*, p. 306). By contrast, studies on $\dot{Q}$T adjustments at the onset and offset of work in humans and intact animals are rather scanty, mostly because of methodological difficulties in measuring $\dot{Q}$T transients. At the onset of exercise, $\dot{Q}$T increased in running dogs, with $t_{1/2}$ = 12–15 s (94, 146, 147, 295), which is somewhat faster than the $t_{1/2}$ of the $\dot{V}_{O_2}$ on-response (147, 330). In humans, the $t_{1/2}$ of the $\dot{Q}$T on-response has been reported to be ~15 s for submaximum dynamic work loads (94, 121, 272). The $\dot{Q}$T adjustment kinetics is definitely faster than the average $t_{1/2}$ of the $\dot{V}_{O_2}$ on-response measured in the upper airways, which, depending on the muscle type involved, the training, and the posture of the subject (see *Pulmonary Gas-Exchange Transients*, p. 314), ranges between 25 and over 100 s and is a function of eLa buildup. If, however, the $\dot{V}_{O_2}$ on-response is determined at the muscle level in the absence of eLa accumulation, the $\dot{Q}$T $t_{1/2}$ and $\dot{V}_{O_2}$ $t_{1/2}$ appear to be very close, suggesting that under these conditions the $\dot{Q}$T adjustment is coupled to $\dot{V}_{O_2}$. The kinetics of the $\dot{Q}$T adjustment at the onset of a sustained (3–5 min) isometric contraction appears to be as fast as that for isotonic work (P. Cerretelli, unpublished observations).

The kinetics of the $\dot{Q}$T off-response is similar to that of the on-response in dynamic exercise, although it appears to be extremely variable after static efforts, which is probably a consequence of the additional chemical drive introduced by the massive release of metabolic intermediates accumulated in the muscle. Thus, in all cases except pathological situations in which the $\dot{Q}$T on-response may be delayed and in cardiac surgical denervation, the $\dot{Q}$T on-response anticipated or paralleled the $\dot{V}_{O_2}$ transient.

Both in humans and in dogs the kinetics of adjustment of muscle blood flow at the onset of a square-wave dynamic exercise (running, arm cranking, or leg pedaling) is very fast and a new steady state is usually reached within 9–30 s, depending on the muscle involved, the muscle-specific training level, and the work load (84, 102). Experiments by Tibes et al. (475–477) indicate that also in the human, blood-flow adjustments in limb muscles correlate satisfactorily with muscle metabolic factors, particularly with extracellular $[K^+]$, which is also involved in the control of HR and perhaps of ventilation at the onset of exercise. By contrast, according to Honig's group (248–252) the control of muscle vasodilation at exercise is initiated by the intrinsic nerves whose cell bodies lie within the walls of the arterioles; the metabolic factors intervene with a delay on the order of minutes.

In conclusion, the picture emerging from this survey of the literature is still controversial. It appears, however, that, as for steady-state exercise, cardiovascular changes (HR, $\dot{Q}$T, muscle blood flow) are coupled to oxidative metabolism, and the fine adjustments during the on-transients are modulated by fast-responding neurohumoral factors.

Control and Kinetics of Gas Exchange in Muscle

At the onset of exercise, the rate of ATP splitting changes suddenly, dictated by motoneuron discharge. However, the [ATP] is substantially unchanged, because ATP is immediately rephosphorylated at the expense of PC

$$PC + ADP \rightleftharpoons ATP + Cr \qquad (23)$$

The net result of the process is the splitting of PC into inorganic phosphate (P_i) and free creatine (Cr).

However, the [PC] in muscle is low, so that the reaction in Equation 23 would only postpone the drop of [ATP] were it not for the intervention of glycolysis and/or oxidative phosphorylation, the net result of which is the resynthesis of ATP from ADP and P_i

$$\text{glycogen} + \text{ADP} + P_i \rightharpoonup \text{ATP} + \text{La} \qquad (24)$$

$$\text{glycogen and/or fat} + O_2 + \text{ADP} + P_i \rightharpoonup \text{ATP} + CO_2 + H_2O \qquad (25)$$

Under a wide variety of conditions, the reaction rate of Equation 25, which is proportional to $\dot{V}_{O_2}$, seems to be controlled by the biochemical counterpart of the alactic O_2 debt ($V_{PC_{O_2}}$ in Eq. 20) (140, 141). In fact, $\dot{V}s_{O_2}$ is linearly related to $V_{PC_{O_2}}$ both in exercising humans and in the dog gastrocnemius in situ (see Eq. 20). Consistent with this hypothesis, both in humans and intact animals, the O_2 deficit, which under a given set of conditions is proportional to $V_{PC_{O_2}}$, *1)* depends only on work intensity, as it is independent of its duration (289); *2)* does not increase once $\dot{V}s_{O_2}$ is attained (496); *3)* bears the same relationship to $\dot{V}s_{O_2}$ in hypoxia as in normoxia (396); and *4)* is unaffected by changes in ventilatory dynamics (30, 77).

Furthermore, in the dog gastrocnemius in situ, at the onset and offset of square-wave exercises and under conditions in which both eLa and ΔVst_{O_2} (see Eq. 17) are negligible, $\dot{V}_{O_2}$ changes according to monoexponential functions, with $t_{1/2} = 15$–19 s (see OXYGEN DEBT-DEFICIT, p. 317). Similarly, in frog sartorius at 20°C after short tetani, $\dot{V}_{O_2}$ decreases according to monoexponential functions of time, albeit with a much longer $t_{1/2}$ (~2.6 min) (327). Because the rate of ATP hydrolysis undergoes a sudden step change under these conditions, the above findings suggest that the rate of $\dot{V}_{O_2}$ is coupled to ATP hydrolysis by a single reaction with apparent first-order kinetics, the velocity constant of which is identical with that of the $\dot{V}_{O_2}$ changes at the muscle level, i.e., of the $V_{PC_{O_2}}$ contraction and payment (k_{al} in Eq. 20) (140, 141, 327).

This analysis leads to an attempt to identify the precise biochemical nature of *a)* the factor(s) hidden under the term $V_{PC_{O_2}}$ and *b)* the first-order reaction, the time constant of which is reflected by k_{al}. As to *a*, the most obvious candidate is among those substances the concentration of which is a linear function of $V_{PC_{O_2}}$ and hence of $\dot{V}s_{O_2}$: essentially PC, P_i, and Cr (381). In the past P_i has been attributed a preferential role (137, 140, 141). According to Mahler (329, 329a), however, the most likely candidate seems to be Cr, and the rate-limiting reaction (*b*) can be identified with the intramitochondrial production of ADP (see ref. 495).

The remainder of this section is a discussion of Mahler's model. This model, which is derived from previous semiquantitative models (6, 50a, 187, 263, 264, 426), will be completed to account for the transient La production (eLa) that is often observed at the onset of exercise (see AEROBIC EXERCISE, p. 314). According to the model (Fig. 12), *1)* on muscle contraction, [ATP] and [ADP] changes are prevented

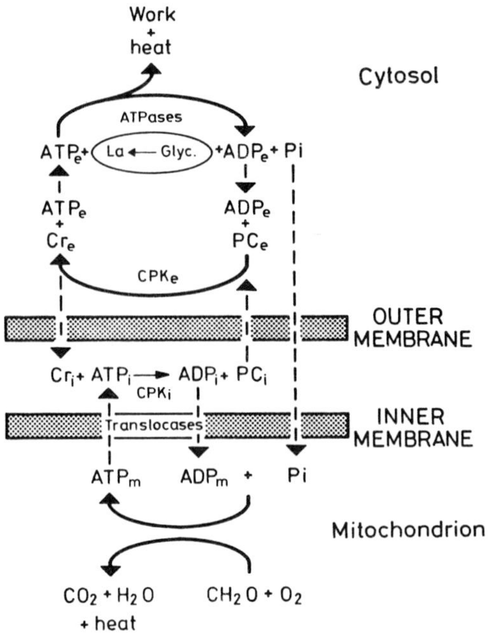

FIG. 12. Model for control of muscle $\dot{V}_{O_2}$ via mitochondrial creatinephosphokinase (CPK). Subscripts: e, extramitochondrial; i, intramitochondrial; m, mitochondrial. Glyc., glycogen. [Adapted from Mahler (329, 329a).]

by the extramitochondrial creatine phosphokinase (CPK_e) reaction; *2)* the resulting increase in [Cr] leads to ADP production within the mitochondrial membrane via intramitochondrial creatine phosphokinase (CPK_i); *3)* the ADP so produced reaches the mitochondrial matrix to be reconverted to ATP at the expense of oxidative phosphorylation; and *4)* finally, closing the cycle, ATP reacts with Cr within the membrane. Hence the mitochondrion as a whole couples the $\dot{V}_{O_2}$ to the phosphorylation of Cr (329). In addition, *1a)* the $\dot{V}_{O_2}$ in the matrix is limited by the mitochondrial membrane production of ADP via the CPK_i reaction, *2a)* the rate of this reaction changes linearly with ΔCr (329a, 495), *3a)* ADP is transported into the mitochondrial matrix as fast as it is produced via the CPK_i reaction, and *4a)* the outer mitochondrial membrane must be highly permeable to both PC and Cr. If the system is to operate at steady state, the net fluxes of the CPK_e and CPK_i reactions must be equal but in opposite directions. These net fluxes are

$$k_1[\text{ADP}]_e[\text{PC}]_e - k_2[\text{ATP}]_e[\text{Cr}]_e \qquad (26)$$

and

$$k_2[\text{ATP}]_i[\text{Cr}]_i - k_1[\text{ADP}]_i[\text{PC}]_i \qquad (27)$$

where e and i are extra- and intramitochondrial (intramembrane) and k_1 and k_2 are the velocity constants of the forward and backward reactions, respectively. Thus in order to attain flow equality

$$[\text{PC}]_e[\text{ADP}]_e - ([\text{ATP}]_e[\text{Cr}]_e)/K_e = ([\text{ATP}]_i[\text{Cr}]_i)/K_i - [\text{PC}]_i[\text{ADP}]_i \qquad (28)$$

where $K_e = (k_1/k_2)$ and $K_i = (k_1/k_2)_i$ are the equilibrium constants in the extra- and intramitochondrial compartments. At the steady state the right and left terms of Equation 28 must be *1)* equal and *2)* larger, the heavier the exercise. These conditions at first seem incompatible with the great permeability of the outer membrane to PC and Cr, which imposes that $[PC]_e \sim [PC]_i$ and $[Cr]_e \sim [Cr]_i$. However, the equilibrium constant of the CPK reaction is probably different in the two compartments, specifically $K_e > K_i$. In fact, Harris et al. (216) have shown that the equilibrium constant of the CPK reaction in human muscle homogenates is a decreasing function of pH

$$\log K = 17.6 - 2.4 \text{ pH} \tag{29}$$

On this basis, and assuming intramitochondrial pH = 7.4 and cytosol pH = 6.9 (2a), then $K_i = 0.7$ and $K_e = 11$. If this is the case, ATP formation at the expense of PC and ADP would be favored in the cytosol, while the opposite would be true inside the mitochondrial membrane (Fig. 12). An additional feature could also favor the appropriate fluxes to be maintained, i.e., that extramitochondrial CPK must be bound in juxtaposition to the relevant ATPases, so that the net rate of the CPK_e reaction can be displaced toward ATP and Cr further than would be predicted from average concentrations of reactants.

No further discussion of the Cr control model is made here (see refs. 329a and 495). Suffice it to say that, besides being supported by experimental data (160a, 160b, 425a, 426), this model is consistent with the observations that muscle $\dot{V}_{O_2}$ is linearly related to ΔCr and that step changes in muscle ATP utilization lead to monoexponential changes of both $\dot{V}_{O_2}$ and ΔCr (137, 327–329, 381), with $t_{1/2} \sim 15$ s in the dog gastrocnemius in situ (381, 384).

In exercising humans, the analysis of the $\dot{V}_{O_2}$ kinetics at the onset and offset of exercise is complicated by O_2-stores changes, eLa production, and circulatory delay (see *Pulmonary Gas-Exchange Transients*, p. 314). However, the O_2 deficit corrected for O_2-stores changes and eLa production ($V_{PC_{O_2}}$; see Eq. 17) is linearly related to $\dot{V}_{S_{O_2}}$, the proportionality constant (k_{al}) being in all cases ~0.045 s^{-1} (see OXYGEN DEBT-DEFICIT, p. 317), i.e., close to the values observed in isolated dog gastrocnemius in situ.

When eLa > 0 the energy sources for ATP resynthesis (in addition to PC breakdown) are $\dot{V}_{O_2}$ and transient La production (eLa); consequently, before a steady state is attained the amount of accumulated Cr may be less than if eLa = 0 because a fraction of ATP is resynthesized bypassing the CPK reaction (see Fig. 12). If this is true, because eLa is not a constant fraction of the energy requirement but decreases with time, attaining zero when a true steady state is reached, the $\dot{V}_{O_2}$ kinetics must be slower than if eLa = 0 throughout the working period. At steady state, however, the relationship between ΔCr (or $V_{PC_{O_2}}$) and $\dot{V}_{S_{O_2}}$ must again conform with Equation 20. In conclusion, also in these conditions, $\dot{V}_{O_2}$ is controlled by ΔCr, as is true when eLa = 0; the accumulation of Cr, however, is slowed because of the concomitant La production. This results in a slower and not necessarily monoexponential $\dot{V}_{O_2}$ on-response, as was experimentally found (see AEROBIC EXERCISE, p. 314). This can be formally shown as follows.

At the onset of square-wave aerobic exercise, the rate of extramitochondrial ATP utilization ($\overrightarrow{\dot{ATP}_e}$) increases from the very beginning and is proportional to work load and $\dot{V}_{S_{O_2}}$. At the expense of extramitochondrial PC breakdown ($\overrightarrow{\dot{PC}_e}$) and anaerobic glycolysis, ATP is immediately rephosphorylated, so that $[ATP]_e$ and $[ADP]_e$ remain essentially unchanged. Thus if La production is zero throughout (eLa = 0)

$$\overrightarrow{\dot{ATP}_e} = \overrightarrow{\dot{PC}_e} = c\dot{V}_{S_{O_2}} = \text{constant} \tag{30}$$

where $c = dPC/dV_{O_2} = dATP/dV_{O_2} = -dCr/dV_{O_2}$ is the amount of high-energy phosphate (~P) resynthesized per unit O_2 consumed, i.e., the P/O ratio. The rate of intramitochondrial ATP resynthesis ($\overleftarrow{\dot{ATP}_i}$) that is proportional to $\dot{V}_{O_2}$ equals intramembrane ADP production (or PC resynthesis), in turn controlled by an increase in free [Cr] (Δ[Cr]), assumed to be equal in the intra- and extramitochondrial space. If this is so

$$\overleftarrow{\dot{ATP}_i} = \overleftarrow{\dot{PC}_i} = k_{al}\,\Delta[Cr] = c\dot{V}t_{O_2} \tag{31}$$

where $\dot{V}t_{O_2}$ is the O_2 consumption at time t and k_{al} is the velocity constant of intramembrane CPK reaction. At steady state ($\dot{V}t_{O_2} = \dot{V}_{S_{O_2}}$), Equations 30 and 31 must be equal so that

$$\dot{V}_{S_{O_2}} = k_{al}\,\frac{\Delta[Cr]}{c} = k_{al}V_{PC_{O_2}} \tag{32}$$

where Δ[Cr]/c is the increase in free Cr expressed in O_2 units, i.e., the alactic O_2 debt ($V_{PC_{O_2}}$). Thus k_{al}, the apparent velocity constant of intramitochondrial ADP production, equals the ratio $\dot{V}_{S_{O_2}}/V_{PC_{O_2}}$ and at the onset and offset of square-wave changes in $\overrightarrow{\dot{ATP}_e}$, $\dot{V}t_{O_2}$ changes according to monoexponential functions of time. In fact

$$\Delta[\dot{Cr}] = \overrightarrow{\dot{PC}_e} - \overleftarrow{\dot{PC}_i} \tag{33}$$

and, substituting Equations 30 and 31 into Equation 33

$$\Delta[\dot{Cr}] = c(\dot{V}_{S_{O_2}} - \dot{V}t_{O_2}) \tag{34}$$

Since $\Delta[Cr] = c\dot{V}t_{O_2}/k_{al}$ (Eq. 31), substituting into Equation 34

$$\ddot{V}t_{O_2} = k_{al}(\dot{V}_{S_{O_2}} - \dot{V}t_{O_2}) \tag{35}$$

Hence the rate of change of Δ[Cr] and of $\dot{V}t_{O_2}$ at any given time t is proportional to $\dot{V}_{S_{O_2}} - \dot{V}t_{O_2}$.

In the initial exercise period a transient La production may occur ($\dot{e}La$). If this is the case, Equation 30 must be modified to take into account also the ATP resynthesized at the expense of anaerobic glycolysis, bypassing the CPK reaction

$$\overrightarrow{A\dot{T}P_e} = \overrightarrow{P\dot{C}_e} + b(e\dot{L}a) = c\dot{V}s_{O_2} \tag{36}$$

where b = dATP/dLa is the amount of ~P resynthesized per unit La produced. As the exercise proceeds, $e\dot{L}a$ decreases progressively to attain zero at $\dot{V}s_{O_2}$, so that the steady state is again described by Equation 32. However, at any time t before the steady state, $\dot{V}t_{O_2}$ is less than when eLa = 0. In fact, as from Equation 33, the amount of Cr accumulated at time t is given by

$$\begin{aligned}\Delta[\text{Cr}]_t &= \int_0^t \Delta[\dot{\text{C}}\text{r}]dt \\ &= \int_0^t (\overrightarrow{P\dot{C}_e} - \overleftarrow{P\dot{C}_i})dt\end{aligned} \tag{37}$$

Thus if eLa = 0, because (from Eq. 30) $\overrightarrow{P\dot{C}_e} = \overrightarrow{A\dot{T}P_e}$ = constant, substituting in Equation 37 it follows that

$$\Delta[\text{Cr}]_t = \overrightarrow{A\dot{T}P_e}\cdot t - \int_0^t \overleftarrow{P\dot{C}_i}\, dt \tag{38}$$

By contrast, if $e\dot{L}a > 0$, because (from Eq. 36) $\overrightarrow{P\dot{C}_e} = \overrightarrow{A\dot{T}P_e} - b(e\dot{L}a)$ and $\overrightarrow{A\dot{T}P_e}$ is constant, substituting in Equation 38, it follows that

$$\Delta[\text{Cr}]_t = \overrightarrow{A\dot{T}P_e}\cdot t - b\int_0^t e\dot{L}a\, dt - \int_0^t \overleftarrow{P\dot{C}_i}\, dt \tag{39}$$

Thus, for a given exercise intensity ($\overrightarrow{A\dot{T}P_e}$) and for a time t shorter than required to attain $\dot{V}s_{O_2}$, $\Delta[\text{Cr}]_t$ in the case of Equation 39 is less than for Equation 38 by the amount $b \int_0^t e\dot{L}a\, dt = b(eLa)$. It necessarily follows that a transient La production at the onset of exercise leads to a slowing of $\dot{V}_{O_2}$ on-kinetics.

The hypothesis that the rate of V_{O_2} is controlled by the biochemical counterpart of $V\text{PC}_{O_2}$ is also consistent with the following findings. *1)* At the onset of very heavy supramaximum exercise, $\dot{V}_{O_2}$ increases according to the "usual" time course, tending asymptotically to the level required by the exercise, although this is greater than $\dot{V}max_{O_2}$ (see Fig. 11). Obviously this increase stops abruptly when $\dot{V}max_{O_2}$ is attained (335). In fact the rate of accumulation of $\dot{C}r$ (and of $V\text{PC}_{O_2}$) and hence the $\dot{V}_{O_2}$ on-kinetics is imposed by the actual energy requirement of the exercise, irrespective of whether it is above or below $\dot{V}max_{O_2}$. *2)* At the offset of supramaximum exercise, $\dot{V}_{O_2}$ remains at its maximum level until a substantial fraction of $V\text{PC}_{O_2}$ has been paid (142). In these conditions the O_2 delivery at the tissue level is limited at $\dot{V}max_{O_2}$ and the rate of ATP resynthesis cannot proceed as would be required by the actual free [Cr]. Consequently, before $\dot{V}_{O_2}$ can decrease below its maximum value, a certain amount of Cr must be rephosphorylated to PC at the expense of oxidations and delayed La production. The net $V\text{PC}_{O_2}$ paid after this type of exercise may reach, in nonathletic subjects, maximum values of 30–32 ml O_2/kg (142, 406) instead of ~18 ml O_2/kg, as observed after exercising at $\dot{V}max_{O_2}$ (Eq. 20), indicating that the amount of ~P split is ~1.8 times larger than after maximum aerobic exercise (see Fig. 11).

The energy charge of the adenylate pool, (ATP + 0.5 ADP)/(ATP + ADP + AMP), has also been suggested as a possible factor controlling muscle $\dot{V}_{O_2}$ (29, 422). However, this hypothesis and the traditional model of Chance et al. (99), which views muscle $\dot{V}_{O_2}$ as regulated by tissue [ADP], do not easily account for the exponential rise and decline of $\dot{V}_{O_2}$ at the onset and offset of exercise nor for the linear relationship found at steady state between $\dot{V}_{O_2}$ on one hand and [PC], [Cr], and [P_i] on the other (329). A more precise estimate of the latter metabolites in vivo, as obtained by nuclear magnetic resonance at steady state and during exercise transients (124a, 357a, 468a), may shed some light on this debated and interesting problem.

In conclusion, the traditional concept, which views the O_2 debt-deficit as caused by the delay of the circulatory and respiratory systems, must be modified. A given amount of the O_2 debt-deficit ($V\text{PC}_{O_2}$) must be incurred to drive muscle metabolism at a certain rate and is therefore dictated by the energy requirement of the exercise. The remaining fraction (eLa and O_2-stores changes; see Eq. 17) depends, on the contrary, on the interplay of central and peripheral circulatory adaptations as well as on muscle fiber myoglobin and enzyme composition, so that the kinetics of the gas exchange in the upper airways is inevitably slower than, and distorted in comparison with, the events taking place at the muscle level.

CONCLUSIONS

This review of the numerous factors that regulate muscle metabolism and gas exchange during exercise tempts us to extrapolate some of the above concepts to the regulation of other basic physiological functions, such as pulmonary ventilation and cardiovascular adjustments.

It is generally assumed that the sudden rise (drop) of $\dot{V}E$ at the onset (offset) of exercise is due to neural stimuli (e.g., see refs. 17, 127, 131), whereas the secondary, more gradual changes of $\dot{V}E$ are under the control of humoral undefined metabolic factors. According to Tibes et al. (473–476) (see also *Cardiovascular Transients*, p. 321), the metabolic control of $\dot{V}E$ and of cardiovascular adjustments at exercise may depend on the activation of muscle receptors sensitive to the concentration changes of metabolites (mostly extracellular K^+) induced by exercise. This hypothesis, however, at least as far as ventilation is concerned, is not supported by the data of Weissman et al. (489), who observed that the $\dot{V}E$ responses ($t_{1/2}$ ~ 30 s) to hindlimb stimulation in anesthetized cats are unaffected by spinal cord section. This chapter is not a review of the different features of the respiratory control; the interested reader is referred to the chapter by Wasserman, Whipp, and Casaburi (485a) in the 1986 edition of the *Handbook* section on the control of breathing. It is tempting, however, to identify the central metabolic controller with V_{PCO_2} (or with its biochemical counterpart). If this is true the other factors known to affect ventilation (e.g., pH, P_{CO_2}, P_{O_2}) as well as circulation (e.g., K^+, P_i, H^+) would intervene only as modulators, with the aim of finely tuning the responses according to the specific requirements of the exercise and/or of the environmental conditions. Note also that the HR control during exercise has been viewed similarly by Stegemann and Kenner (455).

Thus the alactic O_2 debt, or rather its biochemical counterpart, may be a possible central factor for the control of gas exchange, ventilation, and circulation during exercise; this is a tentative working hypothesis that is largely speculative.

We are most grateful to Dr. Claudio Marconi from the Centro di Studi di Fisiologia del Lavoro Muscolare del Consiglio Nazionale delle Ricerche, Milan, Italy, for his collaboration in the selection of the bibliography. We also deeply appreciate the invaluable secretarial work of Sylvie Ferioli and thank Olivier Zulauf for his help with the figures.

This work was supported partly by the Fonds National Suisse de la Recherche Scientifique Grants 3.383.0.78 and 3.364.0.82 and by the Consiglio Nazionale delle Ricerche of Italy.

REFERENCES

1. ACHAR, M. V. S. Effects of injection of Locke solution with higher concentration of potassium on blood pressure in cats. *J. Physiol. Lond.* 198: 115–116, 1968.
2. ADARO, F., M. MEYER, AND R. S. SIKAND. Rebreathing and single breath pulmonary CO diffusing capacity in man at rest and exercise studied by $C^{18}O$ isotope. *Bull. Eur. Physiopathol. Respir.* 12: 747–756, 1976.

2a. ADDANKI, S., F. D. CAHILL, AND J. F. SOTOS. Determination of intramitochondrial pH and intramitochondrial-extramitochondrial pH gradient of isolated heart mitochondria by the use of 5,5-dimethyl-2,4-oxazolidinedione. I. Changes during respiration and adenosine triphosphate-dependent transport of Ca^{2+}, Mg^{2+}, and Zn^{2+}. *J. Biol. Chem.* 243: 2337–2348, 1968.

3. AGHEMO, P., F. PIÑERA-LIMAS, AND G. SASSI. Maximal aerobic power in primitive Indians. *Int. Z. Angew. Physiol. Einschl. Arbeitsphysiol.* 29: 337–342, 1971.
4. AGOSTONI, E., E. J. M. CAMPBELL, AND S. FREEDMAN. The mechanical work of breathing. In: *Respiratory Muscles: Mechanics and Neural Control* (2nd ed.), edited by E. J. M. Campbell, E. Agostoni, and J. Newsom Davis. London: Lloyd-Luke, 1970, p. 115–137.
5. ALAM, M., AND F. H. SMIRK. Observations in man upon a blood pressure raising reflex arising from the voluntary muscles. *J. Physiol. Lond.* 89: 372–383, 1937.
6. ALTSCHULD, R. A., A. J. MEROLA, AND G. P. BRIERLEY. The permeability of heart mitochondria to creatine. *J. Mol. Cell. Cardiol.* 7: 451–462, 1975.
7. AMBROSOLI, G., P. CERRETELLI, P. MAGRASSI, AND E. RESPIGHI. Il bilancio energetico del miocardio durante ischemia. *Rend. Accad. Naz. Lincei (Ser. VIII)* 46: 619–626, 1969.
8. ANDERSEN, K. L. Respiration recovery from muscular exercise of short duration. *Acta Physiol. Scand. Suppl.* 168: 1–102, 1960.
9. ANDERSEN, K. L., A. BOLSTAD, Y. LØYNING, AND L. IRVING. Physical fitness of Artic Indians. *J. Appl. Physiol.* 15: 645–648, 1960.
10. ANDERSEN, P., AND J. HENRIKSSON. Capillary supply of the quadriceps femoris muscle of man: adaptive response to exercise. *J. Physiol. Lond.* 270: 677–690, 1977.
11. ANDERSON, T. W., AND R. J. SHEPHARD. The effects of hyperventilation and exercise upon the pulmonary diffusing capacity. *Respiration* 25: 465–484, 1968.
12. ANDERSON, T. W., AND R. J. SHEPHARD. Physical training and exercise diffusing capacity. *Int. Z. Angew. Physiol. Einschl. Arbeitsphysiol.* 25: 198–209, 1968.
13. ANDREW, G. M, AND L. BAINES. Relationship of pulmonary diffusing capacity (DL) and cardiac output ($\dot{Q}c$) in exercise. *Eur. J. Appl. Physiol. Occup. Physiol.* 33: 127–137, 1974.
14. APTHORP, G. H., AND R. MARSHALL. Pulmonary diffusing capacity, a comparison of breath-holding and steady state methods using carbon monoxide. *J. Clin. Invest.* 40: 1775–1784, 1961.

14a. ARMSTRONG, R. B., M. D. DELP, AND M. H. LAUGHLIN. Cardiac output distribution in miniature swine during locomotory exercise to $\dot{V}O_2$ (Abstract). *Federation Proc.* 45: 282, 1986.

15. ASMUSSEN, E. Ventilation at transition from rest to exercise. *Acta Physiol. Scand.* 89: 68–78, 1973.
16. ASMUSSEN, E., AND E. H. CHRISTENSEN. Die Mittelkapazität der Lungen bei erhöhtem O_2-Bedarf. *Skand. Arch. Physiol.* 82: 201–211, 1939.
17. ASMUSSEN, E., S. H. JOHANSEN, H. JORGENSEN, AND M. NIELSEN. On the nervous factors controlling respiration and circulation during exercise. *Acta Physiol. Scand.* 63: 343–350, 1965.
18. ASMUSSEN, E., AND M. NIELSEN. Studies on the initial changes in respiration at the transition from rest to work and from work to rest. *Acta Physiol. Scand.* 16: 270–285, 1948.
19. ASMUSSEN, E., AND M. NIELSEN. Physiological dead space and alveolar gas pressures at rest and during muscular exercise. *Acta Physiol. Scand.* 38: 1–21, 1956.
20. ASMUSSEN, E., AND M. NIELSEN. Alveolo-arterial gas exchange at rest and during work at different O_2 tensions. *Acta Physiol. Scand.* 50: 153–166, 1960.
21. ASMUSSEN, E., M. NIELSEN, AND G. WIETH-PEDERSEN. On the regulation of circulation during muscular work. *Acta Physiol. Scand.* 6: 353–358, 1943.
22. ÅSTRAND, I. Aerobic work capacity in men and women with special reference to age. *Acta Physiol. Scand. Suppl.* 169: 1–92, 1960.
23. ÅSTRAND, I. Circulatory responses to arm exercise in different work positions. *Scand. J. Clin. Lab. Invest.* 27: 293–297, 1971.
24. ÅSTRAND, P.-O. *Experimental Studies of Physical Working Capacity in Relation to Sex and Age.* Copenhagen: Munksgaard, 1952.
25. ÅSTRAND, P.-O. Human physical fitness with special reference to sex and age. *Physiol. Rev.* 36: 307–335, 1956.
26. ÅSTRAND, P.-O., T. E. CUDDY, B. SALTIN, AND J. STENBERG. Cardiac output during submaximal and maximal work. *J. Appl. Physiol.* 19: 268–274, 1964.
27. ÅSTRAND, P.-O., AND B. SALTIN. Oxygen uptake during the first minutes of heavy muscular exercise. *J. Appl. Physiol.* 16: 971–976, 1961.
28. ÅSTRAND, P.-O., AND B. SALTIN. Plasma and red cell volume after prolonged severe exercise. *J. Appl. Physiol.* 19: 829–832, 1964.
29. ATKINSON, D. E. The energy charge of the adenylate pool as regulatory parameter. Interaction with feedback modifiers. *Biochemistry* 7: 4030–4034, 1968.
30. AUCHINCLOSS, J. H., JR., R. GILBERT, AND G. H. BAULE.

Effect of ventilation on oxygen transfer during early exercise. *J. Appl. Physiol.* 21: 810–818, 1966.

31. BACHOFEN, H., H. J. HOBI, AND M. SCHERRER. Alveolar-arterial N_2 gradients at rest and during exercise in healthy men of different ages. *J. Appl. Physiol.* 34: 137–142, 1973.
32. BAILIE, M. D., S. ROBINSON, H. H. ROSTORFER, AND J. L. NEWTON. Effects of exercise on heart output of the dog. *J. Appl. Physiol.* 16: 107–111, 1961.
33. BANNISTER, R. G., J. E. COTES, R. S. JONES, AND F. MEADE. Pulmonary diffusing capacity on exercise in athletes and non-athletic subjects (Abstract). *J. Physiol. Lond.* 152: 66P–67P, 1960.
34. BANNISTER, R. G., AND D. J. C. CUNNINGHAM. The effects on the respiration and performance during exercise of adding oxygen to the inspired air. *J. Physiol. Lond.* 125: 118–137, 1954.
35. BARLETT, H. L., J. KOLLIAS, J. L. HODGSON, AND E. R. BUSKIRK. A possible explanation for exercise DL_{CO} based on estimations of SA_L and τ_h. *Respir. Physiol.* 19: 333–343, 1973.
36. BAR-OR, O., R. J. SHEPHARD, AND C. L. ALLEN. Cardiac output of 10- to 13-year-old boys and girls during submaximal exercise. *J. Appl. Physiol.* 30: 219–223, 1971.
37. BARR, P. O., M. BECKMAN, J. BJURSTEDT, J. BRISMAR, C. M. HESSER, AND G. MATELL. Time courses of blood gas changes provoked by light and moderate exercise in man. *Acta Physiol. Scand.* 60: 1–17, 1964.
38. BARTELS, H., R. BEER, E. FLEISCHER, H. J. HOFFHEINZ, J. KRALL, G. RODEWALD, J. WENNER, AND I. WITT. Bestimmung von Kurzschlussdurchblutung und Diffusionskapazität der Lunge bei Gesunden und Lungenkranken. *Pfluegers Arch.* 261: 99–132, 1955.
39. BARTELS, H., R. BEER, H. P. KOEPCHEN, J. WENNER, AND I. WITT. Messung der alveolär-arteriellen O_2-Druckdifferenz mit verschiedenen Methoden am Menschen bei Ruhe und Arbeit. *Pfluegers Arch.* 261: 133–151, 1955.
40. BARTLETT, R. G., JR., H. F. BRUBACH, AND H. SPECHT. Oxygen cost of breathing. *J. Appl. Physiol.* 12: 413–424, 1958.
41. BATES, D. V., N. G. BOUCOT, AND A. E. DORMER. The pulmonary diffusing capacity in normal subjects. *J. Physiol. Lond.* 129: 237–252, 1955.
42. BATES, D. V., AND J. F. PEARCE. The pulmonary diffusing capacity: a comparison of methods of measurement and a study of the effect of body position. *J. Physiol. Lond.* 132: 232–238, 1956.
43. BATES, D. V., C. J. VARVIS, R. E. DONEVAN, AND R. V. CHRISTIE. Variations in the pulmonary capillary blood volume and membrane diffusion component in health and disease. *J. Clin. Invest.* 39: 1401–1412, 1960.
44. BEAUMONT, W. VAN. Red cell volume with changes in plasma osmolarity during maximal exercise. *J. Appl. Physiol.* 35: 47–50, 1973.
45. BEAUMONT, W. VAN, J. C. STRAND, J. S. PETROFSKY, S. G. HIPSKIND, AND J. E. GREENLEAF. Changes in total plasma content of electrolytes and proteins with maximal exercise. *J. Appl. Physiol.* 34: 102–106, 1973.
46. BEAUMONT, W. VAN, S. UNDERKOFLER, AND S. VAN BEAUMONT. Erythrocyte volume, plasma volume, and acid-base changes in exercise and heat dehydration. *J. Appl. Physiol.* 50: 1255–1262, 1981.

46a. BEAVER, W. L., N. LAMARRA, AND K. WASSERMAN. Breath-by-breath measurement of true alveolar gas exchange. *J. Appl. Physiol.* 51: 1662–1675, 1981.

47. BEAVER, W. L., AND K. WASSERMAN. Transients in ventilation at start and end of exercise. *J. Appl. Physiol.* 25: 390–399, 1968.
48. BEDELL, G. N., AND R. W. ADAMS. Pulmonary diffusing capacity during rest and exercise. A study of normal persons and persons with atrial septal defect, pregnancy, and pulmonary disease. *J. Clin. Invest.* 41: 1908–1914, 1962.
49. BENNETT, F. M., P. REISCHL, F. S. GRODINS, S. M. YAMASHIRO, AND W. E. FORDYCE. Dynamics of ventilatory response to exercise in humans. *J. Appl. Physiol.* 51: 194–203, 1981.
50. BERG, W. E. Individual differences in respiratory gas exchange during recovery from moderate exercise. *Am. J. Physiol.* 149: 597–610, 1947.

50a. BESSMAN, S. P., AND P. G. GEIGER. Transport of energy in muscle: the phosphorylcreatine shuttle. *Science Wash. DC* 211: 448–452, 1981.

51. BEVEGÅRD, S., U. FREYSCHUSS, AND T. STRANDELL. Circulatory adaptation to arm and leg exercise in supine and sitting position. *J. Appl. Physiol.* 21: 37–46, 1966.
52. BINAK, K., N. HARMANCI, N. SIRMACI, N. ATAMAN, AND H. OGAN. Oxygen extraction rate of the myocardium at rest and on exercise in various conditions. *Br. Heart J.* 29: 422–427, 1966.
53. BING, R. J. The coronary circulation in health and disease as studied by coronary sinus catheterization. *Bull. NY Acad. Med.* 27: 407–424, 1951.
54. BITTERLI, J., H. BACHOFEN, K. KYD, AND M. SCHERRER. Repeated measurements of pulmonary O_2-diffusing capacity in man during graded exercise. In: *Pulmonary Diffusing Capacity on Exercise*, edited by M. Scherrer. Bern: Huber, 1971, p. 139–149.
55. BJURE, J. Pulmonary diffusing capacity for carbon monoxide in relation to cardiac output in man. *Scand. J. Clin. Lab. Invest. Suppl.* 81: 1–113, 1965.
56. BJURE, J., G. GRIMBY, AND N. J. NILSSON. Pulmonary gas exchange during submaximal and maximal exercise in healthy middle-aged men. In: *Pulmonary Diffusing Capacity on Exercise*, edited by M. Scherrer. Bern: Huber, 1971, p. 107–131.
57. BJURSTEDT, H., C. M. HESSER, G. LILJESTRAND, AND G. MATELL. Effects of posture on alveolar-arterial CO_2 and O_2 differences and on alveolar dead space in man. *Acta Physiol. Scand.* 54: 65–82, 1962.
58. BLAIR, D. A., W. E. GLOVER, AND I. C. RODDIE. Vasomotor responses in the human arm during leg exercise. *Circ. Res.* 9: 264–274, 1961.
59. BLOMQVIST, G., R. L. JOHNSON, JR., AND B. SALTIN. Pulmonary diffusing capacity limiting human performance at altitude. *Acta Physiol. Scand.* 76: 284–287, 1969.
60. BOHR, C. Über die spezifische Tätigkeit der Lungen bei der respiratorischen Gasaufnahme und ihr Verhalten zu der durch die Alveolarwand stattfindenden Gasdiffusion. *Skand. Arch. Physiol.* 22: 221–280, 1909.
61. BØJE, O. Uber die Grösse der Lungendiffusion des Menschen während Ruhe und körperlicher Arbeit. *Arbeitsphysiologie* 7: 157–166, 1933.
62. BONDE-PETERSEN, F., A. L. MORK, AND E. NIELSEN. Local muscle blood flow and sustained contractions of human arm and back muscles. *Eur. J. Appl. Physiol. Occup. Physiol.* 34: 43–50, 1975.
63. BORST, C., A. P. HOLLANDER, AND L. N. BOUMAN. Cardiac acceleration elicited by voluntary muscle contractions of minimal duration. *J. Appl. Physiol.* 32: 70–77, 1972.
64. BRADLEY, J., C. BYE, S. P. HAYDEN, AND D. T. HUGHES. Normal values of transfer factor and transfer coefficients in healthy males and females. *Respiration* 38: 221–226, 1979.
65. BRADLEY, S. E. Hepatic blood flow. Effect of posture and exercise upon blood flow through the liver. In: *Trans. Conf. Liver Injury, 7th*, edited by F. W. Hoffbauer. New York: Josiah Macy, Jr. Found., 1948, p. 53–56.
66. BRAUMANN, K. M., D. BÖNING, AND F. TROST. Oxygen dissociation curves in trained and untrained subjects. *Eur. J. Appl. Physiol. Occup. Physiol.* 42: 51–60, 1979.
67. BRAUNWALD, E. Control of myocardial oxygen consumption. Physiological and clinical considerations. *Am. J. Cardiol.* 27: 416–432, 1971.
68. BRAUNWALD, E., J. ROSS, JR., AND E. H. SONNENBLICK. Myocardial energetics. In: *Mechanisms of Contraction of the Normal and Failing Heart* (2nd ed.). Boston, MA: Little, Brown, 1976, p. 166–199.
69. BROMAN, S., AND O. WIGERTZ. Transient dynamics of ventilation and heart rate with step changes in work load from different load levels. *Acta Physiol. Scand.* 81: 54–74, 1971.

70. BROOKS, G. A., K. J. HITTELMAN, J. A. FAULKNER, AND R. E. BEYER. Temperature, skeletal muscle mitochondrial functions, and oxygen debt. *Am. J. Physiol.* 220: 1053–1059, 1971.
71. BROTHERHOOD, J., B. BROZOVIĆ, AND L. G. C. E. PUGH. Haematological status of middle- and long-distance runners. *Clin. Sci. Mol. Med.* 48: 139–145, 1975.
72. BRYAN, A. C., L. G. BENTIVOGLIO, F. BEEREL, H. MACLEISH, A. ZIDULKA, AND D. V. BATES. Factors affecting regional distribution of ventilation and perfusion in the lung. *J. Appl. Physiol.* 19: 395–402, 1964.
73. BUICK, F. J., N. GLEDHILL, A. B. FROESE, L. SPRIET, AND E. C. MEYERS. Effect of induced erythrocythemia on aerobic work capacity. *J. Appl. Physiol.* 48: 636–642, 1980.
74. BURROWS, B., J. E. KASIK, A. H. NIDEN, AND W. R. BARCLEY. Clinical usefulness of the single-breath pulmonary diffusing capacity test. *Am. Rev. Respir. Dis.* 84: 789–806, 1961.
75. CANDER, L., AND E. G. HANOWELL. Effects of fever on pulmonary diffusing capacity and pulmonary mechanics in man. *J. Appl. Physiol.* 18: 1065–1070, 1963.
76. CANFIELD, R. E., AND H. RAHN. Arterial-alveolar N_2 gas pressure differences due to ventilation-perfusion variations. *J. Appl. Physiol.* 10: 165–172, 1957.
77. CASABURI, R., M. L. WEISSMAN, D. J. HUNTSMAN, B. J. WHIPP, AND K. WASSERMAN. Determinants of gas exchange kinetics during exercise in the dog. *J. Appl. Physiol.* 46: 1054–1060, 1979.
78. CASABURI, R., B. J. WHIPP, K. WASSERMAN, W. L. BEAVER, AND S. N. KOYAL. Ventilatory and gas exchange dynamics in response to sinusoidal work. *J. Appl. Physiol.* 42: 300–311, 1977.
79. CERRETELLI, P. Limiting factors to oxygen transport on Mount Everest. *J. Appl. Physiol.* 40: 658–667, 1976.
80. CERRETELLI, P. Metabolismo ossidativo ed anaerobico nel soggetto acclimatato all'altitudine. *Minerva Aerosp.* 67: 11–26, 1976.
81. CERRETELLI, P. Gas exchange at altitude. In: *Pulmonary Gas Exchange. Organism and Environment*, edited by J. B. West. New York: Academic, 1980, vol. II, p. 97–147.
82. CERRETELLI, P. Energy metabolism during exercise at altitude. In: *Medicine and Sport. Physiological Chemistry of Exercise and Training*, edited by P. E. di Prampero and J. R. Poortmans. Basel: Karger, 1981, vol. 13, p. 175–190.
83. CERRETELLI, P., P. AGHEMO, AND E. ROVELLI. Aspetti fisiologici dell'adolescente in relazione alla pratica dell'esercizio fisico. *Med. Sport Turin* 21: 400–406, 1968.
84. CERRETELLI, P., M. BLAU, D. PENDERGAST, C. EISENHARDT, D. W. RENNIE, J. STEINBACH, AND G. ENTINE. Cadmium telluride ^{133}Xe clearance detector for muscle flow studies. *IEEE Trans. Nucl. Sci.* NS-25: 620–623, 1978.
85. CERRETELLI, P., AND I. BRAMBILLA. Cinetica della contrazione di un debito di O_2 nell'uomo. *Boll. Soc. Ital. Biol. Sper.* 34: 679–682, 1958.
86. CERRETELLI, P., J. C. CRUZ, L. E. FARHI, AND H. RAHN. Determination of mixed venous O_2 and CO_2 tensions and cardiac output by a rebreathing method. *Respir. Physiol.* 1: 258–264, 1966.
87. CERRETELLI, P., P. E. DI PRAMPERO, AND D. W. RENNIE. Measurement of mixed venous oxygen tension by a modified rebreathing procedure. *J. Appl. Physiol.* 28: 707–711, 1970.
88. CERRETELLI, P., C. MARCONI, D. PENDERGAST, M. MEYER, N. HEISLER, AND J. PIIPER. Blood flow in exercising muscles by xenon clearance and by microsphere trapping. *J. Appl. Physiol.* 56: 24–30, 1984.
89. CERRETELLI, P., D. PENDERGAST, W. C. PAGANELLI, AND D. W. RENNIE. Effects of specific muscle training on $\dot{V}O_2$ on-response and early blood lactate. *J. Appl. Physiol.* 47: 761–769, 1979.
90. CERRETELLI, P., J. PIIPER, F. MANGILI, F. CUTTICA, AND B. RICCI. Circulation in exercising dogs. *J. Appl. Physiol.* 19: 29–32, 1964.
91. CERRETELLI, P., J. PIIPER, F. MANGILI, AND B. RICCI. Aerobic and anaerobic metabolism in exercising dogs. *J. Appl. Physiol.* 19: 25–28, 1964.
92. CERRETELLI, P., AND P. RADOVANI. Il massimo consumo di O_2 in atleti olimpionici di varie specialità. *Boll. Soc. Ital. Biol. Sper.* 36: 1871–1872, 1960.
93. CERRETELLI, P., D. SHINDELL, D. P. PENDERGAST, P. E. DI PRAMPERO, AND D. W. RENNIE. Oxygen uptake transients at the onset and offset of arm and leg work. *Respir. Physiol.* 30: 81–97, 1977.
94. CERRETELLI, P., R. SIKAND, AND L. E. FARHI. Readjustments in cardiac output and gas exchange during onset of exercise and recovery. *J. Appl. Physiol.* 21: 1345–1350, 1966.
95. CERRETELLI, P., R. S. SIKAND, AND L. E. FARHI. Effect of increased airway resistance on ventilation and gas exchange during exercise. *J. Appl. Physiol.* 27: 597–600, 1969.
96. CERRETELLI, P., A. VEICSTEINAS, M. FUMAGALLI, AND L. DELL'ORTO. Energetics of isometric exercise in man. *J. Appl. Physiol.* 41: 136–141, 1976.
97. CERRETELLI, P., A. VEICSTEINAS, M. SAMAJA, AND E. ROVELLI. Effets de l'entraînement physique sur la courbe de dissociation de l'oxyhémoglobine (CDO) (Abstract). *J. Physiol. Paris* 76: 45A, 1980.
98. CERRETELLI, P., A. VEICSTEINAS, J. TEICHMANN, H. MAGNUSSEN, AND J. PIIPER. Estimation by a rebreathing method of pulmonary O_2 diffusing capacity in man. *J. Appl. Physiol.* 37: 526–532, 1974.
99. CHANCE, B., G. MAURIELLO, AND X. AUBERT. ADP arrival at muscle mitochondria following a twitch. In: *Muscle as a Tissue*, edited by K. Rodahl and S. M. Horvath. New York: McGraw-Hill, 1962, p. 128–145.
100. CHASSIN, P. S., C. R. TAYLOR, N. C. HEGLUND, AND H. J. SEEHERMAN. Locomotion in lions: energetic cost and maximum aerobic capacity. *Physiol. Zool.* 49: 1–10, 1976.
101. CHATONNET, J., AND Y. MINAIRE. Comparison of energy expenditure during exercise and cold exposure in the dog. *Federation Proc.* 25: 1348–1350, 1966.
102. CLAUSEN, J. P. Effect of physical training on cardiovascular adjustments to exercise in man. *Physiol. Rev.* 57: 779–815, 1977.
103. CLAUSEN, J. P., K. KLAUSEN, B. RASMUSSEN, AND J. TRAP-JENSEN. Central and peripheral circulatory changes after training of the arms or legs. *Am. J. Physiol.* 225: 675–682, 1973.
104. CLAUSEN, J. P., AND N. A. LASSEN. Muscle blood flow during exercise in normal man studied by the ^{133}Xenon clearance method. *Cardiovasc. Res.* 5: 245–254, 1971.
105. COFFMAN, J. D., AND D. E. GREGG. Blood flow and oxygen debt from coronary artery occlusion. *Clin. Res.* 8: 179, 1960.
106. COHN, J. E., D. G. CARROLL, B. W. ARMSTRONG, R. H. SHEPARD, AND R. L. RILEY. Maximal diffusing capacity of the lung in normal male subjects of different ages. *J. Appl. Physiol.* 6: 588–597, 1954.
107. CONVERTINO, V. A., P. J. BROCK, L. C. KEIL, E. M. BERNAUER, AND J. E. GREENLEAF. Exercise training-induced hypervolemia: role of plasma albumin, renin, and vasopressin. *J. Appl. Physiol.* 48: 665–669, 1980.
108. COOTE, J. H., AND J. F. PÉREZ-GONZÁLES. The response of some sympathetic neurones to volleys in various afferent nerves. *J. Physiol. Lond.* 208: 261–278, 1970.
109. COSTILL, D. L., L. BRANAM, D. EDDY, AND W. FINK. Alterations in red cell volume following exercise and dehydration. *J. Appl. Physiol.* 37: 912–916, 1974.
109a. COYLE, E. F., W. H. MARTIN III, D. R. SINACORE, M. J. JOYNER, J. M. HAGBERG, AND J. O. HOLLOSZY. Time course of loss of adaptations after stopping prolonged intense endurance training. *J. Appl. Physiol.* 57: 1857–1864, 1984.
110. CRAIG, F. N. Oxygen uptake at the beginning of work. *J. Appl. Physiol.* 33: 611–615, 1972.
111. CRAYTON, S. C., R. AUNG-DIN, D. E. FIXLER, AND J. H. MITCHELL. Distribution of cardiac output during induced isometric exercise in dogs. *Am. J. Physiol.* 236 (*Heart Circ. Physiol.* 5): H218–H224, 1979.
112. CROPP, G. J. A., AND J. H. COMROE, JR. Role of mixed venous

blood P_{CO_2} in respiratory control. *J. Appl. Physiol.* 16: 1029–1033, 1961.

113. Cross, C. E., H. Gong, C. J. Kurpershoek, J. R. Gillespie, and R. W. Hyde. Alterations in distribution of blood flow to the lung's diffusion surfaces during exercise. *J. Clin. Invest.* 52: 414–421, 1973.
114. Cruz, J. C. Mechanics of breathing in high altitude and sea level subjects. *Respir. Physiol.* 17: 146–161, 1973.
115. Cugell, D. W., A. Marks, M. F. Ellicott, T. L. Badger, and E. A. Gaensler. Carbon monoxide diffusing capacity during steady exercise. Comparison of physiological and histological findings in patients with pulmonary fibrosis and granulomatosis. *Am. Rev. Tuberc. Pulm. Dis.* 74: 317–342, 1956.
116. Daly, W. J. Pulmonary diffusing capacity for carbon monoxide and topography of perfusion during changes in alveolar pressure in man. *Am. Rev. Respir. Dis.* 99: 548–553, 1969.
117. Daly, W. J., and J. W. Roe. The effect of a Valsalva manoeuvre on the pulmonary diffusing capacity for carbon monoxide in man. *Clin. Sci. Lond.* 23: 405–409, 1962.
118. D'Angelo, E., and G. Torelli. Neural stimuli increasing respiration during different types of exercise. *J. Appl. Physiol.* 30: 116–121, 1971.
119. Danzer, L. A., J. E. Cohn, and F. W. Zechman. Relationship of D_M and V_C to pulmonary diffusing capacity during exercise. *Respir. Physiol.* 5: 250–258, 1968.
120. Davies, C. T. M., C. Barnes, R. H. Fox, R. O. Ojikutu, and A. S. Samueloff. Ethnic differences in physical working capacity. *J. Appl. Physiol.* 33: 726–732, 1972.
121. Davies, C. T. M., P. E. di Prampero, and P. Cerretelli. Kinetics of cardiac output and respiratory gas exchange during exercise and recovery. *J. Appl. Physiol.* 32: 618–625, 1972.
122. Davies, C. T. M., and A. J. Sargeant. Indirect determination of maximal aerobic power output during work with one or two limbs. *Eur. J. Appl. Physiol. Occup. Physiol.* 32: 207–215, 1974.
123. Davies, C. T. M., and J. P. M. Van Haaren. Maximum aerobic power and body composition in healthy East African older male and female subjects. *Am. J. Phys. Anthropol.* 39: 395–401, 1973.
124. Davis, J. A., M. H. Frank, B. J. Whipp, and K. Wasserman. Anaerobic threshold alterations caused by endurance training in middle-aged men. *J. Appl. Physiol.* 46: 1039–1046, 1979.
124a. Dawson, M. J., D. G. Gadian, and D. R. Wilkie. Studies of the biochemistry of contracting and relaxing muscle by the use of ^{31}P n.m.r. in conjunction with other techniques. *Philos. Trans. R. Soc. Lond. B Biol. Sci.* 289: 445–455, 1980.
125. Dechoux, J., and C. Pivoteau. La capacité de diffusion alvéolo-capillaire. Sa mesure chez le sujet normal et le silicotique. *Rev. Tuberc. Pneumol.* 24: 267–282, 1960.
126. DeGraff, A. C., Jr., R. F. Grover, R. L. Johnson, Jr., J. W. Hammond, Jr., and J. M. Miller. Diffusing capacity of the lung in Caucasians native to 3,100 m. *J. Appl. Physiol.* 29: 71–76, 1970.
127. Dejours, P. La régulation de la ventilation au cours de l'exercice musculaire chez l'homme. *J. Physiol. Paris* 51: 163–261, 1959.
128. Dejours, P. The regulation of breathing during muscular exercise in man—a neuro-humoral theory. In: *The Regulation of Human Respiration*, edited by D. J. C. Cunningham and B. B. Lloyd. Oxford: Blackwell, 1963, p. 335–347.
129. Dejours, P. Neurogenic factors in the control of ventilation during exercise. *Circ. Res.* 20: 146–153, 1967.
130. Dejours, P., R. Flandrois, R. Lefrançois, and A. Teillac. Etude de la régulation de la ventilation au cours de l'exercice musculaire chez l'homme (Abstract). *J. Physiol. Paris* 53: 321, 1961.
131. Dejours, P., J. Raynaud, C. L. Cuenod, and Y. Labrousse. Modifications instantanées de la ventilation au début et à l'arrêt de l'exercice musculaire. Interprétation. *J. Physiol. Paris* 47: 155–159, 1955.
132. Demedts, M., and N. R. Anthonisen. Effects of increased external airway resistance during steady-state exercise. *J. Appl. Physiol.* 35: 361–366, 1973.
133. De Moor, J. C. Individual differences in oxygen debt curves related to mechanical efficiency and sex. *J. Appl. Physiol.* 6: 460–466, 1954.
133a. Dempsey, J. A., P. G. Hanson, and K. S. Henderson. Exercise-induced arterial hypoxaemia in healthy human subjects at sea level. *J. Physiol. Lond.* 355: 161–175, 1984.
134. Dempsey, J. A., W. G. Reddan, M. L. Birnbaum, H. V. Forster, J. S. Thoden, R. F. Grover, and J. Rankin. Effects of acute through life-long hypoxic exposure on exercise pulmonary gas exchange. *Respir. Physiol.* 13: 62–89, 1971.
135. Dempsey, J. A., J. M. Thomson, H. V. Forster, F. C. Cerny, and L. W. Chosey. HbO_2 dissociation in man during prolonged work in chronic hypoxia. *J. Appl. Physiol.* 38: 1022–1029, 1975.
136. Diamond, L. B., R. Casaburi, K. Wasserman, and B. J. Whipp. Kinetics of gas exchange and ventilation in transitions from rest or prior exercise. *J. Appl. Physiol.* 43: 704–708, 1977.
137. Di Prampero, P. E. Energetics of muscular exercise. *Rev. Physiol. Biochem. Pharmacol.* 89: 143–222, 1981.
137a. Di Prampero, P. E. The control of muscle oxygen consumption after heavy exercise. *Boll. Soc. Ital. Biol. Sper.* 40 Suppl. 3: 80–81, 1984.
137b. Di Prampero, P. E. Metabolic and circulatory limitations to $\dot{V}_{O_2}$max at the whole animal level. *J. Exp. Biol.* 115: 319–331, 1985.
138. Di Prampero, P. E., and P. Cerretelli. Maximal muscular power (aerobic and anaerobic) in African natives. *Ergonomics* 12: 51–59, 1969.
139. Di Prampero, P. E., C. T. M. Davies, P. Cerretelli, and R. Margaria. An analysis of O_2 debt contracted in submaximal exercise. *J. Appl. Physiol.* 29: 547–551, 1970.
140. Di Prampero, P. E., and R. Margaria. Relationship between O_2 consumption, high energy phosphates and the kinetics of O_2 debt in exercise. *Pfluegers Arch.* 304: 11–19, 1968.
141. Di Prampero, P. E., and R. Margaria. Mechanical efficiency of phosphagen (ATP + CP) splitting and its speed of resynthesis. *Pfluegers Arch.* 308: 197–202, 1969.
142. Di Prampero, P. E., L. Peeters, and R. Margaria. Alactic O_2 debt and lactic acid production after exhausting exercise in man. *J. Appl. Physiol.* 34: 628–632, 1973.
143. Di Prampero, P. E., F. Piñera-Limas, and G. Sassi. Maximal muscular power, aerobic and anaerobic, in 116 athletes performing at the XIXth Olympic Games in Mexico. *Ergonomics* 13: 665–674, 1970.
144. Doll, E. J., J. Keul, C. Maiwald, and H. Reindell. Das Verhalten von Sauerstoffdruck, Kohlensäuredruck, pH, Standardbicarbonat und Base Excess im arteriellen Blut bei verschiedenen Belastungsformen. *Int. Z. Angew. Physiol. Einschl. Arbeitsphysiol.* 22: 327–355, 1966.
145. Donald, D. E., and D. Ferguson. Response of heart rate, oxygen consumption and arterial blood pressure to graded exercise in dogs. *Proc. Soc. Exp. Biol. Med.* 121: 626–630, 1966.
146. Donald, D. E., S. E. Milburn, and J. T. Shepherd. Effect of cardiac denervation on the maximal capacity for exercise in the racing greyhound. *J. Appl. Physiol.* 19: 849–852, 1964.
147. Donald, D. E., and J. T. Shepherd. Initial cardiovascular adjustment to exercise in dogs with chronic cardiac denervation. *Am. J. Physiol.* 207: 1325–1329, 1964.
148. Donald, K. W., A. R. Lind, G. W. McNicol, P. W. Humphreys, S. H. Taylor, and H. P. Staunton. Cardiovascular response to sustained (static) contractions. *Circ. Res.* 20: 15–30, 1967.
149. Donevan, R. E., W. H. Palmer, C. J. Varvis, and D. V. Bates. Influence of age on pulmonary diffusing capacity. *J. Appl. Physiol.* 14: 483–492, 1959.
149a. Donovan, C. M., and G. A. Brooks. Endurance training affects lactate clearance, not lactate production. *Am. J. Physiol.* 244 (*Endocrinol. Metab.* 7): E83–E92, 1983.
150. Eaton, J. W., J. A. Faulkner, and G. J. Brewer. Increased

2,3-diphosphoglycerate (DPG) in the human red blood cell during muscular exercise (Abstract). *Physiologist* 12: 212, 1969.

151. Ekblom, B. Effect of physical training on oxygen transport system in man. *Acta Physiol. Scand. Suppl.* 328: 1–45, 1969.
152. Ekblom, B., P.-O. Åstrand, B. Saltin, J. Stenberg, and B. Wallström. Effect of training on circulatory response to exercise. *J. Appl. Physiol.* 24: 518–528, 1968.
153. Ekblom, B., A. N. Goldbarg, and B. Gullbring. Response to exercise after blood loss and reinfusion. *J. Appl. Physiol.* 33: 175–180, 1972.
154. Ekblom, B., A. N. Goldbarg, A. Kilbom, and P.-O. Åstrand. Effects of atropine and propranolol on the oxygen transport system during exercise in man. *Scand. J. Clin. Lab. Invest.* 30: 35–42, 1972.
155. Ekblom, B., and L. Hermansen. Cardiac output in athletes. *J. Appl. Physiol.* 25: 619–625, 1968.
156. Ekblom, B., and R. Huot. Response to submaximal exercise at different levels of carboxyhemoglobin. *Acta Physiol. Scand.* 86: 474–482, 1972.
157. Ekblom, B., R. Huot, E. M. Stein, and A. T. Thorstensson. Effect of changes in arterial oxygen content on circulation and physical performance. *J. Appl. Physiol.* 39: 71–75, 1975.
158. Ekblom, B., G. Wilson, and P.-O. Åstrand. Central circulation during exercise after venesection and reinfusion of red blood cells. *J. Appl. Physiol.* 40: 379–383, 1976.
159. Ekelund, L. G. Circulatory and respiratory adaptation during prolonged exercise in the supine position. *Acta Physiol. Scand.* 68: 382–396, 1966.
160. Epstein, S. E., B. F. Robinson, R. L. Kahler, and E. Braunwald. Effects of beta-adrenergic blockade on cardiac response to maximal and submaximal exercise in man. *J. Clin. Invest.* 44: 1745–1753, 1965.

160a. Erickson-Viitanen, S., P. J. Geiger, P. Viitanen, and S. P. Bessman. Compartmentation of mitochondrial creatine phosphokinase. II. The importance of the outer mitochondrial membrane for mitochondrial compartmentation. *J. Biol. Chem.* 257: 14405–14411, 1982.

160b. Erickson-Viitanen, S., P. Viitanen, P. J. Geiger, W. C. T. Yang, and S. P. Bessman. Compartmentation of mitochondrial creatine phosphokinase. I. Direct demonstration of compartmentation with the use of labeled precursors. *J. Biol. Chem.* 257: 14395–14404, 1982.

161. Eriksson, B. O., G. Grimby, and B. Saltin. Cardiac output and arterial blood gases during exercise in pubertal boys. *J. Appl. Physiol.* 31: 348–352, 1971.
162. Fagraeus, L., J. Karlsson, D. Linnarsson, and B. Saltin. Oxygen uptake during maximal work at lowered and raised ambient air pressures. *Acta Physiol. Scand.* 87: 411–421, 1973.
163. Fagraeus, L., and D. Linnarsson. Autonomic origin of heart rate fluctuations at the onset of muscular exercise. *J. Appl. Physiol.* 40: 679–682, 1976.
164. Farhi, L. E. Ventilation-perfusion relationship and its role in alveolar gas exchange. In: *Advances in Respiratory Physiology*, edited by C. G. Caro. London: Arnold, 1966, p. 148–197.
165. Farhi, L. E., and H. Rahn. A theoretical analysis of the alveolar-arterial O_2 difference with special reference to the distribution effect. *J. Appl. Physiol.* 7: 699–703, 1955.
166. Farney, R. J., A. H. Morris, R. M. Gardner, and J. D. Armstrong, Jr. Rebreathing pulmonary capillary and tissue volume in normals after saline infusion. *J. Appl. Physiol.* 43: 246–253, 1977.
167. Faulkner, J. A., G. J. Brewer, and J. W. Eaton. Adaptation of the red blood cell to muscular exercise. *Adv. Exp. Med. Biol.* 6: 213–217, 1970.
168. Filley, G. F., F. Gregoire, and G. W. Wright. Alveolar and arterial oxygen tension and the significance of the alveolar-arterial oxygen tension difference in normal man. *J. Clin. Invest.* 33: 517–529, 1954.
169. Filley, G. F., D. J. MacIntosh, and G. W. Wright. Carbon monoxide uptake and pulmonary diffusing capacity in normal subjects at rest and during exercise. *J. Clin. Invest.* 33: 530–539, 1954.
170. Fixler, D. E., J. M. Atkins, J. H. Mitchell, and L. D. Horwitz. Blood flow to respiratory, cardiac, and limb muscles in dogs during graded exercise. *Am. J. Physiol.* 231: 1515–1519, 1976.
171. Flandrois, R., J. R. Lacour, J. P. Charbonnier, M. Gressier, and J. Genety. Capacité aérobie chez l'athlète français. *Med. Sport Paris* 47: 186–189, 1973.
172. Flandrois, R., R. Puccinelli, Y. Houdas, and R. Lefrançois. Comparison des consommations maximales d'oxygène mesurée et théorique d'une population française. *J. Physiol. Paris* 54: 301–302, 1962.
173. Flatley, F. J., H. Constantine, R. M. McCredie, and P. N. Yu. Pulmonary diffusing capacity and pulmonary capillary blood volume in normal subjects and in cardiac patients. *Am. Heart J.* 64: 159–168, 1962.
174. Forsberg, A., P. Tesch, B. Sjödin, A. Thorstensson, and J. Karlsson. Skeletal muscle fibers and athletic performance. In: *Biomechanics V*, edited by P. V. Komi. Baltimore, MD: University Park, 1976, vol. A, p. 112–117. (Int. Ser. Biomech.)
175. Forster, R. E. Can alveolar P_{CO_2} exceed pulmonary end-capillary CO_2? No. *J. Appl. Physiol.* 42: 323–328, 1977.
176. Forster, R. E., F. J. W. Roughton, L. Cander, W. A. Briscoe, and F. Kreuzer. Apparent pulmonary diffusing capacity for CO at varying alveolar O_2 tensions. *J. Appl. Physiol.* 11: 277–289, 1957.
177. Frayser, R., J. C. Ross, H. S. Levin, J. V. Messer, and J. Pines. Effect of increased environmental temperature on pulmonary diffusing capacity. *J. Appl. Physiol.* 21: 147–150, 1966.
178. Freedman, S. Sustained maximum voluntary ventilation. *Respir. Physiol.* 8: 230–244, 1970.
179. Freyschuss, U. Cardiovascular adjustment to somatomotor activation. *Acta Physiol. Scand. Suppl.* 342: 1–63, 1970.
180. Freyschuss, U., and A. Holmgren. On the variation of $D_{L_{CO}}$ with increasing oxygen uptake during exercise in healthy ordinarily trained young men and women. *Acta Physiol. Scand.* 65: 193–206, 1965.
181. Freyschuss, U., and T. Strandell. Limb circulation during arm and leg exercise in supine position. *J. Appl. Physiol.* 23: 163–170, 1967.
182. Freyschuss, U., and T. Strandell. Circulatory adaptation to one- and two-leg exercise in supine position. *J. Appl. Physiol.* 25: 511–515, 1968.
183. Gaensler, E. A., and A. A. Smith. Attachment for automated single breath diffusing capacity measurement. *Chest* 63: 136–145, 1973.
184. Garman, R. F., R. W. Hyde, A. B. Fischer, and R. E. Forster. The single breath O_2 diffusing capacity ($D_{L_{O_2}}$) at rest and exercise; its use in determining pulmonary diffusion/perfusion relationships (Abstract). *Physiologist* 13: 200, 1970.
185. Gebert, G. Messung der K^+- und Na^+-Aktivität mit Mikroglaselektroden im Extrazellulärraum des Kaninchenskelettmuskels bei Muskelarbeit. *Pfluegers Arch.* 331: 204–214, 1972.
186. Georges, R., G. Saumon, and A. Loiseau. The relationship of age to pulmonary membrane conductance and capillary blood volume. *Am. Rev. Respir. Dis.* 117: 1069–1078, 1978.
187. Gerlach, E. Stoffwechsel der Skelettmuskulatur. *Wien. Klin. Wochenschr.* 13: 229–234, 1967.
188. Geyssant, A., J. Denis, J. Coudert, J. Riffat, D. Dormois, and J. R. Lacour. Effet de l'entraînement à l'exercice de longue durée sur l'affinité de l'hémoglobine pour l'oxygène (Abstract). *J. Physiol. Paris* 75: 54A, 1979.
189. Gibbs, C. L., and J. B. Chapman. Cardiac energetics. In: *Handbook of Physiology. The Cardiovascular System. The Heart*, edited by R. M. Berne and N. Sperelakis. Bethesda, MD: Am. Physiol. Soc., 1979, sect. 2, vol. I, chapt. 22, p. 775–804.

189a. Giezendanner, D., P. Cerretelli, and P. E. di Prampero. Breath-by-breath alveolar gas exchange. *J. Appl. Physiol.* 55: 583–590, 1983.

190. GILBERT, R., J. H. AUCHINCLOSS, JR., AND G. H. BAULE. Metabolic and circulatory adjustments to unsteady-state exercise. *J. Appl. Physiol.* 22: 905–912, 1967.
191. GLEDHILL, N., A. B. FROESE, F. J. BUICK, AND A. C. BRYAN. $\dot{V}A/\dot{Q}$ inhomogeneity and $AaDO_2$ in man during exercise: effect of SF_6 breathing. *J. Appl. Physiol.* 45: 512–515, 1978.
192. GLICK, Z., AND E. SHVARTZ. Physical working capacity of young men of different ethnic groups in Israel. *J. Appl. Physiol.* 37: 22–26, 1974.
193. GOLLNICK, P. D., R. B. ARMSTRONG, B. SALTIN, C. W. SAUBERT IV, W. L. SEMBROWICH, AND R. E. SHEPHERD. Effect of training on enzyme activity and fiber composition of human skeletal muscle. *J. Appl. Physiol.* 34: 107–111, 1973.
194. GOLLNICK, P. D., P. J. STRUCK, R. G. SOULE, AND J. R. HEINRICK. Effect of exercise and training on the blood of normal and splenectomized rats. *Int. Z. Angew. Physiol. Einschl. Arbeitsphysiol.* 21: 169–178, 1965.
195. GONG, H., C. J. KURPERSHOEK, AND C. E. CROSS. $^{18}O_2$ diffusing capacity measured by a rebreathing method in normal man (Abstract). *Clin. Res.* 20: 195, 1972.
196. GONG, H., C. J. KURPERSHOEK, D. B. MEYER, AND C. E. CROSS. Effects of cardiac output on $^{18}O_2$ lung diffusion in normal resting man. *Respir. Physiol.* 16: 313–316, 1972.
197. GONG, H., D. MEYER, R. HYDE, J. GILLESPIE, AND C. E. CROSS. $^{18}O_2$ diffusing capacity at rest and during exercise in normal man (Abstract). *Clin. Res.* 18: 484, 1970.
198. GOODWIN, G. M., D. I. MCCLOSKEY, AND J. H. MITCHELL. Cardiovascular and respiratory responses to changes in central command during isometric exercise at constant muscle tension. *J. Physiol. Lond.* 226: 173–190, 1972.
199. GORESKY, C. A., J. W. WARNICA, J. H. BURGESS, AND B. E. NADEAU. Effect of exercise on dilution estimates of extravascular lung water and on carbon monoxide diffusing capacity in normal adults. *Circ. Res.* 37: 379–389, 1975.
200. GRAHAM, T. P., J. W. COVELL, E. H. SONNENBLICK, J. ROSS, AND E. BRAUNWALD. Control of myocardial oxygen consumption: relative influence of contractile state and tension development. *J. Clin. Invest.* 47: 375–385, 1968.
201. GRANATH, A., B. JONSSON, AND T. STRANDELL. Circulation in healthy old men, studied by right heart catheterization at rest and during exercise in supine and sitting position. *Acta Med. Scand.* 176: 425–446, 1964.
202. GRIMBY, G. Renal clearances during prolonged supine exercise at different loads. *J. Appl. Physiol.* 20: 1294–1298, 1965.
203. GRIMBY, G., E. HÄGGENDAL, AND B. SALTIN. Local xenon 133 clearance from the quadriceps muscle during exercise in man. *J. Appl. Physiol.* 22: 305–310, 1967.
204. GULERIA, J. S., J. N. PANDE, P. K. SETHI, AND S. B. ROY. Pulmonary diffusing capacity at high altitude. *J. Appl. Physiol.* 31: 536–543, 1971.
205. GURTNER, G. H. Can alveolar P_{CO_2} exceed pulmonary end-capillary CO_2? Yes. *J. Appl. Physiol.* 42: 323–328, 1977.
206. GUYTON, A. C., C. E. JONES, AND T. G. COLEMAN. Cardiac output in muscular exercise. In: *Circulatory Physiology: Cardiac Output and its Regulation* (2nd ed.). Philadelphia, PA: Saunders, 1973, p. 436–450.
207. GUZMAN, C. A., AND E. D. SUMMERS. Pulmonary diffusing capacity during exercise in women. *Chest* 64: 678–682, 1973.
208. HAAB, P., C. PERRET, AND J. PIIPER. La capacité de diffusion pulmonaire pour l'oxygène chez l'homme normal jeune. *Helv. Physiol. Pharmacol. Acta* 23: C23–C25, 1965.
209. HAGBERG, J. M., R. C. HICKSON, A. A. EHSANI, AND J. O. HOLLOSZY. Faster adjustment to and recovery from submaximal exercise in the trained state. *J. Appl. Physiol.* 48: 218–224, 1980.
210. HAGBERG, J. M., J. P. MULLIN, AND F. J. NAGLE. Oxygen consumption during constant-load exercise. *J. Appl. Physiol.* 45: 381–384, 1978.
211. HAGBERG, J. M., F. J. NAGLE, AND J. L. CARLSON. Transient O_2 uptake response at the onset of exercise. *J. Appl. Physiol.* 44: 90–92, 1978.
212. HAMILTON, L. H., AND D. J. KERSTING. A study of gas analysis for measurement of pulmonary diffusing capacity for carbon monoxide by chromatographic techniques. *Am. Rev. Respir. Dis.* 102: 916–920, 1970.
213. HANSON, J. S., AND B. S. TABAKIN. Carbon monoxide diffusing capacity in normal male subjects, age 20–60, during exercise. *J. Appl. Physiol.* 15: 402–404, 1960.
214. HANSON, J. S., B. S. TABAKIN, AND A. M. LEVY. Exercise arterial blood gas and end-tidal gas changes during acute airway obstruction. *Respir. Physiol.* 3: 64–77, 1967.
215. HARRIS, R. C., R. H. T. EDWARDS, E. HULTMAN, L.-O. NORDESJÖ, B. NYLIND, AND K. SAHLIN. The time course of phosphoryl-creatine resynthesis during recovery of the quadriceps muscle in man. *Pfluegers Arch.* 367: 137–142, 1976.
216. HARRIS, R. C., K. SAHLIN, AND E. HULTMAN. Phosphagen and lactate contents of m. quadriceps femoris of man after exercise. *J. Appl. Physiol.* 43: 852–857, 1977.
217. HARTLEY, L. H., G. GRIMBY, Å. KILBOM, N. J. NILSSON, I. ÅSTRAND, J. BJURE, B. EKBLOM, AND B. SALTIN. Physical training in sedentary middle-aged and older men. III. Cardiac output and gas exchange at submaximal and maximal exercise. *Scand. J. Clin. Lab. Invest.* 24: 335–344, 1969.
218. HEATH, G. W., J. M. HAGBERG, A. A. EHSANI, AND J. O. HOLLOSZY. A physiological comparison of young and older endurance athletes. *J. Appl. Physiol.* 51: 634–640, 1981.
219. HENRIKSSON, J. Training induced adaptation of skeletal muscle and metabolism during submaximal exercise. *J. Physiol. Lond.* 270: 661–675, 1977.
220. HENRIKSSON, J., AND J. S. REITMAN. Quantitative measures of enzyme activities in type I and type II muscle fibres of man after training. *Acta Physiol. Scand.* 97: 392–397, 1976.
221. HENRIKSSON, J., AND J. S. REITMAN. Time course of changes in human skeletal muscle succinate dehydrogenase and cytochrome oxidase activities and maximal oxygen uptake with physical activity and inactivity. *Acta Physiol. Scand.* 99: 91–97, 1977.
222. HENRY, F. M. Aerobic oxygen consumption and alactic debt in muscular work. *J. Appl. Physiol.* 3: 427–438, 1951.
223. HENRY, F. M., AND W. E. BERG. Physiological and performance changes in athletic conditioning. *J. Appl. Physiol.* 3: 103–111, 1950.
224. HENRY, F. M., AND J. DEMOOR. Metabolic efficiency of exercise in relation to work load at constant speed. *J. Appl. Physiol.* 2: 481–487, 1950.
225. HENRY, F. M., AND J. DEMOOR. Lactic and alactic oxygen consumption in moderate exercise of graded intensity. *J. Appl. Physiol.* 8: 608–614, 1956.
226. HERMANSEN, L., AND K. L. ANDERSEN. Aerobic work capacity in young Norwegian men and women. *J. Appl. Physiol.* 20: 425–431, 1965.
227. HERMANSEN, L., B. EKBLOM, AND B. SALTIN. Cardiac output during submaximal and maximal treadmill and bicycle exercise. *J. Appl. Physiol.* 29: 82–86, 1970.
228. HERMANSEN, L., AND I. STENSVOLD. Production and removal of lactate during exercise in man. *Acta Physiol. Scand.* 86: 191–201, 1972.
229. HESSER, C. M., D. LINNARSSON, AND L. FAGRAEUS. Pulmonary mechanics and work of breathing at maximal ventilation and raised air pressure. *J. Appl. Physiol.* 50: 747–753, 1981.
230. HESSER, C. M., AND G. MATELL. Effect of light and moderate exercise on alveolar-arterial O_2 tension difference in man. *Acta Physiol. Scand.* 63: 247–256, 1965.
231. HICKSON, R. C., H. A. BOMZE, AND J. O. HOLLOSZY. Faster adjustment of O_2 uptake to the energy requirement of exercise in the trained state. *J. Appl. Physiol.* 44: 877–881, 1978.
232. HILL, A. V., C. N. H. LONG, AND H. LUPTON. Muscular exercise, lactic acid and the supply and utilization of oxygen. Pt. IV. *Proc. R. Soc. Lond. B. Biol. Sci.* 97: 84–95, 1924.
233. HIRCHE, H., H. SCHUMACHER, AND H. HAGEMANN. Extracellular K^+ concentration and K^+ balance of the gastrocnemius muscle of the dog during exercise. *Pfluegers Arch.* 387: 231–

237, 1980.

234. HNÍK, P., M. HOLAS, I. KREKULE, N. KŘIŽ, J. MEJSNAR, V. SMIEŠKO, E. UJEC, AND F. VYSKOČIL. Work-induced potassium changes in skeletal muscle and effluent venous blood assessed by liquid ion-exchanger microelectrodes. *Pfluegers Arch.* 362: 85–94, 1976.
235. HNÍK, P., O. HUDLICKÁ, J. KUČERA, AND R. PAYNE. Activation of muscle afferents by nonproprioceptive stimuli. *Am. J. Physiol.* 217: 1451–1458, 1969.
236. HOLLAND, J., J. MILIC-EMILI, P. T. MACKLEM, AND D. V. BATES. Regional distribution of pulmonary ventilation and perfusion in elderly subjects. *J. Clin. Invest.* 47: 81–92, 1968.
237. HOLLAND, R. A. B., AND R. B. BLACKET. The carbon monoxide diffusing capacity of the lung in normal subjects. *Australas. Ann. Med.* 7: 192–203, 1958.
238. HOLLANDER, A. P., AND L. N. BOUMAN. Cardiac acceleration in man elicited by a muscle-heart reflex. *J. Appl. Physiol.* 38: 272–278, 1975.
239. HOLLOSZY, J. O., AND F. W. BOOTH. Biochemical adaptations to endurance exercise in muscle. *Annu. Rev. Physiol.* 38: 273–291, 1976.
240. HOLLOSZY, J. O., M. J. RENNIE, R. C. HICKSON, R. K. CONLEE, AND J. M. HAGBERG. Physiological consequences of the biochemical adaptation to endurance exercise. *Ann. NY Acad. Sci.* 301: 440–450, 1977.
241. HOLMBERG, S., W. SERZYSKO, AND E. VARNAUSKAS. Coronary circulation during heavy exercise in control subjects and patients with coronary heart disease. *Acta Med. Scand.* 190: 465–480, 1971.
242. HOLMGREN, A. Circulatory changes during muscular work in man: with special reference to arterial and central venous pressures in the systemic circulation. *Scand. J. Clin. Lab. Invest. Suppl.* 24: 1–97, 1956.
243. HOLMGREN, A. On the reproducibility of steady state DL_{CO} measurements during exercise in man. *Scand. J. Clin. Lab. Invest.* 17: 110–116, 1965.
244. HOLMGREN, A. On the variation of DL_{CO} with increasing oxygen uptake during exercise in healthy young men and women. *Acta Physiol. Scand.* 65: 207–220, 1965.
245. HOLMGREN, A. Experience of measuring the diffusing capacity during exercise with the steady state method of Filley, modified by Linderholm. In: *Pulmonary Diffusing Capacity on Exercise*, edited by M. Scherrer. Bern: Huber, 1971, p. 65–84.
246. HOLMGREN, A., AND P.-O. ÅSTRAND. DL and the dimensions and functional capacities of the O_2 transport system in humans. *J. Appl. Physiol.* 21: 1463–1470, 1966.
247. HOLMGREN, A., AND H. LINDERHOLM. Oxygen and carbon dioxide tensions of arterial blood during heavy and exhaustive exercise. *Acta Physiol. Scand.* 44: 203–215, 1958.
248. HONIG, C. R. Contributions of nerves and metabolites to exercise vasodilation: a unifying hypothesis. *Am. J. Physiol.* 236 (*Heart Circ. Physiol.* 5): H705–H719, 1979.
249. HONIG, C. R., AND J. L. FRIERSON. Neurons intrinsic to arterioles initiate postcontraction vasodilation. *Am. J. Physiol.* 230: 493–507, 1976.
250. HONIG, C. R., AND J. L. FRIERSON. Role of adenosine in exercise vasodilation in dog gracilis muscle. *Am. J. Physiol.* 238 (*Heart Circ. Physiol.* 7): H703–H715, 1980.
251. HONIG, C. R., AND T. E. J. GAYESKI. Capillary recruitment and de-recruitment in exercise: relation to control mechanisms, and tissue Po_2 (Abstract). *Proc. Int. Congr. Physiol. Sci., 28th, Budapest, 1980*, vol. 14, p. 23.
252. HONIG, C. R., C. L. ODOROFF, AND J. L. FRIERSON. Capillary recruitment in exercise: rate, extent, uniformity, and relation to blood flow. *Am. J. Physiol.* 238 (*Heart Circ. Physiol.* 7): H31–H42, 1980.
253. HORSTMAN, D. H., M. GLESER, D. WOLFE, T. TRYON, AND J. DELEHUNT. Effects of hemoglobin reduction on $\dot{V}o_{2\,max}$ and related hemodynamics in exercising dogs. *J. Appl. Physiol.* 37: 97–102, 1974.
254. HUBBARD, J. L. The effect of exercise on lactate metabolism. *J. Physiol. Lond.* 231: 1–18, 1973.
255. HUDLICKÁ, O. Effect of training on macro- and microcirculatory changes in exercise. *Exercise Sport Sci. Rev.* 5: 181–230, 1978.
255a. HUGHSON, R. L., AND M. MORRISSEY. Delayed kinetics of respiratory gas exchange in the transition from prior exercise. *J. Appl. Physiol.* 52: 921–929, 1982.
256. HULTMAN, E., J. BERGSTRÖM, AND N. MCLENNON ANDERSON. Break-down and resynthesis of phosphorylcreatine and adenosine-triphosphate in connection with muscular work in man. *Scand. J. Clin. Lab. Invest.* 19: 56–66, 1967.
257. HULTMAN, E., AND K. SAHLIN. Acid-base balance during exercise. *Exercise Sport Sci. Rev.* 8: 41–128, 1980.
258. HYDE, R. W., R. E. FORSTER, G. G. POWER, J. NAIRN, AND R. RYNES. Measurement of O_2 diffusing capacity of the lungs with a stable O_2 isotope. *J. Clin. Invest.* 45: 1178–1193, 1966.
259. HYDE, R. W., M. G. MARIN, R. I. RYNES, G. KARREMAN, AND R. E. FORSTER. Measurement of uneven distribution of pulmonary blood flow to CO diffusing capacity. *J. Appl. Physiol.* 31: 605–612, 1971.
260. HYDE, R. W., R. J. M. PUY, W. F. RAUB, AND R. E. FORSTER. Rate of disappearance of labelled carbon dioxide from the lungs of humans during breath holding: a method for studying the dynamics of pulmonary CO_2 exchange. *J. Clin. Invest.* 47: 1535–1552, 1968.
261. INGJER, F. Maximal aerobic power related to the capillary supply of the quadriceps femoris muscle in man. *Acta Physiol. Scand.* 104: 138–140, 1978.
262. IVY, J. L., D. L. COSTILL, AND B. D. MAXWELL. Skeletal muscle determinants of maximum aerobic power in man. *Eur. J. Appl. Physiol. Occup. Physiol.* 44: 1–8, 1980.
263. JACOBS, H. A., H. W. HELDT, AND M. KLINGENBERG. High activity of creatine-kinase in mitochondria from heart and brain and evidence for a separate mitochondrial isoenzyme of creatine kinase. *Biochem. Biophys. Res. Commun.* 16: 516–524, 1964.
264. JACOBUS, W. E., AND A. L. LEHNINGER. Coupling of creatine phosphorylation to electron transport. *J. Biol. Chem.* 248: 4803–4810, 1973.
265. JEBAVÝ, P., J. HURYCH, AND J. WIDIMSKÝ. Relations of pulmonary diffusing capacity to ventilation and haemodynamics in healthy subjects. *Respiration* 34: 152–161, 1977.
266. JEBAVÝ, P., AND J. WIDIMSKÝ. Lung-transfer factor at maximal effort in healthy men. *Respiration* 30: 297–310, 1973.
267. JOHNSON, P. C. The microcirculation, and local and humoral control of the circulation. In: *Cardiovascular Physiology I*, edited by A. C. Guyton and C. E. Jones. Baltimore, MD: University Park, 1974, vol. 1, p. 163–195. (Int. Rev. Physiol. Ser.)
268. JOHNSON, R. L., JR., AND J. M. MILLER. Distribution of ventilation, blood flow, and gas transfer coefficients in the lung. *J. Appl. Physiol.* 25: 1–15, 1968.
269. JOHNSON, R. L., JR., W. S. SPICER, J. M. BISHOP, AND R. E. FORSTER. Pulmonary capillary blood volume, flow and diffusing capacity during exercise. *J. Appl. Physiol.* 15: 893–902, 1960.
270. JONES, N. L., G. J. R. MCHARDY, A. NAIMARK, AND E. J. M. CAMPBELL. Physiological dead space and alveolar-arterial gas pressure differences during exercise. *Clin. Sci. Lond.* 31: 19–29, 1966.
271. JONES, N. L., D. G. ROBERTSON, AND J. W. KANE. Difference between end-tidal and arterial Pco_2 in exercise. *J. Appl. Physiol.* 47: 954–960, 1979.
272. JONES, W. B., R. N. FINCHUM, R. O. RUSSELL, JR., AND T. J. REEVES. Transient cardiac output response to multiple levels of supine exercise. *J. Appl. Physiol.* 28: 183–189, 1970.
273. KAIJSER, L. Limiting factors for aerobic muscle performance. *Acta Physiol. Scand. Suppl.* 346: 1–96, 1970.
274. KAIJSER, L., B. W. LASSERS, M. L. WAHLQVIST, AND L. A. CARLSON. Myocardial lipid and carbohydrate metabolism in fasting men during prolonged exercise. *J. Appl. Physiol.* 32:

847–858, 1972.
275. KARLSSON, J. Lactate and phosphagen concentrations in working muscle of man. *Acta Physiol. Scand. Suppl.* 358: 1–72, 1971.
276. KARLSSON, J., L.-O. NORDESJÖ, L. JORFELDT, AND B. SALTIN. Muscle lactate, ATP, and CP levels during exercise after physical training in man. *J. Appl. Physiol.* 33: 199–203, 1972.
277. KARLSSON, J., AND B. SALTIN. Lactate, ATP, and CP in working muscles during exhaustive exercise in man. *J. Appl. Physiol.* 29: 598–602, 1970.
278. KATCH, V. L. Kinetics of oxygen uptake and recovery for supramaximal work of short duration. *Int. Z. Angew. Physiol. Einschl. Arbeitsphysiol.* 31: 197–207, 1973.
279. KEUL, J., E. DOLL, H. STEIM, U. FLEER, AND H. REINDELL. Ueber den Stoffwechsel des menschlichen Herzens. III. Der oxydative Stoffwechsel des menschlichen Herzens unter verschiedenen Arbeitsbedingungen. *Pfluegers Arch.* 282: 43–53, 1965.
280. KITAMURA, K., C. R. JORGENSEN, F. L. GOBEL, H. L. TAYLOR, AND Y. WANG. Hemodynamic correlates of myocardial oxygen consumption during upright exercise. *J. Appl. Physiol.* 32: 516–522, 1972.
281. KJELLBERG, S. R., U. RUDHE, AND T. SJÖSTRAND. Increase of the amount of hemoglobin and blood volume in connection with physical training. *Acta Physiol. Scand.* 19: 146–151, 1949.
282. KJELLMER, I. The potassium ion as a vasodilator during muscular exercise. *Acta Physiol. Scand.* 63: 460–468, 1965.
283. KLEIN, J. P., H. V. FORSTER, R. D. STEWART, AND A. WU. Hemoglobin affinity for oxygen during short-term exhaustive exercise. *J. Appl. Physiol.* 48: 236–242, 1980.
284. KLISSOURAS, V. Heritability of adaptive variation. *J. Appl. Physiol.* 31: 338–344, 1971.
285. KLISSOURAS, V., F. PIRNAY, AND J.-M. PETIT. Adaptation to maximal effort: genetics and age. *J. Appl. Physiol.* 35: 288–293, 1973.
286. KLOCKE, F. J., E. BRAUNWALD, AND J. ROSS, JR. Oxygen cost of electrical activation of the heart. *Circ. Res.* 18: 357–365, 1966.
287. KLOCKE, F. J., R. C. KOBERSTEIN, D. E. PITTMAN, I. L. BUNNEL, D. G. GREENE, AND D. R. ROSIG. Effects of heterogeneous myocardial perfusion on coronary venous H_2 desaturation curves and calculations of coronary flow. *J. Clin. Invest.* 47: 2711–2724, 1968.
288. KNUTTGEN, H. G. Oxygen debt, lactate, pyruvate, and excess lactate after muscular work. *J. Appl. Physiol.* 17: 639–644, 1962.
289. KNUTTGEN, H. G. Oxygen debt after submaximal physical exercise. *J. Appl. Physiol.* 29: 651–657, 1970.
290. KNUTTGEN, H. G., F. BONDE-PETERSEN, AND K. KLAUSEN. Oxygen uptake and heart rate responses to exercise performed with concentric and eccentric muscle contractions. *Med. Sci. Sports* 3: 1–15, 1970.
291. KNUTTGEN, H. G., AND K. KLAUSEN. Oxygen debt in short-term exercise with concentric and eccentric muscle contractions. *J. Appl. Physiol.* 30: 632–635, 1971.
292. KNUTTGEN, H. G., AND B. SALTIN. Oxygen uptake, muscle high energy phosphates, and lactate in exercise under acute hypoxic conditions in man. *Acta Physiol. Scand.* 87: 368–376, 1973.
293. KOBAYASHI, K., K. KITAMURA, M. MIURA, H. SODEYAMA, Y. MURASE, M. MIYASHITA, AND H. MATSUI. Aerobic power as related to body growth and training in Japanese boys: a longitudinal study. *J. Appl. Physiol.* 44: 666–672, 1978.
294. KOMI, P. V., AND J. KARLSSON. Physical performance, skeletal muscle enzyme activities and fibre types in monozygous and dizygous twins of both sexes. *Acta Physiol. Scand. Suppl.* 462: 1–28, 1979.
295. KRASNEY, J. A., M. G. LEVITZKY, AND R. C. KOEHLER. Sinoaortic contribution to the adjustment of systemic resistance in exercising dogs. *J. Appl. Physiol.* 36: 679–685, 1974.
296. KREUKNIET, J., AND B. F. VISSER. Die Diffusionskapazität der Lungen für Kohlenmonoxid berechnet mit Hilfe des arteriellen und des alveolären Kohlensäuredruckes bei Patienten mit Verteilungsstörungen. *Pfluegers Arch.* 277: 585–602, 1963.
297. KREUZER, F., AND P. VAN LOOKEREN CAMPAGNE. Resting pulmonary diffusing capacity for CO and O_2 at high altitude. *J. Appl. Physiol.* 20: 519–524, 1965.
298. KROGH, A. The diffusion of gases through the lungs of man. *J. Physiol. Lond.* 49: 271–300, 1915.
299. KROGH, A., AND J. LINDHARD. The regulation of respiration and circulation during the initial stages of muscular work. *J. Physiol. Lond.* 47: 112–136, 1913.
300. KRUHØFFER, P. Studies on the lung diffusion coefficient for carbon monoxide in normal subjects by means of ^{14}CO. *Acta Physiol. Scand.* 32: 106–123, 1954.
301. KRUMHOLZ, R. A., L. H. KING, JR., AND J. C. ROSS. Effect of pulmonary vascular engorgement on DL during and immediately after exercise. *J. Appl. Physiol.* 18: 1180–1182, 1963.
302. KUNSKI, H., AND M. SZTOBRYN. The effect of physical exercise on 2,3-diphosphoglycerate (2,3-DPG) concentration in erythrocytes. *Acta Physiol. Pol.* 27: 293–299, 1976.
303. LACOUR, J. R., AND R. FLANDROIS. Le rôle du métabolisme aérobie dans l'exercice intense de longue durée. *J. Physiol. Paris* 73: 89–130, 1977.
304. LAMMERT, O. Maximal aerobic power and energy expenditure of Eskimo hunters in Greenland. *J. Appl. Physiol.* 33: 184–188, 1972.
305. LASSEN, N. A., I. F. LINDBJERG, AND O. MUNCK. Measurement of blood flow through skeletal muscle by intramuscular injection of ^{133}Xenon. *Lancet* 1: 686–689, 1964.
306. LASSERS, B. W., M. L. WAHLQVIST, L. KAIJSER, AND L. A. CARLSON. Effect of nicotinic acid on myocardial metabolism in man at rest and during exercise. *J. Appl. Physiol.* 33: 72–80, 1972.
307. LAURENT, D., C. BOLENE-WILLIAMS, F. L. WILLIAMS, AND L. N. KATZ. Effects of heart rate on coronary flow and cardiac oxygen consumption. *Am. J. Physiol.* 185: 355–364, 1956.
308. LAVALLÉE, H., G. LARIVIÈRE, AND R. J. SHEPHARD. Correlation between field tests of performance and laboratory measurements of fitness. Results in the 10-year-old school child. *Acta Paediatr. Belg.* 28, Suppl.: 29–39, 1974.
309. LAWSON, W. H., JR. Rebreathing measurements of pulmonary diffusing capacity for CO during exercise. *J. Appl. Physiol.* 29: 896–900, 1970.
310. LAWSON, W. H., JR. Effect of drugs, hypoxia, and ventilatory maneuvers on lung diffusion for CO in man. *J. Appl. Physiol.* 32: 788–794, 1972.
311. LEARY, W. P., AND C. H. WYNDHAM. The capacity for maximum physical effort of Caucasian and Bantu athletes of international class. *S. Afr. Med. J.* 39: 651–655, 1965.
312. LECHNER, A. J. The scaling of maximal oxygen consumption and pulmonary dimensions in small mammals. *Respir. Physiol.* 34: 29–44, 1978.
313. LEVINE, M. J., AND R. J. WAGMAN. Energetics of the human heart. *Am. J. Cardiol.* 9: 372–383, 1962.
314. LEWIS, B. M., E. J. HAYFORD-WELSING, A. FURUSHO, AND L. C. REED, JR. Effect of uneven ventilation on pulmonary diffusing capacity. *J. Appl. Physiol.* 16: 679–683, 1961.
315. LEWIS, B. M., T. H. LIN, F. E. NOE, AND E. J. HAYFORD-WELSING. The measurement of pulmonary diffusing capacity for carbon monoxide by a rebreathing method. *J. Clin. Invest.* 38: 2073–2086, 1959.
316. LEWIS, B. M., T. H. LIN, F. E. NOE, AND R. KOMISARUK. The measurement of pulmonary capillary blood volume and pulmonary membrane diffusing capacity in normal subjects: the effects of exercise and position. *J. Clin. Invest.* 37: 1061–1070, 1958.
317. LILIENTHAL, J. L., JR., R. L. RILEY, D. D. PROEMMEL, AND R. E. FRANKE. An experimental analysis in man of the oxygen pressure gradient from alveolar air to arterial blood during rest and exercise at sea level and at altitude. *Am. J. Physiol.* 147: 199–216, 1946.
318. LILJESTRAND, G. Untersuchungen über die Atmungsarbeit. *Skand. Arch. Physiol.* 35: 199–293, 1918.

319. LIND, A. R., AND G. W. MCNICOL. Local and central circulatory responses to sustained contractions and the effect of free or restricted arterial inflow on post-exercise hyperaemia. *J. Physiol. Lond.* 192: 575–593, 1967.
320. LIND, A. R., AND G. W. MCNICOL. Circulatory responses to sustained hand-grip contractions performed during other exercise, both rythmic and static. *J. Physiol. Lond.* 192: 595–607, 1967.
321. LIND, A. R., S. H. TAYLOR, P. W. HUMPHREYS, B. M. KENNELLY, AND K. W. DONALD. The circulatory effects of sustained voluntary muscle contraction. *Clin. Sci. Lond.* 27: 229–244, 1964.
322. LINDERHOLM, H. On the significance of CO tension in pulmonary capillary blood for determination of pulmonary diffusing capacity with the steady state CO method. *Acta Med. Scand.* 156: 413–427, 1957.
323. LINDERHOLM, H. Diffusing capacity of the lungs as a limiting factor for physical working capacity. *Acta Med. Scand.* 163: 61–84, 1959.
324. LINNARSSON, D. Dynamics of pulmonary gas exchange and heart rate changes at start and end of exercise. *Acta Physiol. Scand. Suppl.* 415: 1–68, 1974.
325. LUCAS, A., A. THERMINARIAS, AND M. TANCHE. Maximum oxygen consumption in dogs during muscular exercise and cold exposure. *Pfluegers Arch.* 388: 83–87, 1980.
326. MAGEL, J. R., AND K. LANGE-ANDERSEN. Pulmonary diffusing capacity and cardiac output in young trained Norwegian swimmers and untrained subjects. *Med. Sci. Sports* 1: 131–139, 1969.
327. MAHLER, M. Kinetics of oxygen consumption after a single isometric tetanus of frog sartorius muscle at 20°C. *J. Gen. Physiol.* 71: 559–580, 1978.
328. MAHLER, M. The relationship between initial creatine phosphate breakdown and recovery oxygen consumption for a single isometric tetanus of the frog sartorius muscle at 20°C. *J. Gen. Physiol.* 73: 159–174, 1979.
329. MAHLER, M. Kinetics and control of oxygen consumption in skeletal muscle. In: *Exercise Bioenergetics and Gas Exchange*, edited by P. Cerretelli and B. J. Whipp. Amsterdam: Elsevier, 1980, p. 53–66.
329a. MAHLER, M. First-order kinetics of muscle oxygen consumption, and equivalent proportionality between Q_{O_2} and phosphorylcreatine level. Implications for the control of respiration. *J. Gen. Physiol.* 86: 135–165, 1985.
330. MARCONI, C., AND P. CERRETELLI. Gas exchange adjustments in running dogs. *Prog. Respir. Res.* 16: 311–313, 1981.
331. MARGARIA, R. Aerobic and anaerobic energy sources in muscular exercise. In: *Exercise at Altitude*, edited by R. Margaria. Amsterdam: Excerpta Med., 1967, p. 15–32.
332. MARGARIA, R., E. CAMPORESI, P. AGHEMO, AND G. SASSI. The effect of O_2 breathing on maximal aerobic power. *Pfluegers Arch.* 336: 225–235, 1972.
333. MARGARIA, R., P. CERRETELLI, S. MARCHI, AND L. ROSSI. Maximum exercise in oxygen. *Int. Z. Angew. Physiol. Einschl. Arbeitsphysiol.* 18: 465–467, 1961.
334. MARGARIA, R., H. T. EDWARDS, AND D. B. DILL. The possible mechanisms of contracting and paying the oxygen debt and the rôle of lactic acid in muscular contraction. *Am. J. Physiol.* 106: 689–715, 1933.
335. MARGARIA, R., F. MANGILI, F. CUTTICA, AND P. CERRETELLI. The kinetics of the oxygen consumption at the onset of muscular exercise in man. *Ergonomics* 8: 49–54, 1965.
336. MARGARIA, R., G. MILIC-EMILI, J. M. PETIT, AND G. CAVAGNA. Mechanical work of breathing during muscular exercise. *J. Appl. Physiol.* 15: 354–358, 1960.
337. MARKS, A., D. W. CUGELL, J. B. CADIGAN, AND E. A. GAENSLER. Clinical determination of the diffusion capacity of the lungs. Comparison of methods in normal subjects and patients with "alveolar-capillary block" syndrome. *Am. J. Med.* 22: 51–73, 1957.
338. MARSHALL, R. A comparison of methods for measuring the diffusing capacity of the lungs for carbon monoxide. Investigation by fractional analysis of the alveolar air. *J. Clin. Invest.* 37: 394–408, 1958.
339. MARTIN, B. J., E. J. MORGAN, C. W. ZWILLICH, AND J. V. WEIL. Control of breathing during prolonged exercise. *J. Appl. Physiol.* 50: 27–31, 1981.
340. MATELL, G. Time-courses of changes in ventilation and arterial gas tensions in man induced by moderate exercise. *Acta Physiol. Scand. Suppl.* 206: 1–53, 1963.
341. MCCLOSKEY, D. I., P. B. C. MATTHEWS, AND J. M. MITCHELL. Absence of appreciable cardiovascular and respiratory responses to muscle vibration. *J. Appl. Physiol.* 33: 623–626, 1972.
342. MCCLOSKEY, D. I., AND J. M. MITCHELL. Reflex cardiovascular and respiratory responses originating in exercising muscle. *J. Physiol. Lond.* 224: 173–186, 1972.
343. MCCLOSKEY, D. I., AND K. A. STREATFEILD. Muscular reflex stimuli to cardiovascular system during isometric contractions of muscle groups of different mass. *J. Physiol. Lond.* 250: 431–441, 1975.
344. MCGRATH, M. W., AND M. L. THOMSON. The effect of age, body size and lung volume change on alveolar-capillary permeability and diffusing capacity in man. *J. Physiol. Lond.* 146: 572–582, 1959.
345. MCKERROW, C. B., AND A. B. OTIS. Oxygen cost of hyperventilation. *J. Appl. Physiol.* 9: 375–379, 1956.
346. MESSER, J. V., AND W. A. VEILL. The oxygen supply of the human heart. *Am. J. Cardiol.* 9: 384–394, 1962.
347. MESSER, J. V., R. J. WAGMAN, H. J. LEVINE, W. A. VEILL, N. KRASNOW, AND R. GORLIN. Patterns of human myocardial oxygen extraction during rest and exercise. *J. Clin. Invest.* 41: 725–742, 1962.
348. MEYER, M. Analyse des alveolär-kapillären Gasaustausches in der Lunge. Untersuchung der Diffusionskapazität der Lunge mit stabilen Isotopen. Göttingen, FRG: Georg-August-Universität, 1980. Habilitations Dissertation.
349. MEYER, M., P. SCHEID, G. RIEPL, H.-J. WAGNER, AND J. PIIPER. Pulmonary diffusing capacities for O_2 and CO measured by a rebreathing technique. *J. Appl. Physiol.* 51: 1643–1650, 1981.
350. MICHELI, J. L., AND P. HAAB. Estimation de la capacité de diffusion pulmonaire pour l'oxygène chez l'homme au repos par la méthode du rebreathing hypoxique. *J. Physiol. Paris* 62, Suppl. 1: 194–195, 1970.
351. MILIC-EMILI, G., J. M. PETIT, AND R. DEROANNE. The effects of respiratory rate on the mechanical work of breathing during muscular exercise. *Int. Z. Angew. Physiol. Einschl. Arbeitsphysiol.* 18: 330–340, 1960.
352. MILIC-EMILI, G., J. M. PETIT, AND R. DEROANNE. Mechanical work of breathing during exercise in trained and untrained subjects. *J. Appl. Physiol.* 17: 43–46, 1962.
353. MILLER, J. M., AND R. L. JOHNSON. Effect of lung inflation on pulmonary diffusing capacity at rest and exercise. *J. Clin. Invest.* 45: 493–500, 1966.
354. MINAIRE, Y. Origine et destinée du lactate plasmatique. *J. Physiol. Paris* 66: 229–257, 1973.
355. MITCHELL, J. H., F. C. PAYNE, B. SALTIN, AND B. SCHIBYE. The role of muscle mass in the cardiovascular response to static contractions. *J. Physiol. Lond.* 309: 45–54, 1980.
356. MITCHELL, J. H., AND K. WILDENTHAL. Static (isometric) exercise and the heart: physiological and clinical considerations. *Annu. Rev. Med.* 25: 369–381, 1974.
357. MOGNONI, P., M. G. CLEMENT, C. MARCONI, F. SAIBENE, AND G. AGUGGINI. Estimate of the cost of breathing in dog at maximal exercise (Abstract). *Proc. Int. Congr. Physiol. Sci., 27th, Paris, 1977*, vol. 13, p. 521.
357a. MOLÉ, A. P., R. L. COULSON, J. R. CATON, B. G. NICHOLS, AND T. J. BARSTOW. In vivo ^{31}P-NMR in human muscle: transient patterns with exercise. *J. Appl. Physiol.* 59: 101–104, 1985.
358. MORRISON, P., F. A. RYSER, AND A. R. DAWE. Studies on the physiology of the masked shrew *Sorex cinereus*. *Physiol. Zool.* 32: 256–271, 1959.

359. MOSTYN, E. M., S. HELLE, J. B. L. GEE, L. G. BENTIVOGLIO, AND D. V. BATES. Pulmonary diffusing capacity of athletes. *J. Appl. Physiol.* 18: 687–695, 1963.
360. NAIRN, J. R., G. G. POWER, R. W. HYDE, R. E. FORSTER, C. J. LAMBERTSEN, AND J. DICKSON. Diffusing capacity and pulmonary capillary blood flow at hyperbaric pressures. *J. Clin. Invest.* 44: 1591–1599, 1965.
361. NEWTH, C. J. L., D. J. COTTON, AND J. A. NADEL. Pulmonary diffusing capacity measured at multiple intervals during a single exhalation in man. *J. Appl. Physiol.* 43: 617–625, 1977.
362. NIELSEN, M., AND O. HANSEN. Maximale körpliche Arbeit bei O_2-reicher Luft. *Skand. Arch. Physiol.* 76: 37–59, 1937.
363. OGILVIE, C. M., R. E. FORSTER, W. S. BLAKEMORE, AND J. W. MORTON. A standardized breath holding technique for the clinical measurement of the diffusing capacity of the lung for carbon monoxide. *J. Clin. Invest.* 36: 1–17, 1957.
364. OLAFSSON, S., AND R. E. HYATT. Ventilatory mechanics and expiratory flow limitation during exercise in normal subjects. *J. Clin. Invest.* 48: 564–573, 1969.
365. OLSSON, R. A. Local factors regulating cardiac and skeletal muscle blood flow. *Annu. Rev. Physiol.* 43: 385–395, 1981.
366. OPIE, L. H. Metabolism of the heart in health and disease. II. *Am. Heart J.* 77: 100–122, 1969.
367. OSCAI, L. B., B. T. WILLIAMS, AND B. A. HERTIG. Effects of exercise on blood volume. *J. Appl. Physiol.* 24: 622–624, 1968.
368. OSMAN, H., R. FLANDROIS, J. R. LACOUR, S. QUARD, M. A. DANJOU, AND C. NATTON. Modifications de la ventilation et de la fréquence cardiaque au cours d'exercices musculaires de différentes puissances chez le chien. *J. Physiol. Paris* 61: 363–364, 1969.
369. OTIS, A. B. The work of breathing. *Physiol. Rev.* 34: 449–458, 1954.
370. PASQUIS, P., A. LACAISSE, AND P. DEJOURS. Maximal oxygen uptake in four species in small mammals. *Respir. Physiol.* 9: 298–309, 1970.
371. PATCH, L. D., AND G. A. BROOKS. Effects of training on $\dot{V}O_{2\,max}$ and $\dot{V}O_2$ during two running intensities in rats. *Pfluegers Arch.* 386: 215–219, 1980.
372. PAULEV, P.-E. Cardiac rate and ventilatory volume rate reactions to a muscle contraction in man. *J. Appl. Physiol.* 34: 578–583, 1973.
373. PENDERGAST, D., P. CERRETELLI, AND D. W. RENNIE. Aerobic and glycolytic metabolism in arm exercise. *J. Appl. Physiol.* 47: 754–760, 1979.
373a. PENDERGAST, D. R., J. A. KRASNEY, A. ELLIS, B. MCDONALD, C. MARCONI, AND P. CERRETELLI. Cardiac output and muscle blood flow in exercising dogs. *Respir. Physiol.* 61: 317–326, 1985.
374. PÉREZ-GONZÁLEZ, J. F., AND J. H. COOTE. Activity of muscle afferents and reflex circulatory responses to exercise. *Am. J. Physiol.* 223: 138–143, 1972.
375. PETRO, J. K., A. P. HOLLANDER, AND L. N. BOUMAN. Instantaneous cardiac acceleration in man induced by a voluntary muscle contraction. *J. Appl. Physiol.* 29: 794–798, 1970.
376. PETROFSKY, J. S., C. A. PHILLIPS, M. N. SAWKA, D. HANPETER, A. R. LIND, AND D. STAFFORD. Muscle fiber recruitment and blood pressure response to isometric exercise. *J. Appl. Physiol.* 50: 32–37, 1981.
377. PIIPER, J. Variations of ventilation and diffusing capacity to perfusion determining the alveolar-arterial O_2 difference: theory. *J. Appl. Physiol.* 16: 507–510, 1961.
378. PIIPER, J. Apparent increase of the O_2 diffusing capacity with increased O_2 uptake in inhomogeneous lungs: theory. *Respir. Physiol.* 6: 209–218, 1969.
379. PIIPER, J., P. CERRETELLI, F. CUTTICA, AND F. MANGILI. Energy metabolism and circulation in dogs exercising in hypoxia. *J. Appl. Physiol.* 21: 1143–1149, 1966.
380. PIIPER, J., P. CERRETELLI, D. W. RENNIE, AND P. E. DI PRAMPERO. Estimation of the pulmonary diffusing capacity for O_2 by a rebreathing procedure. *Respir. Physiol.* 12: 157–162, 1971.
381. PIIPER, J., P. E. DI PRAMPERO, AND P. CERRETELLI. Oxygen debt and high-energy phosphates in gastrocnemius muscle of the dog. *Am. J. Physiol.* 215: 523–531, 1968.
382. PIIPER, J., M. MEYER, C. MARCONI, AND P. SCHEID. Alveolar-capillary equilibration kinetics of $^{13}CO_2$ in human lungs studied by rebreathing. *Respir. Physiol.* 42: 29–41, 1980.
382a. PIIPER, J., D. R. PENDERGAST, C. MARCONI, M. MEYER, N. HEISLER, AND P. CERRETELLI. Blood flow distribution in dog gastrocnemius muscle at rest and during stimulation. *J. Appl. Physiol.* 58: 2068–2074, 1985.
383. PIIPER, J., AND P. SCHEID. Blood-gas equilibrium in lungs. In: *Pulmonary Gas Exchange. Ventilation, Blood Flow, and Diffusion*, edited by J. B. West. New York: Academic, 1980, vol. 1, p. 131–171.
384. PIIPER, J., AND P. SPILLER. Repayment of O_2 debt and resynthesis of high-energy phosphates in gastrocnemius muscle of the dog. *J. Appl. Physiol.* 28: 657–662, 1970.
385. PIRNAY, F., J. DUJARDIN, R. DEROANNE, AND J. M. PETIT. Muscular exercise during intoxication by carbon monoxide. *J. Appl. Physiol.* 31: 573–575, 1971.
386. PIRNAY, F., R. MARECHAL, R. RADERMECKER, AND J. M. PETIT. Muscle blood flow during submaximum and maximum exercise on a bicycle ergometer. *J. Appl. Physiol.* 32: 210–212, 1972.
387. PODLESCH, J., AND M. STEVANOVIC. Die Altersabhängigkeit der Diffusionskapazität der Lunge in Ruhe und während Belastung. *Med. Thorac.* 23: 144–159, 1966.
388. POWER, G. G., AND W. C. BRADFORD. Measurement of pulmonary diffusing capacity during blood-to-gas exchange in humans. *J. Appl. Physiol.* 27: 61–66, 1969.
389. PUGH, L. G. C. E. Blood volume changes in outdoor exercise of 8–10 hour duration. *J. Physiol. Lond.* 200: 345–351, 1969.
390. PUGH, L. G. C. E., M. B. GILL, S. LAHIRI, J. S. MILLEDGE, M. P. WARD, AND J. B. WEST. Muscular exercise at great altitudes. *J. Appl. Physiol.* 19: 431–440, 1964.
391. RAHN, H., AND L. E. FARHI. Ventilation, perfusion, and gas exchange—the $\dot{V}A/\dot{Q}$ concept. In: *Handbook of Physiology. Respiration*, edited by W. O. Fenn and H. Rahn. Washington, DC: Am. Physiol. Soc., 1964, sect. 3, vol. I, chapt. 30, p. 735–766.
392. RAMPULLA, C., C. MARCONI, G. BEULCKE, AND S. AMADUCCI. Correlations between lung-transfer factor, ventilation, and cardiac output during exercise. *Respiration* 33: 405–415, 1976.
393. RAMSAY, A. G. Effects of metabolism and anesthesia on pulmonary ventilation. *J. Appl. Physiol.* 14: 102–104, 1959.
394. RAND, P. W., J. M. NORTON, N. BARKER, AND M. LOVELL. Influence of athletic training on hemoglobin-oxygen affinity. *Am. J. Physiol.* 224: 1334–1337, 1973.
395. RAVEN, P. B., B. L. DRINKWATER, R. O. RUHLING, N. BOLDUAN, S. TAGUCHI, J. GLINER, AND S. M. HORVATH. Effect of carbon monoxide and peroxyacetyl nitrate on man's maximal aerobic capacity. *J. Appl. Physiol.* 36: 288–293, 1974.
396. RAYNAUD, J., J. P. MARTINEAUD, J. BORDACHAR, M. C. TILLOUS, AND J. DURAND. Oxygen deficit and debt in submaximal exercise at sea level and high altitude. *J. Appl. Physiol.* 37: 43–48, 1974.
397. REGAN, T. M., C. TIMMIS, M. GRAY, K. BINAK, AND H. K. HELLEMS. Myocardial oxygen consumption during exercise in fasting and lipemic subjects. *J. Clin. Invest.* 40: 624–630, 1962.
398. REMMERS, J. E., AND J. C. MITHOEFER. The carbon monoxide diffusing capacity in permanent residents at high altitudes. *Respir. Physiol.* 6: 233–244, 1969.
399. RENNIE, D. W. Exercise physiology. In: *Eskimos of Northwestern Alaska: A Biological Perspective*, edited by P. L. Jamison, S. L. Zegura, and F. A. Milan. Stroudsburg, PA: Dowden, Hutchinson & Ross, 1978, p. 198–216.
400. RENNIE, D. W., P. E. DI PRAMPERO, AND P. CERRETELLI. Effects of water immersion on cardiac output, heart rate, and stroke volume of man at rest and during exercise. *Med. Sport Turin* 24: 223–228, 1971.
401. RENNIE, D. W., P. E. DI PRAMPERO, R. W. FITTS, AND L.

SINCLAIR. Physical fitness and respiratory function of Eskimos of Wainwright, Alaska. *Arct. Anthropol.* 2: 73–82, 1970.

402. REUSCHLEIN, P. S., W. G. REDDAN, J. BURPEE, J. B. L. GEE, AND J. RANKIN. Effect of physical training on the pulmonary diffusing capacity during submaximal work. *J. Appl. Physiol.* 24: 152–158, 1968.
403. RIEPL, G., AND P. HILPERT. Der Einfluss funktioneller Inhomogenitäten auf die Single-breath-CO-Diffusionskapazität (DL_{CO-SB}). *Respiration* 31: 60–70, 1974.
404. RILEY, R. L., J. L. LILIENTHAL, JR., D. D. PROEMMEL, AND R. E. FRANKE. On the determination of the physiologically effective pressures of oxygen and carbon dioxide in alveolar air. *Am. J. Physiol.* 147: 191–198, 1946.
405. RILEY, R. L., R. H. SHEPARD, J. E. COHN, D. G. CARROLL, AND B. W. ARMSTRONG. Maximal diffusing capacity of the lungs. *J. Appl. Physiol.* 6: 573–587, 1954.
406. ROBERTS, D. A., AND A. A. MORTON. Total and alactic oxygen debts after supramaximal work. *Eur. J. Appl. Physiol. Occup. Physiol.* 38: 281–289, 1978.

406a. ROBERTSON, R. J., R. GILCHER, K. F. METZ, C. J. CASPERSEN, T. G. ALLISON, R. A. ABBOTT, G. S. SKRINAR, J. R. KRAUSE, AND P. A. NIXON. Hemoglobin concentration and aerobic work capacity in women following induced erythrocythemia. *J. Appl. Physiol.* 57: 568–575, 1984.

406b. ROBERTSON, R. J., R. GILCHER, K. F. METZ, G. S. SKRINAR, T. G. ALLISON, H. T. BAHNSON, R. A. ABBOTT, R. BECKER, AND J. E. FALKEL. Effect of induced erythrocythemia on hypoxia tolerance during physical exercise. *J. Appl. Physiol.* 53: 490–495, 1982.

407. ROBINSON, S. Experimental studies of physical fitness in relation to age. *Arbeitsphysiologie* 10: 251–323, 1938.
408. ROBINSON, S., D. B. DILL, R. D. ROBINSON, S. P. TZANKOFF, AND J. A. WAGNER. Physiological aging of champion runners. *J. Appl. Physiol.* 41: 46–51, 1976.
409. RODE, A., AND R. J. SHEPHARD. Cardiorespiratory fitness of an Arctic community. *J. Appl. Physiol.* 31: 519–526, 1971.
410. ROMO-SALAS, F., L. AQUIN, J. M. SEARLES, JR., AND N. BANCHERO. Oxygen cost of breathing in dogs. *Respiration* 35: 186–191, 1978.
411. ROSE, G. L., S. S. CASSIDY, AND R. L. JOHNSON, JR. Diffusing capacity at different lung volumes during breath holding and rebreathing. *J. Appl. Physiol.* 47: 32–37, 1979.
412. ROSENBERG, E., AND L. D. MACLEAN. Effect of high oxygen tensions on diffusing capacity for CO and Krogh's K. *J. Appl. Physiol.* 23: 11–17, 1967.
413. ROSENMANN, M., AND P. MORRISON. Maximum oxygen consumption and heat loss facilitation in small homeotherms by $He-O_2$. *Am. J. Physiol.* 226: 490–495, 1974.
414. ROSENMANN, M., P. MORRISON, AND D. FEIST. Seasonal changes in the metabolic capacity of red-backed voles. *Physiol. Zool.* 48: 303–310, 1975.
415. ROSS, J. C., R. FRAYSER, AND J. B. HICKAM. A study of the mechanisms by which exercise increases the pulmonary diffusing capacity for carbon monoxide. *J. Clin. Invest.* 38: 916–932, 1959.
416. ROSS, J. C., R. W. REINHART, J. F. BOXELL, AND L. H. KING, JR. Relationship of increased breath-holding diffusing capacity to ventilation in exercise. *J. Appl. Physiol.* 18: 794–797, 1963.
417. ROWELL, L. B. Circulation. *Med. Sci. Sports* 1: 15–22, 1969.
418. ROWELL, L. B. Human cardiovascular adjustments to exercise and thermal stress. *Physiol. Rev.* 54: 75–159, 1974.
419. ROWELL, L. B., H. J. MARX, R. A. BRUCE, R. D. CONN, AND F. KUSUMI. Reductions in cardiac output, central blood volume, and stroke volume with thermal stress in normal men during exercise. *J. Clin. Invest.* 45: 1801–1816, 1966.
420. SACKNER, M. A., G. GREENELTCH, M. S. HEIMAN, S. EPSTEIN, AND N. ATKINS. Diffusing capacity, membrane diffusing capacity, capillary blood volume, pulmonary tissue volume, and cardiac output measured by a rebreathing technique. *Am. Rev. Respir. Dis.* 111: 157–165, 1975.
421. SACKNER, M. A., M. M. RASKIN, P. J. JULIEN, AND W. G. AVERY. Effect of lung volume on steady state pulmonary membrane diffusing capacity and pulmonary capillary blood volume. *Am. Rev. Respir. Dis.* 104: 408–417, 1971.
422. SAHLIN, K., G. PALMSKOG, AND E. HULTMAN. Adenine nucleotide and IMP contents of the quadriceps muscle in man after exercise. *Pfluegers Arch.* 374: 193–198, 1978.
423. SAIBENE, F. Work of breathing at altitude. In: *Medicine and Sport. Physiological Chemistry of Exercise and Training*, edited by P. E. di Prampero and J. R. Poortmans. Basel: Karger, 1981, vol. 13, p. 191–198.
424. SAIBENE, F., P. MOGNONI, G. AGUGGINI, AND M. G. CLEMENT. Work of breathing in dog during exercise. *J. Appl. Physiol.* 50: 1087–1092, 1981.
425. SAIBENE, F., P. MOGNONI, C. LAFORTUNA, AND R. MOSTARDI. Oronasal breathing during exercise. *Pfluegers Arch.* 378: 65–69, 1978.

425a. SAKS, V. A., V. V. KUPRIYANOV, G. V. ELIZAROVA, AND W. E. JACOBUS. Studies of energy transport in heart cells. The importance of creatine kinase localization for the coupling of mitochondrial phosphorylcreatine production to oxidative phosphorylation. *J. Biol. Chem.* 255: 755–763, 1980.

426. SAKS, V. A., N. V. LIPINA, V. N. SMIRNOV, AND E. I. CHASOV. Studies of energy transport in heart cells. The functional coupling between mitochondrial creatine phosphokinase and ATP-ADP translocase: kinetic evidence. *Arch. Biochem. Biophys.* 173: 34–41, 1976.
427. SALTIN, B. The interplay between peripheral and central factors in the adaptive response to exercise and training. *Ann. NY Acad. Sci.* 301: 224–231, 1977.
428. SALTIN, B., AND P.-O. ÅSTRAND. Maximal oxygen uptake in athletes. *J. Appl. Physiol.* 23: 353–358, 1967.
429. SALTIN, B., C. G. BLOMQVIST, R. C. MITCHELL, R. L. JOHNSON, K. WILDENTHAL, AND C. B. CHAPMAN. Response to exercise after bed rest and after training. *Circulation* 38, Suppl. 7: 1–78, 1968.
430. SALTIN, B., R. F. GROVER, C. G. BLOMQVIST, L. H. HARTLEY, AND R. L. JOHNSON, JR. Maximal oxygen uptake and cardiac output after 2 weeks at 4,300 m. *J. Appl. Physiol.* 25: 400–409, 1968.
431. SALTIN, B., K. NAZAR, D. L. COSTILL, E. STEIN, E. JANSSON, B. ESSÉN, AND P. D. GOLLNICK. The nature of the training response: peripheral and central adaptations to one-legged exercise. *Acta Physiol. Scand.* 96: 289–305, 1976.
432. SAMAJA, M., A. VEICSTEINAS, AND P. CERRETELLI. Oxygen affinity of blood in altitude Sherpas. *J. Appl. Physiol.* 47: 337–341, 1979.
433. SARNOFF, S. J., E. BRAUNWALD, G. H. WELCH, JR., R. B. CASE, W. N. STAINSBY, AND R. MACRUZ. Hemodynamic determinants of oxygen consumption of the heart with special reference to the tension time-index. *Am. J. Physiol.* 192: 148–156, 1958.
434. SAVITZ, D. V., W. SIDEL, AND A. K. SOLOMON. Osmotic properties of human red cells. *J. Gen. Physiol.* 48: 79–94, 1965.
435. SCHEID, P., AND J. PIIPER. Blood/gas equilibrium of carbon dioxide in lungs. A critical review. *Respir. Physiol.* 39: 1–31, 1980.
436. SCHMIDT, W., G. THEWS, AND K. H. SCHNABEL. Results of distribution analysis of ventilation, perfusion and O_2 diffusing capacity in the human lung. *Respiration* 29: 1–16, 1972.

436a. SCHUMACKER, P. T., B. GUTH, A. J. SUGGETT, P. D. WAGNER, AND J. B. WEST. Effects of transfusion-induced polycythemia on O_2 transport during exercise in the dog. *J. Appl. Physiol.* 58: 749–758, 1985.

436b. SEALS, D. R., J. M. HAGBERG, B. F. HURLEY, A. A. EHSANI, AND J. O. HOLLOSZY. Endurance training in older men and women. I. Cardiovascular responses to exercise. *J. Appl. Physiol.* 57: 1024–1029, 1984.

436c. SEALS, D. R., B. F. HURLEY, J. SCHULTZ, AND J. M. HAGBERG. Endurance training in older men and women. II. Blood lactate response to submaximal exercise. *J. Appl. Physiol.* 57: 1030–1033, 1984.

437. SEEHERMAN, H. J., C. R. TAYLOR, AND G. M. O. MALOIY. Maximum aerobic power and anaerobic glycolysis during running in lions, horses and dogs (Abstract). *Federation Proc.* 35: 797, 1976.
438. SEEHERMAN, H. J., C. R. TAYLOR, G. M. O. MALOIY, AND R. B. ARMSTRONG. Design of the mammalian respiratory system. II. Measuring maximum aerobic capacity. *Respir. Physiol.* 44: 11–23, 1981.
439. SHAPPELL, S. D., J. A. MURRAY, A. J. BELLINGHAM, R. D. WOODSON, J. C. DETTER, AND C. LENFANT. Adaptation to exercise: role of hemoglobin affinity for oxygen and 2,3-diphosphoglycerate. *J. Appl. Physiol.* 30: 827–832, 1971.
440. SHEPARD, R. H., E. VARNAUSKAS, H. B. MARTIN, H. A. WHITE, S. PERMUTT, J. E. COTES, AND R. L. RILEY. Relationship between cardiac output and apparent diffusing capacity of the lung in normal men during treadmill exercise. *J. Appl. Physiol.* 13: 205–210, 1958.
441. SHEPHARD, R. J. "Breath-holding" measurements of carbon monoxide diffusing capacity. Comparison of a field test with steady-state and other methods of measurements. *J. Physiol. Lond.* 141: 408–419, 1958.
442. SHEPHARD, R. J. The oxygen cost of breathing during vigorous exercise. *Q. J. Exp. Physiol.* 51: 336–350, 1966.
443. SHEPHARD, R. J. Cardio-respiratory fitness—a new look at maximum oxygen intake. In: *Advances in Exercise Physiology*, edited by E. Jokl, R. L. Anand, and H. Stoboy. Basel: Karger, 1976, vol. 9, p. 61–84.
444. SHEPHARD, R. J., C. ALLEN, O. BAR-OR, C. T. M. DAVIES, S. DEGRE, R. HEDMAN, K. ISHII, M. KANEKO, J. R. LACOUR, P. E. DI PRAMPERO, AND V. SELIGER. The working capacity of Toronto schoolchildren. Pt. I. *Can. Med. Assoc. J.* 100: 560–566, 1969.
445. SIDNEY, K. H., AND R. J. SHEPHARD. Maximum and submaximum exercise tests in men and women in the seventh, eighth, and ninth decades of life. *J. Appl. Physiol.* 43: 280–287, 1977.
446. SIEBENS, A. A., N. R. FRANK, D. C. KENT, M. M. NEWMAN, R. A. RAUF, AND B. L. VESTAL. Measurements of the pulmonary diffusing capacity for oxygen during exercise. *Am. Rev. Respir. Dis.* 80: 806–824, 1959.
447. SMITH, J. R., AND L. H. HAMILTON. DL_{CO} measurements with gas chromatography. *J. Appl. Physiol.* 17: 856–860, 1962.
448. SMITH, R. J. Rethinking allometry. *J. Theor. Biol.* 87: 97–111, 1980.
449. SØLVSTEEN, P. Measurement of lung diffusing capacity by means of $C^{14}O$ in a closed system. *J. Appl. Physiol.* 19: 59–74, 1964.
450. SONNENBLICK, E. H., E. BRAUNWALD, J. F. WILLIAMS, JR., AND G. GLICK. Effects of exercise on myocardial force-velocity relations in intact unanesthetized man: relative roles of changes in heart rate, sympathetic activity, and ventricular dimensions. *J. Clin. Invest.* 44: 2051–2062, 1965.
451. SPARKS, H. V., JR., AND F. L. BELLONI. The peripheral circulation: local regulation. *Annu. Rev. Physiol.* 40: 67–92, 1978.
451a. SPRIET, L. L., N. GLEDHILL, A. B. FROESE, D. L. WILKES, AND E. C. MEYERS. The effect of induced erythrocythemia on central circulation and oxygen transport during maximal exercise (Abstract). *Med. Sci. Sports Exercise* 12: 122, 1980.
452. SPROULE, B. J., J. H. MITCHELL, AND W. F. MILLER. Cardiopulmonary physiological responses to heavy exercise in patients with anemia. *J. Clin. Invest.* 39: 378–388, 1960.
453. STAUB, N. C. Alveolar-arterial oxygen tension gradient due to diffusion. *J. Appl. Physiol.* 18: 673–680, 1963.
454. STEGALL, H. F. Muscle pumping in the dependent leg. *Circ. Res.* 19: 180–190, 1966.
455. STEGEMANN, J., AND T. KENNER. A theory on heart rate control by muscular metabolic receptors. *Arch. Kreislaufforsch.* 64: 185–214, 1971.
456. STEINHAGEN, G., H. HIRCHE, N. W. NESTLE, U. BOVENKAMP, AND I. HOSSELMANN. The interstitial pH of the working gastrocnemius muscle of the dog. *Pfluegers Arch.* 367: 151–156, 1976.
457. STENBERG, J., B. EKBLOM, AND R. MESSIN. Hemodynamic response to work at simulated altitude, 4,000 m. *J. Appl. Physiol.* 21: 1589–1594, 1966.
458. STEPLOCK, D. A., A. VEICSTEINAS, AND M. MARIANI. Maximal aerobic and anaerobic power and stroke volume of the heart in a subalpine population. *Int. Z. Angew. Physiol. Einschl. Arbeitsphysiol.* 29: 203–214, 1971.
459. STRØMME, S. B., F. INGJER, AND H. D. MEEN. Assessment of maximal aerobic power in specifically trained athletes. *J. Appl. Physiol.* 42: 833–837, 1977.
460. SUNDSTRÖM, G. Influence of body position on pulmonary diffusing capacity in young and old men. *J. Appl. Physiol.* 38: 418–423, 1975.
461. SUNDSTRÖM, G. Influence of ventilation, exercise, and body position on techniques for determining steady state diffusing capacity. *Scand. J. Respir. Dis. Suppl.* 92: 1–74, 1975.
462. SUNDSTRÖM, G., C. W. ZAUNER, AND M. ARBORELIUS, JR. Decrease in pulmonary diffusing capacity during lipid infusion in healthy men. *J. Appl. Physiol.* 34: 816–820, 1973.
463. SUSKIND, M., R. A. BRUCE, M. E. MCDOWELL, P. N. G. YU, AND F. W. LOVEJOY, JR. Normal variations in end-tidal air and arterial blood carbon dioxide and oxygen tensions during moderate exercise. *J. Appl. Physiol.* 3: 282–290, 1950.
464. SWENSON, E. R., AND T. H. MAREN. A quantitative analysis of CO_2 transport at rest and during maximal exercise. *Respir. Physiol.* 35: 129–159, 1978.
465. TAUNTON, J. E., E. W. BANISTER, T. R. PATRICK, P. OFORSAGD, AND W. R. DUNCAN. Physical work capacity in hyperbaric environments and conditions of hyperoxia. *J. Appl. Physiol.* 28: 421–427, 1970.
466. TAUNTON, J. E., C. A. TAUNTON, AND E. W. BANISTER. Alterations in 2,3-DPG and P_{50} with maximal and submaximal exercise. *Med. Sci. Sports* 6: 238–241, 1974.
467. TAYLOR, C. R., AND V. J. ROWNTREE. Running on two or on four legs: which consumes more energy? *Science Wash. DC* 179: 186–187, 1973.
468. TAYLOR, C. R., AND E. R. WEIBEL. Design of the mammalian respiratory system. I. Problem and strategy. *Respir. Physiol.* 44: 1–10, 1981.
468a. TAYLOR, D. J., M. CROWE, P. J. BORE, P. STYLES, D. L. ARNOLD, AND G. K. RADDA. Examination of the energetics of aging skeletal muscle using nuclear magnetic resonance. *Gerontology* 30: 2–7, 1984.
469. TENNEY, S. M., AND R. E. REESE. The ability to sustain great breathing efforts. *Respir. Physiol.* 5: 187–201, 1968.
470. THODEN, J. S., J. A. DEMPSEY, W. G. REDDAN, M. L. BIRNBAUM, H. V. FORSTER, R. F. GROVER, AND J. RANKIN. Ventilatory work during steady state response to exercise. *Federation Proc.* 28: 1316–1321, 1969.
471. THOMAS, D. P., AND G. F. FREGIN. Cardiorespiratory and metabolic responses to treadmill exercise in the horse. *J. Appl. Physiol.* 50: 864–868, 1981.
472. THOMSON, J. M., J. A. DEMPSEY, L. W. CHOSY, N. T. SHAHIDI, AND W G. REDDAN. Oxygen transport and oxyhemoglobin dissociation during prolonged muscular work. *J. Appl. Physiol.* 37: 658–664, 1974.
473. TIBES, U. Neurogenic control of ventilation in exercise. In: *Exercise Bioenergetics and Gas Exchange*, edited by P. Cerretelli and B. J. Whipp. Amsterdam: Elsevier, 1980, p. 149–158.
474. TIBES, U., E. HABERKORN-BUTENDEICH, AND F. HAMMERSEN. Effect of contraction on lymphatic, venous, and tissue electrolytes and metabolites in rabbit skeletal muscle. *Pfluegers Arch.* 368: 195–202, 1977.
475. TIBES, U., B. HEMMER, AND D. BÖNING. Heart rate and ventilation in relation to venous [K^+], osmolality, pH, PCO_2, PO_2, [orthophosphate], and [lactate] at transition from rest to exercise in athletes and non-athletes. *Eur. J. Appl. Physiol. Occup. Physiol.* 36: 127–140, 1977.
476. TIBES, U., B. HEMMER, D. BÖNING, AND U. SCHWEIGART. Relationships of femoral venous [K^+], [H^+], PO_2, osmolality, and [orthophosphate] with heart rate, ventilation, and leg blood flow during bicycle exercise in athletes and non-athletes.

Eur. J. Appl. Physiol. Occup. Physiol. 35: 201–214, 1976.
477. TIBES, U., B. HEMMER, U. SCHWEIGART, D. BÖNING, AND D. FOTESCU. Exercise acidosis as cause of electrolyte changes in femoral venous blood of trained and untrained man. *Pfluegers Arch.* 347: 145–158, 1974.
478. TURINO, G. M., E. H. BERGOFSKY, R. M. GOLDRING, AND A. P. FISHMAN. Effect of exercise on pulmonary diffusing capacity. *J. Appl. Physiol.* 18: 447–456, 1963.
479. TURINO, G. M., M. BRANDFONBRENER, AND A. P. FISHMAN. The effects of changes in ventilation and pulmonary blood flow on the diffusing capacity of the lung. *J. Clin. Invest.* 38: 1186–1201, 1959.
480. VATNER, S. F., C. B. HIGGINS, S. WHITE, T. PATRICK, AND D. FRANKLIN. The peripheral vascular response to severe exercise in untethered dogs before and after complete heart block. *J. Clin. Invest.* 50: 1950–1960, 1971.
481. VAUGHAN, T R., E. M. DEMARINO, AND N. C. STAUB. Indicator dilution lung water and capillary blood volume in prolonged heavy exercise in normal men. *Am. Rev. Respir. Dis.* 113: 757–762, 1976.
482. VEICSTEINAS, A., H. MAGNUSSEN, M. MEYER, AND P. CERRETELLI. Pulmonary O_2 diffusing capacity at exercise by a modified rebreathing method. *Eur. J. Appl. Physiol. Occup. Physiol.* 35: 79–88, 1976.
482a. VEICSTEINAS, A., M. SAMAJA, M. GUSSONI, AND P. CERRETELLI. Blood O_2 affinity and maximal O_2 consumption in elite bicycle racers. *J. Appl. Physiol.* 57: 52–58, 1984.
483. VOGEL, J. A., AND M. A. GLESER. Effect of carbon monoxide on oxygen transport during exercise. *J. Appl. Physiol.* 32: 234–239, 1972.
484. WAGNER, J. A., S. M. HORVATH, AND T. E. DAHMS. Cardiovascular, respiratory, and metabolic adjustments to exercise in dogs. *J. Appl. Physiol.* 42: 403–407, 1977.
485. WAGNER, P. D., R. W. MAZZONE, AND J. B. WEST. Diffusing capacity and anatomic dead space for carbon monoxide ($C^{18}O$). *J. Appl. Physiol.* 31: 847–852, 1971.
485a. WASSERMAN, K., B. J. WHIPP, AND R. CASABURI. Respiratory control during exercise. In: *Handbook of Physiology. The Respiratory System. Control of Breathing*, edited by N. S. Cherniack and J. G. Widdicombe. Bethesda, MD: Am. Physiol. Soc., 1986, sect. 3, vol. II, pt. 2, chapt. 17, p. 595–619.
486. WASSERMAN, K., B. J. WHIPP, R. CASABURI, AND A. OREN. Coupling of ventilation to metabolism during exercise. In: *Exercise Bioenergetics and Gas Exchange*, edited by P. Cerretelli and B. J. Whipp. Amsterdam: Elsevier, 1980, p. 159–173.
487. WEBER, G., W. KARTODIHARDJO, AND V. KLISSOURAS. Growth and physical training with reference to heredity. *J. Appl. Physiol.* 40: 211–215, 1976.
488. WEIBEL, E. R., AND C. R. TAYLOR (editors). Design of the mammalian respiratory system. *Respir. Physiol.* 44: 1–164, 1981.
489. WEISSMAN, M. L., B. J. WHIPP, D. J. HUNTSMAN, AND K. WASSERMAN. Role of neural afferents from working limbs in exercise hyperpnea. *J. Appl. Physiol.* 49: 239–248, 1980.
490. WELCH, H. G., AND P. K. PEDERSEN. Measurement of metabolic rate in hyperoxia. *J. Appl. Physiol.* 51: 725–731, 1981.
491. WEST, J. B. Diffusing capacity of the lung for carbon monoxide at high altitude. *J. Appl. Physiol.* 17: 421–426, 1962.
492. WEST, J. B. Distribution of gas and blood in the normal lungs. *Br. Med. Bull.* 19: 53–58, 1963.
493. WEST, J. B., AND C. T. DOLLERY. Distribution of blood flow and ventilation-perfusion ratio in the lung, measured with radioactive CO_2. *J. Appl. Physiol.* 15: 405–410, 1960.
494. WHIPP, B. J. Rate constant for the kinetics of oxygen uptake during light exercise. *J. Appl. Physiol.* 30: 261–263, 1971.
495. WHIPP, B. J., AND M. MAHLER. Dynamics of pulmonary gas exchange during exercise. In: *Pulmonary Gas Exchange. Organism and Environment*, edited by J. B. West. New York: Academic, 1980, vol. 2, p. 33–96.
496. WHIPP, B. J., C. SEARD, AND K. WASSERMAN. Oxygen deficit-oxygen debt relationships and efficiency of anaerobic work. *J. Appl. Physiol.* 28: 452–456, 1970.
496a. WHIPP, B. J., S. A. WARD, N. LAMARRA, J. A. DAVIS, AND K. WASSERMAN. Parameters of ventilatory and gas exchange dynamics during exercise. *J. Appl. Physiol.* 52: 1506–1513, 1982.
497. WHIPP, B. J., AND K. WASSERMAN. Alveolar-arterial gas tension differences during graded exercise. *J. Appl. Physiol.* 27: 361–365, 1969.
498. WHIPP, B. J., AND K. WASSERMAN. Oxygen uptake kinetics for various intensities of constant-load work. *J. Appl. Physiol.* 33: 351–356, 1972.
499. WHIPP, B. J., K. WASSERMAN, R. CASABURI, C. JURATSCH, M. L. WEISSMANN, AND L. W. STREMEL. Ventilatory control characteristics of conditions resulting in isocapnic hyperpnea. In: *Control of Respiration During Sleep and Anesthesia*, edited by R. Fitzgerald, S. Lahiri, and H. Gautier. New York: Plenum, 1978, p. 355–365.
500. WHIPP, B. J., K. WASSERMAN, A J. DAVIS, N. LAMARRA, AND S. A. WARD. Determinants of O_2 and CO_2 kinetics during exercise in man. In: *Exercise Bioenergetics and Gas Exchange*, edited by P. Cerretelli and B. J. Whipp. Amsterdam: Elsevier, 1980, p. 175–185.
501. WIGERTZ, O. Dynamics of ventilation and heart rate in response to sinusoidal work load in man. *J. Appl. Physiol.* 29: 208–218, 1970.
502. WIGERTZ, O. Dynamics of respiratory and circulatory adaptation to muscular exercise in man. *Acta Physiol. Scand. Suppl.* 363: 1–32, 1971.
503. WILDENTHAL, K., D. S. MIERZWIAK, N. S. SKINNER, JR., AND J. H. MITCHELL. Potassium-induced cardiovascular and ventilatory reflexes from the dog hindlimb. *Am. J. Physiol.* 215: 542–548, 1968.
504. WILLIAMS, M. H., A. R. GOODWIN, R. PERKINS, AND J. BOCRIE. Effect of blood reinjection upon endurance capacity and heart rate. *Med. Sci. Sports* 5: 181–186, 1973.
505. WILLIAMS, M. H., M. LINDHEJM, AND R. SCHUSTER. The effect of blood infusion upon endurance capacity and ratings of specified exertion. *Med. Sci. Sports* 10: 113–118, 1978.
506. WOODSON, R. D., R. E. WILLS, AND C. LENFANT. Effect of acute and established anemia on O_2 transport at rest, submaximal and maximal work. *J. Appl. Physiol.* 44: 36–43, 1978.
507. WYNDHAM, C. H. The physiology of exercise under heat stress. *Annu. Rev. Physiol.* 35: 193–220, 1973.
508. WYNDHAM, C. H., N. B. STRYDOM, J. F. MORRISON, J. PETER, C. G. WILLIAMS, G. A. G. BREDELL, AND A. JOFFE. Differences between ethnic groups in physical working capacity. *J. Appl. Physiol.* 18: 361–366, 1963.
509. WYNDHAM, C. H., N. B. STRYDOM, A. J. VAN RENSBURG, AND G. G. ROGERS. Effects on maximal oxygen intake of acute changes in altitude in a deep mine. *J. Appl. Physiol.* 29: 552–555, 1970.
510. YOUNG, D. R., R. MOSHER, P. ERVE, AND H. SPECTOR. Energy metabolism and gas exchange during treadmill running in dogs. *J. Appl. Physiol.* 14: 834–838, 1959.
511. ZEDDA, S. Steady-state diffusing capacity for CO during exercise in normal subjects. *Respiration* 30: 127–131, 1973.
512. ZELIS, R., AND J. LONGHURST. The circulation in congestive heart failure. In: *The Peripheral Circulations*, edited by R. Zelis. New York: Grune & Stratton, 1975, p. 286–289.
513. ZELIS, R., D. T. MASON, AND E. BRAUNWALD. Partition of blood flow to the cutaneous and muscular beds of the forearm at rest and during leg exercise in normal subjects and in patients with heart failure. *Circ. Res.* 24: 799–806, 1969.
514. ZUNTZ, N., AND O. HAGEMANN. Untersuchungen über den Stoffwechsel des Pferdes bei Ruhe und Arbeit. *Landwirtsch. Jahrb.* 27, Suppl. 3: 1–438, 1898. (Cited in *Circ. Res.* 23: 8, 1968.)

CHAPTER 17

Gas exchange in pregnancy

JAMES METCALFE
JOHN M. BISSONNETTE

Departments of Medicine and Obstetrics and Gynecology, Oregon Health Sciences University, Portland, Oregon

CHAPTER CONTENTS

The young creature, separate individuality as it is, finds the newly prepared nest ready for it, and occupies it. Ensconced there it thrusts thence suckers into the maternal tissue, and draws from the circulation of the mother nutriment, and in effect breathes through its mother's circulation.

C. Sherrington (72)

SUCCESSFUL VIVIPARITY entails modifications of maternal physiology, i.e., shifts of equilibria from the nonpregnant state. Some of these shifts involve respiration. Their importance is emphasized by evidence that the changes in maternal respiration accompanying gestation are essential for normal development of the fetus. Weinberger and colleagues (86) recently reviewed the pulmonary components of respiration in pregnancy.

PULMONARY GAS EXCHANGE

Ventilation

SHAPE OF THORAX. The configuration of the thorax changes during human pregnancy. Thomson and Cohen (78) found that the transverse diameter of the chest was increased by an average of 2.1 cm at its maximum in late pregnancy. This was accompanied by an increase in diaphragmatic height, averaging 4 cm near term, and a progressive increase in the subcostal angle, from 68.5° in early pregnancy to 103.5° in late pregnancy. These changes, derived from measurements of chest roentgenograms, were attributed to increasing intra-abdominal pressure resulting from uterine enlargement. However, the increase in subcostal angle occurred earlier than would be predicted from this explanation. Diaphragmatic movement is not limited by the increased upward pressure from the enlarging uterus. In fact, diaphragmatic excursion is greater during pregnancy than in the puerperium (47), according to an analysis of radiographs. The same study contradicted the persistent idea that intercostal rather than diaphragmatic breathing is favored during pregnancy.

LUNG VOLUMES. Decreases in expiratory reserve volume and residual volume occur in the second half of pregnancy. Consequently, functional residual capacity (FRC) at term averages ~20% less than its nonpregnant value (18). However, the decrease in FRC is accompanied by an increase in inspiratory capacity, so vital capacity is essentially unchanged in both upright and supine subjects (18). As a result, total lung capacity at term is diminished by an average of 4% (175 ml), a statistically insignificant amount. These changes are summarized in Figure 1. The alterations in lung volume, like those in thoracic configuration, are generally attributed to the diaphragmatic elevation caused by uterine enlargement: upward pressure on the diaphragm decreases FRC but, because the strength of the diaphragm and thoracic musculature is not affected, vital capacity remains unchanged.

Measurements of lung volumes made within 2 wk after delivery showed decreases in vital and inspiratory capacities and an increase in residual volume (18). These changes were attributed to the inability of the subjects to cooperate because of fatigue, pain, breast binders, and abdominal or perineal supports. These observations are important when evaluating the

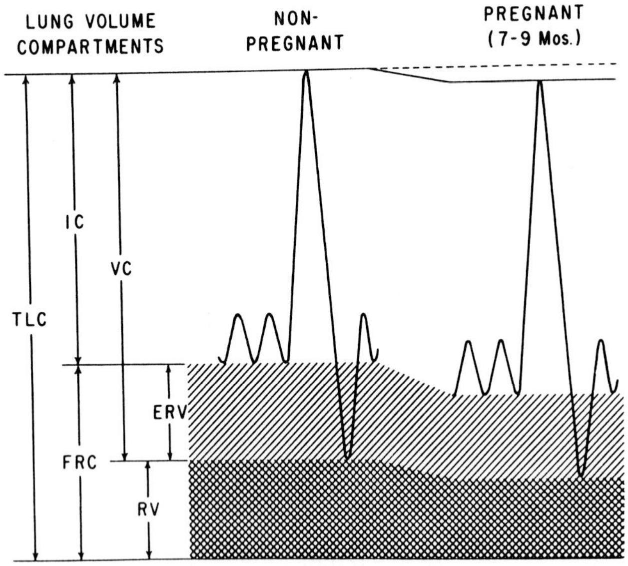

FIG. 1. Changes in lung volumes in women 7–9 months pregnant compared with changes in nonpregnant women. TLC, total lung capacity; IC, inspiratory capacity; FRC, functional residual capacity; VC, vital capacity; RV, residual volume; ERV, expiratory reserve volume. [From Novy and Edwards (58).]

older literature: measurements made in the early puerperium should not be used as control values for data obtained during pregnancy.

Total blood volume increases by an average of 40% during pregnancy (36). Radiological evidence of increased pulmonary blood volume has been reported by some observers (29) and denied by others (79). Although most of the increased blood volume of pregnancy is probably contained in the veins of the lower extremities and the broad ligament when the woman is standing or sitting, lateral recumbency might be accompanied by an increase in intrathoracic blood volume and a consequent decrease in total lung volume.

AIRWAYS. Total airway resistance to flow declines in late pregnancy (67). This change is attributed to relaxation of smooth muscle in the tracheobronchial tree, analogous to the well-documented changes in venous tone (90), generally considered to be due to the action of progesterone. The attribution of the cause of these changes to airway dilation is strengthened by the finding that respiratory dead space increases during pregnancy. The mean value obtained from studies of 12 subjects in the last 10 wk of pregnancy was 186 ml; the mean value 12 wk postpartum was 125 ml (61).

Measurements of closing volume in pregnant women near term show that closure of small airways begins nearer to FRC than it does in nonpregnant women. Indeed, some data suggest that airway closure begins during tidal breathing in pregnant women near term (10), but this has not been uniformly found (17). The fact that small airway closure begins nearer to (or above) the FRC is explainable, at least partly, by the decrease in FRC that results from compression of the lung bases by diaphragmatic elevation. Thus in pregnant women the finding is not evidence of a change in the small airways. If airway closure occurs above FRC, i.e., during tidal breathing, it might explain the widened difference between alveolar and arterial O_2 tensions ($P_{A_{O_2}} - P_{a_{O_2}}$) (6) that has been found near term (see VENTILATION-PERFUSION RELATIONSHIPS, p. 344).

DYNAMICS. The volume of air that can be expired in 1 s from maximum inspiratory capacity [forced expiratory volume in 1 s (FEV_1)] is not altered by pregnancy, indicating that large airway function is not impaired (2, 8, 18). The ratio of FEV_1 to the forced vital capacity does not change, and maximum expiratory flow-volume curves show no evidence of peripheral airway dysfunction (8, 26).

The maximum breathing capacity (MBC) averaged 102 liters/min in 19 subjects studied when they were not pregnant, compared with 96 liters/min at term. The difference was not statistically significant, and 5 of the 19 subjects showed a greater MBC during pregnancy than postpartum (18). The calculated air velocity index (percent of predicted MBC/percent of predicted vital capacity) increased from a mean of 0.94 at term to a mean of 1.04 postpartum. However, as pointed out originally by Cugell et al. (18), this result is difficult to interpret because, as body weight increases during pregnancy, predicted values for MBC increase. This illustrates the fallacy of expressing values of physiological functions during pregnancy in terms of body surface area. To our knowledge the surface area of a pregnant woman has not been measured. Pregnant women were not included among the subjects whose measurements form the basis for DuBois' formula (21). Expression of physiological variables in terms of body weight during pregnancy (or of surface area calculated from body weight) is misleading because the progressive increase in weight during pregnancy can be attributed to fluid retention as well as to the growth of the metabolically active fetus. For these reasons, corrections for differences in body size should probably be based on the nonpregnant weight of the mother.

LUNG COMPLIANCE AND WORK OF BREATHING. Measurements of intraesophageal balloon pressure in the last trimester of pregnancy demonstrated no change in lung compliance, compared with postpartum studies (27). Despite the unaltered lung compliance and the decreased resistance to airflow in the airways, the O_2 cost of ventilation increases progressively during pregnancy (7), reaching a value at term ~50% above nonpregnant controls. Apparently the work of depressing the diaphragm and expanding the thoracic cage becomes greater as the uterus enlarges.

MINUTE VENTILATION AT REST. Hyperventilation occurs during the progestational phase of each menstrual cycle (compared with the preovulatory phase) (24, 28). Subjects in the luteal phase of the cycle show a higher mouth occlusion pressure as well as an increase in both hypoxic and hypercapnic ventilatory responses (69). When pregnancy occurs the hyperventilation of the progestational phase continues and, according to some studies (44, 61), increases as gestation advances. The change in expired minute ventilation ($\dot{V}_E$) is due to an increase in tidal volume without a change in respiratory frequency (18, 38, 62, 64, 87).

Many observations have documented the maternal hyperventilation of pregnancy. In one study (18) $\dot{V}_E$ was 42% greater near term than postpartum, but O_2 consumption ($\dot{V}_{O_2}$) averaged 32% more during pregnancy, so the ventilatory equivalent for O_2 (liters $\dot{V}_E$/100 ml $\dot{V}_{O_2}$) increased only 10%, from 3.0 in the nonpregnant state to 3.3 near term. Alveolar ventilation ($\dot{V}_A$) averaged 7.4 liters/min near term in 12 subjects seated at rest on a bicycle. In the same subjects the average value was 5.1 liters/min when measured 12 wk postpartum under the same conditions (61), and resting end-tidal partial pressure of CO_2 (P_{CO_2}) averaged 28 Torr in the last month of pregnancy compared with 33 Torr postpartum. Arterial partial pressure of CO_2 (Pa_{CO_2}) values below 30 Torr were found under carefully controlled resting conditions in pregnant women near term (44).

In light of the close relationship recently reported between CO_2 production and ventilation (63), we have reexamined the data obtained at rest and during exercise by Pernoll and co-workers (61, 62). In 12 subjects during pregnancy, $\dot{V}_A$ (liters/min) = 0.0048 + 26.196 $\dot{V}_{CO_2}$ (liters/min), $r = 0.99$, where $\dot{V}_{CO_2}$ is CO_2 production. For the same subjects postpartum, $\dot{V}_A = -0.0207 + 23.267\ \dot{V}_{CO_2}$, $r = 0.98$. Thus the magnitude of the increase in $\dot{V}_A$ for a given increase in CO_2 production is significantly greater than during pregnancy. The 13% increase in $\dot{V}_A/\dot{V}_{CO_2}$ that occurred in late pregnancy paralleled the simultaneous 15% fall in resting end-tidal P_{CO_2}.

The hyperventilation of pregnancy seems to be adequately explained by the gradually increasing level of progesterone in blood. Progesterone concentration averages 25 ng/ml at 6 wk of pregnancy and rises to 150 ng/ml in the last month of gestation (93). Ventilation increases in nonpregnant subjects within a few hours after the intramuscular injection of progesterone (45). The curve of ventilatory response to an increasing end-tidal CO_2 concentration has a steeper slope (61), as does the curve of respiratory response to CO_2 inhalation (45), in pregnant women compared with postpartum women. Skatrud et al. (74) found that medroxyprogesterone given orally resulted in a significant fall in alveolar partial pressure of CO_2 ($P_{A_{CO_2}}$) within 48 h with a maximum decline (5 Torr) at 7 days. They also reported no change in respiratory drive measured with CO_2 breathing at rest; there was, however, an increase during exercise. Some work (88) suggests an auxiliary role for estrogens in the increased ventilation of pregnancy. [For additional discussion of hormonal effects on the control of respiration, see the chapter by Dempsey, Olson, and Skatrud (18a) in volume II of the *Handbook* section on respiration.]

Although the increase in ventilation with pregnancy is well established in women, its occurrence in animals is much less prevalent. In a cross-sectional study (different animals at different times), a significant fall in maternal Pa_{CO_2} was found in the 5th through 9th mo of gestation in cows (25). In pygmy goats, Pa_{CO_2} at 19–21 wk of pregnancy was 32.3 ± 1.2 Torr (mean ± SE) compared with 38.3 ± 1.0 in the same animals 4–6 wk postpartum (31). These animals, however, showed a prepartum value of 32.7 ± 1.2 Torr. In a subsequent study from the same laboratory with procedures less likely to cause agitation in the animals, maternal Pa_{CO_2} was 38.6 ± 1.0 Torr in late pregnancy (11). In the awake rhesus monkey (*Macaca mulatta*) maternal Pa_{CO_2} during the last third of pregnancy has been reported as 31.4 ± 2.4 Torr (mean ± SD) (59). This can be compared with 40.5 ± 8.4 Torr in nonpregnant monkeys of unspecified sex (40). No clear-cut ventilatory response to progesterone has been found in the rat and pony (74) or rabbit and goat (75). However, hyperventilation has been induced in nonpregnant guinea pigs by the administration of progesterone (30b). Simultaneous administration of estradiol in these guinea pigs did not result in a greater degree of hyperventilation compared to the animals that received progesterone alone. More recently (30a), it has been shown that estrogen and progesterone are independently capable of stimulating ventilation in male guinea pigs and that hypoventilation occurs in the castrated male animals. Brodeur et al. (12a), using rats as experimental animals, showed that the number of progesterone receptors in the uterus (and by inference, in the medulla) was increased by estradiol administration. Estradiol by itself in these rats did not induce hyperventilation. When medroxyprogesterone was administered after estradiol pretreatment, hyperventilation occurred and the number of uterine progesterone receptors was increased. However, medroxyprogesterone injected without estrogen pretreatment did not cause hyperventilation and the rats had a low number of progesterone receptors in their uterine tissue.

Moore et al. (55a) have demonstrated in human subjects that the magnitude of the ventilatory response to hypoxia increases progressively during pregnancy. The increased sensitivity is observed at rest and during exercise. The degree of response to a given hypoxic stimulus has previously been shown to be related to metabolic rate; Moore et al. (55a) calculated that approximately half of the increased hypoxic response observed in pregnant women might be explained by the increased metabolic rate of pregnancy. The remainder of the stimulus is unexplained, but the magnitude of the ventilatory response did not correlate with serum concentrations of estradiol or progesterone.

Predictably, intrapulmonary mixing of inhaled gases appears to improve during pregnancy, probably because of hyperventilation. The percentage of N_2 remaining in the alveolar air at the end of 7 min of breathing pure O_2 averaged 0.46% in 19 women studied at term compared with 0.56% in the same subjects when not pregnant (18), but the difference was statistically insignificant.

The respiratory alkalosis created by the hyperventilation of pregnancy evokes a compensatory bicarbonate diuresis. As a result, arterial blood pH rose to a mean of only 7.47 (44) when Pa_{CO_2} had fallen to 28 Torr; standard bicarbonate fell from 27 to 21 meq/liter during the course of pregnancy. By 6 wk postpartum, Pa_{CO_2} had returned to a mean value of 37 Torr (4).

Hyperventilation is accentuated during labor. In one study (91), ventilation rose sharply in the first stage of labor from an average of 12 liters/min to 20 liters/min, then increased to 23 liters/min at delivery. Peak values of 40 liters/min were observed in several instances. Respiratory minute volumes approaching the patient's MBC were recorded during labor by Bonica (12). Ventilation decreased promptly after delivery. Some of the maternal hyperventilation during labor is undoubtedly caused by anxiety and pain; extradural analgesia diminished the degree of hyperventilation associated with uterine contractions (46). The magnitude of the hyperventilation is emphasized by the observation that Pa_{CO_2} fell to levels below 20 Torr during uterine contractions (4). Concurrently, arterial pH rose to 7.52, with a calculated base excess of 8.5 meq/liter.

VENTILATION-PERFUSION RELATIONSHIPS. The hyperventilation of pregnancy is associated with an increase in Pa_{O_2}. Mean values lie between 105 and 110 Torr in the first trimester (3, 76). A lower mean value for Pa_{O_2} was obtained in the third trimester and the $PA_{O_2} - Pa_{O_2}$ averaged 14 Torr near term in sitting subjects (6). These findings may be explained by the closure of small airways near the end of expiration or by a general ventilation-perfusion imbalance, which is discussed in *Pulmonary Blood Flow* (this page). Whatever its cause, the widened $PA_{O_2} - Pa_{O_2}$ that occurs near term is particularly evident in residents of high altitude (55, 56) and in obese women (23).

Diffusing Capacity

Measurements of pulmonary diffusing capacity have shown inconsistent changes during pregnancy. Single-breath pulmonary diffusing capacity of CO showed a transient increase during the first trimester, a fall at midgestation, and a slightly decreased value in the last month of pregnancy compared with postpartum measurements (54). When the pulmonary diffusing capacity of CO was divided into its components, a slight decrease in membrane diffusing capacity occurred without a change in pulmonary capillary blood volume (26). These latter studies showed, however, no significant change in total diffusing capacity.

If the decreased diffusing capacity near term is confirmed by subsequent studies, the most likely explanation would probably be compression of the lung bases and perhaps airway closure secondary to diaphragmatic elevation.

Pulmonary Blood Flow

The importance of pulmonary blood flow with regard to maternal respiration depends on its changes during pregnancy and specifically on how these changes are related in time and magnitude to changes in $\dot{V}A$. Therefore we confine our review of cardiac output in pregnancy to those species for which data on $\dot{V}A$ are available.

Cardiac output has been measured during human pregnancy by a number of methods with varied experimental protocols for patient selection. When the same patients are studied serially by the indicator-dilution method, a significant increase in cardiac output is detectable by the end of the first trimester, i.e., by the 12th wk of gestation (19, 41, 66, 84). Most workers (19, 41, 84) have found that cardiac output reaches its peak by the end of the first trimester. However, Roy et al. (66) noted that the maximum increment was reached between 16 and 24 wk.

There appears to be general agreement that the supine position causes cardiac output to decrease in late pregnancy (41, 81). This partially explains the earlier observations that maternal cardiac output returns to near the nonpregnant value in late pregnancy (1, 19, 66, 84). Whether cardiac output declines in late pregnancy in other body positions is an unsettled question. Lees et al. (41) noted no change in measurements at 34–37 wk compared with 24–27 wk with subjects in the lateral position. In contrast, Ueland and his colleagues (81) found that maternal cardiac output measured in lateral recumbency fell from 7.0 liters/min at 26–34 wk to 5.7 liters/min at 38–40 wk (these women had a cardiac output of 5.0 liters/min when studied at 6–8 wk postpartum). As shown in Table 1, the absolute values measured in late pregnancy are similar in both of these studies; the difference occurs in midpregnancy, at which time Ueland et al. (81) found higher values. Because neither report gives the weights of the subjects and because Lees et al. (41) did not make any determinations for nonpregnant subjects, we are unable to speculate on the basis for the discrepancy.

The magnitude of the rise in cardiac output in human pregnancy has ranged from 25% (84) to 50% (19). Average values for nonpregnant subjects in these studies ranged from 4.8 to 6.3 liters/min (1, 19, 41, 66, 81, 84), and the maximum values ranged from 6.1 to 7.6 liters/min. Measurements in pregnant pygmy

TABLE 1. *Pulmonary Ventilation-Perfusion Ratios During Pregnancy*

	Weeks of Pregnancy			Postpartum	Ref.
	20–24	28–32	38–40		
Perfusion*	5.9†	6.2	5.9		41
	6.9	7.0	5.7	5.2	81
Alveolar ventilation	7.1	7.5	8.2	5.6	61, 62
Ventilation-perfusion	1.20	1.21	1.39		41, 61, 62
ratio	1.03	1.07	1.44	1.08	61, 62, 81
Ventilation-O_2 consumption ratio	25.7	25.3	26.3	22.2	61, 62
Ventilation-CO_2 elimination ratio	34.0	34.7	35.2	30.7	61, 62
Perfusion-O_2	21.3	20.9	18.9		41, 61, 62
consumption ratio	24.9	23.6	18.3	20.6	61, 62, 81
Perfusion-CO_2	28.2	28.6	25.3		41, 61, 62
elimination ratio	33.0	32.3	24.5	28.4	61, 62, 81

Perfusion and alveolar ventilation measured in liters/min. *Measured with subjects in lateral recumbency. †Measured at 11–13 wk.

goats (31, 32) showed a gradual increase in maternal cardiac output over the first two-thirds of gestation, when it rose from a nonpregnant value of 3.3 to 3.8 liters/min. A sharp rise occurred during the final third of gestation, reaching 5.3 liters/min near term. Although the relative magnitude of the rise in pygmy goats is comparable to that in humans, the timing with respect to gestational length is quite different.

Serial data on $\dot{V}_A$ in human pregnancy are available from a single group of experiments (61, 62). Knuttgen and Emerson (38) noted a constant increase in $\dot{V}_E$ at rest throughout pregnancy. They began their studies as early as the 10th wk, but no serial data are presented and they did not measure $\dot{V}_A$. Pernoll and associates (61, 62) did not measure $\dot{V}_A$ until midpregnancy, so we cannot compare it to the early rise in pulmonary blood flow. They reported a gradual increase in $\dot{V}_A$ from 19–22 wk to 39–42 wk, reaching a maximum of 8.2 liters/min in late pregnancy compared with a postpartum value of 5.6 liters/min. Thus the time course of the change in $\dot{V}_A$ during pregnancy differs from that of pulmonary blood flow in that a progressive increase occurs. The magnitude of the increment in $\dot{V}_A$ (46%) is within the range of reported change in cardiac output but is higher than the 35%–40% found by most workers.

The effects of these concurrent changes in $\dot{V}_A$ and pulmonary blood flow on pulmonary gas exchange are examined in Table 1. We have used the two reports (41, 81) in which maternal cardiac output was measured in the lateral position. It is clear that the ventilation-perfusion ratio ($\dot{V}_A/\dot{Q}$) increases significantly in the last weeks of human pregnancy. This rise in $\dot{V}_A/\dot{V}$ would tend to cause an increase in $P_{A_{O_2}}$ and provides an alternative explanation to the increase of small airway closure for the widening of the $P_{A_{O_2}} - Pa_{O_2}$ that has been observed in late pregnancy. The changes in $\dot{V}_A/\dot{V}_{O_2}$, $\dot{V}_A/\dot{V}_{CO_2}$, $\dot{Q}/\dot{V}_{O_2}$, and $\dot{Q}/\dot{V}_{CO_2}$ that would be predicted from an increase in $\dot{V}_A/\dot{Q}$ (see chapter by Farhi in this *Handbook*) have been observed in late pregnancy (Table 1). The calculations in Table 1 are based on the assumption that the maternal lung is a single unit. Examining the possibility of the distribution of $\dot{V}_A/\dot{Q}$ and intrapulmonary shunting in late pregnancy with inert-gas methods would be very interesting (82, 83).

PERIPHERAL GAS EXCHANGE

Oxygen Consumption and Carbon Dioxide Production

A study of basal $\dot{V}_{O_2}$ in six women (13) showed a progressive increase during the last two trimesters of pregnancy. The $\dot{V}_{O_2}$ per minute was 15% greater at term than postpartum. The $\dot{V}_{O_2}$ of resting (but not basal) women increases proportionately more during pregnancy than does the basal value, an average of 33% over the postpartum mean when measurements are made with the subject sitting quietly on a bicycle ergometer. The decline in $\dot{V}_{O_2}$ in the postpartum period is proportionately greater than the weight loss: postabsorptive subjects at bed rest showed a 30% decline of $\dot{V}_{O_2}$ after delivery compared with a weight loss of only 15% (38).

The respiratory exchange ratio under postabsorptive resting conditions was significantly higher in 13 prepartum subjects than in the same women postpartum (0.83 compared with 0.76) (38). Adequate procedures were followed to assure a steady state of gas exchange, so the higher ratio was attributed to an increased utilization of carbohydrates during pregnancy.

Respiratory Gas Transport by Maternal Blood

The best teleological justification for maternal hyperventilation is its effect on Pa_{CO_2}. Because transfer of CO_2 from fetal to maternal blood requires that fetal arterial blood have a higher Pa_{CO_2} than maternal arterial blood, hyperventilation by the mother allows the fetus to develop at physiological Pa_{CO_2} values.

The respiratory alkalosis that accompanies mammalian pregnancy encourages 2,3-diphosphoglycerate formation and lowers the O_2 affinity of maternal blood (10a), facilitating O_2 release in peripheral tissues and O_2 diffusion from maternal to fetal blood across the placental membrane (48). Total maternal blood volume increases by an average of 40% above nonpregnant values during pregnancy (36). The 50% expansion of plasma volume (34) occurs mainly between the 6th and 24th wk of pregnancy (65). Total red cell volume, in contrast, increases progressively throughout pregnancy, the rate of rise accelerating somewhat after the 28th wk when plasma volume has stabilized (70). The maximum increment in total red cell volume averages from 20% to 30% in various studies (35). The differences in the magnitude and time course of the changes in plasma and red cell volume result in hemodilution, which is most pronounced in midpregnancy. The hematocrit may fall to as low as 33% (35). Blood hemoglobin concentration reached an average low value of 11.4 g/dl at 16–22 wk of pregnancy in women with "proven iron stores and normal folate status" (70). Hematocrit and blood hemoglobin concentration rise near term as plasma volume stabilizes and total red cell volume continues to increase. The mechanism that allows dilution anemia has not been adequately studied. The erythropoietic activity that would be required to prevent dilution anemia does not exceed the capacity of the healthy bone marrow. The maternal hyperventilation and the renal hyperemia of gestation (14) may depress erythropoietin production.

Organ Distribution of Increased Oxygen Consumption

The only organ for which there are quantitative data with respect to the distribution of the increased maternal $\dot{V}_{O_2}$ is the uterus. Uterine $\dot{V}_{O_2}$ is usually expressed with respect to the weight of the uterus and its contents (fetus and placenta but not amniotic fluid). This convention arose because many workers have used diffusional equilibrium of an inert gas or solute to measure uterine blood flow.

Uterine $\dot{V}_{O_2}$ has been measured in human pregnancy at cesarean section near term with N_2O as the diffusible gas. The two reports give a wide range of uterine $\dot{V}_{O_2}$, from 5 $ml \cdot min^{-1} \cdot kg^{-1}$ (53) to 19 $ml \cdot min^{-1} \cdot kg^{-1}$ (5). Much more literature exists for animal pregnancy. The results in large animals that were unanesthetized at the time of measuring uterine O_2 uptake are given in Table 2. Under these conditions there is remarkable interspecies consistency.

TABLE 2. *Uterine Blood Flow and Oxygen Consumption*

Species	Blood Flow, $ml \cdot min^{-1} \cdot kg^{-1}$	$Ca_{O_2} - C\bar{v}_{O_2}$, ml/dl	O_2 Uptake, $ml \cdot min^{-1} \cdot kg^{-1}$	Ref.
Sheep	248 ± 11	4.2 ± 0.2	10.4 ± 0.4	33
	231*	3.5 ± 0.1	8.1 ± 0.3	57
	262 ± 18	3.5*	9.3 ± 0.3	15
Goat, nubian	346 ± 21	2.3*	8.3 ± 0.2	16
Goat, pygmy	349 ± 48	2.4 ± 0.1	9.3 ± 1.3	11
Horse	315 ± 14	2.7*	8.5 ± 0.3	73
Cow	312 ± 20	2.6*	8.1 ± 0.7	73

$Ca_{O_2} - C\bar{v}_{O_2}$, arteriovenous O_2 concentration difference. *Data not reported independently and calculated from the other two parameters.

If we assume that uterine $\dot{V}_{O_2}$ is 8–10 $ml \cdot min^{-1} \cdot kg^{-1}$, then in women with a 3.5-kg fetus at term, 0.5-kg placenta, and 1.0-kg uterus, 40–50 ml O_2 per minute will be consumed by the uterus. Thus approximately two-thirds of the increased maternal $\dot{V}_{O_2}$ is used by the uterus and its contents. The pygmy goat has a resting $\dot{V}_{O_2}$ of 175 ml/min in late pregnancy (20) compared with 143 ml/min postpartum, a difference of 32 ml/min. Calculated uterine $\dot{V}_{O_2}$ in the pygmy goat approximates 30 ml/min (11), accounting for all of the increase in maternal $\dot{V}_{O_2}$. Although accurate data are not available, it seems likely that several maternal tissues increase their O_2 requirements during normal pregnancy. Prominent among these tissues are the muscles of respiration. In addition to the work of hyperventilation, the volume of the physiological dead space (62) and the O_2 cost for each liter of ventilation are increased during pregnancy compared with nonpregnant controls (7). Even at rest, hyperventilation would require an extra 10 ml of O_2 per minute at the end of pregnancy.

Similar calculations can be made with regard to myocardial $\dot{V}_{O_2}$. If we assume (neglecting any changes in contractility and afterload) that the percentage increase in $\dot{V}_{O_2}$ by the heart is the product of the percentage changes in heart rate, diastolic size, and ventricular mass, a 35% increase in resting myocardial $\dot{V}_{O_2}$ can be calculated from echocardiographic data (37). About 10 ml/min of the increased maternal $\dot{V}_{O_2}$ can be attributed to the increased needs of the myocardium.

The respiratory costs of reproduction are not satisfied when the mammalian fetus is delivered. Measurements of mammary blood flow and $\dot{V}_{O_2}$ have been made in goats (42). The $\dot{V}_{O_2}$ of the nonlactating mammary gland of nonpregnant goats averaged ~1 $ml \cdot 100\ g^{-1} \cdot min^{-1}$ and did not rise during pregnancy. During lactation, however, mammary blood flow rose from ~30 to ~50 $ml \cdot 100\ g^{-1} \cdot min^{-1}$ and the arteriovenous O_2 difference increased from 3.7 to 4.9 ml/dl. In some goats, total udder blood flow reached 1.5 liters/min during peak lactation, varying by only ~10% per hour (43). The total mammary $\dot{V}_{O_2}$ of the lactating goat may, therefore, exceed 75 ml/min. If the relationship of mammary blood flow to milk yield, which has been established in goats, pertains to humans, and if the arteriovenous O_2 difference is the same in both species, milk production of 850 ml/day for a lactating woman (89) would require a mammary blood flow of ~300 ml/min and a mammary $\dot{V}_{O_2}$ of 17 ml/min.

EXERCISE IN PREGNANCY

The hyperventilation observed in resting pregnant human subjects persists during moderate exercise. After a steady state had been achieved during 50-W bicycle exercise, end-tidal P_{CO_2} was significantly lower in 12 normal women near term than in the same women postpartum (61).

A breath-by-breath analysis of $\dot{V}_{O_2}$, CO_2 production, and $\dot{V}_E$ showed that the speed of these respiratory responses at the onset of exercise was increased during pregnancy (22). The hypothesis proposed to explain the observed acceleration is that the rate of venous return to the lungs at the onset of exercise is increased. The inferior vena cava and veins of the lower extremities are more distended with blood because of the expanded blood volume of pregnancy and also because the gravid uterus obstructs venous return while the woman is sitting on the bicycle before exercise. Oxygen uptake and CO_2 elimination increase as soon as the flow rate of venous blood to the lungs increases. This occurs within a few seconds after the leg muscles begin to compress the distended leg veins. The mechanism is analogous to suddenly opening further the faucet at the proximal end of a host that is already filled and emitting a trickle of water from its distal end; the flow of water (and, in the case of blood, its contained CO_2 and deoxygenated hemoglobin) will increase almost at once. The initial increase in ventilation promptly follows the increased flow of blood and CO_2 to the lungs and chemoreceptors (85, 92).

Pregnancy also affects $\dot{V}_{O_2}$ during exercise. In the case of weight-bearing exercise, women have higher rates of $\dot{V}_{O_2}$ when pregnant than they do postpartum at the same speed and inclination of the treadmill (38, 77, 87). In this situation the subjects carry more weight as pregnancy progresses and, as a result, there is a steady increase in the amount of work they perform at the same treadmill settings. Bicycle ergometer exercise has been employed to study the effects of pregnancy on the O_2 requirement for performing a standard workload. One study with this design compared a group of pregnant women with a group of nonpregnant women. No significant difference was found between the pregnant and nonpregnant groups in the total $\dot{V}_{O_2}$ (including O_2 debt) required for a standard bout of exercise (71). A subsequent study (38) took advantage of the possibility of using postpartum values in the same women as controls for studies performed during pregnancy; no significant difference in $\dot{V}_{O_2}$ during the steady state of bicycle exercise was observed. In contrast, two studies (62, 80) have found that the rate of $\dot{V}_{O_2}$ in the steady state of bicycle exercise is higher in pregnant women compared with values obtained from the same individuals performing the same exercise postpartum. The steady-state rate of $\dot{V}_{O_2}$ at a 50-W work load increased progressively as pregnancy advanced and the difference between exercising and resting values rose (62). In other words, the O_2 cost of standard bicycle exercise increased during pregnancy. Oxygen consumption during steady-state 50-W exercise averaged 1,200 ml/min near term compared with a value of 1,020 ml/min 3 mo postpartum, and the O_2 cost of exercise (difference between steady-state exercise and steady-state rest) averaged 840 ml/min at term compared with 770 ml/min 3 mo postpartum. Furthermore, the O_2 debt incurred by this relatively mild exercise also increased during pregnancy, reaching a value of 1,060 ml/min near term in contrast with a postpartum value of 762 ml/min. The same investigators (22) have subsequently reported similar studies of women enrolled in a regular exercise program during pregnancy. These subjects showed no difference in either O_2 debt or steady-state $\dot{V}_{O_2}$ when data near term were compared with postpartum results. The differences in the two groups of subjects are attributed to the increased efficiency of muscular exercise observed with training (68). The augmented ventilatory response to hypoxia that is observed during the luteal phase of the menstrual cycle is less pronounced in athletic women than in nonathletes (69), raising the possibility that training diminishes respiratory work during pregnancy.

PREGNANCY AT HIGH ALTITUDE

Some interesting and important observations concerning respiratory physiology during pregnancy have been made on persons residing at high altitude. The hyperventilation that accompanies pregnancy is superimposed on the hyperventilation caused by the hypoxia of high altitude (30). In contrast with the situation at sea level, hyperventilation causes a leftward shift in blood O_2 affinity by the Bohr effect (55). Blood hemoglobin concentration is higher in women residing at high altitude than in their sea-level counterparts, although the hematocrit in Leadville, Colorado (altitude 3,100 m) women declined significantly during pregnancy, from 42.9% to 39.9% (55). As a result of these two compensatory adjustments, the O_2 content of arterial blood was as high in many women during gestation at an altitude of 3,100 m as in sea-level women.

We know of no measurements of maternal cardiac output during high-altitude pregnancy, but studies of pregnant sheep in Morococha, Peru (altitude 4,500 m), gave evidence of an increased maternal uterine blood flow (51). These and other adaptations (52) apparently provide an intrauterine climate for fetal development, which in healthy women is similar to that of the fetuses of normal women at sea level.

MATERNAL RESPIRATION AND FETAL DEVELOPMENT

The importance of the maternal physiological adjustments to the health of the developing fetus is suggested by several lines of evidence. Leadville, Colorado women who delivered babies weighing less than 2,900 g at birth showed relatively less hyperventilation during gestation than Leadville women who delivered babies weighing more than 3,500 g (56); the mothers of the smaller babies also had a greater fall in blood hemoglobin concentration during pregnancy. On the basis of these findings, Moore and her colleagues (56) have postulated that when maternal arterial O_2 content is not adequately maintained during pregnancy, fetal growth is jeopardized. A possible alternative explanation is that some other defect, such as inadequate progesterone production by the placenta, is associated with both retarded fetal growth and relative maternal hypoventilation.

The possible importance of maternal hyperventilation during pregnancy is supported by studies of methadone addicts (49). Methadone diminishes the hyperventilation of pregnancy, an effect that persists for more than 24 h after an oral dose. Methadone addiction is also associated with retarded fetal growth, resulting in low-birth-weight infants and a high incidence of sudden infant death syndrome. The offspring of methadone addicts also show delayed maturation of the ventilatory response to CO_2 (60).

The well-established effect of maternal cigarette smoking in retarding fetal growth may be due, at least partly, to the effects of CO on blood O_2 affinity and the O_2 content of maternal arterial blood (39). Bauer et al. (9) have experimentally retarded fetal growth in rats by increasing the O_2 affinity of maternal blood near term.

The evidence that fetal growth is jeopardized by limiting maternal O_2 supply to the uterus, coupled with the knowledge that the mammalian fetus normally develops with blood O_2 tensions much lower than those found in adults of the same species, leads to speculation concerning the role of O_2 in the regulation of fetal growth. Experimental methods for chronically increasing fetal blood O_2 tension in mammals have not been developed; however, the growth rate of the chick embryo can be accelerated by incubating hens' eggs in 60% O_2 (50).

REFERENCES

1. ADAMS, J. Q. Cardiovascular physiology in normal pregnancy: studies with the dye dilution technique. *Am. J. Obstet. Gynecol.* 67: 741–759, 1954.
2. ALAILY, A. B., AND K. B. CARROL. Pulmonary ventilation in pregnancy. *Br. J. Obstet. Gynaecol.* 85: 518–524, 1978.
3. ANDERSEN, G. J., G. B. JAMES, N. P. MATHERS, E. L. SMITH, AND J. WALKER. The maternal oxygen tension and acid-base status during pregnancy. *J. Obstet. Gynaecol. Br. Commonw.* 76: 16–19, 1969.
4. ANDERSEN, G. J., AND J. WALKER. The effect of labour on the maternal blood-gas and acid-base status. *J. Obstet. Gynaecol. Br. Commonw.* 77: 289–293, 1970.
5. ASSALI, N. S., R. A. DOUGLASS, JR., W. W. BAIRD, D. B. NICHOLSON, AND R. SUYEMOTO. Measurement of uterine blood flow and uterine metabolism. IV. Results in normal pregnancy. *Am. J. Obstet. Gynecol.* 66: 248–253, 1953.
6. AWE, R. J., M. B. NICOTRA, T. D. NEWSOM, AND R. VILES. Arterial oxygenation and alveolar-arterial gradients in term pregnancy. *Obstet. Gynecol.* 53: 182–186, 1979.
7. BADER, R. A., M. E. BADER, AND D. J. ROSE. The oxygen cost of breathing in dyspnoeic subjects as studied in normal pregnant women. *Clin. Sci. Lond.* 18: 223–235, 1959.
8. BALDWIN, G. R., D. S. MOORTHI, J. A. WHELTON, AND K. F. MACDONNELL. New lung functions and pregnancy. *Am. J. Obstet. Gynecol.* 127: 235–239, 1977.
9. BAUER, C., W. JELKMANN, AND W. MOLL. High oxygen affinity of maternal blood reduces fetal weight in rats. *Respir. Physiol.* 43: 169–177, 1981.
10. BEVAN, D. R., A. HOLDCROFT, L. LOH, W. G. MACGREGOR, J. C. O'SULLIVAN, AND M. K. SYKES. Closing volume and pregnancy. *Br. Med. J.* 1: 13–15, 1974.

10a. BILLE-BRAHE, N. E., AND M. RØRTH. Red cell 2,3-diphosphoglycerate in pregnancy. *Acta Obstet. Gynecol. Scand.* 58: 19–21, 1979.

11. BISSONNETTE, J. M., J. METCALFE, A. R. HOHIMER, M. L. PERNOLL, J. E. WELCH, AND M. S. LAWSON. Uterine oxygen uptake in the pregnant pygmy goat. *Respir. Physiol.* 42: 373–381, 1980.
12. BONICA, J. J. Maternal physiological changes during pregnancy and anesthesia. In: *The Anesthesiologist, Mother and Newborn,* edited by S. M. Shnider and F. Moya. Baltimore, MD: Williams & Wilkins, 1974, p. 3–19.

12a. BRODEUR, P., M. B. MOCKUS, AND L. G. MOORE. Progestin receptors and ventilatory stimulation by progestin (Abstract). *Clin. Respir. Physiol.* 33: 76A, 1985.

13. BURWELL, C. S., W. D. STRAYHORN, D. FLICKINGER, M. B. CORLETTE, E. P. BOWERMAN, AND J. A. KENNEDY. Circulation during pregnancy. *Arch. Intern. Med.* 62: 979–1003, 1938.
14. CHESLEY, L. C., AND G. M. DUFFUS. Preeclampsia, posture and renal function. *Obstet. Gynecol.* 38: 1–5, 1971.
15. CLAPP, J. F., III. Cardiac output and uterine blood flow in the pregnant ewe. *Am. J. Obstet. Gynecol.* 130: 419–423, 1978.
16. COTTER, J. R., J. N. BLECHNER, AND H. PRYSTOWSKY. Blood flow and oxygen consumption of pregnant goats. *Am. J. Obstet. Gynecol.* 103: 1098–1101, 1969.
17. CRAIG, D. B., AND M. A. TOOLE. Airway closure in pregnancy. *Can. Anaesth. Soc. J.* 22: 665–672, 1975.
18. CUGELL, D. W., N. R. FRANK, E. A. GAENSLER, AND T. L. BADGER. Pulmonary function in pregnancy. I. Serial observations in normal women. *Am. Rev. Tuberc. Pulm. Dis.* 67: 568–597, 1953.

18a. DEMPSEY, J. A., E. B. OLSON, JR., AND J. B. SKATRUD. Hormones and neurochemicals in the regulation of breathing. In: *Handbook of Physiology. The Respiratory System. Control of Breathing,* edited by N. S. Cherniack and J. G. Widdicombe. Bethesda, MD: Am. Physiol. Soc., 1986, sect. 3, vol. II, pt. 1, chapt. 7, p. 181–221.

19. DE SCHWARCZ, S. B., P. ARAMENDIA, AND A. C. TAQUINI. Variaciones hemodinamicas en el embarazo normal. *Medicina Buenos Aires* 24: 113–118, 1964.
20. DHINDSA, D. S., J. METCALFE, AND D. H. HUMMELS. Responses to exercise in the pregnant pygmy goat. *Respir. Physiol.* 32: 299–311, 1978.
21. DUBOIS, E. F. *Basal Metabolism in Health and Disease* (3rd ed.). Philadelphia, PA: Lea & Febiger, 1936, p. 134.
22. EDWARDS, M. J., J. METCALFE, M. J. DUNHAM, AND M. S. PAUL. Accelerated respiratory response to moderate exercise in late pregnancy. *Respir. Physiol.* 45: 229–241, 1981.
23. ENG, M., J. BUTLER, AND J. J. BONICA. Respiratory function in pregnant obese women. *Am. J. Obstet. Gynecol.* 123: 241–245, 1975.
24. ENGLAND, S. J., AND L. E. FARHI. Fluctuations in alveolar CO_2 and in base excess during the menstrual cycle. *Respir. Physiol.* 26: 157–161, 1976.
25. GAHLENBECK, H., H. FRERKING, A. M. RATHSCHLAG-SCHAEFER, AND H. BARTELS. Oxygen and carbon dioxide exchange across the cow placenta during the second part of pregnancy. *Respir. Physiol.* 4: 119–131, 1968.
26. GAZIOGLU, K., N. L. KALTREIDER, M. ROSEN, AND P. N. YU. Pulmonary function during pregnancy in normal women and in patients with cardiopulmonary disease. *Thorax* 25: 445–450, 1970.
27. GEE, J. B. L., B. S. PACKER, J. E. MILLEN, AND E. D. ROBIN. Pulmonary mechanics during pregnancy. *J. Clin. Invest.* 46: 945–952, 1967.
28. GOODLAND, R. L., AND W. T. POMMERENKE. Cyclic fluctuations of the alveolar carbon dioxide tension during the normal menstrual cycle. *Fertil. Steril.* 3: 394–401, 1952.
29. HARRIS, G. B. C. Non-obstetric diagnostic radiology during pregnancy. *Clin. Obstet. Gynecol.* 9: 59–70, 1966.

30. HELLEGERS, A., J. METCALFE, W. E. HUCKABEE, H. PRYSTOWSKY, G. MESCHIA, AND D. H. BARRON. Alveolar P_{CO_2} and P_{O_2} in pregnant and nonpregnant women at high altitude. *Am. J. Obstet. Gynecol.* 82: 241–245, 1961.
30a. HOHIMER, A. R., M. V. HART, AND J. A. RESKO. The effect of castration and sex steroids on ventilatory control in male guinea pigs. *Respir. Physiol.* 61: 383–390, 1985.
30b. HOSENPUD, J. D., M. V. HART, M. J. MORTON, A. R. HOHIMER, AND J. A. RESKO. Progesterone-induced hyperventilation in the guinea pig. *Respir. Physiol.* 52: 259–264, 1983.
31. HOVERSLAND, A. S., J. METCALFE, AND J. T. PARER. Adjustments in maternal blood gases, acid-base balance, and oxygen consumption in the pregnant pygmy goat. *Biol. Reprod.* 10: 589–595, 1974.
32. HOVERSLAND, A. S., J. T. PARER, AND J. METCALFE. Hemodynamic adjustments in the pygmy goat during pregnancy and early postpartum. *Biol. Reprod.* 10: 578–588, 1974.
33. HUCKABEE, W. E., M. C. CRENSHAW, L. B. CURET, AND D. H. BARRON. Uterine blood flow and oxygen consumption in the unrestrained pregnant ewe. *Q. J. Exp. Physiol. Cogn. Med. Sci.* 57: 12–23, 1972.
34. HYTTEN, F. E., AND I. LEITCH. *The Physiology of Human Pregnancy* (2nd ed.). Oxford, UK: Blackwell, 1971, p. 12–13.
35. HYTTEN, F. E., AND I. LEITCH. *The Physiology of Human Pregnancy* (2nd ed.). Oxford, UK: Blackwell, 1971, p. 32–33.
36. HYTTEN, F. E., AND D. B. PAINTIN. Increase in plasma volume during normal pregnancy. *J. Obstet. Gynaecol. Br. Commonw.* 70: 402–407, 1963.
37. KATZ, R., J. S. KARLINER, AND R. RESNIK. Effects of a natural volume overload state (pregnancy) on left ventricular performance in normal human subjects. *Circulation* 58: 434–441, 1978.
38. KNUTTGEN, H. G., AND K. EMERSON, JR. Physiological response to pregnancy at rest and during exercise. *J. Appl. Physiol.* 36: 549–553, 1974.
39. LANDESMAN-DWYER, S., AND I. EMANUEL. Smoking during pregnancy. *Teratology* 19: 119–126, 1979.
40. LEES, M. H., R. H. HERR, J. D. HILL, C. L. MORGAN, A. J. OCHSNER III, C. THOMAS, AND D. L. VAN FLEET. Distribution of systemic blood flow of the rhesus monkey during cardiopulmonary bypass. *J. Thorac. Cardiovasc. Surg.* 61: 570–586, 1971.
41. LEES, M. M., S. H. TAYLOR, D. B. SCOTT, AND M. G. KERR. A study of cardiac output at rest throughout pregnancy. *J. Obstet. Gynaecol. Br. Commonw.* 74: 319–328, 1967.
42. LINZELL, J. L. Mammary-gland blood flow and oxygen, glucose and volatile fatty acid uptake in the conscious goat. *J. Physiol. Lond.* 153: 492–509, 1960.
43. LINZELL, J. L. Mammary blood flow and methods of identifying and measuring precursors of milk. In: *Lactation, A Comprehensive Treatise: The Mammary Gland/Development and Maintenance*, edited by B. L. Larson and V. R. Smith. New York: Academic, 1974, vol. 1, p. 143–225.
44. LUCIUS, H., H. GAHLENBECK, H.-O. KLEINE, H. FABEL, AND H. BARTELS. Respiratory functions, buffer system, and electrolyte concentrations of blood during human pregnancy. *Respir. Physiol.* 9: 311–317, 1970.
45. LYONS, H. A., AND R. ANTONIO. The sensitivity of the respiratory center in pregnancy and after the administration of progesterone. *Trans. Assoc. Am. Physicians* 72: 173–180, 1959.
46. MARX, G. F., A. S. MACATANGAY, A. V. COHEN, AND H. SCHULMAN. Effect of pain relief on arterial blood gas values during labor. *NY State J. Med.* 69: 819–822, 1969.
47. MCGINTY, A. P. The comparative effects of pregnancy and phrenic nerve interruption on the diaphragm and their relation to pulmonary tuberculosis. *Am. J. Obstet. Gynecol.* 35: 237–248, 1938.
48. METCALFE, J., H. BARTELS, AND W. MOLL. Gas exchange in the pregnant uterus. *Physiol. Rev.* 47: 782–838, 1967.
49. METCALFE, J., M. J. DUNHAM, G. D. OLSEN, AND M. A. KRALL. Respiratory and hemodynamic effects of methadone in pregnant women. *Respir. Physiol.* 42: 383–393, 1980.
50. METCALFE, J., I. E. MCCUTCHEON, D. L. FRANCISCO, A. B. METZENBERG, AND J. E. WELCH. Oxygen availability and growth of the chick embryo. *Respir. Physiol.* 46: 81–88, 1981.
51. METCALFE, J., G. MESCHIA, A. HELLEGERS, H. PRYSTOWSKY, W. HUCKABEE, AND D. H. BARRON. Observations on the placental exchange of the respiratory gases in pregnant ewes at high altitude. *Q. J. Exp. Physiol. Cogn. Med. Sci.* 47: 74–92, 1962.
52. METCALFE, J., M. J. NOVY, AND E. N. PETERSON. Reproduction at high altitudes. In: *Comparative Aspects of Reproductive Failure*, edited by K. Benirschke. New York: Springer-Verlag, 1967, p. 447–457.
53. METCALFE, J., S. L. ROMNEY, L. H. RAMSEY, D. E. REID, AND C. S. BURWELL. Estimation of uterine blood flow in normal human pregnancy at term. *J. Clin. Invest.* 34: 1632–1638, 1955.
54. MILNE, J. A., R. J. MILLS, J. R. T. COUTTS, M. C. MACNAUGHTON, F. MORAN, AND A. I. PACK. The effect of human pregnancy on the pulmonary transfer factor for carbon monoxide as measured by the single-breath method. *Clin. Sci. Mol. Med.* 53: 271–276, 1977.
54a. MOORE, L. G., P. BRODEUR, O. CHUMBE, J. D'BROT, S. HOFMEISTER, AND C. MONGE. Maternal ventilation, hypoxic ventilatory response and infant birth weight during high altitude pregnancy (Abstract). *Federation Proc.* 43: 434, 1984.
55. MOORE, L. G., D. JAHNIGEN, S. S. ROUNDS, J. T. REEVES, AND R. F. GROVER. Maternal hyperventilation helps preserve arterial oxygenation during high altitude pregnancy. *J. Appl. Physiol.: Respirat. Environ. Exercise Physiol.* 52: 690–694, 1982.
55a. MOORE, L. G., R. E. MCCULLOUGH, AND J. V. WEIL. Maternal hypoxic ventilatory response increases during pregnancy (Abstract). *Federation Proc.* 44: 833, 1985.
56. MOORE, L. G., S. S. ROUNDS, D. JAHNIGEN, R. F. GROVER, AND J. T. REEVES. Infant birth weight is related to maternal arterial oxygenation at high altitude. *J. Appl. Physiol.: Respirat. Environ. Exercise Physiol.* 52: 695–699, 1982.
57. MORRISS, F. H., JR., C. R. ROSENFELD, R. RESNIK, G. MESCHIA, E. L. MAKOWSKI, AND F. C. BATTAGLIA. Growth of uterine oxygen and glucose uptakes during pregnancy in sheep. *Gynecol. Obstet. Invest.* 5: 230–241, 1974.
58. NOVY, M. J., AND M. J. EDWARDS. Respiratory problems in pregnancy. *Am. J. Obstet. Gynecol.* 99: 1024–1045, 1967.
59. NOVY, M. J., G. J. PIASECKI, J. D. HILL, AND B. T. JACKSON. Cardiorespiratory measurements in fetal monkeys obtained by chronic catheters. *J. Appl. Physiol.* 31: 788–791, 1971.
60. OLSEN, G. D., AND M. H. LEES. Ventilatory response to carbon dioxide of infants following chronic prenatal methadone exposure. *J. Pediatr.* 96: 983–989, 1980.
61. PERNOLL, M. L., J. METCALFE, P. A. KOVACH, R. WACHTEL, AND M. J. DUNHAM. Ventilation during rest and exercise in pregnancy and postpartum. *Respir. Physiol.* 25: 295–310, 1975.
62. PERNOLL, M. L., J. METCALFE, T. L. SCHLENKER, J. E. WELCH, AND J. A. MATSUMOTO. Oxygen consumption at rest and during exercise in pregnancy. *Respir. Physiol.* 25: 285–293, 1975.
63. PHILLIPSON, E. A., J. DUFFIN, AND J. D. COOPER. Critical dependence of respiratory rhythmicity on metabolic CO_2 load. *J. Appl. Physiol.: Respirat. Environ. Exercise Physiol.* 50: 45–54, 1981.
64. PLASS, E. D., AND F. W. OBERST. Respiration and pulmonary ventilation in normal nonpregnant, pregnant and puerperal women: with an interpretation of the acid-base balance during normal pregnancy. *Am. J. Obstet. Gynecol.* 35: 441–452, 1938.
65. PRITCHARD, J. A. Changes in the blood volume during pregnancy and delivery. *Anesthesiology* 26: 393–399, 1965.
66. ROY, S. B., P. K. MALKANI, R. VIRIK, AND M. L. BHATIA. Circulatory effects of pregnancy. *Am. J. Obstet. Gynecol.* 96: 221–225, 1966.
67. RUBIN, A., N. RUSSO, AND D. GOUCHER. The effect of pregnancy upon pulmonary function in normal women. *Am. J. Obstet. Gynecol.* 72: 963–969, 1956.
68. SCHEUER, J., AND C. M. TIPTON. Cardiovascular adaptations to physical training. *Annu. Rev. Physiol.* 39: 221–251, 1977.
69. SCHOENE, R. B., H. T. ROBERTSON, D. J. PIERSON, AND A. P. PETERSON. Respiratory drives and exercise in menstrual cycles

of athletic and nonathletic women. *J. Appl. Physiol.: Respirat. Environ. Exercise Physiol.* 50: 1300–1305, 1981.
70. SCOTT, D. E. Anemia in pregnancy. In: *Obstetrics and Gynecology Annual: 1972*, edited by R. M. Wynn. New York: Appleton-Century-Crofts, 1972, p. 219–244.
71. SEITCHIK, J. Body composition and energy expenditure during rest and work in pregnancy. *Am. J. Obstet. Gynecol.* 97: 701–713, 1967.
72. SHERRINGTON, C. *Man on His Nature.* New York: Doubleday, 1953, p. 65.
73. SILVER, M., AND R. S. COMLINE. Transfer of gases and metabolites in the equine placenta: a comparison with other species. *J. Reprod. Fertil. Suppl.* 23: 589–594, 1975.
74. SKATRUD, J. B., J. A. DEMPSEY, AND D. G. KAISER. Ventilatory response to medroxyprogesterone acetate in normal subjects: time course and mechanism. *J. Appl. Physiol.: Respirat. Environ. Exercise Physiol.* 44: 939–944, 1978.
75. SMITH, C. A., AND R. H. KELLOGG. Ventilatory response of rabbits and goats to chronic progesterone administration. *Respir. Physiol.* 39: 383–391, 1980.
76. TEMPLETON, A., AND G. R. KELMAN. Maternal blood-gases, ($PA_{O_2} - Pa_{O_2}$), physiological shunt and VD/VT in normal pregnancy. *Br. J. Anaesth.* 48: 1001–1004, 1976.
77. TERUOKA, G. Labour physiological studies on pregnant women. *Arbeitsphysiologie* 7: 259–279, 1933.
78. THOMSON, K. J., AND M. E. COHEN. Studies on the circulation in pregnancy. II. Vital capacity observations in normal pregnant women. *Surg. Gynecol. Obstet.* 66: 591–603, 1938.
79. TURNER, A. F. The chest radiograph in pregnancy. *Clin. Obstet. Gynecol.* 18: 65–74, 1975.
80. UELAND, K., M. J. NOVY, AND J. METCALFE. Cardiorespiratory responses to pregnancy and exercise in normal women and patients with heart disease. *Am. J. Obstet. Gynecol.* 115: 4–10, 1973.
81. UELAND, K., M. J. NOVY, E. N. PETERSON, AND J. METCALFE. Maternal cardiovascular dynamics. IV. The influence of gestational age on the maternal cardiovascular response to posture and exercise. *Am. J. Obstet. Gynecol.* 104: 856–864, 1969.
82. WAGNER, P. D., R. B. LARAVUSO, R. R. UHL, AND J. B. WEST. Continuous distributions of ventilation-perfusion ratios in normal subjects breathing air and 100% O_2. *J. Clin. Invest.* 54: 54–68, 1974.
83. WAGNER, P. D., H. A. SALTZMAN, AND J. B. WEST. Measurement of continuous distributions of ventilation-perfusion ratios: theory. *J. Appl. Physiol.* 36: 588–599, 1974.
84. WALTERS, W. A., W. G. MACGREGOR, AND M. HILLS. Cardiac output at rest during pregnancy and the puerperium. *Clin. Sci. Lond.* 30: 1–11, 1966.
85. WASSERMAN, K., B. J. WHIPP, S. N. KOYAL, AND W. L. BEAVER. Anaerobic threshold and respiratory gas exchange during exercise. *J. Appl. Physiol.* 35: 236–243, 1973.
86. WEINBERGER, S. E., S. T. WEISS, W. R. COHEN, J. W. WEISS, AND T. S. JOHNSON. Pregnancy and the lung. *Am. Rev. Respir. Dis.* 121: 559–581, 1980.
87. WIDLUND, G. The cardio-pulmonal function during pregnancy. *Acta Obstet. Gynecol. Scand.* 25: 1–125, 1945.
88. WILBRAND, U., C. PORATH, P. MATTHAES, AND R. JASTER. Der Einfluss der Ovarialsteroide auf die Funktion des Atemzentrums. *Arch. Gynaekol.* 191: 507–531, 1959.
89. WILLIAMS, S. R. (editor). *Nutrition and Diet Therapy* (3rd ed.). St. Louis, MO: Mosby, 1977, p. 371–389.
90. WOOD, J. E., III, AND S. M. GOODRICH. Dilation of the veins with pregnancy or with oral contraceptive therapy. *Trans. Am. Clin. Climatol. Assoc.* 76: 174–180, 1964.
91. WULF, K. H., W. KUNZEL, AND V. LEHMANN. Clinical aspects of placental gas exchange. In: *Respiratory Gas Exchange and Blood Flow in the Placenta*, edited by L. D. Longo and H. Bartels. Bethesda, MD: U. S. Dept. of Health, Education, and Welfare, 1972, p. 505–521. (Publ. no. 73-361.)
92. YAMAMOTO, W. S., AND M. W. EDWARDS, JR. Homeostasis of carbon dioxide during intravenous infusion of carbon dioxide. *J. Appl. Physiol.* 15: 807–818, 1960.
93. YANNONE, M. E., J. R. MCCURDY, AND A. GOLDFIEN. Plasma progesterone levels in normal pregnancy, labor, and the puerperium. II. Clinical data. *Am. J. Obstet. Gynecol.* 101: 1058–1061, 1968.

CHAPTER 18

Respiratory gas exchange in the placenta

LAWRENCE D. LONGO | *Division of Perinatal Biology, Departments of Physiology and Obstetrics and Gynecology, School of Medicine, Loma Linda University, Loma Linda, California*

CHAPTER CONTENTS

---

neither is there occasion for returning and refining this blood [of the fetus] in the lungs of the mother, because that office is sufficiently performed in the placenta until the foetus is delivered, when its own lungs are put to their proper use.

William Smellie (315)

THE PLACENTA

A distinguishing feature of development of the mammalian conceptus is the provision of nutrients from the maternal organism. Adequate exchange of respiratory gases and substrates across the placenta between the maternal and fetal circulations of eutherian mammals is essential for normal fetal growth and differentiation. The placenta is unique in its function

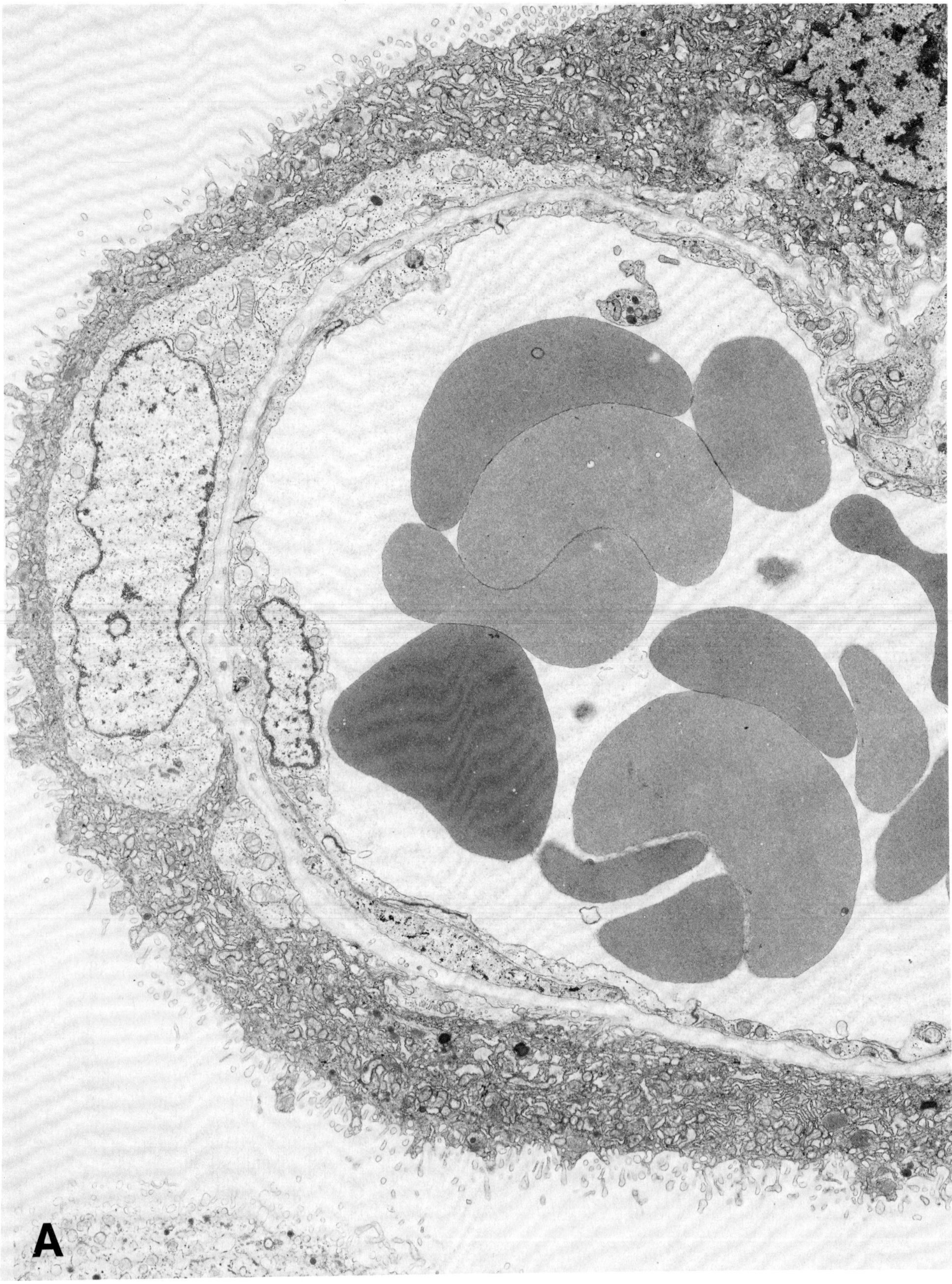

FIG. 1*A*. Near-term human placental villus showing well-differentiated syncytiotrophoblast with its border folded with tufts of microvilli facing maternal intervillous space. Large cytotrophoblast cell is on left and fetal capillary contains several erythrocytes. × 7,350. (Courtesy of B. F. King.)

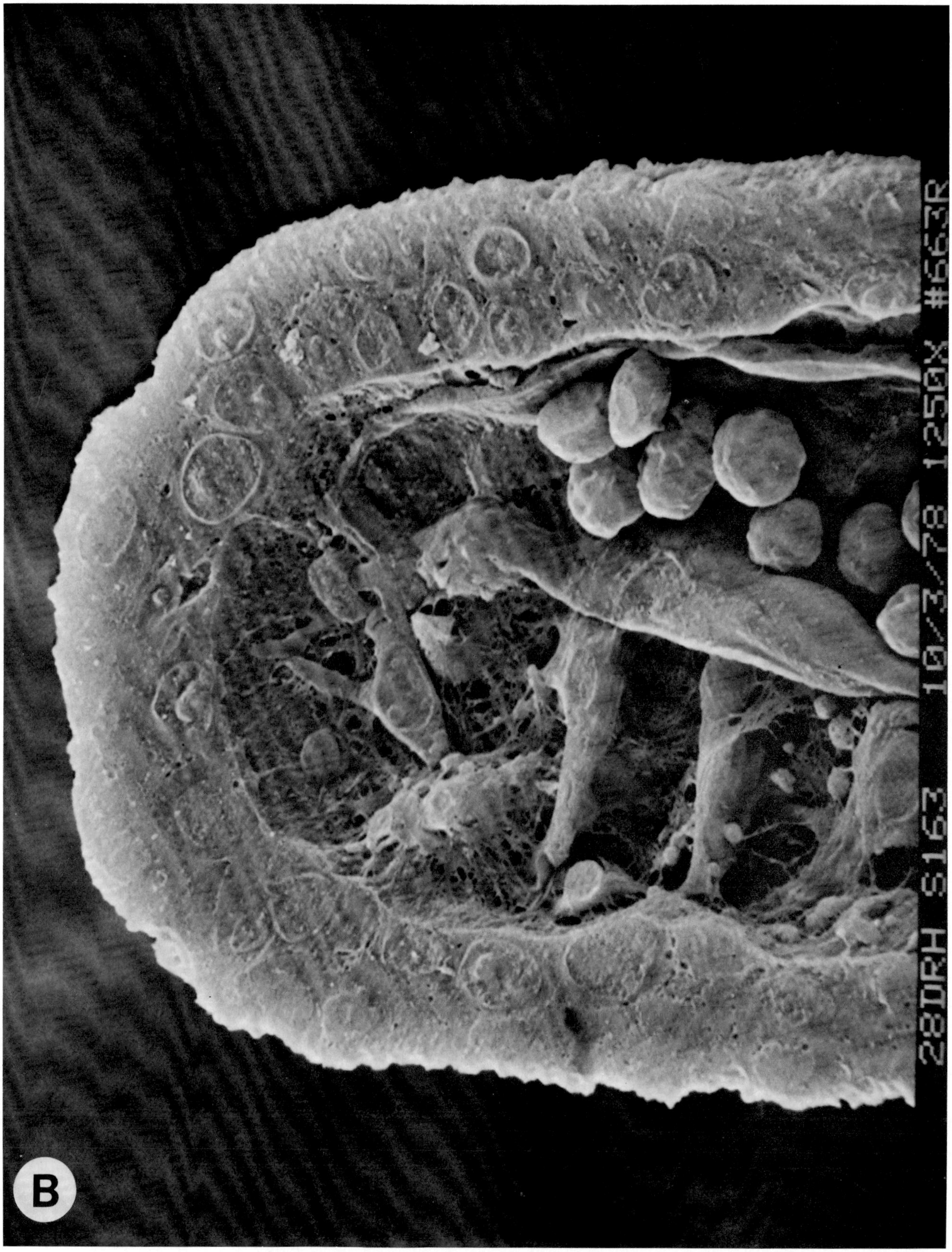

FIG. 1*B*. Scanning electron micrograph of 28-day rhesus monkey villus with fetal capillary containing erythrocytes. × 2,250. (Courtesy of B. F. King.)

from several points of view. Its lifetime is short relative to that of the fetus, and its size and function change continually during the course of gestation. For the fetus the placenta serves not only as the lung but also as the gastrointestinal tract, kidney, liver, and polyendocrine gland. Its morphology changes during gestation in ways that would only be considered pathological in any other organ. Finally, whereas respiratory gases diffuse between the maternal and fetal circulations, other substances exchange by facilitated diffusion, active transport, pinocytosis, and bulk flow.

At least from the time of William Smellie (315) and John and William Hunter (155) in the mid-eighteenth century, it has been recognized that the maternal and fetal placental circulations are separate and that blood continuously perfuses these two conducting systems so that the various nutrients can exchange through the intervening membranes (Fig. 1). Placental vascular anatomy varies widely among mammals, and perhaps no other mammalian organ displays as much diversity in its gross and microscopic structure. Although placental O_2 and CO_2 exchanges have been studied in several species, generalizing the results is difficult because of major species differences. Figure 2 summarizes some of these differences in terms of functional efficiency for gas exchange and the morphology of the placental barrier. Rabbits (18, 248), guinea pigs, and cats (323) have efficient placentas with relatively thin hemochorial barriers that consist of a fetal endothelial layer, mesenchymal tissue, and chorionic membranes arranged in a labyrinthine pattern. Fetal venous partial pressure of O_2 ($P_{V_{O_2}}$) in the umbilical vein can exceed uterine $P_{V_{O_2}}$ (101), suggesting a countercurrent-type exchange pattern for O_2, although this does not seem to explain the CO_2 measurements.

Sheep and other ruminants have less efficient placentas with thicker epitheliochorial barriers. Although the vascular anatomy suggests a crosscurrent (221) or even countercurrent (14) pattern, functionally it is useful to treat these placentas as having concurrent flow patterns. This is because the sizable partial pressure of O_2 (P_{O_2}) difference between exiting maternal and fetal blood suggests either a large diffusion barrier or the presence of sizable shunting of blood past the exchange region in both maternal and fetal circulations.

Human and other primate placentas appear to be intermediate in efficiency. The microvascular structure is hemochorial, similar to that found in guinea pigs, but the vascular pattern may be described as a maternal pool with fetal vessels dipping into it, form-

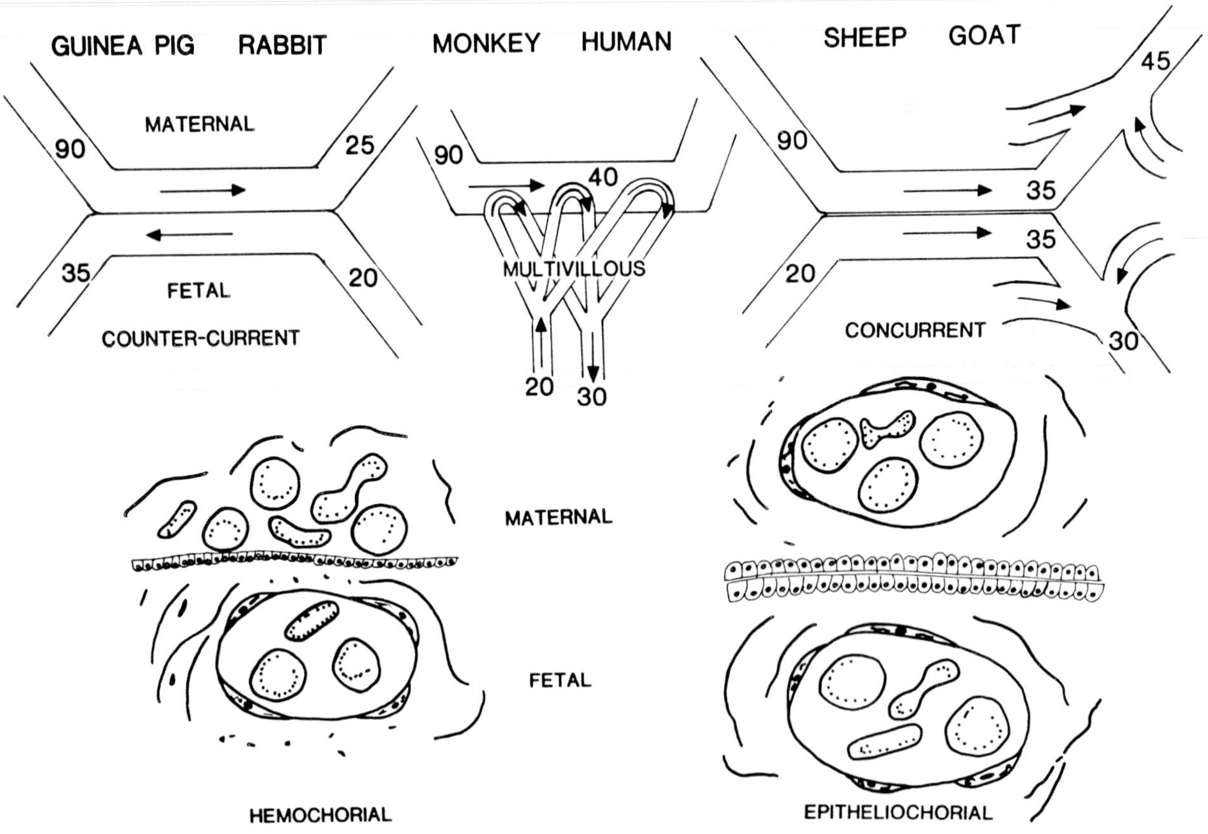

FIG. 2. Schematic illustration of functional anatomy and morphology of placental barrier of several species. Numerical values indicate typical O_2 tensions (P_{O_2}, Torr) for inflowing and outflowing maternal and fetal blood.

ing a multivillous arrangement (26). Maternal blood flows through the spiral endometrial arteries, which in the human open into the intervillous space. Blood is propelled by the *vis a tergo* toward the chorionic villi in fairly discrete spurts. As the momentum of the incoming stream is spent, the blood spreads laterally, eventually draining into the endometrial veins (288, 289). Unfortunately little information is available on the explicit relations of placental flow and respiratory gas exchange.

Placental Exchange and Fetal Oxygenation

Several considerations of the relation of placental O_2 transfer ($\dot{V}_{O_2}$) to fetal oxygenation are relevant. The developing fetus presents a paradox of sorts. On the one hand, its arterial O_2 tension (Pfa_{O_2}) is only 20–30 Torr, compared with adult values of ~100 Torr (see Table 1 for normal values). In addition, its rate of O_2 consumption ($\dot{V}f_{O_2}$) is twice that of the adult per unit weight (8 vs. 4 $ml \cdot min^{-1} \cdot kg^{-1}$), and its O_2 reserve is only enough to meet its metabolic needs for 1–2 min. On the other hand, fetal blood O_2 affinity in humans and many other species exceeds that of the mother. Also, its blood O_2 capacity (O_2Cap) is greater than that of the mother (at least during the final third of pregnancy), so that despite its much lower P_{O_2} and an oxyhemoglobin saturation ([HbO_2] or Sa_{O_2}) that is ~25% lower (75% vs. 98%), the O_2 concentration (Cfa_{O_2}) of arterial blood flowing to its brain and heart is greater than that of maternal arterial blood (16.5 vs. 15.4 $ml \cdot dl^{-1}$). In addition, both maternal and fetal blood flows to the placental exchange area must be reasonably well matched for optimal O_2 transfer.

Because the integrity of fetal neural and other vital cells demands a relatively uninterrupted O_2 supply, the processes whereby O_2 cascades by convection and diffusion from the mother's ambient environment to the cristae of the fetal mitochondria must be exquisitely regulated at each step (Fig. 3). A critical link in this chain of sequential events is the placenta, where

TABLE 1. *Normal Values of O_2, CO_2, and pH in Human Maternal and Fetal Blood*

	Maternal Uterine		Fetal Umbilical	
	Artery	Vein	Vein	Artery
P_{O_2}, Torr	95	38	30	22
HbO_2, % saturation	98	72	75	50
O_2 content, $ml \cdot dl^{-1}$	16.4	11.8	16.2	10.9
O_2 content, mM	7.3	5.3	7.2	4.5
Hb, $g \cdot dl^{-1}$	12.0	12.0	16.0	16.0
O_2 capacity, $ml \cdot dl^{-1}$	16.4	16.4	21.9	21.9
O_2 capacity, mM	7.3	7.3	9.8	9.8
P_{CO_2}, Torr	32	40	43	48
CO_2 content, mM	19.6	21.8	25.2	26.3
HCO_3^-,	18.8	20.7	24.0	25.0
pH	7.42	7.35	7.38	7.34

P_{O_2} and P_{CO_2}, partial pressures of O_2 and CO_2, respectively; Hb, hemoglobin.

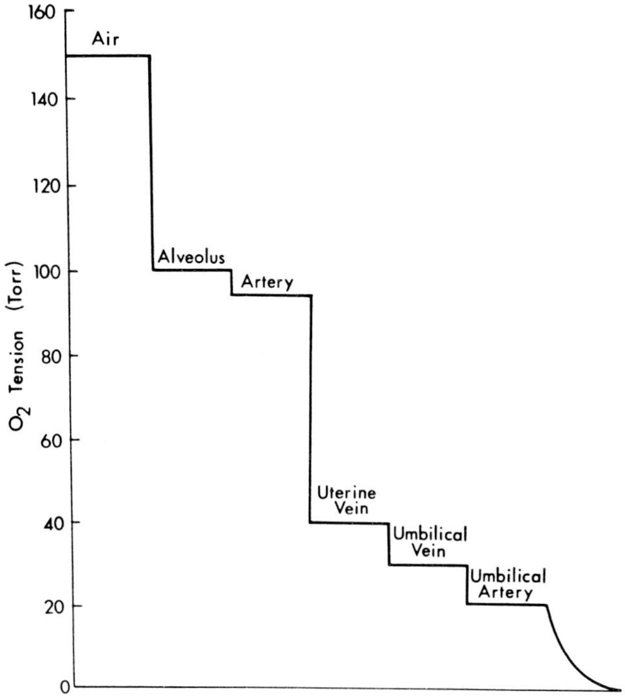

FIG. 3. Cascade of P_{O_2} from air to alveolar gas, arterial and uterine venous blood of maternal organism, fetal umbilical venous and arterial blood, and cristae of fetal mitochondria.

sufficient O_2 to supply fetal needs must diffuse across the membranes from maternal to fetal blood during the short time the two circulations are in proximity. This process is a function of a number of variables. Table 2 lists some of the most important of these: maternal and fetal arterial O_2 partial pressure (Pa_{O_2}), maternal and fetal Hb-O_2 affinities, maternal and fetal placental Hb flow rates, the diffusing capacity of the placenta, the vascular relations between maternal and fetal vessels, and the amount of CO_2 exchanged (200). Each of these variables in turn is a function of other factors.

Questions to Consider

The interactions, dynamics, and specific regulatory mechanisms whereby these and other factors affect and limit placental O_2 and CO_2 exchange are of fundamental physiological and clinical importance. Although recent years have witnessed new approaches, based largely on experimental studies in chronically instrumented animals and theoretical inquiry with mathematical models, to gain increased understanding of these problems, there has been no major review of the subject since that of Metcalfe et al. (237).

This overview synthesizes into a coherent whole many of the isolated findings reported during the past two decades. Specific questions that I address include the following. *1)* What changes in maternal blood O_2 affinity and capacity occur during pregnancy, and what is their effect on placental O_2 exchange? *2)* How

TABLE 2. *Principal Factors Affecting Placental O_2 Transfer*

Variable	Associated Components
Placental diffusing capacity (Dp)	Membrane diffusing capacity (area, thickness, solubility, diffusivity of tissues), capillary blood volume, diffusing capacity of blood (O_2 capacity, Hb reaction rates, concentration of reduced Hb)
Maternal arterial P_{O_2} (Pma_{O_2})	Inspired P_{O_2}, alveolar ventilation, mixed venous P_{O_2}, pulmonary blood flow, pulmonary diffusing capacity
Fetal arterial P_{O_2} (Pfa_{O_2})	Maternal arterial P_{O_2}, maternal placental Hb flow, placental diffusing capacity, umbilical venous P_{O_2}, fetal O_2 consumption, peripheral blood flow
Maternal Hb-O_2 affinity (Pm_{50})	pH, temperature, P_{CO_2}, 2,3-diphosphoglycerate concentration, CO concentration
Fetal Hb-O_2 affinity (Pf_{50})	pH, temperature, P_{CO_2}, 2,3-diphosphoglycerate concentration, CO concentration
Maternal placental Hb flow rate ($\dot{Q}m_{Hb}$)	Arterial pressure, placental resistance to blood flow, venous pressure, blood O_2 capacity
Fetal placental Hb flow rate ($\dot{Q}f_{Hb}$)	Umbilical artery blood pressure, umbilical venous blood pressure (or maternal vascular pressure under conditions of sluice flow), placental resistance to blood flow, O_2 capacity of blood
Spatial relation of maternal to fetal flow	
Amount of CO_2 exchange ($\dot{V}_{CO_2}$)	

P_{O_2} and P_{CO_2}, partial pressures of O_2 and CO_2, respectively; Hb, hemoglobin. [Adapted from Longo et al. (200).]

do variations in fetal blood O_2 affinity and capacity affect $\dot{V}_{O_2}$? *3*) How is placental respiratory function quantified? *4*) How do physiological or pathological alterations affect $\dot{V}_{O_2}$? *5*) What is the role of placental O_2 consumption in limiting $\dot{V}_{O_2}$? *6*) What is the relation of maternal and fetal Pa_{O_2} values to $\dot{V}_{O_2}$? *7*) What factors limit CO_2 exchange? *8*) To what extent do maternal and fetal placental blood flows affect O_2 and CO_2 transfer? *9*) What are the normal relations of maternal and fetal placental blood flows, and how does the distribution of these flows affect respiratory gas exchange? *10*) To what extent do O_2 and CO_2 exchange in the placenta compare with that in the lung? A number of these topics are controversial, presumably representing areas of ignorance. This review makes no attempt to consider the interrelations of respiratory gas exchange and transplacental fluxes of metabolites and water or the fetal consequences of decreased placental O_2 exchange.

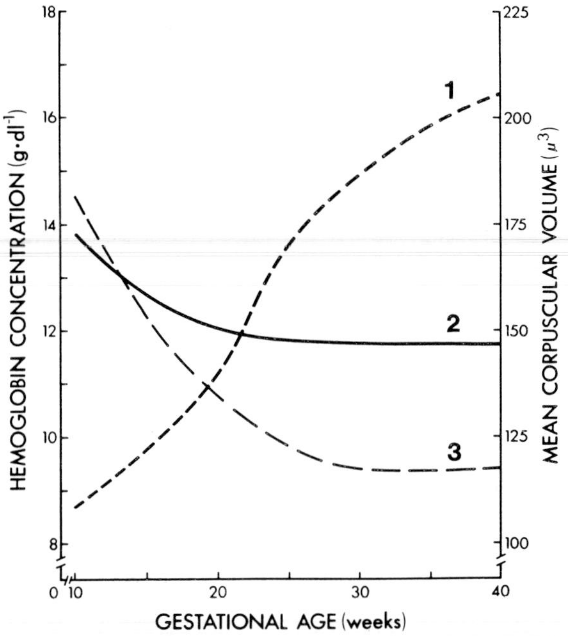

FIG. 4. Changes in human maternal (*line 2*) and fetal (*line 1*) hemoglobin (Hb) concentrations and fetal mean corpuscular volume (*line 3*) during course of gestation.

MATERNAL BLOOD O_2 AFFINITY AND CAPACITY

Hemoglobin

The blood of a normal near-term pregnant woman contains ~12 $g \cdot dl^{-1}$ (2 mM) Hb [Fig. 4; (281)], and her blood volume (assuming 72-kg wt) is ~5.7 liters, i.e., 79 $ml \cdot kg^{-1}$ (198). In contrast to adult Hb [Hb A or A_1, designated $\alpha_2^A\beta_2^A$ (where superscript denotes Hb source of chain and subscript has usual chemical significance), and Hb A_2, designated $\alpha_2^A\Delta_2^A$], human fetal Hb (Hb F, designated $\alpha_2^A\gamma_2^F$) contains two γ-chains combined with the two α-chains. Each mole of Hb can combine with 4 mol of O_2 for a normal blood O_2Cap of ~8 mM or 1.368 $ml \cdot g^{-1}$ (308).

Blood O_2 Affinity and HbO_2 Saturation Curve

The HbO_2 saturation curve is approximated by the equation

$$Y/100 = (kP_{O_2}^n)/(1 + kP_{O_2}^n) \quad (1)$$

where Y is the percent saturation with O_2 and k is an equilibrium constant. The exponent n represents the number of Fe atoms per Hb molecule, which for normal Hb approximates 2.9. Figure 5 depicts the HbO_2 saturation curve for normal adult blood [blood O_2 affinity (P_{50}) = 26.5 Torr] under standard conditions [pH = 7.4, CO_2 partial pressure (P_{CO_2}) = 40 Torr, and 37°C]. Hemoglobin in solution without the influence of intracellular factors such as H^+ and 2,3-diphosphoglycerate (DPG) has a P_{50} of 19.7 Torr.

Because pregnancy is associated with a number of maternal respiratory, cardiovascular, hematological, endocrinological, and metabolic changes, the question arises as to what extent blood O_2 affinity is altered.

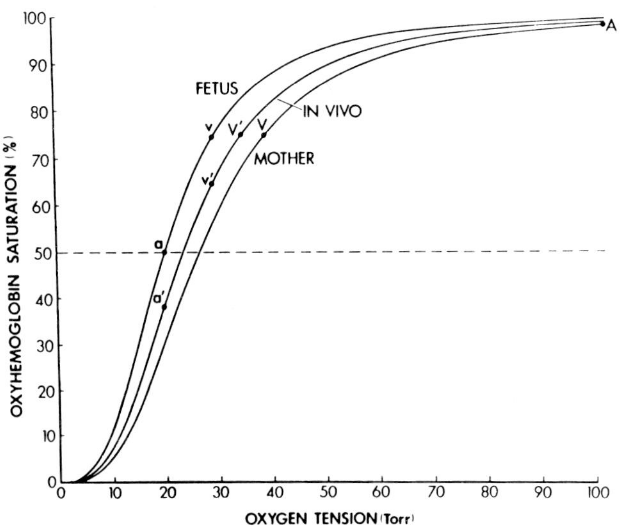

FIG. 5. HbO_2 saturation curves for human maternal and near-term fetal blood. Maternal and fetal Hb-O_2 affinities (P_{50}) are 26.5 and 20 Torr, respectively. A and V, maternal arterial and venous values, respectively, under standard conditions; a and v, umbilical arterial and venous values, respectively; V′, a′, and v′, probable in vivo maternal venous, umbilical arterial, and umbilical venous values, respectively.

Most studies have indicated that a pregnant woman's P_{50} (Pm_{50}) varies by no more than 1 Torr from that of her nonpregnant sister (33, 78, 86, 135, 213, 219, 283, 314, 327). Some workers have suggested that for women P_{50} = 28.3 Torr, whereas for men P_{50} = 26.3 Torr (154). Bauer et al. (30, 31) reported that the difference is even greater, with Pm_{50} = 31 Torr under standard conditions. Although the pregnant women in these studies had 10% greater [2,3-DPG] than controls, this factor alone could account for <1 Torr increase of Pm_{50}. However, Bauer et al. (30, 31) also showed that dialyzed pregnant and nonpregnant Hb solutions possessed identical O_2 affinities (P_{50} = 19.7 Torr) and that during pregnancy intraerythrocyte concentrations of the dialyzable substances Na^+, K^+, carbonic anhydrase, and ATP (all of which tend to shift the curve to the right) increase (31). Rørth and Bille-Brahe (303) reported a similarly increased Pm_{50} during pregnancy; however, their sample size was small, some subjects may have been anemic with elevated [2,3-DPG], and there was a wide scatter in results. A subsequent report from these authors substantiated the increase in [2,3-DPG] from the third month of gestation onward. A potential problem with both of these studies is that they were cross-sectional (31, 320); i.e., comparisons were based on values obtained from different pregnant women in each trimester of pregnancy.

In contrast, longitudinal studies in which serial determinations of O_2 transport variables were made in the same individual during the course of pregnancy have shown little change in Pm_{50}. For instance, Madsen and Ditzel (219) reported that, although [2,3-DPG] increased 15% (from 14.8 to 17 $\mu M \cdot g\ Hb^{-1}$) during pregnancy, Pm_{50} was not significantly different from nonpregnant values (27 Torr) (219). This agrees with other studies in humans (213, 314) and guinea pigs (228) that reported no significant change.

The possible influence of base deficit on maternal blood O_2 affinity also bears examination. Early in the course of pregnancy, hyperventilation secondary to increased progesterone levels (133) decreases maternal arterial P_{CO_2} (Pma_{CO_2}) from a nonpregnant value of 40 Torr to ~32 Torr. With increased renal HCO_3^- excretion, plasma [HCO_3^-] decreases from 26 to ~23 $meq \cdot liter^{-1}$, and the subject continues through pregnancy with a compensated respiratory alkalosis. This base deficit of ~3 $meq \cdot liter^{-1}$ would shift the HbO_2 curve to the left only ~0.5 Torr, however. In vivo the maternal HbO_2 saturation curve lies to the left of that measured under standard conditions because of the lowered P_{CO_2} and slightly elevated pH.

In summary, with few exceptions studies indicate no significant alteration of a woman's blood O_2 affinity during pregnancy.

Blood O_2 Capacity

From a knowledge of its molecular weight, it can be calculated that 1 g of Hb can theoretically bind 1.39 ml of O_2. However, the value of this constant may be 1.34 (152) or 1.368 (308); the exact value varies slightly depending on the amount of methemoglobin and carboxyhemoglobin (HbCO) present (85).

In the normal nonpregnant female the [Hb] and O_2Cap are ~14 $g \cdot dl^{-1}$ and 19.1 $ml \cdot dl^{-1}$, respectively (Fig. 4). During the course of gestation, erythrocyte mass increases 25%–30%, whereas plasma volume increases 40%–50% (198). Thus, because of hemodilution, [Hb] progessively decreases to ~12 $g \cdot dl^{-1}$ with a O_2Cap of 16.4 $ml \cdot dl^{-1}$ (281).

FETAL BLOOD O_2 AFFINITY AND CAPACITY

Fetal Hb

The role of fetal Hb and the manner in which it differs from that of the adult have intrigued investigators for a century or more. In 1866, von Körber (171) first noted that blood from human newborn umbilical vessels denatured less readily in alkaline or acid solutions than did blood from adults, the difference being most pronounced in alkali. This observation was confirmed by others (173–175, 336). The demonstration that the difference in alkaline denaturation resides in the Hb globin chains (131) and the discovery that fetal blood O_2 affinity differed from that of the adult (153) gave impetus to the search for fetal Hb. In 1935, Brinkman and Jonxis (53) first definitely demonstrated the existence of a human fetal Hb, and Kleihauer et al. (167) demonstrated Hb F with both light and electron microscopy (182). Schroeder et al. (313) first demonstrated the difference in amino acid sequences of human β- and γ-globin chains. These workers also recorded that the 141 residues of the Hb F α-chain have the same amino acid sequence as the α-chain of human Hb A (312), whereas the non-α- (γ-) chains both contain 146 amino acids but differ by the replacement of 39 amino acids with four isoleucine residues and other residues. Hemoglobin F contains three types of γ-chains, two of which differ at amino acid position 136: one contains an alanine residue and the other a glycine residue (311). The third type of γ-chain is characterized by a threonyl residue that replaces isoleucine at position 75.

Also in contrast to adult erythrocytes, those of the fetus are larger (145), have a shorter life span (113), and differ in ultrastructure (270). They also vary in their mechanical (50), osmotic (293), temperature (38), and acid (166) fragilities, electrophoretic mobility (306), and membrane structure (143).

Early in gestation, human embryos and fetuses contain Hbs other than Hb F (91, 112, 125–127, 150, 151). Near term, a demand for accelerated erythropoiesis leads preferentially to synthesis of Hb A. Blood of the newborn infant contains 65%–75% Hb F and an additional 15% Hb F_1, which is characterized by acetylation of the NH_2-terminal of the γ-chain (310). Thus the near-term infant has ~80%–90% fetal and 10%–20% adult Hb. The reported values vary somewhat because of inaccuracies both in estimating gestational age and in quantifying Hb F (54, 163). The mechanisms regulating the subcellular events (such as transcription and translation) responsible for switching from synthesis of γ- (Hb F) to β- (Hb A) chains remain to be elucidated but appear to be determined by a developmental clock inherent to the hematopoietic stem cells (349).

Despite the attention given to the importance of Hb F in humans, this Hb is not required to survive intrauterine life in all species. To date no specific fetal Hb has been detected in the horse (116, 320), dromedary camel (295), hamster (116), several breeds of dogs (183, 252), cat (260), lion, or pig (325). In the fetal elephant, P_{50} (Pf_{50}) changes in an unexpected manner. At 5-mo gestation (term, 22 mo) it has the same O_2 affinity as the mother (Pm_{50} = 23 Torr), but at 12 mo (when it has no fetal Hb) Pf_{50} decreases to 17 Torr (294). In contrast, the 7-mo-old fetal camel, which does not have a distinct Hb F, shows a characteristic higher O_2 affinity than that of the mother (295).

Blood O_2 Affinity

A question of recurring interest concerns the relation of fetal blood O_2 affinity to that of the mother. In 1927 Huggett (153) first demonstrated that the HbO_2 curve of fetal blood differs from that of the adult but mistakenly held that fetal goat blood possessed a lower O_2 affinity (P_{50} = ~40 Torr) than that of the adult. Eastman et al. (95) first measured the fetal dissociation curve under near-standard conditions and concluded that the curve for the fetus was similar to that for the nonpregnant adult (P_{50} = 24 Torr), whereas that for the mother had a lower affinity (P_{50} = 32 Torr). Barcroft (12) determined that in the goat the fetal and maternal curves lay to the left and right, respectively, of normal adult values. During the subsequent decade, several workers depicted the fetal curve relatively correctly in its relation to that of the mother (78, 184, 298, 299).

Figure 5 portrays this relationship for the human, in which Pf_{50} = 20 ± 1 (mean ± SE) Torr under standard conditions (135, 263, 334). Human embryonic erythrocytes have an O_2 affinity essentially the same as those of the fetus (149). In contrast, in embryonic mouse red cells the O_2 affinity is high (339), whereas in the rabbit (159) and rat (115) it is low. The value of n (Eq. 1) for fetal blood is the same as that in the adult (13). The Pf_{50} value progressively increases during the course of gestation, approximating the maternal curve as the concentration of Hb A increases relative to that of Hb F (12, 34, 129, 163, 298).

The question arises as to the mechanism(s) responsible for the increased O_2 affinity of fetal blood. Hall (128) first suggested that this might result from a specific difference in Hb. In solution, Hb F possesses an even higher O_2 affinity than in erythrocytes (128); however, this is slightly lower than that of the adult P_{50} (13.2 vs. 12.6 Torr at pH = 6.8) (5, 218, 333). This relationship is reversed in the erythrocyte as a result of different responses to 2,3-DPG and other organic phosphates and does not result from structural differences of the Hb molecules (5, 30).

Several groups have independently demonstrated the role of 2,3-DPG in the modulation of fetal O_2 affinity (30, 83, 331). The 2,3-DPG stabilizes deoxyhemoglobin A by binding to four positively charged residues on the β-chain. Despite almost equal [2,3-DPG] in human maternal and fetal blood, Hb F interacts less than does Hb A with this organic phosphate because its γ-chains lack one binding site for 2,3-DPG. For instance, after addition of 2,3-DPG to dialyzed solutions of Hb F and of Hb A, P_{50} shifted from 19.7 to 22.4 and 29.4 Torr, respectively (30). The two most important influences of fetal blood O_2 affinity are the percentage of Hb A and [2,3-DPG], and Orzalesi and Hay (262) have defined the term *functional DPG fraction* to describe the product of these variables. Changes in fetal and postnatal blood O_2 affinity correlate better with the functional DPG fraction than with either [Hb A] or [2,3-DPG] alone.

Table 3 lists the blood O_2 affinities of various mammals. In human fetuses and to a certain extent in rhesus monkey fetuses (238, 324), the weak interactions of 2,3-DPG and Hb F account for the higher O_2 affinity. Ungulate (goat and sheep) fetal Hb possesses

TABLE 3. *Relation of Fetal to Maternal Blood O_2 Capacities and Affinities*

Species	O_2 Capacity M	O_2 Capacity F	Sum of O_2 Capacities	P_{50}, Torr M	P_{50}, Torr F	P_{50} Difference	Ref.
Weddell seal	32	28	60	29	21	8	185
				27	21	6	286
Human							
Nonpregnant female	20			27			219
Pregnant female	17	22	39	30	23	7	31
				26	22	4	238
	16			28			213
	15	22	37	26	22	4	33
Rabbit	17	20	37				348
				30	20	10	159
	15	14	29	31	27	4	22
Elephant	20	17	37	23	17	6	294
				24	21	3	294
Pig	19	16	35				348
				35	22	13	329
	13	13	26	33	23	10	238
Llama	14	19	33	21	18	3	234
Monkey (*Macaca mulatta*)	15	18	33	32	19	13	134
Baboon				31	25	6	268
Cat	16	17	33				348
				36	36	0	260
Rat	16	16	32	40	25	15	132
				38	28	10	238
Camel	15	17	32	21	16	5	295
Guinea pig	16	16	32	30	19	11	22
Sheep	15	17	32				19
				34	17	17	23
				27–37*	17	10–20*	232
Hamster	12	12	24	36	36	0	238
Cow	15	12	27	31	22	9	111
				32	19	13	317
Chicken	14	12	26	49	34	15	24
Goat	13	12	25	30	19	11	22
Dog				31	21	10	238
				31	20	11	252

M, maternal values; F, fetal values; P_{50}, Hb-O_2 affinity. * P_{50} for maternal sheep equals 27 Torr for Hb A and 37 Torr for Hb B. [Adapted from Bartels (21) and Metcalfe et al. (238).]

a high O_2 affinity per se, and its interaction with intraerythrocyte phosphates is reduced (238). In the dog, horse, pig, and Weddell seal, intraerythrocyte [2,3-DPG] is low before birth, producing a relatively high O_2 affinity (286). After birth, [2,3-DPG] rapidly increases to adult levels with a resultant decrease in O_2 affinity (32, 72, 84, 252, 259, 329, 330). In contrast, the fetal cat, which also has no Hb F, represents an exception to the rule that fetal blood always possesses a higher O_2 affinity than that of the mother; the P_{50} values of the two are essentially the same (260).

Blood O_2 Capacity

Near term, human fetal blood O_2Cap exceeds that of the mother by ~50%, but during much of fetal life the reverse situation holds (see Fig. 4). At ~10-wk gestation the fetal [Hb] ([Hb]f) is ~8.5 $g \cdot dl^{-1}$ (263, 337), whereas that of the mother ([Hb]m) is ~13 $g \cdot dl^{-1}$. As pregnancy progresses, [Hb]f rises, reaching a value of ~16.5 $g \cdot dl^{-1}$ at term, whereas [Hb]m decreases to ~11.5 $g \cdot dl^{-1}$ (see Fig. 4). These reciprocal changes have also been demonstrated in the goat (96), cat, dog, pig, rabbit, rat (347, 348), and sheep (14). The fetal erythrocyte count and packed cell volume also increase during the course of gestation. In contrast, the mean corpuscular volume (ratio of packed cell volume to erythrocyte count) and erythrocyte Hb content (ratio of [Hb] to erythrocyte count) decrease.

A recurring question is whether the greater O_2Cap of fetal blood reflects relative hypoxemia, as does that at high altitude (8, 14, 21, 337). Barcroft reported that fetal O_2Cap varied inversely as a function of umbilical arterial [HbO_2] (14). However, more recent studies in chronically catheterized animals reveal no evidence of [HbO_2] changes of the magnitude that he described (194, 222). This relative erythrocytosis is seen only near term in the human, it is not common to many species, there is no evidence of anerobic metabolism, and fetal O_2Cap at sea level is much lower than that of an adult at high altitude with an equivalent Pa_{O_2} (22 $ml \cdot dl^{-1}$ in fetus at sea level vs. 32 $ml \cdot dl^{-1}$ in adult at 18,000–21,000 ft). These facts suggest that the normal fetus is not hypoxemic.

An additional question regards whether fetal blood binds less O_2 per gram of Fe, i.e., has a lower specific O_2 capacity (11). Although one group reported a lower specific O_2 capacity (322), other authors have reported that this value is normal (1, 172), and there is no good evidence to the contrary.

INTERRELATIONS OF MATERNAL AND FETAL BLOOD O_2 AFFINITY AND CAPACITY

General Considerations

In this section, I consider how maternal and fetal blood O_2 affinities and capacities are interrelated in humans and other species. Figure 5 depicts the HbO_2 curves for human maternal and near-term fetal blood, and Figure 6 shows the O_2 content as a function of P_{O_2} for these bloods. The HbO_2 curves can be described by

$$\log P_{O_2} = k_1 - k_2(\text{pH} - 7.4) + k_3 \log([HbO_2]/100 - [HbO_2]) \quad (2)$$

Alternatively this relation may be expressed

$$[HbO_2] = 100/\{P_{O_2}/[10^{k_1 - k_2(\text{pH} - 7.4)}]^{-1/k_3} + 1\} \quad (3)$$

where for human maternal blood $k_1 = 1.421$, $k_2 = 0.456$, and $k_3 = 0.373$ and for human fetal blood $k_1 = 1.302$, $k_2 = 0.464$, and $k_3 = 0.395$ (140).

Figure 6 demonstrates that in the fetus, despite Pfa_{O_2} being only one-fifth to one-third that of the adult and because of its high O_2Cap and affinity, arterial [O_2] is actually greater (16.5 vs. 15.4 $ml \cdot dl^{-1}$) and [HbO_2] is only ~25% lower (75% vs. 98%) than

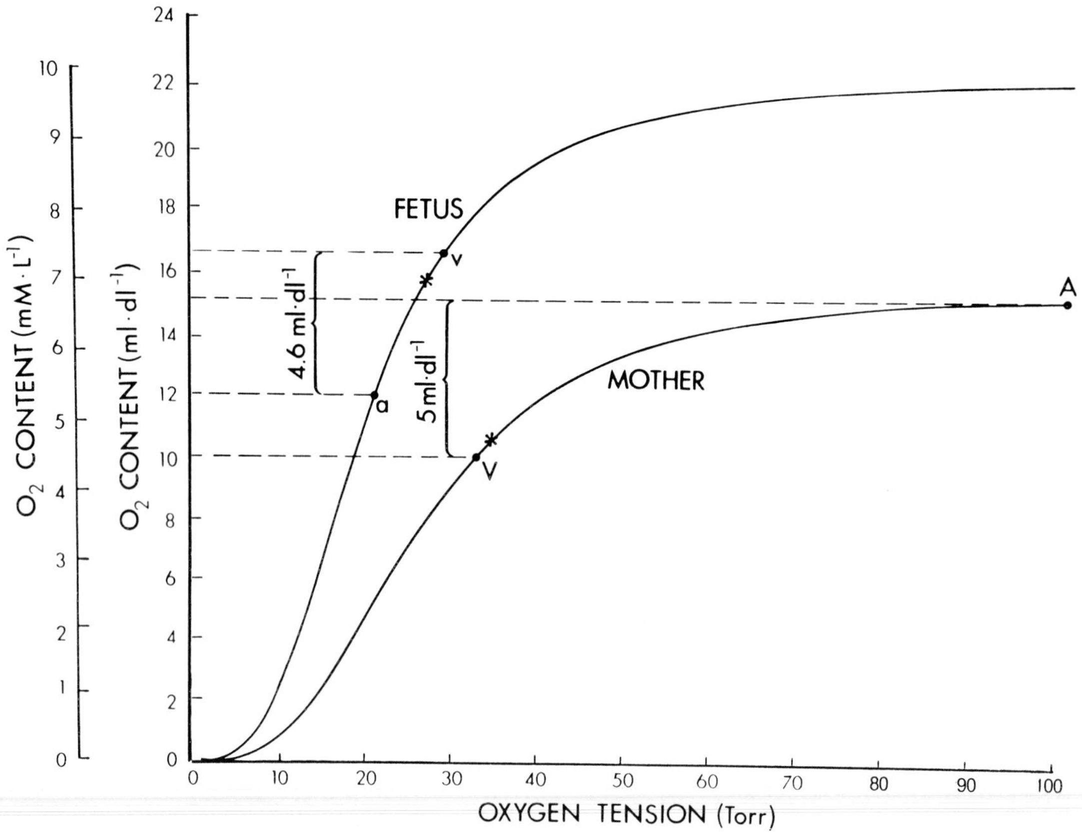

FIG. 6. Blood O_2 content as function of P_{O_2} for maternal ([Hb]m = 12 g·dl^{-1} and Pm_{50} = 26.5 Torr) and near-term fetal ([Hb]f = 16.5 g·dl^{-1} and Pf_{50} = 20 Torr) blood. *Asterisks*, maternal and fetal $\bar{P}_{O_2}$; A and V, maternal arterial and venous values; a and v, umbilical arterial and venous values.

in the adult. Thus the greater O_2 affinity of fetal blood permits a relatively high [HbO_2] at relatively low P_{O_2} values, whereas its acute slope permits a major decrement in [O_2] for a small P_{O_2} decrease.

An additional consideration is the actual [HbO_2] curve in vivo as blood flows through the placental exchange capillaries. In contrast to the saturation curves under standard conditions, maternal arterial blood is slightly alkalotic (pH = 7.42) and hypocarbic (P_{CO_2} = 32 Torr), whereas the fetal blood is slightly acidotic (pH = 7.35) and hypercarbic (P_{CO_2} = 45 Torr) (see Table 1). As fetal blood courses through the exchange vessels it gives up H^+ and CO_2 with a rise in pH. The opposite changes occur in the maternal exchange vessels. Thus in vivo the maternal and fetal [HbO_2] curves may be almost superimposed, as indicated in Figure 5. Although this double Bohr effect in the placenta has been credited with significantly augmenting $\dot{V}_{O_2}$, theoretical studies suggest that this accounts for only 8% of the total O_2 transferred (139). In contrast, the placental double Haldane effect accounts for 46% of the effect of O_2 on CO_2 exchange [see PLACENTAL CO_2 EXCHANGE, p. 378; (139)].

With CO_2 titration the Bohr factor ($\Delta\log P_{50}/\Delta pH$) has a value of −0.41 for maternal and −0.44 for fetal sheep blood at 50% [HbO_2] (142). The maternal value increases in magnitude at lower saturations, and both maternal and fetal values decrease at higher saturations. In contrast, with fixed acid titration the Bohr factor of fetal blood (−0.36) is significantly greater than that of maternal blood (−0.27), and these values appear to be independent of [HbO_2] (142). Nonetheless the magnitude of the saturation dependence of the Bohr factor is apparently not great enough to have physiological significance on $\dot{V}_{O_2}$ (61).

An additional factor tending to shift the in vivo fetal dissociation curve to the right is the temperature of the fetus, which exceeds that of the mother by 0.5°C–1.0°C. The changes in maternal and fetal temperature during hyperthermia may affect $\dot{V}_{O_2}$ (see RESPONSES TO MATERNAL EXERCISE, p. 366).

Species Differences

Among eutherian mammals the relation of fetal to maternal blood O_2Cap and affinity varies widely. An increase in either maternal or fetal O_2Cap will promote $\dot{V}_{O_2}$ (21, 200). All other factors remaining the same, the larger the sum of maternal and fetal blood O_2Cap, the more O_2 will be exchanged. Table 3 summarizes the blood O_2Cap of a number of species. Figure 7 depicts the relation of fetal to maternal blood O_2Cap

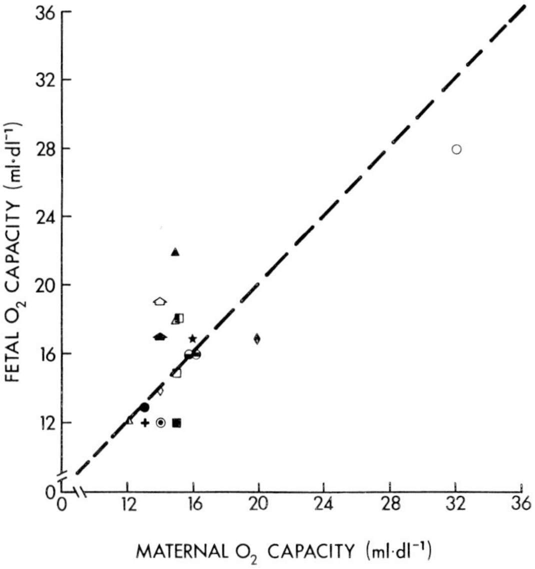

FIG. 7. Relation of blood O_2 capacity of fetus to that of mother in various species. □, Camel; ★, cat; ◉, chicken; ■, cow; ♦, elephant; +, goat; ◒, guinea pig; ◭, hamster; ▲, human; ⌓, llama; ●, pig; ◇, rabbit; ⊖, rat; △ and ◧, rhesus monkey; ○, seal; ☗, sheep. Line of identity is shown.

in these species. Generally fetal O_2Cap exceeds the maternal value by 10%–20%. However, in many species (e.g., rat, guinea pig, sheep) the values are about equal, and in others (e.g., cow, goat, pig, rabbit) fetal O_2Cap is less than in the mother. Generally the sum of maternal and fetal O_2Cap is proportional to the ratio of fetal to maternal body weights; however, the biological meaning of this relation is unclear.

Among almost all mammalian species, fetal blood O_2 affinity exceeds that of the mother (see Table 3). Many workers have considered that the larger the difference between maternal and fetal P_{50} values, the more efficient is placental O_2 exchange. This concept is not completely valid (see next section). Figure 8 depicts Pf_{50} as a function of Pm_{50} for the species listed in Table 3; Pf_{50} is inversely proportional to the log of fetal weight, but again the biological meaning of this relation is not evident.

TRANSPLACENTAL DIFFUSION

Mean Maternal-to-Fetal O_2 Tension Differences

At the level of greatest subdivision each unit of the fetal placental vascular network intimately contacts the smallest subdivision of the maternal placental vessels or, in the case of humans and other species with a hemochorial placenta, the intervillous space. The dimensions are so small that a metabolically inert gas such as N_2O will reach 95% equilibration between the two bloodstreams in <10 ms (197). The human placenta provides an exchange area of 5 (201) to 17 (227) m^2 in a volume of ~0.5 liters, a relatively compact organ.

As noted in Table 2, placental O_2 exchange depends on a number of factors, including the $\bar{P}_{O_2}$ difference between maternal and fetal exchange vessels. A logical question is what are the P_{O_2} values in maternal and fetal blood that account for this exchange? Unfortunately this answer is not readily available. Ideally one would like to study the exchange process by sampling inflowing and end-capillary blood within a single exchange unit, i.e., in humans in the maternal intervillous space and individual fetal placental capillaries. However, this presents formidable problems.

As a first step to understanding the exchange process, early investigators measured the P_{O_2} values of uterine and umbilical arteries and veins [Fig. 9; Table 1; (7, 14, 153, 298, 299)]. These workers then calculated a maternal-to-fetal $\bar{P}_{O_2}$ difference of 40–50 Torr, which suggested a significant barrier to O_2 diffusion (16, 17). Subsequent studies in rabbits (18) and humans (282) yielded only slightly smaller values. Several problems with these studies are now evident. The human measurements were made on patients at the time of vaginal delivery, with umbilical P_{O_2} values that now would be regarded as abnormally low, and the blood samples thought to represent the intervillous space may instead have been from a uterine vein (107). Because of these and other difficulties, it became apparent that indirect measures must be used to determine this P_{O_2} difference and the diffusing capacity.

Placental Diffusing Capacity

GENERAL CONSIDERATIONS. According to Fick's first law, diffusion from a region of high concentration to

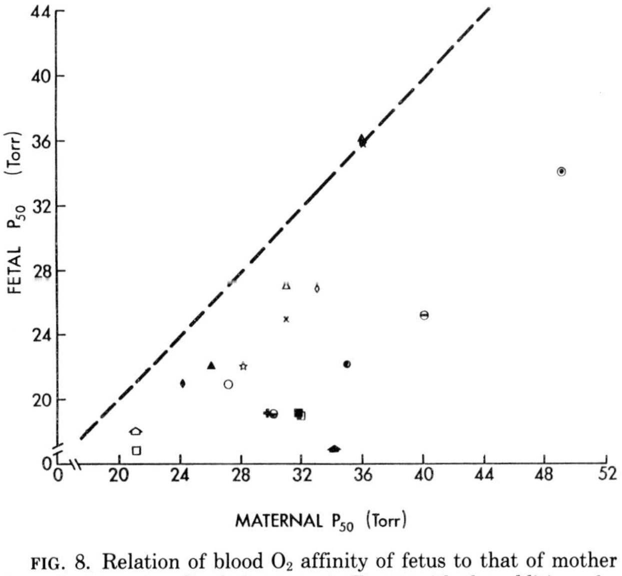

FIG. 8. Relation of blood O_2 affinity of fetus to that of mother in various species. Symbols are as in Fig. 7, with the addition of × for baboon and ☆ for dog.

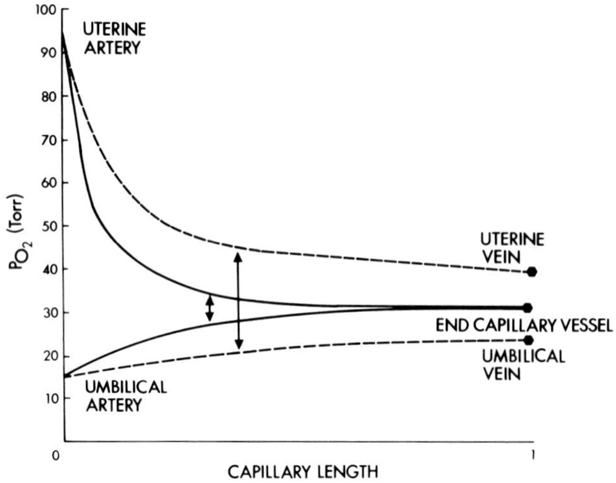

FIG. 9. Diagrammatic representation of time course of change in P_{O_2} in maternal and fetal blood during single transit in placental exchange vessels. *Dashed lines*, values assuming that P_{O_2} values in uterine and umbilical veins are the same as those of maternal and fetal end capillaries, which is probably incorrect; *long arrow*, average maternal-to-fetal P_{O_2} difference of ~30 Torr calculated on this basis. *Solid lines*, time courses of changes in P_{O_2} values in maternal and fetal placental exchange vessels calculated from measurements of placental CO diffusing capacity; *short arrow*, probable true maternal-to-fetal $\bar{P}_{O_2}$ difference of 5–7 Torr based on calculations of placental diffusing capacity for CO (Dp_{CO}); under these conditions, P_{O_2} values in maternal and fetal blood probably reach near equilibrium in end-capillary vessels.

one of lower concentration may be described by

$$\delta J/\delta t = -(APD\delta C)/x \quad (4)$$

where $\delta J/\delta t$ is the differential rate of movement of substance J across an area A of an infinite plane under a concentration gradient δC, P is the membrane permeability, D is the gas diffusivity (or diffusion coefficient), and x is the membrane thickness. For a complex structure such as the placental membranes, which have variable thickness and permeability, the area, permeability, diffusivity, and thickness are constants and may be combined into a single term that expresses the membrane diffusion characteristics

$$Dp = \delta J/\delta t(\bar{P}m - \bar{P}f) \quad (5)$$

where Dp is the diffusing capacity of the placenta in $ml \cdot min^{-1} \cdot Torr^{-1}$. For respiratory gases the Bunsen solubility coefficient (α) and $\bar{P}m - \bar{P}f$ are used rather than the concentration difference.

The term *diffusing capacity* has been used in reference to the lung and is well entrenched in the physiological literature; therefore its application to the placenta seems reasonable. Nonetheless the term may be confusing because what is measured is not necessarily the maximum exchange possible. In addition, Dp is as much a measure of the maternal and fetal placental capillary blood volumes and rate of chemical reaction of ligand gas with Hb as it is a measure of the diffusion characteristics of the placental membranes per se.

Barcroft and Barron (14) first attempted to quantify $\dot{V}_{O_2}$ from uterine and umbilical arterial and venous P_{O_2} values of sheep (see *Mean Maternal-to-Fetal O_2 Tension Differences*, p. 361). By using a graphical analysis, they calculated the mean maternal-to-fetal P_{O_2} difference to be ~50 Torr and the diffusion constant to be ~0.08 $ml \cdot min^{-1} \cdot Torr^{-1} \cdot kg$ fetal wt^{-1}. Subsequently Barron and co-workers (17, 19) used an interpolation method and Lamport (180) used a modified Bohr integration technique to calculate this constant (0.17 $ml \cdot min^{-1} \cdot Torr^{-1} \cdot kg^{-1}$). Figure 9 depicts the P_{O_2} values in the placental vessels, the time course of changes during a capillary transit, and the value of the $\bar{P}_{O_2}$ difference calculated by Barron's approach. A critical assumption of those calculations was that the blood gas values in uterine and umbilical veins represented the values at the end of a capillary transit. Thus it was concluded that the $\bar{P}_{O_2}$ difference between the uterine and umbilical veins represents a lack of O_2 equilibration between maternal and fetal blood. More recent studies suggest that this assumption was incorrect and that the observed difference probably results from a combination of vascular shunts, nonuniform distribution of maternal-to-fetal placental blood flows, nonuniform distribution of Dp to blood flows, and placental O_2 consumption. Several facets of these factors are detailed below.

CARBON MONOXIDE DIFFUSING CAPACITY. How then is one to determine the true maternal-to-fetal P_{O_2} difference and Dp? Because significant amounts of O_2 are consumed by the placenta and $\dot{V}_{O_2}$ is limited by blood flow rather than diffusion, Dp could not be determined from O_2 measurements. Rather, a gas whose exchange is limited by diffusion (e.g., CO) must be used instead. Longo et al. (205) first measured maternal-fetal CO exchanges in sheep and dogs to calculate Dp for CO (Dp_{CO}), using Equation 5 and the Haldane relation

$$P_{CO} = ([HbCO]P_{O_2})/([HbO_2]M) \quad (6)$$

where P_{CO} is the CO partial pressure and M is the relative affinity of Hb for CO and O_2. Although these values change during the course of a single capillary transit, the ratio of P_{O_2} to $[HbO_2]$ changes only to the extent that the HbO_2 saturation curve deviates from a straight line through the origin (see Fig. 5); i.e., it changes much less than the values of either P_{O_2} or $[HbO_2]$ per se. These workers calculated that Dp_{CO} was ~0.5 $ml \cdot min^{-1} \cdot Torr^{-1} \cdot kg^{-1}$, that Dp for O_2 (Dp_{O_2}) was ~0.9 $ml \cdot min^{-1} \cdot Torr^{-1} \cdot kg^{-1}$, and that the maternal-to-fetal $\bar{P}_{O_2}$ difference was only ~7 Torr, rather than the much greater values previously reported [Fig. 9; (205)]. Values of Dp_{CO} in chronically catheterized sheep (194) and macaque monkeys (42) are essentially the same, but in unanesthetized rabbits (297) and guinea pigs (43, 114) Dp_{CO} is 2–3 $ml \cdot min^{-1} \cdot Torr^{-1} \cdot kg^{-1}$ and the $\bar{P}_{O_2}$ difference is only 1–2 Torr (Table 4).

TABLE 4. *Placental CO Diffusing Capacity in Various Species*

Species	No.	Placenta		CO Diffusing Capacity		
		Vascular morphology	Ultrastructure (cell layers)	Fetal wt, g × 10^3	Placental wt, g × 10^3	Ref.
				ml·min⁻¹·Torr⁻¹·g⁻¹		
Guinea pig	9	Labyrinthine	Hemomonochorial (2)	3.27 ± 0.10	50.5 ± 2.1	114
				2.28 ± 0.13	45.3 ± 4.9	43
Rabbit	18	Labyrinthine	Hemodichorial (3)	2.33 ± 0.21	11.6 ± 1.5	297
Rat	12	Labyrinthine	Hemotrichorial (4)	1.73 ± 0.33	9.0 ± 1.0	*
Dog	5	Labyrinthine	Endotheliochorial (4)	0.57 ± 0.8		205
Sheep	26†	Villous	Epitheliochorial (5)	0.55 ± 0.02	3.0 ± 0.4	194
Monkey	9‡	Villous	Hemomonochorial (3)	0.65 ± 0.06	1.6 ± 0.2	42
Human	4	Villous	Hemomonochorial (3)	2.70	16.2	82

Results are means ± SE. Numbers in parentheses are cell layers. * L. D. Longo, B. J. Koos, and R. D. Gilbert, unpublished observations. † 26 measurements in 10 sheep. ‡ 9 measurements in 7 monkeys.

These results suggest that the placenta does not constitute a significant barrier to diffusion, and the maternal-to-fetal $\bar{P}_{O_2}$ difference is of the same magnitude as the pulmonary alveolar-to-capillary difference. Using a mathematical model, Hill et al. (138) calculated that maternal and fetal P_{O_2} values reach near equilibrium during the course of a capillary transit. Thus under normal conditions $\dot{V}_{O_2}$ is limited by the rate of blood flows rather than by diffusion through the membranes. Figure 9 depicts these concepts. Within ~50% of a capillary transit, P_{O_2}values have reached 95% equilibrium, which is essentially complete at ~31 Torr by the end of the capillary transit.

About the same time that the Dp_{CO} studies were reported, several other groups suggested that placental O_2 exchange is limited by blood flow rather than by diffusion. Adapting classic clearance concepts to the placenta, Meschia et al. (229) calculated the placental clearance of several metabolically inert molecules and extrapolated their results on blood flow limitation to respiratory gases. In turn, Faber and Hart (101, 102) calculated the placental permeability

$$P = \dot{Q}f(Cfa - Cfv)/(Cfa \cdot wt) \tag{7}$$

where P is the permeability in ml·min^{-1}·g^{-1}, $\dot{Q}f$ is the fetal placental blood flow in ml·min^{-1}, Cfa and Cfv are the concentrations in the umbilical artery and vein, respectively, in mg·ml^{-1}, and wt is the placental weight in grams. Faber and Hart (101, 102) found the permeability to acetylene and O_2 to be similar and large, despite their differences in solubility and molecular weights, and concluded that their exchange was flow limited. Additional evidence that the placental membranes fail to limit O_2 exchange comes from the in vitro demonstration that human chorion laeve offers no greater resistance to O_2 diffusion than does a water layer of similar thickness (160).

Role of Hb Reaction Rates

Despite this evidence that the placental membranes probably do not limit diffusion, the question arises as to the relative resistances to O_2 diffusion of the membranes per se as opposed to the effective resistances of maternal and fetal blood. In fetal placental exchange vessels, O_2 combines with deoxyhemoglobin by the reaction

$$Hb + O_2 \underset{k_c}{\overset{k_c'}{\rightleftharpoons}} HbO_2 \tag{8}$$

where k_c' and k_c are the respective overall association- and dissociation-reaction rate constants. The reverse reaction occurs in maternal blood. Because of the finite values of these rate constants, the dissociation and association reactions offer an effective resistance to diffusion.

The relative resistances offered by the placental membranes and maternal and fetal blood may be derived by the following considerations. The total partial pressure difference between maternal and fetal blood equals the sum of several pressure differences: *1*) between the interior of the maternal erythrocyte and the maternal plasma, *2*) between the maternal plasma, across the placental membranes, and fetal plasma, and *3*) between fetal plasma and the interior of the fetal erythrocyte (Fig. 10). In turn, the reciprocal of the diffusing capacity, the total resistance to diffusion, equals the sum of several resistances: *1*) that of the maternal blood, *2*) that of the placental membranes, and *3*) that of the fetal blood (206). These resistances may be expressed as

$$1/Dp = 1/\theta mVm + 1/Dmem + 1/\theta fVf \tag{9}$$

where θm and θf are the diffusing capacities in ml·ml^{-1}·min^{-1}·Torr^{-1} of maternal and fetal blood, respectively, Vm and Vf are the blood volumes in milliliters in the maternal and fetal exchange vessels, respectively, and Dmem is the diffusing capacity of the placental membranes in ml·min^{-1}·Torr^{-1}. Although Dmem remains constant, Dp varies along the capillary as θm and θf vary. The diffusing capacity of the red blood cells (θ) is a function of both the rate of combination of O_2 with Hb, which increases at higher P_{O_2}, and the concentration of reduced Hb, which decreases at increased P_{O_2}. At low [HbO_2], θ is relatively constant but decreases rapidly at saturations >80%.

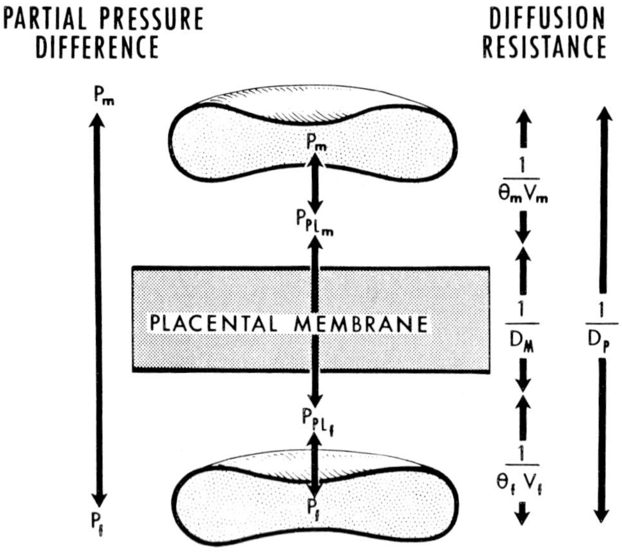

FIG. 10. Schematic representation of maternal-to-fetal partial pressure differences and resistance to diffusion. Total pressure difference ($P_m - P_f$) consists of *1*) difference between interior of maternal erythrocyte and plasma ($P_m - P_{PL_m}$), *2*) difference across membrane between maternal and fetal plasma ($P_{PL_m} - P_{PL_f}$), and *3*) difference between fetal plasma and interior of fetal erythrocyte ($P_{PL_f} - P_f$). Overall resistance to diffusion ($1/D_P$) is sum of individual resistances: *1*) effective resistance of maternal blood to diffusion ($1/\theta_m V_m$), *2*) resistance of placental membrane per se ($1/D_M$), and *3*) resistance of fetal blood ($1/\theta_f V_f$).

From measurements of Dp_{CO} under hyperbaric conditions, Longo et al. (206) observed that this value varied as a function of Pa_{O_2}. By plotting the reciprocal of Dp_{CO} as a function of the reciprocal of the diffusing capacities of maternal and fetal red blood cells ($1/\theta m + 1/\theta f$), the slope gave the reciprocal of the maternal and fetal capillary blood volumes, and the intercept equaled the reciprocal of Dmem (206). The value calculated for both the maternal and fetal placental capillary blood volumes in the exchange area was ~10 ml, whereas Dmem was 2.6 $ml \cdot min^{-1} \cdot Torr^{-1}$. For CO, these authors calculated that the placental membranes comprised ~60% of the overall resistance, whereas the maternal and fetal erythrocytes accounted for ~40%. For O_2, these values were 73% and 27%, respectively (206).

Longo et al. (206) also calculated that the placental exchange area was ~5 m^2, a value similar to that of Dodds (89). However, stereologic analysis has suggested that the functional exchange area is greater, i.e., 12 m^2 (178) and 7–17 m^2 (227). Multiple-isotope indicator-dilution studies by Bissonnette (39) suggest that the volumes of maternal and fetal placental exchange vessels equal ~45 ml each, whereas morphometric studies have given values for the volumes of fetal villous capillary and maternal intervillous space ranging from 30 and 110 ml, respectively (178), to 44 and 176 ml, respectively (227). The larger the existing vascular volumes, the smaller the value of Dmem (and thus the greater the relative resistance of the membranes), which would be compatible with measurements of Dp.

Additional evidence that the diffusion resistance of placental membranes does not limit O_2 or CO_2 exchange was derived from a study of the simultaneous exchange of two metabolically inert gases with very different molecular weights: H_2 (mol wt, 2) and SF_6 (mol wt, 156) (197). In dogs, blood equilibrated with these gases was perfused into either the fetal umbilical artery or the maternal uterine artery, and the uterine and umbilical venous blood was analyzed for these gases. If the placental membranes significantly limited diffusion, P_{SF_6} would have decreased relative to that for H_2 in the venous effluent from the side opposite that in which it was infused. That the ratios of SF_6 to H_2 were essentially the same in both outflowing vessels suggested no significant barrier to diffusion of the larger molecule (197). These calculations assumed that the membrane solubilities of the two molecules equaled the lipid solubilities in vitro, an assumption that may not have been justified. To definitely settle this question it would be edifying to compare the diffusion of one set of molecules with the same solubilities but different molecular weights with another set with identical molecular weights but dissimilar solubilities. Because end-capillary equilibration depends on the ratio of Dp to the effective solubility of the gas in blood rather than on Dp alone (335) and because of the large capacity of blood for O_2 and CO_2, these gases may demonstrate some diffusion limitation even though SF_6 does not.

From a morphometric analysis of the exchange area in 18 term human placentas, Laga et al. (178) calculated the resistances and diffusing capacities of various segments of the diffusion path between maternal and fetal placental erythrocytes. Despite a number of simplifying assumptions and the failure to consider the Hb reaction rates, the agreement with the CO calculations was striking.

Possible Facilitated O_2 Transport

Classically it has been assumed that O_2 diffusion in the lung, placenta, and other tissues occurs passively in response to P_{O_2} gradients. However, from studies of the relation of O_2 uptake to surface P_{O_2} in liver and brain slices, Longmuir et al. (188, 189) suggested that a carrier such as cytochrome *P*-450 facilitated diffusion. If true for the placenta, this would imply that calculations of Dp_{O_2} from measurements of Dp_{CO} may be invalid, as would be the use of Equation 9 to calculate Dmem, Vm, and Vf.

Gurtner and Bruns (123, 124) explored the hypothesis of Longmuir et al. (188, 189) for the placenta, comparing transplacental fluxes of O_2, Ar (123, 124), and N_2O (124) before and after administration of compounds known to inhibit cytochrome P-450. The

$\dot{V}_{O_2}$ they calculated was of such a magnitude that it could be accounted for only by a carrier molecule; they concluded that cytochrome P-450 inhibitors reduced $\dot{V}_{O_2}$ without affecting inert gas transfer (122, 124). In addition, measurements of Dp_{CO} at various concentrations of fetal HbCO (44) showed an inverse relation of Dp_{CO} to [HbCO]f, which suggested saturation kinetics. An alternative explanation for these findings is that Dp_{CO} decreased because less fetal Hb was available to bind CO. Also, human placental microsomes contain only ~10% the concentration of cytochrome P-450 as those of the liver (353), and placentas of some other species contain almost no detectable cytochrome P-450 (114). Because Dp_{O_2} computed from Dp_{CO} fully accounts for measured transplacental O_2 fluxes, postulation of a carrier under these circumstances is unnecessary.

Alterations in Placental Diffusing Capacity

THEORETICAL CONSIDERATIONS. From the preceding discussion it might be thought that considerable data are available on how Dp affects the overall exchange process, but that is not the case. In an attempt to understand the effects of these changes, Longo et al. (200) used a mathematical model in which the value of a given parameter could be altered independently of compensating changes in other factors. Figure 11 shows that increased Dp_{CO} does not affect O_2 transfer during a single capillary transit because even with normal values the P_{O_2} of end-capillary blood reaches near equilibrium (i.e., <1 Torr). Even with a 50% decrease in Dp_{CO}, $\dot{V}_{O_2}$ is predicted to decrease only 12% and fetal end-capillary P_{O_2} is predicted to decrease ~7%. However, under steady-state conditions, fetal end-capillary P_{O_2} should decrease ~22% to 23 Torr, and, as Dp_{CO} is decreased further, fetal end-capillary P_{O_2} should decrease precipitously because further lowering of Pfa_{O_2} can no longer serve to maintain normal O_2 exchange rates (200).

HYPOXIA AND EMBOLIZATION. In an effort to determine the placental and fetal adaptations to long-term hypoxia, Gilbert et al. (114) exposed guinea pigs to an inspired O_2 fraction (FI_{O_2}) of 12% from day 15 to day 62 of gestation. Fetal body weight decreased 30%. In contrast, although placental weight decreased only 5%, Dp_{CO} increased 63% (from 3.3 ± 0.1 to 5.3 ± 0.1 $ml \cdot min^{-1} \cdot Torr^{-1} \cdot kg^{-1}$). Placental microsomal cytochrome P-450 concentrations were low in control animals, did not increase with hypoxia, and thus could not explain the rise in Dp_{CO}. These authors postulated that this higher Dp_{CO} value resulted from an increased functional exchange area or decreased diffusion distance (114). To further explore the relation of Dp_{CO} to placental structure, they exposed guinea pigs to 12%–14% O_2 as in the previous study and used stereological techniques to quantify certain structural details that influence Dp (9). They also used the stereological measurements in a mathematical model to predict Dp. In the hypoxemic animals, measured Dp_{CO} increased 27% (from 2.3 ± 0.2 to 3.3 ± 0.2 $ml \cdot min^{-1} \cdot Torr^{-1} \cdot kg^{-1}$). By comparison, the model predicted a 38% increase in Dp. In these hypoxemic animals, total placental vascular volume (i.e., effective exchange area) increased 12% ± 3%, and diffusion distance decreased 18% ± 5%; these results strongly suggest the dependence of Dp_{CO} on placental structure (9).

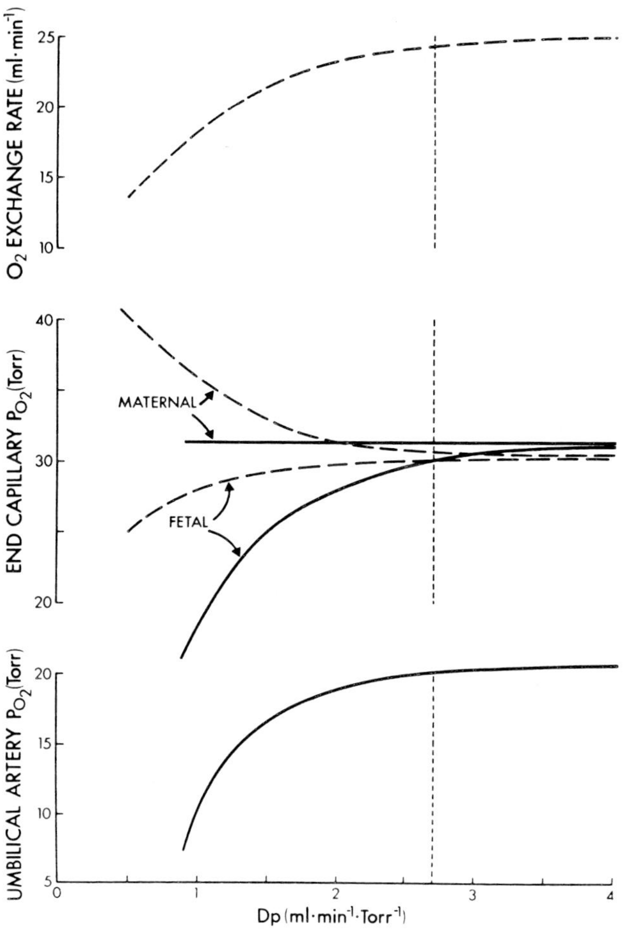

FIG. 11. Calculated changes in transient O_2 exchange rate and maternal and fetal placental end-capillary P_{O_2} values (*dashed curves*) and steady-state maternal and fetal end-capillary P_{O_2} (*solid curves*) as functions of Dp. *Vertical dashed lines*, assumed normal value of Dp. During steady-state conditions, a normal $\dot{V}_{O_2}$ may be maintained within limits by decreases of fetal arterial P_{O_2} (*bottom panel*).

In an effort to stress placental diffusion reserves and to determine whether fetal growth retardation in association with placental embolization (75) results from decreased Dp or from decreased blood flow, Boyle et al. (51) injected 1–2 million 25-μm microspheres into the uteroplacental circulation of the pregnant ewe. Embolization resulted in an immediate 25%–30% drop in uterine arterial flow ($\dot{Q}m$), P_{O_2}, and [O_2], whereas P_{CO_2} and [H^+] increased. Blood gases and $\dot{Q}m$ recovered to ~85% of control values within 30 min after injection. A linear relation existed between $\dot{Q}m$ and Pfa_{O_2}; P_{CO_2} and $[H^+]$ rapidly increased when $\dot{Q}m$ decreased below 150 $ml \cdot min^{-1} \cdot kg^{-1}$, and Dp_{CO} increased 117%. Thus these authors concluded that embolization of the uteroplacental vasculature decreased blood flow rather than affecting the exchange area (51).

Another approach to stressing placental diffusion reserves has been to increase $\dot{V}f_{O_2}$. In the chronically catheterized sheep fetus, norepinephrine infusion for 50 min increased $\dot{V}f_{O_2}$ by 25% (208), whereas triiodothyronine administration for 5 days increased it by 28% (209). Nonetheless fetal blood gas levels and Dp_{CO} remained constant, suggesting that the placental diffusion reserves were not exceeded.

RESPONSES TO MATERNAL EXERCISE. Both the magnitude and distribution of maternal and fetal placental blood flows, as well as the respective Hb concentrations, markedly affect $\dot{V}_{O_2}$. In near-term sheep, acute exercise for 40 min at 70% maximum O_2 consumption ($\dot{V}max_{O_2}$) did not affect Dp_{CO} (211). Despite a 26% decrease in $\dot{Q}m$ in these studies, because of a 20% increase in [Hb]m, uterine O_2 delivery was unchanged (211). However, this did not exclude the possibility that $\dot{V}_{O_2}$ was reduced during exercise because fetal O_2 levels decreased slightly.

In guinea pigs that exercised on a treadmill for 15–60 min throughout gestation, Gilbert et al. (114) and Nelson et al. (254) observed Dp_{CO} values that were as much as 34% lower than those in controls; the decrease was proportional to the exercise duration. In other chronically exercised guinea pigs, Smith et al. (316) demonstrated an inverse relation between exercise duration and both Dp_{CO} and the surface area of maternal lacunae in the peripheral placental labyrinth. In turn, Dp_{CO} was proportional to both the maternal and fetal surface areas of a given volume of placenta as well as to the exchange area of the entire placenta (316). The reason for the smaller areas in chronically exercised guinea pigs is unknown. Also, although theoretically $\dot{V}_{O_2}$ is affected by the decrease in surface area, it remains unclear whether O_2 limitation caused the reduced birth weight that was observed in these fetuses.

Fetal body temperature exceeds that of the mother by ~0.5°C, but the implications of the fetal-to-maternal temperature differences for $\dot{V}_{O_2}$ have not been thoroughly investigated. For example, during maternal exercise for 40 min at 70% $\dot{V}max_{O_2}$, maternal temperature increased ~1.5°C ± 0.5°C. The fetal temperature increased a similar amount but over a slower time course. Fetal P_{O_2} and $[O_2]$ appeared to decrease rather strikingly, but when corrected for the temperature effect the changes were less, ~3 Torr and 1.5 $ml \cdot dl^{-1}$, respectively. The failure to correct for a 1°C temperature increase will result in about a 1.9 and 2.7 Torr underestimate of fetal P_{O_2} and P_{CO_2}, respectively,

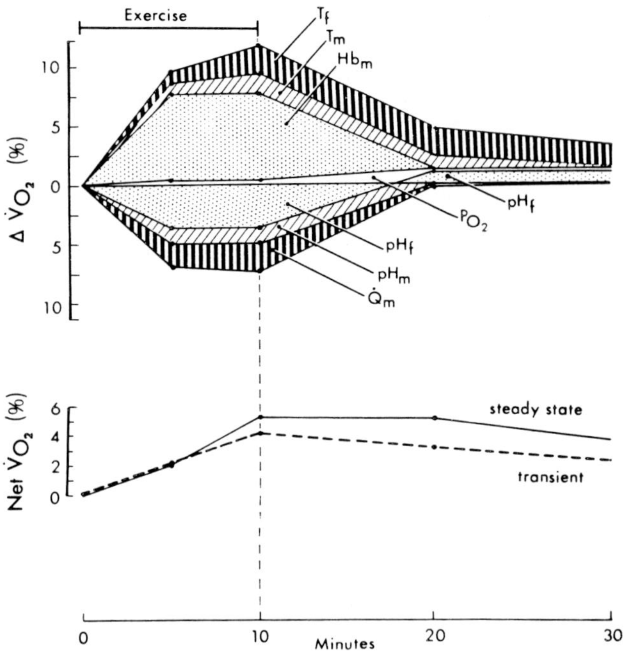

FIG. 12. Theoretical effects of maternal exercise on placental O_2 transfer. *Top*, contribution of individual factors to net $\dot{V}_{O_2}$. *Bottom*, net effect of these changes on transient and steady-state O_2 transfer rates. T_f, fetal temperature; T_m, maternal temperature; Hb_m, maternal Hb concentration; P_{O_2}, maternal arterial P_{O_2}; pH_f, fetal arterial pH; pH_m, maternal arterial pH; $\dot{Q}_m$, uteroplacental blood flow.

whereas the calculated pH will be 0.015 units too high (211).

With the use of a mathematical model, Koos et al. (170) examined the effects of a number of variables that determine placental O_2 transfer during exercise (Fig. 12). Values for each variable were taken for control, exercise, and recovery periods for sheep exercising on a treadmill for 10 min at 70% $\dot{V}max_{O_2}$ (210, 211). The $\dot{V}_{O_2}$ was predicted to be favorably affected by several factors. During both exercise and early recovery, increased [Hb]m accounts for ~60% of this rise, whereas elevated maternal and fetal temperatures are responsible for ~15% and 20%, respectively. Later during the recovery period, $\dot{V}_{O_2}$ is still favored, principally as a result of increased fetal temperatures. Other factors tend to reduce $\dot{V}_{O_2}$. The small increase in fetal arterial pH was predicted to contribute 50% of the total negative effect during exercise and early recovery, whereas decreased $\dot{Q}m$ contributed 30%. The increase in maternal pH also tended to reduce $\dot{V}_{O_2}$. The net exercise effect on transient $\dot{V}_{O_2}$ changes is shown by the broken line in Figure 12. During short-term exercise, $\dot{V}_{O_2}$ is predicted to increase, peaking at the end of the exercise period and gradually declining during the recovery phase (170).

CLINICAL IMPLICATIONS. Throughout the course of gestation the placental mass and exchange area increase to meet the demands of the developing conceptus (4). The exchange area increases both as the placental tissues grow and as the fetal villous capillaries increase in complexity. During the first third of gestation the membranes that separate maternal and fetal blood are relatively thick, but as pregnancy proceeds they become thinner and fetal capillaries approach the surface of the chorionic villi. This is indicated from both morphological studies and the fact that after 35–36 wk placental DNA content remains constant (346) while the surface area continues to increase (4). Thus, during the last third of gestation, although fetal weight increases three- to fivefold (from 1,000 to 3,500 g) and placental weight doubles (from 280 to 500 g), so that the ratio of placental to fetal weight decreases considerably (from 0.22 to 0.14) (119), Dp_{CO} calculated in terms of placental weight increases (40, 194). However, when calculated in terms of fetal weight, which is more common, Dp_{CO} remains remarkably constant (42, 194).

The Dp_{CO} value may decrease in clinical conditions such as diabetes mellitus or syphilis, in which the placental membranes are thickened, or in association with intrauterine growth retardation (4). In addition, Dp_{CO} is probably lowered in conditions associated with decreased blood volume or [Hb] in the placental exchange vessels. However, none of these clinical associations has been established and the development of a method to measure readily Dp_{CO} in humans is needed.

Placental O_2 Consumption

THEORETICAL CONSIDERATIONS. As noted above, a portion of the P_{O_2} difference between the uterine and umbilical veins may result from O_2 consumption by placental tissue ($\dot{V}p_{O_2}$), but the role of this factor in the maternal-to-fetal Pv_{O_2} difference or in limiting fetal O_2 availability is not known. The sites of $\dot{V}p_{O_2}$ could have several anatomical relations to the vascular bed. On one hand, all of the O_2 could be derived from maternal blood in the area of O_2 exchange per se. Alternatively, it could derive from fetal blood in a two-step process in which the O_2 first diffuses into fetal exchange vessels and then backdiffuses into placental tissue. Both of these alternatives would fit an in-parallel pattern (79). An in-series pattern, in which O_2 is consumed from maternal and/or fetal blood after it has left the exchange area, is also possible. Obviously this latter arrangement would contribute to a significant maternal-to-fetal Pv_{O_2} difference. Morphological evidence suggests that a considerable fraction of $\dot{V}p_{O_2}$ derives from blood in the exchange vessels, with an unknown fraction deriving from that in post-exchange vessels. The question of the contribution of $\dot{V}p_{O_2}$ to the maternal-to-fetal venous and mean P_{O_2} differences is important because an increase in the calculated $\bar{P}_{O_2}$ difference would decrease the calculated value of Dp_{O_2}.

Hill et al. (138) used a mathematical model in an attempt to explore this problem. Assuming that $\dot{V}p_{O_2}$ = 10 ml·min^{-1}·kg placenta^{-1} (64) and that this O_2 was derived from maternal and fetal blood in proportion to the P_{O_2} difference between capillary blood and the surrounding tissue, they predicted an end-capillary P_{O_2} difference of <1 Torr; i.e., $\dot{V}p_{O_2}$ would have a negligible effect on uterine and umbilical mixed venous P_{O_2}. This algorithm also predicted that, although net O_2 exchange would be decreased during the early part of a capillary transit (because P_{O_2} gradient was lower) and the continuing loss would lower the P_{O_2} values along the length of the capillary, the maternal-to-fetal end-capillary P_{O_2} difference would be essentially the same as in the absence of $\dot{V}p_{O_2}$. Assumptions about other configurations (e.g., that O_2 supplied to placenta is derived equally from fetal and maternal blood) resulted in similar results. Only if all $\dot{V}p_{O_2}$ were derived from fetal blood, an unlikely possibility, would it contribute to the maternal-to-fetal Pv_{O_2} difference (138).

EXPERIMENTAL STUDIES. Campbell et al. (64) determined $\dot{V}p_{O_2}$ in vivo by replacing the sheep fetus with a pump to perfuse the umbilical circulation. By thus eliminating $\dot{V}f_{O_2}$, P_{O_2} values of umbilical arterial and venous blood became equal at ~50 Torr. From the maternal arteriovenous C_{O_2} difference, these authors calculated $\dot{V}p_{O_2}$ = 10 ml·min^{-1}·kg^{-1} (64), which agrees with most other in vivo and in vitro measurements but slightly exceeds that for the fetus, which approximates 8 ml·min^{-1}·kg^{-1} (for review see ref. 207). These workers obtained similar $\dot{V}p_{O_2}$ values when they retained the fetus in utero, respiring it with O_2 so that Pfa_{O_2} = Pfv_{O_2}. They also estimated that $\dot{V}p_{O_2}$ accounted for 30% of uterine $\dot{V}_{O_2}$ near term. Other estimates of the fraction of total $\dot{V}_{O_2}$ accounted for by $\dot{V}p_{O_2}$ range from 20% in rabbits (101) to 45% in rhesus monkeys (265) and 50% in sheep (231). Earlier in pregnancy, when placental tissue constitutes a greater proportion of the total, $\dot{V}p_{O_2}$ accounts for a proportionally larger fraction, especially as $\dot{V}p_{O_2}$ of human placental slices is twice as great early in gestation as during the latter half (328). Although $\dot{V}p_{O_2}$ may limit fetal O_2 availability during periods of short- or long-term hypoxemia, the extent to which this occurs is not known.

Summary

Placental O_2 and CO_2 exchange in experimental animals can be quantified by measuring diffusing capacity or permeability. For O_2 these values are relatively large, with no significant barrier to diffusion. Thus the true maternal-to-fetal P_{O_2} differences are relatively small, and P_{O_2} values in maternal and fetal placental blood probably equilibrate during the course of a capillary transit. Of the overall resistance to O_2

diffusion, a significant fraction results from the effective resistance caused by Hb reaction rates. No convincing evidence demonstrates that O_2 diffusion is carrier mediated. There are a number of aspects of diffusion about which we are ignorant. We do not know the mechanism whereby Dp and effective exchange area increase in response to long-term hypoxemia or decrease in association with repetitive maternal exercise. We also do not know to what extent Dp is affected by changes in vascular pressure, various pharmacological agents, or different disease states. Furthermore we do not know a precise value for Dp_{CO} in humans, whether it changes during the course of gestation, or whether its measurement will ever be useful as a clinical test.

VARIATIONS IN MATERNAL AND FETAL O_2 TENSIONS

Theoretical Considerations

In light of the above background, one may ask to what extent placental O_2 exchange varies as a function of changes in Pma_{O_2} or Pfa_{O_2} values. Ideally the effects of various factors on $\dot{V}_{O_2}$ should be studied by sampling the inflowing and end-capillary blood within a single exchange unit. Presently this is not technically possible. Therefore, although the placenta has measurable maternal and fetal arterial inputs and mixed venous outputs, it may be compared to a black box in which the dynamics of the exchange process per se remain obscured. Uterine and umbilical venous outflow, rather than representing blood from a single exchange unit, consists of blood from numerous compartments with differing values of O_2 and CO_2 tensions and contents. This probably results from a combination of nonuniform distribution of maternal and fetal placental blood flows, nonuniform distribution of diffusing capacity to blood flow, vascular shunts, and $\dot{V}p_{O_2}$ (see *Distribution of Maternal and Fetal Placental Flows*, p. 385). An additional problem for the investigator is that when one experimentally changes a given variable in an attempt to stress the system, various physiological compensations can mask the effect of this change.

Because of these problems and others, it is useful to model the exchange process mathematically, exploring the effects of variations in individual factors on $\dot{V}_{O_2}$ and calculating their relative importance in comparison with other factors (138, 200). In turn, carefully designed experiments can test these theoretical predictions or obtain more refined values for certain functions (204).

Figure 13 shows the dependence of $\dot{V}_{O_2}$ and end-capillary P_{O_2} values on Pma_{O_2}. Uncompensated decreases in Pma_{O_2} to ~70 Torr (from normal value of 95–100 Torr) have relatively little effect. However, a further decrease to 50 Torr reduces transient $\dot{V}_{O_2}$ by ~25% (from 24 to 18 $ml \cdot min^{-1}$) and fetal end-capillary P_{O_2} by ~10% (from 30 to 27 Torr). Figure 13 also

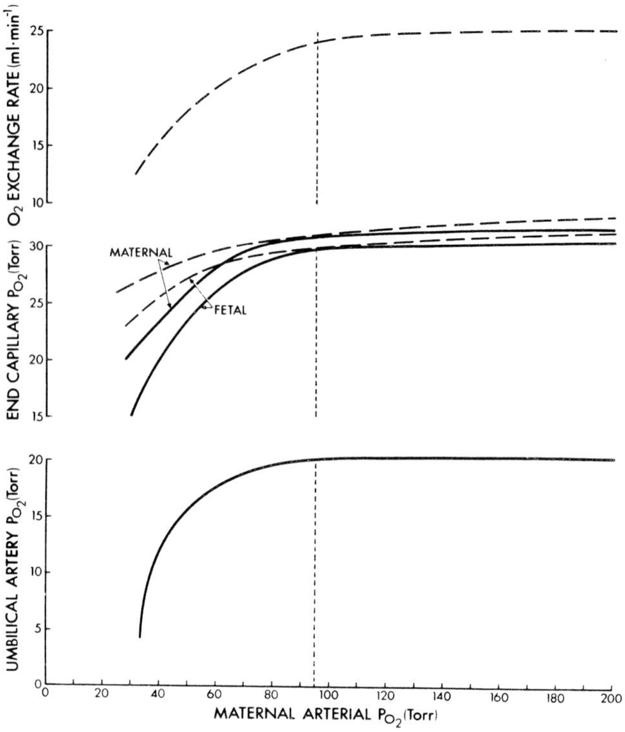

FIG. 13. Calculated effects of changes in maternal arterial P_{O_2} (Pma_{O_2}) on transient maternal and fetal end-capillary P_{O_2} values and O_2 exchange rate (*dashed curves*) and steady-state end-capillary P_{O_2} values and fetal arterial P_{O_2} (Pfa_{O_2}) (*solid curves*). Moderate increases in Pma_{O_2} above normal values (95 Torr, *vertical dashed lines*) increase end-capillary P_{O_2} and transient $\dot{V}_{O_2}$ only slightly, whereas decreases in Pma_{O_2} produce substantial decreases in $\dot{V}_{O_2}$ and end-capillary P_{O_2} values. Decreases in Pfa_{O_2} alone cannot maintain normal $\dot{V}_{O_2}$ when Pma_{O_2} is below ~40 Torr.

shows changes under steady-state conditions of both end-capillary P_{O_2} values and the Pfa_{O_2} changes necessary to maintain normal $\dot{V}_{O_2}$. For example, if Pma_{O_2} decreased to 50 Torr, placental end-capillary P_{O_2} should fall to 22 Torr, whereas Pfa_{O_2} should decrease to ~15 Torr. Although the rate of $\dot{V}f_{O_2}$ would remain normal, its tissues would be perfused with blood at a lower P_{O_2}. With even more severe maternal hypoxemia (Pma_{O_2} < 50 Torr), compensations such as the decrease in Pfa_{O_2} (with increased maternal-to-fetal $\bar{P}_{O_2}$ difference) would become inadequate, as shown by the steep slope of the solid line (Fig. 13). In addition, as Pfv_{O_2} falls dangerously low it may be inadequate to maintain normal $\dot{V}f_{O_2}$ (200).

Raising Pma_{O_2} to 200 or 600 Torr by breathing 100% O_2 would increase fetal placental end-capillary P_{O_2} only 2 or 5 Torr, respectively. These changes would be similar under both transient and steady-state conditions. Although these increases may seem insignificant, they would result in a higher Pf_{O_2}, which could be beneficial during hypoxemia. The fetal placental end-capillary P_{O_2} and Pfa_{O_2} values could not rise to much higher levels because despite the relatively high Pma_{O_2} the amount of additional physically dissolved O_2 in maternal blood would be only 1–2 $ml \cdot dl^{-1}$ (200).

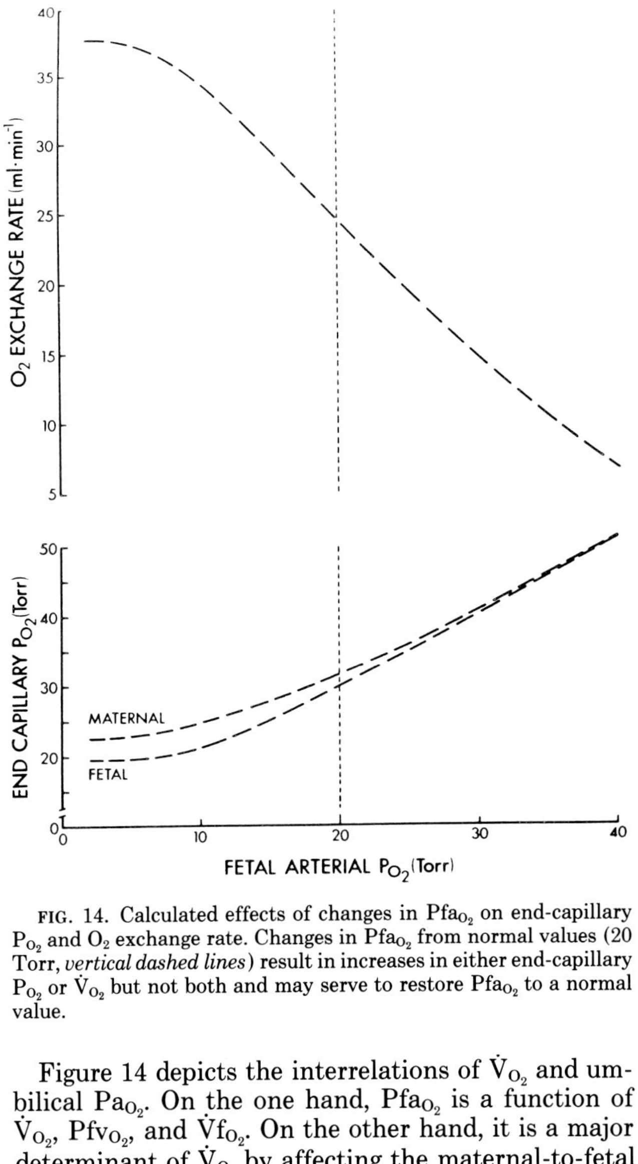

FIG. 14. Calculated effects of changes in Pfa_{O_2} on end-capillary P_{O_2} and O_2 exchange rate. Changes in Pfa_{O_2} from normal values (20 Torr, *vertical dashed lines*) result in increases in either end-capillary P_{O_2} or $\dot{V}_{O_2}$ but not both and may serve to restore Pfa_{O_2} to a normal value.

Figure 14 depicts the interrelations of $\dot{V}_{O_2}$ and umbilical Pa_{O_2}. On the one hand, Pfa_{O_2} is a function of $\dot{V}_{O_2}$, Pfv_{O_2}, and $\dot{V}f_{O_2}$. On the other hand, it is a major determinant of $\dot{V}_{O_2}$ by affecting the maternal-to-fetal P_{O_2} difference. As Pfa_{O_2} decreases, the end-capillary P_{O_2} values fall, but $\dot{V}_{O_2}$ increases as the maternal-to-fetal $\bar{P}_{O_2}$ difference widens (Fig. 14). Alternatively, as Pfa_{O_2} increases, fetal end-capillary P_{O_2} rises and $\dot{V}_{O_2}$ falls. End-capillary P_{O_2} and $\dot{V}_{O_2}$ are more sensitive to a given percentage change in Pfa_{O_2} than to a similar percentage change in any other variable [see Fig. 35; (200)].

Several points of difference may be noted for the intact fetus with blood recirculating between the placenta and peripheral tissues. If $\dot{V}f_{O_2}$ exceeds the rate of $\dot{V}_{O_2}$ and Pfa_{O_2} decreases, the maternal-to-fetal $\bar{P}_{O_2}$ difference increases and $\dot{V}_{O_2}$ increases. Thus $\dot{V}_{O_2}$ rises to match the rate of $\dot{V}f_{O_2}$ and the blood gases will attain new steady-state values (Fig. 14). However, with profound decreases in Pfa_{O_2}, adequate compensation by this passive mechanism could not occur, and placental end-capillary P_{O_2} values would fall below those levels required for optimal respiration of fetal cells.

A caveat is in order. This mathematical paradigm cannot accurately represent the complexity of placental O_2 exchange in vivo nor substitute for experimental studies. The predictions should be subject to testing and insofar as the model fails should be revised. Thus ideally the theoretical predictions should suggest innovative experiments, the results of which will help to refine the model. It is hoped that the system will eventually be well-enough understood for reliance on the predictive capacity of the model alone, but this appears unlikely in the near future.

Experimental Studies

The theoretical studies above suggest that $\dot{V}_{O_2}$ should be particularly sensitive to changes in maternal or fetal Pa_{O_2} values. Variations of these factors are difficult to explore experimentally because, when a given variable such as P_{O_2} is altered, changes in other factors (vascular resistance, blood flow, etc.) obscure the consequences of the variation under study, causing the investigator to misjudge the role of that factor in affecting $\dot{V}_{O_2}$ (see previous section). Also, because uterine and umbilical venous blood represent a mixture from many placental exchange units with varying O_2 values, changes of a given factor may not be reflected accurately by the mixed venous O_2 values.

Surprisingly, few studies have systemically explored the relation of fetal to maternal P_{O_2} values. The experimental conditions of most reports have varied widely, and in only a few instances were attempts made to control the many variables. In sheep, Power and Jenkins (276) perfused the umbilical vessels of an isolated placental cotyledon in situ at controlled flow rates with blood of known P_{O_2}. Figure 15 shows the effect of experimentally varying Pma_{O_2} on the outflow P_{O_2} and $\dot{V}_{O_2}$. As Pma_{O_2} increased from 90 to 300 Torr, Pfv_{O_2} rose from 29 to 34 Torr and $\dot{V}_{O_2}$ rose ~45%, from 5.0 to 7.4 ml·min^{-1}. As Pma_{O_2} fell below ~70 Torr, both Pfv_{O_2} and $\dot{V}_{O_2}$ declined sharply (276). The results predicted by the model are also shown in Figure 15 (solid curves) for comparison. Because certain assumptions (such as value of $\dot{Q}m$) were unknown, any agreement between experimental and theoretical curves is not meaningful in absolute terms, although in general they concurred reasonably well (276).

Power and Jenkins (276) also tested the effects of isolated changes in umbilical Pa_{O_2} on $\dot{V}_{O_2}$ (Fig. 16). Both the outflowing P_{O_2} and $\dot{V}_{O_2}$ showed marked sensitivity to small changes in Pfa_{O_2}. For example, a 20% fall in Pfa_{O_2} resulted in an 18% decrease in outflow P_{O_2} and a 13% increase in $\dot{V}_{O_2}$ (276). These results agree with the theoretical studies that indicate Pfa_{O_2} is the factor to which $\dot{V}_{O_2}$ is most sensitive (200). They also suggest that the small day-to-day (70) or minute-to-minute (158) changes in umbilical Pa_{O_2} and Pv_{O_2}

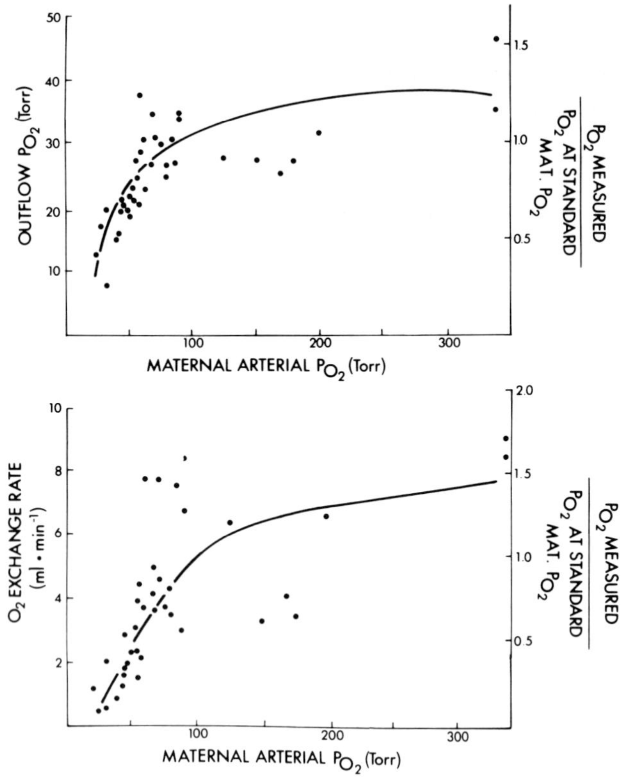

FIG. 15. Effects of experimentally varying Pma_{O_2} on O_2 transfer rate and Pfv_{O_2}. *Solid lines*, theoretical curves. [Adapted from Power and Jenkins (276).]

measured in unanesthetized sheep are probably associated with quantifiable variations in $\dot{V}_{O_2}$.

Changes in Pfa_{O_2} alter both $\dot{V}_{O_2}$ and outflow P_{O_2}, with the responses occurring in opposite directions. Thus decreases in Pfa_{O_2} increase $\dot{V}_{O_2}$, but at the cost of lowering Pfv_{O_2}. Conversely, increases in Pfa_{O_2} increase Pfv_{O_2} at the expense of lowering $\dot{V}_{O_2}$ (200). A similar type of divergent response is noted with changes in umbilical flow rates (see VARIATIONS IN RATE OF MATERNAL AND FETAL PLACENTAL HB AND O_2 FLOWS, p. 381). Indeed, apparently only a more uniform maternal-to-fetal flow pattern would be able to increase both outflow P_{O_2} and $\dot{V}_{O_2}$ simultaneously.

Clinical Implications

MATERNAL O_2 INHALATION. Since the early 1930s, numerous authors have reported increased fetal O_2 levels after maternal O_2 inhalation (94, 216, 338). Figure 17 summarizes data of Pfa_{O_2} versus Pma_{O_2} from several studies. Unfortunately the various reports are somewhat difficult to compare because the samples were obtained from different vessels, and in some instances the reported values were for O_2 or $[HbO_2]$ rather than P_{O_2}.

Because of the shape of the HbO_2 saturation curve, under most conditions relatively large increases in Pma_{O_2} result in only small increases in fetal O_2 tension and content. For instance, raising Pma_{O_2} from 100 Torr (breathing air) to 600 Torr (breathing 100% O_2) increases maternal $[O_2]$ 1.5 $ml \cdot dl^{-1}$ from 16 to 17.5 $ml \cdot dl^{-1}$. In sheep, Pma_{O_2} had to be raised ~200 Torr for Pfv_{O_2} to increase 4 Torr [Fig. 17; (296)]. Similar results were noted in humans when fetal blood was obtained by scalp sampling (162). In women who breathed O_2 during cesarean section, Pfv_{O_2} and Pfa_{O_2} rose 8 and 5 Torr, respectively (352). In women undergoing vaginal delivery, Newman and colleagues (256) reported the empirical relation

$$\text{fetal scalp blood } P_{O_2} \text{ (Torr)} = 17.69 + 0.06\, Pma_{O_2} \tag{10}$$

Fetal P_{O_2} changes relatively rapidly after a change in maternal FI_{O_2}. For instance, in pregnant ewes an increase in FI_{O_2} to 100% increased Pma_{O_2} in ~6 s, reaching a new steady-state value in ~4 min. Fetal Pv_{O_2} rose at 13 s, increasing 5 Torr during the first 10 min and continuing to increase during the next 20

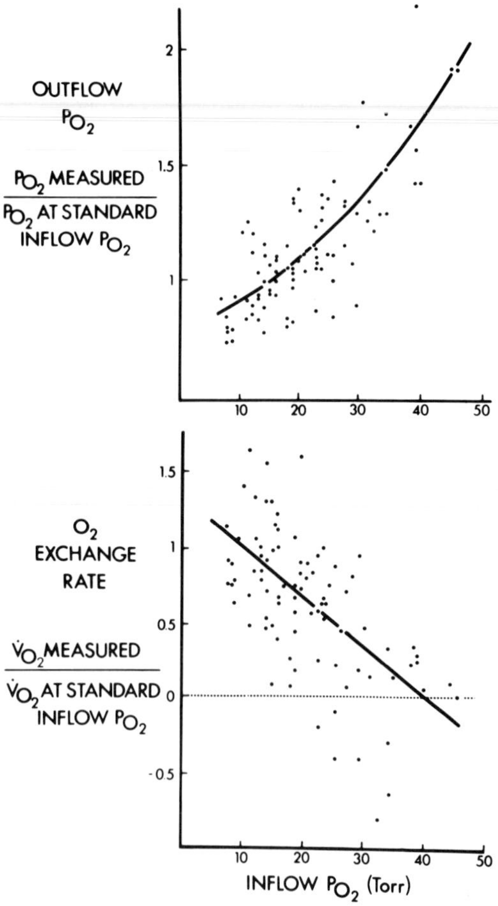

FIG. 16. Effects of varying Pfa_{O_2} on $\dot{V}_{O_2}$ and outflowing umbilical P_{O_2}. *Solid lines*, theoretical curves. [Adapted from Power and Jenkins (276).]

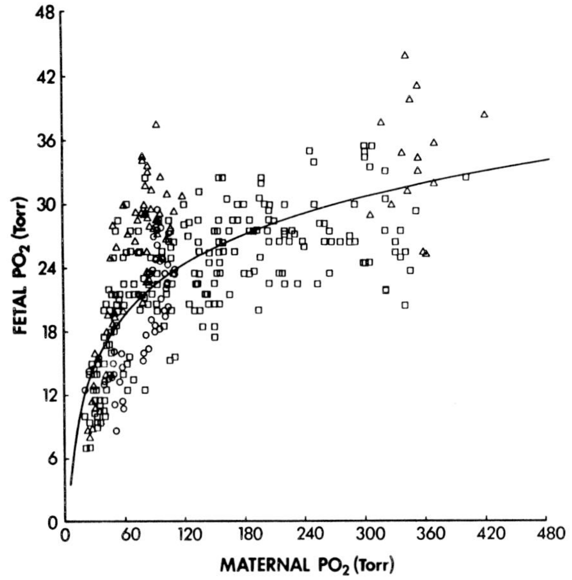

FIG. 17. Relation of Pfa_{O_2} to that of mother in chronically catheterized sheep (□) and monkeys (△) and acutely anesthetized sheep (○).

min (69, 267). In humans, fetal scalp P_{O_2} rose 4–6 Torr within 15 min of maternal O_2 inhalation (162).

Because relatively small changes in Pf_{O_2} follow large changes in maternal O_2 levels when Pma_{O_2} exceeds 80 Torr, the question arises whether O_2 administration to the mother during labor or delivery improves $\dot{V}_{O_2}$ and fetal oxygenation. In normal sheep, increasing FI_{O_2} to 100% results in no significant change in $\dot{V}_{O_2}$ (195). In instances of fetal distress, any increase in fetal O_2 levels decreases the chance of damage to the brain and other vital structures. Thus, although one cannot be certain that maternal O_2 administration will be of benefit, there is no justification for withholding it.

HYPERBARIC OXYGENATION. Because O_2 therapy at pressures >1 atm can be useful in several clinical conditions, it might be queried whether hyperbaric oxygenation affects $\dot{V}_{O_2}$ and has potential for alleviating fetal hypoxemia. Longo et al. (206) first investigated the effects of hyperbaric pressures on $\dot{V}_{O_2}$ and Dp. Above 3.5 atm, the maternal arteriovenous P_{O_2} difference was relatively constant at 1,200 Torr (or 2.6 $ml \cdot dl^{-1}$), and all O_2 exchanged was derived from that amount physically dissolved in maternal blood (Fig. 18). Fetal Pv_{O_2} increased as a function of increasing pressure to ~650 Torr at 5 atm, whereas Pfa_{O_2} rose to only 40 Torr. Subsequently, Kirschbaum et al. (165) demonstrated small but insignificant decreases in $\dot{Q}m$ and $\dot{Q}f$ at 3 atm, with no significant change in $\dot{V}f_{O_2}$.

Although hyperbaric oxygenation might be considered of value in treating fetal hypoxemia, it presently has no clinical role because of the danger of maternal O_2 toxicity. During maternal inhalation of 100% O_2 at 3 atm, coma, convulsions, and death may occur within 10–15 min (179). In near-term rabbits, prolonged maternal hyperoxia resulted in an increased incidence of prematurity, stillbirths, neonatal deaths, and eye abnormalities (108).

ACUTE DECREASE IN INSPIRED O_2 TENSION. Probably the earliest study of the effects of hypoxia on the developing mammal was Robert Boyle's demonstration in 1670 that one-day-old "Kitlings . . . continued three times longer in the exhausted receiver than other animals of that bigness would probably have done" (52). Since then many studies have verified that fetal and newborn animals are more resistant to hypoxemia than are adults. Although numerous studies have explored various aspects of fetal hypoxemia, I review only those contributing to an understanding of transplacental O_2 exchange.

In a study of anesthetic-induced asphyxia neonatorum, Eastman (93) reported a rather startling human experiment. Inspired O_2 concentrations as low as 5% were given for 5–21 min to pregnant mothers during vaginal delivery or cesarean section. When the women inspired an 80% N_2O-20% O_2 mixture, umbilical venous and arterial [HbO_2] averaged 41% and 22%, respectively. Assuming pH values of 7.35 and 7.32, these saturations correspond to ~18 and 12 Torr, respectively. In nine subjects who breathed 15% O_2, maternal [HbO_2] averaged 79% (Pma_{O_2} = 43 Torr), and the umbilical venous and arterial [HbO_2] were 32% and 16%, respectively, corresponding to P_{O_2} values of 16 and 11 Torr, respectively. In three patients who breathed 10% O_2, maternal [HbO_2] was 67% (Pma_{O_2} = 33 Torr), and umbilical venous [HbO_2] and

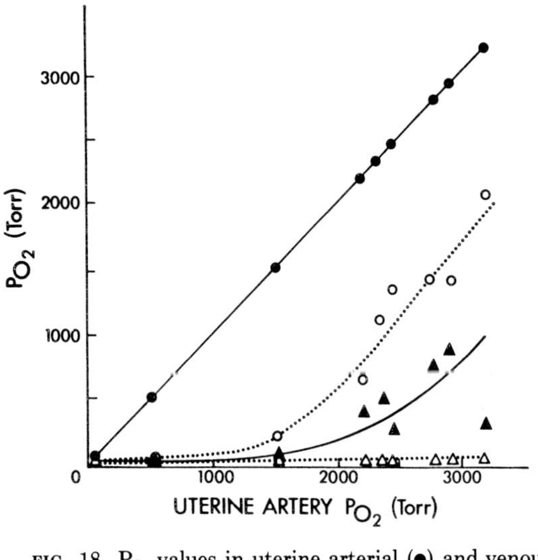

FIG. 18. P_{O_2} values in uterine arterial (●) and venous (○) blood and in umbilical arterial (△) and venous (▲) blood as function of Pma_{O_2}. When Pmv_{O_2} was >200 Torr, uterine venous HbO_2 was completely saturated and O_2 crossing the placenta was almost entirely from that physically dissolved in maternal plasma. In all cases, Pfv_{O_2} was <Pmv_{O_2}.

P_{O_2} were 12% and 9 Torr, respectively. Two of these mothers were slightly cyanotic, and the newborn infants showed evidence of asphyxia. In seven subjects who breathed only 5% O_2 for up to 20 min, [HbO_2] was 59% (Pma_{O_2} = 29 Torr), and umbilical venous [HbO_2] was 8.6% (P_{O_2} = 7 Torr). The umbilical arteries of most of these latter infants were collapsed, presumably due to inadequate perfusion. All of the newborns were asphyxiated: 5 were apneic for 5–25 min, and 2 died despite resuscitative efforts. The hypoxemic fetuses had shown decreased respiratory movements in utero. Eastman (93) concluded by warning physicians of the extreme danger of using <15% FI_{O_2} in conjunction with N_2O anesthesia.

Numerous subsequent reports have shown a drop in Pf_{O_2} with decreased Pma_{O_2}. Figures 15 and 17 demonstrate this relation and the relative stability of Pfv_{O_2} despite large changes in Pma_{O_2} when the latter is >70 Torr. Although this constancy results from the shape of the HbO_2 curves, it also follows from maternal and fetal circulatory compensations to maintain $\dot{V}_{O_2}$ as near normal as possible. During mild maternal hypoxemia, $\dot{Q}m$ remains constant (97, 195) or decreases slightly (223), but [Hb] increases so that uterine Hb flow increases slightly (195, 223).

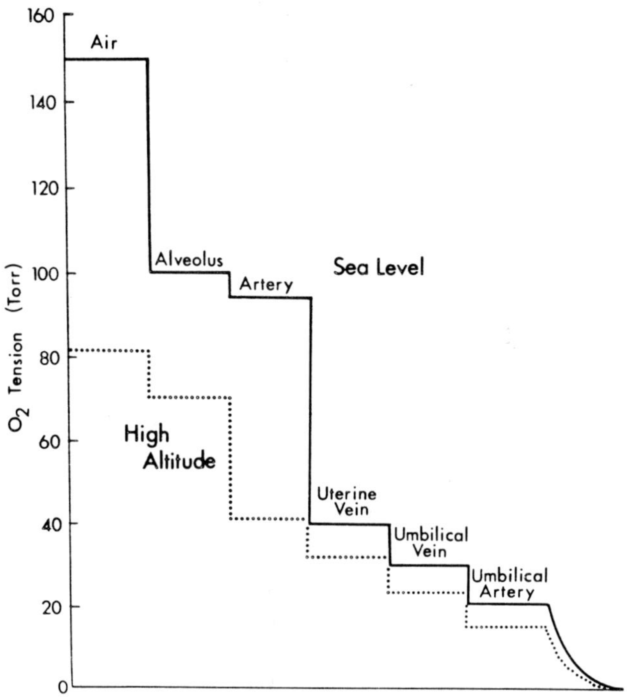

FIG. 19. Cascade of P_{O_2} from ambient air to maternal and fetal blood at ~5,000 m (*dotted line*) as compared with that at sea level (*solid line*).

CHRONIC DECREASE IN MATERNAL INSPIRED O_2 TENSION—HIGH ALTITUDE. Despite the hypoxia associated with high altitude, many individuals live at elevations over 3,000 m, and in the Andes permanent residents live higher than 4,600 m. Because Pfa_{O_2} at sea level approximates that of an adult at ~5,000 m, one would anticipate that the P_{O_2} values of a fetus at high altitude would be much lower than normal. Surprisingly, such is not the case (Fig. 19), and it is instructive to examine the blood gas values reported at various altitudes. Near 1,525 m, Pma_{O_2} is ~80 Torr in humans and 70–75 Torr in sheep (45, 222). Values of Pfv_{O_2} and Pfa_{O_2} at these altitudes range from 20 to 29 and 16 to 21 Torr, respectively. The higher values were from acclimatized sheep (222), whereas the lower ones were obtained in sheep acutely exposed to simulated altitudes (45).

At ~3,100 m, pregnant women both hyperventilate and elevate [Hb] to help maintain arterial [O_2] at a value comparable to that at sea level (224, 245). The infant birth weights of such women apparently reflect their level of oxygenation, which is a function of both ventilation rate and arterial [O_2]. Howard et al. (147) reported that, before the onset of respiration in newborn infants at this altitude, umbilical arterial [HbO_2] averaged ~50% at 3,100 m as compared with 58% at 1,525 m. For sheep and goats acutely exposed to a simulated altitude of 3,050 m, Pma_{O_2}, Pfv_{O_2}, and Pfa_{O_2} were 47, 15, and 11 Torr, respectively (45).

Considerable data about altitude effects on placental O_2 transfer were derived from the studies by Barron and his colleagues (234, 239, 285) in the Peruvian Andes at elevations near 4,575 m. In acclimatized sheep, Pma_{O_2} was 38–40 Torr, depending on whether the ewes had Hb type A or B, and Pfv_{O_2} and Pfa_{O_2} averaged 22 and 12 Torr, respectively (239). In acutely anesthetized and surgically operated llamas at these elevations, P_{O_2} and [HbO_2] averaged 38 Torr and 85%, respectively, in the maternal artery, 20 Torr and 49%, respectively, in the umbilical vein, and 7 Torr and 5%, respectively, in the umbilical artery (234). In sheep in a hypobaric pressure chamber at similar PI_{O_2} (4,940 m), Kaiser et al. (161) recorded a 30% increase in [Hb]f.

In chronically catheterized sheep acutely exposed to hypobaric conditions, Blechner et al. (45) subsequently reported lower P_{O_2} values in the various vessels; i.e., Pma_{O_2}, Pfv_{O_2}, and Pfa_{O_2} were 34, 13, and 9 Torr, respectively. The differences between results in acclimatized and nonacclimatized animals are more readily understandable in light of blood gas values after the ewes had been transported from ~1,525 m to 4,300 m (222). Initially umbilical venous and arterial [HbO_2] fell from normal values of 74% and 61%, respectively, to 45% and 28%, respectively, during the first few days at the new elevation. Then, over a period of 6–18 days, [HbO_2] increased to values similar to those at the lower altitude (222).

Apparently the only study of human fetal blood gas values at high elevations is from Cerro de Pasco, Peru (4,200 m), where during labor fetal scalp P_{O_2} averaged 19 Torr, which is only slightly less than the sea-level value of 22 Torr (318).

Although humans do not reside for prolonged periods much above 4,500 m, at a simulated altitude of 5,490 m for 10 days the P_{O_2} and [HbO_2] values in four pregnant sheep averaged 35 Torr and 50%, respectively, in the maternal artery, 21 Torr and 60%, respectively, in the umbilical vein, and 8 Torr and 30%, respectively, in the umbilical artery (161). At 6,100-m equivalent altitude, Pma_{O_2} and [HbO_2] averaged 32 Torr and 43%, respectively. In a single fetus, umbilical venous and arterial [HbO_2] were 66% and 18%, respectively. One ewe as well as the fetuses of two other ewes died at this diminished pressure (161).

Taken together, these results indicate that at high altitude various physiological mechanisms operate to maintain $\dot{V}_{O_2}$ at a rate close to that at sea level. Unfortunately the maternal and fetal adaptations that serve to maintain $\dot{V}_{O_2}$ under these conditions are not known.

CHRONIC MATERNAL HYPOXEMIA—CYANOTIC CONGENITAL HEART DISEASE. Women with cyanotic heart disease are chronically hypoxemic and develop compensatory adjustments, such as increased blood O_2Cap and decreased O_2 affinity, to maintain their tissue O_2 requirements. The numbers of abortions and perinatal loss in these patients are proportional to their hematocrit and [Hb], undoubtedly reflecting compromised fetal O_2 delivery. In such women, newborn weight varies inversely with maternal hematocrit (15, 27, 261), but little is known about the specific maternal and fetal physiological compensatory mechanisms.

VARIATIONS IN MATERNAL AND FETAL O_2 AFFINITY

Theoretical Considerations

Blood O_2 affinity may differ from normal in a number of disease states and in the presence of abnormal hemoglobins. However, few studies have rigorously explored the relations of either maternal or fetal blood O_2 affinity to $\dot{V}_{O_2}$ under such conditions. Using the mathematical model described in *Theoretical Considerations* (p. 368), one may examine the effect of an isolated change in either maternal or fetal blood O_2 affinity on $\dot{V}_{O_2}$ (200). With Pm_{50} increases above the normal value of 26.5 Torr, both transient $\dot{V}_{O_2}$ and P_{O_2} in maternal and fetal end-capillary vessels should increase, provided no compensatory adjustments occur. A decreased Pm_{50} should demonstrate the opposite effect. This trend is similar even for compensatory adjustments under steady-state conditions, such as an increased $\dot{V}_{O_2}$ due to the lowered Pfa_{O_2} (200).

Theory predicts that variations in Pf_{50} should also affect transient $\dot{V}_{O_2}$ and end-capillary P_{O_2} as well as steady-state P_{O_2} values (200). Raising Pf_{50} (e.g., by transfusing fetus with maternal blood) should lower $\dot{V}_{O_2}$ only slighly (<2%), and fetal end-capillary P_{O_2} should remain essentially constant. In contrast, decreasing Pf_{50} to 15 Torr or less should significantly decrease the transient $\dot{V}_{O_2}$, whereas the end-capillary P_{O_2} should rise significantly. Thus normal maternal and fetal P_{50} values apparently are not greatly different from those that are optimal for O_2 transfer (200).

Decrease in Fetal Blood O_2 Affinity by Intrauterine Transfusion

During the late 1960s and 1970s, intrauterine transfusion for erythroblastosis fetalis developed as a lifesaving procedure in instances of Rh incompatibility (187). Several investigators have examined the effects of transfusion of blood with different O_2 affinities in experimental animals. Battaglia et al. (28) exchange transfused six singleton chronically catheterized fetal lambs with type B maternal sheep blood (P_{50} = 37 Torr) so that the O_2 affinity decreased (Pf_{50} values not given) and O_2Cap remained constant. Fetal Pv_{O_2} increased ~4 Torr (from 27 to 31 Torr), and in three fetuses this value reached 36 Torr. Despite this increased P_{O_2}, [HbO_2] decreased 28% from 79% to 51%. Although Battaglia et al. (28) had no adequate explanation for the rise in Pfv_{O_2}, it is entirely reasonable on the basis of the theoretical considerations detailed above [see p. 368; (200)]. In these animals the maternal-to-fetal Pv_{O_2} difference decreased, and there was no significant change in $\dot{Q}f$ or $\dot{V}_{O_2}$ (230), again results that would be predicted. That the decreased blood O_2 affinity had no deleterious effect on fetal survival was attested by the continuance of pregnancy for 1–5 wk in five of the six animals (28). Of course, during this time fetal erythrocytes gradually replaced the transfused maternal cells. These findings were confirmed in acutely anesthetized sheep (164). In contrast, other workers have reported that exchange transfusion in fetal sheep resulted in increases in Pfa_{O_2} as described above, but they also reported decreases in $\dot{Q}f$ and $\dot{V}f_{O_2}$ of 49% and 44%, respectively (156). Based on the results of intrauterine transfusion in human fetuses with hemolytic disease, it is apparent that fetuses can tolerate fairly wide variations in blood O_2 affinity (226, 257, 258).

The manner in which greater-than-normal fetal O_2 affinity affects $\dot{V}_{O_2}$ can be clarified with an illustration. Because of the dogma that the difference in positions of the maternal and fetal HbO_2 curves accounts for the major P_{O_2} difference resulting in placental O_2 diffusion, it may not be readily apparent how an adequate amount of O_2 exchanges if the HbO_2 curves are superimposed. In Figure 20, O_2 content is plotted as a function of P_{O_2} for maternal and fetal blood, both of which have a P_{50} value of 26.5 Torr. Under these circumstances the maternal and fetal end-capillary P_{O_2} values would equilibrate at 30 Torr, and Pfa_{O_2} and Pfv_{O_2} would be ~20 and 28 Torr, respectively. These later values give a fetal arteriovenous C_{O_2} difference of 4.6 ml·dl^{-1} ($\dot{Q}m$ and $\dot{Q}f$ are considered equal and blood O_2Cap is assumed to be 15 and 22 ml·dl^{-1},

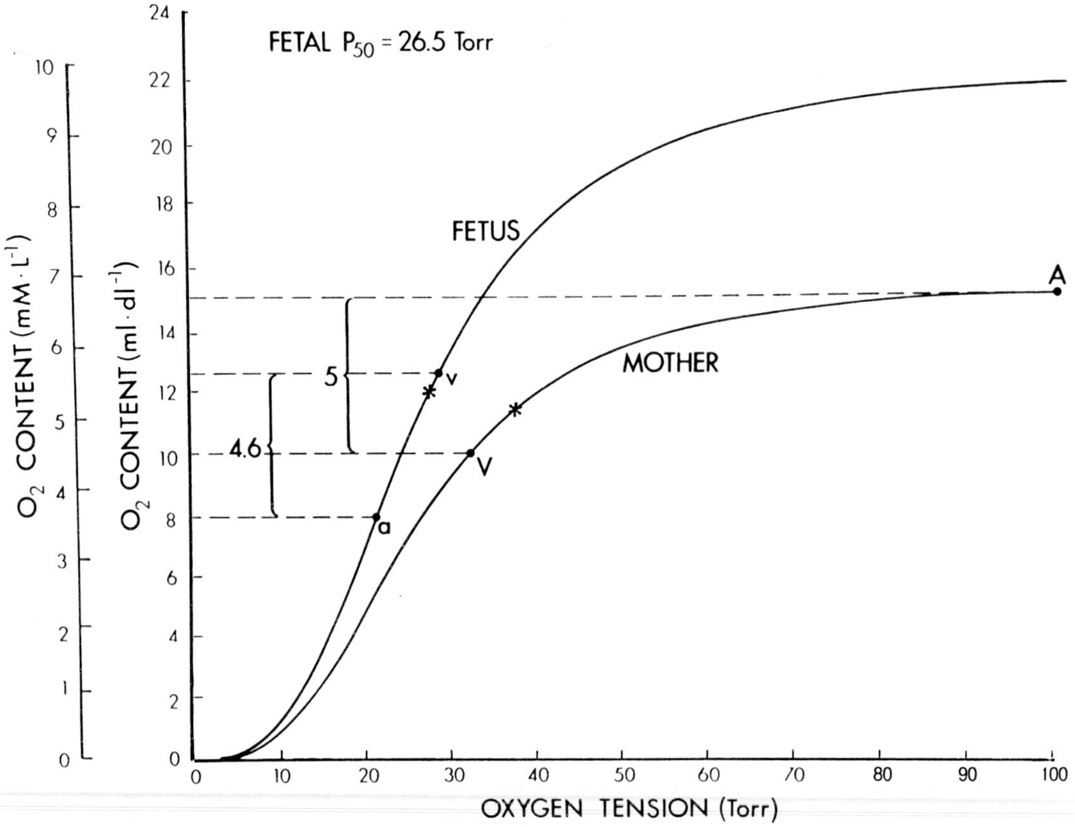

FIG. 20. Calculated maternal and fetal blood O_2 contents as function of P_{O_2} when relative positions of maternal and fetal HbO_2 saturation curves are identical; i.e., both Pm_{50} and Pf_{50} are 26.5 Torr. *Asterisks*, $\bar{P}m_{O_2}$ and $\bar{P}f_{O_2}$; A and V, maternal arterial and venous values; a and v, umbilical arterial and venous values.

respectively, for mother and fetus). The $\bar{P}_{O_2}$ values in the exchange vessels are indicated (Fig. 20, asterisks) and the maternal-to-fetal $\bar{P}_{O_2}$ difference is 9 Torr. Figure 20 also depicts the role of fetal blood O_2Cap in allowing for ample $[O_2]$ despite its lowered P_{O_2}.

Changes in O_2 Affinity Due to Hemoglobinopathies

Human Hb presents an almost bewildering diversity: the structure of nearly 300 variants has been described (58). By amino acid substitution or deletion the genetic mutation responsible for these variants may affect the α-, β-, or γ-chains or other chains and affect blood O_2 affinity by changes in the normal areas of contact between the Hb subunits. These alterations result in P_{50} values ranging from 10 Torr in Hb McKees Rocks and 12 Torr in Hb Ranier and Hb Yakima to ~70 Torr in Hb Kansas. Apparently, in an attempt to optimize tissue O_2 delivery, blood with a low P_{50} generally develops a high O_2Cap. The maintenance of a relatively normal $\dot{V}_{O_2}$ despite such hemoglobinopathies in mothers and/or fetuses is attested by numerous case reports (2, 65, 246, 264).

Several groups have examined the effects of experimentally lowering Pm_{50} of pregnant rats to a value similar to Pf_{50} (~25 Torr) by incubating the erythrocytes with sodium cyanate (29, 132). Between 19- and 22-days gestation, fetal weight decreased 10%–18%, and in one of the studies the placental weight increased 21% compared with that of controls (132). These changes, coupled with a 10% increase in the maternal hematocrit (and slight increase in that of fetus), suggest some hypoxemia.

The manner in which altered maternal or fetal blood O_2 affinity affects $\dot{V}_{O_2}$ is illustrated by two contrasting situations. First, in Figure 21, a pregnant woman with Hb A carries a fetus in which Hb Kansas (P_{50} = 70 Torr) rather than Hb A replaces Hb F. Because Hb A normally constitutes ~25% of the total Hb near term, we assume that Hb Kansas would comprise the same fraction so that Pf_{50} would be ~35 Torr (whereas values for other factors would be the same as those for Fig. 20). In this case the maternal and fetal end-capillary P_{O_2} values would equilibrate at 31 Torr, and Pfv_{O_2} and Pfa_{O_2} would be ~28 and 20 Torr, respectively (Fig. 21). The maternal-to-fetal $\bar{P}_{O_2}$ difference would be ~9 Torr, and $\dot{V}_{O_2}$ would be normal.

Second, in Figure 22, a pregnant woman with Hb Ranier (Pm_{50} = 12 Torr) carries an infant with Hb F. The [Hb] of such patients usually increases so that blood O_2Cap is ~15 $ml \cdot dl^{-1}$. Under these conditions

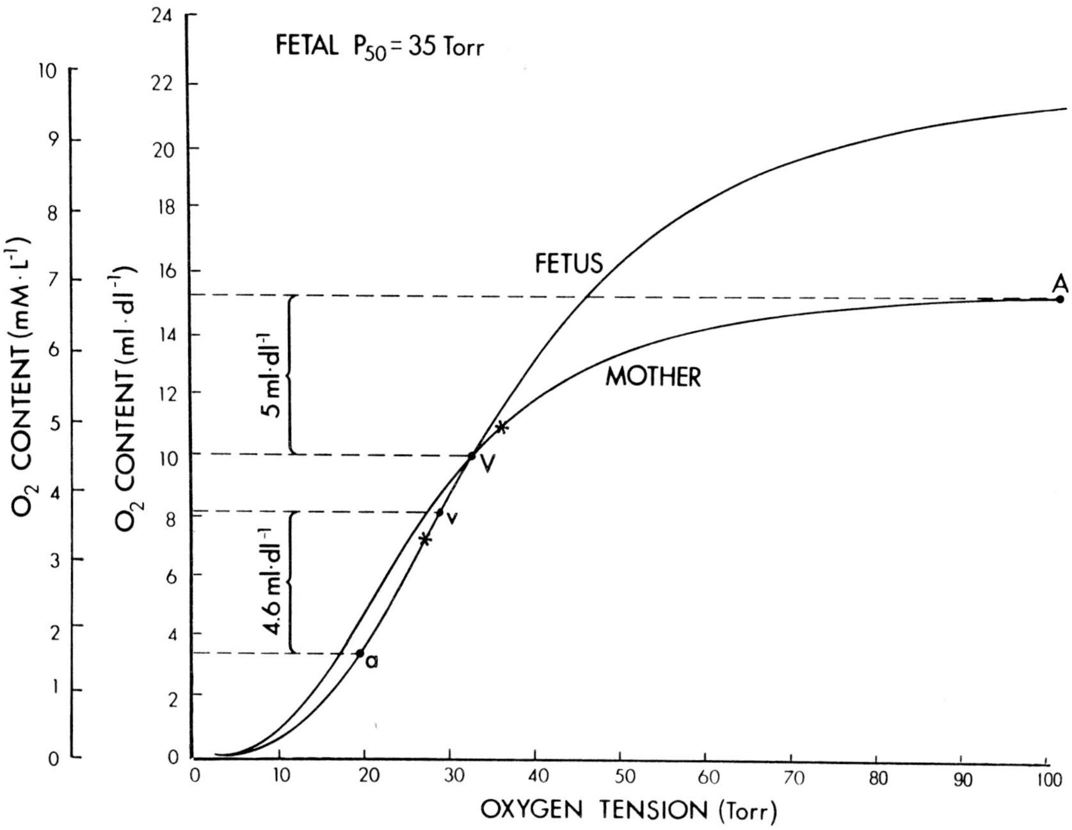

FIG. 21. Maternal and fetal blood O_2 contents as function of P_{O_2} when relative positions of maternal and fetal HbO_2 saturation curves are reversed. In this instance, affinity of maternal blood is normal (Pm_{50} = 26.5 Torr), whereas that of fetus is increased (Pf_{50} = 35 Torr) due to Hb Kansas replacing Hb A. Symbols are as in Fig. 20.

the maternal and fetal end-capillary P_{O_2} values would equilibrate at 19 Torr, and Pfv_{O_2} and $P\bar{f}a_{O_2}$ would be ~18 and 11 Torr, respectively (Fig. 22). Again, the maternal-to-fetal $\bar{P}_{O_2}$ difference and $\dot{V}_{O_2}$ would be normal. Although these examples help to emphasize that the normal positions of the dissociation curves are not absolutely essential for normal $\dot{V}_{O_2}$, this is not to say that altered P_{50} values are not accompanied by physiological adaptions to help maintain adequate $\dot{V}_{O_2}$. Unfortunately, however, essentially nothing is known of these compensations.

A minor variant of Hb A, Hb A_{1C}, which is distinguished by the presence of a glucose molecule covalently bound to the NH_2-terminal β-chain, has attracted interest as an index of control in diabetic patients (59, 60). This glycohemoglobin comprises 4%–6% of the total Hb of normal individuals but correlates with mean blood glucose level (340, 341) and may be elevated twofold in diabetics (220, 340, 341). Although the O_2 affinity of this variant is only slightly greater than normal (Pm_{50} = 24 Torr), several authors have suggested that in association with diabetes $\dot{V}_{O_2}$ might be compromised (88, 341). However, the reported small changes of Pm_{50} in vivo during the third trimester and the lack of relation between Pm_{50} and [Hb A_{1C}] (220, 340) suggest minimal, if any, effects on $\dot{V}_{O_2}$. Nonetheless, significant increases in either maternal or fetal O_2 affinity that decrease the amount of O_2 released as blood traverses a capillary and that result in tissue hypoxia at the venous end of the vessel (87), in combination with thickened placental membranes, increased aggregation and reduced deformability of erythrocytes, and microangiopathy, may result in altered placental blood flows and $\dot{V}_{O_2}$.

Maternal Hyperventilation

Maternal blood O_2 affinity is also affected by changes in blood acid-base balance. For instance, with hyperventilation during labor, Pma_{CO_2} can decrease from 30 to 26 Torr with increases in pH to 7.6. Although it might be argued that the associated leftward shift in the maternal dissociation curve would decrease $\dot{V}_{O_2}$, this effect is probably slight (200).

During the 1960s rather extreme hyperventilation during cesarean section for "hypocapnic enhancement" of the anesthetic agent became popular for a brief period (68, 74). However, problems associated with respiratory alkalosis became apparent. Several patients who experienced forced hyperventilation developed severe respiratory alkalosis with $Pma_{CO_2} < 17$ Torr and pH > 7.66. The newborn infants of these

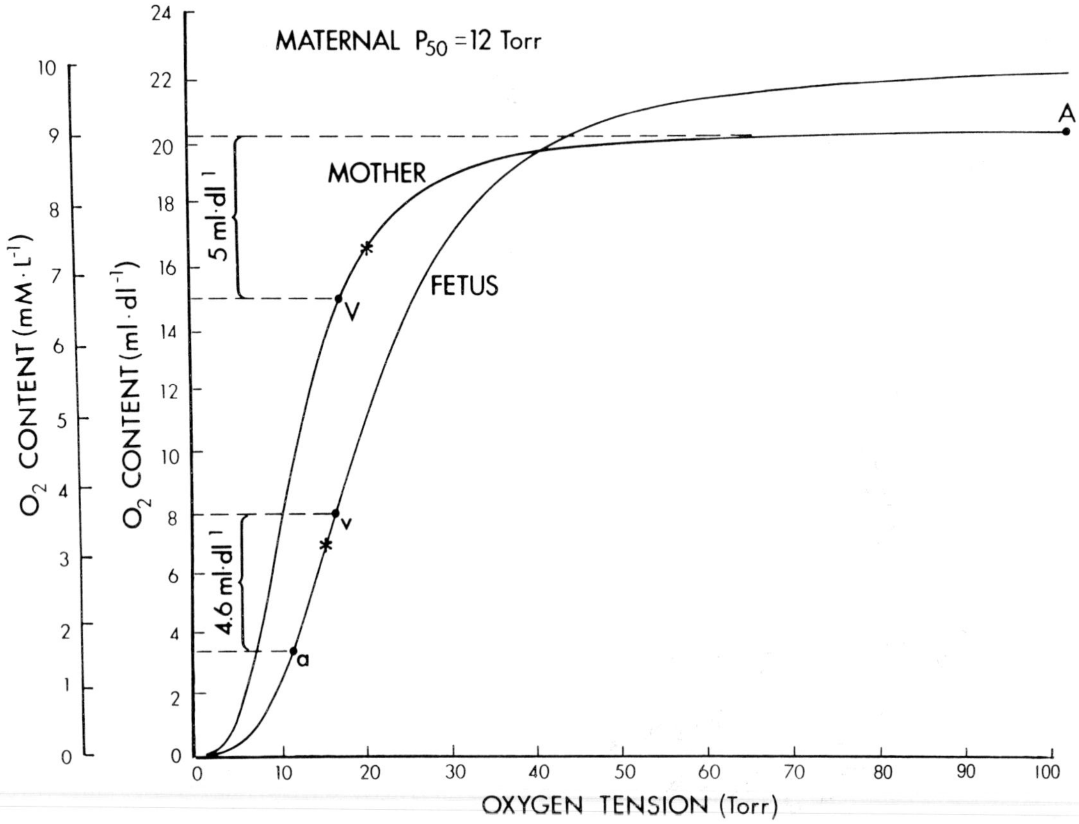

FIG. 22. Maternal and fetal blood O_2 contents as function of P_{O_2} when maternal and fetal HbO_2 saturation curves are reversed. In this instance, Pm_{50} = 12 Torr and [Hb]m = 15 $g \cdot dl^{-1}$, whereas Pf_{50} = 20 Torr. Symbols are as in Fig. 20.

patients experienced severe metabolic acidosis (i.e., umbilical venous pH = 7.10 and P_{CO_2} = 73 Torr) with abnormally low [HbO_2] and Apgar scores (251).

In hyperventilated guinea pigs, fetal pH varied inversely with maternal arterial pH, such that maternal pH values >7.5 were associated with fetal hypoxemia, acidosis, and increased P_{CO_2}. At Pma_{CO_2} values <20 Torr, maternal hypotension and low Apgar scores in the newborn piglets were observed (247). In hyperventilated ewes, Pfv_{O_2} and Pfa_{O_2} values of exteriorized lambs were proportional to maternal arterial P_{CO_2} and [H^+] (250). Furthermore the fetal changes appeared to be associated with decreases in maternal [H^+] and $\dot{Q}$m rather than with changes in P_{CO_2} per se (250). Hyperventilation without altered pH or P_{CO_2} produced no significant effect (249, 250).

Several groups have attempted to elucidate the mechanisms responsible for these changes, demonstrating significant decreases in $\dot{Q}$f, $\dot{V}_{O_2}$ (250), and the coefficient of O_2 utilization (Ca_{O_2} − Cv_{O_2}/Ca_{O_2}) (269). Uterine blood flow decreased as much as 25% from the mechanical effects of severe hyperventilation alone, presumably by impeding venous return rather than from changes in blood gas values (186).

In spontaneously hyperventilating pregnant women, data on the interrelations of fetal O_2 and maternal CO_2 levels are limited. A positive relation has been shown by several groups (242, 249, 269, 301), whereas others have reported only a minor influence (103, 215). Several groups have reported small but significant decreases in scalp blood P_{O_2} in humans during hyperventilation that was unaccompanied by O_2 debt or fetal acidosis (212, 242). Several animal studies have also shown only small decrements in Pfv_{O_2} after maternal hyperventilation, with no significant decrease in $\dot{V}_{O_2}$ (35, 266) or acidosis (10).

In conclusion, hyperventilation is relatively common during pregnancy, particularly during labor and delivery, but evidence does not exist that it alters $\dot{V}_{O_2}$. During anesthesia, forced hyperventilation may lower maternal arterial P_{CO_2} and [H^+] sufficiently to interfere with $\dot{Q}$m and $\dot{V}_{O_2}$. Despite several reports of alterations in fetal P_{O_2} and pH with spontaneous hyperventilation, the overwhelming evidence is to the contrary.

Carbon Monoxide Effects

Carbon monoxide also affects blood O_2 affinity, as described in the chapter by Coburn and Forman in this *Handbook*, and it may be asked how elevated [HbCO] affects $\dot{V}_{O_2}$. If one assumes that under steady-state conditions the P_{CO} values in maternal and fetal blood are equal, the Haldane equation (90)

$$[HbCO]/[HbO_2] = (P_{CO}M)/P_{O_2} \quad (11)$$

which is Equation 5 rearranged, may be equated for maternal and fetal blood and be rearranged

$$[HbCO]f/[HbCO]m = ([HbO_2]f \cdot Pm_{O_2} \cdot Mf)/(Pf_{O_2} \cdot [HbO_2]m \cdot Mm) \quad (12)$$

The $[HbO_2]/P_{O_2}$ ratios for maternal and fetal blood are the O_2 affinities of these bloods, and Mf and Mm are the relative affinities for CO as compared with O_2 of fetal and maternal blood, respectively. Therefore during the steady state the ratio of [HbCO]f to [HbCO]m depends on the relative O_2 affinities of fetal and maternal blood as well as on the ratio of Mf to Mm.

As shown in Figure 23, CO markedly shifts the $[HbO_2]$ curves to the left, altering their shapes to a more hyperbolic form so that Pm_{50} and Pf_{50} decrease. For instance, at 10% [HbCO], Pm_{50} decreases from 26.5 to 23 Torr and Pf_{50} decreases from 20.5 to 17.3 Torr. The physiological implications of these increases in O_2 affinity have been discussed elsewhere (192). Normally the ratio of human [HbCO]f to [HbCO]m is 1.1; i.e., [HbCO]f exceeds [HbCO]m by 10%–15%. Of course for other mammals the steady-state ratios of [HbCO]f to [HbCO]m will vary because of the different affinities of fetal and maternal blood for O_2 and CO (190).

The CO-induced leftward shift of the HbO_2 curve requires that the blood P_{O_2} must decrease to lower-than-normal values before a given amount of O_2 will dissociate. Figure 24 shows the basis for understanding the consequences of CO-O_2 interactions in maternal and fetal blood (136, 191). An elevated [HbCO]m (in this instance 9.4%) decreases maternal O_2Cap and shifts the curve to the left. Although Pmv_{O_2} remains essentially unchanged, the maternal arterial $[O_2]$ decreases ~1.6 ml·dl^{-1}, whereas Pmv_{O_2} decreases ~7 Torr [Fig. 24; (191)].

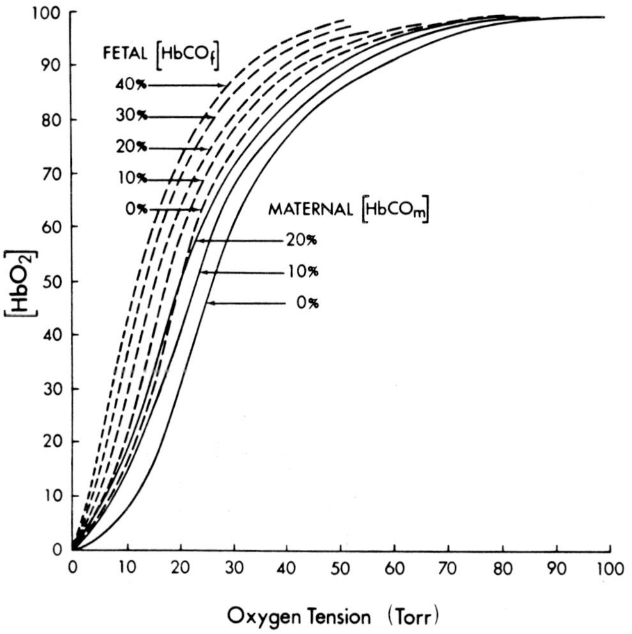

FIG. 23. Human maternal and fetal HbO_2 saturation curves showing CO effects. The HbO_2 saturation ($[HbO_2]$) is that percentage of Hb not bound as HbCO.

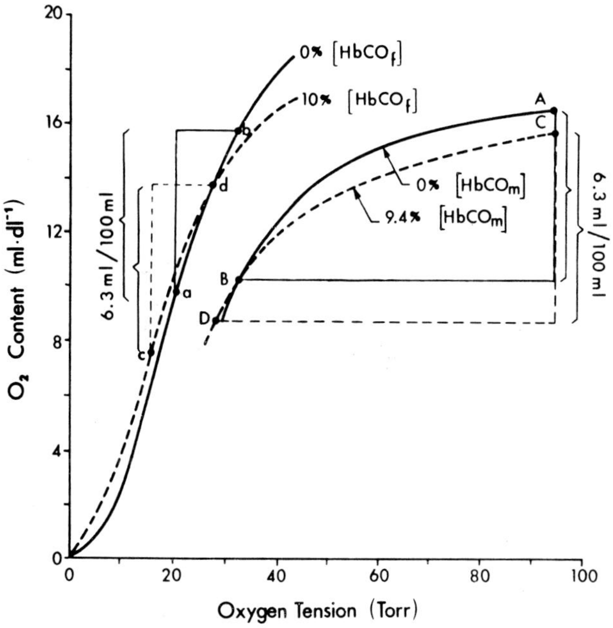

FIG. 24. Calculated O_2 content vs. P_{O_2} of human blood with [HbCO]f = 0% and 10% and [HbCO]m = 0% and 9.4%. [Hb]m and [Hb]f are assumed to be 12 and 16.5 g·dl^{-1}, respectively. Normal arteriovenous O_2 difference of 5 ml·dl^{-1} is assumed for both the uterus and its contents and the fetus. Figure depicts mechanism accounting for reduction of umbilical artery and vein O_2 tensions and contents resulting from elevated [HbCO].

Under normal circumstances, Pfv_{O_2} is ~28 Torr and $[O_2]$ is ~12 ml·dl^{-1}, whereas Pfa_{O_2} is 20 Torr. With elevated [HbCO]f (in this instance 10%), both Pfv_{O_2} and Pfa_{O_2} decrease. (This contrasts with the case in the adult, in whom Pa_{O_2} remains normal, because fetal blood equilibrates with lowered P_{O_2} values in maternal placental capillaries.) With a normal $\dot{V}f_{O_2}$, Pfv_{O_2} would decrease to 15 Torr and mixed venous (inferior vena caval) P_{O_2} would decrease from a normal value of ~16 Torr to 11 Torr (191).

Using chronically catheterized near-term fetal sheep, Longo (191) examined the effects of elevated [HbCO] on maternal and fetal O_2 levels. The regression equations for the relations of maternal and fetal P_{O_2} values were Pmv_{O_2} (Torr) = 43 − 0.5[HbCO]m (r = −0.96) and Pfa_{O_2} = 21.1 − 0.4[HbCO]f (r = −0.94) (191).

Clinically, although greatly elevated [HbCO] sufficient to affect maternal and fetal blood O_2 affinity and capacity occurs with acute CO poisoning during pregnancy, even much lower concentrations, such as those associated with maternal smoking or excessive air pollution, can result in significant effects on fetal O_2 levels (192).

PLACENTAL CO_2 EXCHANGE

Carbon dioxide must be eliminated from the fetus by diffusing across the placenta into maternal blood. Despite a number of studies on placental CO_2 exchange ($\dot{V}_{CO_2}$), most observations have consisted of rather descriptive accounts of CO_2 levels in maternal and fetal blood under a variety of circumstances. Several vital problems relating to this process remain unresolved.

Forms of CO_2

As noted in the chapter by Klocke in this *Handbook*, CO_2 is present in blood in several forms, including dissolved gas, bicarbonate ion, carbonate ion, carbonic acid, and carbaminohemoglobin. The concentrations of carbonic acid and carbonate ion are negligible and are ignored in this discussion. The major reactions of CO_2 in maternal and placental blood are similar to those elsewhere.

Table 1 gives the concentrations of various forms of CO_2 and the pH in maternal and fetal arterial and venous placental blood. Table 5 summarizes the P_{CO_2} values reported for several species. Surprisingly, although the uterine-to-umbilical $P_{V_{O_2}}$ difference varies greatly among species, the corresponding P_{CO_2} difference is 4 or 5 Torr in all species listed except humans, in which it is only 1–2 Torr. In addition, why placentas such as those of the guinea pig and rabbit, which show efficient exchange for O_2, do not demonstrate similarly efficient CO_2 exchange is puzzling. It has been suggested that the CO_2 difference results from relatively low carbonic anhydrase concentrations in fetal blood (26); however, the reduced enzyme levels could explain only a small fraction of this difference (see *Umbilical-to-Uterine Venous CO_2 Tension Differences*, p. 380).

TABLE 5. *Summary of Maternal and Fetal CO_2 Tensions in Various Species*

Species	Maternal Artery	Uterine Vein	Umbilical Vein	Umbilical Artery	Umbilical Vein − Uterine Vein	Ref.
Sheep	34	38	42	46	4	70
	36	40	43	48	3*	70
		38	43		5*	233
	27	36	40	46	4*	19
	34	40	45	55	5*	161
	34	38	40	47	2*	10
Goat	36	39	46	49	7*	161
		43	50		7*	22
	29	33	40	42	7	45
Cow	33	37	41	48	4	111
	36	40	44	49	4	72
	35	38	39	46	1	71
	38	42	43	50	1	72
Pig	36	41	45	52	4*	72
Rabbit		43	48		5*	22
Guinea pig		57	60		3*	22
Human	26	29†	33	39	4†‡	57
		37†	40	49	3†‡	300
		37†	42	46	5*†	284
	30	33	42		9	319
	36	46	49	60	3*	350

Values are expressed in Torr. * Anesthetized subjects. † Sample from intervillous space rather than uterine vein. ‡ Samples from newborn. [Adapted from Hill and Longo (137).]

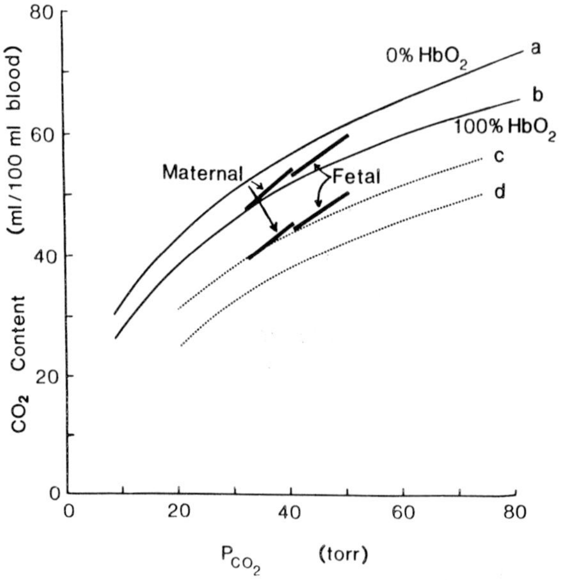

FIG. 25. Dissociation curves for CO_2 in human maternal and fetal blood showing effects of O_2 saturation and base deficit. *a*, Adult deoxygenated blood; *b*, adult oxygenated blood; *c*, pregnant women and fetuses; *d*, fetal blood. *Heavy lines*, positions expected for maternal and fetal blood based on degree of oxygenation. [Adapted from Eastman et al. (95).]

Carbon Dioxide Dissociation Curves

Figure 25 shows CO_2 dissociation curves for human adult deoxygenated and oxygenated blood and indicates the positions one would expect for maternal and fetal blood on the basis of their degree of oxygenation [heavy lines; (137)]. On that basis, the total fetal end-capillary CO_2 would be less than that of maternal end capillaries because the left-shifted fetal dissociation curve produces a higher fetal than maternal [HbO_2] at the same P_{O_2}. However, this effect is probably minor compared with other factors that affect the CO_2 dissociation curves. First, the pregnant woman hyperventilates, producing a respiratory alkalosis that when compensated leads to a base deficit and reduces the total CO_2 (Fig. 25, curve c). One may also consider the effect of a lowered [Hb] in the pregnant woman relative to the normal adult, which allows less carbaminohemoglobin, thereby decreasing the CO_2 content slightly. In contrast, because total [HCO_3^-] is inversely related to hematocrit, it should be elevated by the hematocrit effect. Of all these effects, the most important is almost certainly that due to the base deficit produced by hyperventilation.

The fetal CO_2 curve is also shifted relative to the adult curve. Fetal blood is acidotic, with a base deficit of 1–6 meq·liter^{-1} (56, 300, 319). Eastman et al. (95) reported a fetal CO_2 dissociation curve considerably below that of pregnant women (Fig. 25, curve d), but that blood (with base deficit of 6 meq·liter^{-1}) was obtained from the umbilical cord after delivery when there may have been considerable hypoxia. More recent data indicate an average fetal base deficit of ~4 meq·liter^{-1}, which would place the fetal dissociation curve close to that of the mother (Fig. 25, curve c). Again, one might consider the effects of the high hematocrit of fetal blood in producing more carbaminohemoglobin but less HCO_3^- than blood with a lower hematocrit. The net result of all these considerations is that the maternal and fetal curves are probably nearly superimposed (Fig. 25, curve c). Total CO_2 and [HCO_3^-] are higher due to the higher average P_{CO_2} values in the fetus but are not significantly different on the basis of acid-base status.

Transplacental CO_2 Exchange

Because P_{CO_2} in the fetus is greater than that in the mother, on entering the exchange vessels CO_2 begins to diffuse across the placental membranes from fetal to maternal plasma. This disturbs the equilibriums throughout the system, CO_2 diffuses from fetal erythrocytes into the plasma, additional CO_2 is formed from HCO_3^-, etc. Because CO_2 is highly lipid soluble it is believed to diffuse rapidly through placental membranes. However, it is not known to what extent HCO_3^- contributes to $\dot{V}_{CO_2}$. In unanesthetized sheep and goats, Blechner et al. (46) reported that, although the fetal [HCO_3^-] bore little relation to that of the mother, Pfa_{CO_2} was 17–19 Torr higher than Pma_{CO_2}, irrespective of the maternal CO_2 or [HCO_3^-]. Even after NH_4Cl infusion into the ewe's circulation, with lowering of [HCO_3^-] to 9 meq·liter^{-1}, Pf_{CO_2} values followed those of the mother (46).

To establish whether CO_2 or [HCO_3^-] is the major species diffusing across the placenta, Longo et al. (196) studied $\dot{V}_{CO_2}$ in fetal sheep in response to either inhibition of carbonic anhydrase or marked lowering of [HCO_3^-]. After fetal acetazolamide administration, Pfa_{CO_2} values rose ~22 ± 2 Torr to 75 ± 3 Torr. Neither fetal [HCO_3^-] nor maternal carbonic anhydrase activity changed significantly. Thus primarily physically dissolved CO_2 exchanged because CO_2 diffusing out of the fetal placental capillaries could not be replenished from [HCO_3^-] (196).

Perhaps more convincing evidence that molecular CO_2 is the major species that exchanges was obtained by these workers during tromethamine infusion into the fetus (196). Under these circumstances Pfa_{CO_2} fell 16 ± 3 Torr to 35 ± 6 Torr. In several instances this reversed the normal fetal-to-maternal P_{CO_2} gradient as well as the umbilical artery–to–umbilical vein CO_2 difference. Under these circumstances CO_2 could diffuse from maternal to fetal blood against an [HCO_3^-] gradient.

In an effort to gain a more complete understanding of fetal-to-maternal CO_2 exchanges, Hill et al. (139) developed a mathematical model to calculate the time course of CO_2 and O_2 changes along the exchange vessels, overall transfer rates, end-capillary values, and the importance of interactions of CO_2 with O_2 and [H^+]. Their theoretical results predicted that the overall rate of CO_2 exchange is not much faster than that of O_2. This finding was somewhat unexpected because the almost 20-fold greater solubility of CO_2 in lipid membranes as compared with O_2 suggested a more rapid CO_2 equilibration. Nonetheless, the overall exchange rate of CO_2 depends on the series of chemical reactions, including those for O_2. Thus CO_2 and O_2 exchange are linked so that during a capillary transit 90% of the CO_2 and O_2 exchanges occur within 0.95 and 1.0 s, respectively (139).

Haldane and Bohr Effects

Hill et al. (139) also simulated the importance of CO_2 and O_2 interactions in placental gas exchange. The CO_2 and O_2 total exchange rates were calculated in both the presence and absence of simultaneous transfer of the other gas. To estimate the importance of the Bohr effect, $\dot{V}_{O_2}$ was calculated allowing for no P_{CO_2} or pH change. Only 2 ml·min^{-1} additional O_2 was transferred in the presence of CO_2 exchange, indicating that the Bohr effect accounts for only ~8% of total O_2 exchange. Equilibration occurred at the same P_{O_2} regardless of the Bohr effect because of the shifts of the dissociation curves (139).

In a similar manner these workers calculated the enhancement of CO_2 transfer by the oxygenation of fetal Hb and deoxygenation of maternal Hb, i.e., the Haldane effect (139). When O_2 transfer was disallowed, $\dot{V}_{CO_2}$ was only 11 ml·min^{-1}. Comparison of this value with the normal value of 20.4 ml·min^{-1} in the presence of simultaneous O_2 exchange indicated that the Haldane effect accounts for ~46% of total $\dot{V}_{CO_2}$. The contribution of the various forms of CO_2 to the Haldane effect was also calculated: increased HCO_3^- transport and the carbamino changes accounted for ~60% and 40%, respectively (139).

Importance of Various Factors on CO_2 Exchange

Because CO_2 is even more diffusible than O_2, one would expect CO_2 exchange to also be limited by blood flow rather than diffusion. As with O_2, CO_2 exchange depends on several factors (umbilical and uterine Pa_{CO_2}, umbilical and uteroplacental blood flow rates, buffering capacity, and O_2 exchange), which Hill et al.

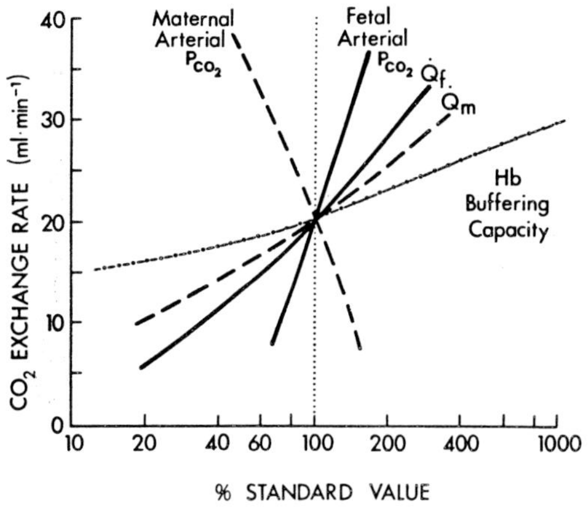

FIG. 26. Effect of changes in various factors on transient placental CO_2 transfer rate. To facilitate comparison, values are plotted as percent changes from assumed normal values. Slope of each curve at 100% may be used as index of relative sensitivity of CO_2 transfer to that factor. [Adapted from Hill et al. (139).]

(139) analyzed in an attempt to determine those most likely to be important in limiting CO_2 exchange.

To compare the importance of the various factors on $\dot{V}_{CO_2}$ and to eliminate differences in units, Figure 26 shows the values plotted as percentages of their assumed normal values. Placental CO_2 exchange is most sensitive to changes in Pfa_{CO_2} and is somewhat less sensitive to Pma_{CO_2}, $\dot{Q}m$, $\dot{Q}f$, and the amount of O_2 exchanged. Changes in Hb buffering capacity and Dp_{CO} demonstrate minor effects in the physiological range (139).

Umbilical-to-Uterine Venous CO_2 Tension Differences

Many investigators have interpreted the uterine-to-umbilical Pv_{O_2} and Pv_{CO_2} differences to result from diffusion limitation (180, 237), and the extent of end-capillary equilibration has remained controversial. Although H_2 and SF_6 equilibrate to the same extent (197), equilibration depends on the ratio of Dp to effective solubility of the gas in the blood rather than on Dp alone (335). Thus, because of the large capacity of blood for O_2 and CO_2, it is possible that these gases may be diffusion limited, even though SF_6 is not.

Relying on measurements of Dp_{CO}, Hill et al. (139) predicted CO_2 equilibration rates during a placental capillary transit (Fig. 27). These calculations suggest that P_{CO_2} rapidly equilibrates between maternal and fetal capillary blood, but that slow chemical reactions continue after blood leaves the exchange area because plasma does not contain carbonic anhydrase. The reactions that continue in the veins produce the P_{CO_2} shifts in a manner similar to the slow chemical reactions postulated in the pulmonary system [Fig. 27, *right*; (105, 140)]. Although the physiological importance of these slow chemical reactions is still in dispute, this effect can produce at most a 1-Torr umbilical-to-uterine Pv_{CO_2} difference. These calculations were initially made by assuming that fetal erythrocytes had sufficient carbonic anhydrase activity to catalyze the CO_2 hydration rate by a factor of 6,500 (compared with a factor of 13,000 in adult red cells). However, even if the fetal catalysis factor is as low as 800 (36, 144), the calculations indicate a postcapillary P_{CO_2} change of only ~1 Torr. This agrees with studies in the lung, which indicate that at rest catalysis can be reduced substantially without interfering with gas exchange (321).

Some of the vein-to-vein difference may be accounted for by placental vascular shunts, which have been estimated to range from nearly 0% in rabbits and guinea pigs (243) to ~20% in sheep and goats (236, 292). A 20% shunt in both circulations of the sheep placenta can explain a uterine-to-umbilical Pv_{O_2} difference of 15 Torr. This degree of shunting would also produce an umbilical-to-uterine Pv_{CO_2} difference of 3 Torr, which approximates that difference experimentally observed.

It is also likely that measurements previously interpreted as indicating large shunts were actually the result of nonuniform distribution of maternal and fetal blood flows (see *Distribution of Maternal and Fetal Placental Flows*, p. 385). Power et al., using radioactive-labeled macroaggregates of albumin (279) and microspheres (273), measured the distributions of maternal and fetal blood flows in sheep placentas. Calculations based on those results indicate that the degree of mismatching of blood flows can explain a maternal-to-fetal Pv_{O_2} difference of 12 Torr and a fetal-to-maternal Pv_{CO_2} difference of 5 Torr, thus accounting for most of the differences observed experimentally (201).

Another possible explanation of the vein-to-vein P_{O_2} and P_{CO_2} differences is placental tissue metabolism. Hill et al. (139) examined this effect for CO_2 production as well as for O_2 consumption. However, regardless of whether one assumes that the CO_2 is

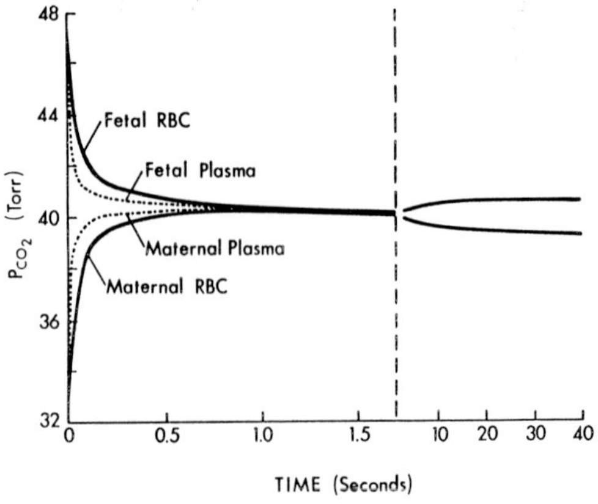

FIG. 27. Time course of P_{CO_2} during single transit through exchange vessels. *Solid lines*, P_{CO_2} values within erythrocytes; *broken lines*, P_{CO_2} values in plasma. Changes occurring after blood leaves exchange area are plotted on *right* with scale compressed 40 times. [Adapted from Hill et al. (139).]

added to the fetal capillary blood or to maternal capillary blood (or some to both), P_{CO_2} equilibration occurs at a higher P_{CO_2} but is still complete by the end of the capillary transit, and postcapillary chemical reactions can account for at most a 1-Torr P_{CO_2} difference. A larger vein-to-vein CO_2 difference would occur if the CO_2 from placental metabolism were added to the venous blood after it left the exchange area.

Interrelations of Placental CO_2 and H_2O Exchange

Wilbur et al. (342) investigated the possibility that CO_2 and HCO_3^- differences between fetal and maternal blood might influence transplacental water balance. Using a mathematical model, they calculated changes in O_2 and CO_2 along the capillary transit, as well as the movement of water in response to osmotic-pressure differences produced by the concentrations of the several ions and metabolites. Initially the osmotic gradient tends to move water into the fetus, but later during the capillary transit this gradient reverses and water returns to the mother (342). This analysis suggests a possible mechanism for the regulation of both fetal O_2 delivery and weight gain. Fetal metabolism with CO_2 production increases fetal $[HCO_3^-]$, hence altering osmotic balance and transplacental water movement. The fetal water gain can thus increase fetal blood volume, venous return, cardiac output, peripheral flow, and O_2 delivery to return $[HCO_3^-]$ to normal (202).

Conclusions

Despite major species differences in placental architecture, morphology, and patterns of maternal and fetal blood flows, the fetal-to-maternal P_{CO_2} difference of 4–5 Torr is remarkably constant. Although maternal blood has a lower [Hb] and higher $[HCO_3^-]$ than that of the fetus, their CO_2 dissociation curves appear to be superimposed. Postexchange capillary P_{CO_2} changes, a matter of theoretical interest, probably account for no more than a 1-Torr difference between umbilical and uterine venous blood, whereas placental CO_2 production probably accounts for none of this difference. Most of the difference can be explained on the basis of uneven distributions of maternal and fetal blood flows, at least in sheep. Carbon dioxide apparently crosses the placenta as molecular CO_2 rather than HCO_3^-. In addition to its role as a buffer, CO_2 helps establish fetal homeostasis because the $[HCO_3^-]$ appears to play an important role in transplacental water movements, the maintenance of optimal fetal blood volume, cardiac output, and fetal O_2 delivery.

VARIATIONS IN RATE OF MATERNAL AND FETAL PLACENTAL HB AND O_2 FLOWS

General Considerations

Perhaps one of the most fundamental aspects of uterine blood flow is that it exists not only to supply nutrients to the uterus per se but to meet the metabolic demands of the growing conceptus so that at term $\dot{Q}m$ accounts for 20%–25% of maternal cardiac output. Perhaps even more remarkable, umbilical blood flow rapidly increases in magnitude and at term represents 40%–50% of fetal cardiac output. Early in gestation, when the ratio of placental to fetal weight is relatively great, the placenta may receive an even larger fraction of fetal cardiac output. These flows have profound physiological effects on the placental transfer of O_2, CO_2, and other substances the exchange of which is flow-limited.

A question of both physiological and clinical importance is the extent to which changes in maternal and fetal blood O_2Cap or placental flow rates affect $\dot{V}_{O_2}$. Blood flow and O_2Cap can be considered together because they exert a similar influence on $\dot{V}_{O_2}$. For instance, consider the Fick principle

$$\dot{V}_{O_2} = \dot{Q}(Cma_{O_2} - Cmv_{O_2}) \qquad (13)$$

where $\dot{V}_{O_2}$ is the amount of O_2 transported ($ml \cdot min^{-1}$), $\dot{Q}$ is the rate of flow ($ml \cdot min^{-1}$), and $Cma_{O_2} - Cmv_{O_2}$ is the maternal arteriovenous content difference (ml $O_2 \cdot$ ml blood^{-1}). In this equation both blood flow and O_2 content (or capacity, its dependent function) determine the amount of O_2 transported. Because the product of $\dot{Q}$ and $[O_2]$ defines the amount of O_2 transported, it is useful to consider them together as Hb or O_2 flow (200, 223).

Hemoglobin flow ($\dot{Q}_{Hb}$) (in $g \cdot min^{-1}$) is simply the product of blood flow rate and [Hb]

$$\dot{Q}_{Hb} = \dot{Q} \cdot [Hb] \qquad (14)$$

Alternatively, one may consider the rate at which O_2 flows in the exchange vessels. Oxygen flow ($\dot{Q}_{O_2}$) is the product of blood flow and Ca_{O_2} (in $ml \cdot ml^{-1}$)

$$\dot{Q}_{O_2} = \dot{Q} \cdot Ca_{O_2} \qquad (15)$$

This can also be expressed

$$\dot{Q}_{O_2} = [HbO_2][Hb](1.368 \times 10^{-2}) \qquad (16)$$

where 1.368 is the milliliters of O_2 that can combine with each gram of Hb.

In a consideration of the transfer of inert substances, Bartels and Moll (25) developed the concept of blood "transport capacity," the product of solubility ($ml \cdot ml^{-1}$) and placental flow ($ml \cdot min^{-1}$). In the linear portion of the HbO_2 saturation curve, O_2 can be regarded as a gas with a high solubility, and the terms *transport capacity* and *O_2 flow* are nearly equivalent.

Although the equivalency of O_2Cap and $\dot{Q}$ is a convenient approximation, it is only that for several reasons. First, changes in [Hb] affect the blood buffer capacity, which in turn influences $\dot{V}_{O_2}$ by the Bohr effect. In addition, [Hb] affects Dp slightly (205). Finally, alterations in [Hb] probably affect the distribution of flow within the placental vessels because of viscosity effects. However, these effects are probably minor and should not detract from the conceptual usefulness of $\dot{Q}_{Hb}$ or $\dot{Q}_{O_2}$.

Little information is available on the explicit relations of $\dot{Q}m$ and $\dot{V}_{O_2}$. Numerous studies in many species with a wide variety of techniques have examined the rate of blood flow per se (particularly near term), its changes during gestation, the relation of flow to blood pressure, and the effects of a myriad of chemical compounds of physiological and pharmacological interest. Early studies in anesthetized, acutely operated, or even exteriorized preparations were hampered by alterations in the measurement one was attempting to make. During recent times the use of relatively noninvasive techniques in chronically catheterized awake animals has minimized this problem (233, 235).

In 1933, Barcroft (12), using a venous outflow technique in sheep, first measured an increase in $\dot{Q}m$ and $\dot{V}_{O_2}$ in proportion to fetal size. More recent studies in sheep indicate that $\dot{Q}m$ increases from ~30 $ml \cdot min^{-1}$ at 40-days gestation to 1,500 $ml \cdot min^{-1}$ at term (304). Calculated per kilogram fetal weight, flow decreased during this period from 9,000 to 250 $ml \cdot min^{-1} \cdot kg^{-1}$ (148, 241). During this same time, flow per gram of maternal placental cotyledons increased from 0.4 $ml \cdot min^{-1} \cdot g^{-1}$ at 90 days to 3 $ml \cdot min^{-1} \cdot g^{-1}$ at term. Power et al. (279) first determined that ~90% of maternal placental flow perfuses the placenta in sheep, whereas the balance supplies the endometrium and myometrium. Similar findings have been reported by others (92, 224).

In humans and other species with hemochorial placentas, the fetal placental circulation has been somewhat easier to describe than that of the mother because it courses through a well-defined vascular network. Although the maternal and fetal placental circulations are conveniently studied separately, functionally they should be considered together. Not only do they perform in concert in affecting substrate exchange, but interactions of hydrostatic pressures in the two vascular beds probably affect their flow per se.

Much has been written about the geometric relations of the placental exchange vessels, but one must concur with the observation of Fracastoro (106) on the motion of the heart that "it is understood by God alone." Of the possible arrangements for exchange, a countercurrent pattern is most effective. In the human placenta, maternal blood composition probably changes little as it passes a single villus. Because the blood around any one villus is therefore of nearly the same composition on all sides, it should make little difference which way the blood flows in fetal capillaries in reference to the direction of maternal flow. Individual villi, however, may be bathed by maternal blood that is of arterial, venous, or intermediate composition according to their location near an arterial or venous opening or at some point in between. Such a flow pattern functionally acts as a poorly efficient concurrent exchanger (200, 240) and results in the fetal end-capillary P_{O_2} reaching a value less than that of the uterine veins. Despite many studies of $\dot{Q}m$, essentially no experimental data exist on the size or geometry of the flow pathways in the human or primate hemochorial placenta.

Because of its relative inaccessibility, $\dot{Q}f$ has been even more difficult to measure under physiological conditions than has maternal placental flow. Studies in chronically catheterized unanesthetized sheep indicate that $\dot{Q}f$ is ~250 $ml \cdot min^{-1} \cdot kg^{-1}$ (67, 76, 100, 193, 208, 307). Only a few studies have explored in any rigorous manner the relation of these flows to O_2 or CO_2 exchange.

Theoretical Considerations

Figure 28 depicts the predicted effects of changes in $\dot{Q}m$ or [Hb]m on $\dot{V}_{O_2}$ and end-capillary P_{O_2} values under both transient and steady-state conditions. In addition, it shows how these variables should be af-

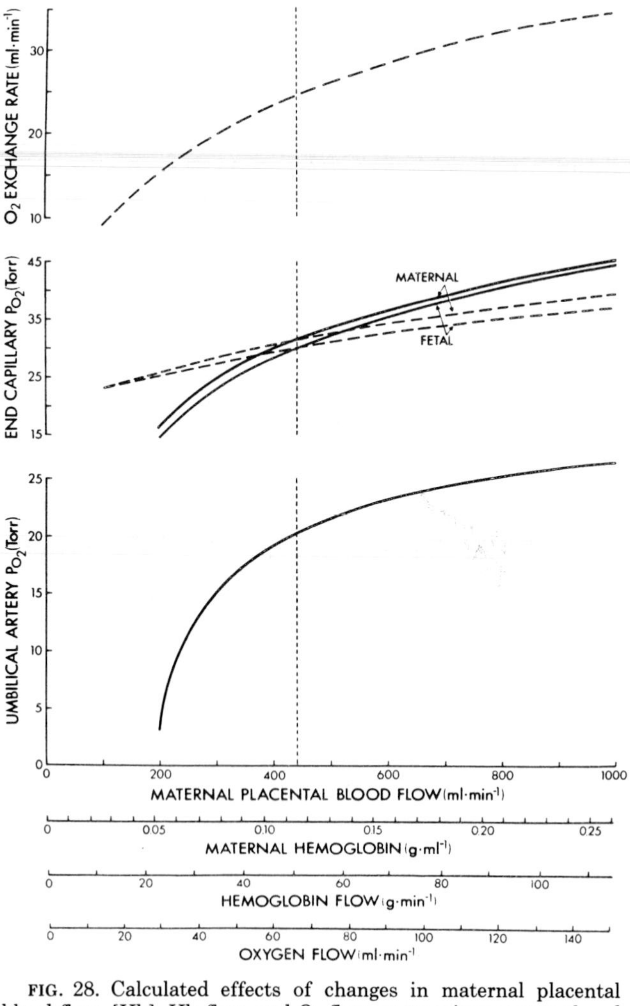

FIG. 28. Calculated effects of changes in maternal placental blood flow, [Hb], Hb flow, and O_2 flow on transient maternal and fetal placental end-capillary P_{O_2} values and $\dot{V}_{O_2}$ (*dashed lines*) and on steady-state end-capillary P_{O_2} values and Pfa_{O_2} (*solid lines*).

fected by altered $\dot{Q}_{Hb}$ or $\dot{Q}_{O_2}$. At high flow rates or [Hb], end-capillary P_{O_2} values approach that of the maternal artery. At lower flow rates the equilibrated P_{O_2} decreases because less O_2 is available for exchange. The transient $\dot{V}_{O_2}$ should follow a trend similar to that of end-capillary P_{O_2} values. When $\dot{Q}$m exceeds ~600 $ml \cdot min^{-1}$, $\dot{V}_{O_2}$ should rise in direct proportion to $\dot{Q}_{Hb}$ or $\dot{Q}_{O_2}$ (120, 200).

With reduced $\dot{Q}_{Hb}$ in steady-state conditions, Pfa_{O_2} falls to low levels (Fig. 28); at flow rates below 200 $ml \cdot min^{-1}$, changes in Pfa_{O_2} alone can no longer maintain normal $\dot{V}_{O_2}$. As noted above, uncompensated decreases in [Hb]m resulted in transient decreases in both $\dot{V}_{O_2}$ and placental end-capillary P_{O_2} (Fig. 28). For example, if [Hb]m were to fall to 0.07 $g \cdot ml^{-1}$ (from normal value of 0.115 $g \cdot ml^{-1}$), $\dot{V}_{O_2}$ would momentarily decrease 27% (from 24 to 17.5 $ml \cdot min^{-1}$) and end-capillary P_{O_2} would fall 17% (from 31.8 to 26.5 Torr). At a constant $\dot{V}f_{O_2}$ this would soon result in a lowered Pfa_{O_2}, an increased maternal-to-fetal $\overline{P}_{O_2}$ difference, and a return to normal of steady-state $\dot{V}_{O_2}$. A fall in Pfa_{O_2} from 20 to 2 Torr would be required to maintain normal O_2 transfer with this degree of anemia.

The lower axes in Figure 28 show the comparable changes in $\dot{Q}_{Hb}$ and $\dot{Q}_{O_2}$ that would result in the changes just described. In summary, it can be seen that both the rate of transplacental O_2 exchange and end-capillary P_{O_2} under either transient or steady-state conditions are proportional to the rates of $\dot{Q}$m, [Hb]m, $\dot{Q}_{Hb}$, and $\dot{Q}_{O_2}$.

The effects of changes in $\dot{Q}$f or [Hb]f on $\dot{V}_{O_2}$ and end-capillary P_{O_2} are shown in Figure 29. This figure also shows how $\dot{V}_{O_2}$ and end-capillary P_{O_2} are affected by changes in $\dot{Q}_{Hb}$ or $\dot{Q}_{O_2}$. As for maternal $\dot{Q}_{Hb}$ or $\dot{Q}_{O_2}$, increases in $\dot{Q}$f allow additional O_2 transport. The transient $\dot{V}_{O_2}$ varies linearly with $\dot{Q}$f over the range from ~200 to 600 $ml \cdot min^{-1}$. Above 600 $ml \cdot min^{-1}$, $\dot{V}_{O_2}$ no longer rises so steeply because additional O_2 is not available from maternal blood.

In contrast to the situation with $\dot{Q}$m, increases in $\dot{Q}$f result in decreased end-capillary P_{O_2}, approaching that of Pfa_{O_2} during a single capillary transit. A maternal-to-fetal end-capillary P_{O_2} difference would become apparent at high $\dot{Q}_{Hb}$ values because of a diffusional limitation (i.e., lower ratio of Dp to $\dot{Q}$) [Fig. 29; (275)]. End-capillary Pf_{O_2} varies inversely with [Hb]f because a higher [Hb]f can combine with more O_2 from the maternal blood. Thus in fetal anemia, end-capillary P_{O_2} increases and $\dot{V}_{O_2}$ decreases. For example, with [Hb]f = 6 $g \cdot dl^{-1}$, end-capillary P_{O_2} increases to 44 Torr and instantaneous $\dot{V}_{O_2}$ decreases to 15 $ml \cdot min^{-1}$, resulting in a 37% decrease in [O_2] of fetal placental end-capillary blood.

During steady-state conditions, decreases in flow are accompanied by a fall in Pfa_{O_2} to maintain normal $\dot{V}_{O_2}$ and end-capillary P_{O_2} (Fig. 29). However, if $\dot{Q}$f decreases below ~200 $ml \cdot min^{-1}$, additional compensations become necessary to maintain normal $\dot{V}_{O_2}$.

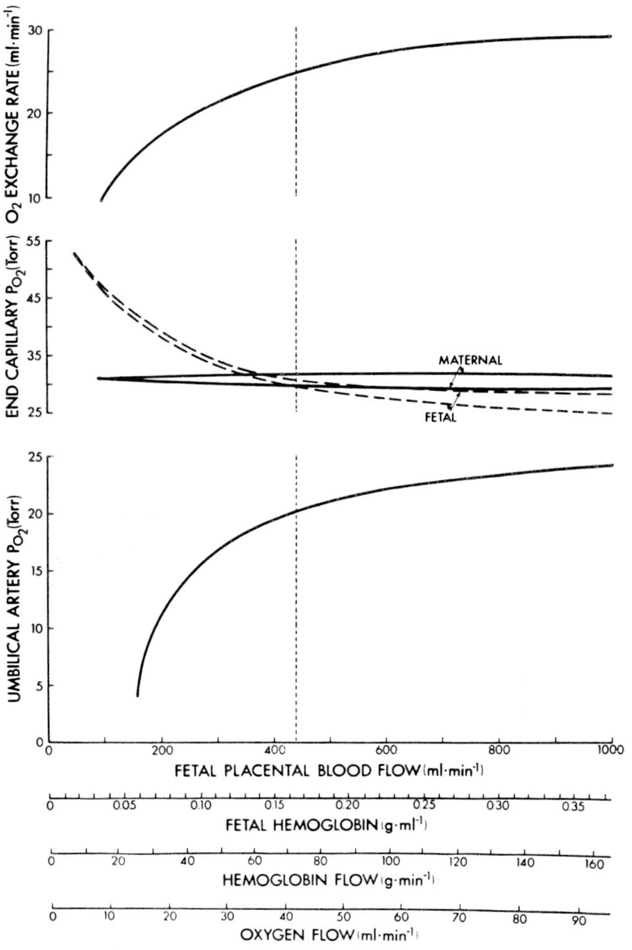

FIG. 29. Calculated effects of changes in fetal placental blood flow, [Hb], Hb flow, and O_2 flow on transient maternal and fetal placental end-capillary P_{O_2} values and $\dot{V}_{O_2}$ (*dashed lines*) and on steady-state end-capillary P_{O_2} values and Pfa_{O_2} (*solid lines*).

Experimental Studies

The above theoretical considerations suggest that $\dot{V}_{O_2}$ should be particularly sensitive to changes in $\dot{Q}m_{Hb}$ or $\dot{Q}f_{Hb}$. Barcroft and Barron (14) recorded that

> if the maternal circulation slows while that in the foetal circulation remains normal, the saturation of oxygen in the umbilical vessels artery and vein will fall. . . . If on the other hand, the circulation is slowed down in the foetus . . . the effect will be to raise the oxygen saturation in the umbilical vein.

Despite this early observation, few studies have explicitly explored these relations. Perhaps this is so because, when a function such as blood flow is altered, other variables may change to mask the consequences of the permutation under study, with the result that the investigator misjudges the role of that factor in affecting $\dot{V}_{O_2}$.

In an effort to circumvent these problems several investigators have studied placental exchange in isolated preparations at accurately controlled flow rates. In the perfused isolated maternal vessels of the sheep uterus in vivo, Fuller et al. (110) determined that near-term $\dot{V}_{O_2}$ averaged 8.1 ± 0.6 ml·min^{-1}·kg uterine contents^{-1}, whereas in midgestation this value averaged 6.3 ± 0.3 ml·min^{-1}·kg^{-1}. In the near-term group, $\dot{V}_{O_2}$ increased parri passu with $\dot{Q}$m, suggesting that O_2 transfer is limited by blood flow rather than by diffusion. In contrast, during midgestation this relation was not apparent at $\dot{Q}$m > 200–250 ml·min^{-1}·kg^{-1}, although the relatively small size of the conceptus and its maximal $\dot{V}f_{O_2}$ in relation to $\dot{Q}$m may have made such a determination difficult. Others have noted the critical dependence of O_2 uptake (177, 344) and placental ethanol clearance (343) on $\dot{Q}$m. In contrast, Clapp (66) reported that the rate of O_2 uptake by the uterus, placenta, and fetus remained relatively constant at $\dot{Q}$m = 100–400 ml·min^{-1}·kg^{-1}, with compensatory changes in the maternal arteriovenous C_{O_2} difference. These latter results have been confirmed by Longo et al. (195) in near-term ewes in which $\dot{V}_{O_2}$ was measured continuously and agree with the theoretical predictions described for steady-state conditions.

To explore the effects of variations of $\dot{Q}$f on $\dot{V}_{O_2}$, Dawes and Mott (81) varied flow in exteriorized immature (79- to 86-day) fetal lambs by constriction of the umbilical vein or aorta or by phlebotomy. Fetal $\dot{V}_{O_2}$ varied as a function of $\dot{Q}$f from 40 to 200 ml·min^{-1}·kg^{-1} but was relatively constant above that highest value. The change in $\dot{V}f_{O_2}$ was greater when flow was altered by hemorrhage than when it was reduced by vessel constriction, perhaps because vessel manipulation resulted in release of catecholamines with increased $\dot{V}f_{O_2}$ (208), tending to offset the expected decrease. Other workers have shown a decrease in $\dot{V}_{O_2}$ as a function of $\dot{Q}$f in both anesthetized and exteriorized (176) and chronically catheterized (157) fetal sheep. In contrast, as with $\dot{Q}$m, Clapp (66) reported that, as $\dot{Q}$f varied from 100 to 400 ml·min^{-1}·kg^{-1}, $\dot{V}_{O_2}$ remained constant with changes in the fetal arteriovenous C_{O_2} difference.

In an effort to examine $\dot{Q}$f effects on $\dot{V}_{O_2}$ while minimizing compensatory changes, Power and Jenkins (276) perfused isolated placental cotyledons in sheep and rabbits. As predicted (Fig. 30), $\dot{V}_{O_2}$ [normalized as (measured O_2 exchange)/(O_2 exchange at standard flow)] rose as $\dot{Q}$f increased, whereas outflowing P_{O_2} tended to increase at low $\dot{Q}$f values. In fact, ignoring $\dot{V}p_{O_2}$, theoretically the P_{O_2} value of fetal outflowing blood should approach that of Pma_{O_2} at low $\dot{Q}$f values. At high rates of $\dot{Q}$f, blood remains in the exchange vessels for a relatively short time, and diffusional limitation to O_2 exchange, if present, should become apparent above a certain critical flow rate by an abrupt decrease in effluent Pf_{O_2} (200). These data give no hint of such a change, supporting the concept that $\dot{V}_{O_2}$ is flow limited.

An additional consideration is the [Hb] in placental exchange vessels, which need not necessarily be the same as that in larger vessels. For instance, Newcomb and Power (255) demonstrated that the hematocrit in the fetal rabbit placental vessels was ~25% as compared with the large-vessel hematocrit of 37%, giving a ratio of placental to large-vessel hematocrit of 0.76. This plasma "skimming" has implications for $\dot{V}_{O_2}$. During a steady state, the volume of erythrocytes and plasma that flows into the placenta must equal the volume that leaves it. Because the hematocrit of blood in placental vessels is apparently less than that in larger vessels, erythrocytes in these vessels have a shorter mean transit time than the plasma, which implies a truncated period for O_2 exchange. For example, the mean transit time in sheep placental capillaries is ~1.7 s (206). Although maternal and fetal P_{O_2} values can equilibrate during a capillary transit of this duration, if the transit times of erythrocytes and plasma were 1.26 and 1.84 s, respectively [values that would agree with results of Newcomb and Power (255)], P_{O_2} values might not equilibrate. In other words, the placental diffusion reserves may not be as great as previously considered, and a small maternal-to-fetal P_{O_2} difference could result from diffusional limitation.

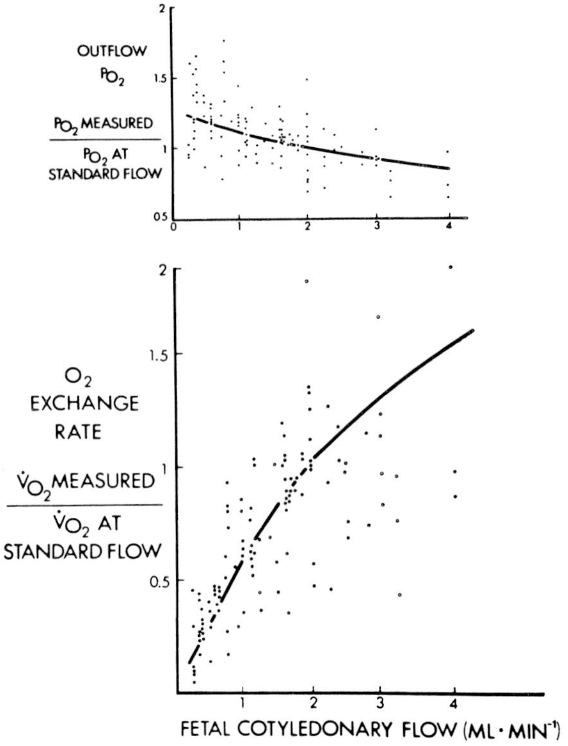

FIG. 30. Relations between venous outflow P_{O_2}, placental O_2 transfer, and fetal cotyledonary flow in perfused isolated sheep and rabbit placentas. *Solid lines*, predicted relations using mathematical model. [Adapted from Power and Jenkins (276).]

Clinical Implications of Altered Placental Flows

Maternal placental blood flow in humans is noto-

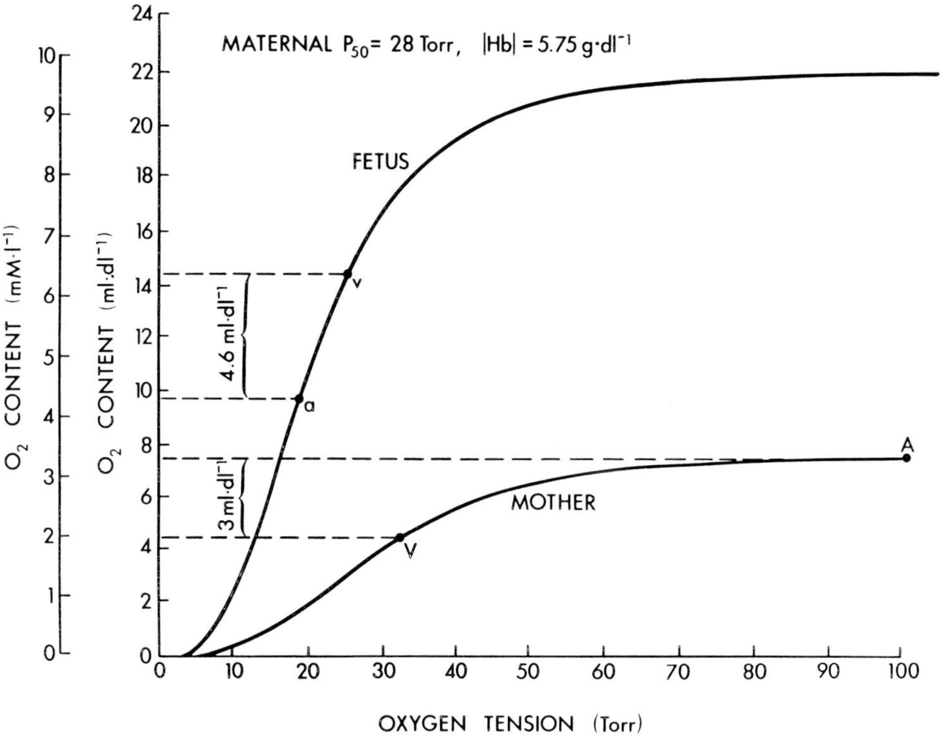

FIG. 31. Calculated blood O_2 content as function of P_{O_2} in presence of maternal anemia ($[Hb]m = 5.75\ g \cdot dl^{-1}$) with associated slight increase in O_2 affinity ($Pm_{50} = 28$ Torr). A and V, maternal arterial and venous values; a and v, umbilical arterial and venous values.

riously difficult to measure, and none of the various techniques that have been employed is satisfactory. Studies with the radioactive inert gases Kr or Xe may prove useful, but the validity of this approach has yet to be established. Most of our knowledge of the changes in $\dot{Q}m$ under various circumstances derives from the experimental animal studies detailed above. Maternal blood O_2Cap can vary from polycythemia to profound anemia under a wide variety of circumstances; changes are associated with alterations of O_2 affinity because intraerythrocyte [2,3-DPG] varies inversely with [Hb] (141, 168, 169, 327, 332).

Figure 31 illustrates some consequences of reduced $\dot{Q}m_{Hb}$ on $\dot{V}_{O_2}$. If $[Hb]m = 5.75\ g \cdot dl^{-1}$ [i.e., 50% anemia with associated slight increase in blood O_2 affinity ($P_{50} = 29$ Torr)], the inevitable result is fetal hypoxemia unless maternal cardiac output increases and $\dot{Q}m$ doubles to maintain $\dot{V}_{O_2}$. Under these circumstances (other variables remaining constant), the maternal arteriovenous C_{O_2} difference would be $\sim 2.5\ ml \cdot dl^{-1}$, and the maternal-to-fetal $\overline{P}_{O_2}$ difference and end-capillary P_{O_2} values should remain normal.

Fetal blood O_2Cap is decreased in association with hemolytic disease and increased in residents at high altitude (285) and in association with intrauterine growth retardation (27). Fetal O_2Cap may rapidly rise in response to acute hypoxemia (49) or asphyxia (3) produced by umbilical cord occlusion. Figure 32 portrays the effects on $\dot{V}_{O_2}$ of uncorrected fetal anemia when [Hb]f is assumed to equal $8.25\ g \cdot dl^{-1}$ rather than a normal value of $16.5\ g \cdot dl^{-1}$. Under these conditions there is no evidence of either a shift in the HbO_2 curve or an increase in $\dot{Q}f$. Thus the maternal-to-fetal $\overline{P}_{O_2}$ difference would be only slightly increased (9.9 Torr), as are the end-capillary P_{O_2} values, and the umbilical fetal arteriovenous C_{O_2} difference would remain at $4.6\ ml \cdot dl^{-1}$; this suggests that despite this degree of anemia fetal oxygenation could be maintained.

INTERRELATIONS OF MATERNAL AND FETAL PLACENTAL FLOWS AND O_2 EXCHANGE

Distribution of Maternal and Fetal Placental Flows

Thus far the discussion of the effects of blood flow changes in $\dot{V}_{O_2}$ assumes a uniform distribution of $\dot{Q}m$ to $\dot{Q}f$. When such flows are evenly matched with respect to one another, $\dot{V}_{O_2}$ is optimized. However, as in the lung with ventilation-perfusion inequalities, there may be inhomogeneity in the relation of $\dot{Q}m$ to $\dot{Q}f$, which can profoundly affect $\dot{V}_{O_2}$. Not only may there be nonuniformity in the distributions of blood flows, but there may be other inhomogeneities, such as the distribution of Dp to flows, the distribution of maternal and fetal placental vascular volumes, and the distribution of $\dot{V}p_{O_2}$ to blood flows. Thus it is

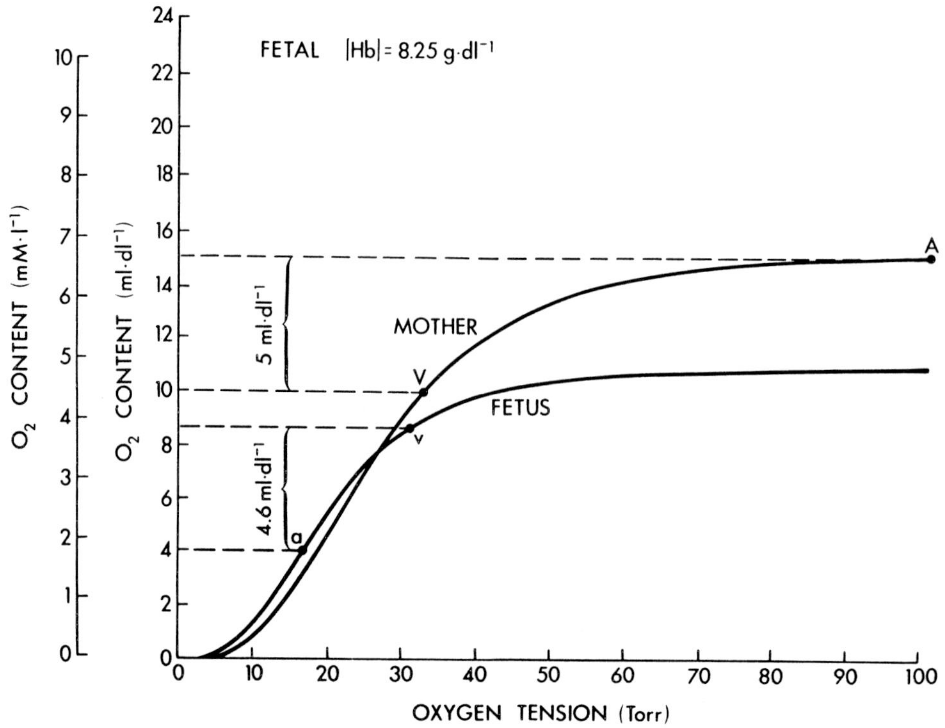

FIG. 32. Calculated blood O_2 content as function of P_{O_2} in presence of fetal anemia ($[Hb]f = 8.25$ g·dl^{-1}). Symbols are as in Fig. 31.

important to consider the consequences of flow distributions on $\dot{V}_{O_2}$.

NONUNIFORM DISTRIBUTION OF MATERNAL AND FETAL BLOOD FLOWS. Several lines of evidence suggest that the distribution of maternal and fetal placental flows is not uniform. For instance, the opening of arteriolar orifices into the human intervillous space is inhomogeneous (55), and cineradioangiography demonstrates intermittent flow in maternal and fetal placental vessels (48, 225, 288). Further evidence derives indirectly from comparison of placental O_2 exchange, which is relatively sensitive to flow distribution, and CO exchange, which is not (205). The most compelling evidence, however, originates from studies of the flow distribution per se. Using radioactive-labeled macroaggregates of albumin in the sheep placenta, Power et al. (279) demonstrated that in 1 g of placental samples both $\dot{Q}m$ and $\dot{Q}f$ were distributed nonuniformly. Moreover, the ratio of $\dot{Q}m$ to $\dot{Q}f$ was markedly uneven: i.e., only ~30% of the placenta had a flow ratio of 50% of the mean value; the remainder displayed a $\dot{Q}m$-$\dot{Q}f$ ratio above or below these limits. In contrast, subsequent studies with radioactive microspheres in chronically catheterized sheep analyzed 5-g portions of placenta and reported a more uniform distribution (224, 291). However, Power et al. (273) demonstrated that the degree of nonuniformity measured critically depends on the size of the placental sample taken. Thus small (40-mg) individual portions display a great deal of nonuniformity. However, as an investigator uses larger tissue samples and therefore integrates the samples and their individual variations, the inhomogeneities evident in the smaller portions tend to be nullified, obscuring the true variation (273).

Another factor that could affect the efficiency of the O_2 exchange process and mimic the effects of an uneven $\dot{Q}m$-$\dot{Q}f$ ratio is the presence of vascular shunts in the maternal and/or fetal placental vascular beds. Some anatomical studies have shown the presence of such shunts in the human placenta (47, 76), but these are not major. Metcalfe et al. (240) estimated the physiological shunt by perfusing in situ sheep umbilical vessels with a CO-saturated dextran solution. They assumed that essentially all the CO in fetal exchange vessels would combine with the Hb in maternal blood and that the CO remaining in the perfusate would be derived from shunts. Using standard equations, they calculated a 20% shunt of $\dot{Q}f$, a fraction that remained constant over the 30 min of perfusion (240). However, in this study the perfusion rate was only 30%–50% of normal values, whereas if the flows had been more nearly normal more exchange vessels might have been perfused and the calculated shunt fraction might have been lower. Nonetheless the reported findings could have resulted from nonuniform distribution of $\dot{Q}m$ to $\dot{Q}f$ rather than from anatomical shunts per se. A similar argument applies to the finding of shunts of 36% and 23% in the CO-saturated dextran–perfused uterine and umbilical circulations, respectively (292).

The distribution of maternal and fetal flows has

profound implications for O_2 and CO_2 exchange. If both flows were distributed perfectly uniformly, the end-capillary P_{O_2} and P_{CO_2} values in all exchange units would be equal (201). On the other hand, nonuniform flow distribution results in equilibration of end capillaries of different exchange units at various P_{O_2} and P_{CO_2} values, which vary with the $\dot{Q}m$-$\dot{Q}f$ ratios (201). For instance, with $\dot{Q}m$-$\dot{Q}f$ ratios of 3 and 0.3, end-capillary P_{O_2} would be ~51 and 21 Torr, respectively (277). Under these conditions maternal blood would leave the first compartment with a C_{O_2} of 12.0 $ml \cdot dl^{-1}$ and exit from the other with a C_{O_2} of 0.34 $ml \cdot dl^{-1}$. The compartment with the higher $\dot{Q}m$-$\dot{Q}f$ ratio and the higher O_2 values would contribute a disproportionately large share to the uterine venous blood, raising its P_{O_2} and C_{O_2} to 41 Torr and 9.9 $ml \cdot dl^{-1}$, respectively. In the fetal vessels the compartment with the low flow ratio and the low O_2 values would contribute a disproportionately large fraction to the umbilical venous blood, decreasing its P_{O_2} and C_{O_2} to 23 Torr and 11.7 $ml \cdot dl^{-1}$, respectively. Thus, despite P_{O_2} equilibration in individual exchange units, a maternal-to-fetal Pv_{O_2} difference of 18 Torr would result. With this type of analysis, the overall O_2 or CO_2 tension and content differences can be calculated for any given pattern of flow distribution (201, 275, 277, 279).

Figure 33 illustrates the contributions of both a

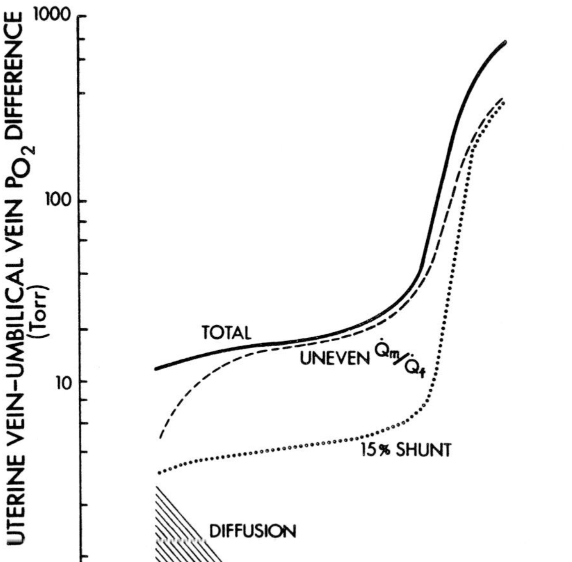

FIG. 33. Total uterine vein–to-umbilical vein P_{O_2} difference at various values of Pma_{O_2} (*solid line*). Contribution of distribution effect is shown over entire range of P_{O_2} values (*dashed line*) assuming that distribution of maternal to fetal flow ($\dot{Q}m/\dot{Q}f$) at higher P_{O_2} values is similar to that during normal oxygenation. Diffusion effect (*shaded area*) is shown to be insignificant when Pma_{O_2} exceeds 100 Torr. *Dotted line*, maternal-to-fetal venous P_{O_2} difference produced by 15% maternal shunt. Sum of various factors must represent total of this difference. [Adapted from Longo and Power (201).]

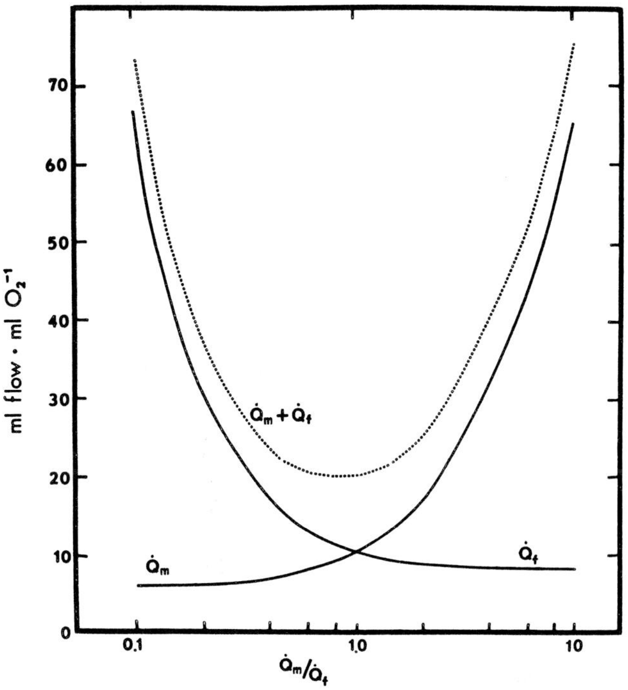

FIG. 34. Volume of maternal ($\dot{Q}m$) and fetal ($\dot{Q}f$) placental flows required to exchange 1 ml of O_2. As ratio of $\dot{Q}m$ to $\dot{Q}f$ increases above 1.0, progressively more $\dot{Q}m$ is required. This occurs because equilibration occurs at higher P_{O_2} and greater saturation of maternal Hb; therefore less O_2 is removed from each milliliter of maternal blood. Similarly, fetal blood undergoes greatest changes in $[O_2]$ with high $\dot{Q}m$-$\dot{Q}f$ ratios; therefore less fetal flow is required. Sum of both curves equals total maternal and fetal flow (*dotted line*). Optimum $\dot{Q}m$-$\dot{Q}f$ ratio for O_2 transport in terms of total flow is ~0.9. [Adapted from Power and Longo (277).]

nonuniform $\dot{Q}m$-$\dot{Q}f$ ratio and diffusion resistance to the total maternal-to-fetal Pv_{O_2} difference over a wide range of Pma_{O_2} values. When the mother breathes room air (Pma_{O_2} = 100 Torr), uneven distribution contributes ~11 Torr to the total maternal-to-fetal Pv_{O_2} difference of 14 Torr (i.e., 80%). Diffusion resistance contributes only ~1 Torr to this difference. When the mother breathes 100% O_2, essentially all of the Pv_{O_2} difference results from nonuniform flow distribution. During maternal hypoxemia (Pma_{O_2} = 50 Torr), uneven distribution contributes relatively less to the Pv_{O_2} difference, whereas diffusion resistance contributes relatively more (201).

A further consideration is the optimal $\dot{Q}m$-$\dot{Q}f$ ratio for efficient O_2 exchange. Figure 34 depicts the amount of $\dot{Q}m$ and $\dot{Q}f$ required to deliver a given amount of O_2 (277). For example, if $\dot{Q}m/\dot{Q}f$ = 3.0, the maternal and fetal blood volumes required would be ~8 ml and 24 ml, respectively. Because both $\dot{Q}m$ and $\dot{Q}f$ are involved in O_2 transport, they can be summed (Fig. 34, dotted line). The minimum value for this total flow represents the optimum flow ratio for O_2 exchange, i.e., ~0.9 (277), which is close to that determined experimentally for highly diffusible molecules (343).

DISTRIBUTION OF PLACENTAL DIFFUSING CAPACITY TO BLOOD FLOWS. Not only may the distribution of blood flows vary, but there may be a nonuniformity in the distribution of Dp to $\dot{Q}$. This is suggested by such morphologic findings as a wide variation in the thickness of placental tissue layers separating the maternal and fetal circulations (214, 351). The value of Dp is a function of exchange surface area, thickness, and exchange vessel volume (see previous section). Thus Dp may vary in different portions of the placenta and may be adequate or inadequate in relation to the ability of fetal blood to transport O_2. That is, the relation of Dp to blood transport capacity rather than the value of Dp per se determines whether $\dot{V}_{O_2}$ proceeds to equilibrium. Power et al. (275) presented a detailed analysis of the theoretical aspects of the distribution of Dp to $\dot{Q}$ on $\dot{V}_{O_2}$; however, at present there is no method to experimentally assess the importance of this phenomenon or other types of inhomogeneities.

"Sluice" or "Waterfall" Flow in Placental Vessels

Because O_2 and CO_2 exchange critically depend on blood flows, anything that affects the flows in turn affects the exchange process. With the juxtaposition of the exchange vessels in maternal and fetal placental circulations, it is reasonable that changes in the dimensions in one vascular bed might affect the size and therefore the vascular resistance in the other, with resultant effects on flow. Although in most organs blood flow is a function of the inflow minus outflow hydrostatic pressure difference, in the lung and some other organs the flow varies as a function of the inflow minus the surrounding pressure. Such a phenomenon also probably exists in the placenta, with flow through the fetal capillaries being affected by the surrounding pressure in the maternal vessels or intervillous space and perhaps vice versa. In isolated perfused sheep cotyledons, Power and Longo (278) first demonstrated that maternal placental surrounding pressure can affect $\dot{Q}f$. For instance, at a constant perfusion rate not only did fetal arterial (inflow) pressure rise when the surrounding pressure in maternal vessels was raised, but inflow pressure remained independent of changes in outflow pressure until that pressure exceeded the surrounding pressure, i.e., ~15 mmHg. Also, umbilical vascular resistance increased or decreased with increments or decrements in placental surrounding pressure (278).

Additional evidence for maternal-fetal vascular interactions derives from the demonstration that fetal placental vascular compliance increased with a decrease in maternal vascular pressure (274). Several other workers exhibited a "sluice" flow phenomenon in the vascular bed of sheep and guinea pig placentas (41, 309). For instance, in the perfused guinea pig placenta, Schröder et al. (309) demonstrated that changes in either maternal or fetal placental flow rates resulted in changes in the volumes both of the particular vascular bed being perfused and of the opposing bed, which showed reciprocal volume changes. A sluice effect may operate in the opposite direction, as shown by increased fetal placental vascular pressure affecting flow through perfused sheep uterine vessels (109).

Results of in vivo studies in chronically catheterized sheep have been contradictory: $\dot{Q}f$ was unaffected by increased uterine venous pressure (326), at least until hypoxemia developed (37); in contrast, both Cottle et al. (73) and Hasaart and de Haan (130) have demonstrated decreased $\dot{Q}m$ in response to umbilical cord compression with increased pressure in the fetal placental vasculature.

Thus, although some evidence exists against the concept of sluice flow in chronically instrumented ewes (37, 326), several potential problems exist with these studies. First, the changes in umbilical vascular resistance were not considered. The sluice effect is relatively small (i.e., 20- to 30-mmHg increase in surrounding pressure results in 3- to 4-mmHg increase in umbilical arterial pressure). In vivo partial umbilical venous occlusion results in both increased umbilical vascular bed pressure and probable resistance changes (secondary to changes in transmural pressure), reduced fetal venous return, and decreased umbilical arterial pressure and flow. The lack of such resistance changes have not been demonstrated. In addition, in one of the negative studies, $\dot{Q}m$ was measured in the common internal iliac artery, which supplies tissues other than the uterus (37).

Uterine Contractions and O_2 Exchange

Up to now only the virtually continuous O_2 exchange during fetal life has been considered. However, during uterine contractions, $\dot{V}_{O_2}$ may decrease or become discontinuous, and fetal distress may become evident. Although the changes associated with labor generally are ascribed to placental insufficiency, these changes undoubtedly have a physiological basis. Studies in primates indicate that uterine contractions result in decreased uterine venous outflow (290) and in some instances in depressed arterial inflow (287, 288). Butler et al. (62, 63) simulated the effects of changes in intrauterine pressure on $\dot{Q}m$, $\dot{Q}f$, and $\dot{V}_{O_2}$. This mathematical model predicted that during a normal contraction (50-mmHg peak intensity, 1-min duration), $\dot{Q}m$ and maternal intervillous space blood volume decreased ~50% and 20%, respectively, Pfv_{O_2} decreased ~36% (from 28 to 18 Torr), and $\dot{V}_{O_2}$ dropped 40% (from 20 to 12 ml·min^{-1}). End-capillary P_{O_2} was most sensitive to the values of contraction intensity and maternal blood pressure and less sensitive to the value of Pma_{O_2}. Contraction duration had essentially no effect on Pfv_{O_2}. Butler et al. (62) derived an empirical relation to predict the minimal Pfv_{O_2} reached during a uterine contraction

$$Pmin_{O_2} = 26.7 - 0.219 \cdot \text{intensity} \qquad (17)$$

where $Pmin_{O_2}$ is minimal P_{O_2} (in Torr) and intensity is in millimeters of Hg.

This model further predicted that if two or more factors changed simultaneously their combined effect would not equal the sum of their individual effects. To illustrate, the interaction between contraction intensity and duration could be expressed by the relation

$$O_2 \text{ deficit} = 0.33 + \text{duration} \cdot [\text{intensity} \cdot (2.04 \times 10^{-3}) - (3 \times 10^{-2})] \quad (18)$$

where O_2 deficit is in milliliters and duration is in seconds. This relation applied in the range of 20- to 60-mmHg intensity and from 0.5- to 2-min duration. For instance, a 50-mmHg contraction lasting for 60 s should produce an O_2 deficit of 4.7 ml, which constitutes ~20% of the normal $\dot{V}f_{O_2}$ for a 3-kg fetus during 1 min (62). With more intense longer contractions, $\dot{V}_{O_2}$ would be compromised even more severely. From measurements of continuous O_2 uptake by the uterus of chronically catheterized sheep, Longo et al. (195) determined that, with both spontaneous and oxytocin-induced uterine contractions, $\dot{Q}m$ decreased ~10%. During spontaneous contractions, amniotic fluid pressure rose to ~11 mmHg, and $\dot{V}_{O_2}$ dropped 4% but then increased 12% near the end of the contraction. Similarly, during oxytocin-induced contractions, amniotic fluid pressure rose to 12 mmHg, but $\dot{V}_{O_2}$ fell 10% with a modest overshoot after the contraction (195). These $\dot{V}_{O_2}$ changes are consistent with those predicted by Butler et al. (62).

During normal labor, $\dot{Q}m$ briefly and repeatedly decreases, but the fetal blood is reoxygenated during the recovery period. Using electromagnetic flowmeters, Greiss and Anderson (117, 118) showed that $\dot{Q}m$ in the ewe decreased as a result of either increased resting uterine tonus or increased frequency and duration of contractions.

In 1940, Windle (345) wrote

> we have observed that the contractions, provided they are not severe, are accompanied by improvement in the color of the umbilical veins and relaxation of the uterus results in darkening of the blood.

In light of these considerations, such a result could only occur if $\dot{Q}f$ decreased without a parallel decrease in $\dot{Q}m$, allowing a longer time for Pfv_{O_2} to approach that of maternal blood (see Fig. 29). In contrast, during a contraction in the rhesus monkey, Dawes et al. (80) demonstrated a 1.5%–9% decrease of $[HbO_2]f$. However, intrauterine pressure was not reported; thus a quantitative relation between pressure and fetal O_2 levels cannot be established. Also, in the fetal monkey, Myers et al. (253) demonstrated decrements in Pfa_{O_2} in association with fetal bradycardia, so-called "late decelerations." In chronically catheterized fetal sheep, Pa_{O_2} decreased 2–3 Torr (158) and 4–6 Torr (217) in response to spontaneous and oxytocin-induced contractions, respectively.

From these considerations, it can be appreciated that vaginal delivery may pose a special problem in humans, in which intrauterine pressure rises to relatively high levels. On the one hand, uterine contractions must be of such intensity and duration as to affect birth of the conceptus. On the other hand, the contractions must not unduly curtail $\dot{Q}m$ and $\dot{V}_{O_2}$ with the resulting development of fetal hypoxemia and central nervous system damage.

Importance of Various Parameters in O_2 Transfer

Figure 35 compares the transient effects of isolated changes in the several factors that affect placental O_2 exchange (200). The values of each of the factors are expressed as percentages of their assumed normal value so that they may be conveniently compared with one another. As in Figure 26, which shows the effects of various factors on CO_2 exchange, the slope of each curve at 100% of normal indicates the sensitivity of $\dot{V}_{O_2}$ to a change in that factor. The O_2 transfer rate is most sensitive to Pfa_{O_2}; it is only slightly less sensitive to the sum of maternal and fetal flows, followed by fetal and maternal Hb flows and fetal and maternal P_{50} values. Changes in diffusing capacity, Pma_{O_2}, or the $\dot{Q}m$-$\dot{Q}f$ ratio have little effect in the physiological range (200).

The importance of a determinant of O_2 transfer as a physiological regulator depends on its physiological range of variation as well as the sensitivity, i.e., the slope of the response curve. Thus it would seem reasonable to exclude several of the factors listed in Table 2 as important physiological regulators of $\dot{V}_{O_2}$. For example, moderate changes in diffusing capacity would not affect $\dot{V}_{O_2}$ appreciably. Normally the range of variation in Pma_{O_2} is not more than a few Torr. There is no known mechanism for [Hb]m to respond to the level of fetal oxygenation. Changes in [Hb]f would require at least several days. Finally, there is little evidence to suggest that either $\dot{Q}m$ or $\dot{Q}f$ changes in a direction that would maintain $\dot{V}_{O_2}$ in response to changing needs.

Surprisingly few factors remain as physiological regulators of O_2 transfer. Fetal Pa_{O_2} is important and, although its level varies only a few Torr from day to day, $\dot{V}_{O_2}$ is more sensitive to it than to any other factor. The distribution of $\dot{Q}m$ to $\dot{Q}f$ may become more uniform during maternal hypoxemia, but there is considerable uncertainty regarding this (279), and other compensations may exist.

Summary Equations

Mathematical modeling has been increasingly used as a powerful tool to understand the dynamics of placental respiratory gas exchange (6, 121, 138, 165, 181, 200, 204). Although such a model is an abstraction that deliberately neglects certain features of a system, it makes possible a rigorous treatment of other features. Properly formulated, the model fulfills several

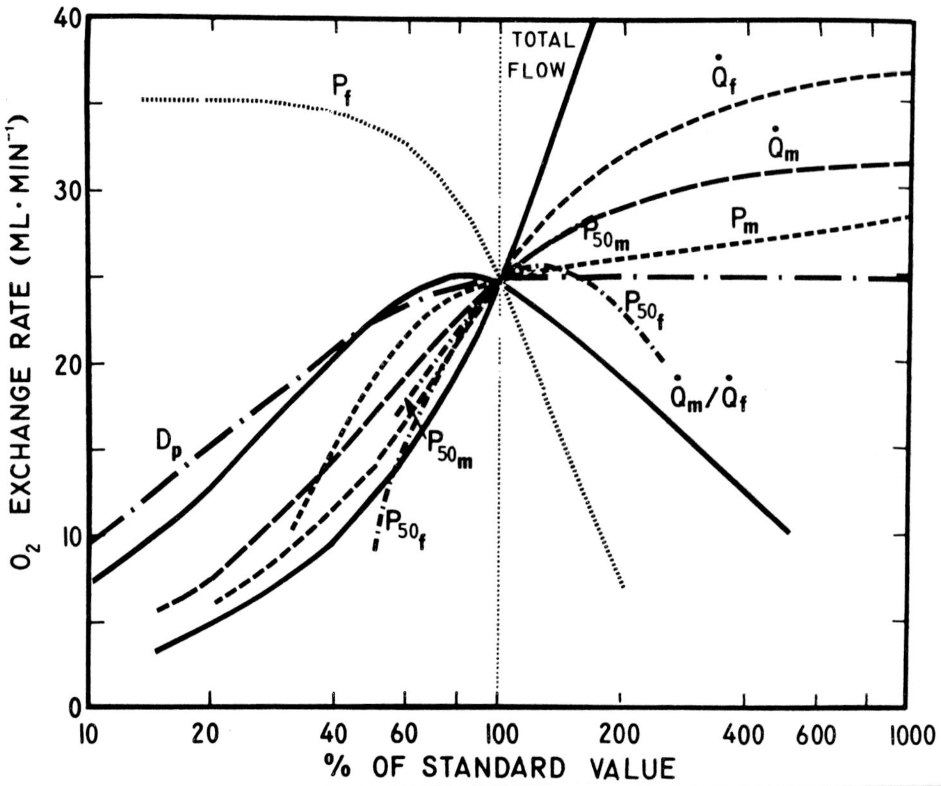

FIG. 35. Effects of changes in various factors on transient placental O_2 exchange rate. Results are normalized by plotting percent change in $\dot{V}_{O_2}$ as function of percent change in assumed normal value of given factor. As in Fig. 26, slope of each curve at 100% of normal value indicates relative sensitivity of O_2 exchange rate to that factor. $\dot{V}_{O_2}$ is most sensitive to umbilical arterial P_{O_2}, followed closely by total, maternal, and fetal flow rates and O_2 affinity of maternal and fetal blood. Curves for maternal and fetal [Hb] are superimposed on Q̇m and Q̇f curves. Pm and Pf, maternal and fetal Pa_{O_2} values; Dp, placental diffusing capacity. [Adapted from Longo et al. (200).]

functions. It approaches an integrated understanding of how the several parts of a complex system, such as $\dot{V}_{O_2}$, interact to result in a given effect. In addition, the very process of constructing the mathematical paradigm can be a heuristic exercise to identify areas of ignorance and relationships that have not been examined and thus to suggest experiments to answer specific questions. Finally, the model makes quantitative predictions that can be experimentally tested. Thus the predictive power of the theoretical analysis can be continually improved to more closely approximate reality by the rigors of experimental verification (204).

Typically these paradigms consist of a system of somewhat complex equations that must be solved numerically for any given set of initial conditions. Thus the investigator interested in using a given model faces the rather formidable task of adapting the algorithm to his computer and circumstances. In an attempt to circumvent these limitations, P. S. Dale and G. G. Power (personal communication) developed four algebraic equations that summarize the results of the model of Hill et al. (138). These equations predict values for $\dot{V}_{O_2}$, fetal placental end-capillary P_{O_2}, and $[HbO_2]$ as a function of nine major determinants of $\dot{V}_{O_2}$. The equations may be used in isolation for the calculation of specific values or may be included in large-scale systems analysis of placental exchange and fetal oxygenation.

For instance, if one of the variables affecting $\dot{V}_{O_2}$ changes from its standard value, the fractional change (f) from its standard value may be calculated as

$$f = A(1 - e^{-k\Delta x}) \qquad (19)$$

where Δx is the absolute change in the variable and A and k are constants. The authors tabulated values for humans as well as sheep. For example, using data for humans, suppose Q̇m were to decrease 50% below an assumed normal value of 430 ml·min^{-1}. The fractional change in $\dot{V}_{O_2}$ could then be estimated as 0.5414[1 − exp(−0.002293)(−215)] or −0.345 (from standard value of 24 ml·min^{-1} for 3-kg fetus to 15.7 ml·min^{-1}). This estimate may be compared with the fractional change of −0.335 (to 15.9 ml·min^{-1}, calculated by solving original equations).

An estimate of the O_2 transfer rate when more than one variable changes is derived by

$$\dot{V}_{O_2} = 24 \prod_{i=1}^{n} (1 + f_i) \qquad (20)$$

For instance, when n of the nine determinant variables deviate from their standard value, Equation 20 is used to calculate f_i for $i = 1$ to n. One is added to each f_i and the results are multiplied, giving the predicted fraction of the standard $\dot{V}_{O_2}$. Standard equations are used to convert $\dot{V}_{O_2}$ to $[HbO_2]$ and P_{O_2}.

Graphical Analysis of Placental O_2 and CO_2 Exchange

In the lung, graphical analysis of O_2 and CO_2 exchange, the so-called Rahn-Fenn diagram, has proven useful in lieu of solving rather complex equations with multiple variables. Ross (305) first applied this approach to placental gas exchange. With the blood gas values of maternal and umbilical arterial bloods as limits, he constructed exchange lines for various values of respiratory exchange ratio. Using values obtained from vaginal deliveries and cesarean section, Ross concluded that most data reported were inconsistent with the constraints imposed by graphical analysis. Furthermore he concluded that fetal and maternal blood probably reach near equilibrium in placental exchange vessels. Finally, he diagramed the effects of varying the $\dot{Q}m$-$\dot{Q}f$ ratio on the exchange process and concluded that such nonuniform flows act functionally as a shunt (305).

In an attempt to concisely describe the diffusion characteristics of the placenta, Faber and Hart (101) applied the theory of heat exchangers to transfer for several models of maternal-to-fetal placental blood flow, reducing several of the chief factors influencing placental exchange to dimensionless variables. A transport function for maternal blood (T) was given by

$$T = (Cma - Cmv)/(Cma - Cfa) \qquad (21)$$

where Cma, Cmv, and Cfa are the concentrations of a substance in the maternal artery and vein and umbilical artery, respectively. They also defined the $\dot{Q}f$-$\dot{Q}m$ ratio (R) and a permeability variable (D) as

$$D = P/(\dot{Q}m fm) \qquad (22)$$

where P is the placental permeability, $\dot{Q}m$ is the rate of maternal placental flow (fetal flow may also be used), and fm is the ratio of the amount of substance contained in a given volume of blood to the amount contained in an equal volume of water (101). They used these formulations to develop empirical exchange diagrams for the various patterns of blood flow with different permeabilities.

In the same study, Faber and Hart (101) perfused the umbilical circulation of rabbits with deoxygenated blood equilibrated with acetylene or oxygenated blood. Their results for the rabbit placenta best fit the predictions for a countercurrent exchanger but also agreed well with predicted results for a crosscurrent pattern. In contrast, data from the literature for the sheep, cow, monkey, and human did not fit this pattern, presumably because of a less-efficient pattern of blood flow or a low value of placental permeability or both.

Faber (98) extended this graphical analytic approach with dimensionless variables, defining a fetal transport function (Tf) as

$$Tf = (Cfv - Cfa)/(Cma - Cfa) \qquad (23)$$

where Cfv is the concentration in the umbilical vein. Again, he used these formulations to develop exchange diagrams for the various transfer patterns and flow ratios. Perfusion of the umbilical vessels of the goat placenta with blood equilibrated with N_2O and acetylene indicated that this placenta behaved either as a concurrent exchanger with moderately uneven distribution of $\dot{Q}m$ to $\dot{Q}f$, or as a countercurrent exchanger with markedly nonuniform distribution of $\dot{Q}m$ to $\dot{Q}f$ (292). A subsequent study has confirmed that the placentas for most species behave as concurrent exchangers with moderately uneven distributions of flows (99).

Power and Longo (277) described an alternative graphical analysis, constructing placental O_2 and CO_2 exchange diagrams by superimposing isopleths for various ratios of $\dot{Q}m$ and $\dot{Q}f$ on a plot relating the maternal and fetal HbO_2 curves. Given Pma_{O_2} and Pfa_{O_2} and assuming diffusion equilibration, the maternal and fetal placental end-capillary P_{O_2} and P_{CO_2} values, $[HbO_2]$, and $[O_2]$ can be read from the diagram for exchange units with various flow ratios. In addition, this approach could analyze the consequences of wide variations in Pma_{O_2} (from hyperbaric oxygenation to hypoxia) and in blood pH (277).

SOME COMPARISONS OF BLOOD FLOW AND GAS EXCHANGE IN THE PLACENTA AND LUNG

Sir Joseph Barcroft (13) first explored the question of how respiratory gas exchange in the placenta compares with that in the lung. Because of the low values of Dp he used, he estimated that the lung is "perhaps twenty times as efficient or more" (13). Of course the outcome of such a comparison will vary, depending on the function being compared. Table 6 presents comparative values for several measures of placental and pulmonary respiratory gas exchange and blood flow.

Despite the similar weights of these organs, 10- to 20-fold more O_2 is exchanged per minute in the lungs than in the term placenta, in rough accord with the mass of the organism supplied. Although in the lungs $\dot{V}_{O_2}$ by parenchymal tissue is an insignificant fraction of the total quantity exchanged, at term 20%–50% or more of the O_2 derived from maternal blood is consumed by placental tissue before it reaches the fetus (231). In both organs, O_2 and CO_2 exchange mutually enhance one another; the placenta shows double Bohr and Haldane effects because these reactions occur in both maternal and fetal blood.

TABLE 6. *Comparisons of Blood Flow and Gas Exchange in Placenta and Lungs*

	Placenta	Lungs
CO diffusing capacity, $ml \cdot min^{-1} \cdot Torr^{-1}$	1.81	25
CO diffusing capacity, $ml \cdot min^{-1} \cdot Torr^{-1} \cdot kg$ body wt^{-1}	0.60	0.42
CO diffusing capacity, $ml \cdot min^{-1} \cdot Torr^{-1} \cdot kg$ organ wt^{-1}	3.6	42
O_2 diffusing capacity, $ml \cdot min^{-1} \cdot Torr^{-1}$	2.3	30
Mean alveolar-to-pulmonary capillary P_{O_2} difference, Torr		8
Mean maternal-to-fetal placental P_{O_2} difference, Torr	8	
O_2 transfer rate, $ml \cdot min^{-1}$	24	300
O_2 transfer per unit blood flow, $ml \cdot min^{-1}$	6	54
Tissue O_2 consumption and CO_2 production	Significant	Insignificant
Interaction of O_2 and CO_2	Double Bohr and double Haldane effects	Bohr and Haldane effects
Fixed acid transfer	Significant	Insignificant
Blood flow	45% of cardiac output	100% of cardiac output
Distribution	Uneven maternal flow/fetal flow	Uneven ventilation/blood flow
Shunt, %	20	2
Type of flow	Sluice (maternal vascular pressure surrounding fetal capillaries)	Sluice (alveolar pressure surrounding pulmonary capillaries)
Regulation	Unknown	Active and precise

Adapted from Power (272).

Both organs receive a generous blood supply. However, in the placenta 20% (240) to 36% (292) of flow functionally bypasses gas-exchange sites, a fraction much larger than that in the lung. Although some of the placental shunts may be anatomical (77), probably most are actually uneven distribution of $\dot{Q}m$ to $\dot{Q}f$ (273, 279), analogous to nonuniform distribution of ventilation to perfusion in the lung. Both organs have flow characterized by a sluice or waterfall phenomenon (271, 278). Although the pulmonary circulation displays active and precise regulation, the regulation of $\dot{Q}m$ or $\dot{Q}f$ remains poorly understood.

Another question concerns the relative efficiency of placental O_2 exchange. A large exchange surface with a small barrier (as expressed by Dp) is advantageous for substrate exchange. In addition, both a uniform distribution of $\dot{Q}m$ to $\dot{Q}f$ and a countercurrent flow pattern optimize exchange. Placental "efficiency" may be considered from several points of view: e.g., the magnitude of Dp, the degree of arterialization of umbilical venous blood, the maternal-to-fetal Pv_{O_2} or Pv_{CO_2} differences, the arteriovenous Pf_{O_2} difference, and the percentage of O_2 extracted from maternal arterial blood. Table 7 presents data on some of these variables for several species. However, data under physiological conditions simply are not available from many of these species. Generally the coefficient of O_2 utilization and Dp correlate fairly well, but insufficient data are available for more than a generalization.

Bartels (21) has described several other measures of placental efficiency. The dimensionless variable "O_2 utilization perfusion quotient" (χ) is defined as

$$\chi = (Cma - Cmv)\dot{Q}T/(Cma\dot{Q}m) \quad (24)$$

where $\dot{Q}T$ is maternal cardiac output. The highest values are in rabbits and guinea pigs, and the lowest are in humans, sheep, and goats (Table 7). Bartels (21) also compared the fetal mass produced per maternal mass per day of gestation. Table 7 presents this "coefficient of fetal/maternal weight gestation duration" for several species. Apparently rats, guinea pigs, and rabbits must have highly efficient placentas because they allow the greatest percentage increase in fetal mass per unit time.

CONCLUSIONS

The purpose of this chapter is to synthesize into a coherent whole many seemingly isolated aspects of placental respiratory gas exchange, thereby deriving an understanding of how the individual factors relate to the whole. A series of questions on the several facets of this topic are proposed, a consideration of which will direct the reader toward such comprehension. These range from the relationship between the structure of fetal Hb and its function to an inquiry into the interrelations of [Hb], blood flow, and O_2 exchange. As is evident, the physiology of placental O_2 and CO_2 exchange is a complex, closely integrated, and fascinating process.

I have assayed many of the developments that have enabled the investigator to monitor under relatively physiological conditions the fetus in its intrauterine "space capsule," which until recently had been about as isolated as that of an astronaut in orbit. However, almost all of the experimental data quoted are from studies in laboratory animals. We know relatively nothing of the events during the course of human gestation. Also, essentially all of the studies were performed near term. We know little of the specific features early in pregnancy. While we are at the portal of understanding the effects of physiological adaptations on $\dot{V}_{O_2}$, we have little knowledge of the deviations caused by pathological alterations. Although impressive progress has been made by the classic analytic or reductionist approach, we are barely on the threshold

TABLE 7. *Comparisons of Placental O_2 Exchange in Several Species*

Species	Duration of Gestation, days	Maternal Wt, kg*	Fetal Wt, kg*	Placental Wt, kg	Litter Size	Fetal-to-Maternal Wt Ratio, %	Coefficient of Fetal Growth†	Uterine Blood Flow, ml/(kg fetus·min)	Uterine Flow as Percent Maternal Cardiac Output	Coefficient of O_2 Utilization‡	O_2 Utilization Perfusion Quotient§	Placental Diffusing Capacity	
												ml/(min Torr·kg fetus)	ml/(min ·Torr·kg placenta)
Human	267	60	3.3	0.5	1	5.5	2.1	150	10	30	3		
Monkey (*Macaca mulatta*)	164	7	0.45	0.13	1	6.4	3.9	145	5	50	10	0.6	1.6
Elephant	624	2,600	93		1	3.6	0.57						
Cow	280	600	40		1	6.6	2.4						
Horse		400	40		1	10							
Seal	270	169	13.6			8	3.0						
Pig	114	90	2		9	20	17.5						
Sheep	150	50	3.5		1.5	10.5	7.0	330	20	30	1.5	0.5	3.0
Goat	147	45	3.5		2	15.5	10.6	325	20	28	1.4		
Dog	63	12	0.3		5							0.6	
Cat	60	2.5	0.1										
Rabbit	31	3.5	0.06		8	13.7	44.2	83	10–15	70	5.6	2.3	11.6
Guinea pig	68	1.3	0.09	0.005	3.9				10–15	80	6.4	3.3	50.5
Hamster	16	0.1	0.002			2.3			9			2.3	45.3
Rat	22	0.3	0.005		7	11.6	53					1.7	9.0
Mouse	21	0.03	0.001										
Opossum	12.5	2	0.013										
Chicken	22	1.1	0.03			3							

* For many species the data are mean values for several breeds. † Calculated as (total fetal wt)/(maternal wt) × (100/duration of gestation) × 100. ‡ Calculated as $(Cma_{O_2} - Cmv_{O_2})(100/Cma_{O_2})$. § Calculated as $[(Cma_{O_2} - Cmv_{O_2})/Cma_{O_2}]/(\dot{Q}m/\dot{Q}_T)$.

of an effective synthesis of these isolated fragments into a unified ensemble of understanding.

Our concepts of the placenta and its role have been markedly altered by the accumulating results of experimental investigation. That remarkable organ has perhaps suffered a loss of reputation in an area or two, but it has certainly gained increased respect in others. Until relatively recently the placenta was believed to be optimally designed to facilitate respiratory gas exchange. We now appreciate, however, that the vascular architecture is not arranged most efficiently, that O_2 consumption and CO_2 production occur in the regions of gas transfer, and that inhomogeneities of several types introduce further inefficiency. Although it was previously thought that the membranes separating maternal and fetal blood constituted a significant barrier to diffusion, we now realize that these tissues constitute only a minor resistance to exchange.

Formerly, the placenta was considered a glorified sieve separating the fetus from the mother. We now know that it performs complex metabolic syntheses in the interplay of hormones between the two organisms and that it serves other metabolic and immunologic functions as vital as respiratory gas exchange. Finally, it is designed for rapid growth during a relatively brief life span. In view of the diversity of placental morphologic types and vascular arrangements that exist among the various mammalian species, it is evident that a wide divergence of architecture is compatible with similar physiological functions. None of this new information denies the fact that the respiratory function of the placenta is of critical importance for optimal fetal development. It does, however, suggest that the respiratory function may be a subsidiary consideration in its design.

Although most of the ideas presented in this essay are firmly grounded in experimental findings, many of the concepts are more theoretical and tentative, and they raise further questions. If some of the perceptions seem unduly speculative, one must recall that without speculation there is no progress.

I thank Francine Artis for helping to prepare this manuscript.

This work was supported by USPHS Grants HD-03807 and HD-13949.

REFERENCES

1. ABRAHAMOV, A., AND C. A. SMITH. Oxygen capacity and affinity of blood from erythroblastotic newborns. I. Effects of plasma environment on erythrocytes containing fetal or adult hemoglobin. *Am. J. Dis. Child.* 97: 375–379, 1959.
2. ADAMSON, J. W., J. T. PARER, AND G. STAMATOYANNOPOULOS. Erythrocytosis associated with hemoglobin Ranier: oxygen equilibria and marrow regulation. *J. Clin. Invest.* 48: 1376–1386, 1969.
3. ADAMSONS, K., R. W. BEARD, AND R. E. MYERS. Comparison of the composition of arterial, venous, and capillary blood of the fetal monkey during labor. *Am. J. Obstet. Gynecol.* 107: 435–440, 1970.
4. AHERNE, W., AND M. S. DUNNILL. Quantitative aspects of placental structure. *J. Pathol. Bacteriol.* 91: 123–139, 1966.
5. ALLEN, D. W., J. WYMAN, JR., AND C. H. SMITH. The oxygen equilibrium of fetal and adult human hemoglobin. *J. Biol. Chem.* 203: 81–87, 1953.
6. ALLEN, W. W., G. G. POWER, AND L. D. LONGO. Fetal O_2

changes in response to hypoxic stress: a mathematical model. *J. Appl. Physiol.* 42: 179–190, 1977.

7. ANSELMINO, K. J., AND F. HOFFMANN. Die Ursachen des Icterus neonatorum. *Arch. Gynaekol.* 143: 447–499, 1930.
8. ANSELMINO, K. J., AND F. HOFFMANN. Die Ursachen des Icterus neonatorum. Bemerkungen zu der vorstehenden Arbeit von Haselhorst und Stromberger, zugleich eine Erweiterung unserer Theorie. *Arch. Gynaekol.* 147: 69–71, 1931.
9. BACON, B. J., R. D. GILBERT, P. KAUFMANN, A. D. SMITH, T. TREVINO, AND L. D. LONGO. Placental anatomy and diffusing capacity in guinea pigs following long-term maternal hypoxia. *Placenta* 5: 475–488, 1984.
10. BAILLIE, P., G. S. DAWES, C. L. MERLET, AND R. RICHARDS. Maternal hyperventilation and foetal hypocapnia in sheep. *J. Physiol. Lond.* 218: 635–650, 1971.
11. BARCROFT, J. *The Respiratory Function of the Blood. Haemoglobin.* Cambridge, UK: Cambridge Univ. Press, 1928, pt. 2, p. 52.
12. BARCROFT, J. The conditions of foetal respiration. *Lancet* 225: 1021–1024, 1933.
13. BARCROFT, J. *Researches on Prenatal Life.* Oxford, UK: Blackwell, 1946, vol. 1.
14. BARCROFT, J., AND D. H. BARRON. Observations upon the form and relations of the maternal and fetal vessels in the placenta of the sheep. *Anat. Rec.* 94: 569–595, 1946.
15. BARNES, A. C. Discussion. Congenital heart disease in pregnancy, by D. E. Cannell and C. P. Vernon. *Am. J. Obstet. Gynecol.* 85: 749–750, 1963.
16. BARRON, D. H. The oxygen pressure gradient between the maternal and fetal blood in pregnant sheep. *Yale J. Biol. Med.* 19: 23–27, 1946.
17. BARRON, D. H., AND G. ALEXANDER. Supplementary observations on the oxygen pressure gradient between the maternal and fetal bloods of sheep. *Yale J. Biol. Med.* 25: 61–66, 1952.
18. BARRON, D. H., AND F. C. BATTAGLIA. The oxygen concentration gradient between the plasmas in the maternal and fetal capillaries of the placenta of the rabbit. *Yale J. Biol. Med.* 28: 197–207, 1955–56.
19. BARRON, D. H., AND G. MESCHIA. A comparative study of the exchange of the respiratory gases across the placenta. *Cold Spring Harbor Symp. Quant. Biol.* 39: 93–103, 1954.
20. BARTELS, H. Carriage of oxygen in the blood of the foetus. In: *Development of the Lung*, edited by A. V. S. de Reuck and R. Porter. Boston, MA: Little, Brown, 1967, p. 276–296. (Ciba Found. Symp.)
21. BARTELS, H. *Prenatal Respiration.* Amsterdam: North-Holland, 1970.
22. BARTELS, H., D. EL YASSIN, AND W. REINHARDT. Comparative studies of placental gas exchange in guinea pigs, rabbits, and goats. *Respir. Physiol.* 2: 149–162, 1967.
23. BARTELS, H., H. HARMS, V. PROBST, K. RIEGEL, AND J. SCHNEIDER. Sauerstoffbindungskurve, fetales Hämoglobin und Erythrocytenmorphologie bei Frühgeborenen und Säuglingen. *Klin. Wochenschr.* 37: 664–665, 1959.
24. BARTELS, H., G. HILLER, AND W. REINHARDT. Oxygen affinity of chicken blood before and after hatching. *Respir. Physiol.* 1: 345–356, 1966.
25. BARTELS, H., AND W. MOLL. Passage of inert substances and oxygen in the human placenta. *Pfluegers Arch.* 280: 165–177, 1964.
26. BARTELS, H., W. MOLL, AND J. METCALFE. Physiology of gas exchange in the human placenta. *Am. J. Obstet. Gynecol.* 84: 1714–1730, 1962.
27. BATTAGLIA, F. C. Intrauterine growth retardation. *Am. J. Obstet. Gynecol.* 106: 1103–1114, 1970.
28. BATTAGLIA, F. C., W. BOWES, H. R. MCGAUGHEY, E. L. MAKOWSKI, AND G. MESCHIA. The effect of fetal exchange transfusions with adult blood upon fetal oxygenation. *Pediatr. Res.* 3: 60–65, 1969.
29. BAUER, C., W. JELKMANN, AND W. MOLL. High oxygen affinity of maternal blood reduces fetal weight in rats. *Respir. Physiol.* 43: 169–178, 1981.
30. BAUER, C., I. LUDWIG, AND M. LUDWIG. Different effects of 2,3-diphosphoglycerate and adenosine triphosphate on the oxygen affinity of adult and foetal human haemoglobin. *Life Sci.* 7: 1339–1343, 1968.
31. BAUER, C., M. LUDWIG, I. LUDWIG, AND H. BARTELS. Factors governing the oxygen affinity of human adult and foetal blood. *Respir. Physiol.* 7: 271–277, 1969.
32. BAUMANN, R., F. TEISCHEL, R. ZOCH, AND H. BARTELS. Changes in red cell 2,3-diphosphoglycerate concentration as cause of the postnatal decrease of pig blood oxygen affinity. *Respir. Physiol.* 19: 153–161, 1973.
33. BEER, R., H. BARTELS, AND H. A. RACZKOWSKI. Die Saüerstoffdissoziationskurve des fetalen Blutes und der Gasaustausch in der menschlichen Placenta. *Pfluegers Arch.* 260: 306–319, 1955.
34. BEER, R., E. DOLL, AND J. WENNER. Die Verschiebung der Säuerstoffdissoziationskurve des Blutes von Säuglingen während der ersten Lebensmonate. *Pfluegers Arch.* 265: 526–540, 1958.
35. BEHRMAN, R. E., J. T. PARER, AND M. J. NOVY. Acute maternal respiratory alkalosis (hyperventilation) in the pregnant rhesus monkey. *Pediatr. Res.* 1: 354–363, 1967.
36. BERFENSTAM, R. Studies in carbonic anhydrase activity in children. I. Enzyme activity in the blood of infants and children of different ages, particularly in premature infants. *Acta Paediatr. Scand.* 41: 32–52, 1952.
37. BERMAN, W., JR., R. C. GOODLIN, M. A. HEYMANN, AND A. M. RUDOLPH. Relationships between pressure and flow in the umbilical and uterine circulations of the sheep. *Circ. Res.* 38: 262–266, 1976.
38. BETKE, K., AND E. KLEIHAUER. Fetaler und bleibender Blutfarbstoff in Erythrozyten und Erythroblasten von menschlichen Feten und Neugeborenen. *Blut* 4: 241–249, 1958.
39. BISSONNETTE, J. M. Control of vascular volume in sheep umbilical circulation. *J. Appl. Physiol.* 38: 1057–1061, 1975.
40. BISSONNETTE, J. M. Regulation of capillary volume in the fetal placental circulation. In: *Fetal and Newborn Cardiovascular Physiology. Fetal and Newborn Circulation*, edited by L. D. Longo and D. D. Reneau. New York: Garland, 1978, vol. 2, p. 69–80.
41. BISSONNETTE, J. M., AND R. C. FARRELL. Pressure-flow and pressure-volume relationships in the fetal placental circulation. *J. Appl. Physiol.* 35: 355–360, 1973.
42. BISSONNETTE, J. M., L. D. LONGO, M. J. NOVY, Y. MURATA, AND C. B. MARTIN, JR. Placental diffusing capacity and its relation to fetal growth. *J. Dev. Physiol. Oxf.* 1: 351–359, 1979.
43. BISSONNETTE, J. M., AND W. K. WICKHAM. Placental diffusing capacity for carbon monoxide in unanesthetized guinea pigs. *Respir. Physiol.* 31: 161–168, 1977.
44. BISSONNETTE, J. M., W. K. WICKHAM, AND W. H. DRUMMOND. Placental diffusing capacities at varied carbon monoxide tensions. *J. Clin. Invest.* 59: 1038–1044, 1977.
45. BLECHNER, J. N., J. R. COTTER, C. M. HINKLEY, AND H. PRYSTOWSKY. Observations on pregnancy at altitude. II. Transplacental pressure differences of oxygen and carbon dioxide. *Am. J. Obstet. Gynecol.* 102: 794–805, 1968.
46. BLECHNER, J. N., C. MESCHIA, AND D. H. BARRON. A study of the acid-base balance of foetal sheep and goats. *Q. J. Exp. Physiol.* 45: 60–71, 1960.
47. BØE, F. Vascular morphology of the human placenta. *Cold Spring Harbor Symp. Quant. Biol.* 19: 29–35, 1954.
48. BORELL, U., I. FERNSTRÖM, AND A. WESTMAN. Eine arteriographische Studie des Plazentarkreislaufs. *Geburtsh. Frauenheilkd.* 18: 1–9, 1958.
49. BORN, G. V. R., G. S. DAWES, AND J. C. MOTT. Oxygen lack and autonomic nervous control of the foetal circulation in the lamb. *J. Physiol. Lond.* 134: 149–166, 1956.
50. BOS, S. E. De mechanische fragiliteit van erythrocyten. *Maandschr. Kindergeneeskd.* 23: 335–348, 1955.
51. BOYLE, J. W., F. K. LOTGERING, AND L. D. LONGO. Acute embolization of the uteroplacental circulation: uterine blood flow and placental CO diffusing capacity. *J. Dev. Physiol. Oxf.*

6: 377–386, 1984.
52. BOYLE, R. New pneumatical experiments about respiration. *Philos. Trans. R. Soc. Lond.* 5: 2011–2031, 1670.
53. BRINKMAN, R., AND J. H. P. JONXIS. The occurrence of several kinds of haemoglobin in human blood. *J. Physiol. Lond.* 85: 117–127, 1935.
54. BRINKMAN, R., A. WILDSCHUT, AND A. WITTERMANS. On the occurrence of two kinds of haemoglobin in normal human blood. *J. Physiol. Lond.* 80: 377–387, 1934.
55. BROSENS, I., AND H. G. DIXON. The anatomy of the maternal side of the placenta. *J. Obstet. Gynaecol. Br. Commonw.* 73: 357–363, 1966.
56. BRUNS, P. D., W. A. BOWES, JR., V. E. DROSE, AND F. C. BATTAGLIA. Effect of respiratory acidosis on the rabbit fetus in utero. *Am. J. Obstet. Gynecol.* 87: 1074–1080, 1963.
57. BRUNS, P. D., W. E. COOPER, AND V. E. DROSE. Maternal-fetal oxygen and acid-base studies and their relationships to hyaline membrane disease in the newborn infant. *Am. J. Obstet. Gynecol.* 82: 1079–1088, 1962.
58. BUNN, H. F., B. G. FORGET, AND H. M. RANNEY. Hemoglobinopathies. *Major Probl. Intern. Med.* 12: 1–291, 1977.
59. BUNN, H. F., K. H. GABBAY, AND P. M. GALLOP. The glycosylation of hemoglobin: relevance to diabetes mellitus. *Science Wash. DC* 200: 21–27, 1978.
60. BUNN, H. F., D. N. HANEY, S. KAMIN, K. H. GABBAY, AND P. M. GALLOP. The biosynthesis of human hemoglobin A_1c. Slow glycosylation of hemoglobin in vivo. *J. Clin. Invest.* 57: 1652–1659, 1976.
61. BURSAUX, E., C. POYART, P. GUESNON, AND B. TEISSEIRE. Comparative effects of CO_2 on the affinity for O_2 of fetal and adult erythrocytes. *Pfluegers Arch.* 378: 197–203, 1979.
62. BUTLER, L. A., L. D. LONGO, AND G. G. POWER. Placental blood flows and oxygen transfer during uterine contractions: a mathematical model. *J. Theor. Biol.* 61: 81–95, 1976.
63. BUTLER, L. A., L. D. LONGO, AND G. G. POWER. A model of placental parameters during labor contractions. In: *Fetal and Newborn Cardiovascular Physiology. Developmental Aspects*, edited by L. D. Longo and D. D. Reneau. New York: Garland, 1978, vol. 1, p. 561–578.
64. CAMPBELL, A. G. M., G. S. DAWES, A. P. FISHMAN, A. I. HYMAN, AND G. B. JAMES. The oxygen consumption of the placenta and the foetal membranes in the sheep. *J. Physiol. Lond.* 182: 439–464, 1966.
65. CHARACHE, S., AND E. A. MURPHY. Is placental oxygen transport normal in carriers of high affinity hemoglobins? *Colloq. INSERM* 70: 285–294, 1977.
66. CLAPP, J. F., III. The relationship between blood flow and oxygen uptake in the uterine and umbilical circulations. *Am. J. Obstet. Gynecol.* 132: 410–413, 1978.
67. CLAPP, J. F., III, R. M. ABRAMS, D. CATON, J. R. COTTER, G. B. JAMES, AND D. H. BARRON. Umbilical blood flow in late gestation: a comparison of simultaneous measurements with two different techniques. *Am. J. Obstet. Gynecol.* 119: 919–923, 1974.
68. COLEMAN, A. J. Absence of harmful effect of maternal hypocapnea in babies delivered at caesarean section. *Lancet* 1: 813–814, 1967.
69. COMLINE, R. S., AND I. A. SILVER. Factors responsible for the stimulation of the adrenal medulla during asphyxia in the fetal lamb. *J. Physiol. Lond.* 178: 211–238, 1965.
70. COMLINE, R. S., AND M. SILVER. Daily changes in foetal and maternal blood of conscious pregnant ewes, with catheters in umbilical and uterine vessels. *J. Physiol. Lond.* 209: 567–586, 1970.
71. COMLINE, R. S., AND M. SILVER. P_{O_2}, P_{CO_2} and pH levels in the umbilical and uterine blood of the mare and ewe. *J. Physiol. Lond.* 209: 587–608, 1970.
72. COMLINE, R. S., AND M. SILVER. A comparative study of blood gas tensions, oxygen affinity and red cell 2,3-DPG concentrations in foetal and maternal blood in the mare, cow and sow. *J. Physiol. Lond.* 242: 805–826, 1974.
73. COTTLE, M. K. W., G. R. VAN PETTEN, AND P. VAN MUYDEN. Depression of uterine blood flow in response to cord compression in sheep. *Can. J. Physiol. Pharmacol.* 60: 825–829, 1982.
74. CRAWFORD, J. S. Anaesthesia for caesarean section: a proposal for evaluation, with analysis of a method. *Br. J. Anaesth.* 34: 179–194, 1962.
75. CREASY, R. K., C. T. BARRETT, M. DESWIET, K. V. KAHANPAA, AND A. M. RUDOLPH. Experimental intrauterine growth retardation in the sheep. *Am. J. Obstet. Gynecol.* 112: 566–573, 1972.
76. CRENSHAW, C., W. E. HUCKABEE, L. B. CURET, L. MANN, AND D. H. BARRON. A method for the estimation of the umbilical blood flow in unstressed sheep and goats with some results of its application. *Q. J. Exp. Physiol.* 53: 65–75, 1968.
77. DANESINO, V. Dispositivi di blocco ed anastomosi arterovenose nei vasi fetali della placenta umana. *Arch. Ostet. Ginecol.* 55: 251–272, 1959.
78. DARLING, R. C., C. A. SMITH, E. ASMUSSEN, AND F. M. COHEN. Some properties of human fetal and maternal blood. *J. Clin. Invest.* 20: 739–747, 1941.
79. DAWES, G. S. *Foetal and Neonatal Physiology.* Chicago, IL: Year Book, 1968.
80. DAWES, G. S., H. N. JACOBSON, J. C. MOTT, AND H. J. SHELLEY. Some observations on foetal and newborn rhesus monkeys. *J. Physiol. Lond.* 152: 271–298, 1960.
81. DAWES, G. S., AND J. C. MOTT. Changes in O_2 distribution and consumption in foetal lambs with variations in umbilical blood flow. *J. Physiol. Lond.* 170: 524–540, 1964.
82. DELIVORIA-PAPADOPOULOS, M., R. F. COBURN, AND R. E. FORSTER II. The placental diffusing capacity of carbon monoxide in pregnant women at term. In: *Respiratory Gas Exchange and Blood Flow in the Placenta*, edited by L. D. Longo and H. Bartels. Bethesda, MD: Natl. Inst. Health, 1972, p. 259–265. (No. NIH 73-361.)
83. DE VERDIER, C.-H., AND GARBY, L. Low binding of 2,3-diphosphoglycerate to haemoglobin F: a contribution to the knowledge of the binding site and an explanation for the high oxygen affinity of fetal blood. *Scand. J. Clin. Lab. Invest.* 23: 149–151, 1969.
84. DHINDSA, D. S., C. J. SEDGWICK, AND J. METCALFE. Comparative studies of the respiratory functions of mammalian blood. VIII. Asian elephant (*Elephas maximus*) and African elephant (*Loxodonta africana*). *Respir. Physiol.* 14: 332–342, 1972.
85. DIJKHUIZEN, P., A. BUURSMA, T. M. E. FONGERS, A. M. GERDING, B. OESEBURG, AND W. G. ZIJLSTRA. The oxygen binding capacity of human haemoglobin. Hüfner's factor redetermined. *Pfluegers Arch.* 36: 223–231, 1977.
86. DILL, D. B., A. GRAYBIEL, A. HURTADO, AND A. TAQUINI. Der Gasaustausch in den Lungen im Alter. *Z. Alternsforsch* 2: 20–33, 1940.
87. DITZEL, J. Changes in red cell oxygen release capacity in diabetes mellitus. *Federation Proc.* 38: 2484–2488, 1979.
88. DITZEL, J., AND E. STANDL. The problem of tissue oxygenation in diabetes mellitus. I. Its relation to the early functional changes in the microcirculation of diabetic subjects. *Acta Med. Scand. Suppl.* 578: 49–58, 1975.
89. DODDS, G. S. The area of the chorionic villi in the full term placenta. *Anat. Rec.* 24: 287–294, 1922/1923.
90. DOUGLAS, C. G., J. S. HALDANE, AND J. B. S. HALDANE. The laws of combination of haemoglobin with carbon monoxide and oxygen. *J. Physiol. Lond.* 44: 275–304, 1912.
91. DRESCHER, H., AND W. KÜNZER. Der Blutfarbstoff des menschlichen Feten. *Klin. Wochenschr.* 32: 92, 1954.
92. DUNCAN, S. L. B., AND B. V. LEWIS. Maternal placental and myometrial blood flow in the pregnant rabbit. *J. Physiol. Lond.* 202: 471–481, 1969.
93. EASTMAN, N. J. Fetal blood studies. V. The role of anesthesia in the production of asphyxia neonatorum. *Am. J. Obstet. Gynecol.* 31: 563–572, 1936.
94. EASTMAN, N. J. Discussion. Oxygen utilization by the human fetus in utero, by S. L. Romney, D. E. Reid, J. Metcalfe, and C. S. Burwell. *Am. J. Obstet. Gynecol.* 70: 791–799, 1955.
95. EASTMAN, N. J., E. M. K. GEILLING, AND A. M. DE LAWDNER.

Foetal blood studies. IV. The oxygen and carbon-dioxide dissociation curves of fetal blood. *Bull. Johns Hopkins Hosp.* 53: 246–254, 1933.
96. ELLIOTT, R. H., F. G. HALL, AND A. ST. G. HUGGETT. The blood volume and oxygen capacity of the foetal blood in the goat. *J. Physiol. Lond.* 82: 160–171, 1934.
97. ELSNER, R., D. D. HAMMOND, AND H. R. PARKER. Circulatory responses to asphyxia in pregnant and fetal animals: a comparative study of Weddell seals and sheep. *Yale J. Biol. Med.* 42: 202–217, 1969–70.
98. FABER, J. J. Application of the theory of heat exchangers to the transfer of inert materials in placentas. *Circ. Res.* 24: 221–234, 1969.
99. FABER, J. J. Steady-state methods for the study of placental exchange. *Federation Proc.* 36: 2640–2646, 1977.
100. FABER, J. J., C. F. GAULT, T. J. GREEN, AND K. L. THORNBURG. Fetal blood volume and fetal placental blood flow in lambs. *Proc. Soc. Exp. Biol. Med.* 142: 340–344, 1973.
101. FABER, J. J., AND F. M. HART. The rabbit placenta as an organ of diffusional exchange. Comparison with other species by dimensional analysis. *Circ. Res.* 19: 816–833, 1966.
102. FABER, J. J., AND F. M. HART. Transfer of charged and uncharged molecules in the placenta of the rabbit. *Am. J. Physiol.* 213: 890–894, 1967.
103. FISHER, A., AND C. PRYS-ROBERTS. Maternal pulmonary gas exchange: a study during normal labour and extradural blockade. *Anaesthesia* 23: 350–356, 1968.
104. FORSTER, R. E., II. Some principles governing maternal-foetal transfer in the placenta. In: *Foetal and Neonatal Physiology*, edited by K. S. Comline, K. W. Cross, G. S. Dawes, and P. W. Nathanielsz. London: Cambridge Univ. Press, 1973, p. 223–237. (Proc. Sir Joseph Barcroft Centenary Symp., Cambridge, July, 1972.)
105. FORSTER, R. E., II, AND E. D. CRANDALL. Time course of exchanges between red cells and extracellular fluid during CO_2 uptake. *J. Appl. Physiol.* 38: 710–718, 1975.
106. FRACASTORO, G. *De sympathia et antipathia rerum liber unus. De contagione et contagiosis morbis et curatione.* Venice: Iuntae, 1546.
107. FUCHS, F., T. SPACKMAN, AND N. S. ASSALI. Complexity and nonhomogeneity of the intervillous space. *Am. J. Obstet. Gynecol.* 86: 226–233, 1963.
108. FUJIKURA, T. Retrolental fibroplasia and prematurity in newborn rabbits induced by maternal hyperoxia. *Am. J. Obstet. Gynecol.* 90: 854–858, 1964.
109. FULLER, E. O., P. M. GALLETTI, D. O. NUTTER, AND R. W. MILLARD. Hemodynamics of the perfused pregnant sheep uterus. *Sci. Abstr. Soc. Gynecol. Invest., 1979*, p. 24.
110. FULLER, E. O., J. W. MANNING, D. O. NUTTER, AND P. M. GALLETTI. A perfused uterine preparation for the study of uterine and fetal physiology. In: *Fetal and Newborn Cardiovascular Physiology. Fetal and Newborn Circulation*, edited by L. D. Longo and D. D. Reneau. New York: Garland, 1978, vol. 2, p. 421–435.
111. GAHLENBECK, H., H. FRERKING, A. M. RATHSCHLAG-SCHAFFNER, AND H. BARTELS. Oxygen and carbon dioxide exchange across the cow placenta during the second part of pregnancy. *Respir. Physiol.* 4: 119–131, 1968.
112. GALE, R. E., J. B. CLEGG, AND E. R. HUEHNS. Human embryonic haemoglobins Gower 1 and Gower 2. *Nature Lond.* 280: 162–164, 1979.
113. GARBY, L., S. SJÖLIN, AND J. C. VUILLE. Studies on erythrokinetics in infancy. V. Estimations of the life span of red cells in the newborn. *Acta Paediatr.* 53: 165–171, 1964.
114. GILBERT, R. D., L. A. CUMMINGS, M. R. JUCHAU, AND L. D. LONGO. Placental diffusing capacity and fetal development in exercising or hypoxic guinea pigs. *J. Appl. Physiol.* 46: 828–834, 1979.
115. GILMAN, J. G. Rat embryonic and foetal erythrocytes. High 2,3-bisphosphoglycerate and ATP and low oxygen affinity in vitro for nucleated embryonic cells. *Biochem. J.* 192: 355–359, 1980.
116. GRATZER, W. B., AND A. C. ALLISON. Multiple haemoglobins. *Biol. Rev. Lond.* 35: 459–506, 1960.
117. GREISS, F. C., JR. Effect of labor on uterine blood flow. Observations on gravid ewes. *Am. J. Obstet. Gynecol.* 93: 917–923, 1965.
118. GREISS, F. C., JR., AND S. G. ANDERSON. Uterine blood flow during labor. *Clin. Obstet. Gynecol.* 11: 96–109, 1968.
119. GRUENWALD, P. Chronic fetal distress and placental insufficiency. *Biol. Neonat.* 5: 215–265, 1963.
120. GUILBEAU, E. J., D. D. RENEAU, AND M. H. KNISELY. A distributed parameter mathematical analysis of oxygen exchange from maternal to fetal blood in the human placenta. In: *Blood Oxygenation*, edited by D. Hershey. New York: Plenum, 1970, p. 218–221. (Proc. Int. Symp. on Blood Oxygenation, Univ. of Cincinnati, December, 1969.)
121. GUILBEAU, E. J., D. D. RENEAU, AND M. H. KNISELY. The effects of placental oxygen consumption and the contractions of labor on fetal oxygen supply. A steady and unsteady state mathematical simulation. In: *Respiratory Gas Exchange and Blood Flow in the Placenta*, edited by L. D. Longo and H. Bartels. Bethesda, MD: Natl. Inst. Health, 1972, p. 297–344. (No. NIH 73-361.)
122. GURTNER, G. H. Evidence for facilitated transport of oxygen and carbon monoxide. In: *Pulmonary Gas Exchange. Organism and Environment*, edited by J. B. West. New York: Academic, 1980, vol. 2, p. 205–239.
123. GURTNER, G. H., AND B. BURNS. Physiological evidence consistent with the presence of a specific O_2 carrier in the placenta. *J. Appl. Physiol.* 39: 728–734, 1975.
124. GURTNER, G. H., AND B. BURNS. Possible facilitated transport of oxygen across the placenta. *Nature Lond.* 240: 473–475, 1972.
125. HALBRECHT, I., AND C. KLIBANSKI. Identification of a new normal embryonic haemoglobin. *Nature Lond.* 178: 794–795, 1956.
126. HALBRECHT, I., C. KLIBANSKI, AND F. BAR ILAN. Co-existence of the embryonic (third normal) haemoglobin fraction with erythroblastosis in the blood of two full-term newborn babies with multiple malformations. *Nature Lond.* 183: 327–328, 1959.
127. HALBRECHT, I., C. KLIBANSKI, H. BRZOZA, AND M. LAHAV. Further studies on the various hemoglobins and the serum protein fractions in early embryonic life. *Am. J. Clin. Pathol.* 29: 340–344, 1958.
128. HALL, F. G. A spectroscopic method for the study of haemoglobin in dilute solutions. *J. Physiol. Lond.* 80: 502–507, 1934.
129. HALL, F. G. Haemoglobin function in the developing chick. *J. Physiol. Lond.* 83: 222–228, 1935.
130. HASAART, T. H. M., AND J. DE HAAN. Depression of uterine blood flow during total umbilical cord occlusion in sheep. *Eur. J. Obstet. Gynecol. Reprod. Biol.* 19: 125–131, 1985.
131. HAUROWITZ, F. Zur Chemie des Blutfarbstoffes. Über das Hämoglobin des Menschen. *Z. Phys. Chem.* 186: 141–147, 1930.
132. HEBBEL, R. P., E. M. BERGER, AND J. W. EATON. Effect of increased maternal hemoglobin oxygen affinity on fetal growth in the rat. *Blood* 55: 969–974, 1980.
133. HEERHABER, I., H. H. LOESCHCKE, AND U. WESTPHAL. Eine Wirkung des Progesterons auf die Atmung. *Pfluegers Arch.* 250: S42–S55, 1948.
134. HELLEGERS, A. E., C. J. HELLER, R. E. BEHRMAN, AND F. C. BATTAGLIA. Oxygen and carbon dioxide transfer across the rhesus monkey placenta (*Macaca mulatta*). *Am. J. Obstet. Gynecol.* 88: 22–31, 1964.
135. HELLEGERS, A. E., AND J. J. P. SCHRUEFER. Nomograms and empirical equations relating oxygen tension, percentage saturation, and pH in maternal and fetal blood. *Am. J. Obstet. Gynecol.* 81: 377–384, 1961.
136. HILL, E. P., J. R. HILL, G. G. POWER, AND L. D. LONGO. Carbon monoxide exchanges between the human fetus and mother: a mathematical model. *Am. J. Physiol.* 232 (*Heart Circ. Physiol.* 1): H311–H323, 1977.
137. HILL, E. P., AND L. D. LONGO. Placental CO_2 exchange. In: *Biophysics and Physiology of Carbon Dioxide*, edited by C.

Bauer, G. Gros, and H. Bartels. Berlin: Springer-Verlag, 1980, p. 379–389.

138. HILL, E. P., G. G. POWER, AND L. D. LONGO. A mathematical model of placental O_2 transfer with consideration of hemoglobin reaction rates. *Am. J. Physiol.* 222: 721–729, 1972.
139. HILL, E. P., G. G. POWER, AND L. D. LONGO. A mathematical model of carbon dioxide transfer in the placenta and its interaction with oxygen. *Am. J. Physiol.* 224: 283–299, 1973.
140. HILL, E. P., G. G. POWER, AND L. D. LONGO. Mathematical simulation of pulmonary O_2 and CO_2 exchange. *Am. J. Physiol.* 224: 904–917, 1973.
141. HJELM, M. The mode of expressing the content of intracellular components of human erythrocytes with special reference to adenine nucleotides. *Scand. J. Haematol.* 6: 56–64, 1969.
142. HLASTALA, M. P., T. A. STANDAERT, R. L. FRANADA, AND H. P. MCKENNA. Hemoglobin-ligand interaction in fetal and maternal sheep blood. *Respir. Physiol.* 34: 185–194, 1978.
143. HOLLÁN, S. R., J. G. SZELÉNYI, J. H. BREUER, G. MEDGYESI, AND V. N. SÖTÉR. Differences between the structure and function of human adult and foetal erythrocytes. *Folia Haematol. Leipz.* 90: 125–133, 1968.
144. HOLLAND, R. A. B. Rate of carbon dioxide uptake by suspension of human fetal red cell. In: *Fetal and Newborn Cardiovascular Physiology. Fetal and Newborn Circulation*, edited by L. D. Longo and D. D. Reneau. New York: Garland, 1978, vol. 2, p. 475–482.
145. HORAN, M. Studies in anaemia of infancy and childhood. The haemoglobin, red cell count, and packed cell volume of normal English infants during the first year of life. *Arch. Dis. Child.* 25: 110–128, 1950.
146. HÖRLEIN, H., AND G. WEBER. Über chronische familiare Methämoglobinamie und eine neue Modifikation des Methämoglobins. *Dtsch. Med. Wochenschr.* 73: 476–478, 1948.
147. HOWARD, R. C., P. D. BRUNS, AND J. A. LICHTY. Studies on babies born at high altitudes. III. Arterial oxygen saturation and hematocrit values at birth. *AMA J. Dis. Child.* 93: 674–678, 1957.
148. HUCKABEE, W. E., AND D. H. BARRON. Factors affecting the determination of uterine blood flow in vivo. *Circ. Res.* 9: 312–318, 1961.
149. HUEHNS, E. R., AND A. M. FAROOQUI. Oxygen dissociation properties of human embryonic red cells. *Nature Lond.* 254: 335–337, 1975.
150. HUEHNS, E. R., F. V. FLYNN, E. A. BUTLER, AND G. H. BEAVEN. Two new haemoglobin variants in a very young human embryo. *Nature Lond.* 189: 496–497, 1961.
151. HUEHNS, E. R., F. HECHT, J. V. KEIL, AND A. G. MOTULSKY. Developmental hemoglobin anomalies in a chromosomal triplication: D_1 trisomy syndrome. *Proc. Natl. Acad. Sci. USA* 51: 89–97, 1964.
152. HÜFNER, C. G. VON. Neue Versuche zur Bestimmung der Sauerstoffcapacitat des Blutfarbstoffs. *Arch. Physiol. Leipz.* 130–176, 1894.
153. HUGGETT, A. ST. G. Foetal blood-gas tensions and gas transfusion through the placenta of the goat. *J. Physiol. Lond.* 62: 373–384, 1927.
154. HUMPELER, E., AND H. AMOR. Sex differences in the oxygen affinity of hemoglobin. *Pfluegers Arch.* 343: 151–156, 1973.
155. HUNTER, J. *Observations on Certain Parts of the Animal Oeconomy.* London: Castle-Street Leicester-Square, 1786.
156. ITSKOVITZ, J., B. W. GOETZMAN, C. ROMAN, AND A. M. RUDOLPH. Effects of fetal-maternal exchange transfusion on fetal oxygenation and blood flow distribution. *Am. J. Physiol.* 247 (*Heart Circ. Physiol.* 16): H655–H660, 1984.
157. ITSKOVITZ, J., E. F. LAGAMMA, AND A. M. RUDOLPH. The effect of reducing umbilical blood flow on fetal oxygenation. *Am. J. Obstet. Gynecol.* 145: 813–818, 1983.
158. JANSEN, C. A. M., E. J. KRANE, A. L. THOMAS, N. F. G. BECK, K. C. LOWE, P. JOYCE, M. PARR, AND P. W. NATHANIELSZ. Continuous variability of fetal P_{O_2} in the chronically catheterized fetal sheep. *Am. J. Obstet. Gynecol.* 134: 776–783, 1979.
159. JELKMANN, W., AND C. BAUER. Oxygen affinity and phosphate compounds of red blood cells during intrauterine development of rabbits. *Pfluegers Arch.* 372: 149–156, 1977.
160. JOHNSON, J. W. C. The diffusivities of oxygen and water in human chorion (Abstract). *Soc. Gynecol. Invest. Program Meet., Denver, March 20–21, 1969*, p. 15.
161. KAISER, I. H., J. N. CUMMINGS, S. R. M. REYNOLDS, AND J. P. MARBARGER. Acclimatization response of the pregnant ewe and fetal lamb to diminished ambient pressure. *J. Appl. Physiol.* 13: 171–178, 1958.
162. KHAZIN, A. F., E. H. HON, AND F. W. HEHRE. Effects of maternal hyperoxia on the fetus. I. Oxygen tension. *Am. J. Obstet. Gynecol.* 109: 628–637, 1971.
163. KIRSCHBAUM, T. H. Fetal hemoglobin composition as a parameter of the oxyhemoglobin dissociation curve of fetal blood. *Am. J. Obstet. Gynecol.* 84: 477–485, 1962.
164. KIRSCHBAUM, T. H., C. R. BRINKMAN III, AND N. S. ASSALI. Effects of maternal-fetal blood exchange transfusion in fetal lambs. *Am. J. Obstet. Gynecol.* 110: 190–202, 1971.
165. KIRSCHBAUM, T. H., AND N. Z. SHAPIRO. A mathematical model of placental oxygen transfer. *J. Theor. Biol.* 25: 380–402, 1969.
166. KLEIHAUER, E. Blutausstrich. *Z. Geburtshilfe Gynaekol.* 159: 79–86, 1962.
167. KLEIHAUER, E., H. BRAUN, AND K. BETKE. Demonstration von fetalem Hämoglobin in den Erythrocyten eines Blutausstrichs. *Klin. Wochenschr.* 35: 637–638, 1957.
168. KLOCKE, R. A. Oxygen transport and 2,3-diphosphoglycerate. *Chest* 62, Suppl.: 79S–85S, 1972.
169. KOCH, H.-H., AND W. SCHRÖTER. Kompensatorische Veränderungen der erythrocytären 2,3-Diphosphoglyceratkionzentration bei Anämien und Polyglobulien. *Monatsschr. Kinderheilkd.* 121: 392–394, 1973.
170. KOOS, B. J., G. G. POWER, AND L. D. LONGO. Placental oxygen transfer with considerations for maternal exercise. In: *Exercise in Pregnancy*, edited by R. Artal and R. A. Wiswell. Baltimore, MD: Williams & Wilkins, 1986, p. 155–180.
171. KÖRBER, E. VON. Über Differenzen des Blutfarbstoffes. Dorpat, Germany, 1866. Inaugural dissertation.
172. KORECKÝ, B., AND B. RAŠKA. A contribution to the question of variability in the specific blood capacity for oxygen. *Physiol. Bohemoslov.* 7: 181–187, 1958.
173. KRÜGER, F. VON. Beobachtungen über die Absorption des Lichtes durch das Oxyhämoglobin. *Z. Biol.* 24: 47–66, 1887.
174. KRÜGER, F. VON. Vergleichende Untersuchungen über die Resistenz das Hämoglobins Verschiedener Tiere. *Z. Vgl. Physiol.* 2: 254–263, 1925.
175. KRÜGER, F. VON, AND W. GERLACH. Weitere Untersuchungen über den Einfluss von Blutentziehungen auf die Resistenz des Blutfarbstoffes. *Z. Gesamte Exp. Med.* 54: 653–660, 1927.
176. KÜNZEL, W., L. J. MANN, A. BHAKTHAVATHSALAN, J. AIROMLOOI, AND M. LIU. The effect of umbilical vein occlusion on fetal oxygenation, cardiovascular parameters, and fetal electroencephalogram. *Am. J. Obstet. Gynecol.* 128: 201–208, 1977.
177. KÜNZEL, W., AND W. MOLL. Uterine O_2 consumption and blood flow of the pregnant uterus. Experiments in pregnant guinea pigs. *Z. Geburtshilfe Perinatol.* 176: 108–117, 1972.
178. LAGA, E. M., S. G. DRISCOLL, AND H. N. MUNRO. Quantitative studies of human placenta. I. Morphometry. *Biol. Neonat.* 23: 231–259, 1973.
179. LAMBERTSEN, C. J. Effects of oxygen at high partial pressure. In: *Handbook of Physiology. Respiration*, edited by W. O. Fenn and H. Rahn. Washington, DC: Am. Physiol. Soc., 1965, sect. 3, vol. II, p. 1027–1046.
180. LAMPORT, H. The transport of oxygen in the sheep's placenta: the diffusion constant of the placenta. *Yale J. Biol. Med.* 27: 26–34, 1954/1955.
181. LARDNER, T. J. A model for placental oxygen exchange. *J. Biomech.* 8: 131–134, 1975.
182. LECKS, H., AND I. J. WOLMAN. Fetal hemoglobin in the human: a review. *Am. J. Med. Sci.* 219: 684–689, 1950.
183. LECRONE, C. N. Absence of special fetal hemoglobin in beagle dogs. *Blood* 35: 451–452, 1970.
184. LEIBSON, R. G., I. I. LIKHNITZKY, AND M. G. SAX. Oxygen

transport of the foetal and maternal blood during pregnancy. *J. Physiol. Lond.* 87: 97–112, 1936.

185. LENFANT, C., R. ELSNER, G. L. KOOYMAN, AND C. M. DRABEK. Respiratory function of blood of the adult and fetus Weddell seal *Leptonychotes weddelli. Am. J. Physiol.* 216: 1595–1597, 1969.
186. LEVINSON, G., S. M. SHNIDER, A. A. DELORIMIER, AND J. L. STEFFENSON. Effects of maternal hyperventilation on uterine blood flow and fetal oxygenation and acid-base balance. *Anesthesiology* 40: 340–347, 1974.
187. LILEY, A. W. Intrauterine transfusion of foetus in haemolytic disease. *Br. Med. J.* 2: 1107–1109, 1963.
188. LONGMUIR, I. S., D. C. MARTIN, H. J. GOLD, AND S. SUN. Nonclassical respiratory activity of tissue slices. *Microvasc. Res.* 3: 125–141, 1971.
189. LONGMUIR, I. S., AND S. SUN. A hypothetical tissue oxygen carrier. *Microvasc. Res.* 2: 287–293, 1970.
190. LONGO, L. D. Carbon monoxide in the pregnant mother and fetus and its exchange across the placenta. *Ann. NY Acad. Sci.* 174: 313–341, 1970.
191. LONGO, L. D. Carbon monoxide: effects on oxygenation of the fetus-in-utero. *Science Wash. DC* 194: 523–525, 1976.
192. LONGO, L. D. The biologic effects of carbon monoxide on the pregnant woman, fetus, and newborn infant. *Am. J. Obstet. Gynecol.* 129: 69–103, 1977.
193. LONGO, L. D., W. W. ALLEN, J. W. H. NISWONGER, K. D. PAGEL, H. C. WIELAND, AND R. D. GILBERT. The interrelations of blood and extracellular fluid volumes and cardiac output in the newborn lamb. In: *Fetal and Newborn Cardiovascular Physiology. Developmental Aspects*, edited by L. D. Longo and D. D. Reneau. New York: Garland, 1978, vol. 1, p. 345–367.
194. LONGO, L. D., AND K. S. CHING. Placental diffusing capacity for carbon monoxide and oxygen in unanesthetized sheep. *J. Appl. Physiol.* 43: 885–893, 1977.
195. LONGO, L. D., P. S. DALE, AND R. D. GILBERT. Uteroplacental O_2 uptake: continuous measurements during uterine quiescence and contractions. *Am. J. Physiol.* 250 (*Regulatory Integrative Comp. Physiol.* 19): R1099–R1116, 1986.
196. LONGO, L. D., M. DELIVORIA-PAPADOPOULOS, AND R. E. FORSTER II. Placental CO_2 transfer after fetal carbonic anhydrase inhibition. *Am. J. Physiol.* 226: 703–710, 1974.
197. LONGO, L. D., M. DELIVORIA-PAPADOPOULOS, G. G. POWER, E. P. HILL, AND R. E. FORSTER II. Diffusion equilibration of inert gases between maternal and fetal placental capillaries. *Am. J. Physiol.* 219: 561–569, 1970.
198. LONGO, L. D., AND J. S. HARDESTY. Maternal blood volume: measurement, hypothesis of control, and clinical considerations. *Rev. Perinat. Med.* 5: 35–59, 1984.
199. LONGO, L. D., E. P. HILL, AND G. G. POWER. Factors affecting placental oxygen transfer. In: *Chemical Engineering in Medicine*, edited by D. D. Reneau. New York: Plenum, 1972, p. 88–129.
200. LONGO, L. D., E. P. HILL, AND G. G. POWER. Theoretical analysis of factors affecting placental O_2 transfer. *Am. J. Physiol.* 222: 730–739, 1972.
201. LONGO, L. D., AND G. G. POWER. Analysis of P_{O_2} and P_{CO_2} differences between maternal and fetal blood in the placenta. *J. Appl. Physiol.* 26: 48–55, 1969.
202. LONGO, L. D., AND G. G. POWER. Long-term regulation of fetal cardiac output. A theory on the role of carbon dioxide. *Gynecol. Invest.* 4: 277–287, 1973.
203. LONGO, L. D., AND G. G. POWER. Problems in the placental transfer of carbon dioxide. In: *The Placenta, Biological and Clinical Aspects*, edited by K. S. Moghissi and E. S. E. Hafez. Springfield, IL: Thomas, 1974, p. 89–125.
204. LONGO, L. D., AND G. G. POWER. Placental oxygen transfer: a systems approach. In: *Reviews in Perinatal Medicine*, edited by E. M. Scarpelli and E. V. Cosmi. Baltimore, MD: University Park, 1976, vol. I, p. 1–34.
205. LONGO, L. D., G. G. POWER, AND R. E. FORSTER II. Respiratory function of the placenta as determined with carbon monoxide in sheep and dogs. *J. Clin. Invest.* 46: 812–828, 1967.
206. LONGO, L. D., G. G. POWER, AND R. E. FORSTER II. Placental diffusing capacity for carbon monoxide at varying partial pressures of oxygen. *J. Appl. Physiol.* 26: 360–370, 1969.
207. LORIJN, R. H. W., AND L. D. LONGO. Clinical and physiological implications of increased fetal oxygen consumption. *Am. J. Obstet. Gynecol.* 136: 451–457, 1980.
208. LORIJN, R. H. W., AND L. D. LONGO. Norepinephrine elevation in the fetal lamb: oxygen consumption and cardiac output. *Am. J. Physiol.* 239 (*Regulatory Integrative Comp. Physiol.* 8): R115–R122, 1980.
209. LORIJN, R. H. W., J. C. NELSON, AND L. D. LONGO. Induced fetal hyperthyroidism: cardiac output and oxygen consumption. *Am. J. Physiol.* 239 (*Heart Circ. Physiol.* 8): H302–H307, 1980.
210. LOTGERING, F. K., R. D. GILBERT, AND L. D. LONGO. Exercise responses in pregnant sheep: oxygen consumption, uterine blood flow, and blood volume. *J. Appl. Physiol.* 55: 834–841, 1983.
211. LOTGERING, F. K., R. D. GILBERT, AND L. D. LONGO. Exercise responses in pregnant sheep: blood gases, temperatures, and fetal cardiovascular system. *J. Appl. Physiol.*: 55: 842–850, 1983.
212. LOW, J. A., R. W. BOSTON, AND F. W. CERVENKO. Effect of low maternal carbon dioxide tension on placental gas exchange. *Am. J. Obstet. Gynecol.* 106: 1032–1043, 1970.
213. LUCIUS, H., H. GAHLENBECK, H. O. KLEINE, H. FABEL, AND H. BARTELS. Respiratory functions, buffer system, and electrolyte concentrations of blood during human pregnancy. *Respir. Physiol.* 9: 311–317, 1970.
214. LUDWIG, K. S. Zur Feinstruktur der maternofetalen Verbindung im Placentom des Schafes (*Ovis avies L.*). *Experientia Basel* 18: 212–213, 1962.
215. LUMLEY, J., P. RENOU, W. NEWMAN, AND C. WOOD. Hyperventilation in obstetrics. *Am. J. Obstet. Gynecol.* 103: 847–855, 1969.
216. LUND, C. J. The recognition and treatment of fetal heart arrhythmias due to anoxia. *Am. J. Obstet. Gynecol.* 40: 946–957, 1940.
217. LYE, S. J., M. E. WLODEK, AND J. R. G. CHALLIS. Relation between fetal arterial P_{O_2} and oxytocin-induced uterine contractions in pregnant sheep. *Can. J. Physiol. Pharmacol.* 62: 1337–1340, 1984.
219. MADSEN, H., AND J. DITZEL. Red cell 2,3-diphosphoglycerate and hemoglobin-oxygen affinity during normal pregnancy. *Acta Obstet. Gynecol. Scand.* 63: 399–402, 1984.
220. MADSEN, H., AND J. DITZEL. Red cell 2,3-diphosphoglycerate and hemoglobin-oxygen affinity during diabetic pregnancy. *Acta Obstet. Gynecol. Scand.* 63: 403–406, 1984.
221. MAKOWSKI, E. L. Maternal and fetal vascular nets in placentas of sheep and goats. *Am. J. Obstet. Gynecol.* 100: 283–288, 1968.
222. MAKOWSKI, E. L., F. C. BATTAGLIA, G. MESCHIA, R. E. BEHRMAN, J. SCHRUEFER, A. E. SEEDS, AND P. D. BRUNS. Effect of maternal exposure to high altitude upon fetal oxygenation. *Am. J. Obstet. Gynecol.* 100: 852–861, 1968.
223. MAKOWSKI, E. L., R. H. HERTZ, AND G. MESCHIA. Effects of acute maternal hypoxia and hyperoxia on the blood flow to the pregnant uterus. *Am. J. Obstet. Gynecol.* 115: 624–631, 1973.
224. MAKOWSKI, E. L., G. MESCHIA, W. DROEGEMUELLER, AND F. C. BATTAGLIA. Distribution of uterine blood flow in the pregnant sheep. *Am. J. Obstet. Gynecol.* 101: 409–412, 1968.
225. MARTIN, C. B., JR., H. S. MCGAUGHEY, JR., I. H. KAISER, M. W. DONNER, AND E. M. RAMSEY. Intermittent functioning of the uteroplacental arteries. *Am. J. Obstet. Gynecol.* 90: 819–823, 1964.
226. MATHERS, N. P., G. B. JAMES, AND J. WALKER. The oxygen affinity of the blood of infants treated by intrauterine transfusion. *J. Obstet. Gynaecol. Br. Commonw.* 77: 648–653, 1970.
227. MAYHEW, T. M., C. F. JOY, AND J. D. HAAS. Structure-function correlation in the human placenta: the morphometric diffusing capacity for oxygen at full term. *J. Anat.* 139: 691–708, 1984.

227a. McCarthy, E. F. The oxygen affinity of human maternal and foetal haemoglobin. *J. Physiol. Lond.* 102: 55–61, 1943.
228. Merlet-Bénichou, C., E. Azoulay, and M. Muffat-Joly. Dependence of 2,3-DPG and oxygen affinity of haemoglobin on sex and pregnancy in the guinea pig. *Pfluegers Arch.* 354: 187–195, 1975.
229. Meschia, G., F. C. Battaglia, and P. D. Bruns. Theoretical and experimental study of transplacental diffusion. *J. Appl. Physiol.* 22: 1171–1178, 1967.
230. Meschia, G., F. C. Battaglia, E. L. Makowski, and W. Droegemueller. Effect of varying umbilical blood O_2 affinity on umbilical vein P_{O_2}. *J. Appl. Physiol.* 26: 410–416, 1969.
231. Meschia, G., J. R. Cotter, E. L. Makowski, and D. H. Barron. Simultaneous measurement of uterine and umbilical blood flows and oxygen uptakes. *Q. J. Exp. Physiol.* 52: 1–18, 1966.
232. Meschia, G., A. Hellegers, J. N. Blechner, A. S. Wolkoff, and D. H. Barron. A comparison of the oxygen dissociation curves of the bloods of maternal, fetal and newborn sheep at various pHs. *Q. J. Exp. Physiol.* 46: 95–100, 1961.
233. Meschia, G., E. L. Makowski, and F. C. Battaglia. The use of uterine and umbilical veins of sheep for a description of fetal acid-base balance and oxygenation. *Yale J. Biol. Med.* 42: 154–165, 1969/1970.
234. Meschia, G., H. Prystowsky, A. Hellegers, W. Huckabee, J. Metcalfe, and D. H. Barron. Observations on the oxygen supply to the fetal llama. *Q. J. Exp. Physiol.* 45: 284–291, 1960.
235. Meschia, G., A. S. Wolkoff, and D. H. Barron. The oxygen, carbon dioxide and hydrogen-ion concentrations in the arterial and uterine venous bloods of pregnant sheep. *Q. J. Exp. Physiol.* 44: 333–342, 1959.
236. Metcalfe, J. Uterine oxygen supply and fetal health. *Yale J. Biol. Med.* 42: 166–179, 1969/1970.
237. Metcalfe, J., H. Bartels, and W. Moll. Gas exchange in the pregnant uterus. *Physiol. Rev.* 47: 782–838, 1967.
238. Metcalfe, J., D. S. Dhindsa, and M. J. Novy. General aspects of oxygen transport in maternal and fetal blood. In: *Respiratory Gas Exchange and Blood Flow in the Placenta*, edited by L. D. Longo and H. Bartels. Bethesda, MD: Natl. Inst. Health, 1972, p. 63–77. (No. NIH 73-361.)
239. Metcalfe, J., G. Meschia, A. Hellegers, H. Prystowsky, W. Huckabee, and D. H. Barron. Observations on the placental exchange of the respiratory gases in pregnant ewes at high altitude. *Q. J. Exp. Physiol.* 47: 74–92, 1962.
240. Metcalfe, J., W. Moll, H. Bartels, P. Hilpert, and J. T. Parer. Transfer of carbon monoxide and nitrous oxide in the artificially perfused sheep placenta. *Circ. Res.* 16: 95–101, 1965.
241. Metcalfe, J., S. L. Romney, J. R. Swartwout, D. M. Pitcairn, A. N. Lethin, Jr., and D. H. Barron. Uterine blood flow and oxygen consumption in pregnant sheep and goats. *Am. J. Physiol.* 197: 929–934, 1959.
242. Miller, F. C., R. H. Petrie, J. J. Arce, R. H. Paul, and E. H. Hon. Hyperventilation during labor. *Am. J. Obstet. Gynecol.* 120: 489–495, 1974.
243. Moll, W., and E. Kastendieck. Transfer of N_2O, CO and HTO in the artificially perfused guinea-pig placenta. *Respir. Physiol.* 29: 283–302, 1977.
244. Moore, L. G., D. Jahnigen, S. S. Rounds, J. T. Reeves, and R. T. Grover. Maternal hyperventilation helps preserve arterial oxygenation during high-altitude pregnancy. *J. Appl. Physiol.* 52: 690–694, 1982.
245. Moore, L. G., S. S. Rounds, D. Jahnigen, R. F. Grover, and J. T. Reeves. Infant birth weight is related to maternal arterial oxygenation at high altitude. *J. Appl. Physiol.* 52: 695–699, 1982.
246. Moore, W. M. O., F. C. Battaglia, and A. E. Hellegers. Whole blood oxygen affinities of women with various hemoglobinopathies. *Am. J. Obstet. Gynecol.* 97: 63–66, 1967.
247. Morishima, H. O., F. Moya, A. C. Bossers, and S. S. Daniel. Adverse effects of maternal hypocapnia on the newborn guinea pig. *Am. J. Obstet. Gynecol.* 88: 524–528, 1964.
248. Mossman, H. W. The rabbit placenta and the problem of placental transmission. *Am. J. Anat.* 37: 433–497, 1926.
249. Motoyama, E. K., G. Rivard, F. Acheson, and C. D. Cook. Adverse effect of maternal hyperventilation on the foetus. *Lancet* 1: 286–288, 1966.
250. Motoyama, E. K., G. Rivard, F. Acheson, and C. D. Cook. The effect of changes in maternal pH and P_{CO_2} of fetal lambs. *Anesthesiology* 28: 891–903, 1967.
251. Moya, F., H. O. Morishima, S. M. Shnider, and L. S. James. Influence of maternal hyperventilation on the newborn infant. *Am. J. Obstet. Gynecol.* 91: 76–84, 1965.
252. Mueggler, P. A., G. Jones, J. S. Peterson, J. M. Bissonnette, R. D. Koler, J. Metcalfe, R. T. Jones, and J. A. Black. Postnatal regulation of canine oxygen delivery: erythrocyte components affecting Hb function. *Am. J. Physiol.* 238 (*Heart Circ. Physiol.* 7): H73–H79, 1980.
253. Myers, R. E., E. Mueller-Heubach, and K. Adamsons. Predictability of the state of fetal oxygenation from a quantitative analysis of the components of late deceleration. *Am. J. Obstet. Gynecol.* 115: 1083–1094, 1973.
254. Nelson, P. S., R. D. Gilbert, and L. D. Longo. Fetal growth and placental diffusing capacity in guinea pigs following long-term maternal exercise. *J. Dev. Physiol. Oxf.* 5: 1–10, 1983.
255. Newcomb, S. L., and G. G. Power. Hematocrit of the fetal rabbit placenta. *Am. J. Physiol.* 229: 1393–1396, 1975.
256. Newman, W., L. McKinnon, L. Phillips, P. Paterson, and C. Wood. Oxygen transfer from mother to fetus during labor. *Am. J. Obstet. Gynecol.* 99: 61–70, 1967.
257. Novy, M. J. Alterations in blood oxygen affinity during fetal and neonatal life. In: *Oxygen Affinity of Hemoglobin and Red Cell Acid Base Status*, edited by M. Rørth and P. Astrup. Copenhagen: Munksgaard, 1972, p. 696–712. (Alfred Benzon Symp. 4.)
258. Novy, M. J., F. D. Frigoletto, C. L. Easterday, I. Umansky, and N. M. Nelson. Changes in umbilical-cord blood oxygen affinity after intrauterine transfusions for erythroblastosis. *N. Engl. J. Med.* 285: 589–596, 1971.
259. Novy, M. J., A. S. Hoversland, D. S. Dhindsa, and J. Metcalfe. Blood oxygen affinity and hemoglobin type in adult, newborn, and fetal pigs. *Respir. Physiol.* 19: 1–11, 1973.
260. Novy, M. J., and J. T. Parer. Absence of high blood oxygen affinity in the fetal cat. *Respir. Physiol.* 6: 144–150, 1969.
261. Novy, M. J., E. N. Peterson, and J. Metcalfe. Respiratory characteristics of maternal and fetal blood in cyanotic congenital heart disease. *Am. J. Obstet. Gynecol.* 100: 821–828, 1968.
262. Orzalesi, M. M., and W. W. Hay. The regulation of oxygen affinity of fetal blood. I. In vitro experiments and results in normal infants. *Pediatrics* 48: 857–864, 1971.
263. Oski, F. A. Hematological problems. In: *Neonatology. Patho-Physiology and Management of the Newborn*, edited by G. B. Avery. Philadelphia, PA: Lippincott, 1975, p. 379–422.
264. Parer, J. T. Oxygen transport in human subjects with hemoglobin variants having altered oxygen affinity. *Respir. Physiol.* 9: 43–49, 1970.
265. Parer, J. T., and R. E. Behrman. The oxygen consumption of the pregnant uterus and fetus of *Macaca mulatta*. *Respir. Physiol.* 3: 288–301, 1967.
266. Parer, J. T., M. Eng, H. Aoba, and K. Ueland. Uterine blood flow and oxygen uptake during maternal hyperventilation in monkeys at cesarean section. *Anesthesiology* 32: 130–135, 1970.
267. Parker, H. R., and M. J. Purves. Some effects of maternal hyperoxia and hypoxia on the blood gas tensions and vascular pressures in the foetal sheep. *Q. J. Exp. Physiol.* 52: 205–221, 1967.
268. Paton, J. B., E. Peterson, D. E. Fisher, and R. E. Behrman. Oxygen dissociation curves of fetal and adult baboons. *Respir. Physiol.* 12: 283–290, 1971.
269. Peng, A. T. C., L. S. Blancato, and E. K. Motoyama. Effect of maternal hypocapnia vs. eucapnia on the foetus during caesarean section. *Br. J. Anaesth.* 44: 1173–1178, 1972.
270. Perk, K., and D. Danon. Comparative structure analysis of

foetal and adult type red cells in newborn and adult cattle. *Res. Vet. Sci.* 6: 442–446, 1965.
271. PERMUTT, S., AND R. L. RILEY. Hemodynamics of collapsible vessels with tone: the vascular waterfall. *J. Appl. Physiol.* 18: 924–932, 1963.
272. POWER, G. G. Some aspects of O_2 and CO_2 transfer in the placenta. *Chest* 61, Suppl.: 22S–24S, 1972.
273. POWER, G. G., P. S. DALE, AND P. S. NELSON. Distribution of maternal and fetal blood flow within cotyledons of the sheep placenta. *Am. J. Physiol.* 241 (*Heart Circ. Physiol.* 10): H486–H496, 1981.
274. POWER, G. G., AND R. D. GILBERT. Umbilical vascular compliance in sheep. *Am. J. Physiol.* 233 (*Heart Circ. Physiol.* 2): H660–H664, 1977.
275. POWER, G. G., E. P. HILL, AND L. D. LONGO. Analysis of uneven distribution of diffusing capacity and blood flow in the placenta. *Am. J. Physiol.* 222: 740–746, 1972.
276. POWER, G. G., AND F. JENKINS. Factors affecting O_2 transfer in sheep and rabbit placenta perfused in situ. *Am. J. Physiol.* 229: 1147–1153, 1975.
277. POWER, G. G., AND L. D. LONGO. Graphical analysis of maternal and fetal exchange of O_2 and CO_2. *J. Appl. Physiol.* 26: 38–47, 1969.
278. POWER, G. G., AND L. D. LONGO. Sluice flow in placenta: maternal vascular pressure effects on fetal circulation. *Am. J. Physiol.* 225: 1490–1496, 1973.
279. POWER, G. G., L. D. LONGO, H. N. WAGNER, JR., D. E. KUHL, AND R. E. FORSTER II. Uneven distribution of maternal and fetal placental blood flow, as demonstrated using macroaggregates, and its response to hypoxia. *J. Clin. Invest.* 46: 2053–2063, 1967.
280. PRITCHARD, J. A. Changes in the blood volume during pregnancy and delivery. *Anesthesiology* 26: 393–399, 1965.
281. PRITCHARD, J. A., AND C. F. HUNT. A comparison of the hematologic responses following the routine prenatal administration of intramuscular and oral iron. *Surg. Gynecol. Obstet.* 106: 516–518, 1958.
282. PRYSTOWSKY, H. Fetal blood studies. VII. The oxygen pressure gradient between the maternal and fetal bloods of the human in normal and abnormal pregnancy. *Bull. Johns Hopkins Hosp.* 101: 48–56, 1957.
283. PRYSTOWSKY, H., A. HELLEGERS, AND P. BRUNS. Fetal blood studies. XIV. A comparative study of the oxygen dissociation curve of nonpregnant, pregnant, and fetal human blood. *Am. J. Obstet. Gynecol.* 78: 489–493, 1959.
284. PRYSTOWSKY, H., A. HELLEGERS, AND P. BRUNS. Fetal blood studies. XV. The carbon dioxide concentration gradient between the fetal and maternal blood of humans. *Am. J. Obstet. Gynecol.* 81: 372–376, 1961.
285. PRYSTOWSKY, H., A. HELLEGERS, G. MESCHIA, J. METCALFE, W. HUCKABEE, AND D. H. BARRON. The blood volume of fetuses carried by ewes at high altitude. *Q. J. Exp. Physiol.* 45: 292–297, 1960.
286. QVIST, J., R. E. WEBER, AND W. M. ZAPOL. Oxygen equilibrium properties of blood and hemoglobin of fetal and adult Weddell seals. *J. Appl. Physiol.* 50: 999–1005, 1981.
287. RAMSEY, E. M. Uteroplacental circulation during labor. *Clin. Obstet. Gynecol.* 11: 78–95, 1968.
288. RAMSEY, E. M., G. W. CORNER, JR., AND M. W. DONNER. Cineradioangiographic visualization of the venous drainage of the primate placenta in vivo. *Science Wash. DC* 141: 909–910, 1963.
289. RAMSEY, E. M., G. W. CORNER, JR., M. W. DONNER, AND H. M. STRAN. Radioangiographic studies of circulation in the maternal placenta of the rhesus monkey: preliminary report. *Proc. Natl. Acad. Sci. USA* 46: 1003–1008, 1960.
290. RAMSEY, E. M., C. B. MARTIN, JR., H. S. MCGAUGHEY, JR., I. H. KAISER, AND M. W. DONNER. Venous drainage of the placenta in rhesus monkeys: radiographic studies. *Am. J. Obstet. Gynecol.* 95: 948–955, 1966.
291. RANKIN, J., G. MESCHIA, E. L. MAKOWSKI, AND F. C. BATTAGLIA. Macroscopic distribution of blood flow in the sheep placenta. *Am. J. Physiol.* 219: 9–16, 1970.
292. RANKIN, J. H. G., AND E. N. PETERSON. Application of the theory of heat exchangers to a physiological study of the goat placenta. *Circ. Res.* 24: 235–250, 1969.
293. REIMANN, F., AND E. YENEN. Der Einfluss von fetalem Hämoglobin auf die Bestimmung der osmotischen Resistenz im Blut des Neugeborenen. *Acta Haematol. Basel* 27: 359–366, 1962.
294. RIEGEL, K., H. BARTELS, I. O. BUSS, P. G. WRIGHT, E. KLEIHAUER, C. P. LUCK, J. T. PARER, AND J. METCALFE. Comparative studies of the respiratory functions of mammalian blood. IV. Fetal and adult African elephant blood. *Respir. Physiol.* 2: 182–195, 1967.
295. RIEGEL, K., H. BARTELS, D. EL YASSIN, J. OUFI, E. KLEIHAUER, J. T. PARER, AND J. METCALFE. Comparative studies of the respiratory functions of mammalian blood. III. Fetal and adult dromedary camel blood. *Respir. Physiol.* 2: 173–181, 1967.
296. RIVARD, G., E. K. MOTOYAMA, F. M. ACHESON, C. D. COOK, AND E. O. R. REYNOLDS. The relation between maternal and fetal oxygen tensions in sheep. *Am. J. Obstet. Gynecol.* 97: 925–930, 1967.
297. ROCCO, E., T. R. BENNETT, AND G. G. POWER. Placental diffusing capacity in unanesthetized rabbits. *Am. J. Physiol.* 228: 465–469, 1975.
298. ROOS, J., AND C. ROMIJN. The oxygen dissociation curve of the cow's blood during pregnancy and the dissociation curve of the blood of the newborn animal in the course of the first time after birth. *Proc. K. Ned. Akad. Wet. Ser. C Biol. Med. Sci.* 40: 803–812, 1937.
299. ROOS, J., AND C. ROMIJN. Some conditions of foetal respiration in the cow. *J. Physiol. Lond.* 92: 249–267, 1938.
300. ROOTH, G., AND S. SJÖSTEDT. The placental transfer of gases and fixed acids. *Arch. Dis. Child.* 37: 366–370, 1962.
301. RORKE, M. J., D. A. DAVEY, AND H. G. DUTOIT. Foetal oxygenation during caesarean section. *Anaesthesia* 23: 585–596, 1968.
302. RØRTH, M., AND N. E. BILLE-BRAHE. 2,3-Diphosphoglycerate and creatinine in the red cell during human pregnancy. *Scand. J. Clin. Lab. Invest.* 28: 271–276, 1971.
303. RØRTH, M., AND N. E. BILLE-BRAHE. 2,3-DPG in human pregnancy. In: *Oxygen Affinity of Hemoglobin and Red Cell Acid Base Status*, edited by M. Rørth and P. Astrup. Copenhagen: Munksgaard, 1972, p. 692–695. (Alfred Benzon Symp. 4.)
304. ROSENFELD, C. R., F. H. MORRISS, JR., E. L. MAKOWSKI, G. MESCHIA, AND F. C. BATTAGLIA. Circulatory changes in the reproductive tissues of ewes during pregnancy. *Gynecol. Invest.* 5: 252–268, 1974.
305. ROSS, B. B. Comparative properties of the lungs and the placenta: a graphical analysis of placental gas exchange. In: *Development of the Lung*, edited by A. V. S. de Reuck and R. Porter. Boston, MA: Little, Brown, 1967, p. 238–257. (Ciba Found. Symp.)
306. ROTTINO, A., AND J. W. ANGERS. Electrophoretic mobility of the red blood cell during human pregnancy. *Am. J. Obstet. Gynecol.* 82: 1302–1306, 1961.
307. RUDOLPH, A. M., AND M. A. HEYMANN. The circulation of the fetus in utero. Methods for studying distribution of blood flow, cardiac output and organ blood flow. *Circ. Res.* 21: 163–184, 1967.
308. SCHERRER, M., AND H. BACHOFEN. The oxygen-combining capacity of hemoglobin (Letter to the editor). *Anesthesiology* 36: 190, 1972.
309. SCHRÖDER, H., W. PAUL, AND H.-P. LEICHTWEISS. Vascular volumes in isolated perfused guinea pig placenta. *Am. J. Physiol.* 241 (*Heart Circ. Physiol.* 10): H73–H77, 1981.
310. SCHROEDER, W. A., J. T. CUA, G. MATSUDA, AND W. D. FENNINGER. Hemoglobin F_1, an acetyl-containing hemoglobin. *Biochim. Biophys. Acta* 63: 532–534, 1962.
311. SCHROEDER, W. A., T. H. J. HUISMAN, J. R. SHELTON, J. B. SHELTON, E. F. KLEIHAUER, A. M. DOZY, AND B. ROBBERSON. Evidence for multiple structural genes for the γ chain of human fetal hemoglobin. *Proc. Natl. Acad. Sci. USA* 60: 537–

544, 1968.
312. SCHROEDER, W. A., J. R. SHELTON, J. B. SHELTON, AND J. CORMICK. The amino acid sequence of the α chain of human fetal hemoglobin. *Biochemistry* 2: 1353–1357, 1963.
313. SCHROEDER, W. A., J. R. SHELTON, J. B. SHELTON, J. CORMICK, AND R. T. JONES. The amino acid sequence of the γ chain of human fetal hemoglobin. *Biochemistry* 2: 992–1008, 1963.
314. SINET, M., E. AZOULAY, AND M. C. BLAYO. Affinité du sang pour l'oxygèn et 2,3-DPG chez l'homme, la femme et la femme enciente. *Bull. Physio-Pathol. Respir.* 10: 419–434, 1974.
315. SMELLIE, W. *A Treatise on the Theory and Practice of Midwifery.* London: Wilson, 1752, p. 140.
316. SMITH, A. D., R. D. GILBERT, R. J. LAMMERS, AND L. D. LONGO. Placental exchange area in guinea pigs following long-term maternal exercise: a stereological analysis. *J. Dev. Physiol. Oxf.* 5: 11–21, 1983.
317. SMITH, R. C., G. J. GARBUTT, R. E. ISAAKS, AND D. R. HARKNESS. Oxygen binding of fetal and adult bovine hemoglobin in the presence of organic phosphates and uric acid ribose. *Hemoglobin* 3: 47–55, 1979.
318. SOBREVILLA, L. A., M. T. CASSINELLI, A. CARCELEN, AND J. M. MALAGA. Human fetal and maternal oxygen tension and acid-base status during delivery at high altitude. *Am. J. Obstet. Gynecol.* 111: 1111–1118, 1971.
319. STENGER, V., D. EITZMAN, T. ANDERSON, C. DE PADUA, I. GESSNER, AND H. PRYSTOWSKY. Observations on the placental exchange of the respiratory gases in pregnant women at cesarean section. *Am. J. Obstet. Gynecol.* 88: 45–47, 1964.
320. STOCKELL, A., M. F. PERUTZ, H. MUIRHEAD, AND S. C. GLAUSER. A comparison of adult and foetal horse haemoglobins. *J. Mol. Biol.* 3: 112–116, 1961.
321. SWENSON, E. R., AND T. H. MAREN. A quantitative analysis of CO_2 transport at rest and during maximal exercise. *Respir. Physiol.* 35: 129–159, 1978.
322. SWIERCZEWSKI, E., AND A. MINKOWSKI. Le pouvoir oxyphorique (ou capacité en oxyène) du sang artériel foetal. *Etud. Neo-Natales* 5: 11–17, 1956.
323. TAFANI, A. La circulation dans le placenta de quelques mammiferes. *Arch. Ital. Biol.* 8: 49–57, 1887.
324. TAKENAKA, O., AND H. MORIMOTO. Oxygen equilibrium characteristics of adult and fetal hemoglobin of Japanese monkey (*Macaca fuscata*). *Biochim. Biophys. Acta* 446: 457–462, 1976.
325. TAUTZ, C., AND E. KLEIHAUER. Gibt es ein fetales Hämoglobin beim Schwein? II. Analysen des Globins. *Res. Exp. Med.* 159: 44–49, 1972.
326. THORNBURG, K. L., J. M. BISSONNETTE, AND J. J. FABER. Absence of fetal placental waterfall phenomenon in chronically prepared fetal lambs. *Am. J. Physiol.* 230: 886–892, 1976.
327. TORRANCE, J., P. JACOBS, A. RESTREPO, J. ESCHBACH, C. LENFANT, AND C. A. FINCH. Intraerythrocytic adaptation to anemia. *N. Engl. J. Med.* 283: 165–169, 1970.
328. TREMBLAY, P. C., S. SYBULSKI, AND G. B. MAUGHAN. Role of the placenta in fetal malnutrition. *Am. J. Obstet. Gynecol.* 91: 597–605, 1965.
329. TWEEDDALE, P. M. Blood oxygen affinities of the adult and foetal large white pig. *Respir. Physiol.* 19: 145–152, 1973.
330. TWEEDDALE, P. M. DPG and the oxygen affinity of maternal and foetal pig blood and haemoglobins. *Respir. Physiol.* 19: 12–18, 1973.
331. TYUMA, I., AND K. SHIMIZU. Different response to organic phosphates of human fetal and adult hemoglobins. *Arch. Biochem. Biophys.* 129: 404–405, 1969.
332. VALERI, C. R., AND N. L. FORTIER. Red-cell 2,3-diphosphoglycerate and creatine levels in patients with red-cell mass deficits or with cardiopulmonary insufficiency. *N. Engl. J. Med.* 281: 1452–1455, 1969.
333. VERSMOLD, H., AND K. P. RIEGEL. The effect of methemoglobin on the equilibrium between oxygen and the hemoglobins F and A_1 at different concentrations of 2,3-diphosphoglycerate (Abstract). *Pediatr. Res.* 8: 140, 1974.
334. VERSMOLD, H., G. SEIFERT, AND K. P. RIEGEL. Blood oxygen affinity in infancy: the interaction of fetal and adult hemoglobin, oxygen capacity, and red cell hydrogen ion and 2,3-diphosphoglycerate concentration. *Respir. Physiol.* 18: 14–25, 1973.
335. WAGNER, P. D. Diffusion and chemical reaction in pulmonary gas exchange. *Physiol. Rev.* 57: 257–312, 1977.
336. WAKULENKO, J. L. Zur Frage nach der Zusammensetzung und den Eigenschaften des Nabelvenenblutes im Momente der Geburt. *Arb. Med. Chem. Lab. K. Univ. Tomsk* 2: 1, 1910.
337. WALKER, J., AND E. P. N. TURNBULL. Haemoglobin and red cells in the human foetus and their relation to the oxygen content of the blood in the vessels of the umbilical cord. *Lancet* 2: 312–318, 1953.
338. WATERS, R. M., AND J. W. HARRIS. Carbon dioxide and oxygen problems in obstetric anesthesia. *Anesth. Analg.* 10: 59–63, 1931.
339. WELLS, R. M. G. Haemoglobin-oxygen affinity in developing embryonic erythroid cells of the mouse. *J. Comp. Physiol.* 129: 333–338, 1979.
340. WIDNESS, J. A., H. C. SCHWARTZ, C. B. KAHN, W. OH, AND R. SCHWARTZ. Glycohemoglobin in diabetic pregnancy: a sequential study. *Am. J. Obstet. Gynecol.* 136: 1024–1029, 1980.
341. WIDNESS, J. A., H. C. SCHWARTZ, D. THOMPSON, C. B. KAHN, W. OH, AND R. SCHWARTZ. Haemoglobin A_{Ic} (glycohaemoglobin) in diabetic pregnancy: an indicator of glucose control and foetal size. *Br. J. Obstet. Gynaecol.* 85: 812–817, 1978.
342. WILBUR, W. J., G. G. POWER, AND L. D. LONGO. Water exchange in the placenta: a mathematical model. *Am. J. Physiol.* 235 (*Regulatory Integrative Comp. Physiol.* 4): R181–R199, 1978.
343. WILKENING, R. B., S. ANDERSON, L. MARTENSSON, AND G. MESCHIA. Placental transfer as a function of uterine blood flow. *Am. J. Physiol.* 242 (*Heart Circ. Physiol.* 11): H429–H436, 1982.
344. WILKENING, R. B., AND G. MESCHIA. Fetal oxygen uptake, oxygenation, and acid-base balance as a function of uterine blood flow. *Am. J. Physiol.* 244 (*Heart Circ. Physiol.* 13): H749–H755, 1983.
345. WINDLE, W. F. *Physiology of the Fetus. Origin and Extent of Function in Prenatal Life.* Philadelphia, PA: Saunders, 1940.
346. WINICK, M., A. COSCIA, AND A. NOBLE. Cellular growth in human placenta. I. Normal placental growth. *Pediatrics* 39: 248–251, 1967.
347. WINTROBE, M. M., AND H. B. SCHUMACKER, JR. Comparison of hematopoiesis in the fetus and during recovery from pernicious anemia. Together with a consideration of the relationship of fetal hematopoiesis to macrocytic anemia of pregnancy and anemia in infants. *J. Clin. Invest.* 14: 837–852, 1935.
348. WINTROBE, M. M., AND H. B. SHUMACKER, JR. Erythrocyte studies in the mammalian fetus and newborn. Erythrocyte counts, hemoglobin and volume of packed red corpuscles, mean corpuscular volume, diameter and hemoglobin content, and proportion of miniature red cells in the blood of fetuses and newborn of the pig, rabbit, cat, dog, and man. *Am. J. Anat.* 58: 313–328, 1936.
349. WOOD, W. G., C. BUNCH, S. KELLY, Y. GUNN, AND G. BRECKON. Control of haemoglobin switching by a developmental clock? *Nature Lond.* 313: 320–323, 1985.
350. WULF, H. Der Gasaustausch in der reifen Placenta des Menschen. *Z. Geburtshilfe Gynaekol.* 158: 117–134, 1962.
351. WYNN, R. M., M. PANIGEL, AND A. H. MACLENNAN. Fine structure of the placenta and fetal membranes of the baboon. *Am. J. Obstet. Gynecol.* 109: 638–648, 1971.
352. YOUNG, D. C., R. POPAT, E. R. LUTHER, K. E. SCOTT, AND W. D. R. WRITER. Influence of maternal oxygen administration of the term fetus before labor. *Am. J. Obstet. Gynecol.* 136: 321–324, 1980.
353. ZACHARIAN, P. K., Q. P. LEE, K. G. SYMMS, AND M. R. JUCHAU. Further studies on the properties of human placental microsomal cytochrome P-450. *Biochem. Pharmacol.* 25: 793–800, 1976.

CHAPTER 19

Gas exchange in hypoxia, apnea, and hyperoxia

STEPHEN M. CAIN | *Department of Physiology and Biophysics, University of Alabama at Birmingham, Birmingham, Alabama*

CHAPTER CONTENTS

THIS CHAPTER FOCUSES on the adaptation of the physiological relationships governing gas exchange at the lung and the tissues to meet the stresses imposed by hypoxia, apnea, and hyperoxia. All responses to stress are not necessarily adaptive. For example, O_2 demand can be increased at the same time that O_2 uptake ($\dot{V}_{O_2}$) is limited during hypoxia. Diving mammals, on the other hand, may be able to shut off O_2-consuming processes temporarily as an adaptive response during apnea, with no consequent stimulation of anaerobiosis or mandatory repayment of O_2 during recovery. As a secondary result of yet another adaptive response, hyperoxia may decrease tissue $\dot{V}_{O_2}$ as blood is diverted through peripheral shunts. This might preserve tissue partial pressure of O_2 (P_{O_2}) within acceptable limits. The question of why tissues use the O_2 that they do, particularly during stress, is the theme of this chapter.

HYPOXIA

Hypoxia is defined in this chapter as any situation in which the supply of O_2 to a cell, tissue, organ, or the whole body is insufficient to meet the O_2 demand. Decreased O_2 supply may be the result of a lowered partial pressure of O_2 in arterial blood (Pa_{O_2}) (hypoxic hypoxia), a decreased rate of transport because of a lesser rate of blood flow (stagnant hypoxia), or a decreased O_2-carrying capacity in blood (anemic hypoxia).

Critical Partial Pressure of O_2

An insufficient supply of O_2 to meet O_2 demand can be quantified as the P_{O_2} at which $\dot{V}_{O_2}$ becomes less than the normoxic control value. This has been called the critical P_{O_2}. At any P_{O_2} above critical, $\dot{V}_{O_2}$ is independent of P_{O_2}, but $\dot{V}_{O_2}$ is directly dependent on P_{O_2} below the critical value. Because of the progressive decrease in P_{O_2} at each step of the O_2 transport chain, critical P_{O_2} depends on the site at which that P_{O_2} is measured in a hypoxic individual.

Oxygen is used in the mitochondrion by the electron transport chain that combines it with protons and in the process phosphorylates available ADP to ATP. This is the principal energy-producing system of the body. Molecular O_2 diffuses to cytochrome *c* oxidase (cytochrome aa_3) in the mitochondrion, where it enters the chain. Therefore the first critical P_{O_2} to consider is the Michaelis constant (K_m) of cytochrome aa_3, which is 0.05 mmHg P_{O_2} (39). Besides having a very great affinity for O_2, cytochrome aa_3 is present in high concentration inside the mitochondrion, so that it seldom becomes a limiting factor in $\dot{V}_{O_2}$ except possibly at maximal rates of energy expenditure (39, 81, 82). For O_2 transport to the tissues, cytochrome aa_3 acts as an infinite "sink" for O_2, so that all available O_2 can be used according to the energy demand. The energy demand, on the other hand, is set by the availability of protons shuttled into the mitochondrion and by the availability of ADP there. Outside the mitochondrion, substrate availability, glycolytic rate, and a sufficient diffusion gradient for O_2 to the mitochondrion may also limit energy production, primarily by the supply of O_2 and protons to cytochrome aa_3.

Cytochrome aa_3 accounts for only ~80% of O_2 consumed at rest. Other oxidases and oxygenases in the body account for the remaining 20% and act on many biochemical functions in both parenchymal cells and smooth muscle cells (39, 103). These activities range from detoxification processes in the liver to a ubiquitous step in catecholamine biosynthesis (tyrosine hydroxylase) that oxidizes tyrosine to dopa. The K_m for tyrosine hydroxylase is 8 mmHg P_{O_2} and other oxidases and oxygenases have K_m values ranging up to 57 mmHg P_{O_2}. Mills and Jöbsis (87) have even described an aberrant cytochrome aa_3 in the carotid body that was fully reduced at P_{O_2} of 7 mmHg. These other oxidative functions, with their much lower affinities for O_2, would decrease activity with the onset of tissue hypoxia well in advance of any slowing of oxidative phosphorylation. Loss of these extramitochondrial functions could be important in local responses to hypoxia, but very little is known about this area. The ~20% of resting $\dot{V}_{O_2}$ devoted to these functions conceivably could be shut off during short-term, acute hypoxia as a form of O_2 conservation with no untoward effects. More experiments are needed in which $\dot{V}_{O_2}$ during hypoxia is closely controlled so that it falls no more than 10% or 20% from the normoxic control level. Then essentiality of all the O_2 that was used could be examined for measurable functions, tissue P_{O_2}, or metabolic consequences, such as lactate production or catecholamine turnover rates. Because of these other ultimate O_2 consumers and their differing affinities, a single value for critical P_{O_2} cannot be defined even at the subcellular level.

If the whole body, a region, or an organ system is considered, a critical P_{O_2} could be measured at the supply side of O_2 delivery as Pa_{O_2}. Arterial P_{O_2} is useful to characterize a P_{O_2} lower than normal in inspired gas or some serious inefficiency of oxygenating venous blood in the lung, but it has no value as a yardstick for the effects of anemia or stagnant hypoxia on $\dot{V}_{O_2}$. Venous P_{O_2}, on the other hand, would represent the lowest vascular P_{O_2} available for a diffusion gradient to supply O_2 to tissues. Tenney (114) evaluated venous P_{O_2} as an estimator of mean tissue P_{O_2} by applying the Krogh model of uniform and unidirectional capillary blood flow supplying cylinders of tissue. He found that venous P_{O_2} is a reasonably close estimator of tissue P_{O_2}, particularly if perfused capillary density increases, but that it can be misleading if density is below the normal range. In his analysis of the various causes of tissue hypoxia, he concluded that venous P_{O_2} would overestimate tissue P_{O_2} in anemic hypoxia but would underestimate it in hypoxic hypoxia.

As an example of the difficulty that can be encountered with the use of mixed venous P_{O_2}, Cain (21) obtained two different critical values in anesthetized dogs during anemic and hypoxic hypoxia. Critical mixed venous P_{O_2} was 45 mmHg in anemic hypoxia and 17 mmHg in hypoxic hypoxia. According to Tenney (114), the critical average tissue P_{O_2} values must have been more widely different. When the percent of control $\dot{V}_{O_2}$ during hypoxia was graphed against the total O_2 transported to the tissue (cardiac output times arterial O_2 content), a single linear relationship was found for the two kinds of hypoxia below a value of 9.8 $ml \cdot kg^{-1} \cdot min^{-1}$. Above that value, $\dot{V}_{O_2}$ was constant and independent of total O_2 transport. The evidence suggested that O_2 transport to tissues in these two forms of hypoxia was not a diffusion-limited process because two very different driving pressures for O_2 diffusion existed when $\dot{V}_{O_2}$ became dependent on supply. Even inert-gas exchange has been shown to be limited by perfusion rather than by diffusion at the tissue level (91), so the idea was not novel. In resting muscle, for example, $\dot{V}_{O_2}$ can be supplied by a P_{O_2} gradient from the capillary of 0.3–1.4 mmHg (39). Capillary recruitment during hypoxia could reduce the necessary gradient to even less because reduction of intercapillary distance is the most effective way to improve tissue oxygenation (114). A reduction of intercapillary distance from 100 μm to 50 μm, for example, decreases the P_{O_2} gradient from the capillary to one-sixth (39). In his comparison of anemic and hypoxic hypoxia, Cain (21) proposed that local feedback control of O_2 transport kept it closely proportional to O_2 demand, once $\dot{V}_{O_2}$ became supply limited. This increased the O_2 extraction from blood by the tissue and accounted for the observed linear relationship between $\dot{V}_{O_2}$ and total O_2 transport. The total O_2 transport is a better index of adequate tissue O_2 supply than the critical P_{O_2}. The slope of the line that relates $\dot{V}_{O_2}$ to total transport is actually the O_2 extraction ratio. Attainment of a maximum extraction ratio then becomes a sign that compensatory adjustments to preserve tissue oxygenation had been fully employed. At that point in experiments on anesthetized dogs, O_2 extraction from arterial blood was >80% complete during both anemic hypoxia (22) and hypoxic hypoxia (23). Comparisons of critical P_{O_2} may be useful, but the physiological significance of a single value for critical P_{O_2} is questionable at best.

Oxygen Demand

As stated earlier (see *Critical Partial Pressure of O_2*, p. 403) the demand for energy, and hence O_2, is set by the availability of ADP and protons under normal conditions of oxygenation. In small mammals such as the rat and cat, however, resting muscle $\dot{V}_{O_2}$ even in normoxia can depend on blood flow. Honig et al. (57) reported that denervation of rat gracilis muscle increased blood flow markedly but kept O_2 extraction constant, so that $\dot{V}_{O_2}$ increased with flow. Whalen et al. (122) varied blood flow in autoperfused soleus and gracilis muscles of cats and found that $\dot{V}_{O_2}$ changed with flow. Others have found no such supply dependency of muscle $\dot{V}_{O_2}$ in dogs during normoxia (40, 110). Honig (56) suggested that O_2 supply dependency of muscle in small mammals is a means of controlling nonshivering thermogenesis and is important in temperature regulation. For small mammals, which have a high ratio of surface area to mass, the ability to control heat production by neural control of blood flow to the periphery may have merit for resting temperature regulation. Even larger mammals, such as the dog, can exhibit supply dependency of resting muscle $\dot{V}_{O_2}$. Durán and Renkin (40) noted that such dependency was found whenever autoregulation of blood flow was absent in muscle. Whalen et al. (122) pointed out that autoregulation was weak or absent in their cat muscle preparation. The reason for this association of lack of autoregulation with supply dependency of muscle $\dot{V}_{O_2}$ is frustratingly obscure. Explanations such as disturbance of cellular architecture or some form of cellular injury by humoral means may vaguely suggest a possible mechanism but are hardly definitive.

Alteration of $\dot{V}_{O_2}$ with flow may have some very real clinical significance if it indicates an alteration in O_2 demand. In a study of the physiological consequences of positive end-expiratory pressure in the treatment of patients with adult respiratory distress syndrome (ARDS), Powers et al. (97) saw that whole-body $\dot{V}_{O_2}$ increased linearly with total O_2 transport to the tissue. This was not just improving O_2 transport, which might have been limiting peripheral O_2 utilization. In these very sick patients, O_2 demand was evidently much higher than expected and no plateau was seen as O_2 transport increased. Danek et al. (33) obtained similar results in ARDS patients. They found a linear increase in $\dot{V}_{O_2}$ with increased O_2 transport; however, in patients without ARDS and over a similar range of $\dot{V}_{O_2}$ and O_2 transport, no such regular relationship was found. The cellular injury that manifests itself as ARDS may have a peripheral effect that causes normal regulation of cellular energy utilization to go awry. The absence of autoregulation and the supply dependency of $\dot{V}_{O_2}$ in muscle preparations and in ARDS patients may have a common link, possibly in mitochondrial function. That common link, if it exists, remains to be demonstrated experimentally. [Cain (21a) has recently reviewed O_2 supply dependency in ARDS more thoroughly.]

The fact that hypoxia itself can alter demand complicates considerations of the balance between O_2 supply and demand in the body. Nahas et al. (90) obtained an early hint of this in paralyzed, mechanically ventilated dogs bled 25 ml/kg. Oxygen uptake increased significantly during the hypovolemic period, but that increase was not observed after treatment with butoxamine or with concurrent hypercapnic acidosis. Both butoxamine and acidosis are known to inhibit the metabolic changes induced by catecholamines (98). The authors attributed the stimulation of $\dot{V}_{O_2}$ to the calorigenic action of catecholamines that are released as a result of sympathoadrenergic responses to hemorrhage.

In another form of hypoxia, Cain (21) found an increase in $\dot{V}_{O_2}$ of anesthetized, pump-ventilated dogs when hematocrit was lowered below 20% by isovolemic hemodilution with dextran. At that time, total O_2 transport to the tissue was approximately halved and mixed venous P_{O_2} was significantly lowered. Part of the increase in $\dot{V}_{O_2}$ was thought to be due to the increased O_2 demand of the heart. There was evidence, however, that some of the increase was also attributable to increased O_2 demand by skeletal muscle (see next section).

One question that arises from the results obtained during hemorrhage and anemia is whether any further increase in $\dot{V}_{O_2}$ was limited by O_2 availability. The tissue requirement for O_2 can no longer be known once $\dot{V}_{O_2}$ becomes limited by the supply of O_2. At that point the energy demand may actually exceed the energy produced. Stimulation of glycolysis and an increase in body lactate levels are consequences of an imbalance between energy supply and demand. As ADP/ATP ratios increase, inhibition of phosphofructokinase activity is relieved and glycolysis proceeds toward lactate. Mitochondrial electron transport chains are slowed by lack of O_2, and pyruvate must act as a proton acceptor to maintain levels of NAD that in turn maintain glycolysis. The pyruvate-lactate redox potential is the lowest in the chain, and lactate accumulates until mitochondrial metabolism is restored to full oxidative potentials. The net result of this anaerobic metabolism is 2 ATP/mol of glucose, which is only ~5% of the ATP realized from the fully oxidized molecule. Anaerobic metabolism as a continuing source of ATP during total anoxia may be important to maintain some cellular functions, but it falls short of normoxic energy requirements. Lactate accumulation therefore has served traditionally as an index of tissue hypoxia and a sign that tissue energy demand has exceeded energy production.

The lactate level in blood is a common index of tissue hypoxia because blood is readily sampled and measured. The lactate level in arterial or mixed venous blood is assumed to parallel the mean tissue level of lactate. This assumption has been challenged for various regional circulations (30). Without global hypoxia, lactate produced by a region of hypoxic tissue could serve as a substrate for a better-oxygenated region. The levels in blood therefore represent the balance between regions producing and using lactate. In global hypoxia, all tissues would presumably produce lactate. Whether or not lactate readily diffuses into blood has also been questioned (30). Evidence that it diffuses freely was obtained from biopsies of the muscles of animals that were exercised until they produced lactate. The lactate levels in venous blood draining the muscle and in the biopsy samples did not differ significantly (108). Therefore, in global hypoxia, the blood lactate levels generally reflect tissue events quite accurately.

Another objection to the use of blood lactate levels to assess imbalance of energy supply and demand is that lactate levels are affected by pH. Respiratory alkalosis will increase arterial lactate levels even though tissue oxygenation remains adequate (46). The mechanism is thought to be a generalized stimulation of glycolysis by pH-sensitive enzymes, such as phosphofructokinase, and a parallel rise in pyruvate is a consequence. For unexplained reasons, the principal source of lactate during respiratory alkalosis appears to be restricted to red blood cells. Regional venous sampling from all major organ systems failed to demonstrate any production of lactate when anesthetized dogs were made alkalotic by hyperventilation (126). Red blood cells, however, increased lactate production even in vitro when pH was increased. This fact helped to explain a set of observations in which rates of increase in blood lactate and a calculated quantity called excess lactate were compared with rates of O_2 deficit accumulation during severe hypoxia (20). Oxygen deficit was calculated as the difference between the $\dot{V}_{O_2}$ during hypoxia and the $\dot{V}_{O_2}$ measured before hypoxia began. Excess lactate (XL) was calculated as the lactate value at time n during hypoxia (L_n) less that which could be accounted for by a mass-action relationship with pyruvate at the same time (P_n) if the prehypoxic value of lactate to pyruvate (L_0/P_0) had not changed [$XL = L_n - P_n(L_0/P_0)$]. Lactate increased more than excess lactate for a given rate of O_2 deficit as a function of increasing pH. The ratio of excess lactate to lactate increase approached unity as pH decreased to 6.9. An argument was developed for excess lactate as a more useful quantifier of an imbalance between tissue energy demand and supply than just the increase in blood lactate because excess lactate corrected for red cell lactate production, which is not affected by O_2 supply but is influenced by pH.

Cain (18) used excess lactate as an index of tissue energy imbalance to show that energy demand actually increased during hypoxic hypoxia severe enough to curtail $\dot{V}_{O_2}$. Even though O_2 deficit accumulated at a linear rate, excess lactate had an upward inflection when >90% of the total O_2 stores had been used and there were no further rapid changes in O_2 stores. The increase in energy demand therefore occurred with the full development of tissue hypoxia. In animals given propranolol to block β-adrenergic receptors, excess lactate maintained a linear relationship with O_2 deficit. The conclusion was that the sympathoadrenal response to fully developed tissue hypoxia caused increased catecholamine calorigenesis that in turn increased energy demand when $\dot{V}_{O_2}$ was already limited by its supply. The calculation of O_2 deficit, with its dependence on extrapolation of the base line for $\dot{V}_{O_2}$ during severe hypoxia, would not measure the actual energy deficit being incurred unless there had been no changes in energy demand. This condition is seldom satisfied in any form of hypoxia unless special measures are taken, such as β-adrenergic blockade, to prevent the calorigenic effect of catecholamines (16).

Another factor that can alter energy demand during hypoxia is the respiratory alkalosis that often results from hypoxic stimulation of ventilation. When pH was elevated, $\dot{V}_{O_2}$ increased in passively hyperventilated dogs in which increased work of breathing was not a factor (17). This helped explain the greater rise in excess lactate associated with a given O_2 deficit in hypocapnic dogs versus hypercapnic dogs that were also hypoxic (15). Excess lactate indicated once again that the energy deficit can be underestimated by the O_2 deficit. Hypoxia stimulates ventilation, causing respiratory alkalosis, and increases sympathoadrenergic activity. Because alkalosis and catecholamines both increase energy demand when oxidative production of energy is limited by O_2 supply, these responses are hardly adaptive to hypoxia.

Regional Gas Exchange During Hypoxia

With a reduction in Pa_{O_2}, the peripheral chemoreceptors (aortic and carotid bodies) are stimulated, which results in vasoconstriction of peripheral areas. Peripheral vascular resistance actually doubled in unanesthetized dogs when carotid chemoreceptors alone were stimulated (127). Initially the heart and brain are perfused at the expense of the periphery during periods when O_2 supply is curtailed, which occurs in diving mammals (see *Aquatic Mammals*, p. 409) to an even greater degree. The different major regions of the body therefore may fare quite differently during hypoxia.

BRAIN. Brain perfusion increased much more in anesthetized rats than did skeletal muscle blood flow while rats were ventilated with a mixture of 10% O_2 in N_2 (118). Brain P_{O_2} consequently fell much less. The addition of 5% CO_2 to the breathing mixture only accentuated the preferential distribution of blood flow to the brain during hypoxia. Kerem and Elsner (68) showed in anesthetized dogs that the critical P_{O_2} for cerebral $\dot{V}_{O_2}$ was lower in hypercapnic hypoxia (asphyxia) than in normocapnic hypoxia. Saggital sinus P_{O_2} was 9 mmHg in asphyxia when brain $\dot{V}_{O_2}$ began to decrease, but it was 13 mmHg if arterial partial pressure of CO_2 (Pa_{CO_2}) was kept near the normoxic level. The vasomotor effects of partial pressure of CO_2 (P_{CO_2}) on cerebral circulation interacted with the effect of brain hypoxia to increase blood flow when P_{CO_2} was raised and to decrease it if P_{CO_2} was decreased by hyperventilation.

In isolated dog brains perfused at a constant rate, Fitzpatrick et al. (45) correlated electroencephalogram (EEG) frequencies with brain $\dot{V}_{O_2}$ as Pa_{O_2} was decreased. The critical venous P_{O_2} in these experiments was ~25 mmHg, but there was no increase of lactate output or glucose uptake as $\dot{V}_{O_2}$ declined (45). Similarly there was no decrease in energy charge or any increase in $NADH/NAD^+$ ratios in anesthetized rats as cerebral venous P_{O_2} was lowered to 10 mmHg by hypoxic hypoxia (84). Bicher (10) found electrical silence in areas of the brain quite distal to a region of localized hypoxia. He postulated a brain tissue O_2 sensor that actively inhibits neuronal firing as a reflex protective and energy conservation mechanism when the brain is challenged by insufficient O_2 supply. This idea was based on his finding that lowering P_{O_2} only in the right cortex of cats produced a period of silence in neuronal activity of the contralateral cortex. He interpreted this as active inhibition emanating from the hypoxic area. The brain consumes O_2 at least five times faster than the whole body per kilogram, and thus a mechanism for shutting off less vital functions in the brain on a local basis makes as much sense as diverting blood flow from skeletal muscle to increase brain O_2 supply. He also noted some increase in glycolytic activity across the brain. The idea that within an organ system, the brain in particular, there could be selective oxygenation or even a facultative decrease in local O_2 demand by a decrease in activity is very attractive. Unfortunately there is little evidence to support this idea.

HEART. The heart extracts ~75% of the O_2 presented to it with the body at rest and in a normoxic state. Its principal response to any decrease in arterial O_2 content therefore is to increase coronary blood flow and to shorten intercapillary distances. In the rat heart, for example, ventilation with hypoxic gas mixtures for as little as 20 s doubled the number of perfused capillaries, and this response was shown to be a direct effect of lowered tissue P_{O_2} (13). The efficacy of shortening intercapillary distance during hypoxia to preserve tissue oxygenation was pointed out earlier in *Critical Partial Pressure of O_2*, p. 403. Maximum O_2 extraction by myocardium of anesthetized dogs was increased to ~85% whether the heart was stressed by decreased coronary blood flow (34) or by isovolemic hemodilution (60). Myocardial $\dot{V}_{O_2}$ decreased and contractile force decreased with each decrement in coronary blood flow. The functional consequence of decreasing coronary blood flow was much more apparent than it was with other means of decreasing O_2 transport to the heart. In experimental hemorrhagic shock to the whole animal, on the other hand, coronary blood flow was maintained despite a lowering of mean aortic pressure to 35 mmHg (12). In those experiments, myocardial $\dot{V}_{O_2}$ was actually increased significantly during the compensatory phase of hemorrhagic shock, an effect attributed to calorigenic effects of catecholamines on the heart.

The demands placed on the heart by the whole body when subjected to a hypoxic challenge are especially noticeable during anemic hypoxia. Primarily as a result of lowered viscosity, cardiac output increases as peripheral vascular resistance decreases (25). In a resting but conscious dog, every lowering of hematocrit increased coronary blood flow, decreased coronary vascular resistance, and increased myocardial $\dot{V}_{O_2}$ (100). The limiting factor in the dog's ability to compensate for the loss of O_2-carrying capacity was in fact the maximal dilation of the coronary bed. This occurred at a hematocrit of ~10%.

The heart's increased O_2 demand during hypoxia may not be related only to an increased work load or to metabolic actions of catecholamines. Powers and Powell (96) reported that when heart rate and cardiac output were controlled in anesthetized dogs during progressive steps of hypoxic hypoxia, myocardial $\dot{V}_{O_2}$ increased as arterial O_2 content was decreased to 6 ml/dl. Below that value, $\dot{V}_{O_2}$ began to fall. The increase, however, did not depend on hemodynamic correlates because tension-time index, left ventricular end-diastolic pressure, left ventricular dP/d*t*, and mean ejection rates either stayed the same or decreased. Similar results were obtained in reserpinized dogs and in nonworking ventricles, which suggested that neither catecholamines nor altered myocardial blood flow distribution was involved in the increased myocardial $\dot{V}_{O_2}$ during hypoxia. The authors were unable to offer any alternative explanation. Apparently in any form of whole-body hypoxia the heart's need for O_2 can only increase, and its ability to satisfy that need may be a crucial factor in the body's capacity to compensate for a decrease in O_2 supply to all other tissues.

VISCERA. When hypoxia creates an energy imbalance, local metabolic factors can modify the initial vasoconstriction seen in many areas of the body other than heart and brain during hypoxic hypoxia. Shepherd (109) tested the metabolic model of intestinal autoregulation by perfusing isolated and denervated loops of canine small bowel with hypoxic blood at constant perfusion pressure. Without any extrinsic neural control of circulation, the gut responded with a prompt decrease in vascular resistance. Extraction of ^{86}Rb by the gut increased from 66% to 79%, which confirmed that the density of perfused capillaries also increased. The responses of both resistance and exchange vessels tended to maintain O_2 delivery to the gut during arterial hypoxia. The same general result was obtained with moderate hemodilution. Reduction of hematocrit to 22% increased gut conductance significantly, but in this case the O_2 extraction ratio changed very little because gut $\dot{V}_{O_2}$ was maintained by increased blood flow (73). The O_2 extraction ratio and effective capillary surface area usually change in parallel. Therefore a more intense anemic hypoxia may cause a greater change in O_2 extraction ratio. With stagnant hypoxia, however, the intestine was never able to extract >75% of the O_2 transported to it (83). The arteriovenous shunts in intestinal villi were thought to account for this lower maximum extraction ratio in the gut.

The liver of intact, anesthetized dogs reduced its lactate uptake whenever hepatic venous P_{O_2} fell below 24 mmHg, whether O_2 delivery was lowered by restricting blood flow or by lowering Pa_{O_2} (112). Unlike the whole body, liver function and $\dot{V}_{O_2}$ appeared to relate better to the hepatic venous P_{O_2} than to total O_2 transport. This may be partially because the liver shows little metabolic regulation of blood flow and relies more on increasing O_2 extraction. Indeed the immediate response to hypoxic hypoxia was to increase vascular resistance and to decrease total blood flow, but not markedly. Within 20 min total blood flow was back to the normoxic control level (59). Most of the changes were in hepatic artery flow, with portal vein flow remaining nearly constant. Similar responses were noted in the liver during anemic hypoxia (73) and during reduced perfusion when the liver's O_2 extraction ratio reached 97% (83). This response of the liver, which is different from that of gut, may be a functional adaptation to its role in the portal transport system. Flow would be largely regulated extrahepatically by the intestinal resistance vessels that show reactive hyperemia. A large increase in portal flow as a result of the intestinal resistance vessels dilating for nutritive reasons would cause a passive hyperemia in the liver, which could efficiently extract sufficient O_2 from the portal venous blood to perform the extra metabolic work required of it. Hepatic $\dot{V}_{O_2}$ never appeared to be stimulated in any form of hypoxia and only decreased as O_2 supply diminished to sufficiently low levels.

MUSCLE. Resting skeletal muscle is another peripheral region that is vasoconstricted by the carotid chemoreceptor reflex during hypoxia, particularly when ventilation is controlled (127). In anesthetized, pump-ventilated dogs, cardiac output increased by 20 min of severe hypoxia (Pa_{O_2} = 26 mmHg), but hindlimb skeletal muscle blood flow did not change until 40 min. During this period of time, $\dot{V}_{O_2}$ was decreased by the supply limitation (23). The sequence of vasoconstriction followed by gradual vasodilation is usually explained by the increased metabolic effect on vasomotor tone in O_2-deprived muscle. The first response to reflex vasoconstriction is in the precapillary sphincters (or their equivalent in skeletal muscle), which are thought to be more sensitive to the state of muscle oxygenation (47). This response increases effective exchange vessel surface area so that O_2 extraction increases without any net change in total blood flow to muscle. With prolonged tissue hypoxia, the proximal flow-controlling arterioles then dilate, so that vascular resistance decreases and flow increases.

Other factors have a role in the hierarchical control of blood flow in skeletal muscle. Cain and Chapler (23) showed that β-adrenergic blockade prevented delayed vasodilation in hypoxic hindlimb of anesthetized dogs. Because tissue hypoxia was just as intense as in the unblocked experiments, the metabolic vasodilatory factors were thought to have been equal in intensity. The difference was the activity of vasodilator β-adrenergic receptors. The same hypoxic stimulus to the peripheral chemoreceptors that causes vasoconstriction in the hindlimb can also stimulate the vasodilator receptors. Vasoconstriction is dominant, but this provides an actively counterpoised system that is more responsive to any additional vasodilator activity that may occur during tissue hypoxia. The O_2 extraction was as complete in the β-blocked dogs as in the unblocked dogs, which suggested that β-adrenergic blockade did not interfere with local control of exchange vessels, even though it affected resistance-vessel responses to severe hypoxia.

Similar responses of blood flow and femoral arterial conductance to the stagnant hypoxia of hemorrhagic shock have been noted (48). Baroreceptor stimulation was presumably responsible for the initial vasoconstriction that decreased as hypotension was prolonged. Granger et al. (47) have called this "autoregulatory escape from adrenergic control," and the process applied to both the more sensitive control over exchange vessels and resistance vessels. The additional vasodilator effect of β-adrenergic receptors was not specifically tested by β-blockade during hemorrhagic shock.

Hindlimb skeletal muscle did not show any tendency toward vasoconstriction during anemic hypoxia (22). Oxygen uptake was maintained despite hemodilution severe enough to decrease whole-body $\dot{V}_{O_2}$. Because the carotid chemoreceptor responds more to lowered P_{O_2} than to lowered O_2 content, it is possible that there was less reflex vasoconstrictor tone for anemic hypoxia than for a similar reduction in total O_2 transport by hypoxic hypoxia. Actually other experiments showed that even increasing vasoconstrictor tone with norepinephrine infusion during dilutional anemia did not increase peripheral vascular resistance (25). The greatly reduced viscosity of the diluted blood evidently masked the resistance change accompanying a change in resistance-vessel caliber. Chapler, Cain, and Stainsby (26) raised the possibility that chemoreceptor stimulation was present during anemic hypoxia as well because of their observation that anemia stimulated muscle $\dot{V}_{O_2}$ and that the stimulation was not seen after β-adrenergic blockade. The most likely mechanism suggested for increased sympathetic activity was the aortic chemoreceptor, which responds to lowered O_2 content in blood.

The response of skeletal muscle to hypoxia will certainly depend on the demand for O_2. Stainsby and Otis (110) showed that the in situ gastrocnemius-plantaris muscle group of the dog had a critical venous P_{O_2} of 25 mmHg at rest but that it decreased to 10 mmHg when the muscle was contracting, so that O_2 demand was increased eightfold. They used the Krogh-Erlanger equation to calculate that capillary density was increased much more by hypoxia when O_2 demand was high. The physiological consequence of that observation was nicely illustrated in experiments in which regional blood flow to respiratory muscles was compared with that in limb muscles of anesthetized rabbits breathing hypoxic gas mixtures. Blood flow to the limb was unchanged, but blood flow to diaphragm and intercostal muscles increased in a direct relationship with the severity of hypoxia (66). In animals paralyzed and ventilated passively, blood flow to respiratory muscle was only 10% of that in normoxic, free-breathing animals and was not changed during hypoxia. This is a reminder that within an organ system and even in the whole animal, regional O_2 supply is proportioned very precisely to O_2 demand during both hypoxia and normoxia when all regulatory systems are intact.

APNEA

Apnea is the cessation of effective respiratory movements, with the consequence that gas exchange between the body and ambient air stops. Breath holding is a voluntary apnea in which the neural drives to breathe are opposed until an involuntary breaking point occurs. Once apnea or breath holding begins, mandatory energy requirements of the body can be met only by using O_2 stores, energy stores such as phosphocreatine, or the inefficient energy production of anaerobic metabolism. Energy stores are relatively fixed anatomically, but O_2 stores can be mobilized and preferentially directed by circulatory control mechanisms. Other possibilities are to reduce energy requirements or to temporarily suspend functions using O_2 that are unnecessary for survival. The success with which these options are managed will govern the size of any energy deficit incurred during apnea and, in involuntary apnea, survival time. Comparisons between aquatic mammals that are specialized breath holders and terrestrial mammals like dogs and humans show the relative utility of the several options.

Aquatic Mammals

The most accomplished breath-holding mammals, such as seals and porpoises, live in aquatic environments. Scholander (107) and more recently Hochachka (53) have described the principal features of the adaptation of these fascinating animals to prolonged breath holds during diving. Gas exchange, as both authors point out, continues during a breath-hold dive, but the specialized aspects of the diving reflex greatly modify the rate of O_2 usage and its distribution in the whole animal. Hochachka explained that during a dive the marine mammal becomes a self-sustaining life-support system (53). The apnea, bradycardia, and peripheral vasoconstriction that are the major components of the diving reflex contribute to conservation of O_2 stores while still supporting vital functions.

Contrary to breath holding on land, lung gas exchange and gas stores are greatly minimized because deep-diving mammals, especially, exhale over half the lung volume before diving (70). The gas remaining in the lung is compressed during descent into the conducting airways, so that between compression and absorption atelectasis the alveolar gas volume is minimal. One practical outcome of this maneuver is the avoidance of compressing N_2 into blood and tissue. In experiments on Weddell, harbor, and elephant seals, Kooyman et al. (70) measured N_2 tensions of arterial and intravertebral venous blood while the animals were made to dive in a pressure chamber. Despite increases in pressure to 14.6 atmospheres absolute (ATA), blood N_2 pressure never exceeded 1.8 ATA, except for a brief peak in arterial blood of <4 ATA.

Ridgeway and Howard (102) found that trained free-diving porpoises (*Tursiops truncatus*) did not experience complete lung collapse until reaching depths below 70 m, based on N_2 washout measurements by an intramuscular mass-spectrometer probe. These same measurements also indicated that muscle perfusion was not decreased to the same extent as was circulation to blubber. Despite being an accomplished breath-hold diver, the porpoise does not seem to utilize lung collapse and peripheral vasoconstriction to avoid decompression sickness to the same extent as seals. How they avoid the untoward consequences of increased N_2 tensions in muscle as they reascend is not completely understood.

If lung O_2 stores do not play a major role in breath-hold diving, what is the magnitude of the nonlung O_2 stores in seals, for example? Packer et al. (92) addressed this question by quantifying exchangeable O_2 stores in the harbor seal using isotopic O_2. They also measured lung volumes and blood volumes, both during and after diving, by appropriate means. The blood volume measurements indicated that at least 95% of total blood volume was available to the central circulation during a dive, so that the bulk of the blood O_2 stores was also available for exchange during the dive. Because of their normally very high hematocrit (60%) and very large blood volume (125 ml/kg), the nonlung O_2 stores are mostly in the blood and are ~2.5 times those found in dogs and humans. The authors point out, however, that maximal diving time of seals is ~5 times that for humans, so that additional factors must still be sought to account for the difference.

Bradycardia and peripheral vasoconstriction are essential components of the O_2 conservation mechanism. In seals that fail to develop an arterial constrictor response or in which it is prevented pharmacologically, death occurs within 4 min of a dive (92). The rate of fall of Pa_{O_2} in another diving mammal, the nutria (*Myocastor coypus*), was more than doubled in the 1st min if the bradycardia was prevented by atropine or vagotomy (44). This also greatly hastened reaching the breaking point of the breath hold, which was a Pa_{O_2} of ~15 mmHg in both normal and vagotomized animals. Using radioactive microspheres, Zapol et al. (125) showed that Weddell seals decreased their cardiac output 86% during a dive. On a regional basis, splanchnic, peripheral, and coronary blood flow decreased 85%–90%. Adrenal blood flow, on the other hand, decreased only 39% and cerebral blood flow remained unchanged during a dive. This highly selective distribution of perfusion ensures the brain an adequate O_2 supply during a dive while reducing the O_2 need of the heart. Tissues that can function anaerobically, muscle especially, are left to do so. An increase in lung radioactivity indicated a large increase of peripheral arteriovenous shunting but may have included an increase of bronchial circulation. An increase in nutritive blood flow to the lung would have been supportive of the metabolic trade-off discussed next.

This metabolic trade-off was described by Murphy et al. (89) in another paper. The lung can be visualized as a mirror image of metabolism in the brain during a dive. By virtue of maintained perfusion and O_2 supply, the lung metabolizes lactate as a preferred carbon source and thus spares blood glucose for the brain. The heart readily utilizes lactate and thereby contributes to the glucose sparing. As Murphy et al. (89) describe it, the central organs are able to facilitate the transition from high-perfusion resting states to low-perfusion diving states by matching enzymatic apparatuses to their specific metabolic need in a cooperative and complementary manner. Their model is based on the metabolism of the three central organs not being O_2 limited. If the central organs are being supported at the expense of the periphery, the size and the nature of the O_2 deficit experienced by the periphery become the next logical concern. A question that can be asked at this point is whether all of the O_2 consumed by the periphery is obligated for preservation of tissue functions.

The results from restrained seals tilted into water to simulate diving have indicated that large amounts of lactate accumulate in the periphery and are washed out during recovery (53, 107). After a dive, there is an initial surge of $\dot{V}_{O_2}$ related to refilling depleted hemoglobin and myoglobin O_2 stores. The gas exchange ratio (R) is initially low as a result. As lactate is washed out by reperfusion of the periphery, CO_2 is released from blood bicarbonate stores and R rises. As recovery proceeds, R returns to the predive value. Kooyman et al. (69) noted in free-diving seals that for dives lasting <5 min, there were no changes in R; for dives of 5–20 min, R peaked by 5 min and returned to predive values by 15 min of recovery; and for dives of 20–70 min, R was still elevated even 30 min later. Similarly they reported that $\dot{V}_{O_2}$ returned rapidly to predive values after short dives but was still elevated 30 min after a dive of 70 min. They calculated the extra O_2 used during recovery and ascribed it to the use of O_2 stores during the dive. Because less O_2 was returned to stores than they calculated was used during the dive, they concluded that $\dot{V}_{O_2}$ during the dive must have been decreased almost 20% from the resting, predive control value. Robin et al. (104) found that only 47% of the O_2 deficit incurred during a 5-min dive by a seal was repaid. Is it possible, as Scholander (107) suggested, that diving mammals such as the seal may actually decrease metabolic energy demand during a dive? Some reduction in O_2 demand should be attributed to decreased work of heart and respiratory muscles during a dive, but that would not seem to be quantitatively sufficient to account for the measured deficit in repayment.

Kooyman et al. (71) extended their series of elegant experiments on free-diving Weddell seals and have provided additional evidence that energy requirement is actually less during a dive than at rest despite increased activity levels. They sampled arterial blood for lactate and measured pulmonary arterial temperature during rest and after dives that lasted up to >1 h. From these and their earlier studies (69, 70), the following picture emerges. The natural diving behavior of Weddell seals is to restrict most dives to <26 min (97.3% of 4,600 observations). For dive durations of <26 min, there was no significant increase of lactate in arterial blood during the dive or recovery period. The calculated O_2 stores or their replacement, as measured during recovery, would have sufficed for this period only if O_2 utilization was decreased. Because no lactate appeared, the decreased $\dot{V}_{O_2}$ must have been facultative rather than dictated by restriction of O_2 supply to the periphery. In other words, the seal apparently can turn off some portion of the metabolic energy chain. This conclusion is supported because core temperature decreased during diving despite less convective heat loss as blood flow to the periphery was restricted, and despite the greater activity entailed in swimming. Shivering was never noted in conjunction with decreases in core temperature. If energy demand were not throttled down, the resultant energy deficit would surely have driven anaerobic metabolism so that lactate would have been increased. Kooyman et al. (69) noted that seals and other aquatic mammals had resting metabolic rates 1.5–3 times those predicted by Kleiber's equation, which relates body size to metabolic rate for terrestrial mammals. They suggested that the seals might always be repaying O_2 debt at some slow, continual rate.

An alternative suggestion is that aquatic mammals generate heat to compensate for losses to the cold aquatic environment and that although they have superior insulative protection, this is not sufficient for thermal balance. Honig (56) made a similar suggestion for small mammals that have large surface areas relative to their mass and thus face a similar problem. The metabolic switch he proposed is the neural control of blood flow to the periphery, where $\dot{V}_{O_2}$ is flow dependent. Perhaps a similar situation is true for aquatic mammals. In both instances, the $\dot{V}_{O_2}$ so controlled is used to generate heat and represents a dispensable fraction of total metabolism that requires little or no repayment for the period that it is decreased. To explore that idea, experiments would have to be done with seals in a warmer environment that perhaps is more nearly thermoneutral than their natural environment. The idea that some portion of metabolism has as its sole purpose the generation of heat is highly speculative but could fit several widely diverse observations such as these for diving mammals.

Humans

Responses resembling the diving reflex in aquatic mammals have been demonstrated in humans, although they are less well developed in humans than in aquatic mammals. Breath holding in air will produce a very mild bradycardia in humans of ~3% reduction in heart rate (93). Face immersion may or may not slightly increase the bradycardia response to breath holding, but cold water has a very pronounced effect on heart rate (55, 65, 93). Divers tend to have a greater bradycardia response than nondivers, but hyperoxia or hypocapnia does not prevent bradycardia (43, 55). The general conclusion is that cold receptors in the face area are most responsible for the human's bradycardia response to immersion breath holding.

Another component of the diving reflex involves redistribution of blood flow away from the periphery to support heart, lungs, and brain. Two groups of workers were able to measure a decrease in forearm blood flow during breath holding by humans. In one study, forearm blood flow correlated with the fall in Pa_{O_2} during immersion breath holding (43). In the other study, breathing 10% O_2 in N_2 elicited the decrease in forearm blood flow with the face immersed or not (50). Lung movements have been reported to alter the effects of chemoreceptors by central interaction of pulmonary stretch receptors (2). Because breathing during immersion did not modify the decrease in forearm blood flow, the chemoreceptor role in the peripheral vasoconstrictor response of humans to breath holding needs to be evaluated further.

The length of a breath hold in humans is governed by the rates at which O_2 stores are used and CO_2 levels are increased. Mithoefer (88) and Hong et al. (54) described gas exchange during a breath hold. The rates of gas exchange between blood and lung and between blood and tissue are separate but linked cycles. The transfer of O_2 from lung to blood decreases progressively until the arteriovenous difference in O_2 content practically disappears by 4 min of breath holding with the lung filled to capacity with air (54). Tissue demands for O_2 are increasingly met by the blood stores of O_2. Initially there is a rapid movement of CO_2 into lung stores, but the arteriovenous P_{CO_2} difference disappears by 30 s. With O_2 still being used from the lung stores, lung volume shrinks and concentrates P_{O_2} and P_{CO_2}. Furthermore, as blood continues to be oxygenated in the lung, the Haldane effect actually reverses the usual gradient of alveolar partial pressure of CO_2 ($P_{A_{CO_2}}$) and Pa_{CO_2} to mixed venous P_{CO_2}. Higher Pa_{CO_2} decreases the transfer of CO_2 from tissue, whereas desaturation of hemoglobin at the tissue depresses tissue-to-blood P_{CO_2} differences. This in turn reinforces the cycle at the lung. If the breath hold occurs during diving, the added compression of lung volumes with descent further decreases the role of lung volume as a store for metabolically produced CO_2. End-tidal P_{CO_2} at the end of diving was significantly lower than that for similar breath holds in air (32).

Lin et al. (78) recognized the potentially more variable results relating P_{CO_2} to the voluntary breaking point of breath holding and used a different end point, which they called the involuntary ventilatory activity (IVA). The time to IVA was identified by esophageal pressure recording and correlated very well with $\dot{V}_{O_2}$, in contrast to the variability found between $\dot{V}_{O_2}$ and the conventional breaking point. The IVA was also considerably shorter than the conventional breaking point, and higher $P_{A_{CO_2}}$ values were found during exercise than at rest. Breath-holding time by IVA multiplied by $\dot{V}_{O_2}$ equaled a constant that was the amount of O_2 consumed during the breath hold. The onset of IVA was prolonged when breathing O_2, so that the amount consumed was greater at that time. The authors considered the IVA to be nonsubjective and dependent on both P_{CO_2} and $\dot{V}_{O_2}$ (78).

If the physiological breaking point represented by IVA is mostly dependent on the rate of $\dot{V}_{O_2}$ during the breath hold, the question may be asked whether O_2 demand is decreased during breath holding in humans as it apparently is in the seal. The same experimental approach has been used. If no O_2 is supplied from outside, then O_2 stores must be used during the breath hold. It is assumed that those stores are refilled during recovery from breath holding to the predive level. The difference between the breath-holding time multiplied by the prehold $\dot{V}_{O_2}$ and the O_2 used to replenish stores during recovery must represent any deficit incurred during the breath hold. Tibes and Stegemann (115) used this approach and observed that 21% of the incurred O_2 deficit during breath holding in air was not repaid during recovery. The deficit was on the average only 10% less during apneic immersion. Breathing while immersed did not decrease $\dot{V}_{O_2}$ (50). Craig and Medd (32) found no evidence that O_2 demand was decreased during apneic diving, but they did measure increased levels of lactate in blood during more active dives, which might have indicated a deficiency of O_2 supply relative to demand. The data are sparse and no firm answers can be given to the question of whether human O_2 demand is altered by breath holding or apneic diving. The literature does not strongly indicate that either O_2 transport limitation or some facultative decrease in $\dot{V}_{O_2}$ occurs in humans.

Other Terrestrial Mammals

Although anesthetized dogs show some semblance to the diving response of aquatic mammals, they display no particular ability to conserve O_2 during apnea or to lower tissue demand for O_2. Lin et al. (79) estimated $\dot{V}_{O_2}$ during 80 s of apnea in anesthetized dogs by measuring cardiac output and rates of change of O_2 content in arterial and mixed venous blood. They found that $\dot{V}_{O_2}$ continued at the same rate as the preapneic value. No measurable effect on $\dot{V}_{O_2}$ was noticed even if the heart worked less because of observed bradycardia.

Cain (19) obtained similar results in anesthetized and paralyzed dogs made apneic or ventilated with N_2. The end point for apnea or N_2 breathing was when arterial blood pressure began to fall rapidly. At that point either the ventilator was turned on again or the animal was again ventilated with room air. The end point was delayed more in apnea than in N_2 breathing because lung O_2 stores were not washed out of the lung during apnea. Despite the different times, arterial lactate levels rose at nearly the same value of mixed venous P_{O_2}. This mixed venous P_{O_2} value was also the value measured when available O_2 stores would have been used up if $\dot{V}_{O_2}$ continued at the same rate measured during the control period. In other words, the stimulation of anaerobic metabolism corresponded to the depletion of O_2 stores and thereby indicated no facultative decrease in O_2 demand. As soon as O_2 supply limited energy production, lactate appeared in the blood.

Cherniack et al. (28) tried to predict Pa_{O_2} and Pa_{CO_2} during apnea in anesthetized and paralyzed dogs and found that behavior of gas stores in the body did not conform to calculations based on metabolic rates, perfusion rates, and buffering capacities of the various compartments. The addition of selective vasoconstriction and increased anaerobic metabolism did not help the prediction model. When a critical P_{O_2} was assumed, below which $\dot{V}_{O_2}$ decreased because of supply limitation, arterial gas tensions were successfully predicted. Once again the need for O_2 appears to be immutable in the anesthetized and apneic dog.

Experiments with anesthetized dogs revealed how regional circulations may differ during apnea. In anesthetized dogs made apneic by clamping the tracheal hose after breathing O_2, the relative distribution of flow to caudal versus cranial areas was quantified by appropriately placed catheters (51). With a continuing source of O_2 during apnea, the Haldane effect minimized the availability of the lung as a CO_2 store and the gradient was quickly reversed so that CO_2 was retained in the tissues. The new information gained from these experiments was that CO_2 was transferred from caudal tissue to cranial tissue. The specific effect of increased P_{CO_2} was to increase cerebral blood flow and thus delay the rise in cranial tissue P_{CO_2}, which created a P_{CO_2} gradient between cranial and caudal regions. With time the cranial tissue actually gained CO_2 content from caudal regions and retained locally produced CO_2.

Kerem and Elsner (68) compared the brain's tolerance to apneic hypoxia and to hypoxic hypoxia in paralyzed dogs. Critical P_{O_2} was defined as the blood value at which reversible but distinctly characteristic signs of hypoxia appeared in the EEG. This critical P_{O_2} proved to be significantly lower in apnea than in hypoxic hypoxia, 9 mmHg versus 13 mmHg in sagittal sinus blood. This was attributed to the higher rates of cerebral blood flow that occurred with elevated Pa_{CO_2} in apnea. No venous-to-arterial difference in lactate was found across the brain, and the critical P_{O_2} for the brain occurred when >80% of O_2 stores had been used. Once again the dog and in particular its brain appear to function in a compulsively aerobic fashion.

Among the common laboratory animals, the rat most resembles aquatic mammals in its cardiovascular responses to head immersion. Lin and Baker (77) used radioactive microspheres in two separate series of experiments; they measured cardiac output in one series and its distribution to tissues in the other. Heart rate and cardiac output decreased >70% as total peripheral resistance increased fourfold. Coronary, cerebral, and bronchial circulations were unchanged, whereas circulations to intestines, spleen, kidney, and skin were decreased >95%. Muscle and liver blood flow were decreased ~50%. The cardiovascular responses of the rat were much closer in intensity and selectivity to those of the seal than those of the dog or human. Unfortunately no metabolic studies have been done. An interesting speculation at this point is whether the rat, like the seal, may be able to dispense with some portion of its O_2 demand when diving. Is that ability part of the full diving reflex?

HYPEROXIA

Hyperoxia is defined as a condition in which inspired P_{O_2} is increased above the tension obtainable breathing air at sea level. The increase can be achieved by enriching the fraction of O_2, by increasing total pressure, or by a combination of these two means. Hyperoxia has been used to measure pulmonary shunting and to study exercise limitation, for example. Hyperoxic effects have been a topic of primary investigation for those interested in diving, space, and hyperbaric medicine. Because the lung is a target organ for O_2 toxicity, all of the studies cited are well within acceptable exposure limits to avoid pulmonary O_2 toxicity (29, 37). These effects of hyperoxia on gas exchange therefore should not be due to any toxic disturbance of the alveolar-capillary membrane.

Effects at Rest

WHOLE BODY. No evidence has been found that resting $\dot{V}_{O_2}$ by the whole body can be increased by increasing P_{O_2} of inspired gas. Whether $\dot{V}_{O_2}$ is supply dependent is discussed earlier, particularly in *Oxygen Demand*, p. 404. Resting skeletal muscle in large mammalian species, such as the dog, displays no supply dependency if normal autoregulation is present (40, 110). In small mammalian species, such as the rat, resting muscle may be supply dependent (57). Because skeletal muscle accounts for 15%–20% of whole-body

$\dot{V}_{O_2}$ at rest, hyperoxia may have some small effect in the rat if the increase in O_2 dissolved in blood increased its transport to tissues. Breathing O_2 at 1 ATA did not alter $\dot{V}_{O_2}$ in humans (62), and no similar study on the rat was found. One other factor should be considered. At 1 and 2 ATA, O_2 has been reported to decrease cardiac output significantly in humans, primarily by a decrease in heart rate (41, 67). That would detract from the gain in dissolved O_2, so that little or no net gain in total O_2 transport may have occurred.

In contrast to results in the awake resting human, Chapler, Cain, and Stainsby (27) found that O_2 at 1 ATA decreased $\dot{V}_{O_2}$ by 7% in anesthetized dogs that were paralyzed and ventilated at constant rates. There was no apparent reason for this finding because O_2 transport should not have been a limiting factor. The authors speculated that peripheral chemoreceptor contribution to sympathetic tone may have been diminished by O_2 breathing, with a consequent small decrease in the calorigenic action of catecholamines. Although CO_2 output was not measured simultaneously in those experiments, it was in others on anesthetized greyhounds in which a 4% decrease was observed (106). Although $\dot{V}_{O_2}$ was not measured at the same time, the two sets of observations corroborate each other because the conditions of a steady state and constant ventilation were the same.

ORGAN SYSTEMS OTHER THAN PULMONARY. Hughes et al. (59) put flow probes around hepatic arteries and veins and portal veins of anesthetized greyhounds. When Pa_{O_2} was raised to 200, 300, and 400 mmHg, liver $\dot{V}_{O_2}$ tended to increase at all levels, but the increase was statistically significant only at 300 mmHg P_{O_2}. The authors suggested that O_2 transport to the liver was marginally inadequate, but that was not consistent with the lesser effect at 400 mmHg. Furthermore in the same study they examined the effects of hypoxia and found that the liver was able to extract more O_2 and increase its blood flow so that its $\dot{V}_{O_2}$ was not significantly decreased until Pa_{O_2} was lowered to 25 mmHg. That ability and its autoregulatory escape from an initial vasoconstrictor response to hypoxia also do not fit with the liver's acceptance of a marginally inadequate O_2 supply during normoxia.

Hindlimb skeletal muscle in the anesthetized dog decreased its blood flow when the animal was ventilated with O_2 at 1 ATA (9, 27). A similar result at both 1 and 2 ATA of O_2 was obtained in the human forearm (11). In one study the denervated but autoperfused dog hindlimb decreased its $\dot{V}_{O_2}$ despite a significant rise in femoral venous P_{O_2} (9).

Cerebral $\dot{V}_{O_2}$ has also been seen to decrease with hyperoxia. Lambertsen et al. (72) found a 12% decrease of cerebral $\dot{V}_{O_2}$ in supine humans during leg exercise while breathing O_2 at 2 ATA. That level of exercise at 1 ATA on air had been shown not to affect cerebral $\dot{V}_{O_2}$. The authors were unwilling to accept a decreased cerebral $\dot{V}_{O_2}$ with hyperoxia and ascribed it to an undetected error in measurement of cerebral blood flow. Jacobson et al. (60) obtained the same result in anesthetized dogs, however.

The depression of whole-body and regional $\dot{V}_{O_2}$ during steady-state conditions of hyperoxia, although by no means common, has been found frequently enough to warrant further comment. Except for toxic effects on enzymes, O_2 does not appear to exert a direct regulatory role on cellular metabolism unless its supply becomes limiting (100). That never occurred in hyperoxia if increased or maintained levels of total O_2 transport and venous P_{O_2} were accepted as proof of supply adequacy. Oxygen depresses respiration of tissue slices at pressures >1 ATA, and the brain was among the most sensitive tissues so tested (49). Such effects have been attributed to toxic actions of O_2 on various dehydrogenase and sulfhydryl enzymes, but those toxic effects were elicited at much higher P_{O_2} levels than that experienced by in vivo tissues in the experiments discussed in this section.

Peripheral shunting of blood flow is one other possible mechanism for the observed decrease in $\dot{V}_{O_2}$, particularly on a regional basis. Either direct or indirect effects of hyperoxia on vascular smooth muscle generally act to constrict arterioles and precapillary sphincters (38) or may more specifically act on terminal arterioles (80). If, in an effort to preserve tissue P_{O_2} at a more acceptable lower level, flow through nutritional vessels is reduced more than in shorter, thoroughfare vessels, then a shuntlike effect is created. That situation could have yielded a higher venous P_{O_2} in the face of a lower tissue $\dot{V}_{O_2}$. If hyperoxia has a physiological effect on regional or whole-body $\dot{V}_{O_2}$ that precedes any toxic effect, then a more complete explanation of its mechanism presents an intriguing challenge.

PULMONARY ORGAN SYSTEM. The lung is regarded as a target organ for O_2 toxicities because the alveolar-capillary membrane is in open communication with elevated P_{O_2} in the environment and consequently is exposed to a higher P_{O_2} than any other vital organ system. Occurrence or therapeutic applications of hyperoxia therefore have caused concern for alterations in the gas-exchange function of the lung. In addition, O_2 has been used to evaluate the contributions of circulatory shunting to alveolar-arterial differences in P_{O_2} ($PA_{O_2} - Pa_{O_2}$). The question has therefore arisen as to whether breathing O_2 itself alters shunting or the relative distributions of ventilation and perfusion in the lung. The toxic effects on the lung can be quantified by measurements of *1*) lung diffusing capacity and *2*) $PA_{O_2} - Pa_{O_2}$ and $Pa_{CO_2} - PA_{CO_2}$. Results have indicated that many of the changes are physiological rather than pathological.

Prolonged hyperoxia, such as O_2 breathing for 6–11 h at 2 ATA or up to 74 h at 1 ATA, caused decreases in lung diffusing capacity for CO (DL_{CO}) as measured by the single-breath method (24, 99). In one case the changes were attributed to alveolar edema formation and alterations in the air-blood barrier. In the other case there was a decrease in pulmonary capillary blood volume that was thought to be secondary to a toxic effect of O_2 on the pulmonary capillaries. In contrast, breathing O_2 at 3 ATA for 1 h increased Krogh's diffusion constant (K). That increase in K was suggested to be the result of an increase in size of the pulmonary capillary bed in direct response to hyperbaric O_2 (105). Either constriction or expansion of the pulmonary capillary bed could be a physiological response to hyperoxia, particularly because the reported changes were reversible. In experiments on anesthetized dogs in which a segment of lung was perfused at constant rate through a wedged catheter, hyperoxic blood (P_{O_2} of 300 mmHg) increased pulmonary vascular resistance ~40%, whereas ventilation with O_2 had no effect (5). This suggested that the site of action was at the arteriolar level. Some of these inconsistencies must be related to time and intensity of hyperoxic exposure. The $D_{L_{CO}}$ was not decreased during the 1st h of hyperoxia, even with hyperbaric oxygenation (24, 99, 105). Early changes in $P_{A_{O_2}} - Pa_{O_2}$ during hyperoxic exposures (discussed next) were therefore probably not attributable to a change in the transfer function of the lung.

Ten investigations of $P_{A_{O_2}} - Pa_{O_2}$ alteration during hyperoxia were selected from many others because the subjects were uniformly young and free of any recognizable cardiopulmonary disease or dysfunction, including any relating to toxic hyperoxic effects (8, 24, 29, 31, 64, 75, 76, 86, 99, 116). Two other important criteria had to be met as well. The means of altering inspired O_2 fraction had to be leak-free, and the measurement of Pa_{O_2} had to avert the several sources of technical error that can vitiate measurements of P_{O_2} above the level at which hemoglobin is fully saturated. These possible errors include alinearity of P_{O_2} electrodes in high ranges of P_{O_2}, the blood-gas differences obtained if gas calibration is used, loss of P_{O_2} by $\dot{V}_{O_2}$ of formed elements of blood, and the solubility of O_2 in components of the electrode and cuvette system.

Even with suitable precautions taken, considerable scatter was evident in the data obtained in these studies. Breathing air at 1 ATA, the average $P_{A_{O_2}} - Pa_{O_2}$ was ~11 mmHg and increased to ~43 mmHg breathing O_2 at 1 ATA. Beyond that the $P_{A_{O_2}} - Pa_{O_2}$ tended to increase only a little more. At the two extremes of changes in $P_{A_{O_2}} - Pa_{O_2}$ as $P_{A_{O_2}}$ increased, one group found a linear increase up to 121 mmHg at 3 ATA (29) and another group reported very little change in $P_{A_{O_2}} - Pa_{O_2}$ between 1 and 3 ATA (86). Several factors could have contributed to both results.

The conditions of the experiment and the precautions taken with respect to time of exposure should have eliminated any limitations of diffusion by hyperoxic effects on the alveolar-capillary membrane. Clark and Lambertsen (29), who reported the linear increase, were able to account for most of the increase by calculating the effect of a widened arteriovenous difference in O_2 content on the $P_{A_{O_2}} - Pa_{O_2}$. They based their calculations on the progressive decrease in cardiac output measured by Whalen et al. (121) in going from 1 to 3 ATA of O_2. Several other investigators also reported decreases in heart rate, cardiac output, or both as hyperoxia progressed to 1 ATA of O_2 and beyond (9, 11, 41, 105). If $\dot{V}_{O_2}$ remains constant and cardiac output decreases, the effect of more desaturated venous blood to increase $P_{A_{O_2}} - Pa_{O_2}$ at a fixed shunt ratio increases almost linearly as Pa_{O_2} exceeds 250 mmHg when hemoglobin is fully saturated. Further venous desaturation as a result of lowered cardiac output, particularly in the range of 1–3 ATA of O_2, would appear to play a substantial role in the modest increase of $P_{A_{O_2}} - Pa_{O_2}$ generally seen at those levels of hyperoxia.

Physiological shunting is another factor to consider in discussing $P_{A_{O_2}} - Pa_{O_2}$ changes with hyperoxia. Venous blood may merge directly with arterial outflow from the heart via anatomical shunts such as thebesian veins in the heart, bronchial circulation, or abnormal defects in circulatory structures. Some anatomic shunting is normally present to a small degree. In addition, blood perfusing poorly ventilated alveoli may not be fully saturated if there is a significant inert-gas fraction. In fact, anatomic shunting is usually quantified by washing out all of the ventilated air spaces with O_2. In this manner only nonventilated alveolar capillary or anatomic shunt could contribute to $P_{A_{O_2}} - Pa_{O_2}$ because even areas with very low alveolar ventilation-perfusion ratios ($\dot{V}A/\dot{Q}$) would still have high enough P_{O_2} to saturate fully the blood passing through them. There is some evidence that hyperoxia itself may alter the number of lung units with zero or indeterminately small $\dot{V}A/\dot{Q}$.

Lenfant (75) measured alveolar-arterial differences in O_2, CO_2, and N_2 in subjects breathing 75% O_2 up to 2.6 ATA. His results were consistent with a bimodal distribution of $\dot{V}A/\dot{Q}$ composed of a large group of well-ventilated alveoli and of a small group of units having an indeterminable $\dot{V}A/\dot{Q}$. Wagner et al. (116) developed newer methods that measured virtually continuous $\dot{V}A/\dot{Q}$ distributions by steady-state elimination of inert gases with different solubilities. Young, semirecumbent subjects breathing air had a virtually log-normal distribution of $\dot{V}A/\dot{Q}$ with very little dispersion. Intrapulmonary shunting ($\dot{V}A/\dot{Q} = 0$) was undetectable. After they breathed O_2 at 1 ATA for 30 min, shunting was found in all subjects. The authors attributed this to atelectasis that developed after denitrogenation. They suggested that hyperoxia might have aggravated the atelectatic process through the release of hypoxic vasoconstriction and the resultant increase in blood flow to areas of already low $\dot{V}A/\dot{Q}$. Later studies failed to demonstrate any change in perfusion with hyperoxia (14). In a theoretical analysis, Dantzker et al. (35) described the conditions under which lung units with low $\dot{V}A/\dot{Q}$ become unstable during O_2 breathing. When the inspired $\dot{V}A/\dot{Q}$ was gradually reduced, a critical value was reached at which inspired ventilation fell to zero. That value increased from 0.001 to 0.1 as inspired gas was changed from air to 100% O_2. Atelectasis need not occur for the shunt effect to be present. A unit with an open airway that receives collateral ventilation sufficient to match gas uptake by blood will have no expired ventilation but eventually must behave as a shunt. That is a small refinement of the well-documented propensity for increased intrapulmonary shunting that occurs even in young, normal subjects breathing 100% O_2 for 30-min periods. Although O_2 breathing decreases any contribution of low $\dot{V}A/\dot{Q}$, it increases the chance that nonventilated units will augment $PA_{O_2} - Pa_{O_2}$. The algebraic summation of opposing factors and the differential effects of hyperoxic exposure time and intensity undoubtedly all contributed to the various results obtained in the 10 selected studies.

An observation related to altered $PA_{O_2} - Pa_{O_2}$ with hyperoxia is that of an altered arterial-alveolar difference in P_{CO_2} ($Pa_{CO_2} - PA_{CO_2}$). In at least two studies, $Pa_{CO_2} - PA_{CO_2}$ increased with hyperoxia (74, 76). Larson and Severinghaus (74) suggested that high $\dot{V}A/\dot{Q}$ units were increased by redistribution of perfusion as hypoxic vasoconstriction was relaxed. That was not the case when perfusion distribution was measured (14). Lenfant (76) also suggested some diversion of flow to dependent areas of the lung and offered an additional mechanism to explain the increase. Hyperoxia constricts cerebral circulation and may further increase tissue P_{CO_2} there if the Haldane effect of increased venous saturation interferes with CO_2 transport of blood. Hyperventilation results and PA_{CO_2} is lowered. The Haldane effect would also cause alveoli with a low $\dot{V}A/\dot{Q}$ to have a higher P_{CO_2}, whereas those with a high $\dot{V}A/\dot{Q}$ would be relatively unaffected (14). Consequently the calculated $Pa_{CO_2} - PA_{CO_2}$ will be greater for breathing O_2 than for air even if $\dot{V}A/\dot{Q}$ distributions are unchanged.

Effects During Exercise

TOTAL O_2 UPTAKE. A long-standing question in exercise physiology has been whether total O_2 transport to working muscle limits the maximum O_2 uptake ($\dot{V}max_{O_2}$) by the whole body. A frequent experimental approach has been to measure $\dot{V}max_{O_2}$ in hyperoxia. The rationale was that some slight gain in arterial O_2 content could be realized as Pa_{O_2} was increased by increasing the O_2 dissolved in blood at the rate of $0.0031\ ml \cdot dl^{-1} \cdot mmHg^{-1}$. In a few instances hyperbaric oxygenation has been used up to 3 ATA, which would increase dissolved O_2 as much as 6.6 ml/dl above the value breathing air at 1 ATA. The effect of hyperoxia on total $\dot{V}_{O_2}$ during exercise, however, has been confused by methodological difficulties in measuring $\dot{V}_{O_2}$ as the inspired O_2 fraction is increased.

The potential pitfalls in measuring $\dot{V}_{O_2}$ by the Douglas bag open-circuit method as the inspired O_2 fraction is increased above ambient have been recognized for many years (52). In open-circuit methods, inspired ventilation is customarily calculated from the expired ventilation measurement and the ratio of inspired and expired inert-gas fraction, usually N_2. As the inspired N_2 fraction becomes very small, the effect of small errors in the measurement of inspired or expired fractions is magnified in its effect on the measurement of $\dot{V}_{O_2}$. If inspired and expired ventilations are measured directly, the measurement must end at precisely the same lung volume because any difference will be reflected as an error in $\dot{V}_{O_2}$ (52). There are also difficulties associated with the direct measurement of inspired ventilation with dry test gas meters because of the intermittent pattern of airflow (120). The contribution of altered gas stores, particularly dissolved gases, to errors in measurement of $\dot{V}_{O_2}$ are relatively small in relation to exercise levels and are readily avoided by having the subject breathe the different gas for 10–20 min (120). Other possible sources of error are contamination of Douglas bag expired gas collections by room air in the dead space of connecting hoses and stopcocks and any contamination from the inspired side by leaks, e.g., at the noseclip, mouthpiece, respiratory valve. The effect of these sources of error in measuring $\dot{V}_{O_2}$ at hyperoxic conditions is always to yield a falsely high value. This must be kept in mind while making any judgment about a transport limitation of $\dot{V}_{O_2}$ during exercise based on a comparison between normoxic and hyperoxic conditions.

Several groups of investigators have measured increases in total $\dot{V}_{O_2}$ of young healthy subjects at both submaximal and maximal work rates in hyperoxia compared with normoxia (42, 85, 95, 113, 124). All the measurements were based on the rates of O_2 removal from inspired ventilation. In two of the studies, however, a closed-circuit method was used that should have avoided the pitfalls just described for open-circuit methods (85, 95); increases of 3% and 8% in $\dot{V}max_{O_2}$ were reported in those cases. However, other equally reliable measurements show no such increases (1, 4).

In a more direct approach to the methodological difficulties, Stanek et al. (111) measured $\dot{V}_{O_2}$ in exercising ponies by the open-circuit method for gas exchange and as the product of cardiac output and arteriovenous O_2 content differences across the lung. The gas analysis indicated significant increases in submaximum $\dot{V}_{O_2}$ during hyperoxia, whereas the blood analysis showed no difference from normoxia. Even in cases where no differences in $\dot{V}_{O_2}$ have been noted, however, either endurance times for exhausting work were extended (1, 6, 85) or blood lactate levels decreased at heavy work loads (3). This suggests that hyperoxia had other metabolic effects that were not detectable as a change in $\dot{V}_{O_2}$.

REGIONAL OR MUSCLE O_2 UPTAKE. Davies and Sargeant (36) compared one- and two-leg exercise by healthy young subjects breathing air or 45% O_2 and found that $\dot{V}max_{O_2}$ was increased by hyperoxia in two-leg exercise but not in one-leg exercise. Because the cardiac output increase was the same for both kinds of exercise, the authors suggested that $\dot{V}max_{O_2}$ was flow limited when the same amount of blood flow had to be distributed to twice the mass of working muscle. Others who studied regional $\dot{V}_{O_2}$ during work by means of deep venous catheters concluded that leg or forearm $\dot{V}max_{O_2}$ values were not flow limited because hyperoxia caused venous P_{O_2} to increase even at maximal work rates (63, 94). Welch et al. (119) measured leg blood flow by dye dilution in similar studies and found that no gain in total O_2 transport was actually realized by working muscle because blood flow decreased 11% when the subjects breathed O_2. Despite that important observation, they too reported leg venous O_2 contents to be significantly greater on O_2, even at heavy work loads. The similarity between these results and those obtained in resting muscle reaffirms the possibility that direct effects of high P_{O_2} on local control of blood flow distribution may have effects on both O_2 demand and vascular control.

Experiments on in situ isolated dog muscles have also yielded mixed results with respect to hyperoxic increases in $\dot{V}max_{O_2}$. In the autoperfused dog gracilis muscle, Horstman et al. (58) found that hyperoxia increased $\dot{V}max_{O_2}$ proportionately to the increase in total O_2 transport. Even though there was an 8% decrease in blood flow, arterial O_2 content in their experiments was increased >17%. Wilson and Stainsby (123), in similar experiments on the dog gastrocnemius-plantaris muscle, found that the decrease in flow compensated for the increase in O_2 content and that $\dot{V}_{O_2}$ was not changed by hyperoxia. In experiments of this kind, however, the presence of vigorous autoregulation in the preparation is not always tested. Durán and Renkin (40) showed that even resting muscle $\dot{V}_{O_2}$ could depend on total O_2 transport if resistance-vessel autoregulation was not present. Whether similar cautions should be extended to working muscle preparations is not clear. Although hyperoxia did not increase $\dot{V}_{O_2}$ in other similar experiments, gastrocnemius muscle tension was maintained at a higher level than in normoxic dogs and blood flow did not decrease to the same extent (7). When flow was maintained by pump perfusion, a result similar to hyperoxia was obtained that suggested that tension maintenance was flow dependent and that the hyperoxic effect was through involvement in the long-term control of blood flow in working muscle.

Most of the information based on blood flow and arteriovenous differences in O_2 content indicated that hyperoxia did not increase $\dot{V}_{O_2}$ of working muscle. Even if true, that conclusion does not obviate the possibility of O_2 transport as the limiting factor in exercise $\dot{V}_{O_2}$ because hyperoxia usually caused a compensatory decrease in blood flow, particularly to skeletal muscle. The inconsistency in the overall findings was that various measures of performance increased in hyperoxia even though $\dot{V}_{O_2}$ was not increased. The question must be *how.* There could be effects of hyperoxia on metabolic control points. Differences in CO_2 output and respiratory exchange ratio have been reported with hyperoxia (111, 123). Decreased lactate production has been attributed to hyperoxic inhibition of glycolytic enzymes (117). Finally, these effects may alter performance indirectly through alterations of intracellular H^+ levels, a suggestion that was made in the past (1, 63) and will be again until a definitive experiment can be designed and accomplished.

SUMMARY

Some disturbance or alteration of gas exchange occurs in all three of the stresses examined in this chapter. During hypoxia, as O_2 transport to tissues is reduced below the level that satisfies demand, reflex mechanisms cause generalized vasoconstriction everywhere except in the brain. The putative function of this response is to maximize O_2 transport to the brain. Other tissues and organ systems resist the vasoconstriction only to the extent necessary to preserve their functional integrity. Active tissues, such as the heart and respiratory muscles, need to overcome vasoconstriction more rapidly in accord with their higher metabolic rate. Resting muscle and gut, on the other hand, can survive longer with supply-limited energy production because of their lower rate of energy use. Eventually their internal environment is sufficiently disturbed so that survival of even these lower-activity regions is threatened. As a result, local vasodilator activity increases and adds to any centrally mediated vasodilator tone already present so that blood flow to the threatened area increases. As this regional process becomes extensive, the brain and more active tissues lose their favored status and must compete on less favorable terms for O_2 transported by blood. At this stage the compensatory responses to hypoxia cease to benefit survival of the whole organism.

During apnea, diving mammals are especially able to utilize reflex mechanisms to conserve O_2 stores, which are greater than in nondiving mammals. By virtue of the pronounced bradycardia associated with the diving reflex, the heart's metabolic rate is lowered toward that of skeletal muscle. Blood is stingily meted out from a central reservoir to maintain oxygenation of heart, lung, and brain. At the same time, glucose is spared for nearly exclusive use of the brain during a dive. In addition to these more specialized responses of the diving mammal, there is some evidence that a portion of $\dot{V}_{O_2}$, used perhaps for thermogenesis, can be temporarily suspended during a dive. In contrast to the very limited ability of nondiving mammals such as the dog to withstand apnea, free-diving seals dive and swim for up to 27 min without incurring any measurable O_2 debt. By way of contrast, any decrease in O_2 transport in the dog appears to stimulate O_2 demand by the body rather than to diminish it and to incur an O_2 debt.

During hyperoxia, the reflex and local control systems act more in parallel with the apparent objective of maintaining the low P_{O_2} usually found in tissues. Slowing of heart rate and peripheral vasoconstriction tend to reduce peripheral blood flow. There is some evidence that regional microcirculatory adjustments might actually shunt blood through nonnutritive vessels. This would raise mixed venous P_{O_2} during hyperoxia, but tissue P_{O_2} would remain normal. The significance of limited observations that $\dot{V}_{O_2}$ actually decreases during hyperoxia remains elusive. It may be related to a decrease in sympathetic tone as hyperoxia decreases peripheral chemoreceptor neural outputs.

For this kind of integrative physiological research, the most rewarding future directions promise to be those that relate local behavior of regions and organ systems to the overall function and integrity of the body. It seems to be a clear case of the whole exceeding the sum of its parts.

This study was supported by National Institutes of Health Grants HL-14693 and HL-26927.

REFERENCES

1. ADAMS, R. P., AND H. G. WELCH. Oxygen uptake, acid-base status, and performance with varied inspired oxygen fractions. *J. Appl. Physiol.* 49: 863–868, 1980.
2. ANGELL JAMES, J. E., AND M. DE B. DALY. Cardiovascular responses in apnoeic asphyxia: role of arterial chemoreceptors and the modification of their effects by a pulmonary vagal inflation reflex. *J. Physiol. Lond.* 201: 87–104, 1969.
3. ASMUSSEN, E., AND M. NIELSEN. Studies on the regulation of respiration in heavy work. *Acta Physiol. Scand.* 12: 171–188, 1946.
4. ASMUSSEN, E., AND M. NIELSEN. The cardiac output in rest and work at low and high oxygen pressures. *Acta Physiol. Scand.* 35: 73–83, 1955.
5. BAIN, W. H., J. R. LANCASTER, AND W. E. ADAMS. Pulmonary vascular changes with increased oxygen tensions. In: *Hyperbaric Oxygenation,* edited by I. M. Lendingham. Edinburgh: Livingstone, 1965.
6. BANNISTER, R. G., AND D. J. C. CUNNINGHAM. The effects on the respiration and performance during exercise of adding oxygen to the inspired gas. *J. Physiol. Lond.* 125: 118–137, 1954.
7. BARCLAY, J. K., C. M. BOULIANNE, B. A. WILSON, AND S. J. TIFFIN. Interaction of hyperoxia and blood flow during fatigue of canine skeletal muscle in situ. *J. Appl. Physiol.* 47: 1018–1024, 1979.
8. BARTELS, H., H.-P. KOEPCHEN, L. LUHNING, M. MOCHIZUKI, AND I. WITT. Die alveolar-arterielle O_2-Druckdifferenz bei Ruhe und arbeit unter Hyperoxie (50% O_2). *Pfluegers Arch. Gesamte Physiol. Menschen Tiere* 261: 534–542, 1955.
9. BERGOFSKY, E. H., AND P. BERTUN. Response of regional circulations to hyperoxia. *J. Appl. Physiol.* 21: 567–572, 1966.
10. BICHER, H. T. Brain oxygen autoregulation: a protective reflex to hypoxia? *Microvasc. Res.* 8: 291–313, 1974.
11. BIRD, A. D., AND A. B. M. TELFER. The effect of oxygen at 1 and 2 atmospheres on resting forearm blood flow. *Surg. Gynecol. Obstet.* 123: 260–268, 1966.
12. BOND, R. F., E. S. MANNING, N. M. GONZALEZ, R. R. GONZALEZ, JR., AND V. E. BECKER. Myocardial and skeletal muscle responses to hemorrhage and shock during α-adrenergic blockade. *Am. J. Physiol.* 225: 247–257, 1973.
13. BOURDEAU-MARTINI, J., C. L. ODOROFF, AND C. R. HONIG. Dual effect of oxygen on magnitude and uniformity of coronary intercapillary distance. *Am. J. Physiol.* 226: 800–810, 1974.
14. BRYAN, A. C., L. G. BENTIVOGLIO, F. BEEREL, H. MACLEISH, A. ZIDULKA, AND D. V. BATES. Factors affecting regional distribution of ventilation and perfusion in the lung. *J. Appl. Physiol.* 19: 395–402, 1964.
15. CAIN, S. M. Effect of P_{CO_2} on the relation of lactate and excess lactate to O_2 deficit. *Am. J. Physiol.* 214: 1322–1327, 1968.
16. CAIN, S. M. Diminution of lactate rise during hypoxia by P_{CO_2} and β-adrenergic blockade. *Am. J. Physiol.* 217: 110–116, 1969.
17. CAIN, S. M. Increased oxygen uptake with passive hyperventilation of dogs. *J. Appl. Physiol.* 28: 4–7, 1970.
18. CAIN, S. M. Relative rates of arterial lactate and oxygen-deficit accumulation in hypoxic dogs. *Am. J. Physiol.* 224: 1190–1194, 1973.
19. CAIN, S. M. Arterial lactate responses in dogs made apneic or breathing nitrogen. *J. Appl. Physiol.* 42: 39–43, 1977.
20. CAIN, S. M. pH effects on lactate and excess lactate in relation to O_2 deficit in hypoxic dogs. *J. Appl. Physiol.* 42: 44–49, 1977.
21. CAIN, S. M. Oxygen delivery and uptake in dogs during anemic and hypoxic hypoxia. *J. Appl. Physiol.* 42: 228–234, 1977.

21a. CAIN, S. M. Supply dependency of oxygen uptake in ARDS: myth or reality? *Am. J. Med. Sci.* 288: 119–124, 1984.

22. CAIN, S. M., AND C. K. CHAPLER. O_2 extraction by hind limb versus whole dog during anemic hypoxia. *J. Appl. Physiol.* 45: 966–970, 1978.
23. CAIN, S. M., AND C. K. CHAPLER. Oxygen extraction by canine hindlimb during hypoxic hypoxia. *J. Appl. Physiol.* 46: 1023–1028, 1979.
24. CALDWELL, P. R. B., W. L. LEE, JR., H. S. SCHILDKRAUT, AND E. R. ARCHIBALD. Changes in lung volume, diffusing capacity, and blood gases in men breathing oxygen. *J. Appl. Physiol.* 21: 1477–1483, 1966.
25. CHAPLER, C. K., AND S. M. CAIN. Blood flow and O_2 uptake in dog hindlimb with anemia, norepinephrine, and propranolol. *J. Appl. Physiol.* 51: 565–570, 1981.
26. CHAPLER, C. K., S. M. CAIN, AND W. N. STAINSBY. Blood flow and oxygen uptake in isolated canine skeletal muscle during acute anemia. *J. Appl. Physiol.* 46: 1035–1038, 1979.
27. CHAPLER, C. K., S. M. CAIN, AND W. N. STAINSBY. The effects of hyperoxia on oxygen uptake during acute anemia. *Can. J. Physiol. Pharmacol.* 62: 809–814, 1984.
28. CHERNIACK, N. S., G. S. LONGOBARDO, F. P. PALERMO, AND M. HEYMANN. Dynamics of oxygen stores changes following an alteration in ventilation. *J. Appl. Physiol.* 24: 809–816, 1968.
29. CLARK, J. M., AND C. J. LAMBERTSEN. Alveolar-arterial O_2 differences in man at 0.2, 1.0, 2.0, and 3.5 Ata inspired P_{O_2}. *J. Appl. Physiol.* 30: 753–763, 1971.
30. COHEN, R. D., AND R. SIMPSON. Lactate metabolism. *Anesthesiology* 43: 661–673, 1975.
31. COLE, R. B., AND J. M. BISHOP. Variation in alveolar-arterial O_2 tension difference at high levels of alveolar O_2 tension. *J. Appl. Physiol.* 22: 685–693, 1967.
32. CRAIG, A. B., JR., AND W. L. MEDD. Oxygen consumption and carbon dioxide production during breath-hold diving. *J. Appl. Physiol.* 24: 190–202, 1968.
33. DANEK, S. J., J. P. LYNCH, J. G. WEG, AND D. R. DANTZKER. The dependence of oxygen uptake on oxygen delivery in the adult respiratory distress syndrome. *Am. Rev. Respir. Dis.* 122: 387–395, 1980.

34. DANIELL, H. B. Coronary flow alterations on myocardial contractility, oxygen extraction, and oxygen consumption. *Am. J. Physiol.* 225: 1020–1025, 1973.
35. DANTZKER, D. R., P. D. WAGNER, AND J. B. WEST. Instability of lung units with low $\dot{V}A/\dot{Q}$ ratios during O_2 breathing. *J. Appl. Physiol.* 38: 886–895, 1975.
36. DAVIES, C. T. M., AND A. J. SARGEANT. Physiological responses to one- and two-leg exercise breathing air and 45% oxygen. *J. Appl. Physiol.* 36: 142–148, 1974.
37. DENEKE, S. M., AND B. L. FANBURG. Normobaric oxygen toxicity of the lung. *N. Engl. J. Med.* 303: 76–86, 1980.
38. DULING, B. R. Microvascular responses to alterations in oxygen tension. *Circ. Res.* 31: 481–489, 1972.
39. DULING, B. R. Oxygen, metabolism, and microcirculatory control. In: *Microcirculation*, edited by G. Kaley and B. M. Altura. Baltimore, MD: University Park, 1978, vol. 2, p. 401–429.
40. DURÁN, W. N., AND E. M. RENKIN. Oxygen consumption and blood flow in resting mammalian skeletal muscle. *Am. J. Physiol.* 226: 173–177, 1974.
41. EGGERS, G. W. N., JR., H. W. PALEY, J. J. LEONARD, AND J. V. WARREN. Hemodynamic responses to oxygen breathing in man. *J. Appl. Physiol.* 17: 75–79, 1962.
42. EKBLOM, B., R. HUOT, E. M. STEIN, AND A. T. THORSTENSSON. Effect of changes in arterial oxygen content on circulation and physical performance. *J. Appl. Physiol.* 39: 71–75, 1975.
43. ELSNER, R., B. A. GOODEN, AND S. M. ROBINSON. Arterial blood gas changes and the diving response in man. *Aust. J. Exp. Biol. Med. Sci.* 49: 435–444, 1971.
44. FERRANTE, F. L. Oxygen conservation during submergence apnea in a diving mammal, the nutria. *Am. J. Physiol.* 218: 363–371, 1970.
45. FITZPATRICK, J. H., JR., D. D. GILBOE, L. R. DREWES, AND A. L. BETZ. Relationship of cerebral oxygen uptake to EEG frequency in isolated canine brain. *Am. J. Physiol.* 231: 1840–1846, 1976.
46. GARCIA, A. C., Y. L. LAI, B. A. ATTEBERY, AND E. B. BROWN, JR. Lactate and pyruvate accumulation during hypocapnia. *Respir. Physiol.* 12: 371–380, 1971.
47. GRANGER, H. J., A. H. GOODMAN, AND D. N. GRANGER. Role of resistance and exchange vessels in local microvascular control of skeletal muscle oxygenation in the dog. *Circ. Res.* 38: 379–385, 1976.
48. HALMAGYI, D. F. J., A. H. GOODMAN, AND I. R. NEERING. Hindlimb blood flow and oxygen usage in hemorrhagic shock. *J. Appl. Physiol.* 27: 508–513, 1969.
49. HAUGAARD, N. Cellular mechanisms of oxygen toxicity. *Physiol. Rev.* 48: 311–373, 1968.
50. HEISTAD, D. D., AND R. C. WHEELER. Simulated diving during hypoxia in man. *J. Appl. Physiol.* 28: 652–656, 1970.
51. HESSER, C. M., B. KATSAROS, AND G. MATELL. Pulmonary and tissue gas exchange during breath holding with oxygen. *Respir. Physiol.* 5: 78–90, 1968.
52. HILL, A. V., C. N. H. LONG, AND H. LUPTON. Muscular exercise, lactic acid, and the supply and utilization of oxygen. Pt. IV. *Proc. R. Soc. Lond. B Biol. Sci.* 97: 84–96, 1924.
53. HOCHACHKA, P. W. *Living Without Oxygen: Closed and Open Systems in Hypoxia Tolerance.* Cambridge, MA: Harvard Univ. Press, 1980, p. 145–169.
54. HONG, S. K., Y. C. LIN, D. A. LALLY, B. J. B. YIM, N. KOMINAMI, P. W. HONG, AND T. O. MOORE. Alveolar gas exchanges and cardiovascular functions during breath holding with air. *J. Appl. Physiol.* 30: 540–547, 1971.
55. HONG, S. K., T. O. MOORE, G. SETO, H. K. PARK, W. R. HIATT, AND E. M. BERNAUER. Lung volumes and apneic bradycardia in divers. *J. Appl. Physiol.* 29: 172–176, 1970.
56. HONIG, C. R. Hypoxia in skeletal muscle at rest and during the transition to steady work. *Microvasc. Res.* 13: 377–398, 1977.
57. HONIG, C. R., J. L. FRIERSON, AND C. N. NELSON. O_2 transport and $\dot{V}O_2$ in resting muscle: significance for tissue-capillary exchange. *Am. J. Physiol.* 220: 357–363, 1971.
58. HORSTMAN, D. H., M. GLESER, AND J. DELEHUNT. Effects of altering O_2 delivery on $\dot{V}O_2$ of isolated, working muscle. *Am. J. Physiol.* 230: 327–334, 1976.
59. HUGHES, R. L., R. T. MATHIE, D. CAMPBELL, AND W. FITCH. Systemic hypoxia and hyperoxia, and liver blood flow and oxygen consumption in the greyhound. *Pfluegers Arch.* 381: 151–157, 1979.
60. JACOBSON, I., A. M. HARPER, AND D. G. MCDOWALL. The effects of oxygen at 1 and 2 atmospheres on the blood flow and oxygen uptake of the cerebral cortex. *Surg. Gynecol. Obstet.* 119: 737–742, 1964.
61. JAN, K. M., J. HELDMAN, AND S. CHIEN. Coronary hemodynamics and oxygen utilization after hematocrit variations in hemorrhage. *Am. J. Physiol.* 239 (*Heart Circ. Physiol.* 8): H326–H332, 1980.
62. JOHNSON, L. F., JR., J. R. NEVILLE, AND R. W. BANCROFT. The effect of decreased barometric pressure on oxygen consumption. *Aerosp. Med.* 34: 97–100, 1963.
63. KAIJSER, L. Limiting factors for aerobic muscle performance. The influence of varying oxygen pressure and temperature. *Acta Physiol. Scand. Suppl.* 346: 1–96, 1970.
64. KARETZKY, M. S., J. F. KEIGHLEY, AND J. C. MITHOEFER. The effect of oxygen administration on gas exchange and cardiopulmonary function in normal subjects. *Respir. Physiol.* 12: 361–370, 1971.
65. KAWAKAMI, Y., B. H. NATELSON, AND A. B. DUBOIS. Cardiovascular effects of face immersion and factors affecting diving reflex in man. *J. Appl. Physiol.* 23: 964–970, 1967.
66. KENDRICK, J. E., S. J. DE HAAN, AND J. D. PARKE. Regulation of blood flow to respiratory muscles during hypoxia and hypercapnia. *Proc. Soc. Exp. Biol. Med.* 166: 157–161, 1981.
67. KENMURE, A. C. F., W. R. MURDOCH, I. HUTTON, AND A. J. V. CAMERON. Hemodynamic effects of oxygen at 1 and 2 Ata pressure in healthy subjects. *J. Appl. Physiol.* 32: 223–226, 1972.
68. KEREM, D., AND R. ELSNER. Cerebral tolerance to asphyxial hypoxia in the dog. *Am. J. Physiol.* 225: 593–600, 1973.
69. KOOYMAN, G. L., D. H. KEREM, W. B. CAMPBELL, AND J. J. WRIGHT. Pulmonary gas exchange in freely diving Weddell seals. *Respir. Physiol.* 17: 283–290, 1973.
70. KOOYMAN, G. L., J. P. SCHROEDER, D. M. DENISON, D. D. HAMMOND, J. J. WRIGHT, AND W. P. BERGMAN. Blood nitrogen tensions of seals during simulated deep dives. *Am. J. Physiol.* 223: 1016–1020, 1972.
71. KOOYMAN, G. L., E. A. WAHRENBRACK, M. A. CASTELLINI, R. W. DAVID, AND E. E. SINNETT. Aerobic and anaerobic metabolism during voluntary diving in Weddell seals: evidence of preferred pathways from blood chemistry and behavior. *J. Comp. Physiol.* 138: 335–346, 1980.
72. LAMBERTSEN, C. J., S. G. OWEN, H. WENDEL, M. W. STROUD, A. A. LURIE, W. LOCHNER, AND G. F. CLARK. Respiratory and cerebral circulatory control during exercise at .21 and 2.0 atmospheres inspired P_{O_2}. *J. Appl. Physiol.* 14: 966–982, 1959.
73. LARETT, W. W. Control of hepatic and intestinal blood flow: effect of isovolaemic haemodilution on blood flow and oxygen uptake in the intact liver and intestines. *J. Physiol. Lond.* 265: 313–326, 1977.
74. LARSON, C. P., JR., AND J. W. SEVERINGHAUS. Postural variations in dead space and CO_2 gradients breathing air and O_2. *J. Appl. Physiol.* 17: 417–420, 1962.
75. LENFANT, C. Measurement of factors impairing gas exchange in man with hyperbaric pressure. *J. Appl. Physiol.* 19: 189–194, 1964.
76. LENFANT, C. Arterial-alveolar difference in P_{CO_2} during air and oxygen breathing. *J. Appl. Physiol.* 21: 1356–1362, 1966.
77. LIN, Y. C., AND D. G. BAKER. Cardiac output and its distribution during diving in the rat. *Am. J. Physiol.* 228: 733–737, 1975.
78. LIN, Y. C., D. A. LALLY, T. O. MOORE, AND S. K. HONG. Physiological and conventional breath-hold breaking points. *J. Appl. Physiol.* 37: 291–296, 1974.
79. LIN, Y. C., T. O. MOORE, J. J. MCNAMARA, AND S. K. HONG.

Oxygen consumption and conservation during apnea in the anesthetized dog. *Respir. Physiol.* 24: 313–324, 1975.

80. LINDBOM, L., R. F. TUMA, AND K. E. ARFORS. Influence of oxygen on perfused capillary density and capillary red cell velocity in rabbit skeletal muscle. *Microvasc. Res.* 19: 197–208, 1980.
81. LÜBBERS, D. W. Tissue oxygen supply and critical oxygen pressure. In: *Oxygen Transport to Tissue*, edited by A. G. B. Kovach, E. Dora, M. Kessler, and I. A. Silver. New York: Pergamon, 1980, vol. 25, p. 3–11. (Proc. Int. Congr. Physiol. Sci., 28th, Budapest, 1980.)
82. LÜBBERS, D. W., AND M. KESSLER. Oxygen supply and rate of tissue respiration. In: *Oxygen Transport in Blood and Tissues*, edited by D. W. Lübbers, U. C. Luft, G. Thews, and E. Witzleb. Stuttgart: Thieme, 1968, p. 90–99.
83. LUTZ, J., H. HENRICH, AND E. BAUEREISEN. Oxygen supply and uptake in the liver and intestine. *Pfluegers Arch.* 360: 7–15, 1975.
84. MACMILLAN, V., AND B. K. SIESJÖ. Critical oxygen tensions in the brain. *Acta Physiol. Scand.* 82: 412–414, 1971.
85. MARGARIA, R., E. CAMPORESI, P. AGHEMO, AND G. SASSI. The effect of O_2 breathing on maximal aerobic power. *Pfluegers Arch.* 336: 225–235, 1972.
86. MCDOWALL, D. G., I. M. LEDINGHAM, AND S. TINDAL. Alveolar-arterial gradients for oxygen at 1, 2, and 3 atmospheres absolute. *J. Appl. Physiol.* 24: 324–329, 1968.
87. MILLS, E., AND F. F. JÖBSIS. Mitochondrial respiratory chain of carotid body and chemoreceptor response to changes in oxygen tension. *J. Neurophysiol.* 35: 405–428, 1972.
88. MITHOEFER, J. C. Breath holding. In: *Handbook of Physiology. Respiration*, edited by W. O. Fenn and H. Rahn. Washington, DC: Am. Physiol. Soc., 1965, sect. 3, vol. II, chapt. 38, p. 1011–1025.
89. MURPHY, B., W. M. ZAPOL, AND P. W. HOCHACHKA. Metabolic activities of heart, lung, and brain during diving and recovery in the Weddell seal. *J. Appl. Physiol.* 48: 596–605, 1980.
90. NAHAS, G. G., L. TRINER, H. S. SMALL, W. M. MANGER, AND D. V. HABIF. Alterations in O_2 uptake following hemorrhage in dogs. *Am. J. Physiol.* 210: 1009–1014, 1966.
91. OHTA, Y., S. H. SONG, A. C. GROOM, AND L. E. FARHI. Is inert gas washout from the tissues limited by diffusion? *J. Appl. Physiol.* 45: 903–907, 1978.
92. PACKER, B. S., M. ALTMAN, C. E. CROSS, H. V. MURDAUGH, JR., J. M. LINTA, AND E. D. ROBIN. Adaptations to diving in the harbor seal: oxygen stores and supply. *Am. J. Physiol.* 217: 903–906, 1969.
93. PAULEV, P. E. Respiratory and cardiovascular effects of breath-holding. *Acta Physiol. Scand. Suppl.* 324: 1–116, 1969.
94. PIRNAY, F., M. LAMY, J. DUJARDIN, R. DEROANNE, AND J. M. PETIT. Analysis of femoral venous blood during maximum muscular exercise. *J. Appl. Physiol.* 33: 289–292, 1972.
95. PIRNAY, F., R. MARECHAL, R. DUJARDIN, M. LAMY, R. DEROANNE, AND J. M. PETIT. Exercise during hyperoxia and hyperbaric oxygenation. *Int. Z. Angew. Physiol. Einschl. Arbeitsphysiol.* 31: 259–268, 1973.
96. POWERS, F. R., AND W. J. POWELL, JR. Effect of arterial hypoxia on myocardial oxygen consumption. *Circ. Res.* 33: 749–756, 1973.
97. POWERS, S. R., JR., R. MANNAL, M. NECLERIO, M. ENGLISH, C. MARR, R. LEATHER, H. UEDA, G. WILLIAMS, W. CUSTEAD, AND R. DUTTON. Physiologic consequences of positive end-expiratory pressure (PEEP) ventilation. *Ann. Surg.* 178: 265–272, 1973.
98. POYART, C., AND G. G. NAHAS. Inhibition of catecholamine-induced calorigenesis and lipolysis by hypercapnic acidosis. *Am. J. Physiol.* 211: 161–168, 1966.
99. PUY, R. J. M., R. W. HYDE, A. B. FISHER, J. M. CLARK, J. DICKSON, AND C. J. LAMBERTSEN. Alterations in the pulmonary capillary bed during early O_2 toxicity in man. *J. Appl. Physiol.* 24: 537–543, 1968.
100. RACKER, E. From Pasteur to Mitchell: a hundred years of bioenergetics. *Federation Proc.* 39: 210–215, 1980.
101. RESTORFF, W. V., B. HOFLING, J. HOLTZ, AND E. BASSENGE. Effect of increased blood fluidity through hemodilution on coronary circulation at rest and during exercise in dogs. *Pfluegers Arch.* 357: 15–24, 1975.
102. RIDGEWAY, S. H., AND R. HOWARD. Dolphin lung collapse and intramuscular circulation during free diving: evidence from nitrogen washout. *Science Wash. DC* 206: 1182–1183, 1979.
103. ROBIN, E. D. Of men and mitochondria: coping with hypoxic dysoxia. *Am. Rev. Respir. Dis.* 122: 517–531, 1980.
104. ROBIN, E. D., H. V. MURDAUGH, JR., W. PYRON, E. WEISS, AND P. SOTERES. Adaptations to diving in the harbor seal—gas exchange and ventilatory response to CO_2. *Am. J. Physiol.* 205: 1175–1177, 1963.
105. ROSENBERG, E., AND L. D. MACLEAN. Effect of high oxygen tensions on diffusing capacity for CO and Krogh's K. *J. Appl. Physiol.* 23: 11–17, 1967.
106. SAUNDERS, K. B., D. M. BAND, P. EBDEN, J. P. VAN DER HOFF, D. J. MABERLEY, AND S. J. G. SEMPLE. Acid-base status and gas exchange in the anesthetized dog breathing pure oxygen. *Respiration* 29: 305–316, 1972.
107. SCHOLANDER, P. F. Animals in aquatic environments: diving mammals and birds. In *Handbook of Physiology. Adaptation to the Environment*, edited by D. B. Dill, and E. F. Adolph. Washington, DC: Am. Physiol. Soc., 1964, sect. 4, chapt. 45, p. 729–739.
108. SEEHERMAN, H. J., C. R. TAYLOR, G. M. O. MALOIY, AND R. B. ARMSTRONG. Design of the mammalian respiratory system. II. Measuring maximum aerobic capacity. *Respir. Physiol.* 44: 11–23, 1981.
109. SHEPHERD, A. P. Intestinal O_2 consumption and ^{86}Rb extraction during arterial hypoxia. *Am. J. Physiol.* 234 (*Endocrinol. Metab. Gastrointest. Physiol.* 3): E248–E251, 1978.
110. STAINSBY, W. N., AND A. B. OTIS. Blood flow, blood oxygen tension, oxygen uptake, and oxygen transport in skeletal muscle. *Am. J. Physiol.* 206: 858–866, 1964.
111. STANEK, K. A., F. J. NAGLE, G. E. BISGARD, AND W. C. BYRNES. Effect of hyperoxia on oxygen consumption in exercising ponies. *J. Appl. Physiol.* 46: 1115–1118, 1979.
112. TASHKIN, D. P., P. J. GOLDSTEIN, AND D. H. SIMMONS. Hepatic lactate uptake during decreased liver perfusion and hypoxemia. *Am. J. Physiol.* 223: 968–974, 1972.
113. TAUNTON, J. E., E. W. BANISTER, T. R. PATRICK, P. OFORSAGD, AND W. R. DUNCAN. Physical work capacity in hyperbaric environments and conditions of hyperoxia. *J. Appl. Physiol.* 28: 421–427, 1970.
114. TENNEY, S. M. A theoretical analysis of the relationship between venous blood and mean tissue oxygen pressures. *Respir. Physiol.* 20: 283–296, 1974.
115. TIBES, U., AND J. STEGEMANN. Das Verhalten der endexpiratorischen Atemgasdrucke, der O_2-Aufnahme, und CO_2-abgabe nach einfacher Apnoe im Wasser, an Land und apnoeischem Tauchen. *Pfluegers Arch.* 311: 300–311, 1969.
116. WAGNER, P. D., R. B. LARARUSO, R. R. UHL, AND J. B. WEST. Continuous distributions of ventilation-perfusion ratios in normal subjects breathing air and 100% O_2. *J. Clin. Invest.* 54: 54–68, 1974.
117. WEGLICKI, W. B., R. E. WHALEN, H. K. THOMPSON, JR., AND H. D. MCINTOSH. Effects of hyperbaric oxygenation on excess lactate production in exercising dogs. *Am. J. Physiol.* 210: 473–477, 1966.
118. WEISS, H. R., J. A. COHEN, AND L. A. MCPHERSON. Blood flow and relative tissue P_{O_2} of brain and muscle: effect of various gas mixtures. *Am. J. Physiol.* 230: 839–844, 1976.
119. WELCH, H. G., F. BONDE-PETERSEN, T. GRAHAM, K. KLAUSEN, AND N. SECHER. Effects of hyperoxia on leg blood flow and metabolism during exercise. *J. Appl. Physiol.* 42: 385–390, 1977.
120. WELCH, H. G., AND P. K. PEDERSEN. Measurement of metabolic rate in hyperoxia. *J. Appl. Physiol.* 51: 725–731, 1981.
121. WHALEN, R. E., H. A. SALTZMAN, D. H. HOLLOWAY, JR., H.

D. McIntosh, H. O. Sieker, and I. W. Brown, Jr. Cardiovascular and blood gas responses to hyperbaric oxygenation. *Am. J. Cardiol.* 15: 638–646, 1965.
122. Whalen, W. J., D. Buerk, and C. A. Thuning. Blood flow-limited oxygen consumption in resting cat skeletal muscle. *Am. J. Physiol.* 224: 763–768, 1973.
123. Wilson, B. A., and W. N. Stainsby. Effects of O_2 breathing on R.Q., blood flow, and developed tension in in situ dog muscle. *Med. Sci. Sports* 10: 167–170, 1978.
124. Wilson, B. A., H. G. Welch, and J. N. Liles. Effects of hyperoxic gas mixtures on energy metabolism during prolonged work. *J. Appl. Physiol.* 39: 267–271, 1975.
125. Zapol, W. M., G. C. Liggins, R. C. Schneider, L. Qvist, M. T. Snider, R. K. Creasy, and P. W. Hochachka. Regional blood flow during simulated diving in the conscious Weddell seal. *J. Appl. Physiol.* 47: 968–973, 1979.
126. Zborowska-Sluis, D. T., and J. B. Dossetor. Hyperlactatemia of hyperventilation. *J. Appl. Physiol.* 22: 746–755, 1967.
127. Zimpfer, M., S. P. Sit, and S. F. Vatner. Effects of anesthesia on the canine carotid chemoreceptor reflex. *Circ. Res.* 48: 400–406, 1981.

Gas exchange in acid-base disturbances

EUGENE E. NATTIE | *Department of Physiology, Dartmouth Medical School, Hanover, New Hampshire*

CHAPTER CONTENTS

THE INTIMACY OF THE EXCHANGE of respiratory gases, O_2 and CO_2, and the importance of CO_2 in mammalian acid-base physiology suggests that acid-base imbalance could affect gas exchange. This chapter examines the effects of acid-base imbalance on gas exchange within the constraints of the definition below.

DEFINITION OF GAS EXCHANGE

The maintenance of normal gas exchange depends on the processes that deliver O_2 from the atmosphere to the cellular oxidative site (46). Carbon dioxide removal as a gas-exchange phenomenon per se is not examined in this chapter. Oxygen delivery includes both convective and diffusive processes. In steps from outside air to cell site, these processes include alveolar ventilation ($\dot{V}_A$), diffusion in the lung, binding of O_2 to Hb and carriage of O_2 by blood, cardiac output ($\dot{Q}_T$), and diffusion of O_2 at the tissue capillary site. The O_2 delivery system can be viewed in terms of a volume supplier of O_2 and in terms of the maintenance of a partial-pressure head for O_2 that ensures an adequate tissue and cell partial pressure of O_2 (P_{O_2}). If the system fails, cell hypoxia develops, which is associated with disorders in cell metabolism and function. The volume supply of O_2 is the product of tissue perfusion and arterial O_2 content, and the average pressure head at the source of O_2 supply to a tissue is regional mean capillary P_{O_2}. Tissue P_{O_2} is more difficult to estimate. In studies on whole animals, the partial pressure of O_2 in mixed venous blood ($P\bar{v}_{O_2}$) has been used to estimate mean body tissue P_{O_2}. Other ways to estimate tissue P_{O_2} are discussed in *Tissues*, p. 427, and *Whole Animal at Rest*, p. 429.

ACID-BASE TERMINOLOGY

The pH or [H^+] in the body is determined by three independent variables: *1*) the partial pressure of CO_2 (P_{CO_2}), *2*) the total weak-acid buffer concentration, and *3*) the strong-ion difference (145). Conventional terminology refers to pH <7.400 as *acidosis* and to pH >7.400 as *alkalosis* in mammals at 37°C. Actually the normal pH of 7.400 is alkaline relative to the neutral pH of water and, as described in COMPARATIVE ASPECTS OF ACID-BASE BALANCE AND POSSIBLE RELATIONSHIP TO O_2 DELIVERY, p. 431, depends on temperature. If an abnormal pH at 37°C is primarily due to an increase or decrease in P_{CO_2} it is called a respiratory acidosis or alkalosis, respectively. If an abnormal pH is primarily due to a change in bicarbonate concentration via an alteration in the strong-ion difference it is called a metabolic acidosis or alkalosis. Mixed disturbances are possible. In any disturbance of acid-base balance there are physiological and chemical mechanisms that tend to minimize the pH change. These defense mechanisms include buffers in blood and in cells, renal and gastrointestinal ionic excretory changes, ionic exchange processes between body compartments, and alterations in $\dot{V}_A$. The presence and capability of these regulatory mechanisms indicate that the maintenance of a normal acid-base balance is one physiological priority in the economy of the body.

This chapter uses these definitions to discuss the effects of acid-base imbalance on the delivery of O_2 to cell oxidative sites in mammals. Each step in the O_2 delivery scheme is examined for possible effects of disordered acid-base balance. Normal ambient O_2 and body temperature conditions are assumed unless otherwise stated.

EFFECTS OF ACID-BASE IMBALANCE ON STEPS IN O_2 DELIVERY PROCESS

Alveolar Ventilation

Changes in acid-base balance can alter the $\dot{V}_A$ level by stimulating chemoreceptors located at the carotid body (12, 84, 96) and centrally in the medulla oblongata (45, 84, 96, 107). A metabolic acidosis stimulates $\dot{V}_A$, which results in a decrease in the partial pressure of CO_2 in arterial blood (Pa_{CO_2}) and, if the lungs are normal, an increase in the partial pressure of O_2 in arterial blood (Pa_{O_2}). In metabolic alkalosis, $\dot{V}_A$ is depressed, Pa_{CO_2} is increased, and Pa_{O_2} is decreased. The response to metabolic acidosis is generally predictable, whereas the response to metabolic alkalosis depends on how the alkalosis is induced (52). The use of buffers or agents that stimulate renal H^+ excretion to produce metabolic alkalosis results in alveolar hypoventilation, whereas the use of agents that stimulate K^+ loss and produce extracellular alkalosis without measurable external H^+ loss results in minimal hypoventilation (52). Little work has been done to clarify the mechanism of the variable ventilatory response to metabolic alkalosis. For example, in some cases of metabolic alkalosis, severe hypercapnia and arterial hypoxemia are reported (85, 156), even though pulmonary function is normal.

Pulmonary Vasculature

Arterial acidosis of any origin results in vasoconstriction in small pulmonary arteries and arterioles and an increase in pulmonary vascular resistance (5, 10, 56, 90, 139). Alkalosis can result in some vasodilation in the pulmonary vascular bed (139), although not all workers have observed this (90). In respiratory acidosis, in addition to the increase in pulmonary vascular resistance, Horwitz et al. (63) observed elevated right and left atrial pressures in unanesthetized dogs, which probably reflect redistribution of blood into the pulmonary bed, a change observed in respiratory acidosis (157) but not in metabolic acidosis (56) unless the acidosis is severe and associated with dehydration (57).

Airways

The responses of tracheobronchial smooth muscle to alterations in acid-base balance involve direct, chemoreflex, and mechanoreflex effects (65, 142, 164). In tracheobronchial smooth muscle with some resting tone the direct effect of an increase in P_{CO_2} is relaxation (99, 104, 138, 143, 161), whereas the direct effect of a decrease in P_{CO_2} is contraction (65, 104, 106, 140, 144). Changes in pH under isocapnic conditions seem to have less effect (104, 164). In the intact animal an increase in Pa_{CO_2} results in bronchoconstriction (65, 99, 134, 164) due to a chemoreflex with a vagal efferent pathway (99). This chemoreflex bronchoconstriction does not depend on peripheral chemoreception in the carotid body (99) and is apparently central in origin (34). Metabolic acidosis under isocapnic conditions has little effect on airway resistance (111). A decrease in Pa_{CO_2} in the intact animal also results in bronchoconstriction, but here the direct constrictor effect of the low P_{CO_2} on tracheobronchial smooth muscle is predominant over the weaker chemoreflex effect (65, 104, 138, 140, 144). Mechanoreceptor reflexes stimulated by increased ventilation can override the respiratory acidosis-induced reflex bronchoconstriction, at least in the isolated trachea, resulting in a return of tracheal smooth muscle tone to normal (134, 144). The presence of these direct and reflex effects of acid-base imbalance makes it difficult to make any summary statement about airways. For gas exchange the importance of any effects of acid-base disturbances on airway tone could be via effects on *1)* dead-space volume (V_{DS}), *2)* distribution of ventilation, and *3)* tidal volume (V_T) if changes in airway resistance alter the ventilatory output in response to a certain amount of respiratory center neural drive.

Pulmonary Gas Exchange

There have been few experimental studies of acid-base imbalance and pulmonary gas exchange. Liljestrand (87) suggested that regional P_{O_2} and P_{CO_2} in the lung could direct flow away from poorly ventilated alveoli. For the entire lung, generalized vasoconstriction can also affect pulmonary gas exchange, at least in some situations. Haas and Bergofsky (53) found that in anesthetized dogs, after 15 min of breathing 5% CO_2, average arterial pH (pH_a) decreased from 7.38 to 7.20 and mean pulmonary artery pressure increased significantly with no significant change in $\dot{Q}_T$ or total O_2 consumption ($\dot{V}_{O_2}$). In addition, Pa_{O_2} increased from 90 to 97 mmHg, whereas the ideal alveolar-arterial difference in P_{O_2} ($PA_{O_2} - Pa_{O_2}$) decreased from 32 to 22 mmHg. This decrease in the $PA_{O_2} - Pa_{O_2}$ gradient was accompanied by a decrease in the ratio of venous admixture to total blood flow ($\dot{Q}_S/\dot{Q}_T$) (from 11.6% to 8.4%) and a decrease in V_{DS}/V_T (from 48% to 30%). Using venous admixture and V_{DS}/V_T as indices of the ventilation-perfusion ratio ($\dot{V}_A/\dot{Q}$) distribution within the lung, the authors found that the small elevation in pulmonary artery pressure improved this distribution and resulted in a lower $PA_{O_2} - Pa_{O_2}$. They also pointed out that mixed venous O_2 saturation, which if increased could increase Pa_{O_2}, was unchanged. Their calculations also showed that any increased Bohr effect in the acidotic venous admixture blood could not contribute enough of an increase in P_{O_2} to the final arterial mixture to account for the observed changes in Pa_{O_2}, venous admixture, and V_{DS}/V_T. These experiments have been performed in supine or laterally positioned anesthetized dogs with control $PA_{O_2} - Pa_{O_2}$ values somewhat higher than those observed in unanesthetized dogs. Thus the proposed improvement in gas exchange by increased pulmonary artery pressure could be less impressive in an unanesthetized preparation.

In another similar experiment in anesthetized dogs, Frans et al. (47) induced metabolic acidosis by infusion of ammonium chloride, and alkalosis by infusion of $NaHCO_3$. The infusion rates were slow, so pulmonary artery pressure, $\dot{Q}T$, venous admixture, and the alveolar dead space were not significantly affected. In acidosis (pH 7.14), Pa_{O_2} increased from 97 to 102 mmHg, and ideal $PA_{O_2} - Pa_{O_2}$ decreased 6 mmHg; in alkalosis (pH 7.54), Pa_{O_2} decreased from 96 to 86 mmHg, and ideal $PA_{O_2} - Pa_{O_2}$ increased 8 mmHg. These workers also reported the degree of change of venous admixture and alveolar dead space as indices of the $\dot{V}A/\dot{Q}$ distribution and concluded that there is no change. Their explanation of the gas-exchange results involved the effect of increased pH on the upper part of the HbO_2 curve (Fig. 1). In acidosis the shift to the right increases the steepness of the upper portion of the HbO_2 curve. For the same ideal end-capillary–to–arterial O_2 content difference, the effect of pH on the HbO_2 dissociation curve is to increase ideal $PA_{O_2} - Pa_{O_2}$ in alkalosis and to decrease it in acidosis (47). The same study also reports a significant effect of acid-base imbalance on $P\bar{v}_{O_2}$. Acidosis increased $P\bar{v}_{O_2}$ ~10 mmHg, whereas alkalosis decreased it 8 mmHg. If these changes in $P\bar{v}_{O_2}$ are accompanied by similar directional changes in mixed venous O_2 content, then, all other factors being equal, ideal $PA_{O_2} - Pa_{O_2}$ would decrease in acidosis and increase in alkalosis.

These limited observations indicate that acidosis tends to improve Pa_{O_2} by lowering $PA_{O_2} - Pa_{O_2}$, and alkalosis tends to decrease Pa_{O_2} by widening $PA_{O_2} - Pa_{O_2}$.

Hemoglobin

In addition to its affinity for O_2, Hb can bind other ligands, and these binding events in turn alter the O_2 affinity. Carbon dioxide, pH, 2,3-diphosphoglycerate (2,3-DPG), and chloride are the most important (6, 82, 153). The Bohr effect (decreased O_2 affinity in association with increased $[H^+]$) as it occurs in tissues is largely attributable to the decreased pH of the blood (15), but there is also a CO_2-specific effect (100) and one due to chloride as well (6, 82).

The metabolite 2,3-DPG also significantly alters O_2 affinity. The [2,3-DPG], a product of erythrocyte glycolysis, is determined by the rate of glycolysis (phosphofructokinase being the rate-limiting enzyme) and the effect of the two enzymes diphosphoglycerate mutase and diphosphoglycerate phosphatase (132, 153). An increase in erythrocyte 2,3-DPG increases the O_2 half-saturation pressure of Hb (P_{50}) (9, 28) by binding 2,3-DPG to HbO_2, thereby altering Hb-O_2 affinity (3, 9, 28), and by changing erythrocyte pH, which then alters Hb-O_2 affinity by the Bohr effect (38). The control of erythrocyte [2,3-DPG] is partly determined

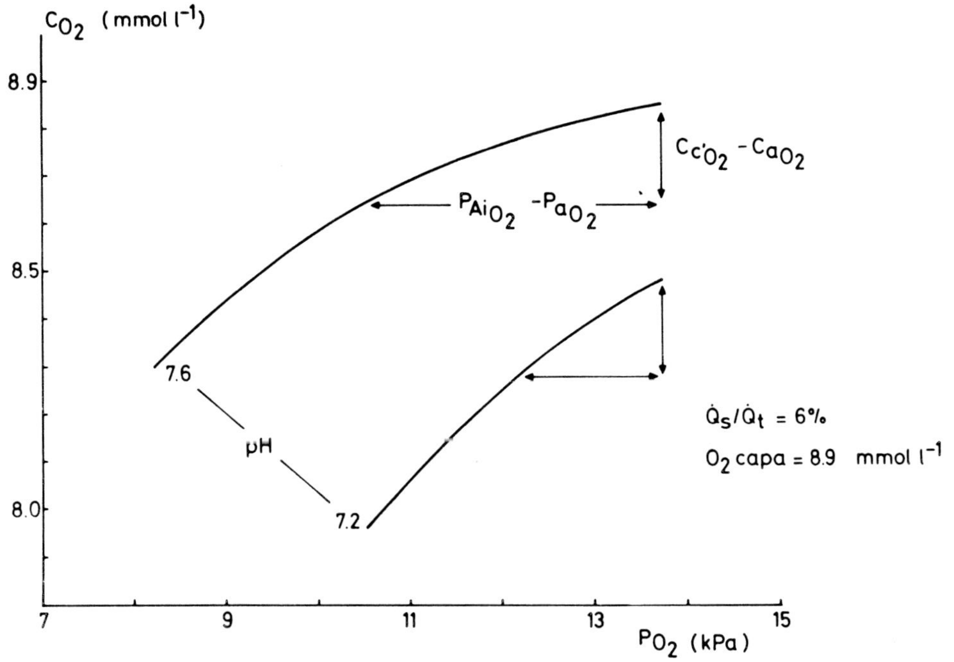

FIG. 1. O_2 concentration (C_{O_2}) shown as a function of partial pressure of O_2 (P_{O_2}) in kPa for 2 values of arterial pH. Degree of venous admixture measured as the ratio of venous admixture to total blood flow ($\dot{Q}S/\dot{Q}T$) and O_2 capacity (O_2 capa) are shown. Only top portion of HbO_2 dissociation curve is represented. For a given ideal end-capillary–to–arterial O_2 content difference ($Cc'_{O_2} - Ca_{O_2}$), the ideal alveolar-arterial difference in P_{O_2} ($PAi_{O_2} - Pa_{O_2}$) is greater in alkalosis than in acidosis. [From Frans et al. (47).]

by pH, probably because of changes in enzyme function (118, 132, 153). Acidosis decreases 2,3-DPG; alkalosis increases it. Thus acidosis decreases Hb-O_2 affinity (increases P_{50}) via the Bohr effect but increases Hb-O_2 affinity (decreases P_{50}) via the decrease in 2,3-DPG. In alkalosis the events occur in the opposite directions.

In many physiological and pathophysiological states the final Hb-O_2 affinity in vivo is determined by the interaction of these and other factors (8, 11, 50, 77, 153). Experimental induction of metabolic acidosis in humans by acetazolamide and ammonium chloride resulted in an initial decrease in P_{50} (measured at pH 7.400 in vitro) over 4 h with no change in 2,3-DPG (Fig. 2). After 4 h, 2,3-DPG levels began to decrease, as did the P_{50} in vitro levels (11). The initial decrease in P_{50}, which occurred independently of 2,3-DPG changes, is attributed to changes in erythrocyte volume and mean corpuscular [Hb]. A decrease in mean corpuscular [Hb] causes Hb interactions within the erythrocyte, which can decrease P_{50}. Thus cell swelling with a resultant decrease in mean corpuscular [Hb] is proposed to account for the initial decrease in P_{50} in vitro during acidosis. If P_{50} is measured under in vivo conditions that do not correct for the Bohr effect, as does the P_{50} in vitro approach, no significant change is observed during the acidosis (Fig. 2). Metabolic alkalosis induced in the same human volunteers by intravenous and oral $NaHCO_3$ resulted in no acute change in 2,3-DPG for 4–5 h. As pH was increased, P_{50} in vitro began to increase, reflecting an increase in mean corpuscular [Hb] (Fig. 2). The net result of the Bohr effect (which decreases P_{50}) and the increase in mean corpuscular [Hb] (which increases P_{50}) is a transient decrease of P_{50} in vivo in metabolic alkalosis. After 4 h, 2,3-DPG levels increased, P_{50} in vitro increased, and P_{50} in vivo was unaltered in steady-state metabolic acidosis and alkalosis. The maintenance of a stable, normal P_{50} in vivo involves direct pH effects (Bohr), changes in mean corpuscular [Hb], and changes in 2,3-DPG induced by pH. Similar results have been reported in dogs: P_{50} in vivo was unchanged,

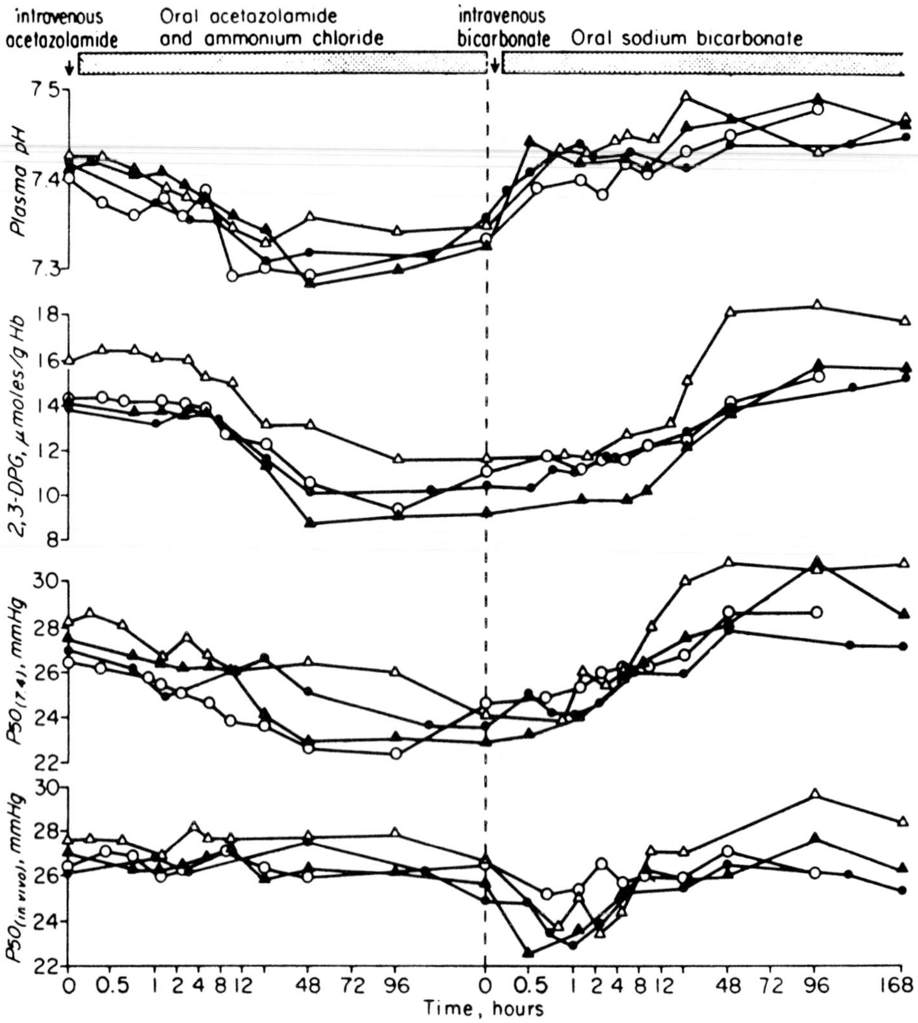

FIG. 2. Plasma pH, erythrocyte 2,3-diphosphoglycerate (2,3-DPG), O_2 half-saturation pressure of Hb (P_{50}) (7.4), and P_{50} (in vivo) in 4 human subjects during acidosis and alkalosis induced by agents noted at *top*. Each symbol represents a different subject. [From Bellingham et al. (8).]

whereas P_{50} in vitro decreased with acid infusion. Here the Bohr effect (to increase P_{50}) and the decrease in 2,3-DPG (to decrease P_{50}) seemed to balance exactly, since no changes in mean corpuscular [Hb] were observed (153).

In diabetic ketoacidosis in which the acidosis develops over some time, the 2,3-DPG levels in erythrocytes are very low (1, 50), raising the question as to whether tissue oxygenation could be impaired. In vitro P_{50} has been reported to be low, 21–23 mmHg (normal = 26–27 mmHg), but in vivo P_{50} is high, 31–33 mmHg (1, 50). This higher in vivo P_{50} would favor tissue O_2 unloading and points out the value of estimating the in vivo P_{50} value. Although there is some inconsistency in the reported data, P_{50} in vivo is generally unchanged or is increased slightly in metabolic acidosis.

In respiratory acidosis a simple increase in P_{CO_2} would increase P_{50} by the Bohr effect. However, in patients with respiratory acidosis, the results have been variable; some workers find a slight increase in P_{50}, others a decrease (153). These patients may have hypoxia, which can increase 2,3-DPG (83), as well as respiratory acidosis, which can decrease 2,3-DPG, an interaction that no doubt contributes to the variability. In addition, changes in [Hb] and in fluid and electrolyte balance, which would alter Hb-O_2 affinity, are not uncommon in these patients.

In summary, although acute changes in pH can alter Hb-O_2 affinity, the secondary responses involving 2,3-DPG and other factors can balance the initial changes so that P_{50} in vivo remains relatively stable. What would be the effect of a change in P_{50} alone on the tissue or capillary P_{O_2}? If $\dot{V}_{O_2}$, blood flow ($\dot{Q}$), and the concentration of O_2 in arterial blood (Ca_{O_2}) are constant, an increased P_{50} must result in an increased $P\bar{v}_{O_2}$. In dogs infused with glycolytic intermediates to decrease Hb-O_2 affinity, P_{50} increased and $P\bar{v}_{O_2}$ was unchanged. However, the arteriovenous O_2 concentration difference ($Ca_{O_2} - C\bar{v}_{O_2}$) increased because of a decrease in $\dot{Q}_T$ (69). Riggs et al. (127) increased P_{50} in anesthetized monkeys by exchange transfusion and observed a decrease in $P\bar{v}_{O_2}$ without a change in $\dot{Q}_T$. When P_{50} was decreased in rats by depletion of 2,3-DPG by prior CO_2 exposure or by exchange transfusion with blood depleted of 2,3-DPG by chemical means (172), a moderate decrease (13 mmHg) was associated with a decrease in the $P\bar{v}_{O_2}$ at rest of 12 mmHg. A smaller decrease in P_{50} had no effect. During exercise, the rats with the greatest decrease in P_{50} had decreased work capability, although compensatory mechanisms seemed to maintain adequate O_2 delivery with lesser changes in Hb-O_2 affinity. Increased Hb-O_2 affinity may be significant in the delivery of O_2, as estimated by $P\bar{v}_{O_2}$ and by work capability.

In addition to Hb-O_2 affinity, the amount of Hb is important in O_2 delivery. The normal blood [Hb] of 15 g/100 ml is maintained by physiological regulatory processes that involve a peptide (erythropoietin) secreted by the kidney. The regulation of circulating Hb mass has been thought to be primarily a function of changes in O_2 demand and availability. Hypoxia results in an increase in erythropoietin and in erythrocyte and Hb mass (78). Anemia also results in an increase in erythropoietin. Genetically abnormal Hb with low P_{50} values can also result in an increased erythropoietin even if $\dot{Q}_T$ and blood [Hb] are normal (78). Some work has examined indirectly the role of acid-base changes on the erythropoietin response to hypoxia. In the rabbit (169), the rat (94), and the human (94), hypoxia induces a respiratory alkalosis due to ventilatory stimulation by the carotid body. Initially P_{50} is decreased, but as 2,3-DPG levels increase, P_{50} returns toward the normal value. Erythropoietin levels are increased initially but tend to decrease as P_{50} returns toward normal. Prevention of respiratory alkalosis by inhalation of CO_2 (93) or the use of the carbonic anhydrase inhibitor acetazolamide (94, 169) prevents or diminishes the initial decrease in P_{50} and the increase in erythropoietin. In these studies the erythropoietin response is determined by the tissue P_{O_2} in the kidney, which reflects the decreased Pa_{O_2} and the respiratory alkalosis because of its effects on P_{50} and perhaps on local perfusion (see next section). Hypercapnia alone at an inspired fraction of O_2 ($F_{I_{O_2}}$) of 0.015–0.05 for 1–4 wk has also been shown to increase the erythrocyte mass (93). The mechanism of this effect is unknown.

Cardiovascular System

In the isolated heart or in the cardiac muscle in vitro, acidosis depresses myocardial contractility (31, 48, 95, 112, 114, 130, 137, 159, 165, 166), slows the heart rate (95, 114, 151), and can participate in the genesis of cardiac arrhythmias (42, 114). The mechanism is not fully understood but probably involves changes in intracellular pH (pH_i) (48, 112, 141) and a competitive interaction of H^+ and Ca^{2+} for important sarcolemmal and intracellular binding sites related to muscle contraction (30, 48, 95, 137, 166). Alkalosis can have a mildly positive inotropic effect (31, 159), presumably by the same contractile mechanisms involving H^+ and Ca^{2+}. Studies of the time course of the changes in pH_i and contractile function support the pH_i hypothesis for the contractile function changes (44, 48, 95, 105, 137). Cardiac muscle exhibits pH_i regulation involving ion exchange, which after an acute decrease in pH_i due to hypercapnia can correct pH_i within minutes to hours (44, 131). As pH_i returns toward normal, so does contractile function (44, 48, 137).

In the intact animal the myocardial contractile response is complicated by the presence of other factors. Acidosis can stimulate the sympathetic nervous system (114, 130, 150, 151, 165), including the release of adrenal cortical and medullary hormones (97, 135, 150, 151). The net results are positive inotropic and chronotropic effects that can, depending on the state of myocardial norepinephrine and adrenal catecholamine stores, override the direct depressant effects of the acidosis (27, 32, 37, 95, 105, 114, 130, 160, 165). The situation is further complicated by the inhibitory effect of acidosis on the norepinephrine mechanism of action at the tissue level (101, 102, 114, 150, 151), although this effect has not always been observed (37).

A similar pattern of acid-base effects occurs in peripheral vessels. Acidosis has a direct effect of relaxation (26, 75), but in vivo this is balanced by the constrictor effect of sympathetic stimulation (160).

Fewer studies have examined alkalosis. Hypocapnic alkalosis in humans results in an initial vasodilation of forearm vessels followed by vasoconstriction (76). In general, the effects seem opposite to those in acidosis but are perhaps of less magnitude (95).

In the intact animal the balance of these direct and indirect effects of acid-base imbalance on the cardiovascular system depends on the degree and type of acid-base disorder and whether or not the animal is anesthetized. In the anesthetized dog, metabolic acidosis produced by bouts of hypoxia with Pa_{CO_2} kept constant by the investigator, resulted in a decrease in plasma pH from 7.40 to 7.20 and a decrease in $\dot{Q}_T$. Increasing Pa_{CO_2} at mild-to-moderate levels of metabolic acidosis improved $\dot{Q}_T$, but with more severe levels of acidosis the hypercapnia further depressed $\dot{Q}_T$ (27). Infusion of lactic acid in anesthetized dogs decreased pH from 7.39 to 7.00, but no change in mean arterial pressure or in mean plasma glucose or catecholamine levels was observed (86). A respiratory acidosis of the same degree in the anesthetized dog increased mean arterial blood pressure, mean plasma glucose, and mean plasma catecholamines (86). In another similar study the respiratory acidosis produced vasoconstriction and an increase in mean arterial pressure while $\dot{Q}_T$ was decreased. Infusion of hexamethonium, a ganglionic blocker, followed by respiratory acidosis resulted in vasodilation, a decrease in mean arterial pressure, and an increase in $\dot{Q}_T$, effects that were not altered by blockade of β-receptors (160). Thus in anesthetized animals a metabolic acidosis without hypercapnia may result in little change in blood pressure or $\dot{Q}_T$ or in slight depression. Respiratory acidosis produces peripheral vasoconstriction and an increase in blood pressure via sympathetic stimulation, but the $\dot{Q}_T$ response may depend on a balance of depression by the direct effect of acidosis and stimulation by reflex sympathetic activity. The degree of sympathetic activity in turn may reflect a balance of CO_2-induced stimulation and baroreceptor-mediated inhibition.

In unanesthetized rats a metabolic acidosis induced by ingestion of ammonium chloride depressed heart rate and $\dot{Q}_T$ (174). At a pH of 6.7 versus a control pH of 7.40, $\dot{Q}_T$ decreased 40%, heart rate decreased 42%, and mean arterial blood pressure decreased 17%. In the conscious dog with respiratory acidosis due to inhalation of 6% CO_2 in air, there was a rapid, transient, but significant decrease in $\dot{Q}_T$, which returned to normal within minutes (63, 105). Brief metabolic acid or base infusion in the unanesthetized dog had little effect (105). In humans, an iatrogenic metabolic acidosis with pH decreasing from 7.42 to 7.34 had no effect on $\dot{Q}_T$ or heart rate [(126); Table 1]. An increase in P_{CO_2} from 40 to 56 mmHg by inhaling 5%–7% CO_2 in air lowered pH from 7.39 to 7.31. Cardiac output increased 45% and stroke volume increased 20%. Mean arterial blood pressure increased from 89 to 105 mmHg, but total peripheral resistance was slightly decreased [(126); Table 1]. Metabolic alkalosis (pH 7.52) also stimulated an increase in $\dot{Q}_T$ (32%) and a decrease in total peripheral resistance, but this experiment is difficult to interpret because of the increase in Pa_{CO_2} from 43 to 48 mmHg, which occurred during the use of $NaHCO_3$ (126). A study of surgical patients with metabolic acidosis found that pH <7.10 is necessary to lower $\dot{Q}_T$, unless other factors like hypoxia or other metabolic derangements are also present (32).

In the unanesthetized animal, severe metabolic acidosis depresses $\dot{Q}_T$ and total peripheral resistance, whereas metabolic alkalosis may enhance $\dot{Q}_T$. Hypercapnia increases stroke volume, heart rate, $\dot{Q}_T$, and blood pressure but results in peripheral vasodilation. Hypocapnia can produce significant peripheral vasoconstriction. In each case, the net effect depends on a balance of direct pH effects mediated largely via changes in pH_i and indirect reflex effects mediated through the sympathoadrenal system.

Tissue Metabolism

Whole-body $\dot{V}_{O_2}$ has been observed to change when acid-base balance is altered. In anesthetized paralyzed dogs, Cain (19) found that passive hyperventilation

TABLE 1. *Cardiovascular Effects of Metabolic and Respiratory Acidosis in the Human*

	n	Arterial pH	Pa_{CO_2}, mmHg	Cardiac Index, liter·min^{-1}·m^{-2}	Peripheral Resistance, mmHg·liter^{-1}·min^{-1}	Heart Rate
Control mean	10	7.42	42	3.6	16.0	77
Metabolic acidosis	10	7.34	40	3.8	14.9	73
		$P < 0.01$	NS	NS	NS	NS
Control mean	16	7.38	42	2.9	16.8	71
Respiratory acidosis	16	7.25	59	4.2	13.1	88
		$P < 0.01$	$P < 0.01$	$P < 0.01$	$P < 0.01$	$P < 0.01$

Values are means. Pa_{CO_2}, partial pressure of CO_2 in arterial blood; n, number of subjects; NS, not significant. [Data from Richardson et al. (126).]

with the development of respiratory alkalosis was associated with an increase in $\dot{V}_{O_2}$, a response that can be prevented if the animals are kept isocapnic. There was a linear relationship between the decrease in P_{CO_2} (or increase in pH) and the increase in $\dot{V}_{O_2}$. In a few animals in which hypercapnia (Pa_{CO_2} = 70 mmHg) was maintained, $\dot{V}_{O_2}$ decreased slightly, but this response was much less reproducible. Others have found that both a metabolic alkalosis and a respiratory alkalosis can increase $\dot{V}_{O_2}$ in intact animals (71, 110).

In respiratory acidosis most mammals, especially smaller ones, respond with a decrease in body temperature (80, 101, 136, 146). The metabolic response varies and depends on the degree of respiratory acidosis, the presence or absence of anesthesia, the species, and whether other stresses are also present, e.g., a change in ambient temperature (101, 136, 146). In unanesthetized rats exposed to 5% or 7% CO_2 in air for up to 3 wk, $\dot{V}_{O_2}$ increased over the first 8 h, then decreased toward normal (80). In unanesthetized guinea pigs exposed to 3% CO_2 in air, $\dot{V}_{O_2}$ increased, but exposure to 15% CO_2 resulted in a decrease in $\dot{V}_{O_2}$ (136). In most animals exposed to CO_2 levels ≥8%, the response is a decrease in $\dot{V}_{O_2}$ (146).

A number of possible mechanisms are involved in the acid-base effects on O_2 utilization. The study of $\dot{V}_{O_2}$ in the isolated hindlimb indicates that alkalosis stimulates $\dot{V}_{O_2}$ (55, 152), but subsequent work has raised the possibility that the anticoagulant used in the experimental system can bind Ca^{2+} and the resultant hypocalcemia caused muscle twitches that produced the increase in $\dot{V}_{O_2}$ (29, 152). Older in vitro tissue studies, however, have found pH effects on $\dot{V}_{O_2}$ (25).

In metabolic pathways many key enzymes are sensitive to pH (101, 103, 125). Acidosis inhibits glycolysis, whereas alkalosis stimulates it (101, 103, 125), most probably via pH effects on the key regulatory enzyme (phosphofructokinase) (154), an effect that can be seen in blood in vitro (66). These pH effects on glucose metabolism have been observed in many tissues (101, 125, 130) but do not necessarily explain the changes in $\dot{V}_{O_2}$ in the whole animal. An alternative possible explanation for the changes in $\dot{V}_{O_2}$ in acidosis involves the role of catecholamines and the sympathoadrenal response to changes in acid-base balance. The catecholamines can increase $\dot{V}_{O_2}$ and lipolysis, causing an increase in plasma free fatty acid (FFA) and glycerol levels (101, 113, 135). In addition, the acidosis can inhibit the peripheral action of the catecholamines (101, 102, 135). The net effect or balance depends on the degree of the acidosis-induced stimulation of catecholamine release versus the degree of inhibition of catecholamine effects in the periphery. Lower levels of CO_2 stimulation result in an increase in whole-body $\dot{V}_{O_2}$, which suggests that catecholamine calorigenesis is predominant over the peripheral inhibition at low levels of hypercapnia.

The metabolic response to respiratory or metabolic alkalosis is more difficult to explain. Most likely the increase in pH that stimulates glycolysis results in some increases in $\dot{V}_{O_2}$ (71). The study of the effects of metabolic acidosis and alkalosis on exercise endurance time and plasma lactate and glycerol levels supports these views (70). In acidosis, endurance time is decreased and plasma lactate, glycerol, and FFA are decreased. Glycolysis and lipolysis are inhibited by the acidosis. In alkalosis, endurance time is prolonged and lactate levels are increased but there is no change in plasma glycerol or FFA levels versus controls.

MEASURED NET EFFECTS OF ACID-BASE IMBALANCE ON O_2 DELIVERY

Tissues

Duling (39) tested the effect of respiratory acidosis and other vasodilators in the hamster cheek pouch preparation on tissue P_{O_2}. Increased P_{CO_2} resulted in a greater increase in tissue P_{O_2} than did other vasodilators. This was ascribed to the dual effect of the increase in P_{CO_2}: vasodilation of the cheek pouch vascular bed and a decrease in the Hb-O_2 affinity in vivo.

The effect of acid-base imbalance on tissue O_2 delivery has also been studied utilizing cerebrospinal fluid (CSF) P_{O_2} as a crude index of mean brain tissue P_{O_2} (14, 40, 67, 68, 73). The CSF P_{O_2} is a function of brain and choroid plexus Pa_{O_2}, Pv_{O_2} (venous blood P_{O_2}), and tissue P_{O_2} values (14, 40, 67, 68, 73); the exact weighting of each of these factors in the determination of CSF P_{O_2} is uncertain. Under normal physiological conditions, the CSF P_{O_2} is less than Pa_{O_2} but greater than brain Pv_{O_2} (14, 40, 67, 68, 73). The CSF P_{O_2} remains relatively stable in the face of changes in Pa_{O_2} (40, 67, 73). Jankowska and Grieb (67) reported that in the anesthetized rabbit, as Pa_{O_2} is decreased to 50 mmHg, the CSF P_{O_2} decreases less than the arterial value and actually becomes greater than the arterial value. They explain this finding by the Bohr effect of H^+ released into choroid plexus capillary blood due to the choroid secretory process. At low P_{O_2} values on the steep part of the HbO_2 dissociation curve, this Bohr effect due to ionic secretion will result in a higher choroid plexus end-capillary P_{O_2}. However, no measurements of the effect of hypoxia on cerebral or choroid plexus blood flow or on brain $\dot{V}_{O_2}$ are provided; these changes could alter the relations of Pa_{O_2}, Pv_{O_2}, and CSF P_{O_2}. If cerebral $Ca_{O_2} - Cv_{O_2}$ decreases because of an increase in the ratio of cerebral blood flow to cerebral metabolism, this also would promote the stability of CSF P_{O_2}, but it would not explain CSF P_{O_2} values above Pa_{O_2}. Regardless of the mechanism, the stability of CSF P_{O_2} in the presence of hypoxemia is an interesting finding with respect to O_2 delivery to the brain.

Laux and Raichle (81) illustrated the intimacy of the relation of the carbonic anhydrase–catalyzed production of H^+ and the Bohr effect on tissue P_{O_2} in the brain. In the lightly anesthetized monkey, total inhibition of carbonic anhydrase activity resulted in an increase in Pa_{CO_2}, an increase in cerebral blood flow greater than that accountable for by the P_{CO_2} change, and a decrease in cerebral $\dot{V}_{O_2}$. The authors contend that the changes in cerebral blood flow and $\dot{V}_{O_2}$ reflect a decrease in tissue P_{O_2} due to the absence of the Bohr effect after total carbonic anhydrase inhibition. This experiment suggests that brain tissue P_{O_2} may be quite sensitive to changes in O_2 delivery produced by acid-base imbalance. This has been further tested in two experiments with acid-base disorders (11, 16).

In uncontrolled diabetes mellitus with ketoacidosis, rapid treatment of the acidosis with $NaHCO_3$ can result in central nervous system (CNS) dysfunction (16, 79). Bureau et al. (16) tested the hypothesis that rapid correction of the acidosis by $NaHCO_3$ infusion abruptly decreases O_2 delivery to the brain. In dogs made acidotic but without ketosis, Pa_{O_2} and CSF P_{O_2} increased initially, but CSF P_{O_2} decreased over the 8-h period of acidosis while Pa_{O_2} remained elevated. Over the latter part of the acidosis, CSF lactate increased, a change associated temporally with the decrease in CSF P_{O_2}. After $NaHCO_3$ therapy, Pa_{O_2} and CSF P_{O_2} both decreased abruptly. In ketoacidosis, CSF lactate was unchanged during the development of the acidosis, and Pa_{O_2} and CSF P_{O_2} were increased. With $NaHCO_3$ therapy, CSF P_{O_2} decreased ~12 mmHg in 1 h, and CSF lactate increased. These workers conclude that the rapid $NaHCO_3$ therapy aggravates CNS hypoxia and results in lactic acid formation. The results support the contention of other workers that rapid correction of diabetic ketoacidosis can cause tissue hypoxia by the immediate leftward Bohr shift of the HbO_2 dissociation curve (1, 8). Bureau et al. (16) acknowledge that in addition to shifts in the HbO_2 dissociation curve, changes in cerebral blood flow during the metabolic acidosis and rapid $NaHCO_3$ therapy could also affect the CSF P_{O_2}. Note that the rapid $NaHCO_3$ therapy also decreased Pa_{O_2} in keeping with the results discussed above of the effects of acid-base changes on ideal $PA_{O_2} - Pa_{O_2}$ (47).

Berthiaume et al. (11) have extended the evaluation of acid-base changes on CSF P_{O_2} by studying the in vitro and in vivo Bohr shift during metabolic acidosis and $NaHCO_3$ therapy in newborn lambs. During acidosis, Pa_{O_2} and CSF P_{O_2} both increased ~7–15 mmHg (Fig. 3). With $NaHCO_3$ therapy, P_{O_2} decreased to control levels in both compartments (Fig. 3). In vitro P_{50} decreased during acidosis and increased with therapy (Fig. 4). In vivo P_{50}, however, increased during acidosis and decreased with therapy. The in vivo decrease in Hb-O_2 affinity during acidosis is correlated with the increase in CSF P_{O_2}. Although Pa_{O_2} also changed, the effects of the changes in Pa_{O_2} on CSF P_{O_2} are small and cannot alone account for the ob-

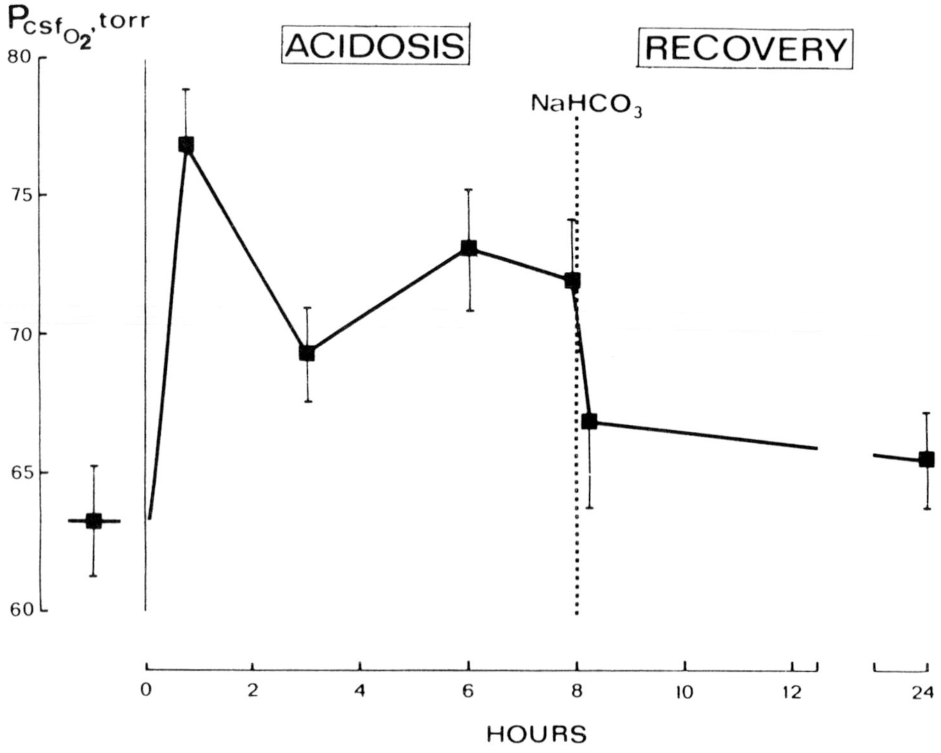

FIG. 3. Cerebrospinal fluid (CSF) P_{O_2} during acidosis and treatment with $NaHCO_3$ in 9-day-old lambs. Plasma pH was decreased from 7.38 to 7.23 over 30 min via HCl infusion and gradually decreased to 7.11 at 8 h. $NaHCO_3$ therapy increased plasma pH to 7.24 at 15 min and to 7.29 after 24 h. [From Berthiaume et al. (11).]

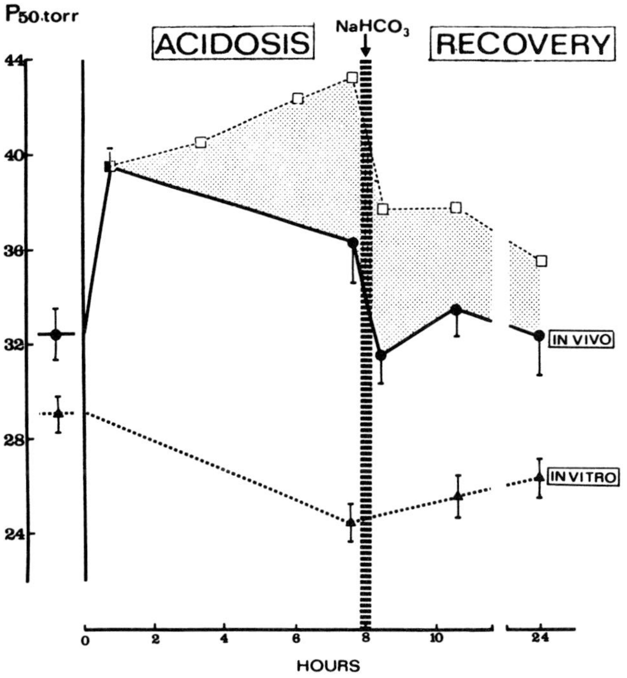

FIG. 4. Values of in vitro P_{50} (7.4 and 37°C) and in vivo P_{50} (pH and animal temperature) during acidosis and $NaHCO_3$ therapy in 9-day-old lambs. (See Fig. 3 for details of plasma pH changes.) *Open squares*, expected P_{50} based only on the Bohr effect. *Shaded areas*, estimated effect of 2,3-DPG decrease that counterbalances the expected P_{50} increase due only to the Bohr effect. [From Berthiaume et al. (11).]

served changes in CSF P_{O_2} (67). In metabolic acidosis, the increase in Pa_{O_2}, the in vivo shift in the HbO_2 dissociation curve, and other unmeasured factors (possibly cerebral blood flow) appear to improve brain tissue O_2 delivery as measured by CSF P_{O_2}. Rapid therapy of the acidosis by $NaHCO_3$ appears in some cases to lower tissue P_{O_2} below normal levels, a result of the decrease in Pa_{O_2}, a leftward Bohr shift in vivo, and perhaps local tissue perfusion alterations. In the hamster cheek pouch and in the brain the net effects of acid-base imbalance on O_2 delivery and utilization, as evaluated by estimates of tissue P_{O_2}, appear to be as predicted.

Whole Animal Stressed by Tissue Hypoxia

In anesthetized paralyzed dogs stressed with hypoxic gas mixtures, Cain (18, 20) studied the effects of acid-base imbalance on O_2 delivery, $\dot{V}_{O_2}$, and hypoxic survival time. In the acidotic group (pH 6.99), hypoxia was induced by ventilation with 9.3% O_2 and 7.1% CO_2 in N_2. The alkalotic group was hyperventilated on an inspired O_2 of 5.2% and infused with 7.5% $NaHCO_3$, so that pH_a was 7.54. The control group was ventilated on 9.1% O_2, so that pH was 7.21. The latter two groups were treated with β-adrenergic blocking agents to inhibit the calorigenic and other effects of sympathoadrenal stimulation. In the respiratory acidotic group this blockade was accomplished by the hypercapnia itself. In all groups the hypoxia was severe enough to depress $\dot{V}_{O_2}$ and mean arterial blood pressure. Hypoxic survival time was defined as the time from the onset of hypoxia until mean arterial blood pressure was <70 mmHg. Although there were differences in $\dot{V}_A$ and $\dot{Q}_T$ among the three experimental groups, total O_2 delivery ($\dot{Q}_T \times Ca_{O_2}$) was the same. The $P\bar{v}_{O_2}$ was the same in the acidotic and normal groups, but in the alkalotic group the $P\bar{v}_{O_2}$ was significantly decreased. Survival time was not significantly affected by the acidosis or alkalosis, although more O_2 is available in acidosis at higher Pa_{O_2} and $P\bar{v}_{O_2}$ values. The $\dot{V}_{O_2}$ decreased in hypoxia but was not correlated with $\dot{Q}_T$, Pa_{O_2}, or $P\bar{v}_{O_2}$. It was correlated linearly and significantly with total O_2 delivery. Irrespective of acid-base status, as total O_2 delivery decreased below a threshold value, $\dot{V}_{O_2}$ was decreased. Cain postulated that the relatively insensitive relationship of $\dot{V}_{O_2}$ to $P\bar{v}_{O_2}$ in these experiments with acid-base imbalance was because the HbO_2 curve in the low P_{O_2} range is relatively insensitive to Bohr shifts. Cain (21) repeated the experiments in anesthetized, paralyzed, and ventilated dogs with diminished O_2 delivery produced by anemia. In this case the acidosis was produced by HCl infusion, and the alkalosis was produced by $NaHCO_3$ infusion. The anemia was severe enough to depress $\dot{V}_{O_2}$, and the hypothesis was that acidosis would shift the anemic HbO_2 curve to the right, aid in unloading, enhance O_2 delivery, and increase $\dot{V}_{O_2}$ for any given degree of anemia. The reverse was expected in alkalosis. The experimental observations were the exact opposite. After anemia induced a depression of $\dot{V}_{O_2}$, alkalosis increased $\dot{V}_{O_2}$ and acidosis further depressed $\dot{V}_{O_2}$. The acidosis (pH 7.1) and alkalosis (pH 7.4) had no significant effect on $P\bar{v}_{O_2}$ or Pa_{O_2}, but acidosis decreased $\dot{Q}_T$, whereas alkalosis enhanced $\dot{Q}_T$. The effects of acid-base imbalance on $\dot{V}_{O_2}$ appeared to be the result not of altered HbO_2 position but of altered $\dot{Q}_T$ and O_2 delivery. In both experiments (20, 21) in which tissue hypoxia was produced followed by acidosis or alkalosis, $\dot{V}_{O_2}$ was decreased as total O_2 delivery was decreased, but $P\bar{v}_{O_2}$ does not appear to be a sensitive indicator of this change. Rather, the volume rate of O_2 delivery seems to be the more important determinant of $\dot{V}_{O_2}$.

Whole Animal at Rest

In a study of the effect of acidosis on tissue gas pressures, Van Liew (158) analyzed published human data and experimentally used the subcutaneous tissue gas pocket technique in unanesthetized rats. Figure 5 shows on an O_2-CO_2 diagram an analysis developed by Van Liew of the effect of metabolic acidosis on tissue P_{O_2} in humans at rest, during diabetic ketoacidosis, and with hyperventilation to lower the Pa_{CO_2} to the same extent as in the ketoacidosis. Measured arterial points are shown on blood gas-exchange lines for a respiratory exchange ratio (R) of 0.7. The numbers on each blood R line represent fractions of normal

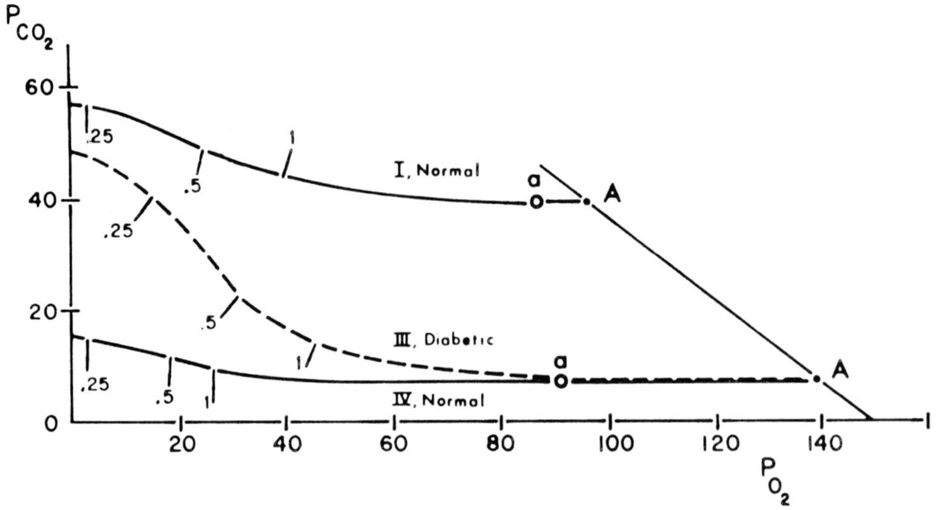

FIG. 5. O_2-CO_2 diagram, P_{CO_2} vs. P_{O_2}. *Line* at *right* with *points* labeled *A*, lung respiratory exchange ratio (R) line of 0.7. *Lines* labeled *I, III,* and *IV*, blood R lines, each with R = 0.7. *I*: normal resting man. *III*: man with diabetic ketoacidosis. *IV*: nonacidotic man hyperventilating as in *III*. *Points* labeled *A*, alveolar points; *points* labeled *a*, arterial points. Numbers on blood R lines, fractions of normal blood flow assuming an arteriovenous O_2 concentration difference of 4.6 ml O_2/100 ml blood. [Data from Henderson (61).]

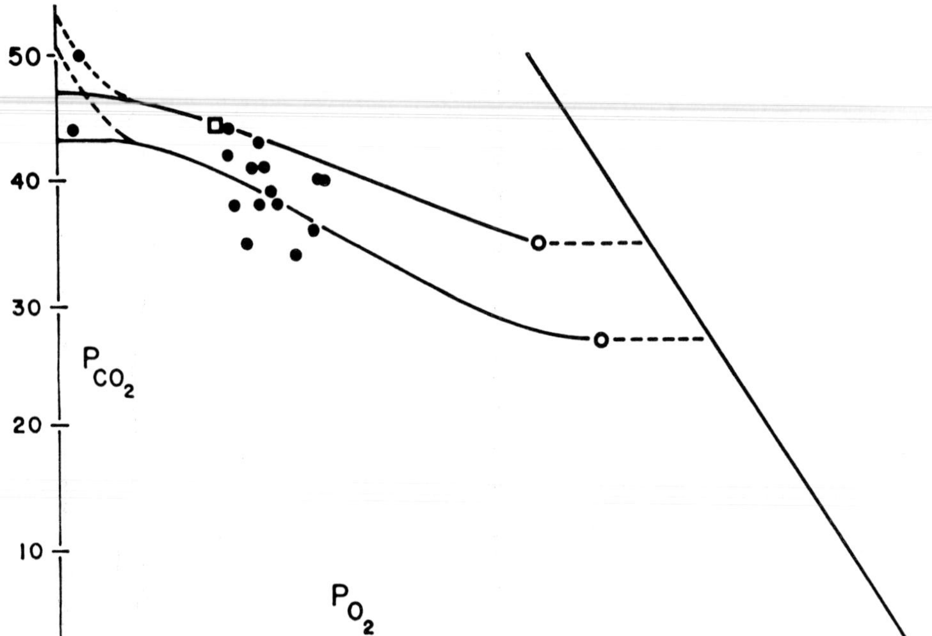

FIG. 6. O_2-CO_2 diagram, P_{CO_2} vs. P_{O_2}. *Line* at *right*, lung R line; *open circles*, arterial points; *dashed lines*, connect arterial points to lung R line at alveolar points. *Open square*, mean control rat subcutaneous gas pocket values. *Solid circles*, gas pocket values obtained in rats made acidotic by NH_4Cl treatment. [From Van Liew (158).]

$\dot{Q}_T$ (1.0, 0.5, 0.25) for constant tissue $\dot{V}_{O_2}$ and CO_2 uptake ($\dot{V}_{CO_2}$). Under normal acid-base balance, as $\dot{Q}_T$ is decreased, $P\bar{v}_{CO_2}$ rises more steeply at low P_{O_2} values. This effect is magnified in metabolic acidosis. In diabetic acidosis, for a given $\dot{Q}_T$, $P\bar{v}_{O_2}$ is higher than in normal humans and than in humans hyperventilating to the same extent as in acidosis. Thus in acidosis the O_2 and CO_2 carriage properties of the blood tend to maintain $P\bar{v}_{O_2}$ (and by inference tissue P_{O_2}) without the necessity of any $\dot{Q}_T$ change.

In the experimental evaluation of these predictions with tissue gas pockets in the rat, pH was decreased from 7.40 to 7.28 by ammonium chloride ingestion. Figure 6 shows tissue P_{O_2} and Pa_{O_2} values. In acidosis, Pa_{O_2} increased and P_{CO_2} decreased compared with control, and $PA_{O_2} - Pa_{O_2}$ decreased. In the tissue gas pocket analysis, the values from acidotic rats are clustered at higher P_{O_2} and lower P_{CO_2} values than in the controls. A derived estimate of local tissue blood flow per unit $\dot{V}_{O_2}$ indicates only a 5% increase. These experimental results show that enhanced O_2 delivery to tissues can occur in metabolic acidosis and that it is due to hyperventilation, a small increase in blood flow, and the physicochemical properties of Hb.

Whole Animal in Exercise

An alternative approach in the experimental study of the effects of acid-base imbalance on O_2 delivery has been the application of endurance time and metabolic substrate utilization in exercise as indices of tissue oxygenation during acidosis and alkalosis (70). In healthy human subjects, acidosis was induced by ingestion of ammonium chloride and alkalosis by ingestion of $NaHCO_3$. Endurance time was measured at 33%, 66%, and 95% of the subject's maximum power output on a bicycle ergometer. Alkalosis (pH 7.44 vs. pH 7.37 in control) significantly increased endurance time at 95% of the maximum power output level from a control mean of 270 s to 438 s. Acidosis (pH 7.20) reduced endurance time to 160 s. The analysis in the previous section and the data on CSF P_{O_2}, both dealing with the resting organism, suggest that acidosis should improve and alkalosis could depress tissue O_2 delivery. Yet in this maximum exercise endurance test, endurance was improved with alkalosis and depressed in acidosis. Analysis of O_2 delivery is limited in this study, but $\dot{V}_{O_2}$, $\dot{V}_{CO_2}$, R (respiratory exchange ratio), and $\dot{Q}_T$ were not different in acidosis versus alkalosis. Surprisingly 2,3-DPG was also not different in acidosis versus alkalosis, although measurements were made in only three subjects. Ventilatory changes were small but ventilation was highest in acidosis and lowest in alkalosis, with corresponding changes in Pa_{CO_2}. Acidosis did result in less of an increase in plasma lactate and less elevation of plasma glycerol and FFA than in controls, whereas alkalosis enhanced these changes. Sutton et al. (147) believed these metabolic changes are due to pH effects on glycolysis and on catecholamine-induced lipolysis. The authors argue that the inhibitory effect of acidosis and the enhancing effect of alkalosis on maximum exercise endurance are due to acid-base effects on metabolism, not on O_2 delivery. Acidosis-related inhibition of lipolysis and glycolysis could diminish energy availability to exercising muscle even if O_2 delivery is adequate. In nonexercising dogs stressed with hypoxia, Cain (18) showed that hypercapnia results in less lactate increase in hypoxia than if P_{CO_2} is allowed to decrease (and pH to increase). This effect has been shown to be due partly to altered glycolysis. Cain proposed that the lactate increase in tissue hypoxia represents a tissue or cellular energy demand satisfied by anaerobic glycolysis. This demand is increased in any conditions of oxygenation if catecholamine calorigenesis is stimulated. Inhibition of glycolysis and catecholamine calorigenesis by acidosis diminishes the excess energy demand due to these mechanisms. In the exercise endurance study, the acidosis-induced inhibition of anaerobic glycolysis and catecholamine calorigenesis via lipolysis could result in less energy availability and in less endurance, even though O_2 delivery may not be inhibited. Presumably the O_2 debt would also have been reduced.

COMPARATIVE ASPECTS OF ACID-BASE BALANCE AND POSSIBLE RELATIONSHIP TO O_2 DELIVERY

At their average body temperature of 37°C, mammals maintain a normal arterial pH of 7.400, Pa_{CO_2} of 40 mmHg, and Pa_{O_2} of 95 mmHg. These normal values are thought to be consistent with optimal physiological function. Yet in ectotherms the normal blood pH and P_{CO_2} are critically dependent on body temperature. A "normal" pH of 7.400 is found only at a single temperature. This temperature dependence of acid-base balance in ectotherms raises important fundamental questions concerning the physiological significance of pH. Why do homeotherms regulate absolute pH so carefully and ectotherms tolerate large changes in pH with temperature? It is clear from the preceding discussion that changes in pH above or below 7.400 or changes in P_{CO_2} above or below 40 mmHg in homeotherms can have significant effects on the processes that determine O_2 delivery and $\dot{V}_{O_2}$. Consideration of the theory of acid-base balance in ectotherms provides some possible insights into mechanisms involved in this physiology.

Temperature and Acid-Base Balance in Ectotherms

Study of a variety of ectotherms, including invertebrates (23, 88, 155), fish (22, 59, 115, 117), and reptiles and amphibians (4, 33, 35, 36, 51, 60, 72, 98, 116, 123, 128), has demonstrated a very similar pattern of decreasing pH (and increasing Pa_{CO_2}) as temperature (T) is increased (Fig. 7). The relation d(pH)/dT ranges from −0.015 to −0.020 pH U/°C. Thus for bullfrogs (*Rana catesbeiana*) at 20°C, normal pH is 7.89, but at 30°C normal pH is 7.74, a difference of 0.15 U. This pH difference in homeotherms resulting from acidosis or alkalosis at 37°C would profoundly alter physiological functions, including gas exchange.

The interpretation of the physiological significance of the relationship of pH to body temperature has developed along two conceptual lines. First, it was noted that the quantitative change in blood pH as a function of temperature is very similar to the change in pH or pOH of neutral water with temperature (64)

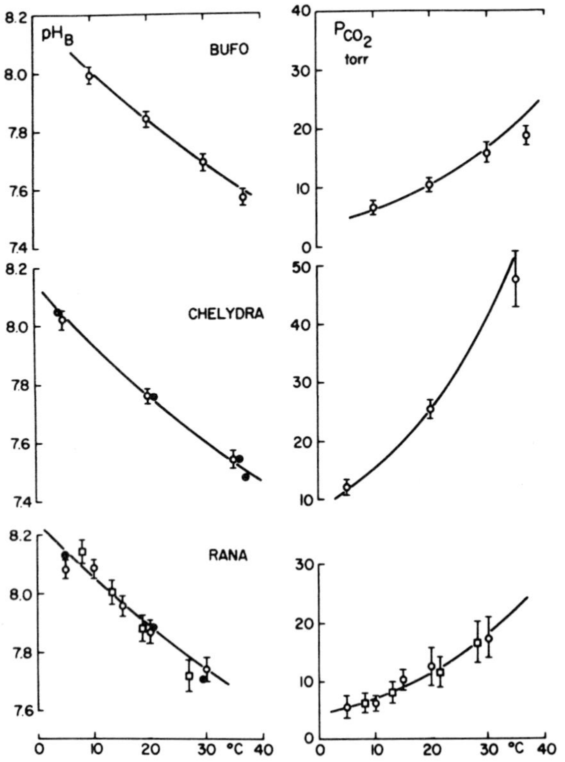

FIG. 7. Blood pH (pH_B) and P_{CO_2} of toads (*Bufo marinus*), snapping turtles (*Chelydra serpentina*), and bullfrogs (*Rana catesbeiana*) shown as function of temperature. *Curves* are drawn from a binary buffer model solution for each animal. *Open circles* are in vivo data and *closed circles* are in vitro data from Howell et al. (64); *open squares* are data from Reeves (120). [From Reeves (123).]

due to the temperature effect on the ionization constant for water (K_w) (159a). This led to the concept of relative alkalinity: it is not the absolute [H^+] or [OH^-] that is biologically important but rather the ratio of their concentrations. The [OH^-]/[H^+] ratios of a simple aqueous solution and of frog, turtle, and toad blood are constant with changing temperature, although the absolute [OH^-]/[H^+] values differ in each case (64). This concept of relative alkalinity, like the observations concerning blood pH at different temperatures, is not new (116, 117) but has been rediscovered and given new emphasis. Its significance in explaining acid-base effects on physiological and biochemical processes has been questioned (131).

Mammalian blood in vitro at constant total [CO_2] has a d(pH)/dT of −0.0157 U/°C, a value very much in the range of those observed in ectotherms (121, 133). Examination of the buffer components of blood indicated that only those with a pK of ~7.0 and an ionization enthalpy of ~7.0 kcal/mol would result in a change in pH with a temperature like that observed in blood (2). Histidine imidazole residues (2, 120, 129), NH_2-terminal α-amino groups (43), and (probably of lesser importance) some sulfhydryl groups (167) fit these criteria. The pK of the most important of the three groups, imidazole (pK_{im}), changes approximately −0.017 U/°C, and this change in pK largely accounts for the change in blood pH studied in a closed system in vitro (120, 123). This effect was demonstrated in a simple in vitro experiment in which three bicarbonate solutions were exposed to different temperatures in a closed system with constant CO_2 content (Fig. 8). A simple bicarbonate buffer solution or a bicarbonate-phosphate buffer solution did not exhibit a d(pH)/dT relationship like that of blood. The combination bicarbonate-imidazole solution, however, has a d(pH)/dT like that of blood in vitro.

Because d(pH)/dT and d(pK_{im})/dT are similar, if not identical, it was deduced that the fractional dissociation of histidine imidazole groups (α-imidazole) will remain constant as pH is changed with temperature (120, 121, 123). The constant fractional dissociation of imidazole with temperature changes further indicates that insofar as dissociable imidazole groups on proteins can determine net protein-charge state and function, temperature-induced pH changes will not alter this function, whereas isothermal pH changes will (the alphastat hypothesis).

Study of intracellular pH with variations in temperature in liver, heart, and muscle of turtle (*Chrysemys scripta*) and frog (*Rana catesbeiana*) has also shown values for d(pH)/dT very smilar to those in blood (89). Because these workers assumed pK_{im} values of intracellular proteins to be like those of blood, an almost constant α-imidazole has also been found. Although the relatively constant intracellular α-imidazole depends on this assumption (23), the finding

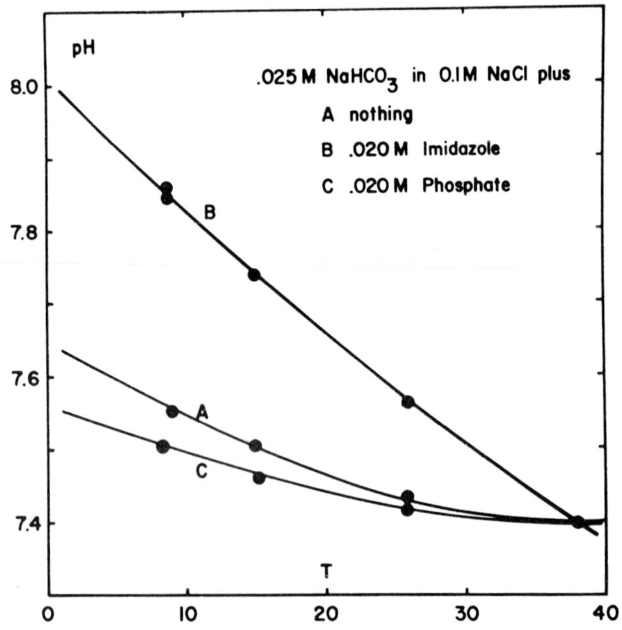

FIG. 8. Values of pH vs. temperature in °C for 3 chemical solutions at constant CO_2 content. *A*, pure carbonic acid-bicarbonate solution; *B*, same as *A* plus 0.020 M imidazole; *C*, same as *A* plus 0.020 M phosphate. *Lines*, theoretical calculations based on model buffer systems. [From Reeves (120).]

that d(pH$_i$)/dT in so many cases is similar to the d(pH)/dT value observed in blood in vitro and in vivo is still a striking observation, especially given the presence inside cells of many buffer groups (128).

The application of the alphastat hypothesis to the study of protein function has been limited. The Cl^- distribution in the erythrocyte remains constant when pH is changed by temperature but changes significantly when pH is changed isothermally (122). Studies of enzyme pH optima at different temperatures in the Na^+-K^+-ATPase of toad skin (*Bufo marinus*) and human erythrocyte ghosts (108), in five soluble and membrane-bound enzymes in rainbow trout (*Salmo gairdneri*) (58), and in M_4-lactate dehydrogenase of six fish and one mammal (173) all support the alphastat hypothesis, as do studies of *p*-aminohippuric acid (109) and glutamine (49) uptake by rat kidney slices. Thus some proteins behave as predicted by the alphastat hypothesis.

However, not all animals studied exhibit this type of d(pH)/dT relationship. The most striking exceptions include hibernating mammals (119), heterothermic mammals (119, 168), and varanid lizards (170, 171). In the estivating bat and in the sloth (mammals with naturally occurring low body temperatures), arterial pH does not increase in hypothermia (119). The Pa_{CO_2} decreases sufficiently to maintain pH almost constant at the value present at 37°C. In the heterothermic mammal (*Perognathus longimembris*, the little pocket mouse), as body temperature is decreased the arterial pH does increase slightly; the d(pH)/dT value is −0.0085 U/°C (168). In varanid lizards, with changing temperature in vivo the observed d(pH)/dT value is −0.005 U/°C (170, 171). The ratio of expired ventilation to $\dot{V}_{CO_2}$ ($\dot{V}E/\dot{V}_{CO_2}$) is constant as temperature is increased; it does not decrease as in other air-breathing ectotherms (74). Three general explanations could apply to these exceptions.

First, if $\dot{V}E/\dot{V}_{O_2}$ were to decrease as temperature (and metabolic demand) increased in an ectothermic species with a high metabolic rate (e.g., *varanids*), then hypoxemia could develop (74, 170, 171). Second, the observed coefficient for blood d(pH)/dT in a species could correlate with similar coefficients for enzyme temperature-pH optima in that species, as suggested for the heterothermic mammal *P. longimembris* (167, 168). Third, variations in cell pH from the predicted value observed in most ectotherms could mean that cell pH in some cases is a regulatory signal, e.g., in hibernation (163) and in many other fundamental cell processes (17).

Significance for Gas Exchange in Homeotherms: Humans

The fundamental significance of the alphastat hypothesis for gas exchange in homeothermic mammals is the same as for other physiological systems. When, where, and if the alphastat hypothesis is relevant, pH changes that occur in isothermal conditions alter function by changing protein structure due to the presence of dissociable imidazole groups. The question is, Where in the system of O_2 delivery and utilization just discussed are there such proteins? The evidence is scanty and indirect, but a few examples are cited.

As mentioned in COMPARATIVE ASPECTS OF ACID-BASE BALANCE AND POSSIBLE RELATIONSHIP TO O_2 DELIVERY, p. 431, human blood exposed in vitro to different temperatures in a closed system behaves as predicted by the ectotherm approach (121, 125, 133). In vivo the problem is more complicated. Humans have significant regional differences in body temperature (e.g., skin vs. core), but overall body temperature is closely regulated. Blayo et al. (13) investigated whether human blood in vivo behaves as predicted by the temperature-pH relationship of ectotherms. In patients made hypothermic for surgery (body temperature = 27°C–28°C), they measured blood pH using electrodes maintained at 37°C. The patients were hyperventilated sufficiently to maintain this 37°C pH at 7.400. Blayo et al. reasoned that if there were no change in the measured [HCO_3^-] then the hyperventilation-induced decrease in P_{CO_2} and increase in pH of the blood in vivo were appropriate for the decrease in temperature, as predicted by the response of human blood in vitro. If the in vitro values for d(pH)/dT and d(P_{CO_2})/dT for human blood do not pertain in vivo, then the degree of hyperventilation that maintains pH at 7.400 measured at 37°C would result in a change in plasma [HCO_3^-]. The plasma [HCO_3^-] remained constant in all cases. These results provide some evidence that the blood of humans in vivo behaves like that of an ectotherm.

Hitzig (62) has linked chemical chemoreceptor function in mammals and turtles to the alphastat hypothesis by analysis of the ventilatory and cerebrospinal fluid pH results obtained in a goat at constant temperature and in the turtle at different temperatures. The similarity of a plot of ventilation versus α-imidazole for both species is interpreted as support for alphastat involvement in central chemoreceptor function.

Hemoglobin-O_2 affinity is affected by both temperature and pH, raising the possibility that temperature-induced pH changes alter O_2 affinity via imidazole groups. Experimental comparison of the changes in P_{50} with temperature in conditions in which total CO_2 was constant (i.e., pH and P_{CO_2} varied with temperature) with those in conditions of constant pH found little difference in the values for d(log P_{50})/dT (124). Thus the temperature effect of Hb-O_2 affinity is largely independent of any temperature-induced acid-base changes. The CO_2 Bohr slopes were also similar at all temperatures, indicating that the Bohr shift in P_{50} is essentially independent of temperature (124). This suggests that changes in pH do not alter Hb-O_2

affinity by an effect on the dissociation of imidazole groups with pK of 7.0 and d(pK_{im})/dT close to −0.0157 U/°C.

Temperature-pH interactions have been reviewed recently with respect to the general issue of the appropriate pH to be maintained during controlled surgical hypothermia (148, 149, 162). This issue is still controversial, although many in the field currently believe that during hypothermia the patient's blood pH should be alkaline at the hypothermic temperature, as predicted by the ectotherm pH model (148, 149, 162). Part of the evidence for this position comes from a few studies of myocardial function during and after hypothermia that compare the effect of pH maintained at an alkaline value at the hypothermic temperature versus pH maintained at 7.4 or lower at the hypothermic temperature. At the alkaline pH values there was less or no depression of myocardial function (7, 14, 91). These results suggest that the function of proteins involved in the relationship of myocardiac contractility and pH is determined in part by dissociable imidazole groups.

CONCLUSIONS

1. Acid-base imbalance can alter each step in the process of O_2 transport from environment to the cell, and it can alter the utilization of O_2.
2. In many cases the net result of acidosis or alkalosis is a balance of opposite effects of [H^+], e.g., stimulation of the sympathoadrenal system by hypercapnia versus inhibition at the end organ of the norepinephrine response. The severity and duration of the changes in [H^+] are important determinants in the balance.
3. A change in [H^+] can have different net results in different conditions. At rest, acidosis, if not too severe, may enhance O_2 transport and increase tissue P_{O_2}. In exercise, however, acidosis decreases endurance time predominantly because of its effects on cell metabolism, not on O_2 transport.
4. Changes in pH produced in isothermal conditions may alter O_2 transport and utilization by effects on certain proteins, as predicted by the alphastat hypothesis. The function of these proteins is determined in part by structural changes caused by dissociation of imidazole groups. Such proteins may be involved in central chemoreception affecting $\dot{V}_A$ and in cardiac contractility affecting output. Many enzymes affecting O_2 utilization may also behave as predicted by this alphastat hypothesis. Other aspects of O_2 transport may involve proteins with these characteristics, but these have not been investigated.

REFERENCES

1. ALBERTI, K. G. M. M., J. H. DARLEY, P. M. EMERSON, AND T. D. R. HOCKADAY. 2,3-Diphosphoglycerate and tissue oxygenation in uncontrolled diabetes mellitus. *Lancet* 2: 391–395, 1972.
2. ALBERY, W. J., AND B. B. LLOYD. Variation of chemical potential with temperature. In: *Development of the Lung*, edited by A. V. S. de Reuck and R. Porter. London: Churchill, 1967. (Ciba Found. Symp.)
3. ARNONE, A. X-ray diffraction study of binding of 2,3-diphosphoglycerate to human deoxyhaemoglobin. *Nature Lond.* 237: 146–149, 1972.
4. AUSTIN, J. H., F. W. SUNDERMAN, AND J. G. CAMACK. The electrolyte composition and the pH of serum of a poikilothermous animal at different temperatures. *J. Biol. Chem.* 72: 677–685, 1927.
5. BARER, G. R., J. R. MCCURRIE, AND J. W. SHAW. Effects of changes in blood pH on the vascular resistance of the normal and hypoxic cat lung. *Cardiovasc. Res.* 5: 490–497, 1971.
6. BARTELS, H., AND R. BAUMANN. Respiratory function of hemoglobin. In: *Respiratory Physiology II*, edited by J. G. Widdicombe. Baltimore, MD: University Park, 1977, vol. 14, p. 107–134. (Int. Rev. Physiol. Ser.)
7. BECKER, H., J. VINTEN-JOHANSON, G. D. BUCKBERG, J. M. ROBERTSON, J. D. LEAF, H. L. LAZAR, AND A. J. MANGANARO. Myocardial damage caused by keeping pH 7.40 during deep systemic hypothermia. *J. Thorac. Cardiovasc. Surg.* 82: 810–820, 1981.
8. BELLINGHAM, A. J., J. C. DETTER, AND C. LENFANT. Regulatory mechanisms of hemoglobin oxygen affinity in acidosis and alkalosis. *J. Clin. Invest.* 50: 700–706, 1971.
9. BENESCH, R., AND R. E. BENESCH. The effect of organic phosphates from the human erythrocyte on the allosteric properties of human hemoglobin. *Biochem. Biophys. Res. Commun.* 26: 162–164, 1967.
10. BERGOFSKY, E. H., D. E. LEHR, AND A. P. FISHMAN. The effect of changes in hydrogen ion concentration on the pulmonary circulation. *J. Clin. Invest.* 41: 1492–1502, 1962.
11. BERTHIAUME, Y., M. A. BUREAU, AND R. BÉGIN. The adaptation of neonatal blood to metabolic acidosis and its effect on cisternal oxygen tension. *Pediatr. Res.* 15: 809–812, 1981.
12. BISCOE, T. J., M. J. PURVES, AND S. R. SAMPSON. The frequency of nerve impulses in single carotid body chemoreceptor afferent fibres recorded in vivo with intact circulation. *J. Physiol. Lond.* 208: 121–131, 1970.
13. BLAYO, M. C., Y. LECOMPTE, AND J. J. POCIDALO. Control of acid-base status during hypothermia in man. *Respir. Physiol.* 42: 287–298, 1980.
14. BLOOR, B. M., J. FRICKER, F. HELLINGER, H. NISHIOKA, AND J. MCCUTCHEN. A study of cerebrospinal fluid oxygen tensions: preliminary clinical and experimental observation. *Arch. Neurol.* 14: 37–47, 1961.
15. BOHR, C., K. HASSELBALCH, AND A. KROGH. Ueber einen in biologischer Beziehung wichtigen Einfluss, den die Kohlen säurespannung des Blutes auf dessen Sauerstoffbindung übt. *Skand. Arch. Physiol.* 16: 402–412, 1904.
16. BUREAU, M. A., R. BÉGIN, Y. BERTHIAUME, D. SHAPCOTT, K. KHOURY, AND N. GAGON. Cerebral hypoxia from bicarbonate infusion in diabetic acidosis. *J. Pediatr.* 96: 968–973, 1980.
17. BUSA, W. B., AND R. NUCCITELLI. Metabolic regulation via intracellular pH. *Am. J. Physiol.* 246 (*Regulatory Integrative Comp. Physiol.* 15): R409–R438, 1984.
18. CAIN, S. M. Diminution of lactate rise during hypoxia by P_{CO_2} and β-adrenergic blockade. *Am. J. Physiol.* 217: 110–116, 1969.
19. CAIN, S. M. Increased oxygen uptake with passive hyperventilation of dogs. *J. Appl. Physiol.* 28: 4–7, 1970.
20. CAIN, S. M. Oxygen delivery and utilization in hypoxic dogs made acidemic and alkalemic. *Adv. Exp. Med. Biol.* 75: 483–489, 1976.

21. CAIN, S. M. Oxygen extraction in severely anemic dogs after infusion of $NaHCO_3$ or HCl. *Adv. Exp. Med. Biol.* 94: 525–530, 1978.
22. CAMERON, J. N. Regulation of blood pH in teleost fish. *Respir. Physiol.* 33: 129–144, 1978.
23. CAMERON, J. N. Acid-base status of fish at different temperatures. *Am. J. Physiol.* 246 (*Regulatory Integrative Comp. Physiol.* 15): R452–R459, 1984.
24. CAMERON, J. N., AND C. V. BATTERTON. Temperature and blood acid-base status in the blue crab, *Callinectes sapidus*. *Respir. Physiol.* 35: 101–110, 1978.
25. CANZANELLI, A., M. GREENBLATT, G. A. ROGERS, AND D. RAPPORT. The effect of pH changes on the in-vitro O_2 consumption of tissues. *Am. J. Physiol.* 127: 290–295, 1939.
26. CARRIER, O., JR., M. COWSERT, J. HANCOCK, AND A. C. GUYTON. Effect of hydrogen ion changes on vascular resistance in isolated artery segments. *Am. J. Physiol.* 207: 169–172, 1964.
27. CARSON, S. A. A., G. E. CHORLEY, F. N. HAMILTON, D. C. LEE, AND L. E. MORRIS. Variation in cardiac output with acid-base changes in the anesthetized dog. *J. Appl. Physiol.* 20: 948–953, 1965.
28. CHANUTIN, A., AND R. R. CURNISH. Effect of organic and inorganic phosphate on the oxygen equilibrium of human erythrocytes. *Arch. Biochem. Biophys.* 121: 96–102, 1967.
29. CHAPLER, C. K., W. N. STAINSBY, AND L. B. GLADDEN. Effect of changes in blood flow, norepinephrine, and pH on oxygen uptake by resting skeletal muscle. *Can. J. Physiol. Pharmacol.* 58: 93–96, 1980.
30. CHAPMAN, R. A., AND D. ELLIS. The existence of Ca^{++} for H^+ exchange across the sarcolemma of frog cardiac muscle cells (Abstract). *J. Physiol. Lond.* 265: 19P–20P, 1977.
31. CLANCY, R. L., H. E. CINGOLANI, R. R. TAYLOR, T. P. GRAHAM, JR., AND J. P. GILMORE. Influence of sodium bicarbonate on myocardial performance. *Am. J. Physiol.* 212: 917–923, 1967.
32. CLOWES, G. H. A., JR., G. A. SABGA, A. KONITAXIS, R. TOMIN, M. HUGHES, AND F. A. SIMEONE. Effects of acidosis on cardiovascular function in surgical patients. *Ann. Surg.* 154: 524–555, 1961.
33. CRAWFORD, E. C., AND R. N. GATZ. Acid-base status of the blood of a desert lizard at different temperatures (Abstract). *Pfluegers Arch.* 343, Suppl.: R3, 1973.
34. DALY, M. DE B., C. J. LAMBERTSEN, AND A. SCHWEITZER. The effects upon bronchial musculature of altering the oxygen and carbon dioxide tensions of the blood perfusing the brain. *J. Physiol. Lond.* 119: 292–341, 1953.
35. DILL, D. B., AND H. T. EDWARDS. Properties of reptilian blood. IV. The alligator (*Alligator mississippiensis*). *J. Cell. Comp. Physiol.* 6: 243–254, 1935.
36. DILL, D. B., H. T. EDWARDS, A. V. BOCK, AND J. H. TALBOTT. Properties of reptilian blood. III. The chuckwalla (*Sauromalus obesus*). *J. Cell. Comp. Physiol.* 6: 37–42, 1935.
37. DOWNING, S. E., N. S. TALNER, AND T. H. GARDNER. Cardiovascular responses to metabolic acidosis. *Am. J. Physiol.* 208: 237–242, 1965.
38. DUHM, J. Effects of 2,3-diphosphoglycerate and other organic phosphate compounds on oxygen affinity and intracellular pH of human erythrocytes. *Pfluegers Arch.* 326: 341–356, 1971.
39. DULING, B. R. Changes in microvascular diameter and oxygen tension induced by carbon dioxide. *Circ. Res.* 32: 370–376, 1973.
40. DUNKIN, R. S., AND S. BONDURANT. The determinants of cerebrospinal fluid P_{O_2}. The effect of oxygen and carbon dioxide breathing in patients with chronic lung disease. *Ann. Intern. Med.* 64: 71–80, 1966.
41. EBERT, P. A., L. J. GREENFIELD, W. G. AUSTEN, AND A. G. MORROW. The relationship of blood pH during profound hypothermia to subsequent myocardial function. *Surg. Gynecol. Obstet.* 114: 357–362, 1962.
42. ELHARRAR, V., AND D. P. ZIPES. Cardiac electrophysiologic alterations during myocardial ischemia. *Am. J. Physiol.* 233 (*Heart Circ. Physiol.* 2): H329–H345, 1977.
43. ELLENBOGEN, E. Dissociation constants of peptides. IV. The isomeric alanylalanines. *J. Am. Chem. Soc.* 78: 369–372, 1956.
44. ELLIS, D., AND R. C. THOMAS. Direct measurement of the intracellular pH of mammalian cardiac muscle. *J. Physiol. Lond.* 262: 755–771, 1976.
45. FENCL, V., T. B. MILLER, AND J. R. PAPPENHEIMER. Studies on the respiratory response to disturbances of acid-base balance, with deductions concerning the ionic composition of cerebral interstitial fluid. *Am. J. Physiol.* 210: 459–472, 1966.
46. FINCH, C. A., AND C. LENFANT. Oxygen transport in man. *N. Engl. J. Med.* 286: 407–415, 1972.
47. FRANS, A., Z. TUREK, H. YOKATA, AND F. KREUZER. Effect of variations in blood hydrogen ion concentration on pulmonary gas exchange of artificially ventilated dogs. *Pfluegers Arch.* 380: 35–39, 1979.
48. FRY, C. H., AND P. A. POOLE-WILSON. Effects of acid-base changes on excitation-contraction coupling in guinea-pig and rabbit cardiac ventricular muscle. *J. Physiol. Lond.* 313: 141–160, 1981.
49. GEORGE, J. P., AND S. SOLOMAN. pH and temperature dependence of glutamine uptake, carbon dioxide, and ammonia production in kidney slices from acidotic rats. *J. Physiol. Lond.* 316: 251–261, 1981.
50. GIBBY, O. M., K. E. A. VEALE, T. M. HAYES, J. G. JONES, AND C. A. J. WALDROP. Oxygen availability from the blood and the effect of phosphate replacement on erythrocyte 2,3-diphosphoglycerate and haemoglobin-oxygen affinity in diabetic ketoacidosis. *Diabetologia* 15: 381–385, 1978.
51. GIORDANO, R. V., AND D. C. JACKSON. The effect of temperature on ventilation in the green iguana (*Iguana iguana*). *Comp. Biochem. Physiol. A Comp. Physiol.* 45: 235–238, 1973.
52. GOLDRING, R. M., P. J. CANNON, H. O. HEINEMANN, AND A. P. FISHMAN. Respiratory adjustment to chronic metabolic alkalosis in man. *J. Clin. Invest.* 47: 188–202, 1968.
53. HAAS, F., AND E. H. BERGOFSKY. Effect of pulmonary vasoconstriction on balance between alveolar ventilation and perfusion. *J. Appl. Physiol.* 24: 491–497, 1968.
55. HARKEN, A. H. Hydrogen ion concentration and oxygen uptake in an isolated canine hindlimb. *J. Appl. Physiol.* 40: 1–5, 1976.
56. HARVEY, R. M., Y. ENSON, R. BETTI, M. L. LEWIS, D. F. ROCHESTER, AND M. I. FEUER. Further observations on the effect of hydrogen ion on the pulmonary circulation. *Circulation* 35: 1019–1027, 1967.
57. HARVEY, R. M., Y. ENSON, M. L. LEWIS, W. B. GREENOUGH, K. M. ALLY, AND R. A. PANNO. Hemodynamic effects of dehydration and metabolic acidosis in Asiatic cholera. *Trans. Assoc. Am. Physicians* 79: 177–186, 1966.
58. HAZEL, J. R., W. S. GARLICK, AND P. A. SELLNER. The effects of assay temperature upon the pH optima of enzymes from poikilotherms: a test of the imidazole alphastat hypothesis. *J. Comp. Physiol.* 123: 97–104, 1978.
59. HEISLER, N. Regulation of the acid-base status in fish. In: *Environmental Physiology of Fishes*, edited by M. A. Ali. New York: Plenum, 1980, p. 123–162.
60. HENDERSON, L. J. Das Gleichgewicht wischen basen and sauren in tierischen Organismus. *Ergeb. Physiol.* 8: 254–325, 1909.
61. HENDERSON, L. J. *Blood: A Study in General Physiology*. New Haven, CT: Yale Univ. Press, 1928.
62. HITZIG, B. M. Temperature-induced changes in turtle CSF pH and central control of ventilation. *Respir. Physiol.* 49: 205–222, 1982.
63. HORWITZ, L. D., V. S. BISHOP, AND H. L. STONE. Effects of hypercapnia on the cardiovascular system of conscious dogs. *J. Appl. Physiol.* 25: 346–348, 1968.
64. HOWELL, B. J., F. W. BAUMGARDNER, K. BONDI, AND H. RAHN. Acid-base balance in cold-blooded vertebrates as a function of body temperature. *Am. J. Physiol.* 218: 600–606, 1970.
65. INGRAM, R. H., JR. Effects of airway versus arterial CO_2

changes on lung mechanics in dogs. *J. Appl. Physiol.* 38: 603–607, 1975.

66. JACEY, M. J., AND K. E. SCHAEFER. The effect of chronic hypercapnia on blood phosphofructokinase activity and the adenine nucleotide system. *Respir. Physiol.* 16: 267–272, 1972.
67. JANKOWSKA, L., AND P. GRIEB. Relationship between arterial and cisternal CSF oxygen tension in rabbits. *Am. J. Physiol.* 236 (*Renal Fluid Electrolyte Physiol.* 5): F220–F225, 1979.
68. JARUM, S., J. LORENZEN, AND E. SKINHØI. Cisternal fluid oxygen tension in man. *Neurology* 14: 703–707, 1964.
69. JOHANSEN, K., AND C. LENFANT. A comparative approach to the adaptability of O_2-Hb affinity. In: *Oxygen Affinity of Hemoglobin and Red Cell Acid-Base Status*, edited by M. Rørth and P. Astrup. Copenhagen: Munksgaard, 1972. (Alfred Benzon Symp., 4th, 1971.)
70. JONES, N. L., J. R. SUTTON, R. TAYLOR, AND C. J. TOEWS. Effect of pH on cardiorespiratory and metabolic responses to exercise. *J. Appl. Physiol.* 43: 959–964, 1977.
71. KARETZKY, M. S., AND S. M. CAIN. Oxygen uptake stimulation following Na-L-lactate infusion in anesthetized dogs. *Am. J. Physiol.* 216: 1486–1490, 1969.
72. KATZ, U. Acid-base status in the toad *Bufo viridis* in vivo. *Respir. Physiol.* 41: 105–115, 1980.
73. KAZEMI, H., R. C. KLEIN, F. N. TURNER, AND D. J. STRIEDER. Dynamics of oxygen transfer in the cerebrospinal fluid. *Respir. Physiol.* 4: 24–31, 1968.
74. KINNEY, J. L., D. T. MATSUURA, AND F. N. WHITE. Cardiorespiratory effects of temperature in the turtle, *Pseudemys floridana*. *Respir. Physiol.* 31: 309–325, 1977.
75. KONTOS, H. A., D. W. RICHARDSON, AND J. L. PATTERSON, JR. Vasodilator effect of hypercapnic acidosis on human forearm blood vessels. *Am. J. Physiol.* 215: 1403–1405, 1968.
76. KONTOS, H. A., D. W. RICHARDSON, A. J. RAPER, Z. UL-HASSAN, AND J. L. PATTERSON, JR. Mechanisms of action of hypocapnic alkalosis on limb blood vessels in man and dog. *Am. J. Physiol.* 223: 1296–1307, 1972.
77. KRALL, M. A., J. D. BRISTOW, J. E. WELCH, AND J. METCALFE. Physiological effects of lowered blood oxygen affinity in dogs. *Respir. Physiol.* 33: 263–270, 1978.
78. KRANTZ, S. G., AND L. O. JACOBSON. *Erythropoietin and the Regulation of Erythropoiesis.* Chicago, IL: Univ. of Chicago Press, 1970.
79. KREISBERG, R. A. Diabetic ketoacidosis: new concepts and trends in pathogenesis and treatment. *Ann. Intern. Med.* 88: 681–695, 1978.
80. LAI, Y.-L., W. J. E. LAMM, AND J. HILDEBRANDT. Ventilation during prolonged hypercapnia in the rat. *J. Appl. Physiol.* 51: 78–83, 1981.
81. LAUX, B. E., AND M. E. RAICHLE. The effect of acetazolamide on cerebral flow and oxygen utilization in the rhesus monkey. *J. Clin. Invest.* 62: 585–592, 1978.
82. LAVER, M. B., E. JACKSON, M. SCHERPEREL, C. TUNG, W. TUNG, AND E. P. RADFORD. Hemoglobin-O_2 affinity regulation: DPG, monovalent anions, and hemoglobin concentration. *J. Appl. Physiol.* 43: 632–642, 1977.
83. LENFANT, C., J. TORRANCE, E. ENGLISH, C. A. FINCH, C. REYNAFARJE, J. RAMOS, AND J. FAURA. Effect of altitude on oxygen binding by hemoglobin and on organic phosphate levels. *J. Clin. Invest.* 47: 2652–2656, 1968.
84. LEUSEN, I. Regulation of cerebrospinal fluid composition with reference to breathing. *Physiol. Rev.* 52: 1–56, 1972.
85. LIFSCHITZ, M. D., R. BRASCH, A. J. CUOMO, AND S. J. MENN. Marked hypercapnia secondary to severe metabolic alkalosis. *Ann. Intern. Med.* 77: 405–409, 1972.
86. LIGOU, J. C., AND G. G. NAHAS. Comparative effects of acidosis induced by acid infusion and CO_2 accumulation. *Am. J. Physiol.* 198: 1201–1206, 1960.
87. LILJESTRAND, G. Chemical control of the distribution of pulmonary blood flow. *Acta Physiol. Scand.* 44: 216–240, 1958.
88. LOEWE, R., AND H. B. DE EGGERT. Blood gas analysis and acid-base status in the hemolymph of a spider (*Eurypelma californicum*). Influence of temperature. *J. Comp. Physiol.* 134: 331–338, 1979.
89. MALAN, A., T. L. WILSON, AND R. B. REEVES. Intracellular pH in cold-blooded vertebrates as a function of body temperature. *Respir. Physiol.* 28: 29–47, 1976.
90. MALIK, A. B., AND B. S. L. KIDD. Independent effects of changes in H^+ and CO_2 concentrations on hypoxic pulmonary vasoconstriction. *J. Appl. Physiol.* 34: 318–323, 1973.
91. MCCONNELL, D. H., F. N. WHITE, R. L. NELSON, S. M. GOLDSTEIN, J. V. MALONEY, E. C. DELAND, AND G. D. BUCKBERG. Importance of alkalosis in maintenance of "ideal" blood pH during hyothermia. *Surg. Forum* 26: 263–265, 1975.
92. MILLER, A. T., JR. Acclimatization to carbon dioxide. *Am. J. Physiol.* 129: 524–531, 1940.
93. MILLER, M. E. The interaction between the regulation of acid-base and erythropoietin production. *Blood Cells* 1: 449–465, 1975.
94. MILLER, M. E., M. RØRTH, H. H. PARVING, D. HOWARD, I. REDDINGTON, C. R. VALERI, AND F. STOHLMAN, JR. pH effect on erythropoietin response to hypoxia. *N. Engl. J. Med.* 288: 706–710, 1973.
95. MITCHELL, J. H., K. WILDENTHAL, AND R. L. JOHNSON, JR. The effects of acid-base disturbances on cardiovascular and pulmonary function. *Kidney Int.* 1: 375–387, 1972.
96. MITCHELL, R. A. The regulation of respiration in metabolic acidosis and alkalosis. In: *Cerebrospinal Fluid and the Regulation of Ventilation*, edited by C. M. Brooks, F. F. Kao, and B. B. Lloyd. Oxford, UK: Blackwell, 1965, p. 109–131.
97. MITTELMAN, A., S. J. DOS, H. G. BARKER, AND G. G. NAHAS. Adrenocortical response during corrected and uncorrected hypercapnic acidosis. *Am. J. Physiol.* 202: 334–336, 1962.
98. MOALLI, R., R. S. MEYERS, G. R. ULTSCH, AND D. C. JACKSON. Acid-base balance and temperature in a predominantly skin-breathing salamander, *Cryptobranchus alleganiensis*. *Respir. Physiol.* 43: 1–11, 1981.
99. NADEL, J. A., AND J. G. WIDDICOMBE. Effect of changes in blood gas tensions and carotid sinus pressure on tracheal volume and total lung resistance to airflow. *J. Physiol. Lond.* 163: 13–33, 1962.
100. NAERAA, N., E. STRANGE PETERSEN, E. BOYE, AND J. W. SEVERINGHAUS. pH and molecular CO_2 components of the Bohr effect in human blood. *Scand. J. Clin. Lab. Invest.* 18: 96–102, 1966.
101. NAHAS, G. G. Mechanisms of carbon dioxide and pH effects on metabolism. In: *Carbon Dioxide and Metabolic Regulation*, edited by G. G. Nahas and K. E. Schaefer. New York: Springer-Verlag, 1974, p. 107–117.
102. NAHAS, G. G., AND C. POYART. Effect of arterial pH alterations on metabolic activity of norepinephrine. *Am. J. Physiol.* 212: 765–772, 1967.
103. NAHAS, G. G., AND O. S. STEINSLAND. Increased rate of catecholamine synthesis during respiratory acidosis. *Respir. Physiol.* 5: 108–117, 1968.
104. NISELL, O. The action of oxygen and carbon dioxide on the bronchioles and vessels of the isolated perfused lungs. *Acta Physiol. Scand. Suppl.* 73: 15–62, 1950.
105. NOBLE, M. I. M., D. TRENCHARD, AND A. GUZ. Effect of changes in Pa_{CO_2} and Pa_{O_2} on cardiac performance in conscious dogs. *J. Appl. Physiol.* 22: 147–152, 1966.
106. O'CAIN, C. F., M. J. HENSLEY, E. R. MCFADDEN, JR., AND R. H. INGRAM, JR. Pattern and mechanism of airway response to hypocapnia in normal subjects. *J. Appl. Physiol.* 47: 8–12, 1979.
107. PAPPENHEIMER, J. R., V. FENCL, S. R. HEISEY, AND D. HELD. Role of cerebral fluids in control of respiration as studied in unanesthetized goats. *Am. J. Physiol.* 208: 436–450, 1965.
108. PARK, Y. S., AND S. K. HONG. Properties of toad skin Na-K-ATPase with special reference to effect of temperature. *Am. J. Physiol.* 231: 1356–1363, 1976.
109. PARK, Y. S., AND S. SOLOMON. pH-temperature dependence of organic acid transport in rat kidney slices. *Am. J. Physiol.* 233 (*Renal Fluid Electrolyte Physiol.* 2): F382–F387, 1977.
110. PATTERSON, R. W., AND S. F. SULLIVAN. Determinants of oxygen uptake during sodium bicarbonate infusion. *J. Appl. Physiol.* 45: 399–402, 1978.

111. PETERS, R. M., E. M. HEDGPETH, JR., AND B. G. GREENBERG. The effect of alterations in acid-base balance on pulmonary mechanics. *J. Thorac. Cardiovasc. Surg.* 57: 303–311, 1969.
112. POPHAM, P. A. B., P. J. OLDERSHAW, AND J. R. CAMERON. Relationship between developed tension and intracellular pH in rat papillary muscle during acute respiratory and metabolic acid-base changes (Abstract). *Clin. Sci. Mol. Med.* 58: 10P, 1980.
113. POYART, C., AND G. G. NAHAS. Inhibition of catecholamine-induced calorigenesis and lipolysis by hypercapnic acidosis. *Am. J. Physiol.* 211: 161–168, 1966.
114. PRICE, H. L. Effects of carbon dioxide on the cardiovascular system. *Anesthesiology* 21: 652–663, 1960.
115. RAHN, H., AND F. W. BAUMGARDNER. Temperature and acid-base regulation in fish. *Respir. Physiol.* 14: 171–182, 1972.
116. RAHN, H., AND B. J. HOWELL. The OH^-/H^{++} concept of acid-base balance: historical development. *Respir. Physiol.* 33: 91–97, 1978.
117. RANDALL, D. J., AND J. N. CAMERON. Respiratory control of arterial pH as temperature changes in rainbow trout *Salmo gairdneri. Am. J. Physiol.* 225: 997–1002, 1973.
118. RAPOPORT, S., AND G. M. GUEST. The decomposition of diphosphoglycerate in acidified blood: its relationship to reactions of the glycolytic cycle. *J. Biol. Chem.* 129: 781–790, 1939.
119. REEVES, R. B. Role of body temperature in determining the acid-base state in vertebrates. *Federation Proc.* 28: 1204–1208, 1969.
120. REEVES, R. B. An imidazole alphastat hypothesis for vertebrate acid-base regulation: tissue carbon dioxide content and body temperature in bullfrogs. *Respir. Physiol.* 14: 219–236, 1972.
121. REEVES, R. B. Temperature-induced changes in blood acid-base status: pH and P_{CO_2} in a binary buffer. *J. Appl. Physiol.* 40: 752–761, 1976.
122. REEVES, R. B. Temperature-induced changes in blood acid-base status: Donnan r_{Cl} and red cell volume. *J. Appl. Physiol.* 40: 762–767, 1976.
123. REEVES, R. B. The interaction of body temperature and acid-base balance in ectothermic vertebrates. *Annu. Rev. Physiol.* 39: 559–586, 1977.
124. REEVES, R. B. The effect of temperature on the oxygen equilibrium curve of human blood. *Respir. Physiol.* 42: 317–328, 1980.
125. RELMAN, S. A. Metabolic consequences of acid-base disorders. *Kidney Int.* 1: 347–359, 1972.
126. RICHARDSON, D. W., A. J. WASSERMAN, AND J. L. PATTERSON. General and regional circulatory responses to change in blood pH and carbon dioxide tension. *J. Clin. Invest.* 40: 31–43, 1961.
127. RIGGS, T. E., A. W. SHAFER, AND C. A. GUENTER. Acute changes in oxyhemoglobin affinity: effects on oxygen transport and utilization. *J. Clin. Invest.* 52: 2660–2663, 1973.
128. ROBIN, E. D. Relationship between temperature and plasma pH and carbon dioxide tension in the turtle. *Nature Lond.* 195: 249–251, 1962.
129. ROBIN, E. D., P. A. BROMBERG, AND C. E. CROSS. Some aspects of the evolution of vertebrate acid-base regulation. *Yale J. Biol. Med.* 41: 448–467, 1969.
130. ROCAMORA, J. M., AND S. E. DOWNING. Preservation of ventricular function by adrenergic influences during metabolic acidosis in the cat. *Circ. Res.* 24: 373–381, 1969.
131. ROOS, A., AND W. F. BORON. Intracellular pH. *Physiol. Rev.* 61: 296–434, 1981.
132. ROSE, I. A. Regulation of human red cell glycolysis: a review. *Exp. Eye Res.* 11: 264–272, 1971.
133. ROSENTHAL, T. B. The effect of temperature on the pH of blood and plasma in vitro. *J. Biol. Chem.* 173: 25–30, 1959.
134. SCARPELLI, E. M., AND E. J. AGASSO. Arterial pH, airway caliber and response to acetylcholine and catecholamines in vivo. *Respir. Physiol.* 38: 235–242, 1979.
135. SCHAEFER, K. E., N. MCCABE, AND J. WITHERS. Stress response in chronic hypercapnia. *Am. J. Physiol.* 214: 543–548, 1968.
136. SCHAEFER, K. E., A. A. MESSIER, C. MORGAN, AND G. T. BAKER III. Effect of chronic hypercapnia on body temperature regulation. *J. Appl. Physiol.* 38: 900–906, 1975.
137. SERUR, J. R., C. L. SKELTON, R. BODEM, AND E. H. SONNENBLICK. Respiratory acid-base changes and myocardial contractility: interaction between calcium and hydrogen ions. *J. Mol. Cell. Cardiol.* 8: 823–836, 1976.
138. SEVERINGHAUS, J. W., E. W. SWENSON, T. N. FINLEY, M. T. LATEGOLA, AND J. WILLIAMS. Unilateral hypoventilation produced in dogs by occluding one pulmonary artery. *J. Appl. Physiol.* 16: 53–60, 1961.
139. SHAPIRO, B. J., D. H. SIMMONS, AND L. M. LINDE. Pulmonary hemodynamics during acute acid-base changes in the intact dog. *Am. J. Physiol.* 210: 1026–1032, 1966.
140. SMITH, L. J., C. R. INNERS, P. B. TERRY, H. A. MENKES, AND R. J. TRAYSTMAN. Effects of methacholine and hypocapnia on airways and collateral ventilation in dogs. *J. Appl. Physiol.* 46: 966–972, 1979.
141. STEENBERGEN, C., G. DELEEUW, T. RICH, AND J. R. WILLIAMSON. Effects of acidosis and ischemia on contractility and intracellular pH of rat heart. *Circ. Res.* 41: 849–858, 1977.
142. STEIN, J. R., AND J. G. WIDDICOMBE. The interaction of chemo- and mechanoreceptor signals in the control of airway calibre. *Respir. Physiol.* 25: 363–376, 1975.
143. STEPHENS, N. L., AND R. W. MITCHELL. Mechanism of action of respiratory acidosis on tracheal smooth muscle. *Am. J. Physiol.* 227: 647–651, 1974.
144. STERLING, G. M. The mechanism of bronchoconstriction due to hypocapnia in man. *Clin. Sci. Lond.* 34: 277–285, 1968.
145. STEWART, P. A. *How to Understand Acid-Base.* New York: Elsevier, 1981.
146. STUPFEL, M. Carbon dioxide and temperature regulation. In: *Carbon Dioxide and Metabolic Regulation*, edited by G. Nahas and K. E. Schaefer. New York: Springer-Verlag, 1974, p. 163–188.
147. SUTTON, J. R., N. L. JONES, AND C. J. TOEWS. Effect of pH on muscle glycolysis during exercise. *Clin. Sci. Lond.* 61: 331–338, 1981.
148. SWAN, H. The hydroxyl-hydrogen ion concentration ratio during hypothermia. *Surg. Gynecol. Obstet.* 155: 897–912, 1982.
149. SWAN, H. The importance of acid-base management for cardiac and cerebral preservation during open heart operations. *Surg. Gynecol. Obstet.* 158: 391–414, 1984.
150. TENNEY, S. M. Sympatho-adrenal stimulation by carbon dioxide and the inhibitory effect of carbonic acid on epinephrine response. *Am. J. Physiol.* 187: 341–346, 1956.
151. TENNEY, S. M. Effects of CO_2 on neurohumoral and endocrine mechanisms. *Anesthesiology* 21: 674–685, 1960.
152. THEYE, R. A., G. A. GRONERT, AND J. J. A. HEFFION. Oxygen uptake of canine whole body and hind limb with hypocapnic alkalosis. *Anesthesiology* 47: 416–422, 1977.
153. THOMAS, H. M., S. S. LEFRAK, R. S. IRWIN, H. W. FRITTS, JR., AND P. R. B. CALDWELL. The oxyhemoglobin dissociation curve in health and disease. *Am. J. Med.* 57: 331–348, 1974.
154. TRIVEDI, B., AND W. H. DANFORTH. Effect of pH on the kinetics of frog muscle phosphofructokinase. *J. Biol. Chem.* 241: 4110–4112, 1966.
155. TRUCHOT, J. P. Temperature and acid-base regulation in the shore crab *Carcinus maenas* (L.). *Respir. Physiol.* 17: 11–20, 1973.
156. TULLER, M. A., AND F. MEHDI. Compensatory hypoventilation and hypercapnia in primary metabolic alkalosis. *Am. J. Med.* 50: 281–290, 1971.
157. TWINING, R. H., V. LOPEZ-MAJANO, H. N. WAGNER, JR., V. CHERNICK, AND R. E. DUTTON. Effect of regional hypercapnia on the distribution of pulmonary blood flow in man. *Johns Hopkins Med. J.* 123: 95–103, 1968.
158. VAN LIEW, H. D. Oxygen and carbon dioxide tensions in tissue and blood of normal and acidotic rats. *J. Appl. Physiol.* 25: 575–580, 1968.
159. VAUGHN-WILLIAMS, E. M. The individual effects of CO_2, bicarbonate and pH on the electrical and mechanical activity

of isolated rabbit auricles. *J. Physiol. Lond.* 129: 90–110, 1955.

159a. WEAST, R. C. (editor). *Handbook of Chemistry and Physics* (46th ed.). Cleveland, OH: CRC, 1965.

160. WENDLING, M. G., J. W. ECKSTEIN, AND F. M. ABBOUD. Cardiovascular responses to carbon dioxide before and after beta-adrenergic blockade. *J. Appl. Physiol.* 22: 223–226, 1967.

161. WEST, J. B. Ventilation-perfusion relationships. *Am. Rev. Respir. Dis.* 116: 919–943, 1977.

162. WHITE, F. N. A comparative physiological approach to hypothermia. *J. Thorac. Cardiovasc. Surg.* 82: 821–831, 1981.

163. WHITE, F. N., AND G. SOMERO. Acid-base regulation and phospholipid adaptations to temperature: time courses and physiological significance of modifying the milieu for protein function. *Physiol. Rev.* 62: 40–90, 1982.

164. WIDDICOMBE, J. G. Regulation of tracheobronchial smooth muscle. *Physiol. Rev.* 43: 1–37, 1963.

165. WILDENTHAL, K., D. S. MIERZWIAK, R. W. MYERS, AND J. H. MITCHELL. Effects of acute lactic acidosis on left ventricular performance. *Am. J. Physiol.* 214: 1352–1359, 1968.

166. WILLIAMSON, J. R., B. SAFER, T. RICH, S. SCHAFFER, AND K. KOBAYASHI. Effects of acidosis on myocardial contractility and metabolism. *Acta Med. Scand. Suppl.* 587: 95–112, 1975.

167. WILSON, T. L. Theoretical analysis of the effects of two pH regulation patterns on the temperature sensitivities of biological systems in nonhomeothermic animals. *Arch. Biochem. Biophys.* 182: 409–419, 1977.

168. WITHERS, P. C. Acid-base regulation as a function of body temperature in ectothermic toads, a heliothermic lizard, and a heterothermic mammal. *J. Therm. Biol.* 3: 163–171, 1978.

169. WOLF-PRIESSNITZ, J., J. C. SCHOOLEY, AND L. J. MAHLMANN. Inhibition of erythropoietin production in unanesthetized rabbits exposed to an acute hypoxic-hypercapnic environment. *Blood* 52: 153–162, 1978.

170. WOOD, S. C., K. JOHANSEN, AND R. N. GATZ. Pulmonary blood flow, ventilation/perfusion ratio, and oxygen transport in a varanid lizard. *Am. J. Physiol.* 233 (*Regulatory Integrative Comp. Physiol.* 2): R89–R93, 1977.

171. WOOD, S. C., K. JOHANSEN, M. L. GLASS, AND R. W. HOYT. Acid-base regulation during heating and cooling in the lizard, *Varanus exanthematicus*. *J. Appl. Physiol.* 50: 779–783, 1981.

172. WOODSON, R. D., B. WRANNE, AND J. C. DETTER. Effects of increased blood oxygen affinity on work performance of rats. *J. Clin. Invest.* 52: 2717–2724, 1973.

173. YANCEY, P. H., AND G. N. SOMERO. Temperature dependence of intracellular pH: its role in the conservation of pyruvate apparent K_m values of vertebrate lactate dehydrogenases. *J. Comp. Physiol.* 125: 129–134, 1978.

174. YUDKIN, J., R. D. COHEN, AND B. SLACK. The haemodynamic effects of metabolic acidosis in the rat. *Clin. Sci. Lond.* 50: 177–184, 1976.

Carbon monoxide toxicity

RONALD F. COBURN
HENRY JAY FORMAN | *Department of Physiology, University of Pennsylvania School of Medicine, Philadelphia, Pennsylvania*

CHAPTER CONTENTS

IT HAS BEEN CLEAR FOR YEARS (118) that exposure to high [CO] in inspired air has extremely deleterious effects on humans and animals. Over the last 20 years the adverse effects of relatively small CO exposures, exposures that can be found in urban, industrial, and household air, have been emphasized (34, 93, 98).

Toxic effects of absorbed CO are a result of the binding of this gas to hemoglobin (Hb) and possibly other proteins. The overall toxic effects are determined by the extent of CO binding and also by complex changes that occur in the circulation and tissue, which can be considered to be adaptations to CO hypoxia. These topics form the basis for understanding CO toxicity. This chapter is a review of possible mechanisms of CO toxicity and adaptation.

Deleterious effects of elevated body CO stores are usually termed *CO hypoxia*, which infers that CO pathophysiology involves inhibition of O_2 transport from blood to tissue, with a resultant fall in tissue partial pressure of O_2 (P_{O_2}). This term is used here. However, inhibition of intracellular oxidoreductases due to CO binding also occurs and may be a component of CO toxicity. Few data in the literature bear on the possibility that a mechanism of CO toxicity is CO binding to oxidoreductases. In this chapter we consider oxidoreductase reactions that CO could potentially inhibit and reactions of CO with O_2-carrier proteins.

Carbon monoxide toxicity is a broad topic. Many important areas that are pertinent to CO effects on humans are not covered here. These topics include sources of CO that pollute our environment, CO levels of air, and factors that influence these levels. Recent reviews have adequately covered these topics (34, 98). The evidence that CO exposures giving concentrations of carboxyhemoglobin (HbCO) as low as 4%–5% saturation have adverse effects on normal humans and on susceptible populations (e.g., the human fetus and/or embryo, patients with atherosclerotic cardiovascular disease or chronic obstructive pulmonary disease) has also been reviewed (34, 93, 98).

The physiologist's interest in CO transcends the importance of CO toxicology. Because CO primarily acts through competition with O_2, studies of CO physiology and biochemistry have helped us understand O_2 physiology and biochemistry. Carbon monoxide measurements have been useful in studies of gas exchange in the lung, placenta, and gills (62, 65, 98); the blood volume (22, 121); body heme turnover (35); mucosal blood flow (17, 41, 111); and tissue oxygenation (38, 40).

BODY CO STORES

Location

The localization of CO in the tissues of humans and animals remains a basic problem for study. This study is pertinent because sites of the CO stores give hints about mechanisms of CO toxicity. Most of the body CO is found in blood chemically bound to Hb. In normal humans, 10%–15% of the total store is located in extravascular tissues (values as high as 25% have been obtained in dogs) (22, 32, 38, 121). Data from muscle biopsy experiments performed on anesthetized dogs suggest that most or all of the extravascular CO may be found in skeletal plus cardiac muscle, presumably bound to myoglobin (Mb) (38, 40). However, a significant fraction of the total stores may be bound to proteins other than Hb or Mb. Less than 1% of the total CO stores is physically dissolved in body tissues because of the low tissue partial pressure of CO (P_{CO}) and low solubility of CO in water and lipid (32).

Mixing of CO in the body stores occurs at the same rate as mixing of labeled erythrocytes in the circulation (102). Therefore equilibrium between intravascular and extravascular CO stores is relatively rapid. Intravascular-to-extravascular exchange of CO depends on tissue blood flow, diffusion between blood and tissue, and reaction rates of CO-binding compounds. For skeletal or cardiac muscle the pertinent reaction rates are those of Hb and of Mb (5, 76). However, the kinetics of blood-muscle CO exchanges have not been rigorously worked out.

It seems unlikely that a significant fraction of the total body CO pool is sequestered at a site that is not in rapid equilibrium with blood CO. As will be discussed in FACTORS THAT DETERMINE CO BINDING, p. 450, extracellular CO stores are determined partly by tissue P_{CO}, which is in equilibrium or in near equilibrium with mean capillary P_{CO}. For a CO store to be isolated from blood CO would require either an area that is devoid of blood flow or combination of CO with an extravascular compound that binds CO irreversibly. The findings of Tobias et al. (165), who detected a persistent ^{13}CO radioactivity over the liver of normal human subjects after the isotope had been eliminated from the blood, may have reflected metabolism to a product other than CO_2. Washout studies of CO during O_2 breathing seem inconsistent with a pool that slowly and reversibly binds CO (35, 129).

Under some experimental conditions the partition of body CO stores between vascular and extravascular space is not constant in an individual human or animal subject. Hypoxic hypoxemia (HH) with arterial P_{O_2} (Pa_{O_2}) < 40 mmHg, or hemorrhagic shock, results in CO shifts out of blood into skeletal and cardiac muscle (38, 40, 42). This finding was the death knell for the use of CO dilution for measurement of blood volume (42). Similar CO shifts can also be seen during exercise at maximum O_2 consumption ($\dot{V}max_{O_2}$) in normal human subjects (28, 173) or during severe vasoconstriction resulting from infused norepinephrine in a canine skeletal muscle preparation (39). The shift appears to result from a fall in intracellular or cytoplasmic P_{O_2}, which allows an increase in the binding of CO to Mb. The lack of the CO shift with less severe falls in Pa_{O_2}, or after hemorrhage giving less severe falls in arterial blood pressure has been interpreted as indicating that autoregulation was able to maintain Mb P_{O_2} near normal levels (38, 40, 42).

Carbon Monoxide Exchanges Between Lung and Body Stores and Processes That Determine HbCO and Body CO Stores

Generally speaking, the body CO stores are determined by pulmonary exchanges between ambient air and the body stores, endogenous production, dilution in the body tissues, and metabolic CO consumption. Early work demonstrated that human subjects exposed to a step increase in ambient [CO] in inspired air absorbed CO into the blood over a period of several hours until "equilibrium" was achieved and CO uptake ceased (69). With a step decrease in inspired [CO], CO was excreted via the lungs until a new equilibrium was achieved. During exercise, CO uptake increased at a given inspired [CO]. The time for equilibrium decreased (63, 72, 125). Uptake of CO was augmented at low inspired P_{O_2} and inhibited at high P_{O_2} (72, 125). Equilibrium times depended on the level of CO exposure; times were shorter at high inspired [CO] (130). Uptake of CO was influenced by alveolar ventilation ($\dot{V}_A$) and by CO diffusion but was largely independent of pulmonary blood flow (72). The time course for CO excretion after exposure to high inspired [CO] is similar to that seen during CO uptake (130).

The development of equations to describe pulmonary CO uptake and the variables that influence the body CO stores and blood [HbCO] was stimulated by studies of the CO diffusing capacity (65). The Coburn-Forster-Kane equation [CFK equation; (36)] considers pulmonary uptake and excretion, endogenous CO production ($\dot{V}_{CO}$), and dilution in the body CO stores. The basic form is

$$\frac{A[\mathrm{HbCO}]_t - B\dot{V}_{CO} - P_{I_{CO}}}{A[\mathrm{HbCO}]_0 - B\dot{V}_{CO} - P_{I_{CO}}} = \exp(-tA/\mathrm{Vb}B)$$

where

$$A = \bar{P}_{C_{O_2}}/M[\mathrm{HbO_2}]$$

$$B = 1/D_{L_{CO}} + P_L/\dot{V}_A$$

Symbols in the above equations are defined here as follows:

$D_{L_{CO}}$	diffusivity of the lungs for CO, milliliters per minute per mmHg
exp	2.7182, the base of natural logarithms raised to the power of the bracketed expression
$[\mathrm{HbCO}]_0$	milliliters of CO per milliliter of blood at beginning of exposure interval
$[\mathrm{HbCO}]_t$	milliliters of CO per milliliter of blood at time t
$[\mathrm{HbO_2}]$	oxyhemoglobin concentration, milliliters of O_2 per milliliter of blood

M	equilibrium constant for reaction of CO with HbO_2
$\bar{P}_{CO_2}$	average partial pressure of O_2 in lung capillaries, mmHg
$P_{I_{CO}}$	partial pressure of CO in inhaled air, mmHg
P_L	barometric pressure minus vapor pressure of water at body temperature, mmHg
t	exposure duration, minutes
$\dot{V}_A$	alveolar ventilation rate, milliliters per minute
Vb	blood volume
$\dot{V}_{CO}$	rate of endogenous CO production, milliliters per minute

The major assumptions are *1)* M is constant over the range of HbO_2 + HbCO encountered during clinical CO poisoning (i.e., perhaps 70%–100%); *2)* CO metabolism is insignificant compared with $\dot{V}_{CO}$; *3)* body CO is rapidly mixed; *4)* $D_{L_{CO}}$ is the same for uptake and for excretion; *5)* $\dot{V}_A/D_{L_{CO}}$ and $P_{A_{O_2}}/D_{L_{CO}}$ ($P_{A_{O_2}}$, alveolar P_{O_2}) are uniform; *6)* mean pulmonary capillary P_{CO} is in chemical equilibrium with mean capillary HbO_2, HbCO, and O_2 as described in the Haldane relationship (69). The $D_{L_{CO}}$ has been shown to be similar for CO uptake or CO excretion (132). The P_{CO} in blood traversing pulmonary capillaries is probably not in complete chemical equilibrium, because P_{CO} increases as P_{O_2} increases. However, this is unlikely to cause significant errors in calculated HbCO because the effect is small. The CFK equation accurately predicted the CO uptake and excretion data in normal human subjects during continuous or discontinuous CO exposures (131). The equation also gave accurate predictions during exercise and is applicable to female and male subjects (131). Calculated steady-state [HbCO] accurately predicted measured [HbCO] in patients with elevated $\dot{V}_{CO}$ (36). These findings are strong evidence that assumptions used in the derivation are not causing major error in patients with normal pulmonary function. It might be predicted that errors would be greater in patients with markedly nonuniform lungs, but this has not been tested.

The CFK equation has been useful in studying relative effects of the various factors that determine HbCO. Figures 1 and 2 illustrate effects of different variables on CO uptake. Calculations with the CFK equation show that the half time for equilibration is a function of the variables listed in the CFK equation,

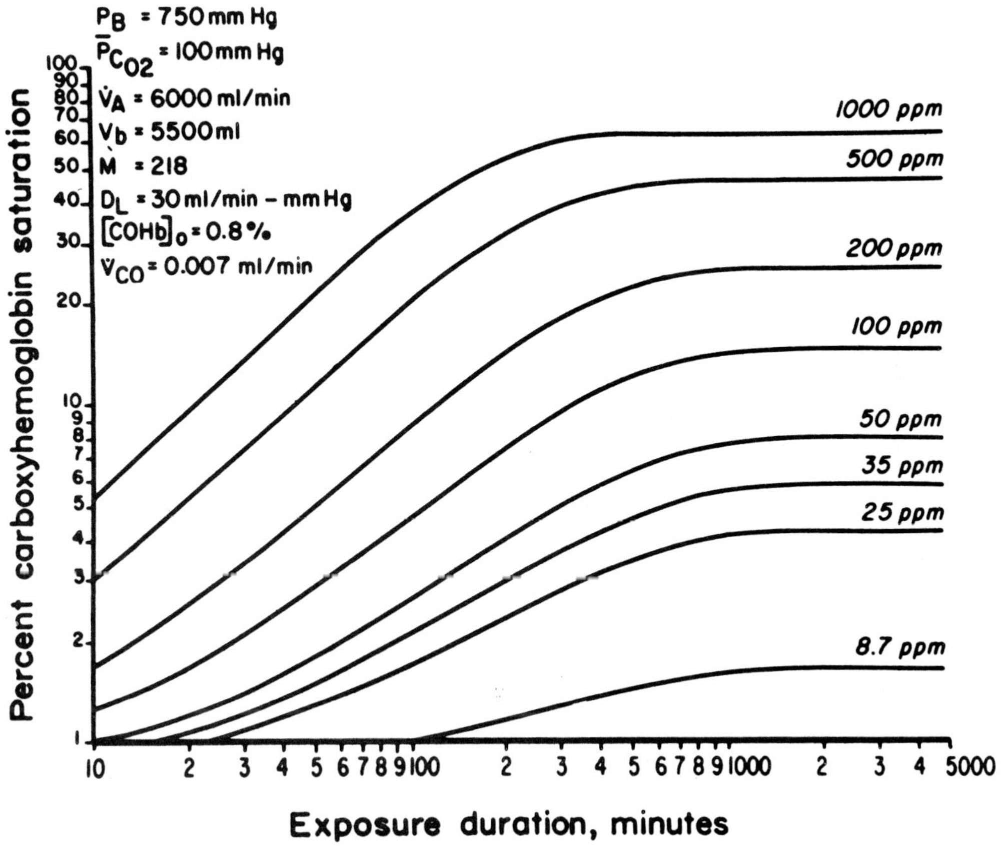

FIG. 1. Carbon monoxide uptake in a normal human subject as a function of inspired [CO]. PB, barometric pressure; $\bar{P}_{CO_2}$, average partial pressure of O_2 in lung capillaries; $\dot{V}_A$, alveolar ventilation rate; Vb, blood volume; M, equilibrium constant; DL, diffusing capacity of the lungs; $[COHb]_0$, control value prior to CO exposure; $\dot{V}_{CO}$, rate of endogenous CO production. Calculated with the Coburn-Forster-Kane (CFK) equation (36). [From Peterson and Stewart (131).]

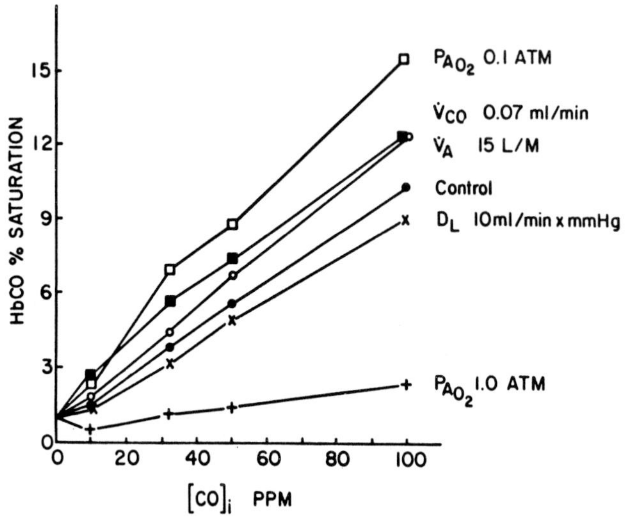

FIG. 2. Effects of alveolar ventilation ($\dot{V}_A$), CO diffusing capacity of the lungs (D_L), alveolar partial pressure of O_2 (P_{AO_2}), and endogenous CO production ($\dot{V}_{CO}$), on uptake of CO. In each case one variable was changed and other variables are the same as in Fig. 1. Data are shown for 8-h exposures. $[CO]_i$, CO in inspired air. [Calculated using the CFK equation (36).]

as had been suspected from earlier studies (36). Figure 3 illustrates processes that influence body CO stores and [HbCO] and gives average values for normal body CO stores in a subject breathing urban air.

It is unlikely that a steady state ever exists in humans where $\dot{V}_{CO}$ equals the rate of excretion of CO and inspired [CO] is in equilibrium with exogenous HbCO in pulmonary capillary blood. Alveolar ventilation, diffusing capacity for CO, and P_{AO_2} vary as a function of physical activity; $\dot{V}_{CO}$ has a diurnal variation; inspired [CO] is variable. Therefore the diurnal variation of HbCO is extremely complex. Figure 4 illustrates a simulated diurnal variation of [HbCO] in a cigarette smoker who also was exposed to a higher ambient CO during the day than was found at night. This simplified case illustrates buildup of the body CO stores during the day with loss during the night.

Endogenous CO Production

MEASUREMENTS AND NORMAL RATES OF CO PRODUCTION. Sjöstrand and his colleagues (153, 154) discovered that patients with hemolytic anemia had elevated venous [HbCO] and that CO was endogenously produced in humans. The quantitation of $\dot{V}_{CO}$ became possible with the application of rebreathing techniques where pulmonary CO excretion was prevented and $\dot{V}_{CO}$ was determined by measuring the rate of increase in the body CO stores (35). This method assumes that CO is not metabolized at a significant rate and that CO dilution in body stores remains constant during the 2-h rebreathing period. Both assumptions have been tested by administering ^{14}CO and measuring $^{14}COHb$ over a period of several hours (102). In normal supine young male subjects at rest who had normal [HbCO], the rate of loss of the isotope from the blood and the rate of appearance of $^{14}CO_2$ was small and can be ignored during the $\dot{V}_{CO}$ measurement (102). In dogs where oxidation of CO occurs at a faster rate, $\dot{V}_{CO}$ can be accurately measured using the tracer and determining the rate of increase in $^{14}CO/^{12}CO$ in venous blood with the animal breathing in a closed system. Skin CO exchanges in the human or dog are insignificant and do not influence the $\dot{V}_{CO}$ measurement with the rebreathing technique (31).

Table 1 lists $\dot{V}_{CO}$ data obtained in various published

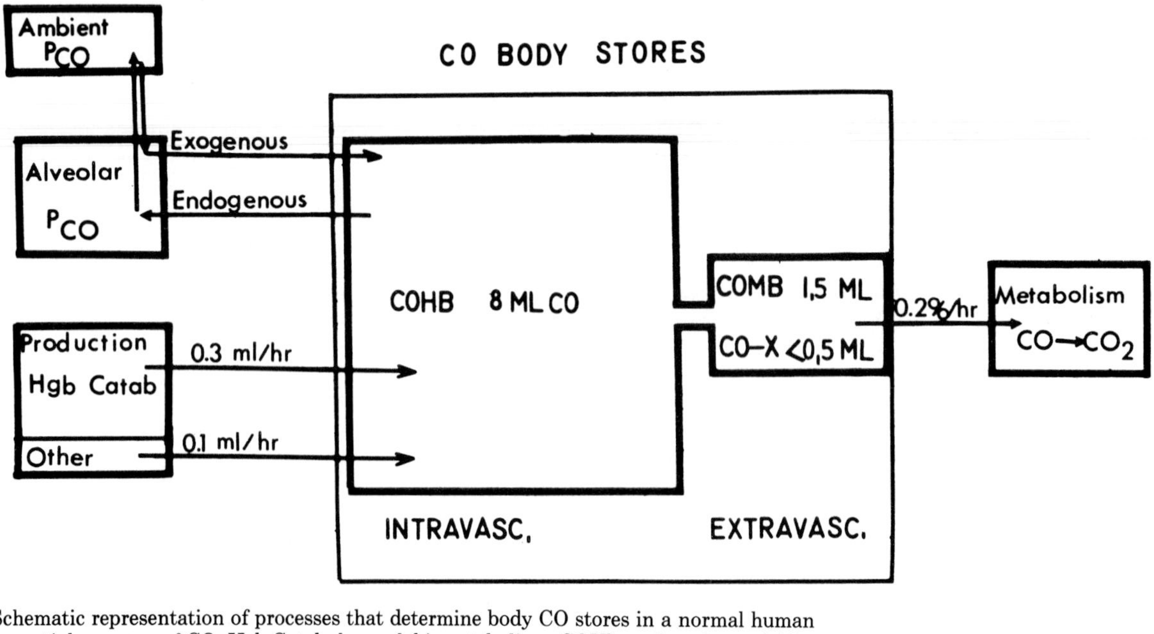

FIG. 3. Schematic representation of processes that determine body CO stores in a normal human subject. P_{CO}, partial pressure of CO; Hgb Catab, hemoglobin catabolism; COHb, carboxyhemoglobin; COMb, carboxymyoglobin; CO-X, CO not explained by CO bound to Hb or Mb; intravasc., intravascular; extravasc., extravascular. [From Coburn (32).]

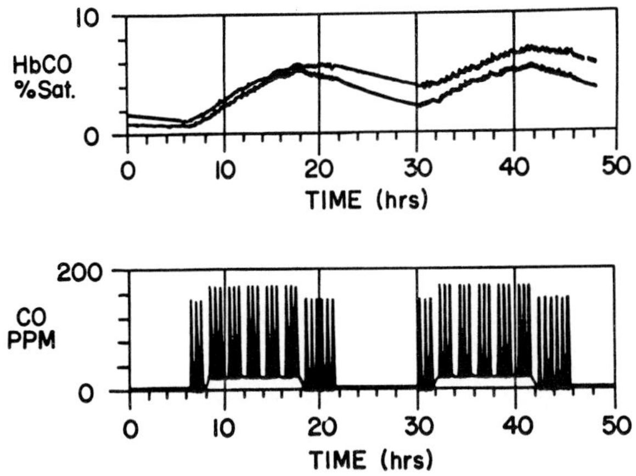

FIG. 4. Diurnal variation in [HbCO]. Data were computed with the CFK equation for a normal subject who was exposed to ambient CO during waking hours and zero inspired [CO] during sleeping hours. *Lower tracing,* [HbCO] was computed with D_L 20, $P_{A_{O_2}}$ 75, $\dot{V}_A$ 6, $\dot{V}_{CO}$ 0.007. *Upper tracing,* D_L 10, $P_{A_{O_2}}$ 50, $\dot{V}_A$ 6, $\dot{V}_{CO}$ 0.07. Note CO exposure included a constant raised environmental level and intermittent 5 min increases in $P_{A_{CO}}$, which is similar to exposures seen with cigarette smokers. [From Coburn et al. (34).]

studies. It has been estimated (36) that of the usual venous blood [HbCO] of 0.7%–1.1% saturation that is seen in humans living in an urban environment, approximately 0.5% saturation originates from endogenous production. The remainder originates from uptake of CO from the ambient air.

Production of CO has been computed from CO measurements in rebreathing gas that is assumed to be in equilibrium with P_{CO} in pulmonary capillary blood (96). This method apparently cannot accurately measure $\dot{V}_{CO}$ because of the many variables that influence rebreathing-gas P_{CO}.

CARBON MONOXIDE PRODUCTION AND HEME CATABOLISM. Carbon monoxide is a catabolic by-product of heme (35, 43, 44, 154). Figure 5 illustrates the conversion of the α-methene carbon atom of heme to CO. Carbon monoxide is formed stoichiometrically during Hb catabolism induced by injection of damaged erythrocytes or Hb solutions (43, 44), including reconstituted Hb where the heme was labeled with ^{14}C but globin was unlabeled (44). Bilirubin and CO are produced in equimolar ratios in humans and under various experimental conditions in animals (13, 92). There is evidence that about 80% of $\dot{V}_{CO}$ is due to catabolism of Hb from senescent erythrocytes in normal humans (35, 43, 175). The remainder may be largely due to catabolism of hepatic heme and bone marrow heme (14). This latter source can be markedly increased in disease (101). Whether $\dot{V}_{CO}$ is increased after injection of drugs that induce hepatic heme turnover is not certain, since results were variable (15, 33, 109). There is some evidence of a biochemical pathway that converts heme to bilirubin in liver without forming CO (14), but this is unlikely to be very large in normal humans in view of the evidence of mole-for-mole $\dot{V}_{CO}$ and bilirubin formation during heme catabolism. Carbon monoxide production has been shown to have a diurnal variation (103, 110), which presumably reflects diurnal variation in heme catabolism.

Heme breakdown to bile pigment and CO is catalyzed by microsomal heme oxygenase (162, 163, 189). This enzyme, which has been isolated from rat liver, has an absolute and stoichiometric requirement for O_2 and NADPH, generates CO in amounts equimolar to bilirubin, is inhibited by CO, and requires cytochrome *P*-450. These findings indicate that this enzyme is a mixed-function oxygenase.

Although there have been reports of CO arising from bacteria (58), there is no strong evidence of a significant source in normal humans of $\dot{V}_{CO}$ other than from heme breakdown. There is evidence that blood in the gastrointestinal tract can be catabolized to CO (21). Peroxidase-catalyzed aerobic oxidations of aromatic pyruvate yield CO (136), but the in vivo significance is unknown. Peroxidation of lipids results in CO formation (187). Whether this is an important source of $\dot{V}_{CO}$ in normal or diseased humans is unknown.

Pulmonary excretion of ^{14}CO has been measured after injection of [2-^{14}C]glycine, a compound that is incorporated into newly synthesized heme, resulting in labeling of the α-methene carbon atom (95, 175). An early peak of ^{14}CO production and excretion is observed 3–8 days after glycine injection, which represents early turnover of heme, either in the bone marrow or liver. A late peak occurring after 100–140 days in normal human subjects represents catabolism of heme from Hb in senescent erythrocytes. This approach has had use in studies of altered heme catabolism in patients with ineffective erythropoiesis and other disease states (95, 175).

Figure 2 illustrates that an increase in $\dot{V}_{CO}$ (which corresponds to the highest $\dot{V}_{CO}$ determined to date) has a major effect on [HbCO] during non-steady-state exposure to exogenous CO. Steady-state [HbCO] levels of nearly 4% saturation have been seen in patients with severe hemolytic media who were breathing urban air containing 0.5–1 ppm CO.

CARBON MONOXIDE PRODUCTION AND HALOMETHANE METABOLISM. Methylene chloride and other dihalomethanes or trihalomethanes, low-boiling organic sol-

TABLE 1. *Endogenous Production Rates of CO in Humans*

	Production Rate		Ref.
	ml/h	$\mu mol \cdot h^{-1} \cdot kg^{-1}$	
Normal young men	0.39–0.44	0.28–0.34	13, 35, 47, 101, 103
Normal young women			
Estrogen phase	0.32–0.35	0.20–0.23	54, 103
Progesterone phase	0.62–0.66	0.35–0.45	
Newborn infants		2.5–3.0	107, 156

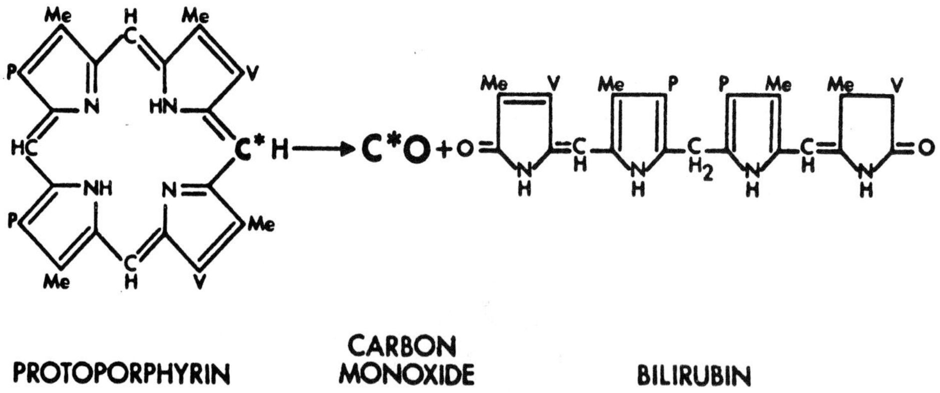

FIG. 5. Degradation of heme to CO plus bilirubin. C*, methene carbon atom that is precursor of the carbon atom in CO. Me:CH_3; V:$CH{=}CH_2$; and P:CH_2COOH.

vents used in industry, seem to be the only known environmental agents that are catabolized forming CO. Workers exposed to methylene chloride developed elevated [HbCO] (89, 157). Rats given this substance had $\dot{V}_{CO}$ 60 times the control rate (137). Isotope studies indicated that methylene chloride acts as a direct substrate for metabolic formation of CO (136). Dihalomethane metabolism utilizes a hepatic mixed-function cytochrome *P*-450–linked oxygenase system. The reaction incorporates molecular O_2, is dependent on NADPH, and is stimulated by glutathione (3, 90, 155).

Carbon Monoxide Metabolism as a CO Sink

Metabolic consumption of CO occurs in skeletal muscle (59), probably in the mitochondria (29). Bovine heart cytochrome-*c* oxidase slowly oxidizes CO to CO_2 (168). Experiments with ^{18}O indicated that molecular O_2 was utilized (191). Oxidation of CO to CO_2 occurred at CO/O_2 ratios as low as 0.1. Azide and CN were effective inhibitors. At least partial reduction of cytochrome-*c* oxidase was necessary for this reaction to occur (191). The mechanism of CO oxidation is still unclear. It may involve a splitting of O_2 atoms by cytochrome-*c* oxidase similar to that in the normal catalytic reaction but with CO rather than a proton acting as an acceptor of one of the O_2 atoms.

Whole-body studies of oxidation of CO to CO_2 have been performed in anesthetized dogs and in resting seated human subjects. The rate of conversion of ^{14}CO to $^{14}CO_2$ in the human subjects averaged 0.16% ± 0.03% of total radioactivity per hour (102). A similar experiment with the dog preparation gave values of 0.03% ± 0.18%/h (102). Metabolism of CO to CO_2 was shown to be a first-order reaction. Therefore the metabolic rate is increased as a function of the body CO stores (presumably as a function of tissue P_{CO}). The data indicate that in resting human subjects the rate of metabolic consumption of CO is insignificant at normal [HbCO]. Even at [HbCO] as high as 20%, the metabolism rate is small compared with $\dot{V}_{CO}$. In dogs metabolic consumption is significant at [HbCO] of 1% saturation and equals $\dot{V}_{CO}$ at [HbCO] of ≅20% saturation.

Some bacteria oxidize CO (52), but no bacteria has been found where the Michaelis constant (K_m) for CO is sufficiently low so that bacterial oxidation of CO could be important in vivo.

CARBON MONOXIDE BINDING TO PROTEINS FOUND IN MAMMALIAN TISSUES

Structure and Reactivity of CO

Carbon monoxide, in competition with O_2, binds to hemoproteins and other iron- or copper-containing proteins. The only known effect of CO binding is interference with O_2 metabolism. This can be brought about by either a fall in tissue P_{O_2} below a critical concentration, which results from CO binding to O_2-carrier proteins, or by direct competition of CO binding with O_2 binding to tissue oxidoreductases. However, the binding to Hb must be the predominant effect.

In view of the competition of CO binding and O_2 binding to various mammalian proteins, it is surprising that the molecular structure of CO more nearly resembles the molecular structure of the inert-gas N_2 than that of O_2. The arrangement of electrons in the formal molecular orbital structure of CO is the same as N_2. This is illustrated by a simple valence bond formulation (50)

$$:N{\equiv}N: \quad :C{\equiv}O:$$

where all occupied orbitals are shared by electron pairs. This configuration helps explain the low propensity for CO to participate in reactions involving formal transfer of electrons (a major difference between O_2 and CO). Like N_2, CO is not easily reduced nor does it accept protons from H_2O. However, in contrast to N_2, CO has a small dipole moment and readily ligands to metals. The following resonance structure illustrates this property of CO (114)

$$\overset{\oplus}{:C}—\overset{\ominus}{\ddot{\underset{..}{O}}}: \leftrightarrow :C{=}\ddot{O}: \leftrightarrow \overset{\ominus}{C}{\equiv}\overset{\oplus}{O}$$

Although CO does not formally accept electrons in liganding to metals, the structure of the complexes can be illustrated as a resonance hybrid (50)

$$\overset{\ominus}{M}—\overset{\oplus}{C}{\equiv}O \leftrightarrow M—C{=}\ddot{O}:$$

The M—C bond has a partial double-bond character, and therefore the metal, carbon, and oxygen atoms will form a linear structure. A more precise molecular orbital description also indicates a tendency for CO to form highly stable linear metal-ligand complexes with various transition metals. In cases where two metals are physically close, it is also possible for CO to form a bridged planar structure somewhat analogous to formaldehyde

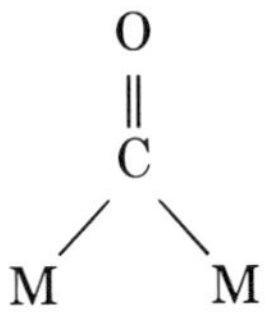

There does not seem to be any indication that CO forms an "end-on" bridged structure in any of its complexes

$$M—C{=}O—M$$

Although CO prefers a linear bond with metals, infrared spectral studies indicate that CO binds to heme proteins (both carriers and oxidoreductases) in a bent configuration (9, 74, 108, 123). The apparent distortion from the linear tendency of this structure has been interpreted to represent the fitting of CO into a tight pocket designed to bind O_2 in its required bent configuration (25). The mechanism for producing this conformational restriction may involve steric blockage of a linear conformation or distortion of the iron orbitals by the ligand on the proximal side of the heme plane.

In contrast to CO, O_2 in its unreacted state is a diradical; i.e., it has two unpaired electrons

$$\dot{\ddot{O}}{\equiv}\dot{\underset{..}{O}}$$

The reactivity of O_2 is produced by this diradical structure and the high electronegativity of the oxygen atoms. In a wide variety of enzymatic (oxidoreductase) as well as nonenzymatic processes that occur in biologic systems, O_2 accepts electrons from substrate forming superoxide radical anion, hydrogen peroxide, or splits to form hydroxyl radical, water, and/or numerous additional products (ketones, alcohols, aldehydes, acids). Some of these reactions are catalyzed by flavin or quinones; many others require binding of O_2 to a metal cofactor. Oxygen ligands to metals in a different manner than does CO, as expected from the difference in electronic structure and reactivity. The most common mode of reaction of O_2 with metal complexes is oxidation of the metal and reduction of O_2. Therefore formation of reversible O_2-metal ligand complexes (such as with the metalloprotein carriers) is the exception. In model stable metal complexes, O_2 binds to two ligand sites

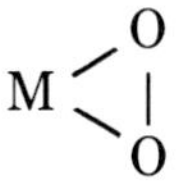

although the chemical and spatial nature of the bonding is not well understood (51). However, in binding to heme iron, in which only one ligand site is available, the nature of the bonding probably involves a tendency toward a bent configuration

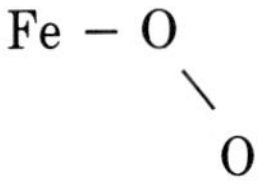

involving an important contribution of electron donation from Fe^{2+} to O_2 (25, 126)

$$Fe^{2+}—O_2 \rightarrow Fe^{3+}—O_2^-$$

The bent configuration is a requirement imposed by the number of electrons (and orbitals) and contrasts with the linear structure preferred, although not required, in CO-metal complexes, in which there are two less electrons.

Carbon Monoxide and O_2 Competition

Although the chemistries of CO and O_2 are markedly different, both CO and O_2 appear to require the same oxidation states of either Fe^{2+} or Cu^{1+} for binding and frequently appear able to bind to the same conformational states of metalloproteins. A basic question is why there are such marked differences in CO affinities relative to O_2 affinities for binding to the various proteins.

In general the competition of CO and O_2 for binding to carrier proteins or oxidoreductases is determined by the nature of the bonds and factors that influence the bonds, including steric and allosteric effects and bending of the metal-ligand bond. Bending of the metal-CO bond may be a major factor in explaining high and low affinity in various CO-binding proteins (9, 25, 74), but Traylor and Berzinis (166), using model heme complexes, could not substantiate this. Perhaps interactions producing variation in the size and shape of the heme pocket in proteins is a better explanation (46). Competition between CO and O_2 is usually given in terms of the CO/O_2 ratio producing 50% CO binding for carrier proteins and a fall in function to 50% of control level for oxidoreductases. (We use the designation $R = CO/O_2$ for 50% binding or fall in rate of oxidoreductase function.)

Competition between CO and O_2 for oxidoreductases is more complex than is the case for liganding to carrier proteins, because the kinetics of substrate oxidation and O_2 reduction affect the apparent affinity of CO relative to the apparent affinity for O_2. Consider the competitive relationship of O_2 and CO in this general model

$$E{-}CO \xrightleftharpoons[k_b]{k_a \; CO} E \xrightleftharpoons[k_d]{k_c \; O_2} E{-}O_2$$

$$\downarrow S$$

$$ES{-}CO \xrightleftharpoons[k_b']{k_a' \; CO} ES \xrightleftharpoons[k_d']{k_c' \; O_2} ESO_2 \xrightarrow{k_e} E$$

+ products

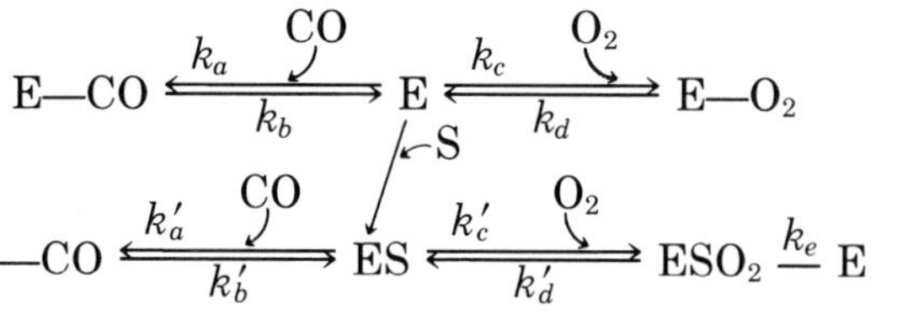

where E is an oxidoreductase, S is an organic substrate, ES is the enzyme-substrate complex, k is the rate constant for binding CO and O_2 to E, and k' is the rate constant for binding CO and O_2 to ES. The association constants $K_{CO} = k_a/k_b$ and $K_{O_2} = k_c/k_d$. The association constants $Ks_{CO} = k_a'/k_b'$ and $Ks_{O_2} = k_c'/k_d'$; k_e is the rate constant for reduction of O_2. (The products of this reaction are not shown in this schema.) The concentration of S and the formation of ES (concentration of ES) influence R because Ks_{CO} and Ks_{O_2} are usually markedly different from K_{CO} and K_{O_2}. In addition the rate of reduction of O_2 has an effect on the apparent affinity for O_2, which equals $[Ks_{O_2} + k_e ESO_2]$ so that increasing O_2 reduction results in an increase in apparent O_2 affinity. In general these effects result in an increase in apparent O_2 affinity and a fall in R so that oxidoreductases are less susceptible to inhibition by CO than are carriers. A comparison of CO binding and R between Hb and cytochrome-c oxidase illustrates this phenomenon. Yoshikawa et al. (190) have determined that K_{CO} for cytochrome-c oxidase is about $\frac{1}{50}$ of that for Hb; however, R for cytochrome-c oxidase is $\frac{1}{1,000}$ that of Hb. With tryptophan dioxygenase, addition of substrate (tryptophan) causes a 28-fold increase in the association constant for CO ($Ks_{CO} = 28\,K_{CO}$) (79). Nevertheless, despite the increased affinity for CO binding, R falls markedly (from near ∞ to 0.55) due to the increase in apparent O_2 affinity.

Carbon Monoxide Binding to Hb

All of the toxic effects of increased body CO stores may be due to alteration in Hb chemistry. Early studies (10, 57, 69, 70) established the high affinity of mammalian Hb for CO and that CO binding to Hb increased the O_2 affinity of this protein. The presence of HbCO shifts the HbO_2 dissociation curve to the left (Fig. 6). Effects of even small concentrations of HbCO on the HbO_2 dissociation curve are not trivial. In a series of blood samples from normal human subjects, considerable variability in the O_2 affinity for Hb was found; HbCO was a major cause of this variation and was more important than was variability of 2,3-diphosphoglycerate (2,3-DPG) (178).

Carbon monoxide binds more slowly to Hb than does O_2, which would tend to decrease the relative affinity of CO for Hb. However, this is more than offset by the extremely slow rate of dissociation of CO

from Hb (143). The HbO_2 and HbCO dissociation curves show similar cooperativity. However, the HbCO dissociation curve is more sigmoid at the bottom (80, 143). The ratio of association constant of O_2 to that of CO (L_1/K_1) for reaction with reduced Hb (Hb_4) is considerably smaller than the ratio L_2/K_2, which approximately equals L_3/K_3 and L_4/K_4 [where O_2 is reacting with $Hb_4(O_2)$, $Hb_4(O_2)_2$, or $Hb_4(O_2)_3$, and CO is reacting with $Hb_4(CO)$, $Hb_4(CO)_2$, or $Hb_4(CO)_3$] (143, 145). The shape of the dissociation curves constructed with CO and O_2 may also vary at the top (143). The kinetic basis for cooperativity differs with O_2 and CO. Oxygen binds to T- and R-state Hb with equal velocity (148) [terminology derived for two-state allosteric model (115)]. Thus for O_2 liganding, cooperativity is due to changes in the off-reaction rate. Carbon monoxide binds to T-state Hb much more slowly than to R-state Hb, and the on rate contributes to the cooperativity phenomenon (7, 74). The binding of CO to Hb is not influenced by tension between heme iron and the base imidazole, which could alter the angle of the heme plane, and the atom of the O_2 molecule forms a hydrogen bond with the imidazole of the distal histidine, pulling this residue farther into the heme pocket (148). The effects of CO and O_2 liganding on the Bohr effect may be different in normal human blood (75), but this is not established (122). Carbon monoxide may bind preferentially to the β-chain of Hb, whereas O_2 binding is random (94).

The equilibrium constant of the reaction of CO and HbO_2 (M) equals $[HbCO][P_{O_2}]/[HbO_2][P_{CO}]$. For practical purposes M can be considered to be constant over the range of $[HbCO] + [HbO_2]$ that is found in normal and CO-poisoned humans and animals (138). In blood from normal adult human subjects, M averages approximately 200 (138). There appears to be significant variation in M in blood from different humans (138). Variation could be explained by technical difficulties, particularly equilibration of gas tensions and ligand binding. In abnormal human Hb, M can be markedly different. An example is Hb Zurich,

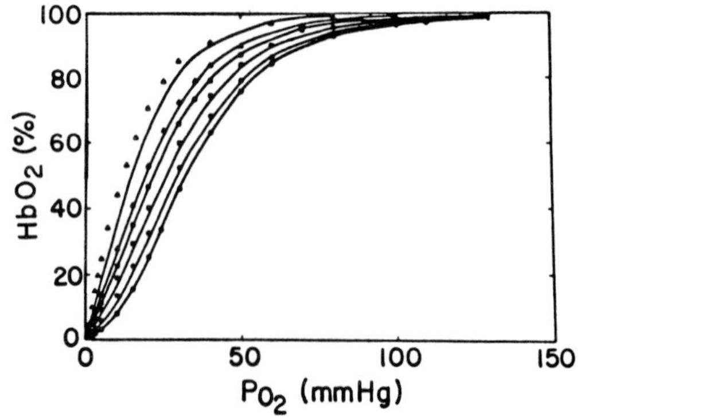

FIG. 6. Observed and calculated effects of HbCO on the HbO_2 dissociation curve. Calculated curves were obtained with the method of Roughton and Darling (144). Percent saturation COHb, *right to left:* 0%, 6.7%, 18.2%, 31%, 40%, and 55.5%. [From Okada et al. (122).]

TABLE 2. *Inhibition Ratio for O_2 Carrier Proteins That Bind CO*

	Source	R*	M†	Temperature, °C	Ref.
Hemoproteins					
Hemoglobin	Human red cell	0.0045	218	37	138
	Roundworm perienteric fluid	13.3	0.07	20	66
	Roundworm body wall	1.2	0.83	20	66
Myoglobin	Sperm whale	0.025–0.04	25–40	25	6
	Horse	0.027	37	25	5
	Aplysia	0.007	143	20	182
Leghemoglobin	Soybean root nodule	0.025	40	20	185
Copper proteins					
Hemocyanin	*Aplysia*	0.81	1.2	20	16
	Horseshoe crab	20	0.05	25	139

* *R* (inhibition ratio) = CO/O_2 at 50% binding, a unit used in biochemical studies. † *M* = O_2/CO at 50% binding, a unit used in physiological literature.

which has an *M* of approximately 300 (192). As expected from the different characteristics of CO and O_2 liganding to Hb, *M* is markedly altered by temperature and pH (4, 80). Table 2 gives some *M* values in blood from different species.

The method of Roughton and Darling (144) for calculating effects of the presence of HbCO on the O_2 dissociation curve assumes that total bound Hb ([HbCO] + [HbO_2]) is determined by the sum of P_{O_2} + MP_{CO}. The method gives accurate predictions over the range of [HbCO] + [HbO_2], where *M* can be considered a constant [Fig. 6; (122)].

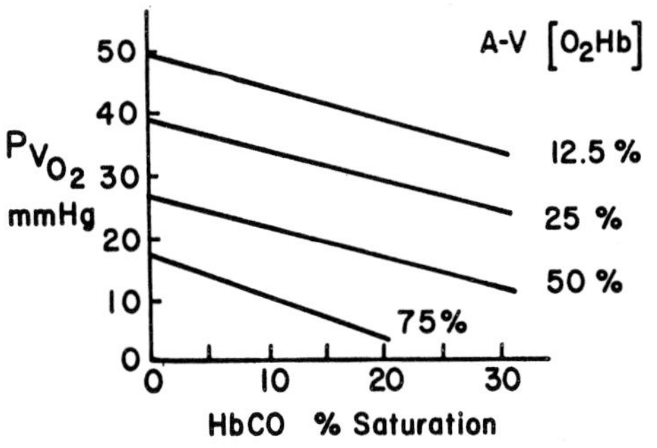

FIG. 7. Calculated venous P_{O_2} (Pv_{O_2}) as a function of [HbCO] at different arteriovenous O_2 saturation differences. In determining A-V[O_2Hb], O_2Hb percent saturation was computed as percent of total Hb, including Hb bound with CO. Lines calculated with the method of Roughton and Darling (144). [From Collier (45).]

Effects of CO Binding to Hb on Oxygenation in Peripheral Tissues

EFFECTS ON CAPILLARY AND TISSUE PARTIAL PRESSURE OF O_2. In normal lungs the presence of HbCO does not alter pulmonary gas exchange. Therefore blood entering peripheral tissues has a normal Pa_{O_2}. In markedly nonuniform lungs this is not the case, since changes in the shape of the HbO_2 dissociation curve will affect the alveolar-arterial oxygen gradient ($PA_{O_2} - Pa_{O_2}$) in the presence of nonuniform ventilation-perfusion ratios ($\dot{V}A/\dot{Q}$) (19).

The effect of the shift to the left and more-hyperbolic shape of the HbO_2 dissociation curve in the presence of HbCO (Fig. 6) is an increased O_2 affinity of Hb for O_2. The increased O_2 affinity affects capillary P_{O_2} in peripheral tissues: for a given O_2 content, P_{O_2} (the driving force for diffusion into tissues) is decreased. Therefore increases in [HbCO] result in decreases in tissue and intracellular P_{O_2}. Figure 7 shows calculated effects of increased [HbCO] on capillary P_{O_2}, as estimated by venous P_{O_2} values. This effect has two components, an anemia effect and an effect due to the leftward shift of the curve.

Several authors have studied effects of elevated [HbCO] on oxygenation of tissue by assessing effects on tissue P_{O_2}. Zorn (194), using a P_{O_2} puncture electrode 1–3 μm in diameter, found that brain tissue P_{O_2} in several different species decreased almost linearly with increases in [HbCO], resulting in a 1.8-mmHg fall per 1% saturation increase in HbCO. Weiss and Cohen (171) failed to find convincing falls in rat muscle or brain tissue P_{O_2} with CO exposures resulting in [HbCO] < 5%. Miller and Wood (112) showed profound falls in rat liver surface P_{O_2} and a smaller effect on brain P_{O_2} after huge CO exposures for 25 h in anesthetized albino rats. The early studies of Campbell (24) documented changes in subcutaneous or abdominal gas pocket P_{O_2} after rabbits were exposed to 1,500 ppm CO. Kleinert et al. (87) found average decreases of heart intracellular P_{O_2} of 4 mmHg (from 75 to 71 mmHg) after CO breathing sufficient to increase [HbCO] to ≅20% saturation.

These approaches have severe limitations and it is difficult to design controls. Despite these problems, these data suggest that a major mechanism for CO toxicity is the effect on capillary P_{O_2}, with resultant falls in tissue P_{O_2}.

ACUTE COMPENSATORY MECHANISMS. Acute hypoxic hypoxemia (HH) has been studied in great detail in a variety of species. Clearly there is a complex interplay of reflex-mediated changes in the circulation and local tissue mechanisms (O_2 autoregulation) that improve the efficiency of gas exchange in vital organs. The discussion of the Krogh model in the chapter by Cain in this *Handbook* illustrates the importance in the regulation of tissue P_{O_2} of the control of diffusion distance between capillary and mitochondria and the control of blood flow. A basic question addressed here is how similar is the response to CO hypoxia (COH) to the response of HH.

There are at least five general components to the cardiovascular response to HH, depending on the severity and duration: *1*) responses due to reflexes initiated by chemoreceptors, *2*) responses due to local O_2 autoregulation, *3*) responses due to release of humoral agents into blood, *4*) effects of altered pH and P_{CO_2}, and *5*) responses that are not related to a regulatory system but due to deleterious effects of hypoxia or anoxia on tissue. Only recently has there been much evidence about COH circulatory reflexes, and the evidence that local autoregulation of the circulation occurs during COH is still fragmentary. Whether autoregulation can be expected to occur during COH depends on whether the P_{O_2} in arteries, arterioles, and precapillary sphincters is a trigger. With COH, unlike HH, Pa_{O_2} is nearly normal.

Circulatory reflexes. The evidence now appears conclusive that small-to-moderate increases in [HbCO] do not stimulate the carotid body. Increases of [HbCO] to 15% saturation did not increase ventilation in cats or normal humans (91, 147). Rates of action potentials in the carotid sinus nerve were not increased with elevated [HbCO], as occurs with falls in Pa_{O_2} (91). Increases of [HbCO] up to 15% saturation did not cause a fall in splanchnic blood flow in rats, but HH had profound effects (141). Effects of COH on heart rate were variable in different studies, but HH always increased cardiac rate and output (1, 7). The COH-induced release of catecholamines was not related to stimulation of the carotid body, whereas HH-evoked catecholamine release was dependent on an intact carotid body (133). The implication of the lack of response of the carotid body to COH is that the major afferent system involved in compensatory changes in the circulation during HH appears to be largely absent during COH.

Although elevated HbCO does not stimulate the carotid body, there is compelling evidence that aortic chemoreceptors are stimulated by HbCO and that these structures are O_2-content sensors (53, 73, 91). However, the function of reflexes initiated by the aortic bodies is obscure. Aortic body receptors do not seem to exert a control on the major organ circulations.

Evidence that autoregulation of circulation occurs during CO hypoxia. Two tissues, skeletal muscle and the myocardium, have been studied most extensively during HH. There appears to be no information in the literature about the skeletal muscle circulation during COH, but many studies of the coronary circulation are relevant. Carboxyhemoglobin as low as 5% resulted in increases in coronary flow (1, 8). Coronary sinus P_{O_2} remained unchanged or only slightly decreased at [HbCO] 10%–20% saturation (8). Myocardial capillary density increased after 6 min of increased [HbCO] (87). These findings suggest that regulatory mechanisms involving resistance vessels as well as "precapillary sphincters" were utilized during COH in this tissue. Because neural control of this circulation is minimal or absent, it is likely that these effects were local (autoregulation). Canine cerebral resistance vessels dilated during COH and HH, and this effect was not influenced by denervation of chemoreceptors (167), suggesting that an autoregulatory mechanism was operative.

We conclude that it is likely that O_2 autoregulation mechanisms of adaptation to hypoxia are intact during COH, at least in the organs and species studied to date.

Blood catecholamines and cortisol. In eucapnic dogs, HH and COH resulted in similar increases in blood catecholamine and cortisol concentrations (159). The effects on adaptation of increases in these agents in blood is unknown.

Effects due to changes in blood pH, partial pressure of CO_2, and ventilation. With HH it is known that effects on the peripheral chemoreceptors are modulated by hyperventilation, possibly by input via pulmonary stretch receptors (159). Whether these effects can be considered an adaptation is unknown, but for COH this component of the hypoxia response is missing since, as discussed in *Circulatory reflexes* (see this page), hyperventilation and the consequent blood P_{CO_2} and pH changes are not seen. Thus adaptation by increasing $P_{A_{O_2}}$ and Pa_{O_2} is absent.

ADAPTATION TO CHRONICALLY ELEVATED BODY CO STORES. In ACUTE COMPENSATORY MECHANISMS, p. 447, we considered acute physiological mechanisms of adaptation to HH or COH. Animals chronically exposed to CO have additional mechanisms that allow them to be exposed to CO concentrations that would kill them if they had not been previously exposed to CO (24, 30, 86, 176, 180). Mice adapted to altitude are also relatively resistant to COH (30). Thus it is likely, as was the case with acute adaptation to COH, that some of the mechanisms of chronic adaptation to HH may also be utilized for chronic adaptation to COH. Similarities include an increased [Hb] and polycythemia (18, 24, 127, 164, 176), increases in myocardial [Mb] and cytochrome-*c* oxidase concentrations (87, 128), and an increase in myocardial capillary density (87). However, there is no increase in erythrocyte [2,3-DPG] (56, 134), which occurs in HH, probably since there may not be as much increase in venous reduced Hb during COH as with HH. Because there is no long-term increase in alveolar ventilation with COH, changes in blood and tissue P_{CO_2} and pH are probably not involved in long-term adaptation mechanisms.

There have been few metabolic studies of chronic COH adaptation. Montgomery and Rubin (117) showed that effects of 1,000 ppm CO on hepatic metabolism of hexobarbital were decreased after adaptation. This apparently was not due to the drug-metabolizing ability of hepatic tissue, the affinity of the hepatic enzyme system for the drug, any alteration in the requirements of the enzyme system for O_2, or affinity of this system for CO. Wilks et al. (176) and Winston and Roberts (180) showed that animals adapted to COH had lower lactate-pyruvate levels in venous blood. Other metabolic studies, however, failed to reveal any differences from those of nonadapted animals.

Extravascular CO-Binding Proteins

The argument that CO toxicity is due only to reaction with Hb is supported only by negative evidence; i.e., no one has shown that CO binding to compounds other than Hb occurs in amounts sufficient to cause deleterious effects. It seems unlikely that physiological changes seen with 3%–5% saturation of HbCO are due entirely to a decrease in capillary P_{O_2} (34). Capillary P_{O_2} decrease is small at these low [HbCO] values, and O_2 autoregulation is expected to completely compensate, as is the case with small falls in Pa_{O_2}. Barcroft (10) observed in the early twentieth century that persons afflicted with anemia and a hematocrit decreased to 50% the normal level were able to work, but persons with a 50% [HbCO] level were completely incapacitated. This may not be entirely explained by the lack of adaptation mechanisms to COH, which are utilized during HH. It could be due partly to CO effects mediated by CO binding to intracellular proteins.

The state of knowledge about binding of CO to intracellular proteins is incomplete. Development of methodology to measure CO binding in vivo under conditions where the circulation is normal and perfused by blood is needed. One must be cautious in claiming a physiological role for any CO inhibition of enzyme activity based on the biochemical studies described next.

HEMOPROTEINS AND "COPPER" PROTEINS. Table 2 lists available information regarding relative CO and O_2 affinities for carrier proteins. Table 3 lists the same information for oxidoreductases that bind CO. These tables include several nonmammalian proteins to indicate the range that can be obtained for *R* and *M*. However, Table 3 does not describe all of the potential sites for CO binding in nature. For example, CO

TABLE 3. *Inhibition Rate for Oxidoreductases That Bind CO*

Hemoproteins	Source	Reaction	*R*	*M*	Temperature, °C	Ref.
Cytochrome-*c* oxidase*	Bovine heart	O_2 + ferrocytochrome-*c* → ferricytochrome-*c* + H_2O	5–15	0.1–0.2	25	174, 186, 188
Tryptophan oxygenase†	*Pseudomonas*	Tryptophan → formylkynurenine	0.55	1.8	25	64, 106
Secondary amine monooxygenase	*Pseudomonas*	$R(CH_3)NH \rightarrow RNH_2 + HCHO$	0.0009	1,100	25	1, 20, 106
Cytochrome *P*-450 or *P*-448						
C-26 hydroxylase	Rat liver mitochondria	Steroid side-chain cleavage at C-26	0.1	10	30	161
Aromatic ring demethylase	Rabbit lung	ρNO_2—ϕOCH_3 → $\rho NO_2\phi$—OH + HCHO	0.5	2	37	61
	Rat liver microsomes	$\phi CH_3 \rightarrow \phi OH + HCH_3$	0.8–1.1	0.9–1.3	25	48
Aromatic ring heme cleavage enzyme, microsomal heme oxygenase	Rat liver microsomes	Heme → biliverdin + CO	0.5	2	30	162
N-hydroxylase	Hamster liver microsomes	Heterocyclic *N*-hydroxylation	4.2–8.0	0.12–0.24	37	100
Side-chain cleavage enzyme	Bovine adrenal mitochondria	Cholesterol → pregnenolone + isocapraldehyde	1.5	0.67	37	71
Heteroaromatic ring hydroxylase	Hamster liver microsomes	Heterocyclic ring C hydroxylation	2.3–8.9	0.11–0.44	37	100
Aromatic ring hydroxylase	Rat liver	Aromatic ring C hydroxylation	9–12	0.8–0.11	37	49
Steroid hydroxylase	Bovine adrenal gland	Steroid side-chain hydroxylation	1.0	1.0	37	49
Polyphenol oxidase, tyrosinase	Mushroom	ϕ—$(OH)_x \rightarrow \phi(OH)_{x+1}$	1–1.7	0.59–1.0	20	83, 84
Dopamine β-hydroxylase	Bovine adrenal gland	Dopamine → norepinephrine	2	0.5		82

R (inhibition ratio) = CO/O_2 at 50% inhibition. *M* = 1/*R*. * Cytochrome-*c* oxidase contains both heme and copper. CO binds to the heme group, but the copper must be reduced for this to occur (168). † Although *R* was not reported for mammalian liver tryptophan oxygenases, Tanaka and Knox (160) have determined that the mammalian and *Pseudomonas* enzymes have very similar kinetics for CO inhibition.

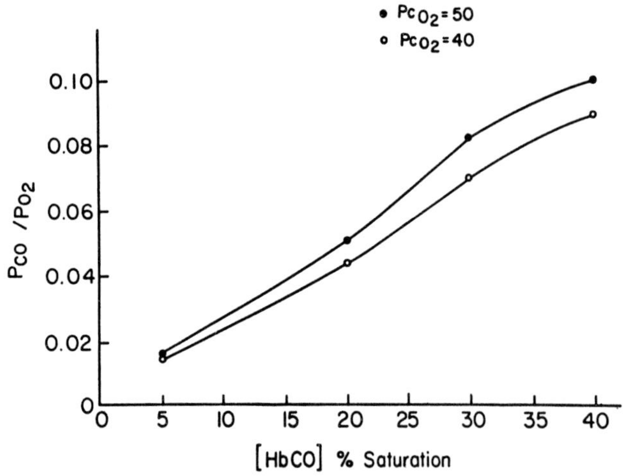

FIG. 8. Calculated tissue P_{CO}/P_{O_2} as a function of blood [HbCO]. Mean tissue P_{CO} is assumed to equal mean capillary P_{CO}, which is calculated with the Haldane equation (70), using mean capillary P_{O_2} values (P_{CO_2}) of 40 or 50 mmHg. The P_{CO}/P_{O_2} ratio was derived with a value for tissue P_{O_2} of 1 mmHg. Errors in this estimate can arise *1)* if CO and O_2 are not in chemical equilibrium with Hb in blood traversing capillaries and *2)* from assumptions about tissue P_{O_2}. The CO/O_2 ratios are probably falsely high due to the low value used for tissue P_{O_2}.

inhibits the heme-containing enzyme horseradish peroxidase in competition with hydrogen peroxide rather than with O_2 (181). Nitrogenase, a molybdenum and nonheme iron-containing enzyme that catalyzes N_2 reduction in bacteria, avidly binds CO, as does hydrogenase, a nonheme iron-containing enzyme that catalyzes H_2 formation from NADH and NADPH in algae and bacteria (88, 124). These two enzymes do not use O_2 but rather are inhibited by O_2. It is likely that other metal-containing oxidoreductases exist that bind CO but have not yet been studied. There has been little exploration of the CO effects on enzymes that do not use O_2 in mammals, although many peroxidases and nonheme iron-containing proteins are present. Oxygen is also utilized in many nonmetal-catalyzed reactions. These oxidoreductases, in which flavin or quinones are the cofactor, do not bind CO.

FACTORS THAT DETERMINE CO BINDING. Because CO binding to various copper proteins and hemoproteins depends on the ratio of P_{CO}/P_{O_2} in proximity, it is pertinent to determine if tissue P_{CO}/P_{O_2} is ever high enough for significant binding to occur.

A plethora of platinum electrode measurements in the literature provide estimates of P_{O_2} profiles in various tissues. Generally these data show very few values less than 5 mmHg and range from 5 to 40 mmHg (the experimental animal respiring ambient air). Because P_{O_2} gradients are unknown in cells and in cell organelles that consume O_2, there is uncertainty about P_{O_2} values at such locations.

Tissue P_{CO} levels have been calculated by computing P_{CO} in mean capillary blood with the Haldane relationship (32). Because the CO metabolic rate is very slow, tissue P_{CO} can be considered to be equilibrated with the P_{CO} in blood in gas-exchange vessels. Figure 8 shows the results of such calculations as a function of blood [HbCO]. Data are given as a CO/O_2 ratio since this is a pertinent physiological variable that determines CO binding to a given CO-binding protein. Because of the uncertainty about P_{O_2} values at the site in the cell of CO-binding protein (so that we cannot precisely compute P_{CO}/P_{O_2}), in Figure 8 we used a relatively low P_{O_2}, 1 mmHg, which probably gives a falsely high CO/O_2 ratio. We compute CO/O_2 for two different mean capillary P_{O_2} values. The results show that tissue P_{CO} and possibly CO/O_2 are a function of the ratio of O_2 uptake/blood flow ($\dot{V}_{O_2}/\dot{Q}$) of tissues. For example, in tissues where $\dot{V}_{O_2}/\dot{Q}$ is low, such as the heart, mean capillary P_{O_2} and P_{CO} are lower than in tissues with higher $\dot{V}_{O_2}/\dot{Q}$. Direct estimates of tissue P_{CO} have been obtained with the gas pocket technique (24, 67) and give data that are consistent with the calculated values listed above.

The above considerations suggest that tissue CO/O_2 may not exceed 0.1 even at very high [HbCO]. However, although a relatively low P_{O_2} was used in these calculations, we cannot be certain that this is an upper limit for CO/O_2 at sites of O_2 consumption. This is particularly true because of recent evidence for steep intracellular P_{O_2} gradients and the possibility that P_{O_2} gradients across organelle membranes may be very large (151). Considering the difficulties in estimating an upper limit for tissue CO/O_2 and in projecting biochemical data such as shown in Table 3 to the in vivo state, we conclude that it is possible that many of the hemoproteins listed are partially inhibited under conditions where HbCO is elevated. The most likely candidates from the intracellular enzymes that have been studied include tryptophan dioxygenase, dopamine β-hydroxylase, the various cytochrome *P*-450– or *P*-448–linked enzymes, and Mb.

CARBON MONOXIDE BINDING TO MB AND CYTOCHROMES AND OTHER CO EFFECTS ON METABOLISM. Of the various extravascular proteins that bind CO (listed in Tables 2 and 3) only Mb, cytochrome-*c* oxidase, and the cytochrome *P*-450–linked enzymes have been studied in intact tissues to determine if CO at the CO/O_2 ratios found in tissue in vivo could cause significant binding or inhibit the function of these proteins. Myoglobin has been found to bind CO in canine hamstring and cardiac muscle (38, 40) even at normal [HbCO]. The [MbCO]/[HbCO] ratios (MbCO, carboxymyoglobin) were approximately unity, and the ratio was unchanged with increases in the body CO stores to [HbCO] of 50% saturation. The quantity of CO bound to Mb under normal conditions, where [HbCO] was 0.8% to 1% saturation, was consistent with a mean CO/O_2 ratio of 0.002–0.005. The significance of CO binding to Mb is unknown. Myoglobin is an O_2-carrier protein that may facilitate O_2 diffusion in the skeletal or cardiac muscle cell or function as an O_2 store in close proximity to mitochondria (2, 183,

184). In either case, inhibition would interfere with oxygenation of the muscle cell. Calculations with the boundary-layer method of Hoofd and Kreuzer (77) predicted that the presence of liganded Mb would inhibit facilitated O_2 diffusion (158). The off-reaction rate of MbCO is slow so that the presence of MbCO effectively would remove Mb from participation as an O_2 carrier. Whether or not CO binding to Mb could contribute to falls in $\dot{V}max_{O_2}$ that have been demonstrated with small increases in the body CO stores (78) is unknown.

Cytochrome *P*-450 and *P*-448 participate in catalysis of reactions known as mixed-function oxidations. In these reactions, several of which appear in Table 3, both O_2 and the substrate are split with formation of an alcohol or phenol and either an aldehyde or water

$$NADPH + R{-}R' + O_2 + H^+ \rightarrow ROH + NADP^+ + RHO$$

$$NADPH + R{-}H + H^+ + O_2 \rightarrow ROH + H_2O + NADP^+$$

Montgomery and Rubin (116, 117) tested the possibility that CO might alter cytochrome *P*-450–linked metabolism in rat liver. After injection of hexobarbital, COH (HbCO ≅ 20% saturation) was less potent or equally potent to an "equivalent" HH in prolonging sleeping times. In an isolated perfused liver, COH and HH had similar effects on drug metabolism (140, 141). Thus the differences in the intact experiments seem related to differences in reflex changes in the splanchnic circulation. In fact, HH was shown to cause a marked fall in liver blood flow, whereas COH had little or no effect (141). Thus [HbCO] values as high as 20% saturation appear to have no effect mediated by binding of CO to cytochrome *P*-450. Effects of CO on *p*-nitrophenol-*O*-demethylation in an isolated perfused rabbit lung are consistent with *R* of about 0.5 for this reaction in intact tissue (60, 61).

As predicted from considerations of tissue CO/O_2 ratios under conditions of elevated [HbCO] and from *R* values given in Table 3, evidence indicates that inhibition of cytochrome-*c* oxidase is probably not a mechanism of CO toxicity, even at high [HbCO]. In isolated mitochondria, CO/O_2 ratios of 5–15 are required for 50% inhibition of O_2 consumption (174, 186). In isolated rabbit aorta (37), isolated perfused rabbit lungs (12, 60), and stomach mucosal membrane (85), CO/O_2 ratios of 12–20 were required for 50% inhibition of oxidative metabolism. Reduction of both cytochrome-*c* oxidase and the invisible copper are required for CO to bind with any affinity (177).

There are a few studies where metabolic effects of CO have been determined in tissues, usually brain. Potentially it might be possible to determine the metabolic site of CO with measurements of appropriate chemical systems. The studies have utilized very high P_{CO} where there must be severe falls in tissue P_{O_2}, and it is likely that effects are dominated by tissue hypoxia or anoxia. Such studies have not shown any difference in severe COH and HH (104, 179, 180).

There are alterations in catecholamine turnover and steady-state levels in rat brains subjected to HH or COH (15%–17% saturation) (119, 120). Increased norepinephrine turnover and decreased steady-state concentrations were seen in the rat hypothalamus. Decreased dopamine turnover and increased steady-state dopamine concentrations were also observed. However, the pattern seems similar with HH and COH, and it is not possible to postulate any mechanisms other than tissue hypoxia resulting from binding of CO to Hb (119, 120).

Bartlett (11) has failed to find effects of elevated [HbCO] on lung growth of rats, such as occur with HH. Thus the HH effect may be due to inhibition of an enzyme that does not bind CO at CO/O_2 ratios found in these experiments.

Carbon monoxide effects mediated by binding to extravascular compounds could be studied in isolated systems where Hb is absent, i.e., tissue culture preparations or tissues perfused by Hb-free solutions. Cultured Purkinje cells (135) showed altered electrical activity at [CO] of 500–1,000 ppm, but CO/O_2 was not determined.

Comparing HH and COH data might give insight about different mechanisms of toxicity. However, as described in CARBON MONOXIDE BINDING TO PROTEINS FOUND IN MAMMALIAN TISSUES, p. 444, the tissue adaptation to hypoxia may utilize different mechanisms than are seen with COH, and it is difficult to determine HH and COH levels that would give equivalent mean capillary P_{O_2}.

CARBON MONOXIDE BINDING TO EXTRAVASCULAR PROTEINS DURING TISSUE HYPOXIA. Under conditions where tissue P_{O_2} falls and CO/O_2 increases, CO binding to proteins should increase. This has been observed for Mb during HH with $Pa_{O_2} < 40$ mmHg or during hemorrhagic shock (38, 40, 42), where 20%–40% of intravascular CO shifted out of the blood into skeletal or myocardial cells. (See *Location*, p. 439, for a discussion of this phenomenon.) These findings imply that during tissue hypoxia the pathophysiology of CO toxicity may be altered so that CO binding to intracellular CO-binding proteins plays a larger role. Therefore, as [HbCO] increases and tissue P_{O_2} falls, extravascular CO-binding proteins may bind significant CO to inhibit their function.

During tissue hypoxia, where cytochrome-*c* oxidase is reduced and reduction of O_2 decreased, the CO affinity may increase to the extent where CO binding might be significant. The off-reaction rate of CO–cytochrome-*c* oxidase is very slow, so that CO binding during transient hypoxia or anoxia might exert a prolonged effect (26).

It can be shown mathematically that O_2 transport in skeletal or cardiac muscle due to diffusion of MbO_2

becomes relatively more important during tissue hypoxia (77). Thus any inhibition of Mb O_2-carrier function due to CO binding may have more significance during tissue hypoxia.

CARBON MONOXIDE AND CARRIER-MEDIATED, FACILITATED DIFFUSION OF O_2. The possibility that Mb may function as an O_2 carrier during transport of O_2 in the muscle cytoplasm has been discussed (see *Extravascular CO-Binding Proteins*, p. 449). It can be shown experimentally that O_2 transport into and out of erythrocytes involves diffusion of HbO_2 as well as O_2 (113). In addition, there is speculation that O_2 transport in the lung, liver, and placenta may, in part, utilize a facilitation mechanism that is inhibited by CO (23, 68, 97). Proposals that this involves inhibition of cytochrome *P*-450 by CO conflict with the present understanding of the mechanisms of the catalytic redox cycle of cytochrome *P*-450, the distribution among cell types of cytochrome *P*-450, and its intracellular location.

This study was supported in part by Grant HL-19173 from the National Heart, Lung, and Blood Institute.

REFERENCES

1. ADAMS, J. D., H. H. ERICKSON, AND H. L. STONE. Myocardial metabolism during exposure to carbon monoxide in the conscious dog. *J. Appl. Physiol.* 34: 238–242, 1973.
2. AGOSTINI, A., R. STABILINI, G. VIGGIANO, M. LUZZANA, AND M. SAMAJA. Influence of capillary and tissue PO_2 on carbon monoxide binding to myoglobin: a theoretical evaluation. *Microvasc. Res.* 20: 81–87, 1980.
3. AHMED, A. E., V. L. KUBIC, AND M. W. ANDERS. Metabolism of haloforms to carbon monoxide. I. In vitro studies. *Drug Metab. Dispos.* 5: 198–204, 1977.
4. ALLEN, T. A., AND W. S. ROOT. Partition of carbon monoxide and oxygen between air and whole blood of rats, dogs and men as affected by plasma pH. *J. Appl. Physiol.* 10: 186–190, 1957.
5. ANTONINI, E. Interrelationship between structure and function in hemoglobin and myoglobin. *Physiol. Rev.* 45: 123–170, 1965.
6. ANTONINI, E., AND M. BRUNORI. *Hemoglobin and Myoglobin and Their Reactions With Ligands.* New York: Elsevier, 1971, p. 174–175.
7. ASMUSSEN, E., AND H. CHIODI. The effect of hypoxemia on ventilation and circulation in man. *Am. J. Physiol.* 132: 426–436, 1941.
8. AYRES, S. M., S. GIANNELLI, JR., AND H. MEULLER. Myocardial and systemic responses to carboxyhemoglobin. *Ann. NY Acad. Sci.* 174: 268–293, 1970.
9. BALDWIN, J. M. The structure of human carbon monoxyhaemoglobin at 2.7 A resolution. *J. Mol. Biol.* 136: 103–128, 1980.
10. BARCROFT, J. *The Respiratory Function of the Blood. Haemoglobin.* London: Cambridge Univ. Press, 1928, pt. II.
11. BARTLETT, D., JR. Postnatal growth of the mammalian lung: lack of influence by carbon monoxide exposure. *Respir. Physiol.* 23: 343–349, 1975.
12. BASSETT, D. J. P., AND A. B. FISHER. Metabolic response to carbon monoxide by isolated rat lungs. *Am. J. Physiol.* 230: 658–663, 1976.
13. BERK, P. D., F. L. RODKEY, T. F. BLASCHKE, H. A. COLLISON, AND J. G. WAGGONER. Comparison of plasma bilirubin turnover and carbon monoxide production in man. *J. Lab. Clin. Med.* 83: 29–37, 1974.
14. BISSELL, D. M., AND P. S. GUZELIAN. Degradation of endogenous hepatic heme by pathways not yielding carbon monoxide. Studies in normal rat liver and in primary hepatocyte culture. *J. Clin. Invest.* 65: 1135–1140, 1980.
15. BLASCHKE, T. F., P. D. BERK, F. L. RODKEY, B. F. SCHARSCHMIDT, H. A. COLLISON, AND J. G. WAGGONER. Drugs and the liver. I. Effects of glutethimide and phenobarbital on hepatic bilirubin clearance, plasma bilirubin turnover and carbon monoxide production in man. *Biochem. Pharmacol.* 23: 2795–2806, 1974.
16. BONAVENTURA, C., B. SULLIVAN, J. BONAVENTURA, AND S. BOURNE. CO binding by hemocyanins of *Limulus polyphemus, Busycon carica,* and *Callinectas sapidus. Biochemistry* 13: 4784–4789, 1974.
17. BOND, J. H., D. G. LEVITT, AND M. D. LEVITT. Use of inert gases and carbon monoxide to study the possible influence of countercurrent exchange on passive absorption from the small bowel. *J. Clin. Invest.* 54: 1259–1265, 1974.
18. BRIEGER, H. Carbon monoxide polycythemia. *J. Ind. Hyg. Toxicol.* 26: 321–327, 1944.
19. BRODY, J. S., AND R. F. COBURN. Carbon monoxide–induced arterial hypoxemia. *Science Wash. DC* 164: 1297–1298, 1969.
20. BROOK, D. F., AND P. J. LARGE. Inhibition by carbon monoxide of the secondary-amine mono-oxygenase of *Pseudomonas aminovorans* and the photochemical action spectrum for its reversal. *Eur. J. Biochem.* 55: 601–609, 1975.
21. BROUILLARD, R. P., M. E. CONRAD, AND T. A. BENSINGER. Effect of blood in the gut on measurements of endogenous carbon monoxide production. *Blood* 45: 67–69, 1975.
22. BROWN, E., J. HOPPER, J. J. SAMPSON, AND C. MUDRICK. Venous congestion of the extremities in relation to blood volume determinations and to mixing curves of carbon monoxide and T1824 in normal human subjects. *J. Clin. Invest.* 30: 1441–1450, 1951.
23. BURNS, B., AND G. H. GURTNER. A specific carrier for oxygen and carbon monoxide in the lung and placenta. *Drug Metab. Dispos.* 1: 374–377, 1973.
24. CAMPBELL, J. A. Tissue oxygen tension and carbon monoxide poisoning. *J. Physiol. Lond.* 68: 81–96, 1929.
25. CAUGHEY, W. S. Carbon monoxide bonding in hemoproteins. *Ann. NY Acad. Sci.* 174: 148–153, 1970.
26. CHANCE, B., M. ERECIŃSKA, AND M. WAGNER. Mitochondrial responses to carbon monoxide toxicity. *Ann. NY Acad. Sci.* 174: 193–204, 1970.
27. CHIODI, H., D. B. DILL, F. CONSOLAZIO, AND S. M. HORVATH. Respiratory and circulatory responses to acute carbon monoxide poisoning. *Am. J. Physiol.* 134: 683–693, 1941.
28. CLARK, B. J., AND R. F. COBURN. Mean myoglobin oxygen tension during exercise at maximal oxygen uptake. *J. Appl. Physiol.* 39: 135–144, 1975.
29. CLARK, R. T., JR. Evidence for conversion of carbon monoxide to carbon dioxide by the intact animal. *Am. J. Physiol.* 162: 560–564, 1950.
30. CLARK, R. T., JR., AND A. B. OTIS. Comparative studies on acclimatization of mice to carbon monoxide and to low oxygen. *Am. J. Physiol.* 169: 285–294, 1952.
31. COBURN, R. F. Endogenous carbon monoxide production and body CO stores. *Acta Med. Scand. Suppl.* 472: 269–281, 1967.
32. COBURN, R. F. The carbon monoxide body stores. *Ann. NY Acad. Sci.* 174: 11–22, 1970.
33. COBURN, R. F. Enhancement by phenobarbital and diphenylhydantoin of carbon monoxide production in normal man. *New Eng. J. Med.* 283: 512–515, 1970.
34. COBURN, R. F., E. R. ALLEN, S. AYRES, D. BARTLETT, JR., S. M. HORVATH, L. H. KULLER, V. LATIES, L. D. LONGO, AND E. P. RADFORD, JR. *Carbon Monoxide.* Washington, DC: Natl. Acad. Sci., 1977.

35. COBURN, R. F., W. S. BLAKEMORE, AND R. E. FORSTER. Endogenous carbon monoxide production in man. *J. Clin. Invest.* 42: 1172–1178, 1963.
36. COBURN, R. F., R. E. FORSTER, AND P. B. KANE. Considerations of the physiological variables that determine the blood carboxyhemoglobin concentration in man. *J. Clin. Invest.* 44: 1899–1910, 1965.
37. COBURN, R. F., B. GRUBB, AND R. D. ARONSON. Effect of cyanide on oxygen tension-dependent mechanical tension in rabbit aorta. *Circ. Res.* 44: 368–378, 1979.
38. COBURN, R. F., AND L. B. MAYERS. Myoglobin O_2 tension determined from measurements of carboxymyoglobin in skeletal muscle. *Am. J. Physiol.* 220: 66–74, 1971.
39. COBURN, R. F., AND M. PENDLETON. Effects of norepinephrine on oxygenation of resting skeletal muscle. *Am. J. Physiol.* 236 (*Heart Circ. Physiol.* 5): H307–H313, 1979.
40. COBURN, R. F., F. PLOEGMAKERS, P. GONDRIE, AND R. ABBOUD. Myocardial myoglobin oxygen tension. *Am. J. Physiol.* 224: 870–876, 1973.
41. COBURN, R. F., M. SWERDLOW, K. J. LUOMANMÄKI, R. E. FORSTER, AND K. POWELL. Uptake of carbon monoxide from the urinary bladder of the dog. *Am. J. Physiol.* 215: 1010–1023, 1968.
42. COBURN, R. F., H. W. WALLACE, AND R. ABBOUD. Redistribution of body carbon monoxide after hemorrhage. *Am. J. Physiol.* 220: 868–873, 1971.
43. COBURN, R. F., W. J. WILLIAMS, AND R. E. FORSTER. Effect of erythrocyte destruction on carbon monoxide production in man. *J. Clin. Invest.* 43: 1098–1103, 1964.
44. COBURN, R. F., W. J. WILLIAMS, P. WHITE, AND S. B. KAHN. The production of carbon monoxide from hemoglobin in vivo. *J. Clin. Invest.* 46: 346–351, 1967.
45. COLLIER, C. R. Oxygen affinity of human blood in presence of carbon monoxide. *J. Appl. Physiol.* 40: 487–490, 1976.
46. COLLMAN, J. P., J. I. BRAUMAN, AND K. M. DOXSEE. Carbon monoxide binding to iron porphyrins. *Proc. Natl. Acad. Sci. USA* 76: 6035–6039, 1979.
47. COLTMAN, C. A., JR., G. M. DUDLEY III, AND S. D. LEVERETT, JR. Measurement of endogenous carbon monoxide production to determine the effect of high $+G_x$ acceleration on the destruction rate of red cells. *Aerosp. Med.* 40: 627–631, 1969.
48. COOPER, D. Y., S. LEVIN, S. NARASIMHULU, O. ROSENTHAL, AND R. W. ESTABROOK. Photochemical action spectrum of the terminal oxidase of mixed function oxidase systems. *Science Wash. DC* 147: 400–402, 1965.
49. COOPER, D. Y., H. SCHLEYER, O. ROSENTHAL, S. LEVIN, A. Y. H. LU, R. KUNTZMAN, AND A. H. CONNEY. Inhibition by CO of hepatic benzo[α]pyrene hydroxylation and its reversal by monochromatic light. *Eur. J. Biochem.* 74: 69–75, 1977.
50. COTTON, F. A., AND G. WILKINSON. *Advanced Inorganic Chemistry. A Comprehensive Text* (3rd ed.). New York: Wiley, 1972, p. 635.
51. COTTON, F. A., AND G. WILKINSON. *Advanced Inorganic Chemistry. A Comprehensive Text* (3rd ed.). New York: Wiley, 1972, p. 684.
52. DANIELS, L., G. FUCHS, R. K. THAUER, AND J. G. ZEIKUS. Carbon monoxide oxidation by methanogenic bacteria. *J. Bacteriol.* 132: 118–126, 1977.
53. DAVIES, R. O., T. NISHINO, AND S. LAHIRI. Sympathectomy does not alter the response of carotid chemoreceptors to hypoxemia during carboxyhemoglobinemia or anemia. *Neurosci. Lett.* 21: 159–163, 1981.
54. DELIVORIA-PAPADOPOULOS, M., R. F. COBURN, AND R. E. FORSTER. Cyclic variation of rate of carbon monoxide production in normal women. *J. Appl. Physiol.* 36: 49–51, 1974.
55. DIEKERT, G. B., AND R. K. THAUER. Carbon monoxide oxidation by *Clostridium thermoaceticum* and *Clostridium formicoaceticum*. *J. Bacteriol.* 136: 597–606, 1978.
56. DINMAN, B. D., J. W. EATON, AND G. L. BREWER. Effects of carbon monoxide on DPG concentrations in the erythrocyte. *Ann. NY Acad. Sci.* 174: 246–251, 1970.
57. DOUGLAS, C. G., J. S. HALDANE, AND J. B. S. HALDANE. The laws of combination of haemoglobin with carbon monoxide and oxygen. *J. Physiol. Lond.* 44: 275–304, 1912.
58. ENGEL, R. R., S. MODLER, J. M. MATSEN, AND Z. J. PETRYKA. Carbon monoxide production from hydroxocobalamin by bacteria. *Biochim. Biophys. Acta* 313: 150–155, 1973.
59. FENN, W. O., AND D. M. COBB. The burning of carbon monoxide by heart and skeletal muscle. *Am. J. Physiol.* 102: 393–401, 1932.
60. FISHER, A. B., AND C. DODIA. Lung as a model for evaluation of critical intracellular P_{O_2} and P_{CO}. *Am. J. Physiol.* 241 (*Endocrinol. Metab.* 4): E47–E50, 1981.
61. FISHER, A. B., N. ITAKURA, C. DODIA, AND R. G. THURMAN. Relationship between alveolar P_{O_2} and the rate of *p*-nitroanisole *O*-demethylation by the cytochrome P-450 pathway in isolated rabbit lungs. *J. Clin. Invest.* 64: 770–774, 1979.
62. FISHER, T. R., R. F COBURN, AND R. E. FORSTER. Carbon monoxide diffusing capacity in the bullhead catfish. *J. Appl. Physiol.* 26: 161–169, 1969.
63. FORBES, W. H., F. SARGENT, AND F. J. W. ROUGHTON. The rate of carbon monoxide uptake by normal men. *Am. J. Physiol.* 143: 594–608, 1945.
64. FORMAN, H. J., AND P. FEIGELSON. Kinetic evidence indicating the absence during catalysis of an unbound ferroprotoporphyrin form of tryptophane oxygenase. *Biochemistry* 10: 760–763, 1971.
65. FORSTER, R. E., W. S. FOWLER, AND D. V. BATES. Considerations on the uptake of carbon monoxide by the lungs. *J. Clin. Invest.* 33: 1128–1168, 1954.
66. GIBSON, Q. H., AND M. H. SMITH. Rates of reaction of ascaris haemoglobins with ligands. *Proc. Soc. Lond. B. Biol. Sci.* 163: 206–214, 1965.
67. GOTHERT, M. Factors influencing the CO content of tissues. *Staub-Reinhalt. Luft* 32: 15–20, 1972.
68. GURTNER, G. H. Evidence for facilitated transport of oxygen and carbon monoxide. In: *Pulmonary Gas Exchange. Organism and Environment*, edited by J. B. West. New York: Academic, 1980, vol. 2, p. 205–239.
69. HALDANE, J., AND J. L. SMITH. The absorption of oxygen by the lungs. *J. Physiol. Lond.* 22: 231–258, 1897.
70. HALDANE, J. S. *Respiration.* New Haven, CT: Yale Univ. Press, 1922.
71. HALL, P. F., J. L. LEWES, AND E. D. LIPSON. The role of mitochondrial cytochrome P-450 from bovine adrenal cortex in side chain cleavage of 20S,22R-dihydroxycholesterol. *J. Biol. Chem.* 250: 2283–2286, 1975.
72. HATCH, T. F. Carbon monoxide uptake in relation to pulmonary performance. *Arch. Ind. Hyg. Occup. Med.* 6: 1–8, 1952.
73. HATCHER, J. D., L. K. CHIU, AND D. B. JENNINGS. Anemia as a stimulus to aortic and carotid chemoreceptors in the cat. *J. Appl. Physiol.* 44: 696–702, 1978.
74. HEIDNER, E. J., R. C. LADNER, AND M. F. PERUTZ. Structure of horse carbon monoxyhemoglobin. *J. Mol. Biol.* 104: 707–722, 1976.
75. HLASTALA, M. P., H. P. MCKENNA, R. L. FRANADA, AND J. C. DETTER. Influence of carbon monoxide on hemoglobin-oxygen binding. *J. Appl. Physiol.* 41: 893–899, 1976.
76. HOLLAND, R. A. B. Rate of O_2 dissociation from O_2Hb and relative combination rate of CO and O_2 in mammals at 37°C. *Respir. Physiol.* 7: 30–42, 1969.
77. HOOFD, L., AND F. KREUZER. Calculation of the facilitation of O_2 or CO transport by Hb or Mb by means of a new method for solving the carrier-diffusion problem. *Adv. Exp. Med. Biol.* 94: 163–168, 1978.
78. HORVATH, S. M., P. B. RAVEN, T. E. DAHMS, AND D. J. GRAY. Maximal aerobic capacity at different levels of carboxyhemoglobin. *J. Appl. Physiol.* 38: 300–303, 1975.
79. ISHIMURA, Y., M. NOZAKI, AND O. HAYAISHI. Evidence for an oxygenated intermediate in the tryptophan pyrrolase reaction. *J. Biol. Chem.* 242: 2574–2576, 1967.
80. JOELS, N., AND L. G. C. E. PUGH. The carbon monoxide dissociation curve of human blood. *J. Physiol. Lond.* 142: 63–77, 1958.

81. JONES, H. A., J. C. CLARK, E. E. DAVIES, R. E. FORSTER, AND J. M. B. HUGHES. Rate of uptake of carbon monoxide at different inspired concentrations in humans. *J. Appl. Physiol.* 52: 109–113, 1982.
82. KAUFMAN, S. D. Coenzymes and hydroxylases: ascorbate and dopamine β-hydroxylase; tetrahydropteridines and phenylalanine and tyrosine hydroxylase. *Pharmacol. Rev.* 18: 61–69, 1966.
83. KEILIN, D., AND T. MANN. Polyphenoloxidase: purification, nature and properties. *Proc. R. Soc. Lond. B Biol. Sci.* 125: 187–204, 1938.
84. KERTESZ, D. The copper of polyphenoloxidase. In: *The Biochemistry of Copper*, edited by J. Peisach, P. Aisen, and W. E. Blumberg. New York: Academic, 1966, p. 359–369.
85. KIDDER, G. W., III. Carbon monoxide insensitivity of gastric acid secretion. *Am. J. Physiol.* 238 (*Gastrointest. Liver Physiol.* 1): G197–G202, 1980.
86. KILLICK, E. M. The nature of the acclimatization occurring during repeated exposure of the human subject to atmospheres containing low concentrations of carbon monoxide. *J. Physiol. Lond.* 107: 27–44, 1948.
87. KLEINERT, H. D., J. L. SCALES, AND H. R. WEISS. Effects of carbon monoxide or low oxygen gas mixture inhalation on regional oxygenation, blood flow, and small vessel blood content of the rabbit heart. *Pfluegers Arch.* 383: 105–111, 1980.
88. KRASNA, A. I. Regulation of hydrogenase activity in enterobacteria. *J. Bacteriol.* 144: 1094–1097, 1980.
89. KUBIC, V. L., AND M. W. ANDERS. Metabolism of dihalomethanes to carbon monoxide. II. In vitro studies. *Drug Metab. Dispos.* 3: 104–112, 1975.
90. KUBIC, V. L., AND M. W. ANDERS. Metabolism of dihalomethanes to carbon monoxide. III. Studies on the mechanism of the reaction. *Biochem. Pharmacol.* 27: 2349–2355, 1978.
91. LAHIRI, S., E. MULLIGAN, T. NISHINO, A. MOKASHI, AND R. O. DAVIES. Relative responses of aortic body and carotid body chemoreceptors to carboxyhemoglobinemia. *J. Appl. Physiol.* 50: 580–586, 1981.
92. LANDAW, S. A., E. W. CALLAHAN, JR., AND R. SCHMID. Catabolism of heme in vivo: comparison of the simultaneous production of bilirubin and carbon monoxide. *J. Clin. Invest.* 49: 914–925, 1970.
93. LATIES, V. Carbon monoxide and behavior. *Arch. Neurol.* 167: 68–126, 1980.
94. LAU, P. W., AND T. ASAKURA. Comparative study of oxygen and carbon monoxide binding by hemoglobin. *J. Biol. Chem.* 255: 1617–1622, 1980.
95. LINDAHL, J. Appearance of [^{14}C]O in expired air and incorporation of ^{14}C in hemoglobin after administration of glycine-2-[^{14}C] in man. *Scand. J. Clin. Lab. Invest.* 33: 353–359, 1979.
96. LOGUE, G. L., W. F. ROSSE, W. T. SMITH, H. A. SALTZMAN, AND L. A. GUTTERMAN. Endogenous carbon monoxide production measured by gas-phase analysis: for estimation of heme catabolic rate. *J. Lab. Clin. Med.* 77: 867–876, 1971.
97. LONGMUIR, I. S., D. C. MARTIN, H. J. GOLD, AND S. SUN. Nonclassical respiratory activity of tissue slices. *Microvasc. Res.* 3: 125–141, 1971.
98. LONGO, L. D. The biological effects of carbon monoxide on the pregnant woman, fetus, and newborn infant. *Am. J. Obstet. Gynecol.* 12: 69–103, 1977.
99. LONGO, L. D., G. G. POWER, AND R. E. FORSTER. Respiratory function of the placenta as determined with carbon monoxide in sheep and dogs. *J. Clin. Invest.* 46: 812–828, 1967.
100. LOTLIKAR, P. D., AND K. ZALESKI. Inhibitory effect of carbon monoxide on the *N*- and ring-hydroxylation of 2-acetamidofluorene by hamster hepatic microsomal preparations. *Biochem. J.* 144: 427–430, 1974.
101. LUNDH, B., E. C. STAHL, AND C. MERCKE. Heme catabolism, carbon monoxide production and red cell survival in anemia. *Acta Med. Scand.* 197: 161–171, 1975.
102. LUOMANMÄKI, K., AND R. F. COBURN. Effects of metabolism and distribution of carbon monoxide on blood and body stores. *Am. J. Physiol.* 217: 354–363, 1969.
103. LYNCH, S. R., AND A. L. MOEDE. Variation in the rate of endogenous carbon monoxide production in normal human beings. *J. Lab. Clin. Med.* 79: 85–95, 1971.
104. MACMILLAN, V. Cerebral carbohydrate metabolism during acute carbon monoxide intoxication. *Brain Res.* 121: 271–286, 1977.
105. MACQUARRIE, R., AND Q. H. GIBSON. Use of a fluorescent analogue of 2,3-diphosphoglycerate as a probe of human hemoglobin conformation during carbon monoxide binding. *J. Biol. Chem.* 246: 5832–5835, 1971.
106. MAENO, H., AND P. FEIGELSON. Studies on the interaction of carbon monoxide with tryptophan oxygenase of *Pseudomonas. J. Biol. Chem.* 243: 301–305, 1968.
107. MAISELS, M. J., A. PATHAK, N. M. NELSON, D. H. NATHAN, AND C. A. SMITH. Endogenous production of carbon monoxide in normal and erythroblastotic newborn infants. *J. Clin. Invest.* 50: 1–8, 1971.
108. MAKINEN, M. W., R. A. HOUTCHENS, AND W. S. CAUGHEY. Structure of carboxymyoglobin in crystals and in solution. *Proc. Natl. Acad. Sci. USA* 76: 6042–6046, 1979.
109. MERCKE, C., E. CAVALLIN-STAHL, AND B. LUNDH. Heme catabolism during short-term treatment with phenobarbital, diazepam and oxazepam. *Acta Med. Scand.* 198: 149–154, 1975.
110. MERCKE, C., E. CAVALLIN-STAHL, AND B. LUNDH. Diurnal variation in endogenous production of carbon monoxide. *Acta Med. Scand.* 198: 161–164, 1975.
111. MICFLIKIER, A. B., J. H. BOND, B. SIRCAR, AND M. D. LEVITT. Intestinal villus blood flow measured with carbon monoxide and microspheres. *Am. J. Physiol.* 230: 916–919, 1976.
112. MILLER, A. T., JR., AND J. J. WOOD. Effects of acute carbon monoxide exposure on the energy metabolism of rat brain and liver. *Environ. Res.* 8: 107–111, 1974.
113. MOCHIZUKI, M., AND R. E. FORSTER. Diffusion of carbon monoxide through thin layers of hemoglobin solution. *Science Wash. DC* 138: 897–898, 1962.
114. MOELLER, T. Carbon monoxide in organic chemistry. In: *An Advanced Textbook.* New York: Wiley, 1952, p. 665.
115. MONOD, J., J. WYMAN, AND J. P. CHANGEUX. On the nature of allosteric transitions: a plausible model. *J. Mol. Biol.* 12: 88–118, 1965.
116. MONTGOMERY, M. R., AND R. J. RUBIN. Oxygenation during inhibition of drug metabolism by carbon monoxide or hypoxic hypoxia. *J. Appl. Physiol.* 35: 505–509, 1973.
117. MONTGOMERY, M. R., AND R. J. RUBIN. Adaptation to the inhibitory effect of carbon monoxide inhalation on drug metabolism. *J. Appl. Physiol.* 35: 601–607, 1973.
118. MORAY, R. A relation of persons killed with subterraneous damps. *Philos. Trans. R. Soc. Lond. A Math. Phys. Sci.* 1: 44–45, 1665.
119. NEWBY, M. B., R. J. ROBERTS, AND R. K. BHATNAGAR. Carbon monoxide- and hypoxia-induced effects on catecholamines in the mature and developing rat brain. *J. Pharmacol. Exp. Ther.* 206: 61–68, 1978.
120. NEWBY-SCHMIDT, B., R. J. ROBERTS, AND R. K. BHATNAGAR. Regional effects of carbon monoxide and hypoxia on catecholamines in the rat brain. *Neurotoxicology Little Rock* 1: 533–540, 1980.
121. NOMOF, N., I. HOPPER, JR., E. BROWN, K. SCOTT, AND R. WENNESLAND. Simultaneous determinations of the total volume of red blood cells by use of carbon monoxide and chromium in breathing and diseased human subjects. *J. Clin. Invest.* 33: 1382–1387, 1954.
122. OKADA, Y., I. TYUMA, Y. UEDA, AND T. SUGIMOTO. Effect of carbon monoxide on equilibrium between oxygen and hemoglobin. *Am. J. Physiol.* 230: 471–475, 1976.
123. O'KEEFE, D. H., R. E. EBEL, J. A. PETERSON, J. C. MAXWELL, AND W. S. CAUGHEY. An infrared spectroscopic study of carbon monoxide bonding to ferrous cytochrome P-450. *Biochemistry* 17: 5845–5852, 1978.
124. ORME-JOHNSON, W. H., E. MUNCK, R. ZIMMERMANN, W. J. BRILL, V. K. SHAH, J. RAWLINGS, M. T. HENZL, B. A. AVERILL, AND N. R. ORME-JOHNSON. On the metal centers

in nitrogenase. In: *Mechanisms of Oxidizing Enzymes,* edited by J. P. Singer and R. N. Ondarza. New York: Elsevier, 1978, p. 165–172.
125. PACE, N., E. STRAJMAN, AND E. L. WALKER. Acceleration of carbon monoxide elimination in man by high pressure oxygen. *Science Wash. DC* 3: 652–654, 1950.
126. PEISACH, J., W. E. BLUMBERG, B. A. WITTENBERG, AND J. B. WITTENBERG. The electronic structure of protoheme proteins. 3. Configuration of the heme and its ligands. *J. Biol. Chem.* 243: 1871–1880, 1968.
127. PENNEY, D. G., AND P. A. BISHOP. Hematological changes in the rat during and after exposure to carbon monoxide. *J. Environ. Pathol. Toxicol.* 2: 407–415, 1978.
128. PENNEY, D. G., R. VAK, AND V. ASHENBRENNER. Carbon monoxide inhalation: effect on heart cytochrome *c* in the neonatal and adult rat. *J. Toxicol. Environ. Health* 12: 395–406, 1983.
129. PETERSON, J. E. Postexposure relationship of carbon monoxide in blood and expired air. *Arch. Environ. Health* 21: 172–173, 1970.
130. PETERSON, J. E., AND R. D. STEWART. Absorption and elimination of carbon monoxide by inactive young men. *Arch. Environ. Health* 21: 165–171, 1970.
131. PETERSON, J. E., AND R. D. STEWART. Predicting the carboxyhemoglobin levels resulting from carbon monoxide exposures. *J. Appl. Physiol.* 39: 633–638, 1975.
132. POWER, G. G., AND W. C. BRADFORD. Measurement of pulmonary diffusing capacity during blood-to-gas exchange in humans. *J. Appl. Physol.* 27: 61–66, 1969.
133. RAFF, H., S. P. TZANKOFF, AND R. S. FITZGERALD. ACTH and cortisol responses to hypoxia in dogs. *J. Appl. Physiol.* 51: 1257–1260, 1981.
134. RAMSEY, J. M., AND P. W. CASPER, JR. Effect of carbon monoxide exposures on erythrocytic 2,3-DPG in rabbits. *J. Appl. Physiol.* 41: 689–692, 1976.
135. RAYBOURN, M. S., C. CORK, W. SCHIMMERLING, AND C. A. TOBIAS. An in vitro electrophysiological assessment of the direct cellular toxicity of carbon monoxide. *Toxicol. Appl. Pharmacol.* 46: 769–779, 1978.
136. RODKEY, F. L., AND H. A. COLLISON. Biological oxidation of [^{14}C]methylene chloride to carbon monoxide and carbon dioxide by the rat. *Toxicol. Appl. Pharmacol.* 40: 33–38, 1977.
137. RODKEY, F. L., AND H. A. COLLISON. Effect of dihalogenated methanes on the in vivo production of carbon monoxide and methane by rats. *Toxicol. Appl. Pharmacol.* 40: 39–47, 1977.
138. RODKEY, F. L., J. D. O'NEAL, H. A. COLLISON, AND D. E. UDDIN. Relative affinity of hemoglobin S and hemoglobin A for carbon monoxide and oxygen. *Clin. Chem.* 20: 83–84, 1974.
139. ROOT, R. W. The combination of carbon monoxide with hemocyanin. *J. Biol. Chem.* 104: 239–244, 1934.
140. ROTH, R. A., AND R. J. RUBIN. Comparison of the effect of carbon monoxide and of hypoxic hypoxia. II. Hexobarbital metabolism in the isolated, perfused rat liver. *J. Pharmacol. Exp. Ther.* 199: 61–66, 1976.
141. ROTH, R. A., JR., AND R. J. RUBIN. Role of blood flow in carbon monoxide and hypoxic hypoxia-induced alterations in hexobarbital metabolism in rats. *Drug Metab. Dispos.* 4: 460–467, 1976.
142. ROUGHTON, F. J. W. The equilibrium between carbon monoxide and sheep haemoglobin at very high percentage saturations. *J. Physiol. Lond.* 126: 369–383, 1954.
143. ROUGHTON, F. J. W. The equilibrium of carbon monoxide with human hemoglobin in whole blood. *Ann. NY Acad. Sci.* 174: 177–188, 1970.
144. ROUGHTON, F. J. W., AND R. C. DARLING. The effect of carbon monoxide on the oxyhemoglobin dissociation curve. *Am. J. Physiol.* 141: 17–31, 1944.
145. ROUGHTON, F. J. W., A. B. OTIS, AND R. L. J. LYSTER. The determination of the individual equilibrium constants of the four intermediate reactions between oxygen and sheep haemoglobin. *Proc. R. Soc. Lond. B Biol. Sci.* 144: 29–54, 1955.
146. ROUGHTON, F. J. W., AND W. S. ROOT. The fate of CO in the body during recovery from mild carbon monoxide poisoning in man. *Am. J. Physiol.* 145: 239–252, 1946.
147. SANTIAGO, T. V., AND N. H. EDELMAN. Mechanism of ventilatory response to carbon monoxide. *J. Clin. Invest.* 57: 977–986, 1976.
148. SHAANAN, B. The structure of human oxyhaemoglobin at 2.1 A resolution. *J. Mol. Biol.* 171: 31–59, 1983.
149. SHARMA, V. S., J. F. GEIBEL, AND H. M. RANNEY. "Tension" on heme by the proximal base and ligand reactivity: conclusions drawn from model compounds for the reaction of hemoglobin. *Proc. Natl. Acad. Sci. USA* 75: 3747–3750, 1978.
150. SHARMA, V. S., M. R. SCHMIDT, AND H. M. RANNEY. Dissociation of CO from carboxyhemoglobin. *J. Biol. Chem.* 251: 4267–4272, 1976.
151. SIES, H. Oxygen gradients during hypoxic steady states in liver: urate oxidases and cytochrome oxidase as intracellular O_2 indicators. *Hoppe-Seyler's Z. Physiol. Chem.* 35: 1021–1032, 1977.
152. SIRS, J. A. The effect of temperature on the reaction of carbon monoxide with oxygenated haemoglobin. *J. Physiol. Lond.* 260: 37–44, 1976.
153. SJÖSTRAND, T. Endogenous formation of carbon monoxide. The CO concentration in the inspired and expired air of hospital patients. *Acta Physiol. Scand.* 22: 137–141, 1950.
154. SJÖSTRAND, T. The in vitro formation of carbon monoxide in blood. *Acta Physiol Scand.* 24: 314–331, 1951.
155. STEVENS, J. L., AND M. W. ANDERS. Metabolism of haloforms to carbon monoxide. III. Studies on the mechanism of the reaction. *Biochem. Pharmacol.* 28: 3189–3194, 1979.
156. STEVENSON, D. K., A. L. BARTOLETTI, C. R. OSTRANDER, AND J. D. JOHNSON. Pulmonary excretion of carbon monoxide in the human newborn infant as an index of bilirubin production. III. Measurement of pulmonary excretion of carbon monoxide after the first post-natal week of premature infants. *Pediatrics* 64: 598–600, 1979.
157. STEWART, R. D., T. N. FISHER, M. H. HOSKO, J. E. PETERSON, E. D. BARTETTA, AND H. C. DODD. Carboxyhemoglobin elevation after exposure to dichloromethane. *Science Wash. DC* 176: 295–296, 1972.
158. SUCHDEO, S. R., J. D. GODDARD, AND J. S. SCHULTZ. An analysis of the competitive diffusion of O_2 and CO through hemoglobin solutions. *Adv. Exp. Med. Biol.* 37: 951–961, 1973.
159. SYLVESTER, J. T., S. M. SCHARF, R. D. GILBERT, R. S. FITZGERALD, AND R. J. TRAYSTMAN. Hypoxic and CO hypoxia in dogs: hemodynamics, carotid reflexes, and catecholamines. *Am. J. Physiol.* 236 (*Heart Circ. Physiol.* 5): H22–H28, 1979.
160. TANAKA, T., AND W. E. KNOX. The nature and mechanism of the tryptophan pyrrolase (peroxidase-oxidase) reaction of *Pseudomonas* and of the rat liver. *J. Biol. Chem.* 234: 1162–1170, 1959.
161. TANIGUCHI, S., N. HOSHITA, AND K. OKUDA. Enzymatic characteristics of CO-sensitive 26-hydroxylase system for 5β-cholestane-3α, 7α, 12α-triol in rat-liver mitochondria and its intramitochondrial localization. *Eur. J. Biochem.* 40: 607–617, 1973.
162. TENHUNEN, R., H. MARVER, N. R. PIMSTONE, F. W. TRAGER, D. Y. COOPER, AND R. SCHMID. Enzymatic degradation of heme. Oxygenative cleavage requiring cytochrome P-450. *Biochemistry* 11: 1716–1720, 1972.
163. TENHUNEN, R., H. S. MARVER, AND R. SCHMID. Microsomal heme oxygenase. Characterization of the enzyme. *J. Biol. Chem.* 244: 6388–6394, 1969.
164. THOMAS, M. F., AND D. G. PENNEY. Hematologic responses to carbon monoxide and altitude: a comparative study. *J. Appl. Physiol.* 43: 365–369, 1977.
165. TOBIAS, C. A., J. H. LAWRENCE, F. J. W. ROUGHTON, W. S. ROOT, AND M. I. GREGERSEN. The elimination of carbon monoxide from the human body with reference to the possible conversion of CO to CO_2. *Am. J. Physiol.* 145: 253–263, 1945.
166. TRAYLOR, T. G., AND A. P. BERZINIS. Binding of O_2 and CO to hemes and hemoproteins. *Proc. Natl. Acad. Sci. USA* 77: 3171–3175, 1980.

167. TRAYSTMAN, R. J., R. S. FITZGERALD, AND S. C. LOSUTOFF. Cerebral circulatory responses to arterial hypoxia in normal and chemodenervated dogs. *Circ. Res.* 42: 649–657, 1978.
168. TZAGOLOFF, A., AND D. C. WHARTON. Studies on the electron transfer system. LXII. The reaction of cytochrome oxidase with carbon monoxide. *J. Biol. Chem.* 240: 2628–2633, 1965.
169. WAGNER, J. A., S. M. HORVATH, AND T. E. DAHMS. Cardiovascular adjustments to carbon monoxide exposure during rest and exercise in dogs. *Environ. Res.* 15: 368–374, 1978.
170. WARBURG, D. *Heavy Metal Prosthetic Groups and Enzyme Action.* London: Oxford Univ. Press, 1949.
171. WEISS, H. R., AND J. A. COHEN. Effects of low levels of carbon monoxide on rat brain and muscle tissue P_{O_2}. *Environ. Physiol. Biochem.* 4: 31–39, 1974.
172. WERNER, B. Inter- and intra-individual variation of carbon monoxide production in young healthy males. *Scand. J. Clin. Lab. Invest.* 38: 199–202, 1978.
173. WERNER B., AND J. LINDAHL. Endogenous carbon monoxide production after bicycle exercise in healthy subjects and in patients with hereditary spherocytosis. *Scand. J. Clin. Lab. Invest.* 40: 319–325, 1980.
174. WHARTON, D. C., AND Q. H. GIBSON. Cytochrome oxidase from *Pseudomonas aeruginosa.* IV. Reaction with oxygen and carbon monoxide. *Biochim. Biophys. Acta* 430: 445–453, 1976.
175. WHITE, P., R. F. COBURN, W. J. WILLIAMS, M. I. GOLDWEIN, M. L. ROTHER, AND B. C. SHAFER. Carbon monoxide production associated with ineffective erythropoiesis. *J. Clin. Invest.* 46: 1986–1988, 1967.
176. WILKS, S. S., J. F. TOMASHEFSKI, AND R. T. CLARK, JR. Physiological effects of chronic exposure to carbon monoxide. *J. Appl. Physiol.* 14: 305–310, 1959.
177. WILSON, D. F., AND Y. MIYATA. Reaction of CO with cytochrome c oxidase. Titration of the reaction site with chemical oxidant and reductant. *Biochim. Biophys. Acta* 461: 218–230, 1977.
178. WINSLOW, R. M., J. M. MORRISSEY, R. L. BERGER, P. D. SMITH, AND C. C. GIBSON. Variability of oxygen affinity of normal blood: an automated method of measurement. *J. Appl. Physiol.* 45: 289–297, 1978.
179. WINSTON, J. M., AND R. J. ROBERTS. Influence of carbon monoxide hypoxic hypoxia or potassium cyanide pretreatment on acute carbon monoxide and hypoxic hypoxia lethality. *J. Pharmacol. Exp. Ther.* 193: 713–719, 1975.
180. WINSTON, J. M., AND R. J. ROBERTS. Glucose catabolism following carbon monoxide or hypoxic hypoxia exposure. *Biochem. Pharmacol.* 27: 377–380, 1978.
181. WITTENBERG, B. A., E. ANTONINI, M. BRUNORI, R. W. NOBLE, J. B. WITTENBERG, AND J. WYMAN. Studies on the equilibria and kinetics of reactions of peroxidases with ligands. III. The dissociation of carbon monoxide from carbon monoxide ferro-horseradish peroxidase. *Biochemistry* 6: 1970–1974, 1967.
182. WITTENBERG, B. A., M. BRUNORI, E. ANTONINI, J. B. WITTENBERG, AND J. WYMAN. Kinetics of the reactions of *Aplysia* myoglobin with oxygen and carbon monoxide. *Arch. Biochem. Biophys.* 111: 576–579, 1965.
183. WITTENBERG, B. A., AND J. B. WITTENBERG. Role of myoglobin in the oxygen supply to red skeletal muscle. *J. Biol. Chem.* 240: 9038–9043, 1975.
184. WITTENBERG, J. B. Myoglobin-facilitated oxygen diffusion: role of myoglobin in oxygen entry into muscle. *Physiol. Rev.* 50: 559–636, 1970.
185. WITTENBERG, J. B., C. A. APPLEBY, AND B. A. WITTENBERG. Kinetics of the reactions of leghemoglobin with oxygen and carbon monoxide. *J. Biol. Chem.* 247: 527–531, 1972.
186. WOHLRAB, H., AND G. B. ORUNMOLA. Carbon monoxide binding studies of cytochrome a_3 hemes in intact rat liver mitochondria. *Biochemistry* 10: 1103–1106, 1971.
187. WOLFF, D. G., AND W. R. BIDLOCK. The formation of carbon monoxide during perioxidation of microsomal lipids. *Biophys. Res. Commun.* 73: 850–855, 1976.
188. YONETANI, T. The a-type cytochromes. In: *The Enzymes*, edited by P. D. Boyer, H. Lary, and K. Myrback. New York: Academic, 1963, vol. 8, p. 42–79.
189. YOSHIDA, T., M. NOGUCHI, AND G. KIKUCHI. The step of carbon monoxide liberation in the sequence of heme degradation catalyzed by the reconstituted microsomal heme oxygenase system. *J. Biol. Chem.* 257: 9345–9348, 1982.
190. YOSHIKAWA, S., M. G. CHOC, M. C. O'TOOLE, AND W. S. CAUGHEY. An infrared study of CO binding to heart cytochrome *c* oxidase and hemoglobin A. Implications re O_2 reactions. *J. Biol. Chem.* 252: 5498–5508, 1977.
191. YOUNG, L. J., M. G. CHOC, AND W. S. CAUGHEY. Role of oxygen and cytochrome *c* oxidase in the detoxification of CO by oxidation to CO_2. In: *Biochemical and Clinical Aspects of Oxygen*, edited by W. S. Caughey. New York: Academic, 1979, p. 355–362.
192. ZINKHAM, W. H., R. A. HOUTCHENS, AND W. S. CAUGHEY. Carboxyhemoglobin level in an unstable hemoglobin disorder (Hb Zürich): effect on phenotypic expression. *Science Wash. DC* 209: 406–408, 1980.
193. ZINNER, K., C. VIDIGAL-MARINELLI, N. DURÁN, A. J. MARSAIOLI, AND G. CILENTO. A new source of carbon oxides in biochemical systems. Implications regarding dioxetane intermediates. *Biochem. Biophys. Res. Commun.* 92: 32–37, 1980.
194. ZORN, H. The partial oxygen pressure in the brain and liver at subtoxic concentrations of carbon monoxide. *Staub-Reinhalt. Luft* 32: 24–29, 1972.

INDEX

Index

QP 6 .H25 sec.3 vol.4
118825

Handbook of physiology (1959
ed.)

Respiratory Mechanics

Main Symbols

C	compliance (capacity in symbols for subdivisions of lung volume)
E	elastance
f	frequency
G	conductance
I	inertance
P	pressure
R	resistance
sG	specific conductance
t	time
V	volume
W	work
$\dot{W}$	power
Z	impedance
$\dot{X}$	dot above any symbol indicates first time derivative; e.g., $\dot{V}$ is flow of gas
$\ddot{X}$	two dots above symbol indicate second time derivative; e.g., $\ddot{V}$ is acceleration of volume

Modifiers

A	alveolar
ab	abdomen
am	ambient
ao	airway opening
aw	airway
B	barometric
bs	body surface
ca	convective acceleration
di	diaphragm
ds	downstream
dyn	dynamic
E	expiratory
el	elastic
es	esophageal
fr	frictional or flow resistive
ga	gastric
I	inspiratory
ia	intercostal/accessory muscles
L	transpulmonary or lung or pulmonary
lam	laminar
m	mouth
max	maximum
mus	muscle
pl	pleural
rc	rib cage
rel	relaxed or relaxation
rs	respiratory system
st	static
ti	tissue
tm	transmural
tur	turbulence
us	upstream
w	chest wall

Subdivisions of Lung Volume

CC	closing capacity
CV	closing volume
ERV	expiratory reserve volume
FRC	functional residual capacity
IC	inspiratory capacity
IRV	inspiratory reserve volume
RV	residual volume
TLC	total lung capacity
VC	vital capacity
VT	tidal volume

Measurements on Forced Respiratory Maneuvers

EPP	equal pressure points
FEF_{x-y}	mean forced expiratory flow between two designated volume points in FVC = $(V_x - V_y)/t$
FET_x	time required to forcibly expire percent of VC, x, from TLC
FEV_t	forced expiratory volume in time interval *t*
$FEV_t/FVC\%$	percent of FVC expired in time interval *t*
FVC	forced vital capacity
IVPF curve	isovolume pressure-flow curve
MEFV curve	maximum expiratory flow-volume curve
MFSR curve	maximum flow–static recoil curve
MIFV curve	maximum inspiratory flow-volume curve
MVV	maximum voluntary ventilation
MVV_t	maximum voluntary ventilation in time interval *t*
PEF	peak expiratory flow
PEFV curve	partial expiratory flow-volume curve
$\dot{V}max_{xx}$	maximum expiratory flow at xx% of VC (note: 100% VC is at TLC; 0% VC is at RV)
$\dot{V}max_{xx,TLC}$	maximum expiratory flow at xx% of TLC

Examples of Combinations

CL	lung compliance
Cst,L	static lung compliance
PA	alveolar pressure
Pao	pressure at the airway opening
$PE,m,max_{xx,TLC}$	maximum expiratory mouth pressure at xx% of TLC
sGaw	specific airway conductance
$\dot{W}di$	diaphragmatic power
WI,el,L	elastic work performed on the lung during inspiration